2018 ICD-10-CM
For Physicians & Hospitals

Are you struggling with the level of ICD-10-CM code specificity required for successful claim submissions?

This invaluable resource will not only get you up to speed with 2018 updates, but will also help you check your coding for medical necessity.

The **ICD-10-CM for Physicians & Hospitals 2018** is brimming with new and revised ICD-10-CM codes and their descriptors, along with expert guidance and the vital features you need for correct coding and reimbursement. And navigation couldn't be simpler!

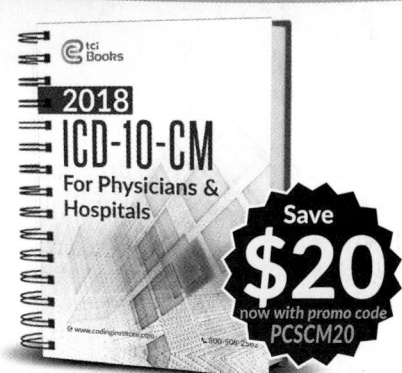

Rely on TCI and avoid unspecified code denials once and for all:

- ⊃ **Complete ICD-10-CM code set**, including its 360 additions, 142 deletions, and 226 revisions
- ⊃ **Full code descriptors** to master new and revised codes
- ⊃ **Official ICD-10-CM Coding Guidelines & Conventions** — Conquer claim denials with guidelines and conventions know-how.
- ⊃ **Official Code Set** — Move swiftly with the Alphabetic Index, Index to External Causes, and Tabular List
- ⊃ **Updated Tables** — Code quicker with the Table of Drugs and Chemicals and Neoplasm Table
- ⊃ **Pre-printed stick-on tabs** to navigate quickly between sections
- ⊃ **Guidelines Tips** for interpreting guidelines from each Tabular List chapter available via the TCI website
- ⊃ **Notes pages** included throughout the book to keep your go-to notes handy
- ⊃ **PLUS!** — Appendix with Z codes for long term use of drugs listed in alphabetical order by drug name
- ⊃ **PLUS!** — Symbol for Z codes used as the first-listed diagnosis
- ⊃ **PLUS!** — Major Complication & Comorbidity (MCC) and Complication & Comorbidity (CC) indicators and exclusions, and alerts for principal diagnosis as its own CC/MCC

Colored Illustrations and Notes, and Alerts:

- ⊃ Symbols for new, revised, and HCC codes
- ⊃ Highlighted alerts for 7th characters
- ⊃ Highlighted MACRA, unspecified codes, other specified codes, and manifestation codes
- ⊃ Colored alert symbols to add 4th, 5th, 6th, 7th characters throughout the Tabular List
- ⊃ Colored full-page anatomical illustrations
- ⊃ Anatomy and physiology with illustrations explained before Tabular List chapters
- ⊃ Color-coded Includes notes, and Excludes1 and Excludes2 notes
- ⊃ **Common sense Color Coding for MCEs** — Color-coding and symbols for Medicare Code Edits (MCEs) for gender, primary diagnosis only, questionable admission, unacceptable principal diagnosis, and age—newborn, pediatric, maternity, and adult
- ⊃ **Official References** — Negotiate intricate coding scenarios with article references from AHA's Coding Clinic®
- ⊃ **Simple Navigation** — Say goodbye to lost t[...] easy dictionary-style head[...] tabs with chapter title, nu[...] ranges on every page.

Stop claim denials and secure revenue with *ICD-10-CM for Physicians & [Hospi]tals 2018!*

To order *ICD-10-CM for Physicians & Hospitals 2018*, call **1-800-508-2582** or visit https://www.codinginstitute.com/books/icd-10-cm-for-physicians-hospitals-2018.html.

Call us: 800-508-2582 | www.codinginstitute.com

The Coding Institute LLC
2222 Sedwick Drive Durham, NC 27713

Service Excellence: Top Patient Relations Strategies for Customer Retention

What's more damaging to a practice than bad word of mouth? NOTHING!

A satisfied customer tells an average of 5 people about good service. A dissatisfied customer tells an average of 20 people about bad service, and then complains online, which has a potential to impact thousands of potential customers.

Can you afford to deliver bad service to even a single patient?

How do you reach for the *exceptional* to retain your patients? The answers and strategies, both doable and transformative, are laid out, step-by-step in *Service Excellence: Top Patient Relations Strategies for Customer Retention.*

TCI experts help you to establish a culture of excellence to retain patients and gain new ones, deliver top-notch customer service, stop patient attrition, and take back control of patient relations:

✓ Learn what quality in healthcare *really* means
✓ Grasp the direct link between quality of healthcare and customer retention
✓ Uphold the golden rules of service and watch your practice grow

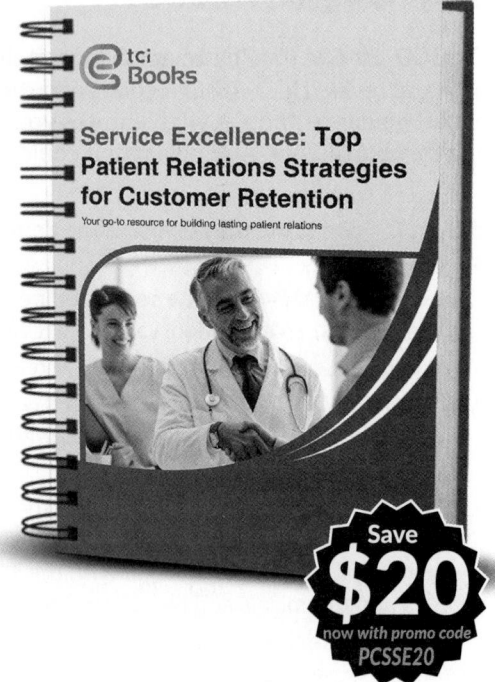

Save $20 now with promo code *PCSSE20*

Master service excellence and avoid traps that send your staff and patients into a tailspin:

✓ Take proactive steps to stop the attrition
✓ Profit from others' real-world service mistakes
✓ Examine "service disasters" and common complaints
✓ Nail down these techniques to improve communications
✓ Bill right the first time

✓ Establish a patient experience improvement team and phase in customer retention strategies
✓ Get the 12-step arsenal to calm angry patients
✓ Learn the ins and outs of patient satisfaction surveys and complaints
✓ Avoid these 30 bad service traps at all costs.
✓ **And much more...**

Say goodbye to humdrum service and hello to outstanding service with this decisive and insightful resource.

To order call 1-800-508-2582
or visit https://www.codinginstitute.com/books/top-patient-relations-strategies-for-customer-retention.html.

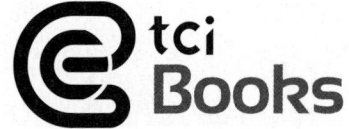

Call us: 800-508-2582 | www.codinginstitute.com
The Coding Institute LLC
2222 Sedwick Drive Durham, NC 27713

HIPAA Handbook 2017

Expert Advice You Need in One Essential Guide

Rest assured, changes this year have meant even tighter HIPAA compliance scrutiny for all practices, no matter how small or large. The HHS Office for Civil Rights (OCR) announced it will ramp up efforts in investigating smaller HIPAA breaches involving fewer than 500 individuals. That means you could be more at risk now than ever before for even unintentional breaches with penalties that could crush your practice.

Having the right resource can make all the difference this year, when the stakes are so high. That's why The Coding Institute has you covered with the *HIPAA Handbook 2017*.

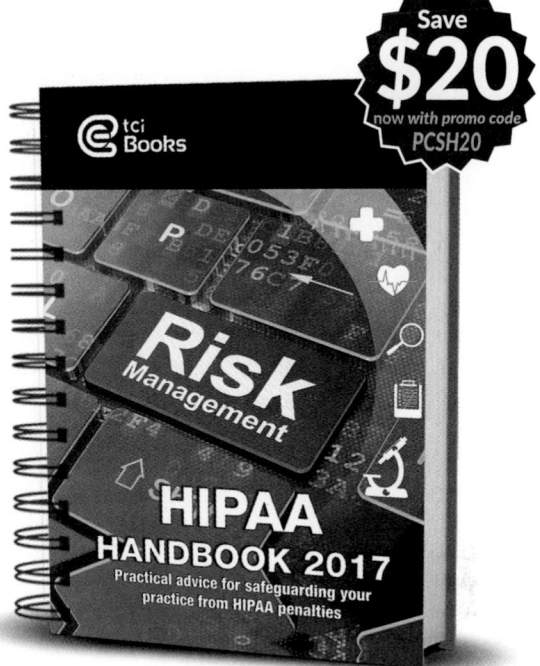

Identify Risk Areas in Your Practice Before the OCR Does

You need to ensure that your breach reporting and other HIPAA compliance efforts are up-to-date and that you're fully equipped for **2017**. Trust the *HIPAA Handbook 2017* to help you master HIPAA compliance.

Here's a sample of the expert analysis you'll get in the HIPAA Handbook 2017:

- ✓ 5 things you need to do to prepare yourself for heightened OCR scrutiny of small breaches.
- ✓ Case study: Your new HIPAA worry: Violations that could put you behind bars.
- ✓ Toolkit: Facts & figures: Here's how to gauge your cybersecurity preparedness.
- ✓ HIPAA phase 2 audits underway — BAs: You're next.
- ✓ What is 'social engineering' & how is it a threat?
- ✓ Nip your 'unaddressed risks' in the bud now — or pay dearly later.
- ✓ Heed 10 expert tips to protect your organization against 'insider threats.'
- ✓ Is 'malvertising' a serious threat to your data security?
- ✓ What's missing in your risk management plan? Here's how to find the gaps.
- ✓ **And much more...**

Don't miss out on the critical HIPAA breach, security, enforcement, and audit topics that could put your practice at risk!

To order call 1-800-508-2582
or visit https://www.codinginstitute.com/books/hipaa-handbook.html.

Call us: 800-508-2582 | www.codinginstitute.com
The Coding Institute LLC
2222 Sedwick Drive Durham, NC 27713

NOTES

2018

ICD-10-PCS

Complete Code Set

Images/Illustrations by the following artists at shutterstock.com:
miucci - 119473492 | ducu59us - 104022683, 125200733 | Alila Medical Media - 228843262, 155445686, 101696095, 96426923, 97755608, 97755611, 147943922, 125899358, 147943910, 155445662, 147943874, 108567068, 106263593, 106263560 | BlueRingMedia - 141162229, 141161560, 141161404 , 149006000, 145028440 | snapgalleria - 142194094 | okili77 - 156466463 | Designua - 180938618, 135935735, 186535475, 165084413 | stockshoppe - 99671552, 180896807, 180896810, 187162247, 187162193, 187162175, 187162163, 187162142, 187162118, 187162106, 187162070, 180896873, 180896855, 180896738, 180896720, 177791516, 177790997 | lotan - 186878060 | sciencepics - 199873508 | Blamb - 24129706 | joshya - 226909492, 261971498 | Della_Liner - 324447776 | Marochkina Anastasiia - 414103342 | Alexander_P - 404964388 | Sylverarts Vectors 552384124

Copyright 2018 © TCI
ISBN (Print): 978-1-63527-145-4
ISBN (eBook): 978-1-63527-146-1

Table of Contents

Preface 2

Changes for 2018 3

List of Features 4

Official Conventions and Additional Conventions Specific to this ICD-10-PCS Book 5

ICD-10-PCS Official Guidelines for Coding and Reporting 7

Anatomical Illustrations 15

Approach Table 43

ICD-10-PCS Index 45

ICD-10-PCS Tables 159

  Medical and Surgical 001-0YW 159

    Central Nervous System and Cranial Nerves 001-00X 159

    Peripheral Nervous System 012-01X 171

    Heart and Great Vessels 021-02Y 181

    Upper Arteries 031-03W 197

    Lower Arteries 041-04W 213

    Upper Veins 051-05W 229

    Lower Veins 061-06W 241

    Lymphatic and Hemic Systems 072-07Y 253

    Eye 080-08X 265

    Ear, Nose, Sinus 090-09W 279

    Respiratory System 0B1-0BY 295

    Mouth and Throat 0C0-0CX 309

    Gastrointestinal System 0D1-0DY............. 321

    Hepatobiliary System and Pancreas 0F1-0FY 341

    Endocrine System 0G2-0GW..................... 351

    Skin and Breast 0H0-0HX 359

    Subcutaneous Tissue and Fascia 0J0-0JX 373

    Muscles 0K2-0KX 391

    Tendons 0L2-0LX 403

    Bursae and Ligaments 0M2-0MX.............. 415

    Head and Facial Bones 0N2-0NW 431

    Upper Bones 0P2-0PW 443

    Lower Bones 0Q2-0QW 457

    Upper Joints 0R2-0RW 469

    Lower Joints 0S2-0SW 485

    Urinary System 0T1-0TY 501

    Female Reproductive System 0U1-0UY 513

    Male Reproductive System 0V1-0VW 529

    Anatomical Regions, General 0W0-0WY 543

    Anatomical Regions, Upper Extremities 0X0-0XY 555

    Anatomical Regions, Lower Extremities 0Y0-0YW 563

  Obstetrics 102-10Y 571

  Placement-Anatomical Regions 2W0-2W6............ 577

  Placement-Anatomical Orifices 2Y0-2Y5 585

  Administration 302-3E1 587

  Measurement and Monitoring 4A0-4B0 603

  Extracorporeal or Systemic Assistance and Performance 5A0-5A2 609

  Extracorporeal or Systemic Therapies 6A0-6AB 611

  Osteopathic 7W0 615

  Other Procedures 8C0-8E0 617

  Chiropractic 9WB 621

  Imaging B00-BY4 623

  Nuclear Medicine C01-CW7 665

  Radiation Therapy D00-DWY 677

  Physical Rehabilitation and Diagnostic Audiology F00-F15 695

  Mental Health GZ1-GZJ 713

  Substance Abuse Treatment HZ2-HZ9 717

  New Technology X2A-XY0...................... 721

    Cardiovascular System X2A-X2R 721

    Skin, Subcutaneous Tissue, Fascia, and Breast XHR 723

    Muscles, Tendons, Bursae, and Ligaments XK0............. 725

    Bones XNS 727

    Joints XR2-XRG 729

    Anatomical Regions XW0 733

    Extracorporeal XY0 735

Appendix A: Root Operations Definitions 737

Appendix B: Body Part Key 743

Appendix C: Device Key 763

Appendix D: Device Aggregation Table 771

Appendix E: Character Meaning 775

Appendix F: Substance Key 845

Appendix G: Combination Clusters 847

Appendix H: Non-OR Not Affecting MS-DRG Assignment 861

Preface

Thank you for your purchase! We are pleased to offer you the 2018 ICD-10-PCS Complete Code Set.

This manual goes beyond the basics to help you code accurately and efficiently. In addition to including the official Alphabetic Index, Tables, and ICD-10-PCS Official Guidelines, we've crafted a select set of bonus features based on requests from coders in the field as well as the recommendations of our core group of veteran coding educators.

Our goal was to apply our unique approach to focusing on the practical application of the codes to this procedure coding manual.

A few of the other features you'll benefit from page after page include the following:

- Full illustrations of body systems at the front of the book so you don't have to search the manual for these large color images of body systems
- An Approach Table at the front of the book listing each approach, its definition, and examples
- Medicare Code Edits, including gender edits and edits for limited coverage, noncovered procedures, HAC-associated procedures, combination clusters, and non-OR procedures affecting MS-DRG assignment

- Intuitive color-coded symbols and alerts identify critical coding and reimbursement issues quickly

See the complete List of Features to learn about everything this manual has to offer.

Rely on Our Combination of Official Sources and Experience

This manual includes the official ICD-10-PCS 2018 Alphabetic Index and Tables. We've also included the 2018 ICD-10-PCS Official Guidelines.

Additionally, our dedicated team drew on their years of experience using coding manuals to develop this manual's user friendly symbols, color coding, and tabs, all designed to help you find the information you need quickly.

Let Us Know What You Think

Our goal for this manual is to support those involved in the business side of healthcare, helping them to do their jobs and do them well. We'd appreciate your feedback, including your suggestions for what you'd like to see in an ICD-10-PCS resource, so we can be sure our manuals serve your needs. Thank you.

Changes for 2018

FY 2018 Update Summary

Change Summary Table

2017 Total	New Codes	Revised Titles	Deleted Codes	2018 Total
75,789	3,562	1,821	646	**78,705**

ICD-10-PCS Code FY 2018 Totals, By Section

Medical and Surgical	68,471
Obstetrics	302
Placement	861
Administration	1,444
Measurement and Monitoring	414
Extracorporeal Assistance and Performance	43
Extracorporeal Therapies	46
Osteopathic	100
Other Procedures	60
Chiropractic	90
Imaging	2,941
Nuclear Medicine	463
Radiation Oncology	1,939
Rehabilitation and Diagnostic Audiology	1,380
Mental Health	30
Substance Abuse Treatment	59
New Technology	62
Total	**78,705**

ICD-10-PCS Changes Highlights

- In the Medical and Surgical section, body part values revised or streamlined for clarity and usefulness as coded data
- Endoscopic approaches added to various tables throughout the system for completeness
- ICD-10-PCS guidelines updated with new and revised guidelines

List of FY 2018 Files

2018 Official ICD-10-PCS Coding Guidelines

- New Guideline B4.1c added in response to public comment.
- Guidelines B3.3, B3.7, and B6.1a revised in response to public comment and internal review.
- Downloadable PDF, file name **pcs_guidelines_2018.pdf**

2018 ICD-10-PCS Code Tables and Index (Zip file)

- Code tables for use beginning October 1, 2017.
- Downloadable PDF, file name is **pcs_2018.pdf**

- Downloadable xml files for developers, file names are **icd10pcs_tables_2018.xml, icd10pcs_index_2018.xml, icd10pcs_definitions_2018.xml**
- Accompanying schema for developers, file names are **icd10pcs_tables_2018.xsd, icd10pcs_index_2018.xsd, icd10pcs_definitions_2018.xsd**

2018 ICD-10-PCS Codes File (Zip file)

- ICD-10-PCS Codes file is a simple format for non-technical uses, containing the valid FY 2018 ICD-10-PCS codes and their long titles.
- File is in text file format, file name is **icd10pcs_codes_2018.txt**
- Accompanying documentation for codes file, file name is **icd10pcsCodesFile.pdf**
- Codes file addenda in text format, file name is **codes_addenda_2018.txt**

2018 ICD-10-PCS Order File (Long and Abbreviated Titles) (Zip file)

- ICD-10-PCS order file is for developers, provides a unique five-digit "order number" for each ICD-10-PCS table and code, as well as a long and abbreviated code title.
- ICD-10-PCS order file name is **icd10pcs_order_2018.txt**
- Accompanying documentation for tabular order file, file name is **icd10pcsOrderFile.pdf**
- Tabular order file addenda in text format, file name is **order_addenda_2018.txt**

2018 ICD-10-PCS Final Addenda (Zip file)

- Addenda files in downloadable PDF, file names are **tables_addenda_2018.pdf, index_addenda_2018.pdf, definitions_addenda_2018.pdf**
- Addenda files also in machine readable text format for developers, file names are **tables_addenda_2018.txt, index_addenda_2018.txt, definitions_addenda_2018.txt**

2018 ICD-10-PCS Conversion Table (Zip file)

- ICD-10-PCS code conversion table is provided to assist users in data retrieval, in downloadable Excel spreadsheet, file name is **icd10pcs_conversion_table_2018.xlsx**
- Conversion table also in machine readable text format for developers, file name is **icd10pcs_conversion_table_2018.txt**
- Accompanying documentation for code conversion table, file name is **icd10pcsConversionTable.pdf**

List of Features

ICD-10-PCS is essential to documenting medical necessity for services rendered, and accurate codes mean better outcomes for the patient, your claims, and your facility.

You can count on this manual to help you choose and report the right ICD-10-PCS code. Unique features, intuitive design, and expert features that coders developed assure this manual will keep your coding on target.

This manual includes the ICD-10-PCS Alphabetic Index and ICD-10-PCS Tables for procedures, effective October 1, 2017 (FY 2018 code set).

To help you make the most of this manual, it also includes the following features:

- ICD-10-PCS Official Conventions and additional conventions and symbols you'll find in this manual
- ICD-10-PCS Official Guidelines for Coding and Reporting, effective October 1, 2017 (FY 2018)

- Approach Table with each approach, definition, and examples listed at the front of the book for quick reference
- Full illustrations of body systems at the front of the book so you don't have to search the manual for these large color images of body systems
- Medicare Code Edits symbols, including gender edits and edits for limited coverage, noncovered procedures, hospital acquired conditions (HAC) associated procedures, combination clusters, and non-OR procedures affecting MS-DRG assignment
- Intuitive color-coded symbols and alerts identify critical coding and reimbursement issues quickly
- Appendices for root operations definitions in alphabetical order, body part key, device key and aggregation table, character meaning, substance key, combination clusters , and non-OR procedures not affecting MS-DRG assignment
- A user-friendly page design, including dictionary-style headers, colored bleed tabs, and legend keys

Official Conventions and Additional Conventions Specific to this ICD-10-PCS Book

This manual includes the procedure code set from the International Classification of Diseases, 10th Revision, Procedure Coding System (ICD-10-PCS). Hospitals and third-party payers use these codes to classify inpatient procedures.

Official Conventions

Index

Refer to the ICD-10-PCS Index to access the Tables in the manual. The Index mirrors the structure of the Tables, so it follows a consistent pattern of organization and use of hierarchies. The Index is organized as an alphabetic lookup.

Two types of main terms are listed in the Index:

- Based on the value of the third character, such as a root operation (excision, insertion)
- Lists common procedure terms

Main terms

For the Medical and Surgical and related sections, the root operation values are used as main terms in the Index. In other sections, the values representing the general type of procedure performed, such as nuclear medicine or imaging type, are listed as main terms.

For the Medical and Surgical and related sections, values such as Excision, Bypass, and Transplantation are included as main terms in the Index. The applicable body system entries are listed beneath the main term and refer to a specific table. For the ancillary sections, values such as Fluoroscopy and Positron Emission Tomography, are listed as main terms.

To find the code to cross-reference to the Tables, search for the root operation for the procedure in the Index, followed by the subterm for the anatomic site or the subterm that further describes the procedure. Locate the partial code, and cross-reference it to the Table that matches the first three characters of the code.

Tables

The Tables are organized in alphanumeric order in a series by Section, which is the first character of a code. Tables that begin with 0 to 9 are listed first, then tables beginning with B-D, then letters F-X, are listed next.

The same convention is followed within each table for the second through the seventh characters—numeric values in order first, followed by alphabetical values in order.

The Medical and Surgical section (first character 0) is organized by body system values. Each body system subdivision in the Medical and Surgical section contains tables that list the valid root operations for that body system. These are the root operation tables that form the system. These tables provide the valid choices of values available to construct a code.

The root operation tables consist of four columns and a varying number of rows, as in the following example of the root operation Insertion, in the Subcutaneous Tissue and Fascia body system.

The values for characters 1 through 3 are provided at the top of each table.

Character 1:   0: MEDICAL AND SURGICAL (Section)
Character 2:   J: SUBCUTANEOUS TISSUE AND FASCIA (Body System)
Character 3:   H: INSERTION: Putting in a nonbiological appliance that monitors, assists, performs, or prevents a physiological function but does not physically take the place of a body part (Root Operation)

Four columns contain the applicable values for characters 4 through 7, given the values in characters 1 through 3:

Body Part	Approach	Device	Qualifier
Character 4	**Character 5**	**Character 6**	**Character 7**
S Subcutaneous Tissue and Fascia, Head and Neck **V** Subcutaneous Tissue and Fascia, Upper Extremity **W** Subcutaneous Tissue and Fascia, Lower Extremity	**0** Open **3** Percutaneous	**1** Radioactive Element **3** Infusion Device	**Z** No Qualifier
T Subcutaneous Tissue and Fascia, Trunk	**0** Open **3** Percutaneous	**1** Radioactive Element **3** Infusion Device **V** Infusion Pump	**Z** No Qualifier

A table may be separated into rows to specify the valid choices of values in characters 4 through 7. A code built using values from more than one row of a table is not a valid code.

Refer to the ICD-10-PCS Official Guidelines for Coding and Reporting in this manual for detailed guidance on assigning ICD-10-PCS codes.

See Reference

The See reference directs you to go elsewhere in the Index to find the root operation that you need.

Use Reference

The Use reference directs you to a character value selection as an additional reference.

Additional Conventions

Additional conventions that you will find in the Tables in this manual include Medicare Code Edits - Symbols and colored font.

Medicare Code Edits – Symbols Applied to 4th Characters

LC Limited Coverage

Procedures that are medically complex and serious in nature that incur extraordinary associated costs. Medicare limits coverage to a portion of the cost.

NC Noncovered

Procedures for which Medicare does not typically reimburse.

HAC HAC-associated Procedure

Procedures that are associated with hospital-acquired conditions (HAC).

CC Combination Cluster

The procedure is part of a procedure code combination, or cluster, listed in Appendix G of this manual. Medicare does not typically pay for these procedures unless you report them with other specific procedures.

DRG Non-OR-Affecting MS-DRG Assignment

Non-operating room procedures which affect MS-DRG assignment for claims reporting.

New/Revised Text in **Orange**

Procedure text was new or revised from the last version of the code set. For new codes, orange text will be shown for all characters in the code. New codes may be shown as their own row in a table and characters 4-7 may be shown in a row that is separate from other characters within that table.

♂ Male

Male procedure only

♀ Female

Female procedure only

Code Lists

Codes that are applicable to each type of symbol in the book are listed after each table.

Notes Pages

Notes pages are included between sections within the Tables.

ICD-10-PCS Official Guidelines for Coding and Reporting

The Centers for Medicare and Medicaid Services (CMS) and the National Center for Health Statistics (NCHS), two departments within the U.S. Federal Government's Department of Health and Human Services (DHHS) provide the following guidelines for coding and reporting using the International Classification of Diseases, 10th Revision, Procedure Coding System (ICD-10-PCS). These guidelines should be used as a companion document to the official version of the ICD-10-PCS as published on the CMS website. The ICD-10-PCS is a procedure classification published by the United States for classifying procedures performed in hospital inpatient health care settings.

These guidelines have been approved by the four organizations that make up the Cooperating Parties for the ICD-10-PCS: the American Hospital Association (AHA), the American Health Information Management Association (AHIMA), CMS, and NCHS.

These guidelines are a set of rules that have been developed to accompany and complement the official conventions and instructions provided within the ICD-10-PCS itself. The instructions and conventions of the classification take precedence over guidelines. These guidelines are based on the coding and sequencing instructions in the Tables, Index and Definitions of ICD-10-PCS, but provide additional instruction. Adherence to these guidelines when assigning ICD-10-PCS procedure codes is required under the Health Insurance Portability and Accountability Act (HIPAA). The procedure codes have been adopted under HIPAA for hospital inpatient healthcare settings. A joint effort between the healthcare provider and the coder is essential to achieve complete and accurate documentation, code assignment, and reporting of diagnoses and procedures. These guidelines have been developed to assist both the healthcare provider and the coder in identifying those procedures that are to be reported. The importance of consistent, complete documentation in the medical record cannot be overemphasized. Without such documentation accurate coding cannot be achieved.

Table of Contents

A. Conventions..8

B. Medical and Surgical Section Guidelines......................................9
   2. Body System 9
   3. Root Operation 9
   4. Body Part 12
   5. Approach 13
   6. Device 13

C. Obstetrics Section Guidelines... 14

D. New Technology Section Guidelines 14

   Selection of Principal Procedure 14

Conventions

A1
ICD-10-PCS codes are composed of seven characters. Each character is an axis of classification that specifies information about the procedure performed. Within a defined code range, a character specifies the same type of information in that axis of classification.

Example: The fifth axis of classification specifies the approach in sections 0 through 4 and 7 through 9 of the system.

A2
One of 34 possible values can be assigned to each axis of classification in the seven-character code: they are the numbers 0 through 9 and the alphabet (except I and O because they are easily confused with the numbers 1 and 0). The number of unique values used in an axis of classification differs as needed.

Example: Where the fifth axis of classification specifies the approach, seven different approach values are currently used to specify the approach.

A3
The valid values for an axis of classification can be added to as needed.

Example: If a significantly distinct type of device is used in a new procedure, a new device value can be added to the system.

A4
As with words in their context, the meaning of any single value is a combination of its axis of classification and any preceding values on which it may be dependent.

Example: The meaning of a body part value in the Medical and Surgical section is always dependent on the body system value.

The body part value 0 in the Central Nervous body system specifies Brain and the body part value 0 in the Peripheral Nervous body system specifies Cervical Plexus.

A5
As the system is expanded to become increasingly detailed, over time more values will depend on preceding values for their meaning.

Example: In the Lower Joints body system, the device value 3 in the root operation Insertion specifies Infusion Device and the device value 3 in the root operation Replacement specifies Ceramic Synthetic Substitute.

A6
The purpose of the alphabetic index is to locate the appropriate table that contains all information necessary to construct a procedure code. The PCS Tables should always be consulted to find the most appropriate valid code.

A7
It is not required to consult the index first before proceeding to the tables to complete the code. A valid code may be chosen directly from the tables.

A8
All seven characters must be specified to be a valid code. If the documentation is incomplete for coding purposes, the physician should be queried for the necessary information.

A9
Within a PCS table, valid codes include all combinations of choices in characters 4 through 7 contained in the same row of the table. In the example below, 0JHT3VZ is a valid code, and 0JHW3VZ is *not* a valid code.

Section: 0 Medical and Surgical

Body System: J Subcutaneous Tissue and Fascia

Operation: H Insertion: Putting in a nonbiological appliance that monitors, assists, performs, or prevents a physiological function but does not physically take the place of a body part

Body Part	Approach	Device	Qualifier
S Subcutaneous Tissue and Fascia, Head and Neck V Subcutaneous Tissue and Fascia, Upper Extremity W Subcutaneous Tissue and Fascia, Lower Extremity	0 Open 3 Percutaneous	1 Radioactive Element 3 Infusion Device	Z No Qualifier
T Subcutaneous Tissue and Fascia, Trunk	0 Open 3 Percutaneous	1 Radioactive Element 3 Infusion Device V Infusion Pump	Z No Qualifier

A10

"And," when used in a code description, means "and/or."

Example: Lower Arm and Wrist Muscle means lower arm and/or wrist muscle.

A11

Many of the terms used to construct PCS codes are defined within the system. It is the coder's responsibility to determine what the documentation in the medical record equates to in the PCS definitions. The physician is not expected to use the terms used in PCS code descriptions, nor is the coder required to query the physician when the correlation between the documentation and the defined PCS terms is clear.

Example: When the physician documents "partial resection" the coder can independently correlate "partial resection" to the root operation Excision without querying the physician for clarification.

Medical and Surgical Section Guidelines (section 0)

B2. Body System

General guidelines

B2.1a

The procedure codes in the general anatomical regions body systems can be used when the procedure is performed on an anatomical region rather than a specific body part (e.g., root operations Control and Detachment, Drainage of a body cavity) or on the rare occasion when no information is available to support assignment of a code to a specific body part.

Examples: Control of postoperative hemorrhage is coded to the root operation Control found in the general anatomical regions body systems.
Chest tube drainage of the pleural cavity is coded to the root operation Drainage found in the general anatomical regions body systems. Suture repair of the abdominal wall is coded to the root operation Repair in the general anatomical regions body system.

B2.1b

Where the general body part values "upper" and "lower" are provided as an option in the Upper Arteries, Lower Arteries, Upper Veins, Lower Veins, Muscles and Tendons body systems, "upper" or "lower "specifies body parts located above or below the diaphragm respectively.

Example: Vein body parts above the diaphragm are found in the Upper Veins body system; vein body parts below the diaphragm are found in the Lower Veins body system.

B3. Root Operation

General guidelines

B3.1a

In order to determine the appropriate root operation, the full definition of the root operation as contained in the PCS Tables must be applied.

B3.1b

Components of a procedure specified in the root operation definition and explanation are not coded separately. Procedural steps necessary to reach the operative site and close the operative site, including anastomosis of a tubular body part, are also not coded separately.

Examples: Resection of a joint as part of a joint replacement procedure is included in the root operation definition of Replacement and is not coded separately.

Laparotomy performed to reach the site of an open liver biopsy is not coded separately. In a resection of sigmoid colon with anastomosis of descending colon to rectum, the anastomosis is not coded separately.

Multiple procedures

B3.2

During the same operative episode, multiple procedures are coded if:
a. The same root operation is performed on different body parts as defined by distinct values of the body part character.
   Examples: Diagnostic excision of liver and pancreas are coded separately.

   Excision of lesion in the ascending colon and excision of lesion in the transverse colon are coded separately.

b. The same root operation is repeated in multiple body parts, and those body parts are separate and distinct body parts classified to a single ICD-10-PCS body part value.
   Examples: Excision of the sartorius muscle and excision of the gracilis muscle are both included in the upper leg muscle body part value, and multiple procedures are coded.

   Extraction of multiple toenails are coded separately.

c. Multiple root operations with distinct objectives are performed on the same body part.
   Example: Destruction of sigmoid lesion and bypass of sigmoid colon are coded separately.

d. The intended root operation is attempted using one approach, but is converted to a different approach.
   Example: Laparoscopic cholecystectomy converted to an open cholecystectomy is coded as percutaneous endoscopic Inspection and open Resection.

Discontinued or incomplete procedures

B3.3
If the intended procedure is discontinued or otherwise not completed, code the procedure to the root operation performed. If a procedure is discontinued before any other root operation is performed, code the root operation Inspection of the body part or anatomical region inspected.

Example: A planned aortic valve replacement procedure is discontinued after the initial thoracotomy and before any incision is made in the heart muscle, when the patient becomes hemodynamically unstable. This procedure is coded as an open Inspection of the mediastinum.

Biopsy procedures

B3.4a
Biopsy procedures are coded using the root operations Excision, Extraction, or Drainage and the qualifier Diagnostic.

Examples: Fine needle aspiration biopsy of fluid in the lung is coded to the root operation Drainage with the qualifier Diagnostic.

Biopsy of bone marrow is coded to the root operation Extraction with the qualifier Diagnostic.

Lymph node sampling for biopsy is coded to the root operation Excision with the qualifier Diagnostic.

Biopsy followed by more definitive treatment

B3.4b
If a diagnostic Excision, Extraction, or Drainage procedure (biopsy) is followed by a more definitive procedure, such as Destruction, Excision or Resection at the same procedure site, both the biopsy and the more definitive treatment are coded.

Example: Biopsy of breast followed by partial mastectomy at the same procedure site, both the biopsy and the partial mastectomy procedure are coded.

Overlapping body layers

B3.5
If the root operations Excision, Repair or Inspection are performed on overlapping layers of the musculoskeletal system, the body part specifying the deepest layer is coded.

Example : Excisional debridement that includes skin and subcutaneous tissue and muscle is coded to the muscle body part.

Bypass procedures

B3.6a
Bypass procedures are coded by identifying the body part bypassed "from" and the body part bypassed "to." The fourth character body part specifies the body part bypassed from, and the qualifier specifies the body part bypassed to.

Example: Bypass from stomach to jejunum, stomach is the body part and jejunum is the qualifier.

B3.6b
Coronary artery bypass procedures are coded differently than other bypass procedures as described in the previous guideline.

Rather than identifying the body part bypassed from, the body part identifies the number of coronary arteries bypassed to, and the qualifier specifies the vessel bypassed from.

Example: Aortocoronary artery bypass of the left anterior descending coronary artery and the obtuse marginal coronary artery is classified in the body part axis of classification as two coronary arteries, and the qualifier specifies the aorta as the body part bypassed from.

B3.6c
If multiple coronary arteries are bypassed, a separate procedure is coded for each coronary artery that uses a different device and/or qualifier.

Example: Aortocoronary artery bypass and internal mammary coronary artery bypass are coded separately.

Control vs. more definitive root operations

B3.7
The root operation Control is defined as, "Stopping, or attempting to stop, postprocedural or other acute bleeding." If an attempt to stop postprocedural or other acute bleeding is initially unsuccessful, and to stop the bleeding requires performing a more definitive root operation, such as Bypass, Detachment, Excision, Extraction, Reposition, Replacement, or Resection, then the more definitive root operation is coded instead of Control.

Example: Resection of spleen to stop bleeding is coded to Resection instead of Control.

Excision vs. Resection

B3.8
PCS contains specific body parts for anatomical subdivisions of a body part, such as lobes of the lungs or liver and regions of the intestine. Resection of the specific body part is coded whenever all of the body part is cut out or off, rather than coding Excision of a less specific body part.

Example: Left upper lung lobectomy is coded to Resection of Upper Lung Lobe, Left rather than Excision of Lung, Left.

Excision for graft

B3.9
If an autograft is obtained from a different procedure site in order to complete the objective of the procedure, a separate procedure is coded.

Example: Coronary bypass with excision of saphenous vein graft, excision of saphenous vein is coded separately.

Fusion procedures of the spine

B3.10a
The body part coded for a spinal vertebral joint(s) rendered immobile by a spinal fusion procedure is classified by the level of the spine (e.g. thoracic). There are distinct body part values for a single vertebral joint and for multiple vertebral joints at each spinal level.

Example: Body part values specify Lumbar Vertebral Joint, Lumbar Vertebral Joints, 2 or More and Lumbosacral Vertebral Joint.

B3.10b
If multiple vertebral joints are fused, a separate procedure is coded for each vertebral joint that uses a different device and/or qualifier.

Example: Fusion of lumbar vertebral joint, posterior approach, anterior column and fusion of lumbar vertebral joint, posterior approach, posterior column are coded separately.

B3.10c
Combinations of devices and materials are often used on a vertebral joint to render the joint immobile. When combinations of devices are used on the same vertebral joint, the device value coded for the procedure is as follows:

- If an interbody fusion device is used to render the joint immobile (alone or containing other material like bone graft), the procedure is coded with the device value Interbody Fusion Device
- If bone graft is the *only* device used to render the joint immobile, the procedure is coded with the device value Nonautologous Tissue Substitute or Autologous Tissue Substitute
- If a mixture of autologous and nonautologous bone graft (with or without biological or synthetic extenders or binders) is used to render the joint immobile, code the procedure with the device value Autologous Tissue Substitute

Examples: Fusion of a vertebral joint using a cage style interbody fusion device containing morselized bone graft is coded to the device Interbody Fusion Device.

Fusion of a vertebral joint using a bone dowel interbody fusion device made of cadaver bone and packed with a mixture of local morselized bone and demineralized bone matrix is coded to the device Interbody Fusion Device.

Fusion of a vertebral joint using both autologous bone graft and bone bank bone graft is coded to the device Autologous Tissue Substitute.

Inspection procedures

B3.11a
Inspection of a body part(s) performed in order to achieve the objective of a procedure is not coded separately.

Example: Fiberoptic bronchoscopy performed for irrigation of bronchus, only the irrigation procedure is coded.

B3.11b
If multiple tubular body parts are inspected, the most distal body part (the body part furthest from the starting point of the inspection) is coded. If multiple non-tubular body parts in a region are inspected, the body part that specifies the entire area inspected is coded.

Examples: Cystoureteroscopy with inspection of bladder and ureters is coded to the ureter body part value.

Exploratory laparotomy with general inspection of abdominal contents is coded to the peritoneal cavity body part value.

B3.11c
When both an Inspection procedure and another procedure are performed on the same body part during the same episode, if the Inspection procedure is performed using a different approach than the other procedure, the Inspection procedure is coded separately.

Example: Endoscopic Inspection of the duodenum is coded separately when open Excision of the duodenum is performed during the same procedural episode.

Occlusion vs. Restriction for vessel embolization procedures

B3.12
If the objective of an embolization procedure is to completely close a vessel, the root operation Occlusion is coded. If the objective of an embolization procedure is to narrow the lumen of a vessel, the root operation Restriction is coded.

Examples : Tumor embolization is coded to the root operation Occlusion, because the objective of the procedure is to cut off the blood supply to the vessel.

Embolization of a cerebral aneurysm is coded to the root operation Restriction, because the objective of the procedure is not to close off the vessel entirely, but to narrow the lumen of the vessel at the site of the aneurysm where it is abnormally wide.

Release procedures

B3.13
In the root operation Release, the body part value coded is the body part being freed and not the tissue being manipulated or cut to free the body part.

Example: Lysis of intestinal adhesions is coded to the specific intestine body part value.

Release vs. Division

B3.14
If the sole objective of the procedure is freeing a body part without cutting the body part, the root operation is Release. If the sole objective of the procedure is separating or transecting a body part, the root operation is Division.

Examples: Freeing a nerve root from surrounding scar tissue to relieve pain is coded to the root operation Release.

Severing a nerve root to relieve pain is coded to the root operation Division.

Reposition for fracture treatment

B3.15
Reduction of a displaced fracture is coded to the root operation Reposition and the application of a cast or splint in conjunction with the Reposition procedure is not coded separately. Treatment of a nondisplaced fracture is coded to the procedure performed.

Examples: Casting of a nondisplaced fracture is coded to the root operation Immobilization in the Placement section.

Putting a pin in a nondisplaced fracture is coded to the root operation Insertion.

Transplantation vs. Administration

B3.16
Putting in a mature and functioning living body part taken from another individual or animal is coded to the root operation Transplantation. Putting in autologous or nonautologous cells is coded to the Administration section.

Example: Putting in autologous or nonautologous bone marrow, pancreatic islet cells or stem cells is coded to the Administration section.

B4. Body Part

General guidelines

B4.1a
If a procedure is performed on a portion of a body part that does not have a separate body part value, code the body part value corresponding to the whole body part.

Example: A procedure performed on the alveolar process of the mandible is coded to the mandible body part.

B4.1b
If the prefix "peri" is combined with a body part to identify the site of the procedure, and the site of the procedure is not further specified, then the procedure is coded to the body part named. This guideline applies only when a more specific body part value is not available.

Examples: A procedure site identified as perirenal is coded to the kidney body part when the site of the procedure is not further specified.
A procedure site described in the documentation as peri-urethral, and the documentation also indicates that it is the vulvar tissue and not the urethral tissue that is the site of the procedure, then the procedure is coded to the vulva body part.

B4.1c
If a procedure is performed on a continuous section of a tubular body part, code the body part value corresponding to the furthest anatomical site from the point of entry.

Example: A procedure performed on a continuous section of artery from the femoral artery to the external iliac artery with the point of entry at the femoral artery is coded to the external iliac body part.

Branches of body parts

B4.2
Where a specific branch of a body part does not have its own body part value in PCS, the body part is typically coded to the closest proximal branch that has a specific body part value. In the cardiovascular body systems, if a general body part is available in the correct root operation table, and coding to a proximal branch would require assigning a code in a different body system, the procedure is coded using the general body part value.

Examples: A procedure performed on the mandibular branch of the trigeminal nerve is coded to the trigeminal nerve body part value. Occlusion of the bronchial artery is coded to the body part value Upper Artery in the body system Upper Arteries, and not to the body part value Thoracic Aorta, Descending in the body system Heart and Great Vessels.

Bilateral body part values

B4.3
Bilateral body part values are available for a limited number of body parts. If the identical procedure is performed on contralateral body parts, and a bilateral body part value exists for that body part, a single procedure is coded using the bilateral body part value. If no bilateral body part value exists, each procedure is coded separately using the appropriate body part value.

Examples: The identical procedure performed on both fallopian tubes is coded once using the body part value Fallopian Tube, Bilateral.
The identical procedure performed on both knee joints is coded twice using the body part values Knee Joint, Right and Knee Joint, Left.

Coronary arteries

B4.4
The coronary arteries are classified as a single body part that is further specified by number of arteries treated. One procedure code specifying multiple arteries is used when the same procedure is performed, including the same device and qualifier values.

Examples: Angioplasty of two distinct coronary arteries with placement of two stents is coded as Dilation of Coronary Artery, Two Arteries with Two Intraluminal Devices.

Angioplasty of two distinct coronary arteries, one with stent placed and one without, is coded separately as Dilation of Coronary Artery, One Artery with Intraluminal Device, and Dilation of Coronary Artery, One Artery with no device.

Tendons, ligaments, bursae and fascia near a joint

B4.5
Procedures performed on tendons, ligaments, bursae and fascia supporting a joint are coded to the body part in the respective body system that is the focus of the procedure. Procedures performed on joint structures themselves are coded to the body part in the joint body systems.

Examples: Repair of the anterior cruciate ligament of the knee is coded to the knee bursa and ligament body part in the bursae and ligaments body system.

Knee arthroscopy with shaving of articular cartilage is coded to the knee joint body part in the Lower Joints body system.

Skin, subcutaneous tissue and fascia overlying a joint

B4.6
If a procedure is performed on the skin, subcutaneous tissue or fascia overlying a joint, the procedure is coded to the following body part:
- Shoulder is coded to Upper Arm
- Elbow is coded to Lower Arm
- Wrist is coded to Lower Arm
- Hip is coded to Upper Leg
- Knee is coded to Lower Leg
- Ankle is coded to Foot

Fingers and toes

B4.7
If a body system does not contain a separate body part value for fingers, procedures performed on the fingers are coded to the body part value for the hand. If a body system does not contain a separate body part value for toes, procedures performed on the toes are coded to the body part value for the foot.

Example: Excision of finger muscle is coded to one of the hand muscle body part values in the Muscles body system.

Upper and lower intestinal tract

B4.8
In the Gastrointestinal body system, the general body part values Upper Intestinal Tract and Lower Intestinal Tract are provided as an option for the root operations Change, Inspection, Removal and Revision. Upper Intestinal Tract includes the portion of the gastrointestinal tract from the esophagus down to and including the duodenum, and Lower Intestinal Tract includes the portion of the gastrointestinal tract from the jejunum down to and including the rectum and anus.

Example: In the root operation Change table, change of a device in the jejunum is coded using the body part Lower Intestinal Tract.

B5. Approach

Open approach with percutaneous endoscopic assistance

B5.2
Procedures performed using the open approach with percutaneous endoscopic assistance are coded to the approach Open.

Example: Laparoscopic-assisted sigmoidectomy is coded to the approach Open.

External approach

B5.3a
Procedures performed within an orifice on structures that are visible without the aid of any instrumentation are coded to the approach External.

Example: Resection of tonsils is coded to the approach External.

B5.3b
Procedures performed indirectly by the application of external force through the intervening body layers are coded to the approach External.

Example: Closed reduction of fracture is coded to the approach External.

Percutaneous procedure via device

B5.4
Procedures performed percutaneously via a device placed for the procedure are coded to the approach Percutaneous.

Example : Fragmentation of kidney stone performed via percutaneous nephrostomy is coded to the approach Percutaneous.

B6. Device

General guidelines

B6.1a
A device is coded only if a device remains after the procedure is completed. If no device remains, the device value No Device is coded. In limited root operations, the classification provides the qualifier values Temporary and Intraoperative, for specific procedures involving clinically significant devices, where the purpose of the device is to be utilized for a brief duration during the procedure or current inpatient stay.

B6.1b
Materials such as sutures, ligatures, radiological markers and temporary post-operative wound drains are considered integral to the performance of a procedure and are not coded as devices.

B6.1c
Procedures performed on a device only and not on a body part are specified in the root operations Change, Irrigation, Removal and Revision, and are coded to the procedure performed.

Example: Irrigation of percutaneous nephrostomy tube is coded to the root operation Irrigation of indwelling device in the Administration section.

Drainage device

B6.2
A separate procedure to put in a drainage device is coded to the root operation Drainage with the device value Drainage Device.

Obstetric Section Guidelines (section 1)

C. Obstetrics Section

Products of conception

C1

Procedures performed on the products of conception are coded to the Obstetrics section. Procedures performed on the pregnant female other than the products of conception are coded to the appropriate root operation in the Medical and Surgical section.

Example: Amniocentesis is coded to the products of conception body part in the Obstetrics section. Repair of obstetric urethral laceration is coded to the urethra body part in the Medical and Surgical section.

Procedures following delivery or abortion

C2

Procedures performed following a delivery or abortion for curettage of the endometrium or evacuation of retained products of conception are all coded in the Obstetrics section, to the root operation Extraction and the body part Products of Conception, Retained. Diagnostic or therapeutic dilation and curettage performed during times other than the postpartum or post-abortion period are all coded in the Medical and Surgical section, to the root operation Extraction and the body part Endometrium.

New Technology Section Guidelines (section X)

D. New Technology Section

General guidelines

D1

Section X codes are standalone codes. They are not supplemental codes. Section X codes fully represent the specific procedure described in the code title, and do not require any additional codes from other sections of ICD-10-PCS. When section X contains a code title which describes a specific new technology procedure, only that X code is reported for the procedure. There is no need to report a broader, non-specific code in another section of ICD-10-PCS.

Example: XW04321 Introduction of Ceftazidime-Avibactam Anti-infective into Central Vein, Percutaneous Approach, New Technology Group 1, can be coded to indicate that Ceftazidime-Avibactam Anti-infective was administered via a central vein. A separate code from table 3E0 in the Administration section of ICD-10-PCS is not coded in addition to this code.

Selection of Principal Procedure

The following instructions should be applied in the selection of principal procedure and clarification on the importance of the relation to the principal diagnosis when more than one procedure is performed:

1. Procedure performed for definitive treatment of both principal diagnosis and secondary diagnosis
   a. Sequence procedure performed for definitive treatment most related to principal diagnosis as principal procedure.

2. Procedure performed for definitive treatment and diagnostic procedures performed for both principal diagnosis and secondary diagnosis.
   a. Sequence procedure performed for definitive treatment most related to principal diagnosis as principal procedure

3. A diagnostic procedure was performed for the principal diagnosis and a procedure is performed for definitive treatment of a secondary diagnosis.
   a. Sequence diagnostic procedure as principal procedure, since the procedure most related to the principal diagnosis takes precedence.

4. No procedures performed that are related to principal diagnosis; procedures performed for definitive treatment and diagnostic procedures were performed for secondary diagnosis
   a. Sequence procedure performed for definitive treatment of secondary diagnosis as principal procedure, since there are no procedures (definitive or nondefinitive treatment) related to principal diagnosis.

Anatomical Illustrations

Circulatory System — Arteries and Veins

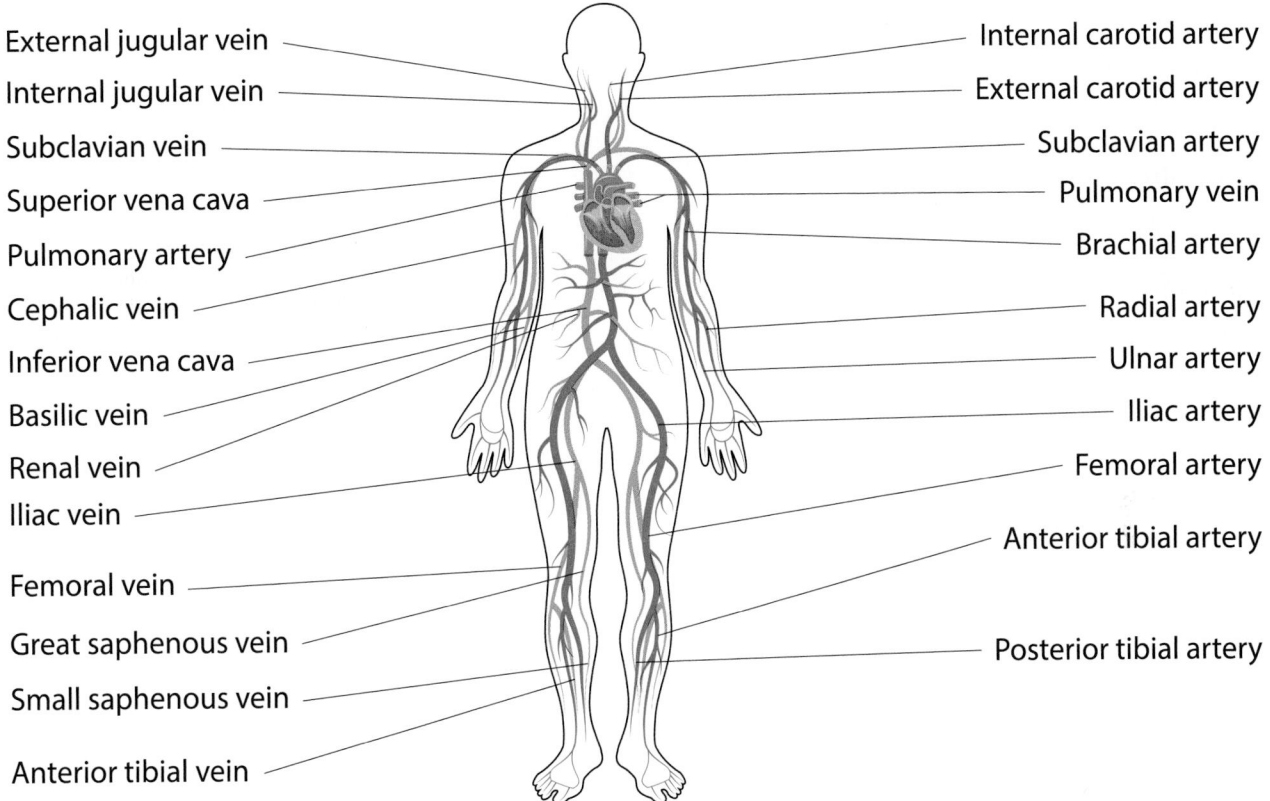

External jugular vein

Internal jugular vein

Subclavian vein

Superior vena cava

Pulmonary artery

Cephalic vein

Inferior vena cava

Basilic vein

Renal vein

Iliac vein

Femoral vein

Great saphenous vein

Small saphenous vein

Anterior tibial vein

Internal carotid artery

External carotid artery

Subclavian artery

Pulmonary vein

Brachial artery

Radial artery

Ulnar artery

Iliac artery

Femoral artery

Anterior tibial artery

Posterior tibial artery

Circulatory System — Artery and Vein Anatomy

Artery

Vein

Adventitia

Blood flow

Smooth muscle

Valve

Internal elastic lamina

Endothelium

Artery

Vein

Circulatory System — Heart Anatomy and Cardiac Cycle

Brachiocephalic trunk
Ascending aorta
Right pulmonary artery
Superior vena cava
Pulmonary trunk
Right pulmonary veins
Right atrium
Right coronary artery
Right ventricle
Inferior vena cava

Left common carotid artery
Left subclavian artery
Aortic arch
Ligamentum arteriosum
Left pulmonary artery
Left pulmonary veins
Left atrium
Circumflex artery
Left coronary artery
Left ventricle
Anterior interventricular artery
Apex

Right atrium
Inferior vena cava
Left atrium
Mitral valve
Aortic valve
Pulmonary valve
Right ventricle

Diastole Ventricular Relaxation and Filling

Superior vena cava
Aorta
Pulmonary artery
Left ventricle
Tricuspid valve

Systole Ventricular Contraction and Ejection

Digestive System — Digestive Organs

Nose
Lips
Genioglossus muscle
Trachea
Liver
Duodenum
Pancreas
Ascending colon
Small intestine
Appendix

Hard palate
Tongue
Hyoid bone
Thyroid cartilage
Esophagus
Stomach
Gallbladder
Spleen
Transverse colon
Large intestine
Rectum
Anus

ANATOMICAL ILLUSTRATIONS

Digestive System — Large Intestine Anatomy

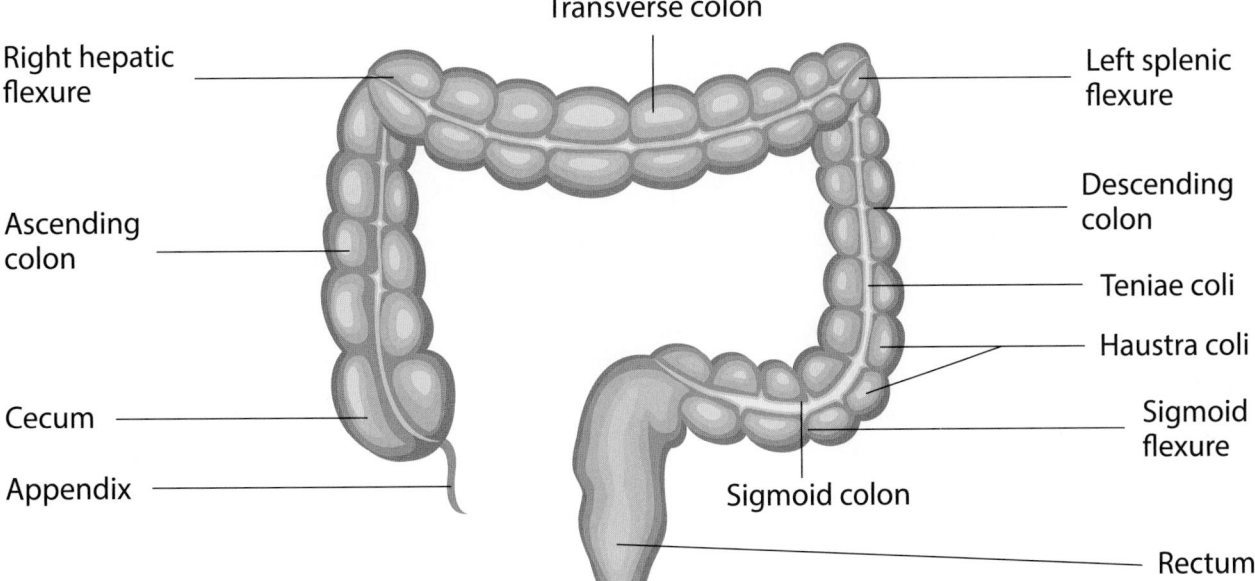

Transverse colon

Right hepatic flexure

Left splenic flexure

Ascending colon

Descending colon

Teniae coli

Haustra coli

Cecum

Sigmoid flexure

Appendix

Sigmoid colon

Rectum

Digestive System — Rectum Anatomy

Rectum

Internal hemorrhoid tissue

Levator ani muscle

Internal anal sphincter

External anal sphincter

External hemorrhoid tissue

Anus

Digestive System — Liver Anatomy

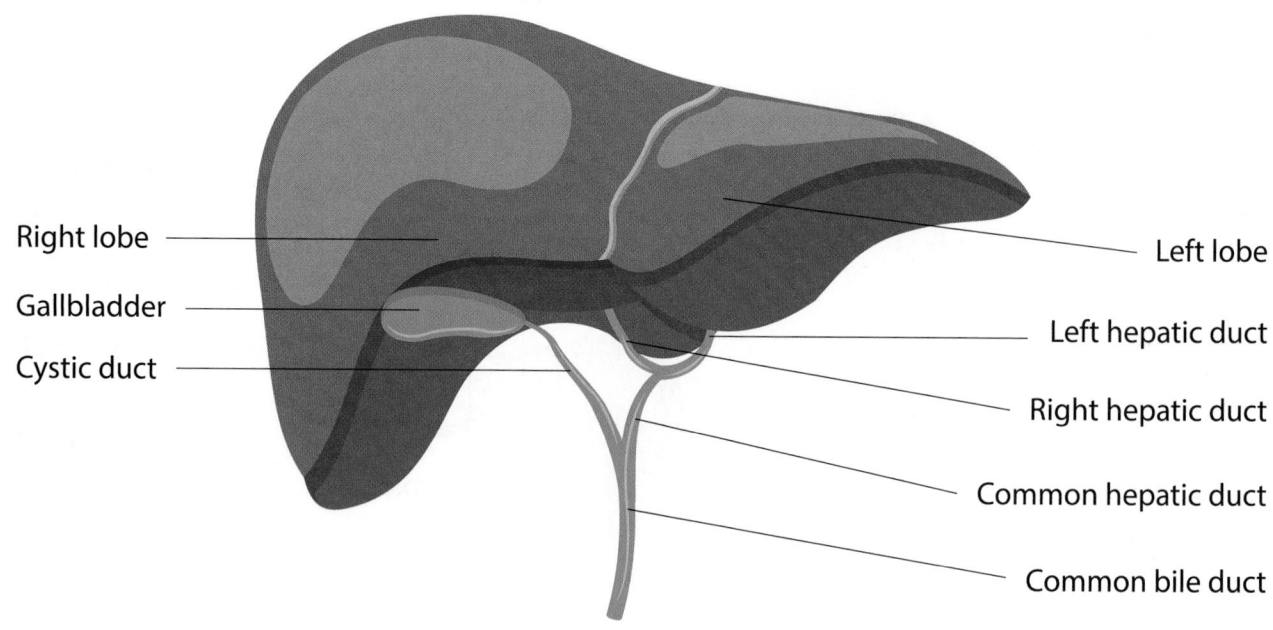

Right lobe

Gallbladder

Cystic duct

Left lobe

Left hepatic duct

Right hepatic duct

Common hepatic duct

Common bile duct

Digestive System — Pancreas Anatomy

Gallbladder

Common bile duct

Stomach

Tail of pancreas

Major duodenal papilla

Pancreatic duct

Duodenum

Body of pancreas

Digestive System — Mouth Anatomy

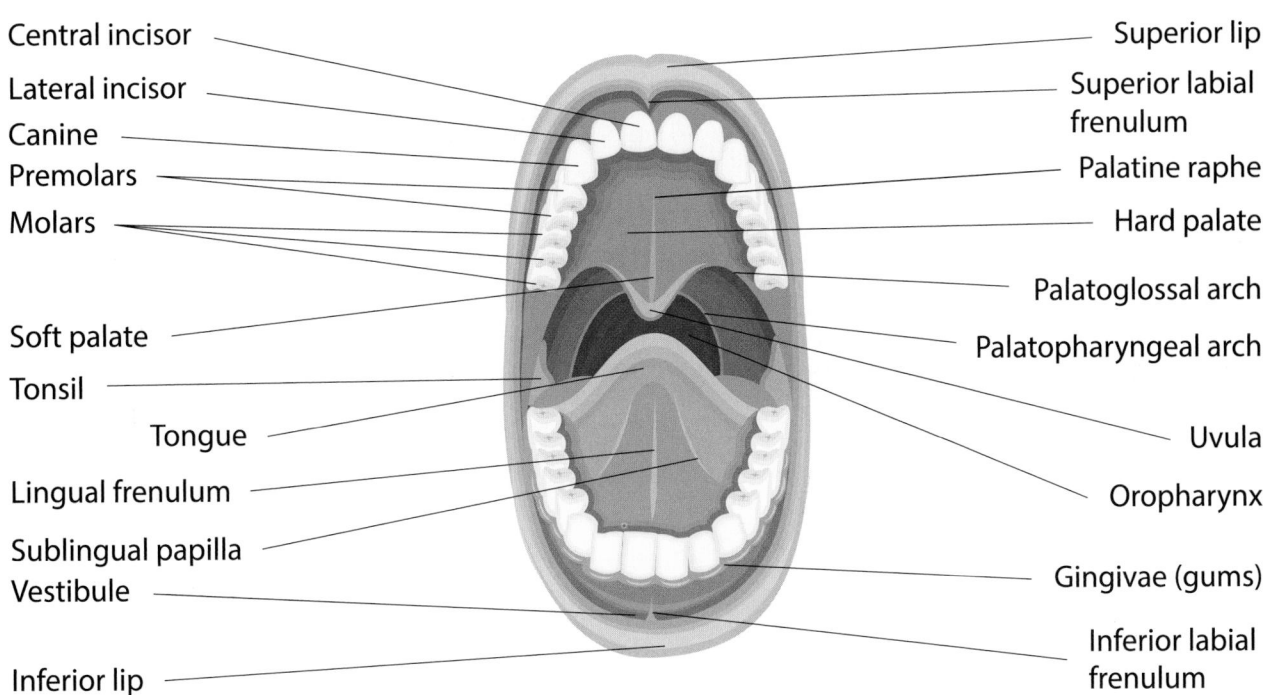

Central incisor
Lateral incisor
Canine
Premolars
Molars

Soft palate
Tonsil
Tongue
Lingual frenulum
Sublingual papilla
Vestibule

Inferior lip

Superior lip
Superior labial frenulum
Palatine raphe
Hard palate
Palatoglossal arch
Palatopharyngeal arch
Uvula
Oropharynx
Gingivae (gums)
Inferior labial frenulum

Digestive System — Tongue Anatomy

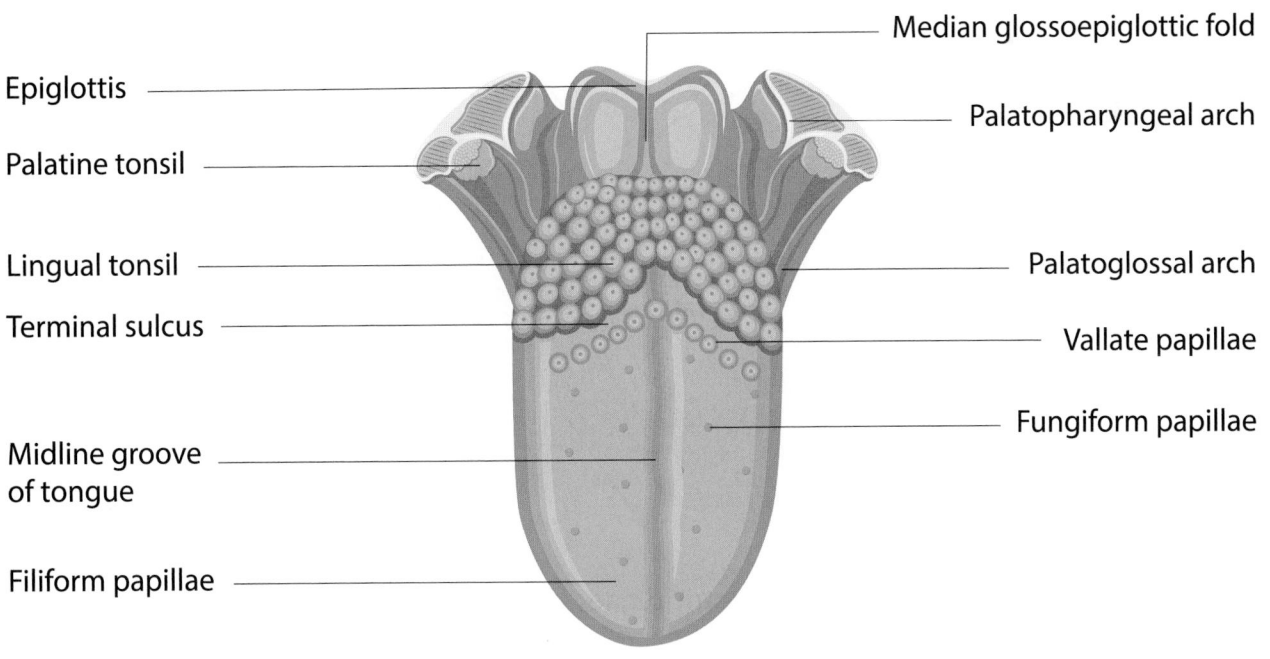

Epiglottis
Palatine tonsil
Lingual tonsil
Terminal sulcus
Midline groove of tongue
Filiform papillae

Median glossoepiglottic fold
Palatopharyngeal arch
Palatoglossal arch
Vallate papillae
Fungiform papillae

Digestive System — Small Intestine Anatomy

Digestive System — Stomach Anatomy

Ear Anatomy

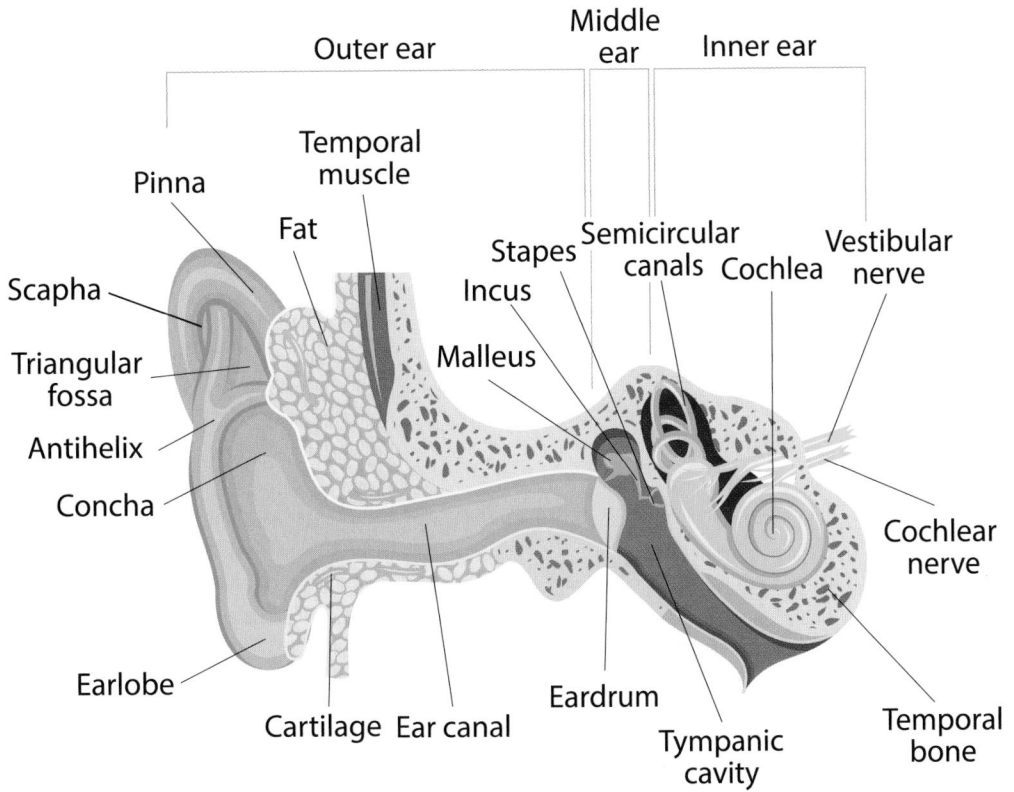

Cochlea Anatomy (Inner Ear)

Endocrine System Anatomy

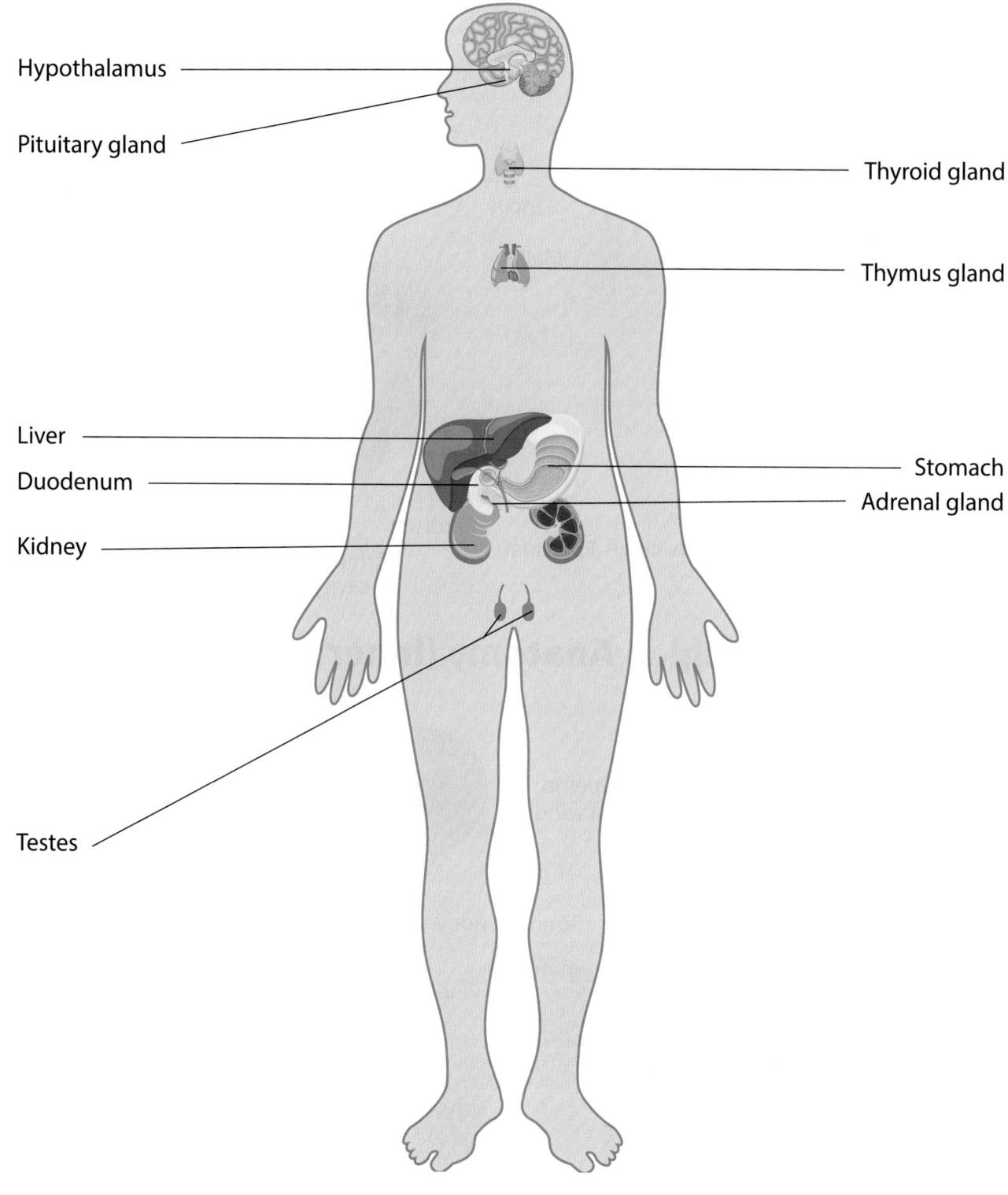

Hypothalamus

Pituitary gland

Thyroid gland

Thymus gland

Liver

Duodenum

Stomach

Adrenal gland

Kidney

Testes

Eye Anatomy

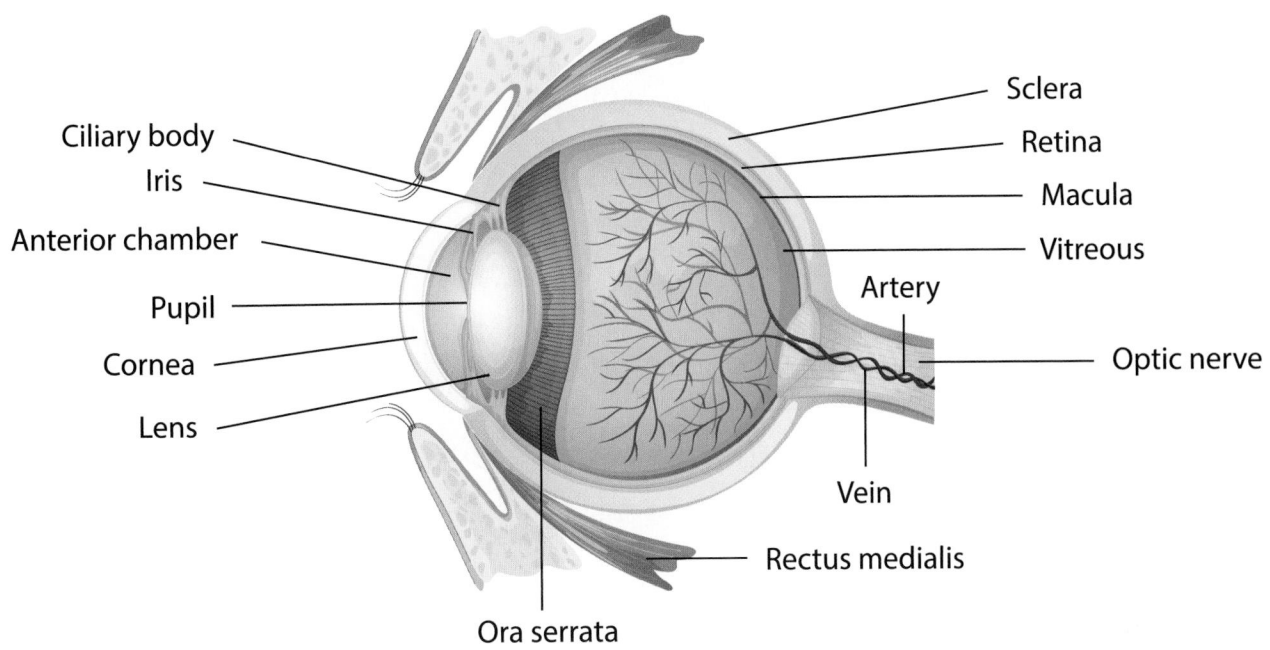

Muscles of the Eye

Female Reproductive System Anatomy

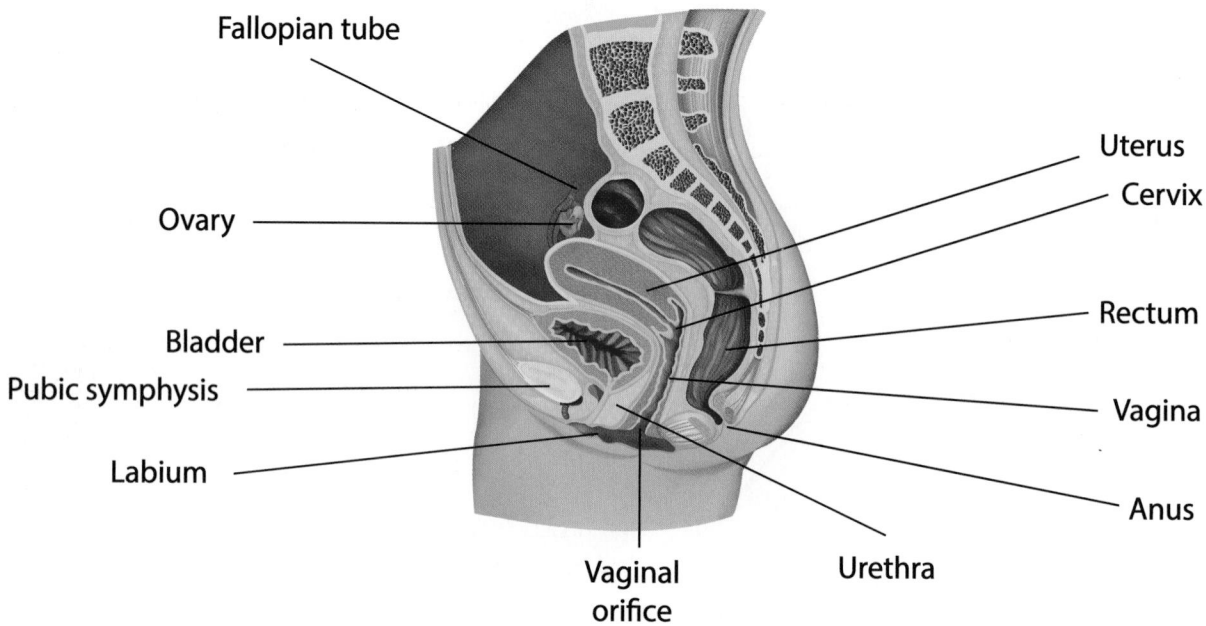

Fallopian tube

Ovary

Bladder

Pubic symphysis

Labium

Vaginal orifice

Uterus

Cervix

Rectum

Vagina

Anus

Urethra

Female Reproductive System — Uterus and Adnexa Anatomy

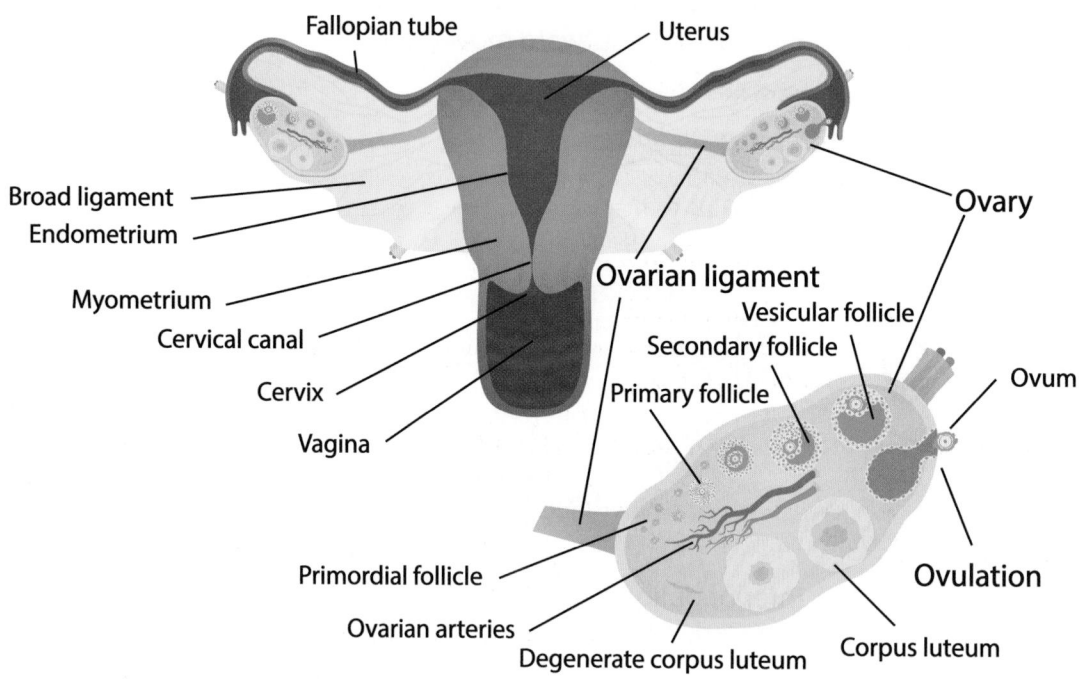

Fallopian tube

Uterus

Broad ligament

Endometrium

Myometrium

Cervical canal

Cervix

Vagina

Ovarian ligament

Ovary

Vesicular follicle

Secondary follicle

Primary follicle

Ovum

Primordial follicle

Ovarian arteries

Degenerate corpus luteum

Corpus luteum

Ovulation

Female Reproductive System — Breast Anatomy

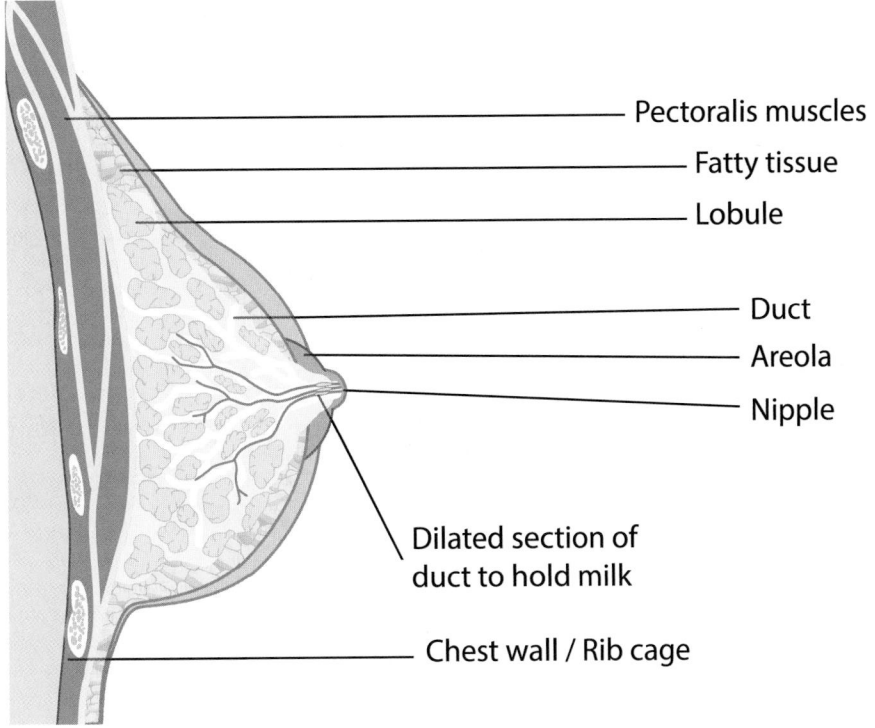

Pectoralis muscles

Fatty tissue

Lobule

Duct

Areola

Nipple

Dilated section of
duct to hold milk

Chest wall / Rib cage

Female Reproductive System — Perineum Anatomy

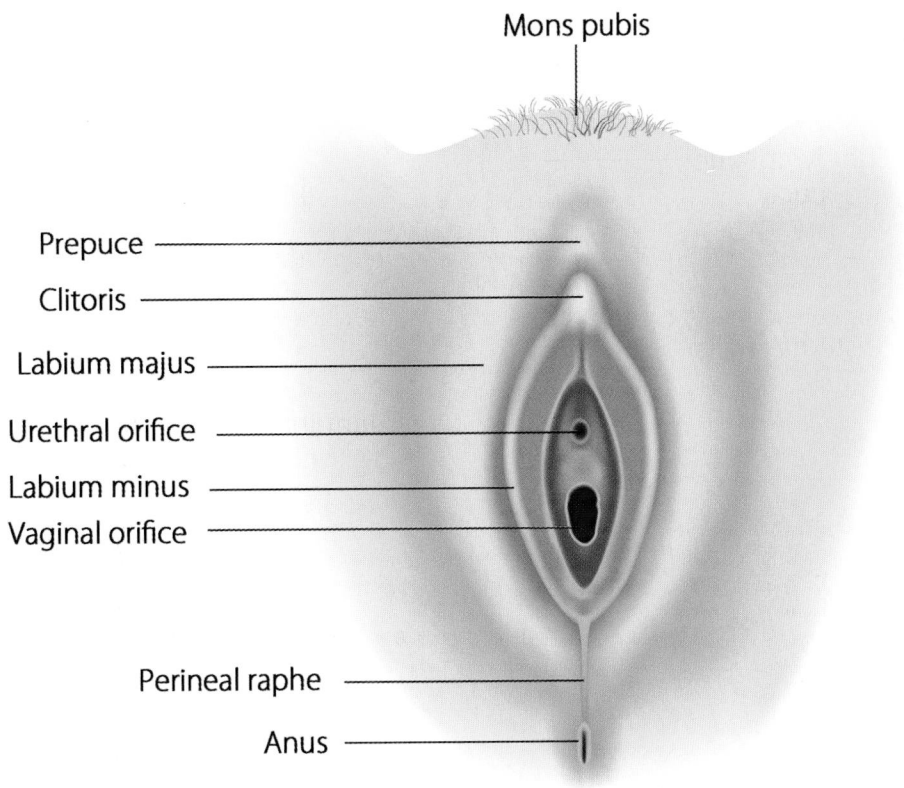

Mons pubis

Prepuce

Clitoris

Labium majus

Urethral orifice

Labium minus

Vaginal orifice

Perineal raphe

Anus

ANATOMICAL ILLUSTRATIONS

Integumentary System Anatomy

Sweat pore

Hair shaft

Meissner's corpuscle

Sweat gland

Stratum corneum (horny cell layer)

Papillary layer

Sebaceous (oil) gland

Arrector pili muscle

Reticular layer

Nerve

Epidermis

Dermis

Subcutaneous tissue

Hair follicle

Artery

Vein

Pacinian corpuscle

Adipose (fat) tissue

Lymphatic System Anatomy

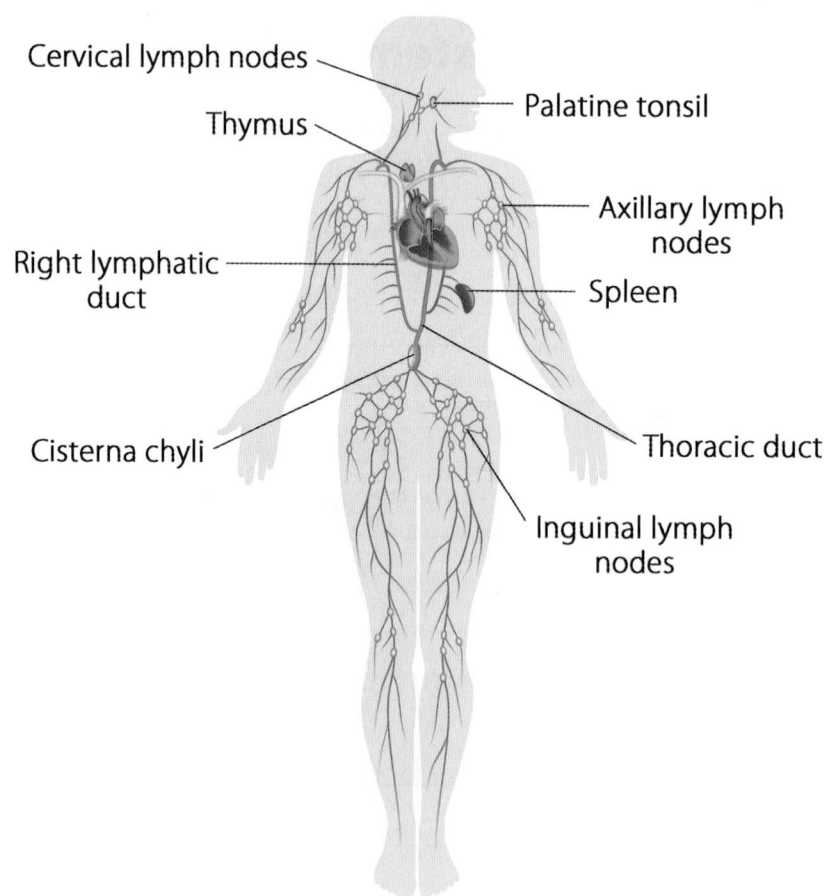

Cervical lymph nodes

Palatine tonsil

Thymus

Axillary lymph nodes

Right lymphatic duct

Spleen

Cisterna chyli

Thoracic duct

Inguinal lymph nodes

Lymphatic System — Humoral Immunity

Lymph Node Anatomy

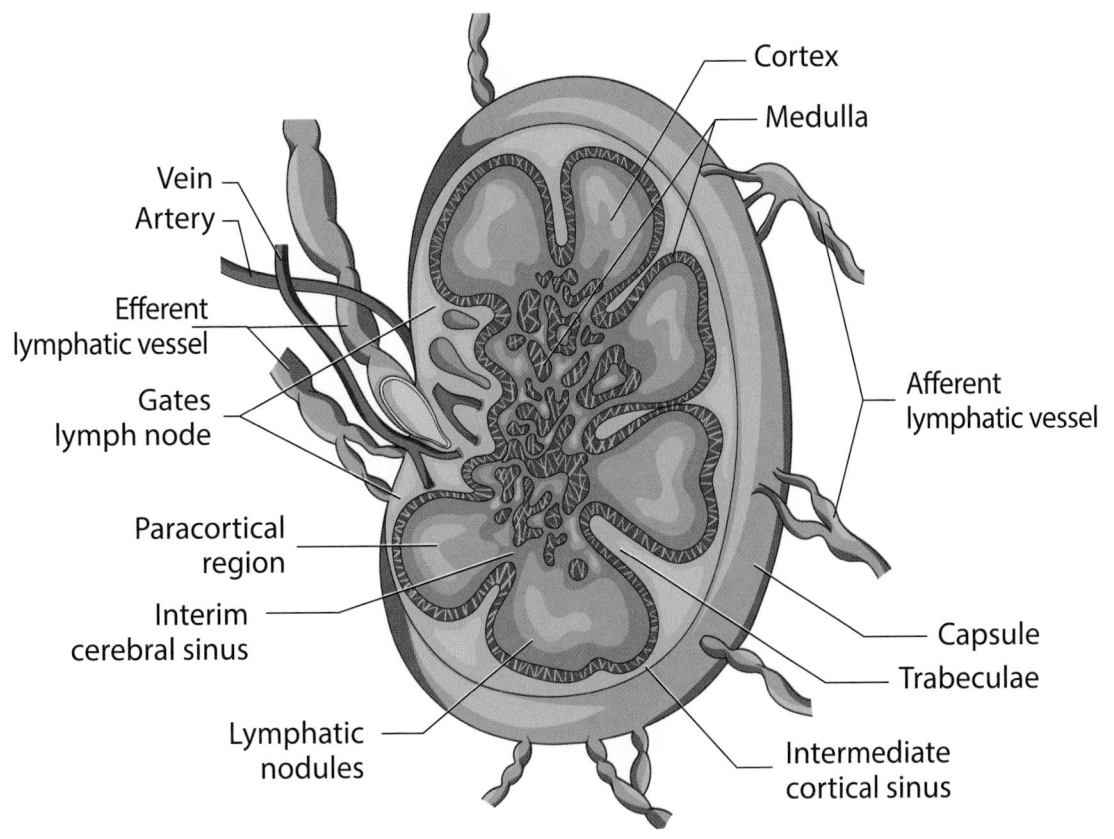

Male Reproductive System Anatomy

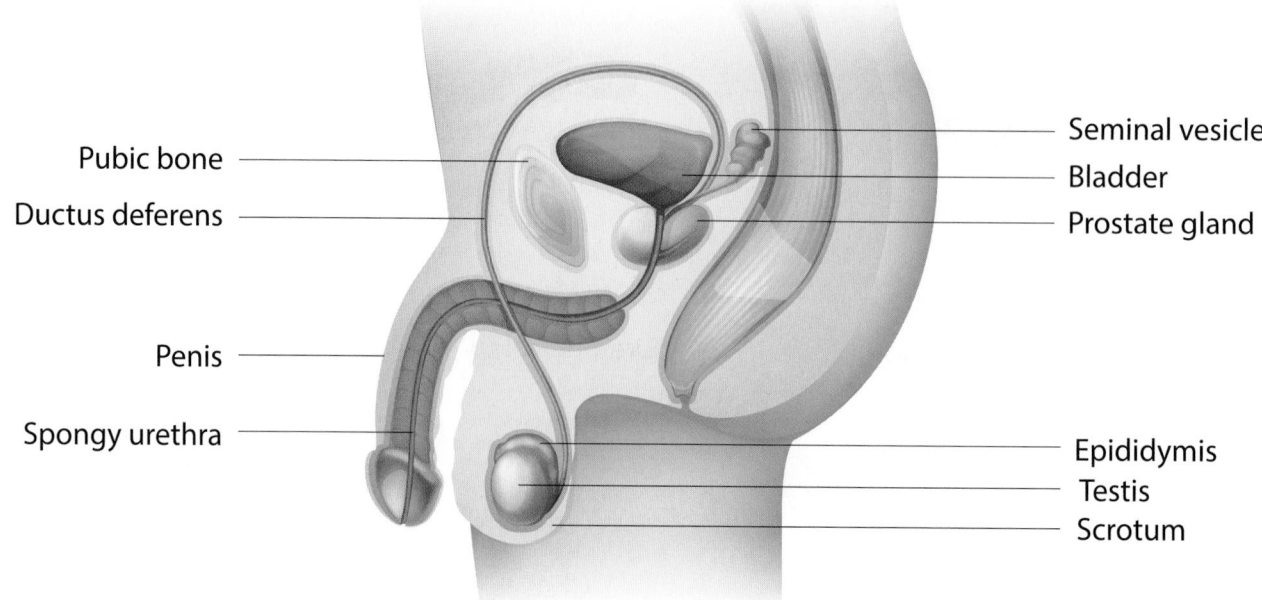

Pubic bone

Ductus deferens

Penis

Spongy urethra

Seminal vesicle

Bladder

Prostate gland

Epididymis

Testis

Scrotum

Male Reproductive System — Testicle Anatomy

Testicular artery

Epididymis

Testis

Pampiniform (venous) plexus

Ductus (vas) deferens

Male Reproductive System — Penis Anatomy

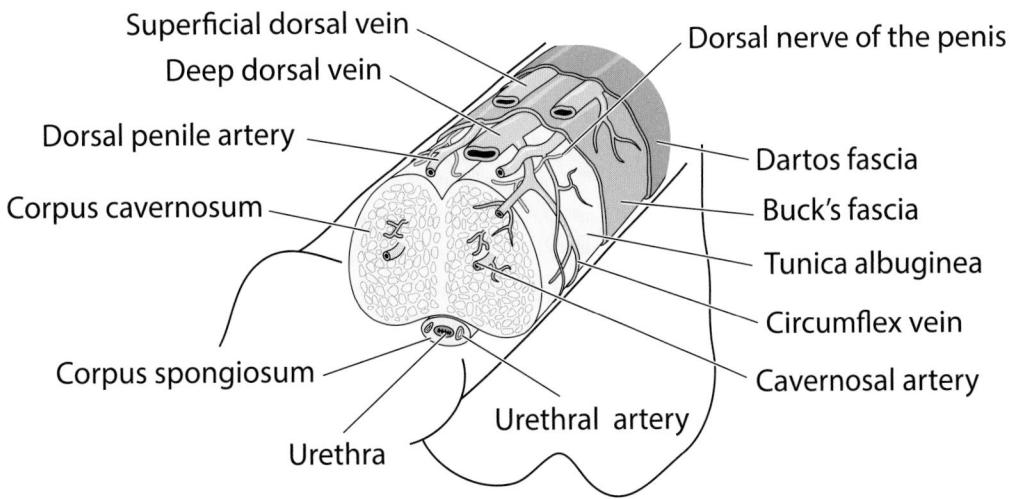

Superficial dorsal vein

Deep dorsal vein

Dorsal penile artery

Corpus cavernosum

Corpus spongiosum

Urethra

Urethral artery

Dorsal nerve of the penis

Dartos fascia

Buck's fascia

Tunica albuginea

Circumflex vein

Cavernosal artery

Muscular System Anatomy

Frontalis

Zygomaticus

Sternocleidomastoid

Deltoid

Pectoralis major

Coracobrachialis

Biceps brachii

Latissimus dorsi

Serratus anterior

External oblique

Gluteus medius

Pectineus

Rectus abdominis

Iliopsoas

Adductor longus

Gracilis

Sartorius

Rectus femoris

Iliotibial band

Vastus lateralis

Vastus medialis

Gastrocnemius

Extensor digitorum longus

Peroneus longus

Tibialis anterior

Extensor hallucis

Muscular System — Forearm Muscles
(Right Arm, Posterior Compartment)

Superficial

Triceps brachii

Brachioradialis

Anconeus

Extensor carpi radialis longus

Flexor carpi ulnaris

Extensor carpi radialis brevis

Extensor carpi ulnaris

Abductor pollicis longus

Extensor digit minimi

Extensor pollicis brevis

Extensor digitorum

Extensor pollicis longus

Extensor retinaculum

Deep

Triceps brachii

Anconeus

Brachioradialis

Extensor carpi radialis longus

Extensor carpi radialis brevis

Flexor carpi

Supinator

Abductor pollicis longus

Extensor pollicis brevis

Extensor pollicis longus

Extensor indicis

Tendons of extensor carpi radialis longus and brevis

Muscular System — Knee Joint Anatomy

Quadriceps femoris muscle

Femur

Quadriceps femoris tendon

Suprapatellar bursa

Prepatellar bursa

Patella

Joint cavity

Articular cartilage

Synovial membrane

Meniscus

Patellar ligament

Joint capsule

Superficial infrapatellar bursa

Deep infrapatellar bursa

Tibia

Muscular System — Shoulder (Rotator Cuff) Muscles

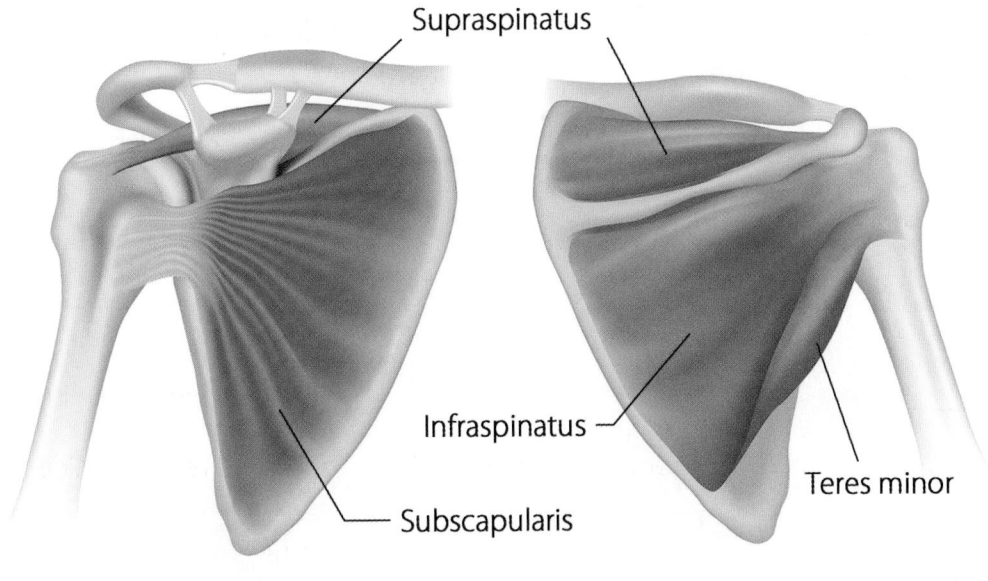

Supraspinatus

Infraspinatus

Subscapularis

Teres minor

Anterior view   **Posterior view**

Nervous System Anatomy

Brachial plexus

Musculocutaneous nerve

Radial nerve

Subcostal nerve

Median nerve

Iliohypogastric nerve

Ulnar nerve

Common peroneal nerve

Deep peroneal nerve

Superficial peroneal nerve

Brain

Cerebellum

Spinal cord

Intercostal nerve

Lumbar plexus

Sacral plexus

Femoral nerve

Pudendal nerve

Sciatic nerve

Saphenous nerve

Tibial nerve

Nervous System — Brain Anatomy

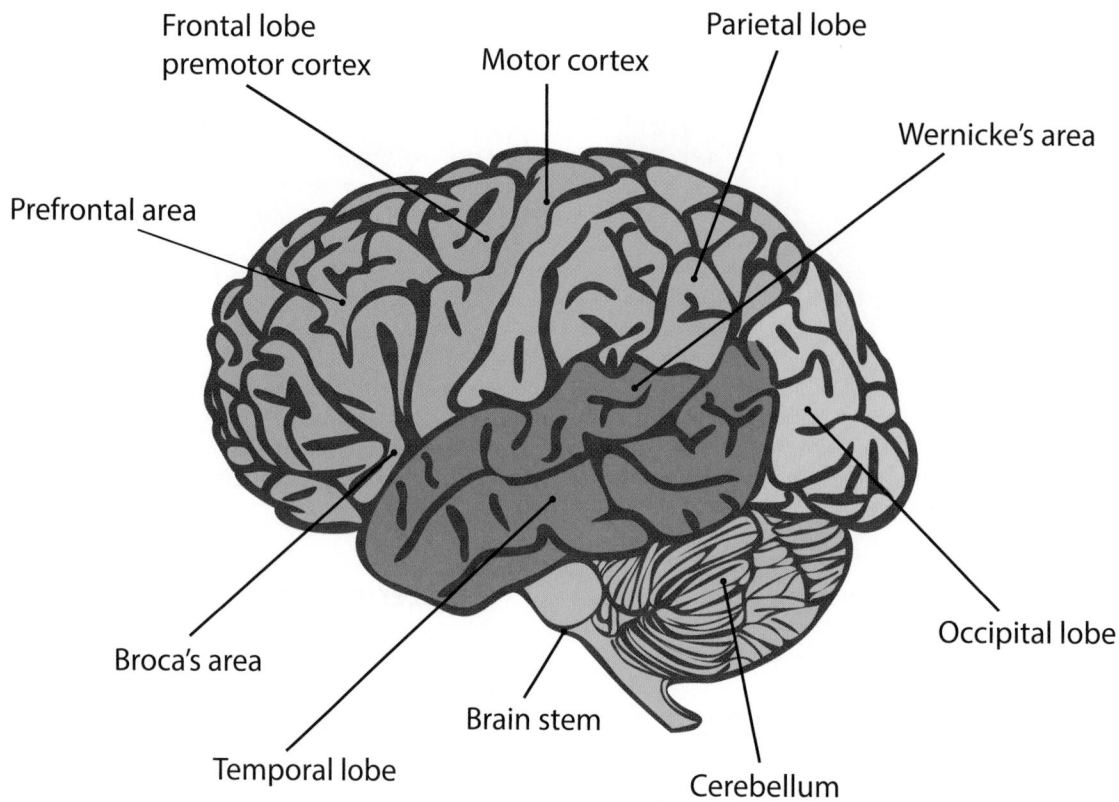

Frontal lobe premotor cortex

Motor cortex

Parietal lobe

Wernicke's area

Prefrontal area

Occipital lobe

Broca's area

Brain stem

Temporal lobe

Cerebellum

Nervous System — Cranial Nerves

Olfactory nerve fibers (I)

Optic nerve (II)

Oculomotor nerve (III)

Trochlear nerve (IV)

Trigeminal nerve (V)

Abducens nerve (VI)

Facial nerve (VII)

Vestibulocochlear nerve (VIII)

Glossopharyngeal nerve (IX)

Vagus nerve (X)

Accessory nerve (XI)

Hypoglossal nerve (XII)

Pons

Medulla

Nervous System — Nerve Anatomy

Spinal nerve

Epineurium

Blood vessels

Perineurium

Unmyelinated nerve fiber

Myelinated nerve fiber

Fascicle

Nerve fibers

Endoneurium

Cross section

Nervous System — Parasympathetic System Anatomy

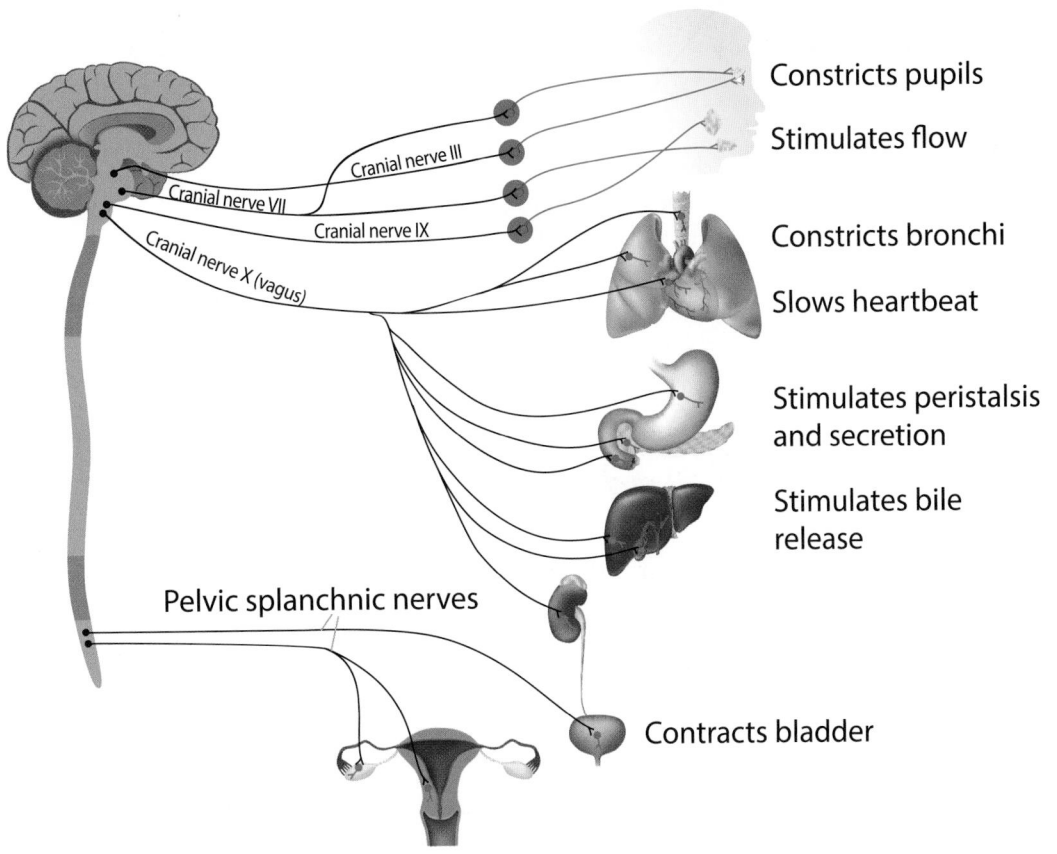

Cranial nerve III

Cranial nerve VII

Cranial nerve IX

Cranial nerve X (vagus)

Pelvic splanchnic nerves

Constricts pupils

Stimulates flow

Constricts bronchi

Slows heartbeat

Stimulates peristalsis and secretion

Stimulates bile release

Contracts bladder

Nervous System — Sympathetic System Anatomy

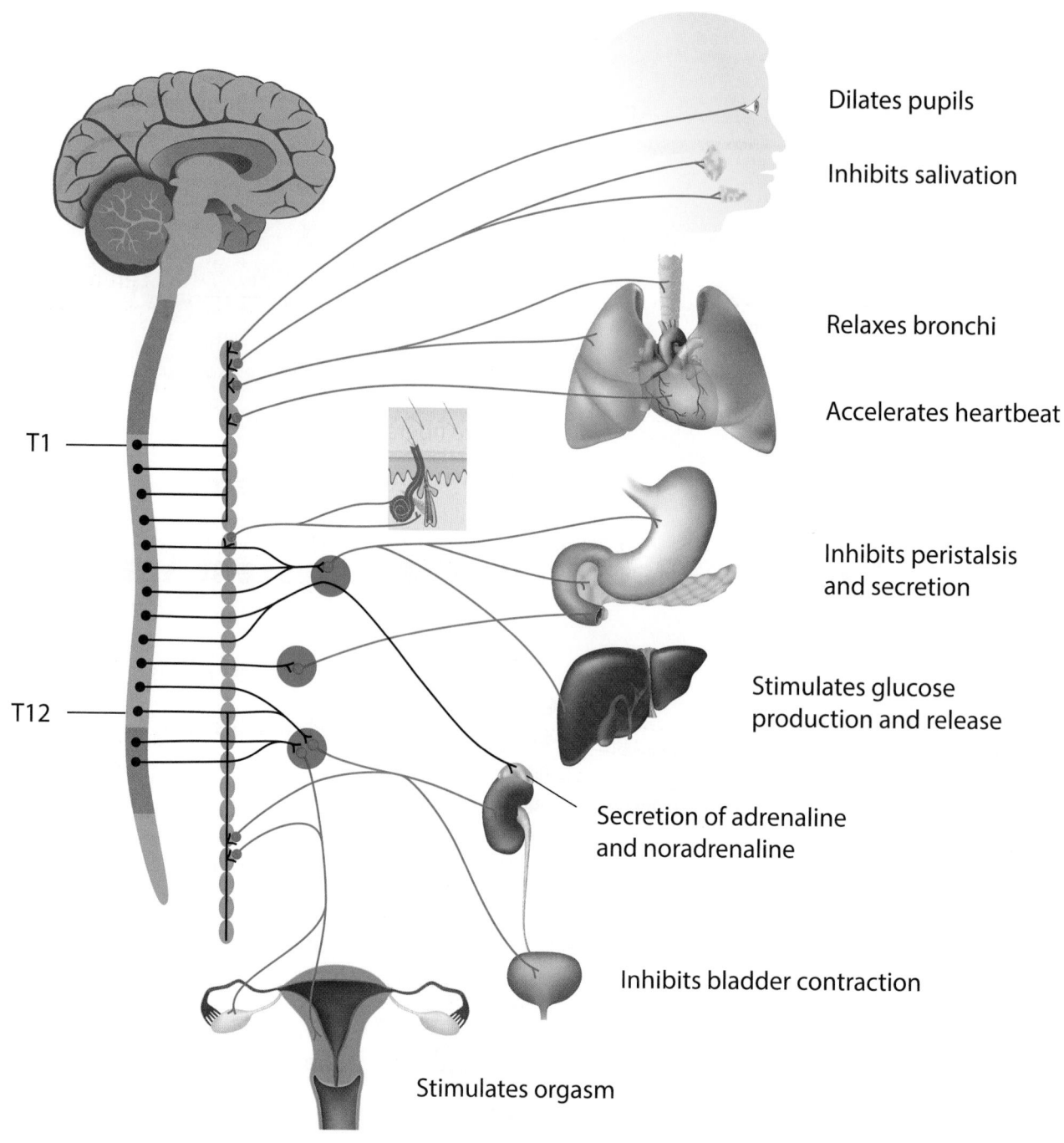

Dilates pupils

Inhibits salivation

Relaxes bronchi

Accelerates heartbeat

Inhibits peristalsis and secretion

Stimulates glucose production and release

Secretion of adrenaline and noradrenaline

Inhibits bladder contraction

Stimulates orgasm

T1

T12

Respiratory System Anatomy

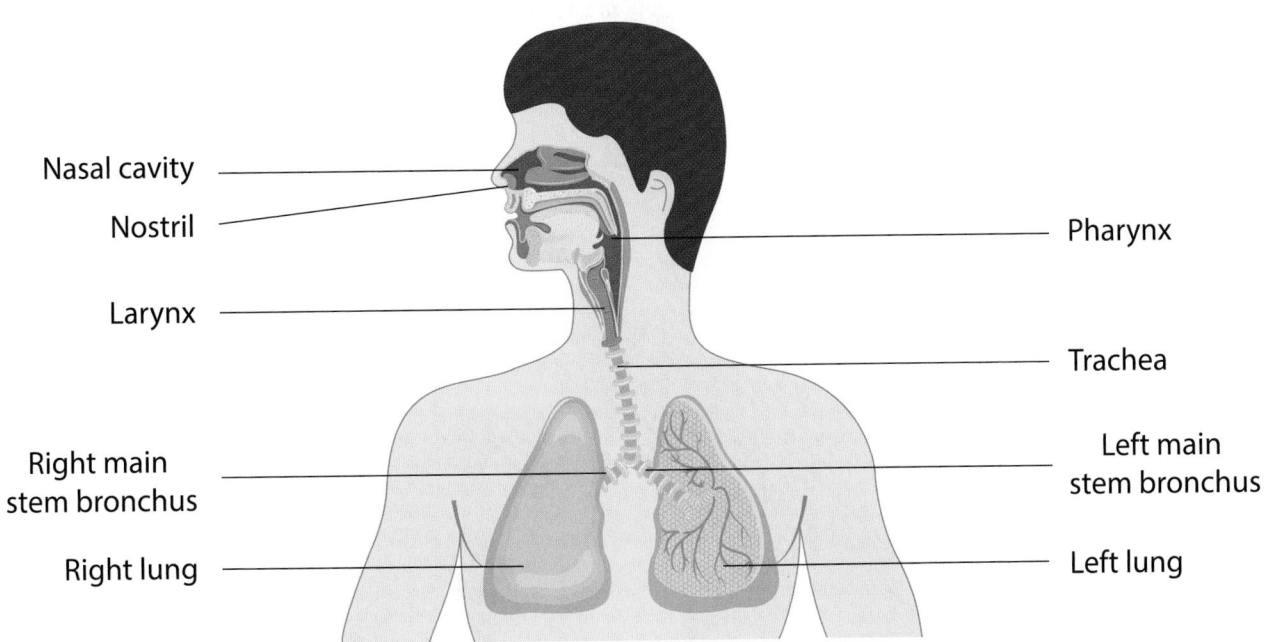

Nasal cavity

Nostril

Larynx

Pharynx

Trachea

Right main
stem bronchus

Left main
stem bronchus

Right lung

Left lung

Respiratory System — Larynx Anatomy

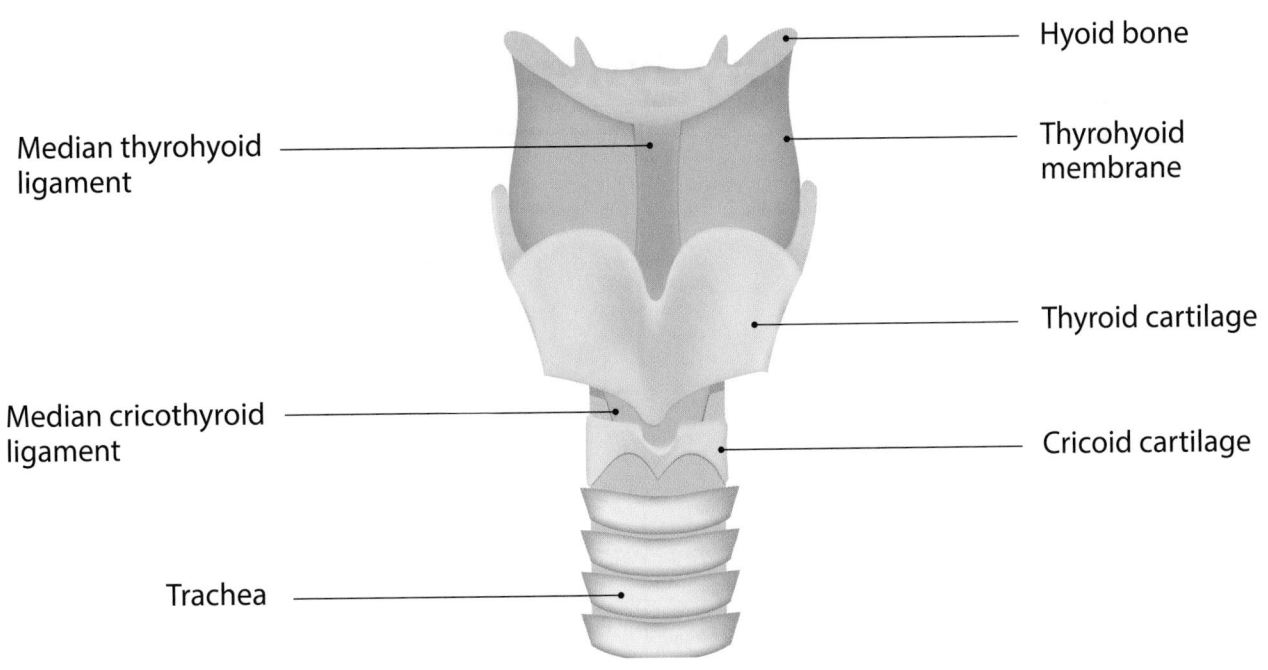

Median thyrohyoid
ligament

Hyoid bone

Thyrohyoid
membrane

Thyroid cartilage

Median cricothyroid
ligament

Cricoid cartilage

Trachea

Respiratory System — Lung Anatomy

Larynx

Trachea (windpipe)

Right superior lobe

Left superior lobe

Bronchial tree

Bronchi

Right middle lobe

Pleura

Right inferior lobe

Left inferior lobe

Diaphragm

Respiratory System Function

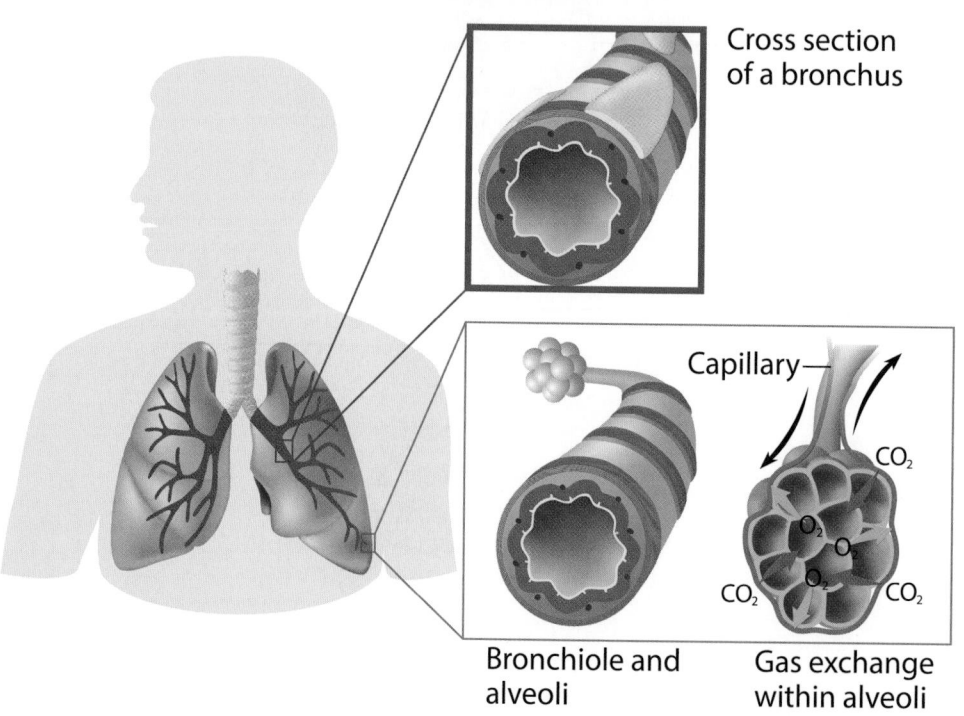

Cross section
of a bronchus

Capillary

CO_2

O_2 O_2 O_2

CO_2 O_2 CO_2

Bronchiole and
alveoli

Gas exchange
within alveoli

Respiratory System — Nose Anatomy

Frontal sinus

Nasal bone

Nasal cavity

Nasal vestibule

Hard palate

Lips

Superior turbinate

Sphenoid sinus

Middle turbinate

Adenoid pad

Inferior turbinate

Soft palate

Respiratory System — Sinus Anatomy

Frontal sinus

Ethmoid sinus

Sphenoid sinus

Maxillary sinus

Respiratory System — Throat Anatomy

Middle turbinate
Superior turbinate
Inferior turbinate
Adenoid
Soft palate
Tongue
Tonsil
Genioglossus muscle
Lingual tonsil
Mandible
Epiglottis
Hyoid bone
Vocal cords
Thyroid cartilage
Esophagus
Trachea

Skeletal System Anatomy

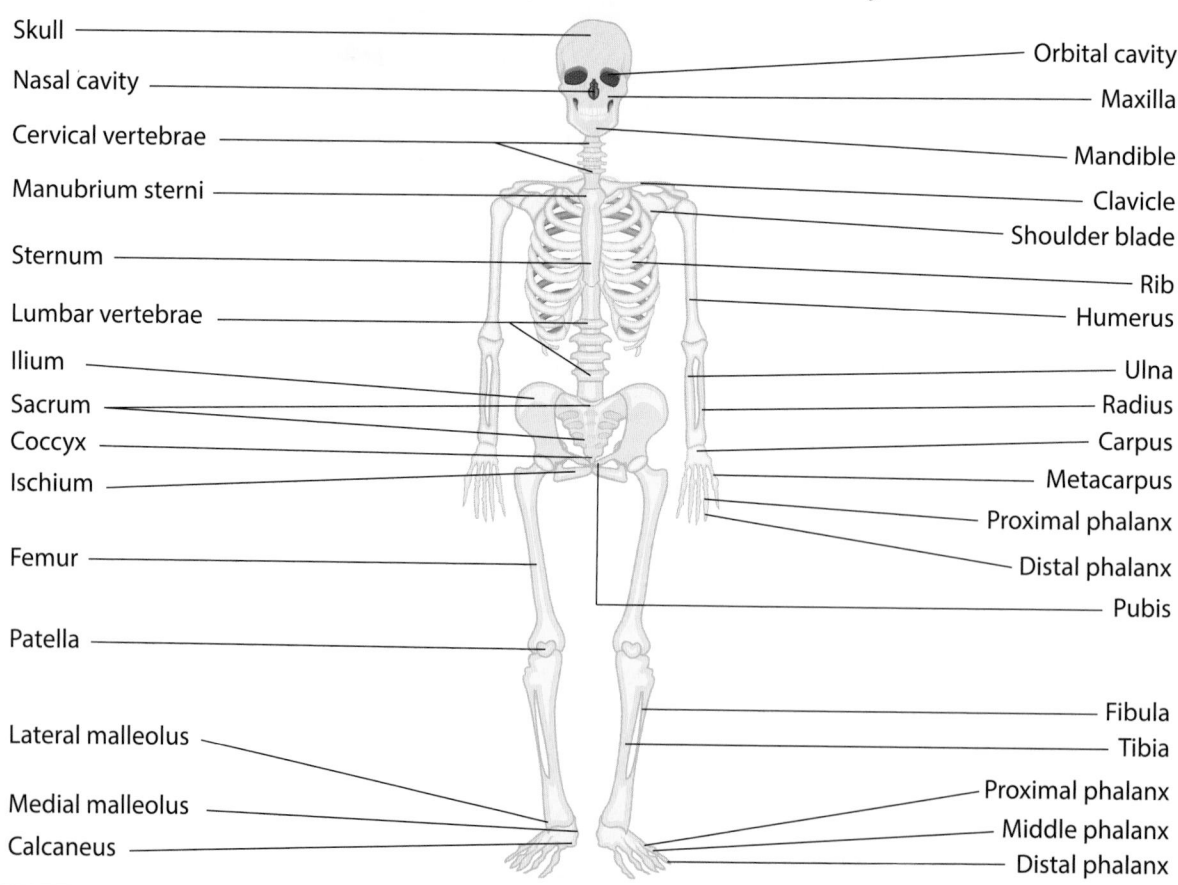

Skull
Orbital cavity
Nasal cavity
Maxilla
Cervical vertebrae
Mandible
Manubrium sterni
Clavicle
Shoulder blade
Sternum
Rib
Humerus
Lumbar vertebrae
Ulna
Ilium
Radius
Sacrum
Carpus
Coccyx
Metacarpus
Ischium
Proximal phalanx
Distal phalanx
Femur
Pubis
Patella
Fibula
Tibia
Lateral malleolus
Proximal phalanx
Medial malleolus
Middle phalanx
Calcaneus
Distal phalanx

Skeletal System — Bone Structure

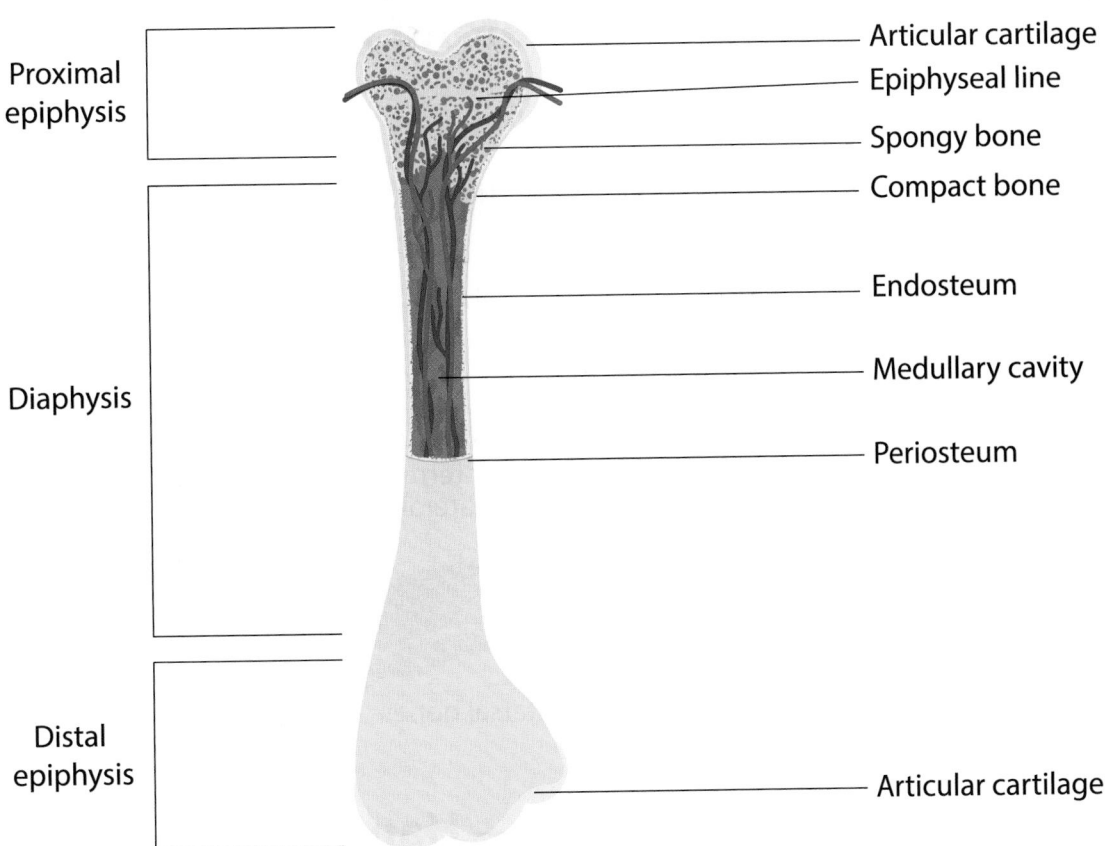

Proximal epiphysis

Diaphysis

Distal epiphysis

Articular cartilage

Epiphyseal line

Spongy bone

Compact bone

Endosteum

Medullary cavity

Periosteum

Articular cartilage

Skeletal System — Cervical, Thoracic, and Lumbar Spine

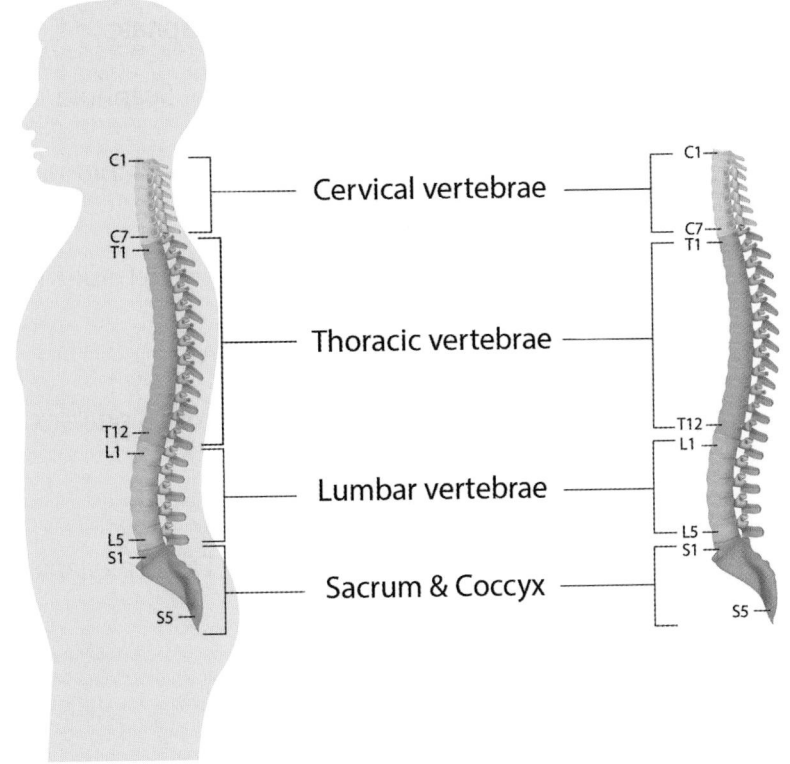

Cervical vertebrae

Thoracic vertebrae

Lumbar vertebrae

Sacrum & Coccyx

Skeletal System — Foot Bones
(Right Foot, Lateral View)

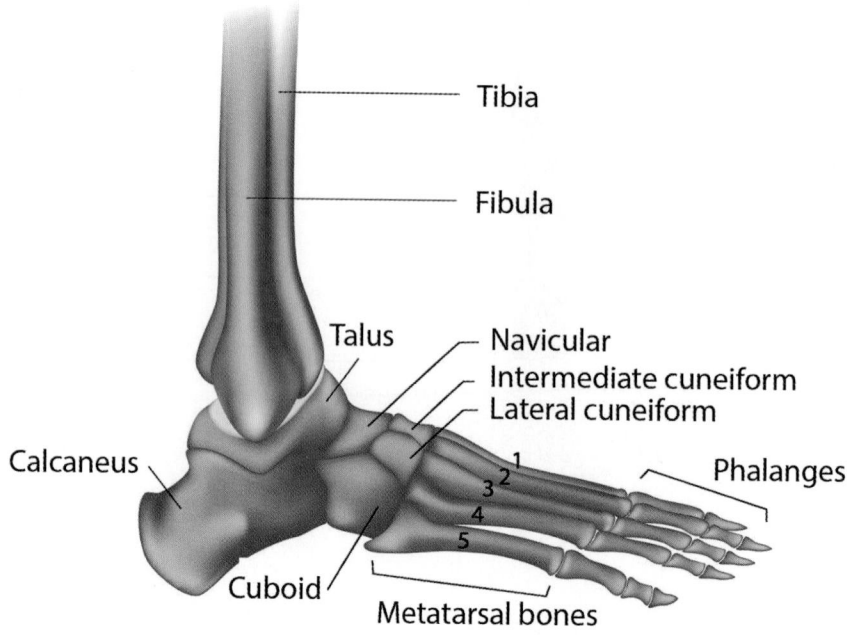

- Tibia
- Fibula
- Talus
- Navicular
- Intermediate cuneiform
- Lateral cuneiform
- Calcaneus
- 1
- 2
- 3
- 4
- 5
- Phalanges
- Cuboid
- Metatarsal bones

Skeletal System — Hand Bones

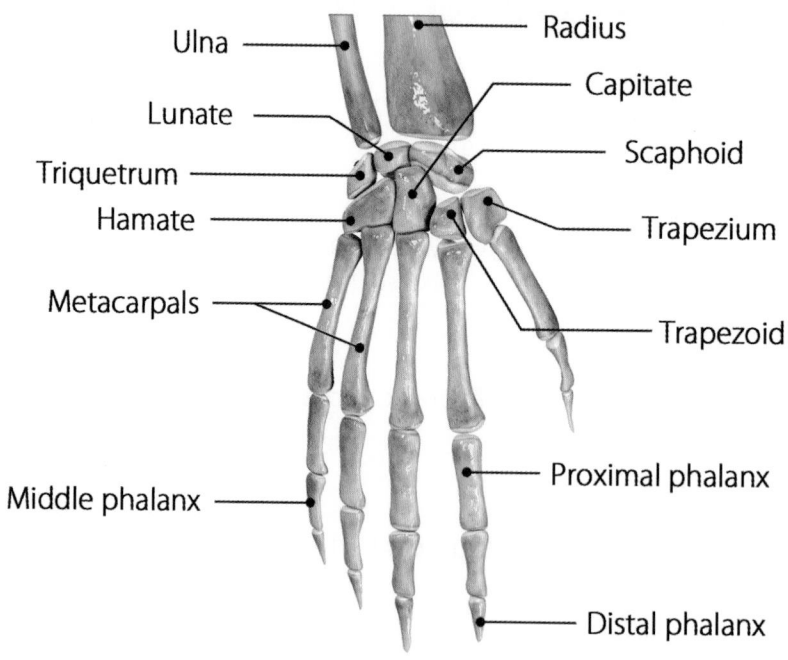

- Ulna
- Radius
- Lunate
- Capitate
- Triquetrum
- Scaphoid
- Hamate
- Trapezium
- Metacarpals
- Trapezoid
- Middle phalanx
- Proximal phalanx
- Distal phalanx

Skeletal System — Skull Anatomy

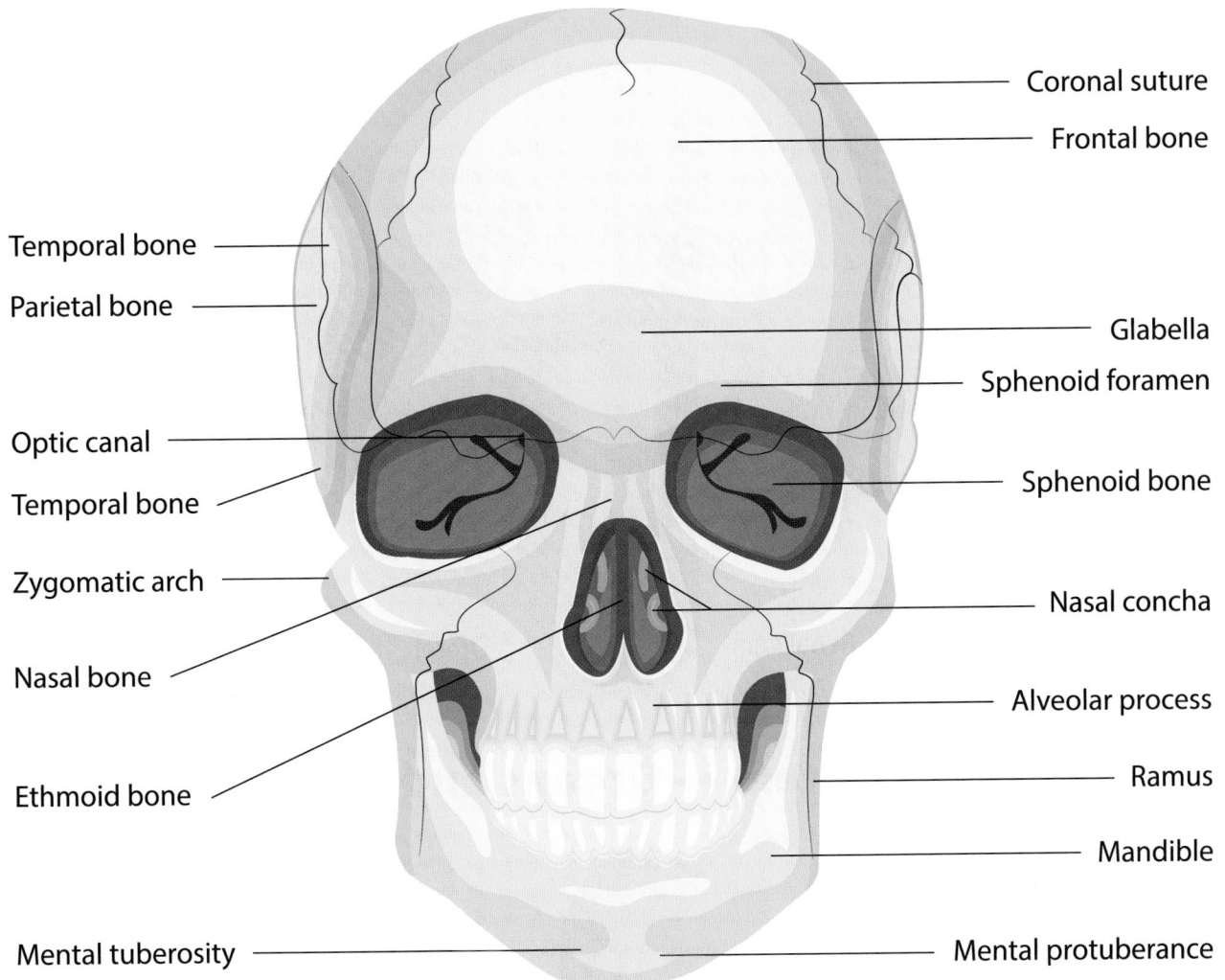

Coronal suture

Frontal bone

Temporal bone

Parietal bone

Glabella

Sphenoid foramen

Optic canal

Temporal bone

Sphenoid bone

Zygomatic arch

Nasal concha

Nasal bone

Alveolar process

Ethmoid bone

Ramus

Mandible

Mental tuberosity

Mental protuberance

Urinary System — Kidney Anatomy

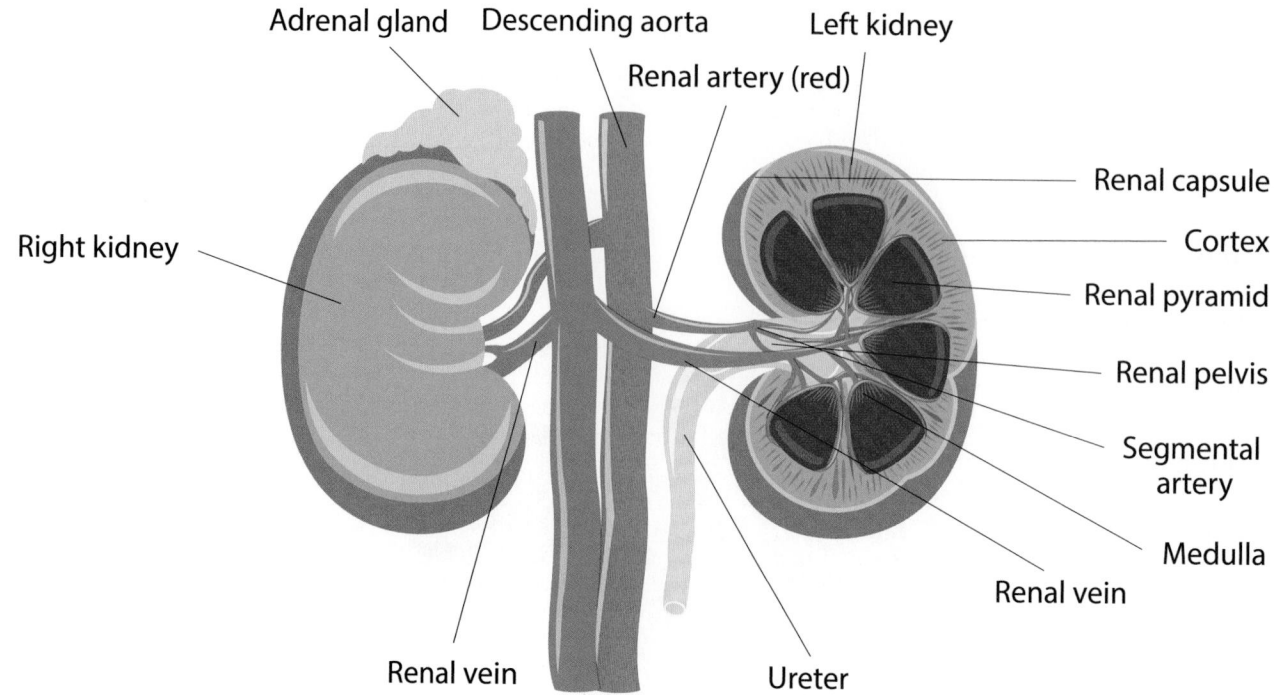

Urinary System — Organs and Structures

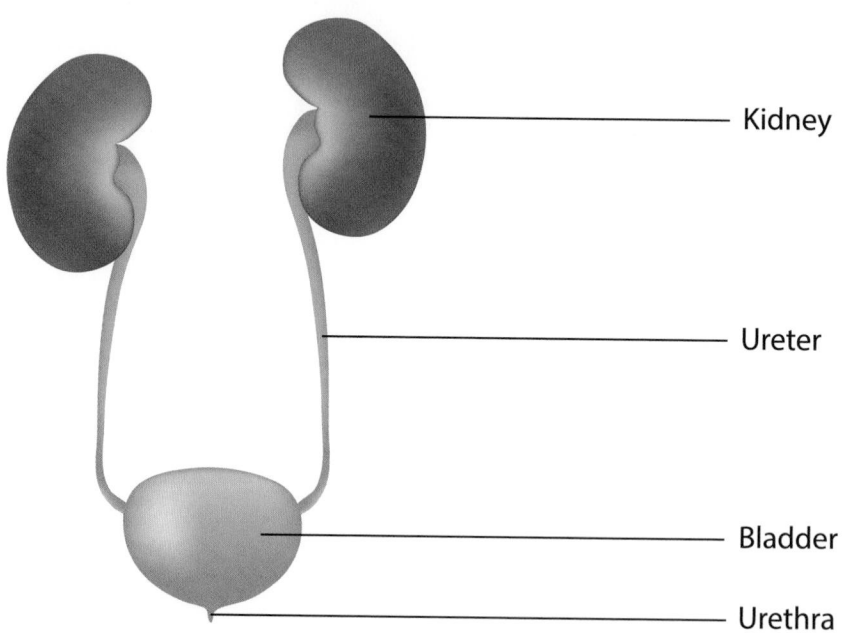

Approach Table

Approach	Definition	Examples
External	Procedures performed directly on the skin or mucous membrane and procedures performed indirectly by the application of external force through the skin or mucous membrane	• Cauterization of epistaxis • Reduction of a dislocated shoulder • Destruction of renal calculi with lithotripsy
Open	Cutting through the skin or mucous membrane and any other body layers necessary to expose the site of the procedure	• Open reduction and internal fixation of a fracture • Abdominal appendectomy • Open coronary artery bypass graft
Percutaneous	Entry, by puncture or minor incision, of instrumentation through the skin or mucous membrane and/or any other body layers necessary to reach the site of the procedure	• Percutaneous paracentesis • Tracheostomy formation with tracheostomy tube placement • Needle biopsy of breast mass
Percutaneous, Endoscopic	Entry, by puncture or minor incision, of instrumentation through the skin or mucous membrane and/or any other body layers necessary to reach and visualize the site of the procedure	• Shoulder arthroscopy • Autograft nerve graft to right median nerve • Mapping of left cerebral hemisphere
Via Natural or Artificial Opening	Entry of instrumentation through a natural or artificial external opening to reach the site of the procedure	• Placement of a Foley catheter • Endotracheal intubation • Transvaginal cervical cerclage
Via Natural or Artificial Opening, Endoscopic	Entry of instrumentation through a natural or artificial external opening to reach and visualize the site of the procedure	• Colonoscopy • Bronchoscopy • Esophagogastroduodenoscopy (EGD)
Via Natural or Artificial Opening, Endoscopic, with Percutaneous Endoscopic Assistance	Entry of instrumentation through a natural or artificial external opening to reach and visualize the site of the procedure, and entry, by puncture or minor incision, of instrumentation through the skin or mucous membrane and any other body layers necessary to aid in the performance of the procedure	• Resections of the female reproductive system • Laparoscopic-assisted vaginal salpingoophrectomy and hysterectomy

This page intentionally left blank

3

3f® (Aortic) Bioprosthesis valve
   use Zooplastic Tissue in Heart and Great Vessels

A

Abdominal aortic plexus
   use Abdominal Sympathetic Nerve
Abdominal esophagus
   use Esophagus, Lower
Abdominohysterectomy
   see Resection, Uterus 0UT9
   see Resection, Cervix 0UTC
Abdominoplasty
   see Alteration, Abdominal Wall 0W0F
   see Repair, Abdominal Wall 0WQF
   see Supplement, Abdominal Wall 0WUF
Abductor hallucis muscle
   use Foot Muscle, Right
   use Foot Muscle, Left
AbioCor® Total Replacement Heart
   use Synthetic Substitute
Ablation
   see Destruction
Abortion
   Products of Conception 10A0
   Abortifacient 10A07ZX
   Laminaria 10A07ZW
   Vacuum 10A07Z6
Abrasion
   see Extraction
Absolute Pro® Vascular (OTW) Self-Expanding Stent System
   use Intraluminal Device
Accessory cephalic vein
   use Cephalic Vein, Right
   use Cephalic Vein, Left
Accessory obturator nerve
   use Lumbar Plexus
Accessory phrenic nerve
   use Phrenic Nerve
Accessory spleen
   use Spleen
Acculink™ (RX) Carotid Stent System
   use Intraluminal Device
Acellular Hydrated Dermis
   use Nonautologous Tissue Substitute
Acetabular cup
   use Liner in Lower Joints
Acetabulectomy
   see Excision, Lower Bones 0QB
   see Resection, Lower Bones 0QT
Acetabulofemoral joint
   use Hip Joint, Right
   use Hip Joint, Left
Acetabuloplasty
   see Repair, Lower Bones 0QQ
   see Replacement, Lower Bones 0QR
   see Supplement, Lower Bones 0QU
Achilles tendon
   use Lower Leg Tendon, Right
   use Lower Leg Tendon, Left
Achillorrhaphy
   see Repair, Tendons 0LQ
Achillotenotomy, achillotomy
   see Division, Tendons 0L8
   see Drainage, Tendons 0L9
Acromioclavicular ligament
   use Shoulder Bursa and Ligament, Right
   use Shoulder Bursa and Ligament, Left

Acromion (process)
   use Scapula, Right
   use Scapula, Left
Acromionectomy
   see Excision, Upper Joints 0RB
   see Resection, Upper Joints 0RT
Acromioplasty
   see Repair, Upper Joints 0RQ
   see Replacement, Upper Joints 0RR
   see Supplement, Upper Joints 0RU
Activa PC® neurostimulator
   use Stimulator Generator, Multiple Array in 0JH
Activa RC® neurostimulator
   use Stimulator Generator, Multiple Array Rechargeable in 0JH
Activa SC® neurostimulator
   use Stimulator Generator, Single Array in 0JH
Activities of Daily Living Assessment F02
Activities of Daily Living Treatment F08
ACUITY™ Steerable Lead
   use Cardiac Lead, Pacemaker in 02H
   use Cardiac Lead, Defibrillator in 02H
Acupuncture
   Breast
      Anesthesia 8E0H300
      No Qualifier 8E0H30Z
   Integumentary System
      Anesthesia 8E0H300
      No Qualifier 8E0H30Z
Adductor brevis muscle
   use Upper Leg Muscle, Right
   use Upper Leg Muscle, Left
Adductor hallucis muscle
   use Foot Muscle, Right
   use Foot Muscle, Left
Adductor longus muscle
   use Upper Leg Muscle, Right
   use Upper Leg Muscle, Left
Adductor magnus muscle
   use Upper Leg Muscle, Right
   use Upper Leg Muscle, Left
Adenohypophysis
   use Pituitary Gland
Adenoidectomy
   see Excision, Adenoids 0CBQ
   see Resection, Adenoids 0CTQ
Adenoidotomy
   see Drainage, Adenoids 0C9Q
Adhesiolysis
   see Release
Administration
   Blood products *see* Transfusion
   Other substance *see* Introduction of substance in or on
Adrenalectomy
   see Excision, Endocrine System 0GB
   see Resection, Endocrine System 0GT
Adrenalorrhaphy
   see Repair, Endocrine System 0GQ
Adrenalotomy
   see Drainage, Endocrine System 0G9
Advancement
   see Reposition
   see Transfer
Advisa (MRI)™
   use Pacemaker, Dual Chamber in 0JH
AFX® Endovascular AAA System
   use Intraluminal Device
AIGISRx Antibacterial Envelope
   use Anti-Infective Envelope
Alar ligament of axis
   use Head and Neck Bursa and Ligament

Alfieri Stitch Valvuloplasty
   see Restriction, Valve, Mitral 02VG
Alimentation
   see Introduction of substance in or on
Alteration
   Abdominal Wall 0W0F
   Ankle Region
      Left 0Y0L
      Right 0Y0K
   Arm
      Lower
         Left 0X0F
         Right 0X0D
      Upper
         Left 0X09
         Right 0X08
   Axilla
      Left 0X05
      Right 0X04
   Back
      Lower 0W0L
      Upper 0W0K
   Breast
      Bilateral 0H0V
      Left 0H0U
      Right 0H0T
   Buttock
      Left 0Y01
      Right 0Y00
   Chest Wall 0W08
   Ear
      Bilateral 0902
      Left 0901
      Right 0900
   Elbow Region
      Left 0X0C
      Right 0X0B
   Extremity
      Lower
         Left 0Y0B
         Right 0Y09
      Upper
         Left 0X07
         Right 0X06
   Eyelid
      Lower
         Left 080R
         Right 080Q
      Upper
         Left 080P
         Right 080N
   Face 0W02
   Head 0W00
   Jaw
      Lower 0W05
      Upper 0W04
   Knee Region
      Left 0Y0G
      Right 0Y0F
   Leg
      Lower
         Left 0Y0J
         Right 0Y0H
      Upper
         Left 0Y0D
         Right 0Y0C
   Lip
      Lower 0C01X
      Upper 0C00X
   Nasal Mucosa and Soft Tissue 090K
   Neck 0W06
   Perineum
      Female 0W0N
      Male 0W0M

Alteration — *continued*
  Shoulder Region
    Left 0X03
    Right 0X02
  Subcutaneous Tissue and Fascia
    Abdomen 0J08
    Back 0J07
    Buttock 0J09
    Chest 0J06
    Face 0J01
    Lower Arm
      Left 0J0H
      Right 0J0G
    Lower Leg
      Left 0J0P
      Right 0J0N
    Neck
      Left 0J05
      Right 0J04
    Upper Arm
      Left 0J0F
      Right 0J0D
    Upper Leg
      Left 0J0M
      Right 0J0L
  Wrist Region
    Left 0X0H
    Right 0X0G
Alveolar process of mandible
  use Mandible, Right
  use Mandible, Left
Alveolar process of maxilla
  use Maxilla
Alveolectomy
  see Excision, Head and Facial Bones 0NB
  see Resection, Head and Facial Bones 0NT
Alveoloplasty
  see Repair, Head and Facial Bones 0NQ
  see Replacement, Head and Facial Bones 0NR
  see Supplement, Head and Facial Bones 0NU
Alveolotomy
  see Division, Head and Facial Bones 0N8
  see Drainage, Head and Facial Bones 0N9
Ambulatory cardiac monitoring 4A12X45
Amniocentesis
  see Drainage, Products of Conception 1090
Amnioinfusion
  see Introduction of substance in or on, Products of Conception 3E0E
Amnioscopy 10J08ZZ
Amniotomy
  see Drainage, Products of Conception 1090
AMPLATZER® Muscular VSD Occluder
  use Synthetic Substitute
Amputation
  see Detachment
AMS 800® Urinary Control System
  use Artificial Sphincter in Urinary System
Anal orifice
  use Anus
Analog radiography
  see Plain Radiography
Analog radiology
  see Plain Radiography
Anastomosis
  see Bypass
Anatomical snuffbox
  use Lower Arm and Wrist Muscle, Right
  use Lower Arm and Wrist Muscle, Left
Andexanet Alfa, Factor Xa Inhibitor Reversal Agent XW0
AneuRx® AAA Advantage®
  use Intraluminal Device
Angiectomy
  see Excision, Heart and Great Vessels 02B

Angiectomy — *continued*
  see Excision, Upper Arteries 03B
  see Excision, Lower Arteries 04B
  see Excision, Upper Veins 05B
  see Excision, Lower Veins 06B
Angiocardiography
  Combined right and left heart *see* Fluoroscopy, Heart, Right and Left B216
  Left Heart *see* Fluoroscopy, Heart, Left B215
  Right Heart *see* Fluoroscopy, Heart, Right B214
  SPY system intravascular fluorescence *see* Monitoring, Physiological Systems 4A1
Angiography
  see Plain Radiography, Heart B20
  see Fluoroscopy, Heart B21
Angioplasty
  see Dilation, Heart and Great Vessels 027
  see Repair, Heart and Great Vessels 02Q
  see Replacement, Heart and Great Vessels 02R
  see Supplement, Heart and Great Vessels 02U
  see Dilation, Upper Arteries 037
  see Repair, Upper Arteries 03Q
  see Replacement, Upper Arteries 03R
  see Supplement, Upper Arteries 03U
  see Dilation, Lower Arteries 047
  see Repair, Lower Arteries 04Q
  see Replacement, Lower Arteries 04R
  see Supplement, Lower Arteries 04U
Angiorrhaphy
  see Repair, Heart and Great Vessels 02Q
  see Repair, Upper Arteries 03Q
  see Repair, Lower Arteries 04Q
Angioscopy
  02JY4ZZ
  03JY4ZZ
  04JY4ZZ
Angiotripsy
  see Occlusion, Upper Arteries 03L
  see Occlusion, Lower Arteries 04L
Angular artery
  use Face Artery
Angular vein
  use Face Vein, Right
  use Face Vein, Left
Annular ligament
  use Elbow Bursa and Ligament, Right
  use Elbow Bursa and Ligament, Left
Annuloplasty
  see Repair, Heart and Great Vessels 02Q
  see Supplement, Heart and Great Vessels 02U
Annuloplasty ring
  use Synthetic Substitute
Anoplasty
  see Repair, Anus 0DQQ
  see Supplement, Anus 0DUQ
Anorectal junction
  use Rectum
Anoscopy 0DJD8ZZ
Ansa cervicalis
  use Cervical Plexus
Antabuse therapy HZ93ZZZ
Antebrachial fascia
  use Subcutaneous Tissue and Fascia, Right Lower Arm
  use Subcutaneous Tissue and Fascia, Left Lower Arm
Anterior (pectoral) lymph node
  use Lymphatic, Right Axillary
  use Lymphatic, Left Axillary
Anterior cerebral artery
  use Intracranial Artery
Anterior cerebral vein
  use Intracranial Vein

Anterior choroidal artery
  use Intracranial Artery
Anterior circumflex humeral artery
  use Axillary Artery, Right
  use Axillary Artery, Left
Anterior communicating artery
  use Intracranial Artery
Anterior cruciate ligament (ACL)
  use Knee Bursa and Ligament, Right
  use Knee Bursa and Ligament, Left
Anterior crural nerve
  use Femoral Nerve
Anterior facial vein
  use Face Vein, Right
  use Face Vein, Left
Anterior intercostal artery
  use Internal Mammary Artery, Right
  use Internal Mammary Artery, Left
Anterior interosseous nerve
  use Median Nerve
Anterior lateral malleolar artery
  use Anterior Tibial Artery, Right
  use Anterior Tibial Artery, Left
Anterior lingual gland
  use Minor Salivary Gland
Anterior medial malleolar artery
  use Anterior Tibial Artery, Right
  use Anterior Tibial Artery, Left
Anterior spinal artery
  use Vertebral Artery, Right
  use Vertebral Artery, Left
Anterior tibial recurrent artery
  use Anterior Tibial Artery, Right
  use Anterior Tibial Artery, Left
Anterior ulnar recurrent artery
  use Ulnar Artery, Right
  use Ulnar Artery, Left
Anterior vagal trunk
  use Vagus Nerve
Anterior vertebral muscle
  use Neck Muscle, Right
  use Neck Muscle, Left
Antigen-free air conditioning
  see Atmospheric Control, Physiological Systems 6A0
Antihelix
  use External Ear, Right
  use External Ear, Left
  use External Ear, Bilateral
Antimicrobial envelope
  use Anti-Infective Envelope
Antitragus
  use External Ear, Right
  use External Ear, Left
  use External Ear, Bilateral
Antrostomy
  see Drainage, Ear, Nose, Sinus 099
Antrotomy
  see Drainage, Ear, Nose, Sinus 099
Antrum of Highmore
  use Maxillary Sinus, Right
  use Maxillary Sinus, Left
Aortic annulus
  use Aortic Valve
Aortic arch
  use Thoracic Aorta, Ascending/Arch
Aortic intercostal artery
  use Upper Artery
Aortography
  see Plain Radiography, Upper Arteries B30
  see Fluoroscopy, Upper Arteries B31
  see Plain Radiography, Lower Arteries B40
  see Fluoroscopy, Lower Arteries B41
Aortoplasty
  see Repair, Aorta, Thoracic, Descending 02QW

Aortoplasty — *continued*
see Repair, Aorta, Thoracic, Ascending/
Arch 02QX
see Replacement, Aorta, Thoracic,
Descending 02RW
see Replacement, Aorta, Thoracic,
Ascending/Arch 02RX
see Supplement, Aorta, Thoracic,
Descending 02UW
see Supplement, Aorta, Thoracic,
Ascending/Arch 02UX
see Repair, Aorta, Abdominal 04Q0
see Replacement, Aorta, Abdominal 04R0
see Supplement, Aorta, Abdominal 04U0
Apical (subclavicular) lymph node
use Lymphatic, Right Axillary
use Lymphatic, Left Axillary
Apneustic center
use Pons
Appendectomy
see Excision, Appendix 0DBJ
see Resection, Appendix 0DTJ
Appendicolysis
see Release, Appendix 0DNJ
Appendicotomy
see Drainage, Appendix 0D9J
Application
see Introduction of substance in or on
Aquapheresis 6A550Z3
Aqueduct of Sylvius
use Cerebral Ventricle
Aqueous humour
use Anterior Chamber, Right
use Anterior Chamber, Left
Arachnoid mater, intracranial
use Cerebral Meninges
Arachnoid mater, spinal
use Spinal Meninges
Arcuate artery
use Foot Artery, Right
use Foot Artery, Left
Areola
use Nipple, Right
use Nipple, Left
AROM (artificial rupture of membranes)
10907ZC
Arterial canal (duct)
use Pulmonary Artery, Left
Arterial pulse tracing
see Measurement, Arterial 4A03
Arteriectomy
see Excision, Heart and Great Vessels 02B
see Excision, Upper Arteries 03B
see Excision, Lower Arteries 04B
Arteriography
see Plain Radiography, Heart B20
see Fluoroscopy, Heart B21
see Plain Radiography, Upper Arteries B30
see Fluoroscopy, Upper Arteries B31
see Plain Radiography, Lower Arteries B40
see Fluoroscopy, Lower Arteries B41
Arterioplasty
see Repair, Heart and Great Vessels 02Q
see Replacement, Heart and Great
Vessels 02R
see Supplement, Heart and Great
Vessels 02U
see Repair, Upper Arteries 03Q
see Replacement, Upper Arteries 03R
see Supplement, Upper Arteries 03U
see Repair, Lower Arteries 04Q
see Replacement, Lower Arteries 04R
see Supplement, Lower Arteries 04U
Arteriorrhaphy
see Repair, Heart and Great Vessels 02Q
see Repair, Upper Arteries 03Q
see Repair, Lower Arteries 04Q

Arterioscopy
see Inspection, Great Vessel 02JY
see Inspection, Artery, Upper 03JY
see Inspection, Artery, Lower 04JY
Arthrectomy
see Excision, Upper Joints 0RB
see Resection, Upper Joints 0RT
see Excision, Lower Joints 0SB
see Resection, Lower Joints 0ST
Arthrocentesis
see Drainage, Upper Joints 0R9
see Drainage, Lower Joints 0S9
Arthrodesis
see Fusion, Upper Joints 0RG
see Fusion, Lower Joints 0SG
Arthrography
see Plain Radiography, Skull and Facial
Bones BN0
see Plain Radiography, Non-Axial Upper
Bones BP0
see Plain Radiography, Non-Axial Lower
Bones BQ0
Arthrolysis
see Release, Upper Joints 0RN
see Release, Lower Joints 0SN
Arthropexy
see Repair, Upper Joints 0RQ
see Reposition, Upper Joints 0RS
see Repair, Lower Joints 0SQ
see Reposition, Lower Joints 0SS
Arthroplasty
see Repair, Upper Joints 0RQ
see Replacement, Upper Joints 0RR
see Supplement, Upper Joints 0RU
see Repair, Lower Joints 0SQ
see Replacement, Lower Joints 0SR
see Supplement, Lower Joints 0SU
Arthroscopy
see Inspection, Upper Joints 0RJ
see Inspection, Lower Joints 0SJ
Arthrotomy
see Drainage, Upper Joints 0R9
see Drainage, Lower Joints 0S9
Artificial anal sphincter (AAS)
use Artificial Sphincter in Gastrointestinal
System
Artificial bowel sphincter (neosphincter)
use Artificial Sphincter in Gastrointestinal
System
Artificial sphincter
Insertion of device in
Anus 0DHQ
Bladder 0THB
Bladder Neck 0THC
Urethra 0THD
Removal of device from
Anus 0DPQ
Bladder 0TPB
Urethra 0TPD
Revision of device in
Anus 0DWQ
Bladder 0TWB
Urethra 0TWD
Artificial urinary sphincter (AUS)
use Artificial Sphincter in Urinary System
Aryepiglottic fold
use Larynx
Arytenoid cartilage
use Larynx
Arytenoid muscle
use Neck Muscle, Right
use Neck Muscle, Left
Arytenoidectomy
see Excision, Larynx 0CBS
Arytenoidopexy
see Repair, Larynx 0CQS

Ascenda Intrathecal Catheter
use Infusion Device
Ascending aorta
use Thoracic Aorta, Ascending/Arch
Ascending palatine artery
use Face Artery
Ascending pharyngeal artery
use External Carotid Artery, Right
use External Carotid Artery, Left
Aspiration, fine needle
fluid or gas *see* Drainage
tissue *see* Excision
Assessment
Activities of daily living *see* Activities
of Daily Living Assessment,
Rehabilitation F02
Hearing *see* Hearing Assessment,
Diagnostic Audiology F13
Hearing aid *see* Hearing Aid Assessment,
Diagnostic Audiology F14
intravascular perfusion, using indocyanine
green (ICG) dye *see* Monitoring,
Physiological Systems 4A1
Motor function *see* Motor Function
Assessment, Rehabilitation F01
Nerve function *see* Motor Function
Assessment, Rehabilitation F01
Speech *see* Speech Assessment,
Rehabilitation F00
Vestibular *see* Vestibular Assessment,
Diagnostic Audiology F15
Vocational *see* Activities of Daily Living
Treatment, Rehabilitation F08
Assistance
Cardiac
Continuous
Balloon Pump 5A02210
Impeller Pump 5A0221D
Other Pump 5A02216
Pulsatile Compression 5A02215
Intermittent
Balloon Pump 5A02110
Impeller Pump 5A0211D
Other Pump 5A02116
Pulsatile Compression 5A02115
Circulatory
Continuous
Hyperbaric 5A05221
Supersaturated 5A0522C
Intermittent
Hyperbaric 5A05121
Supersaturated 5A0512C
Respiratory
24-96 Consecutive Hours
Continuous Negative Airway
Pressure 5A09459
Continuous Positive Airway
Pressure 5A09457
Intermittent Negative Airway
Pressure 5A0945B
Intermittent Positive Airway
Pressure 5A09458
No Qualifier 5A0945Z
Continuous, Filtration 5A0920Z
Greater than 96 Consecutive Hours
Continuous Negative Airway
Pressure 5A09559
Continuous Positive Airway
Pressure 5A09557
Intermittent Negative Airway
Pressure 5A0955B
Intermittent Positive Airway
Pressure 5A09558
No Qualifier 5A0955Z
Less than 24 Consecutive Hours
Continuous Negative Airway
Pressure 5A09359

Assistance — *continued*
  Respiratory — *continued*
    Continuous Positive Airway
      Pressure 5A09357
    Intermittent Negative Airway
      Pressure 5A0935B
    Intermittent Positive Airway
      Pressure 5A09358
    No Qualifier 5A0935Z
Assurant (Cobalt)® stent
  use Intraluminal Device
Atherectomy
  see Extirpation, Heart and Great Vessels 02C
  see Extirpation, Upper Arteries 03C
  see Extirpation, Lower Arteries 04C
Atlantoaxial joint
  use Cervical Vertebral Joint
Atmospheric Control 6A0Z
AtriClip LAA Exclusion System
  use Extraluminal Device
Atrioseptoplasty
  see Repair, Heart and Great Vessels 02Q
  see Replacement, Heart and Great Vessels 02R
  see Supplement, Heart and Great Vessels 02U
Atrioventricular node
  use Conduction Mechanism
Atrium dextrum cordis
  use Atrium, Right
Atrium pulmonale
  use Atrium, Left
Attain Ability® lead
  use Cardiac Lead, Pacemaker in 02H
  use Cardiac Lead, Defibrillator in 02H
Attain StarFix® (OTW) lead
  use Cardiac Lead, Pacemaker in 02H
  use Cardiac Lead, Defibrillator in 02H
Audiology, diagnostic
  see Hearing Assessment, Diagnostic Audiology F13
  see Hearing Aid Assessment, Diagnostic Audiology F14
  see Vestibular Assessment, Diagnostic Audiology F15
Audiometry
  see Hearing Assessment, Diagnostic Audiology F13
Auditory tube
  use Eustachian Tube, Right
  use Eustachian Tube, Left
Auerbach's (myenteric) plexus
  use Abdominal Sympathetic Nerve
Auricle
  use External Ear, Right
  use External Ear, Left
  use External Ear, Bilateral
Auricularis muscle
  use Head Muscle
Autograft
  use Autologous Tissue Substitute
Autologous artery graft
  use Autologous Arterial Tissue in Heart and Great Vessels
  use Autologous Arterial Tissue in Upper Arteries
  use Autologous Arterial Tissue in Lower Arteries
  use Autologous Arterial Tissue in Upper Veins
  use Autologous Arterial Tissue in Lower Veins
Autologous vein graft
  use Autologous Venous Tissue in Heart and Great Vessels
  use Autologous Venous Tissue in Upper Arteries

Autologous vein graft — *continued*
  use Autologous Venous Tissue in Lower Arteries
  use Autologous Venous Tissue in Upper Veins
  use Autologous Venous Tissue in Lower Veins
Autotransfusion
  see Transfusion
Autotransplant
  Adrenal tissue *see* Reposition, Endocrine System 0GS
  Kidney *see* Reposition, Urinary System 0TS
  Pancreatic tissue *see* Reposition, Pancreas 0FSG
  Parathyroid tissue *see* Reposition, Endocrine System 0GS
  Thyroid tissue *see* Reposition, Endocrine System 0GS
  Tooth *see* Reattachment, Mouth and Throat 0CM
Avulsion
  see Extraction
Axial Lumbar Interbody Fusion System
  use Interbody Fusion Device in Lower Joints
AxiaLIF® System
  use Interbody Fusion Device in Lower Joints
Axicabtagene Ciloeucel
  use Engineered Autologous Chimeric Antigen Receptor T-cell Immunotherapy
Axillary fascia
  use Subcutaneous Tissue and Fascia, Right Upper Arm
  use Subcutaneous Tissue and Fascia, Left Upper Arm
Axillary nerve
  use Brachial Plexus

B

BAK/C® Interbody Cervical Fusion System
  use Interbody Fusion Device in Upper Joints
BAL (bronchial alveolar lavage), diagnostic
  see Drainage, Respiratory System 0B9
Balanoplasty
  see Repair, Penis 0VQS
  see Supplement, Penis 0VUS
Balloon atrial septostomy (BAS) 02163Z7
Balloon Pump
  Continuous, Output 5A02210
  Intermittent, Output 5A02110
Bandage, Elastic
  see Compression
Banding
  see Occlusion
  see Restriction
Banding, esophageal varices
  see Occlusion, Vein, Esophageal 06L3
Banding, laparoscopic (adjustable) gastric
  Adjustment/revision 0DW64CZ
  Initial procedure 0DV64CZ
Bard® Composix® (E/X)(LP) mesh
  use Synthetic Substitute
Bard® Composix® Kugel® patch
  use Synthetic Substitute
Bard® Dulex™ mesh
  use Synthetic Substitute
Bard® Ventralex™ hernia patch
  use Synthetic Substitute
Barium swallow
  see Fluoroscopy, Gastrointestinal System BD1

Baroreflex Activation Therapy® (BAT®)
  use Stimulator Lead in Upper Arteries
  use Stimulator Generator in Subcutaneous Tissue and Fascia
Bartholin's (greater vestibular) gland
  use Vestibular Gland
Basal (internal) cerebral vein
  use Intracranial Vein
Basal metabolic rate (BMR)
  see Measurement, Physiological Systems 4A0Z
Basal nuclei
  use Basal Ganglia
Base of Tongue
  use Pharynx
Basilar artery
  use Intracranial Artery
Basis pontis
  use Pons
Beam radiation
  Abdomen DW03
    Intraoperative DW033Z0
  Adrenal Gland DG02
    Intraoperative DG023Z0
  Bile Ducts DF02
    Intraoperative DF023Z0
  Bladder DT02
    Intraoperative DT023Z0
  Bone
    Other DP0C
    Intraoperative DP0C3Z0
  Bone Marrow D700
    Intraoperative D7003Z0
  Brain D000
    Intraoperative D0003Z0
  Brain Stem D001
    Intraoperative D0013Z0
  Breast
    Left DM00
      Intraoperative DM003Z0
    Right DM01
      Intraoperative DM013Z0
  Bronchus DB01
    Intraoperative DB013Z0
  Cervix DU01
    Intraoperative DU013Z0
  Chest DW02
    Intraoperative DW023Z0
  Chest Wall DB07
    Intraoperative DB073Z0
  Colon DD05
    Intraoperative DD053Z0
  Diaphragm DB08
    Intraoperative DB083Z0
  Duodenum DD02
    Intraoperative DD023Z0
  Ear D900
    Intraoperative D9003Z0
  Esophagus DD00
    Intraoperative DD003Z0
  Eye D800
    Intraoperative D8003Z0
  Femur DP09
    Intraoperative DP093Z0
  Fibula DP0B
    Intraoperative DP0B3Z0
  Gallbladder DF01
    Intraoperative DF013Z0
  Gland
    Adrenal DG02
      Intraoperative DG023Z0
    Parathyroid DG04
      Intraoperative DG043Z0
    Pituitary DG00
      Intraoperative DG003Z0
    Thyroid DG05
      Intraoperative DG053Z0

Beam radiation — *continued*
Glands
Salivary D906
Intraoperative D9063Z0
Head and Neck DW01
Intraoperative DW013Z0
Hemibody DW04
Intraoperative DW043Z0
Humerus DP06
Intraoperative DP063Z0
Hypopharynx D903
Intraoperative D9033Z0
Ileum DD04
Intraoperative DD043Z0
Jejunum DD03
Intraoperative DD033Z0
Kidney DT00
Intraoperative DT003Z0
Larynx D90B
Intraoperative D90B3Z0
Liver DF00
Intraoperative DF003Z0
Lung DB02
Intraoperative DB023Z0
Lymphatics
Abdomen D706
Intraoperative D7063Z0
Axillary D704
Intraoperative D7043Z0
Inguinal D708
Intraoperative D7083Z0
Neck D703
Intraoperative D7033Z0
Pelvis D707
Intraoperative D7073Z0
Thorax D705
Intraoperative D7053Z0
Mandible DP03
Intraoperative DP033Z0
Maxilla DP02
Intraoperative DP023Z0
Mediastinum DB06
Intraoperative DB063Z0
Mouth D904
Intraoperative D9043Z0
Nasopharynx D90D
Intraoperative D90D3Z0
Neck and Head DW01
Intraoperative DW013Z0
Nerve
Peripheral D007
Intraoperative D0073Z0
Nose D901
Intraoperative D9013Z0
Oropharynx D90F
Intraoperative D90F3Z0
Ovary DU00
Intraoperative DU003Z0
Palate
Hard D908
Intraoperative D9083Z0
Soft D909
Intraoperative D9093Z0
Pancreas DF03
Intraoperative DF033Z0
Parathyroid Gland DG04
Intraoperative DG043Z0
Pelvic Bones DP08
Intraoperative DP083Z0
Pelvic Region DW06
Intraoperative DW063Z0
Pineal Body DG01
Intraoperative DG013Z0
Pituitary Gland DG00
Intraoperative DG003Z0
Pleura DB05
Intraoperative DB053Z0

Beam radiation — *continued*
Prostate DV00
Intraoperative DV003Z0
Radius DP07
Intraoperative DP073Z0
Rectum DD07
Intraoperative DD073Z0
Rib DP05
Intraoperative DP053Z0
Sinuses D907
Intraoperative D9073Z0
Skin
Abdomen DH08
Intraoperative DH083Z0
Arm DH04
Intraoperative DH043Z0
Back DH07
Intraoperative DH073Z0
Buttock DH09
Intraoperative DH093Z0
Chest DH06
Intraoperative DH063Z0
Face DH02
Intraoperative DH023Z0
Leg DH0B
Intraoperative DH0B3Z0
Neck DH03
Intraoperative DH033Z0
Skull DP00
Intraoperative DP003Z0
Spinal Cord D006
Intraoperative D0063Z0
Spleen D702
Intraoperative D7023Z0
Sternum DP04
Intraoperative DP043Z0
Stomach DD01
Intraoperative DD013Z0
Testis DV01
Intraoperative DV013Z0
Thymus D701
Intraoperative D7013Z0
Thyroid Gland DG05
Intraoperative DG053Z0
Tibia DP0B
Intraoperative DP0B3Z0
Tongue D905
Intraoperative D9053Z0
Trachea DB00
Intraoperative DB003Z0
Ulna DP07
Intraoperative DP073Z0
Ureter DT01
Intraoperative DT013Z0
Urethra DT03
Intraoperative DT033Z0
Uterus DU02
Intraoperative DU023Z0
Whole Body DW05
Intraoperative DW053Z0
Bedside swallow F00ZJWZ
Berlin Heart Ventricular Assist Device
use Implantable Heart Assist System in Heart and Great Vessels
Bezlotoxumab Monoclonal Antibody XW0
Biceps brachii muscle
use Upper Arm Muscle, Right
use Upper Arm Muscle, Left
Biceps femoris muscle
use Upper Leg Muscle, Right
use Upper Leg Muscle, Left
Bicipital aponeurosis
use Subcutaneous Tissue and Fascia, Right Lower Arm
use Subcutaneous Tissue and Fascia, Left Lower Arm

Bicuspid valve
use Mitral Valve
Bililite therapy
see Ultraviolet Light Therapy, Skin 6A80
Bioactive embolization coil(s)
use Intraluminal Device, Bioactive in Upper Arteries
Biofeedback GZC9ZZZ
Biopsy
see Drainage with qualifier Diagnostic
see Excision with qualifier Diagnostic
Bone Marrow *see* Extraction with qualifier Diagnostic
BiPAP
see Assistance, Respiratory 5A09
Bisection
see Division
Biventricular external heart assist system
use Short-term External Heart Assist System in Heart and Great Vessels
Blepharectomy
see Excision, Eye 08B
see Resection, Eye 08T
Blepharoplasty
see Repair, Eye 08Q
see Replacement, Eye 08R
see Reposition, Eye 08S
see Supplement, Eye 08U
Blepharorrhaphy
see Repair, Eye 08Q
Blepharotomy
see Drainage, Eye 089
Blinatumomab Antineoplastic Immunotherapy XW0
Blood glucose monitoring system
use Monitoring Device
Blood pressure
see Measurement, Arterial 4A03
BMR (basal metabolic rate)
see Measurement, Physiological Systems 4A0Z
Body of femur
use Femoral Shaft, Right
use Femoral Shaft, Left
Body of fibula
use Fibula, Right
use Fibula, Left
Bone anchored hearing device
use Hearing Device, Bone Conduction in 09H
use Hearing Device in Head and Facial Bones
Bone bank bone graft
use Nonautologous Tissue Substitute
Bone Growth Stimulator
Insertion of device in
Bone
Facial 0NHW
Lower 0QHY
Nasal 0NHB
Upper 0PHY
Skull 0NH0
Removal of device from
Bone
Facial 0NPW
Lower 0QPY
Nasal 0NPB
Upper 0PPY
Skull 0NP0
Revision of device in
Bone
Facial 0NWW
Lower 0QWY
Nasal 0NWB
Upper 0PWY
Skull 0NW0

Bone marrow transplant
see Transfusion, Circulatory 302
Bone morphogenetic protein 2 (BMP 2)
use Recombinant Bone Morphogenetic Protein
Bone screw (interlocking)(lag)(pedicle) (recessed)
use Internal Fixation Device in Head and Facial Bones
use Internal Fixation Device in Upper Bones
use Internal Fixation Device in Lower Bones
Bony labyrinth
use Inner Ear, Right
use Inner Ear, Left
Bony orbit
use Orbit, Right
use Orbit, Left
Bony vestibule
use Inner Ear, Right
use Inner Ear, Left
Botallo's duct
use Pulmonary Artery, Left
Bovine pericardial valve
use Zooplastic Tissue in Heart and Great Vessels
Bovine pericardium graft
use Zooplastic Tissue in Heart and Great Vessels
BP (blood pressure)
see Measurement, Arterial 4A03
Brachial (lateral) lymph node
use Lymphatic, Right Axillary
use Lymphatic, Left Axillary
Brachialis muscle
use Upper Arm Muscle, Right
use Upper Arm Muscle, Left
Brachiocephalic artery
use Innominate Artery
Brachiocephalic trunk
use Innominate Artery
Brachiocephalic vein
use Innominate Vein, Right
use Innominate Vein, Left
Brachioradialis muscle
use Lower Arm and Wrist Muscle, Right
use Lower Arm and Wrist Muscle, Left
Brachytherapy
Abdomen DW13
Adrenal Gland DG12
Bile Ducts DF12
Bladder DT12
Bone Marrow D710
Brain D010
Brain Stem D011
Breast
Left DM10
Right DM11
Bronchus DB11
Cervix DU11
Chest DW12
Chest Wall DB17
Colon DD15
Diaphragm DB18
Duodenum DD12
Ear D910
Esophagus DD10
Eye D810
Gallbladder DF11
Gland
Adrenal DG12
Parathyroid DG14
Pituitary DG10
Thyroid DG15
Glands, Salivary D916
Head and Neck DW11
Hypopharynx D913

Brachytherapy — continued
Ileum DD14
Jejunum DD13
Kidney DT10
Larynx D91B
Liver DF10
Lung DB12
Lymphatics
Abdomen D716
Axillary D714
Inguinal D718
Neck D713
Pelvis D717
Thorax D715
Mediastinum DB16
Mouth D914
Nasopharynx D91D
Neck and Head DW11
Nerve, Peripheral D017
Nose D911
Oropharynx D91F
Ovary DU10
Palate
Hard D918
Soft D919
Pancreas DF13
Parathyroid Gland DG14
Pelvic Region DW16
Pineal Body DG11
Pituitary Gland DG10
Pleura DB15
Prostate DV10
Rectum DD17
Sinuses D917
Spinal Cord D016
Spleen D712
Stomach DD11
Testis DV11
Thymus D711
Thyroid Gland DG15
Tongue D915
Trachea DB10
Ureter DT11
Urethra DT13
Uterus DU12
Brachytherapy seeds
use Radioactive Element
Broad ligament
use Uterine Supporting Structure
Bronchial artery
use Upper Artery
Bronchography
see Plain Radiography, Respiratory System BB0
see Fluoroscopy, Respiratory System BB1
Bronchoplasty
see Repair, Respiratory System 0BQ
see Supplement, Respiratory System 0BU
Bronchorrhaphy
see Repair, Respiratory System 0BQ
Bronchoscopy 0BJ08ZZ
Bronchotomy
see Drainage, Respiratory System 0B9
Bronchus Intermedius
use Main Bronchus, Right
BRYAN® Cervical Disc System
use Synthetic Substitute
Buccal gland
use Buccal Mucosa
Buccinator lymph node
use Lymphatic, Head
Buccinator muscle
use Facial Muscle
Buckling, scleral with implant
see Supplement, Eye 08U
Bulbospongiosus muscle
use Perineum Muscle

Bulbourethral (Cowper's) gland
use Urethra
Bundle of His
use Conduction Mechanism
Bundle of Kent
use Conduction Mechanism
Bunionectomy
see Excision, Lower Bones 0QB
Bursectomy
see Excision, Bursae and Ligaments 0MB
see Resection, Bursae and Ligaments 0MT
Bursocentesis
see Drainage, Bursae and Ligaments 0M9
Bursography
see Plain Radiography, Non-Axial Upper Bones BP0
see Plain Radiography, Non-Axial Lower Bones BQ0
Bursotomy
see Division, Bursae and Ligaments 0M8
see Drainage, Bursae and Ligaments 0M9
BVS 5000 Ventricular Assist Device
use Short-term External Heart Assist System in Heart and Great Vessels
Bypass
Anterior Chamber
Left 08133
Right 08123
Aorta
Abdominal 0410
Thoracic
Ascending/Arch 021X
Descending 021W
Artery
Axillary
Left 03160
Right 03150
Brachial
Left 03180
Right 03170
Common Carotid
Left 031J0
Right 031H0
Common Iliac
Left 041D
Right 041C
Coronary
Four or More Arteries 0213
One Artery 0210
Three Arteries 0212
Two Arteries 0211
External Carotid
Left 031N0
Right 031M0
External Iliac
Left 041J
Right 041H
Femoral
Left 041L
Right 041K
Foot
Left 041W
Right 041V
Hepatic 0413
Innominate 03120
Internal Carotid
Left 031L0
Right 031K0
Internal Iliac
Left 041F
Right 041E
Intracranial 031G0
Peroneal
Left 041U
Right 041T
Popliteal

Bypass — *continued*
　Artery — *continued*
　　Left 041N
　　Right 041M
　　Pulmonary
　　　Left 021R
　　　Right 021Q
　　Pulmonary Trunk 021P
　　Radial
　　　Left 031C0
　　　Right 031B0
　　Splenic 0414
　　Subclavian
　　　Left 03140
　　　Right 03130
　　Temporal
　　　Left 031T0
　　　Right 031S0
　　Ulnar
　　　Left 031A0
　　　Right 03190
　Atrium
　　Left 0217
　　Right 0216
　Bladder 0T1B
　Cavity, Cranial 0W110J
　Cecum 0D1H
　Cerebral Ventricle 0016
　Colon
　　Ascending 0D1K
　　Descending 0D1M
　　Sigmoid 0D1N
　　Transverse 0D1L
　Duct
　　Common Bile 0F19
　　Cystic 0F18
　　Hepatic
　　　Common 0F17
　　　Left 0F16
　　　Right 0F15
　　Lacrimal
　　　Left 081Y
　　　Right 081X
　　Pancreatic 0F1D
　　　Accessory 0F1F
　Duodenum 0D19
　Ear
　　Left 091E0
　　Right 091D0
　Esophagus 0D15
　　Lower 0D13
　　Middle 0D12
　　Upper 0D11
　Fallopian Tube
　　Left 0U16
　　Right 0U15
　Gallbladder 0F14
　Ileum 0D1B
　Jejunum 0D1A
　Kidney Pelvis
　　Left 0T14
　　Right 0T13
　Pancreas 0F1G
　Pelvic Cavity 0W1J
　Peritoneal Cavity 0W1G
　Pleural Cavity
　　Left 0W1B
　　Right 0W19
　Spinal Canal 001U
　Stomach 0D16
　Trachea 0B11
　Ureter
　　Left 0T17
　　Right 0T16
　Ureters, Bilateral 0T18
　Vas Deferens
　　Bilateral 0V1Q

Bypass — *continued*
　Vas Deferens — *continued*
　　Left 0V1P
　　Right 0V1N
　Vein
　　Axillary
　　　Left 0518
　　　Right 0517
　　Azygos 0510
　　Basilic
　　　Left 051C
　　　Right 051B
　　Brachial
　　　Left 051A
　　　Right 0519
　　Cephalic
　　　Left 051F
　　　Right 051D
　　Colic 0617
　　Common Iliac
　　　Left 061D
　　　Right 061C
　　Esophageal 0613
　　External Iliac
　　　Left 061G
　　　Right 061F
　　External Jugular
　　　Left 051Q
　　　Right 051P
　　Face
　　　Left 051V
　　　Right 051T
　　Femoral
　　　Left 061N
　　　Right 061M
　　Foot
　　　Left 061V
　　　Right 061T
　　Gastric 0612
　　Hand
　　　Left 051H
　　　Right 051G
　　Hemiazygos 0511
　　Hepatic 0614
　　Hypogastric
　　　Left 061J
　　　Right 061H
　　Inferior Mesenteric 0616
　　Innominate
　　　Left 0514
　　　Right 0513
　　Internal Jugular
　　　Left 051N
　　　Right 051M
　　Intracranial 051L
　　Portal 0618
　　Renal
　　　Left 061B
　　　Right 0619
　　Saphenous
　　　Left 061Q
　　　Right 061P
　　Splenic 0611
　　Subclavian
　　　Left 0516
　　　Right 0515
　　Superior Mesenteric 0615
　　Vertebral
　　　Left 051S
　　　Right 051R
　　Vena Cava
　　　Inferior 0610
　　　Superior 021V
　　Ventricle
　　　Left 021L
　　　Right 021K
Bypass, cardiopulmonary 5A1221Z

C

Caesarean section
　see Extraction, Products of
　　Conception 10D0
Calcaneocuboid joint
　use Tarsal Joint, Right
　use Tarsal Joint, Left
Calcaneocuboid ligament
　use Foot Bursa and Ligament, Right
　use Foot Bursa and Ligament, Left
Calcaneofibular ligament
　use Ankle Bursa and Ligament, Right
　use Ankle Bursa and Ligament, Left
Calcaneus
　use Tarsal, Right
　use Tarsal, Left
Cannulation
　see Bypass
　see Dilation
　see Drainage
　see Irrigation
Canthorrhaphy
　see Repair, Eye 08Q
Canthotomy
　see Release, Eye 08N
Capitate bone
　use Carpal, Right
　use Carpal, Left
Capsulectomy, lens
　see Excision, Eye 08B
Capsulorrhaphy, joint
　see Repair, Upper Joints 0RQ
　see Repair, Lower Joints 0SQ
Cardia
　use Esophagogastric Junction
Cardiac contractility modulation lead
　use Cardiac Lead in Heart and Great Vessels
Cardiac event recorder
　use Monitoring Device
Cardiac Lead
　Defibrillator
　　Atrium
　　　Left 02H7
　　　Right 02H6
　　Pericardium 02HN
　　Vein, Coronary 02H4
　　Ventricle
　　　Left 02HL
　　　Right 02HK
　Insertion of device in
　　Atrium
　　　Left 02H7
　　　Right 02H6
　　Pericardium 02HN
　　Vein, Coronary 02H4
　　Ventricle
　　　Left 02HL
　　　Right 02HK
　Pacemaker
　　Atrium
　　　Left 02H7
　　　Right 02H6
　　Pericardium 02HN
　　Vein, Coronary 02H4
　　Ventricle
　　　Left 02HL
　　　Right 02HK
　Removal of device from, Heart 02PA
　Revision of device in, Heart 02WA
Cardiac plexus
　use Thoracic Sympathetic Nerve
Cardiac resynchronization defibrillator pulse generator
　Abdomen 0JH8
　Chest 0JH6

Cardiac Resynchronization Pacemaker Pulse Generator
  Abdomen 0JH8
  Chest 0JH6
Cardiac resynchronization therapy (CRT) lead
  use Cardiac Lead, Pacemaker in 02H
  use Cardiac Lead, Defibrillator in 02H
Cardiac Rhythm Related Device
  Insertion of device in
    Abdomen 0JH8
    Chest 0JH6
  Removal of device from, Subcutaneous Tissue and Fascia, Trunk 0JPT
  Revision of device in, Subcutaneous Tissue and Fascia, Trunk 0JWT
Cardiocentesis
  see Drainage, Pericardial Cavity 0W9D
Cardioesophageal junction
  use Esophagogastric Junction
Cardiolysis
  see Release, Heart and Great Vessels 02N
CardioMEMS® pressure sensor
  use Monitoring Device, Pressure Sensor in 02H
Cardiomyotomy
  see Division, Esophagogastric Junction 0D84
Cardioplegia
  see Introduction of substance in or on, Heart 3E08
Cardiorrhaphy
  see Repair, Heart and Great Vessels 02Q
Cardioversion 5A2204Z
Caregiver Training F0FZ
Caroticotympanic artery
  use Internal Carotid Artery, Right
  use Internal Carotid Artery, Left
Carotid (artery) sinus (baroreceptor) lead
  use Stimulator Lead in Upper Arteries
Carotid glomus
  use Carotid Body, Left
  use Carotid Body, Right
  use Carotid Bodies, Bilateral
Carotid sinus
  use Internal Carotid Artery, Right
  use Internal Carotid Artery, Left
Carotid sinus nerve
  use Glossopharyngeal Nerve
Carotid WALLSTENT® Monorail® Endoprosthesis
  use Intraluminal Device
Carpectomy
  see Excision, Upper Bones 0PB
  see Resection, Upper Bones 0PT
Carpometacarpal ligament
  use Hand Bursa and Ligament, Right
  use Hand Bursa and Ligament, Left
Casting
  see Immobilization
CAT scan
  see Computerized Tomography (CT Scan)
Catheterization
  see Dilation
  see Drainage
  see Insertion of device in
  see Irrigation
  Heart *see* Measurement, Cardiac 4A02
  Umbilical vein, for infusion 06H033T
Cauda equina
  use Lumbar Spinal Cord
Cauterization
  see Destruction
  see Repair
Cavernous plexus
  use Head and Neck Sympathetic Nerve

CBMA (Concentrated Bone Marrow Aspirate)
  use Concentrated Bone Marrow Aspirate
CBMA (Concentrated Bone Marrow Aspirate) injection, intramuscular
  XK02303
Cecectomy
  see Excision, Cecum 0DBH
  see Resection, Cecum 0DTH
Cecocolostomy
  see Bypass, Gastrointestinal System 0D1
  see Drainage, Gastrointestinal System 0D9
Cecopexy
  see Repair, Cecum 0DQH
  see Reposition, Cecum 0DSH
Cecoplication
  see Restriction, Cecum 0DVH
Cecorrhaphy
  see Repair, Cecum 0DQH
Cecostomy
  see Bypass, Cecum 0D1H
  see Drainage, Cecum 0D9H
Cecotomy
  see Drainage, Cecum 0D9H
Ceftazidime-Avibactam Anti-infective XW0
Celiac (solar) plexus
  use Abdominal Sympathetic Nerve
Celiac ganglion
  use Abdominal Sympathetic Nerve
Celiac lymph node
  use Lymphatic, Aortic
Celiac trunk
  use Celiac Artery
Central axillary lymph node
  use Lymphatic, Right Axillary
  use Lymphatic, Left Axillary
Central venous pressure
  see Measurement, Venous 4A04
Centrimag® Blood Pump
  use Short-term External Heart Assist System in Heart and Great Vessels
Cephalogram BN00ZZZ
Ceramic on ceramic bearing surface
  use Synthetic Substitute, Ceramic in 0SR
Cerclage
  see Restriction
Cerebral aqueduct (Sylvius)
  use Cerebral Ventricle
Cerebral Embolic Filtration, Dual Filter
  X2A5312
Cerebrum
  use Brain
Cervical esophagus
  use Esophagus, Upper
Cervical facet joint
  use Cervical Vertebral Joint
  use Cervical Vertebral Joints, 2 or more
Cervical ganglion
  use Head and Neck Sympathetic Nerve
Cervical interspinous ligament
  use Head and Neck Bursa and Ligament
Cervical intertransverse ligament
  use Head and Neck Bursa and Ligament
Cervical ligamentum flavum
  use Head and Neck Bursa and Ligament
Cervical lymph node
  use Lymphatic, Right Neck
  use Lymphatic, Left Neck
Cervicectomy
  see Excision, Cervix 0UBC
  see Resection, Cervix 0UTC
Cervicothoracic facet joint
  use Cervicothoracic Vertebral Joint
Cesarean section
  see Extraction, Products of Conception 10D0

Cesium-131 Collagen Implant
  use Radioactive Element, Cesium-131 Collagen Implant in 00H
Change device in
  Abdominal Wall 0W2FX
  Back
    Lower 0W2LX
    Upper 0W2KX
  Bladder 0T2BX
  Bone
    Facial 0N2WX
    Lower 0Q2YX
    Nasal 0N2BX
    Upper 0P2YX
  Bone Marrow 072TX
  Brain 0020X
  Breast
    Left 0H2UX
    Right 0H2TX
  Bursa and Ligament
    Lower 0M2YX
    Upper 0M2XX
  Cavity, Cranial 0W21X
  Chest Wall 0W28X
  Cisterna Chyli 072LX
  Diaphragm 0B2TX
  Duct
    Hepatobiliary 0F2BX
    Pancreatic 0F2DX
  Ear
    Left 092JX
    Right 092HX
  Epididymis and Spermatic Cord 0V2MX
  Extremity
    Lower
      Left 0Y2BX
      Right 0Y29X
    Upper
      Left 0X27X
      Right 0X26X
  Eye
    Left 0821X
    Right 0820X
  Face 0W22X
  Fallopian Tube 0U28X
  Gallbladder 0F24X
  Gland
    Adrenal 0G25X
    Endocrine 0G2SX
    Pituitary 0G20X
    Salivary 0C2AX
  Head 0W20X
  Intestinal Tract
    Lower 0D2DXUZ
    Upper 0D20XUZ
  Jaw
    Lower 0W25X
    Upper 0W24X
  Joint
    Lower 0S2YX
    Upper 0R2YX
  Kidney 0T25X
  Larynx 0C2SX
  Liver 0F20X
  Lung
    Left 0B2LX
    Right 0B2KX
  Lymphatic 072NX
    Thoracic Duct 072KX
  Mediastinum 0W2CX
  Mesentery 0D2VX
  Mouth and Throat 0C2YX
  Muscle
    Lower 0K2YX
    Upper 0K2XX
  Nasal Mucosa and Soft Tissue 092KX

Change device in — *continued*
Neck 0W26X
Nerve
   Cranial 002EX
   Peripheral 012YX
Omentum 0D2UX
Ovary 0U23X
Pancreas 0F2GX
Parathyroid Gland 0G2RX
Pelvic Cavity 0W2JX
Penis 0V2SX
Pericardial Cavity 0W2DX
Perineum
   Female 0W2NX
   Male 0W2MX
Peritoneal Cavity 0W2GX
Peritoneum 0D2WX
Pineal Body 0G21X
Pleura 0B2QX
Pleural Cavity
   Left 0W2BX
   Right 0W29X
Products of Conception 10207
Prostate and Seminal Vesicles 0V24X
Retroperitoneum 0W2HX
Scrotum and Tunica Vaginalis 0V28X
Sinus 092YX
Skin 0H2PX
Skull 0N20X
Spinal Canal 002UX
Spleen 072PX
Subcutaneous Tissue and Fascia
   Head and Neck 0J2SX
   Lower Extremity 0J2WX
   Trunk 0J2TX
   Upper Extremity 0J2VX
Tendon
   Lower 0L2YX
   Upper 0L2XX
Testis 0V2DX
Thymus 072MX
Thyroid Gland 0G2KX
Trachea 0B21
Tracheobronchial Tree 0B20X
Ureter 0T29X
Urethra 0T2DX
Uterus and Cervix 0U2DXHZ
Vagina and Cul-de-sac 0U2HXGZ
Vas Deferens 0V2RX
Vulva 0U2MX
Change device in or on
Abdominal Wall 2W03X
Anorectal 2Y03X5Z
Arm
   Lower
      Left 2W0DX
      Right 2W0CX
   Upper
      Left 2W0BX
      Right 2W0AX
Back 2W05X
Chest Wall 2W04X
Ear 2Y02X5Z
Extremity
   Lower
      Left 2W0MX
      Right 2W0LX
   Upper
      Left 2W09X
      Right 2W08X
Face 2W01X
Finger
   Left 2W0KX
   Right 2W0JX
Foot
   Left 2W0TX
   Right 2W0SX

Change device in or on — *continued*
Genital Tract, Female 2Y04X5Z
Hand
   Left 2W0FX
   Right 2W0EX
Head 2W00X
Inguinal Region
   Left 2W07X
   Right 2W06X
Leg
   Lower
      Left 2W0RX
      Right 2W0QX
   Upper
      Left 2W0PX
      Right 2W0NX
Mouth and Pharynx 2Y00X5Z
Nasal 2Y01X5Z
Neck 2W02X
Thumb
   Left 2W0HX
   Right 2W0GX
Toe
   Left 2W0VX
   Right 2W0UX
Urethra 2Y05X5Z
Chemoembolization
   see Introduction of substance in or on
Chemosurgery, Skin 3E00XTZ
Chemothalamectomy
   see Destruction, Thalamus 0059
Chemotherapy, Infusion for cancer
   see Introduction of substance in or on
Chest x-ray
   see Plain Radiography, Chest BW03
Chiropractic manipulation
   Abdomen 9WB9X
   Cervical 9WB1X
   Extremities
      Lower 9WB6X
      Upper 9WB7X
   Head 9WB0X
   Lumbar 9WB3X
   Pelvis 9WB5X
   Rib Cage 9WB8X
   Sacrum 9WB4X
   Thoracic 9WB2X
Choana
   use Nasopharynx
Cholangiogram
   see Plain Radiography, Hepatobiliary
     System and Pancreas BF0
   see Fluoroscopy, Hepatobiliary System and
     Pancreas BF1
Cholecystectomy
   see Excision, Gallbladder 0FB4
   see Resection, Gallbladder 0FT4
Cholecystojejunostomy
   see Bypass, Hepatobiliary System and
     Pancreas 0F1
   see Drainage, Hepatobiliary System and
     Pancreas 0F9
Cholecystopexy
   see Repair, Gallbladder 0FQ4
   see Reposition, Gallbladder 0FS4
Cholecystoscopy 0FJ44ZZ
Cholecystostomy
   see Bypass, Gallbladder 0F14
   see Drainage, Gallbladder 0F94
Cholecystotomy
   see Drainage, Gallbladder 0F94
Choledochectomy
   see Excision, Hepatobiliary System and
     Pancreas 0FB
   see Resection, Hepatobiliary System and
     Pancreas 0FT

Choledocholithotomy
   see Extirpation, Duct, Common Bile 0FC9
Choledochoplasty
   see Repair, Hepatobiliary System and
     Pancreas 0FQ
   see Replacement, Hepatobiliary System
     and Pancreas 0FR
   see Supplement, Hepatobiliary System and
     Pancreas 0FU
Choledochoscopy 0FJB8ZZ
Choledochotomy
   see Drainage, Hepatobiliary System and
     Pancreas 0F9
Cholelithotomy
   see Extirpation, Hepatobiliary System and
     Pancreas 0FC
Chondrectomy
   see Excision, Upper Joints 0RB
   see Excision, Lower Joints 0SB
   Knee *see* Excision, Lower Joints 0SB
   Semilunar cartilage *see* Excision, Lower
     Joints 0SB
Chondroglossus muscle
   use Tongue, Palate, Pharynx Muscle
Chorda tympani
   use Facial Nerve
Chordotomy
   see Division, Central Nervous System and
     Cranial Nerves 008
Choroid plexus
   use Cerebral Ventricle
Choroidectomy
   see Excision, Eye 08B
   see Resection, Eye 08T
Ciliary body
   use Eye, Right
   use Eye, Left
Ciliary ganglion
   use Head and Neck Sympathetic Nerve
Circle of Willis
   use Intracranial Artery
Circumcision 0VTTXZZ
Circumflex iliac artery
   use Femoral Artery, Right
   use Femoral Artery, Left
**Clamp and rod internal fixation system
(CRIF)**
   use Internal Fixation Device in Upper Bones
   use Internal Fixation Device in Lower Bones
Clamping
   see Occlusion
Claustrum
   use Basal Ganglia
Claviculectomy
   see Excision, Upper Bones 0PB
   see Resection, Upper Bones 0PT
Claviculotomy
   see Division, Upper Bones 0P8
   see Drainage, Upper Bones 0P9
Clipping, aneurysm
   see Occlusion using Extraluminal Device
   see Restriction using Extraluminal Device
Clitorectomy, clitoridectomy
   see Excision, Clitoris 0UBJ
   see Resection, Clitoris 0UTJ
Clolar®
   use Clofarabine
Closure
   see Occlusion
   see Repair
Clysis
   see Introduction of substance in or on
Coagulation
   see Destruction

COALESCE® radiolucent interbody fusion device
use Interbody Fusion Device, Radiolucent Porous in New Technology

CoAxia NeuroFlo catheter
use Intraluminal Device

Cobalt/chromium head and polyethylene socket
use Synthetic Substitute, Metal on Polyethylene in 0SR

Cobalt/chromium head and socket
use Synthetic Substitute, Metal in 0SR

Coccygeal body
use Coccygeal Glomus

Coccygeus muscle
use Trunk Muscle, Right
use Trunk Muscle, Left

Cochlea
use Inner Ear, Right
use Inner Ear, Left

Cochlear implant (CI), multiple channel (electrode)
use Hearing Device, Multiple Channel Cochlear Prosthesis in 09H

Cochlear implant (CI), single channel (electrode)
use Hearing Device, Single Channel Cochlear Prosthesis in 09H

Cochlear Implant Treatment F0BZ0

Cochlear nerve
use Acoustic Nerve

COGNIS® CRT-D
use Cardiac Resynchronization Defibrillator Pulse Generator in 0JH

COHERE® radiolucent interbody fusion device
use Interbody Fusion Device, Radiolucent Porous in New Technology

Colectomy
see Excision, Gastrointestinal System 0DB
see Resection, Gastrointestinal System 0DT

Collapse
see Occlusion

Collection from
Breast, Breast Milk 8E0HX62
Indwelling Device
  Circulatory System
    Blood 8C02X6K
    Other Fluid 8C02X6L
  Nervous System
    Cerebrospinal Fluid 8C01X6J
    Other Fluid 8C01X6L
Integumentary System, Breast Milk 8E0HX62
Reproductive System, Male, Sperm 8E0VX63

Colocentesis
see Drainage, Gastrointestinal System 0D9

Colofixation
see Repair, Gastrointestinal System 0DQ
see Reposition, Gastrointestinal System 0DS

Cololysis
see Release, Gastrointestinal System 0DN

Colonic Z-Stent®
use Intraluminal Device

Colonoscopy 0DJD8ZZ

Colopexy
see Repair, Gastrointestinal System 0DQ
see Reposition, Gastrointestinal System 0DS

Coloplication
see Restriction, Gastrointestinal System 0DV

Coloproctectomy
see Excision, Gastrointestinal System 0DB
see Resection, Gastrointestinal System 0DT

Coloproctostomy
see Bypass, Gastrointestinal System 0D1
see Drainage, Gastrointestinal System 0D9

Colopuncture
see Drainage, Gastrointestinal System 0D9

Colorrhaphy
see Repair, Gastrointestinal System 0DQ

Colostomy
see Bypass, Gastrointestinal System 0D1
see Drainage, Gastrointestinal System 0D9

Colpectomy
see Excision, Vagina 0UBG
see Resection, Vagina 0UTG

Colpocentesis
see Drainage, Vagina 0U9G

Colpopexy
see Repair, Vagina 0UQG
see Reposition, Vagina 0USG

Colpoplasty
see Repair, Vagina 0UQG
see Supplement, Vagina 0UUG

Colporrhaphy
see Repair, Vagina 0UQG

Colposcopy 0UJH8ZZ

Columella
use Nasal Mucosa and Soft Tissue

Common digital vein
use Foot Vein, Right
use Foot Vein, Left

Common facial vein
use Face Vein, Right
use Face Vein, Left

Common fibular nerve
use Peroneal Nerve

Common hepatic artery
use Hepatic Artery

Common iliac (subaortic) lymph node
use Lymphatic, Pelvis

Common interosseous artery
use Ulnar Artery, Right
use Ulnar Artery, Left

Common peroneal nerve
use Peroneal Nerve

Complete® (SE) stent
use Intraluminal Device

Compression
see Restriction
Abdominal Wall 2W13X
Arm
  Lower
    Left 2W1DX
    Right 2W1CX
  Upper
    Left 2W1BX
    Right 2W1AX
Back 2W15X
Chest Wall 2W14X
Extremity
  Lower
    Left 2W1MX
    Right 2W1LX
  Upper
    Left 2W19X
    Right 2W18X
Face 2W11X
Finger
  Left 2W1KX
  Right 2W1JX
Foot
  Left 2W1TX
  Right 2W1SX
Hand
  Left 2W1FX
  Right 2W1EX
Head 2W10X
Inguinal Region

Compression — *continued*
Inguinal Region — *continued*
  Left 2W17X
  Right 2W16X
Leg
  Lower
    Left 2W1RX
    Right 2W1QX
  Upper
    Left 2W1PX
    Right 2W1NX
Neck 2W12X
Thumb
  Left 2W1HX
  Right 2W1GX
Toe
  Left 2W1VX
  Right 2W1UX

Computer-assisted procedure
Extremity
  Lower
    No Qualifier 8E0YXBZ
    With Computerized Tomography 8E0YXBG
    With Fluoroscopy 8E0YXBF
    With Magnetic Resonance Imaging 8E0YXBH
  Upper
    No Qualifier 8E0XXBZ
    With Computerized Tomography 8E0XXBG
    With Fluoroscopy 8E0XXBF
    With Magnetic Resonance Imaging 8E0XXBH
Head and Neck Region
  No Qualifier 8E09XBZ
  With Computerized Tomography 8E09XBG
  With Fluoroscopy 8E09XBF
  With Magnetic Resonance Imaging 8E09XBH
Trunk Region
  No Qualifier 8E0WXBZ
  With Computerized Tomography 8E0WXBG
  With Fluoroscopy 8E0WXBF
  With Magnetic Resonance Imaging 8E0WXBH

Computerized Tomography (CT Scan)
Abdomen BW20
  Chest and Pelvis BW25
Abdomen and Chest BW24
Abdomen and Pelvis BW21
Airway, Trachea BB2F
Ankle
  Left BQ2H
  Right BQ2G
Aorta
  Abdominal B420
    Intravascular Optical Coherence B420Z2Z
  Thoracic B320
    Intravascular Optical Coherence B320Z2Z
Arm
  Left BP2F
  Right BP2E
Artery
  Celiac B421
    Intravascular Optical Coherence B421Z2Z
  Common Carotid
    Bilateral B325
    Intravascular Optical Coherence B325Z2Z
  Coronary
    Bypass Graft

Computerized Tomography (CT Scan)
— *continued*
  Artery — *continued*
    Multiple B223
      Intravascular Optical
        Coherence B223Z2Z
    Multiple B221
      Intravascular Optical
        Coherence B221Z2Z
    Internal Carotid
      Bilateral B328
        Intravascular Optical
          Coherence B328Z2Z
    Intracranial B32R
      Intravascular Optical
        Coherence B32RZ2Z
    Lower Extremity
      Bilateral B42H
        Intravascular Optical
          Coherence B42HZ2Z
      Left B42G
        Intravascular Optical
          Coherence B42GZ2Z
      Right B42F
        Intravascular Optical
          Coherence B42FZ2Z
    Pelvic B42C
      Intravascular Optical
        Coherence B42CZ2Z
    Pulmonary
      Left B32T
        Intravascular Optical
          Coherence B32TZ2Z
      Right B32S
        Intravascular Optical
          Coherence B32SZ2Z
    Renal
      Bilateral B428
        Intravascular Optical
          Coherence B428Z2Z
      Transplant B42M
        Intravascular Optical
          Coherence B42MZ2Z
    Superior Mesenteric B424
      Intravascular Optical
        Coherence B424Z2Z
    Vertebral
      Bilateral B32G
        Intravascular Optical
          Coherence B32GZ2Z
  Bladder BT20
  Bone
    Facial BN25
    Temporal BN2F
  Brain B020
  Calcaneus
    Left BQ2K
    Right BQ2J
  Cerebral Ventricle B028
  Chest, Abdomen and Pelvis BW25
  Chest and Abdomen BW24
  Cisterna B027
  Clavicle
    Left BP25
    Right BP24
  Coccyx BR2F
  Colon BD24
  Ear B920
  Elbow
    Left BP2H
    Right BP2G
  Extremity
    Lower
      Left BQ2S
      Right BQ2R
    Upper
      Bilateral BP2V

Computerized Tomography (CT Scan)
— *continued*
  Extremity — *continued*
    Left BP2U
    Right BP2T
  Eye
    Bilateral B827
    Left B826
    Right B825
  Femur
    Left BQ24
    Right BQ23
  Fibula
    Left BQ2C
    Right BQ2B
  Finger
    Left BP2S
    Right BP2R
  Foot
    Left BQ2M
    Right BQ2L
  Forearm
    Left BP2K
    Right BP2J
  Gland
    Adrenal, Bilateral BG22
    Parathyroid BG23
    Parotid, Bilateral B926
    Salivary, Bilateral B92D
    Submandibular, Bilateral B929
    Thyroid BG24
  Hand
    Left BP2P
    Right BP2N
  Hands and Wrists, Bilateral BP2Q
  Head BW28
  Head and Neck BW29
  Heart
    Right and Left B226
    Intravascular Optical
      Coherence B226Z2Z
  Hepatobiliary System, All BF2C
  Hip
    Left BQ21
    Right BQ20
  Humerus
    Left BP2B
    Right BP2A
  Intracranial Sinus B522
    Intravascular Optical
      Coherence B522Z2Z
  Joint
    Acromioclavicular, Bilateral BP23
    Finger
      Left BP2DZZZ
      Right BP2CZZZ
    Foot
      Left BQ2Y
      Right BQ2X
    Hand
      Left BP2DZZZ
      Right BP2CZZZ
    Sacroiliac BR2D
    Sternoclavicular
      Bilateral BP22
      Left BP21
      Right BP20
    Temporomandibular, Bilateral BN29
    Toe
      Left BQ2Y
      Right BQ2X
  Kidney
    Bilateral BT23
    Left BT22
    Right BT21
    Transplant BT29

Computerized Tomography (CT Scan)
— *continued*
  Knee
    Left BQ28
    Right BQ27
  Larynx B92J
  Leg
    Left BQ2F
    Right BQ2D
  Liver BF25
  Liver and Spleen BF26
  Lung, Bilateral BB24
  Mandible BN26
  Nasopharynx B92F
  Neck BW2F
  Neck and Head BW29
  Orbit, Bilateral BN23
  Oropharynx B92F
  Pancreas BF27
  Patella
    Left BQ2W
    Right BQ2V
  Pelvic Region BW2G
  Pelvis BR2C
    Chest and Abdomen BW25
  Pelvis and Abdomen BW21
  Pituitary Gland B029
  Prostate BV23
  Ribs
    Left BP2Y
    Right BP2X
  Sacrum BR2F
  Scapula
    Left BP27
    Right BP26
  Sella Turcica B029
  Shoulder
    Left BP29
    Right BP28
  Sinus
    Intracranial B522
      Intravascular Optical
        Coherence B522Z2Z
    Paranasal B922
  Skull BN20
  Spinal Cord B02B
  Spine
    Cervical BR20
    Lumbar BR29
    Thoracic BR27
  Spleen and Liver BF26
  Thorax BP2W
  Tibia
    Left BQ2C
    Right BQ2B
  Toe
    Left BQ2Q
    Right BQ2P
  Trachea BB2F
  Tracheobronchial Tree
    Bilateral BB29
    Left BB28
    Right BB27
  Vein
    Pelvic (Iliac)
      Left B52G
        Intravascular Optical
          Coherence B52GZ2Z
      Right B52F
        Intravascular Optical
          Coherence B52FZ2Z
    Pelvic (Iliac) Bilateral B52H
      Intravascular Optical
        Coherence B52HZ2Z
    Portal B52T
      Intravascular Optical
        Coherence B52TZ2Z

Computerized Tomography (CT Scan)
— continued
Vein — continued
Pulmonary
Bilateral B52S
Intravascular Optical
Coherence B52SZ2Z
Left B52R
Intravascular Optical
Coherence B52RZ2Z
Right B52Q
Intravascular Optical
Coherence B52QZ2Z
Renal
Bilateral B52L
Intravascular Optical
Coherence B52LZ2Z
Left B52K
Intravascular Optical
Coherence B52KZ2Z
Right B52J
Intravascular Optical
Coherence B52JZ2Z
Splanchnic B52T
Intravascular Optical
Coherence B52TZ2Z
Vena Cava
Inferior B529
Intravascular Optical
Coherence B529Z2Z
Superior B528
Intravascular Optical
Coherence B528Z2Z
Ventricle, Cerebral B028
Wrist
Left BP2M
Right BP2L
Concentrated Bone Marrow Aspirate (CBMA) injection, intramuscular XK02303
Concerto® II CRT-D
use Cardiac Resynchronization Defibrillator Pulse Generator in 0JH
Condylectomy
see Excision, Head and Facial Bones 0NB
see Excision, Upper Bones 0PB
see Excision, Lower Bones 0QB
Condyloid process
use Mandible, Right
use Mandible, Left
Condylotomy
see Division, Head and Facial Bones 0N8
see Drainage, Head and Facial Bones 0N9
see Division, Upper Bones 0P8
see Drainage, Upper Bones 0P9
see Division, Lower Bones 0Q8
see Drainage, Lower Bones 0Q9
Condylysis
see Release, Head and Facial Bones 0NN
see Release, Upper Bones 0PN
see Release, Lower Bones 0QN
Conization, cervix
see Excision, Cervix 0UBC
Conjunctivoplasty
see Repair, Eye 08Q
see Replacement, Eye 08R
CONSERVE® PLUS Total Resurfacing Hip System
use Resurfacing Device in Lower Joints
Construction
Auricle, ear see Replacement, Ear, Nose, Sinus 09R
Ileal conduit see Bypass, Urinary System 0T1
Consulta® CRT-D
use Cardiac Resynchronization Defibrillator Pulse Generator in 0JH

Consulta CRT-P
use Cardiac Resynchronization Pacemaker Pulse Generator in 0JH
Contact Radiation
Abdomen DWY37ZZ
Adrenal Gland DGY27ZZ
Bile Ducts DFY27ZZ
Bladder DTY27ZZ
Bone, Other DPYC7ZZ
Brain D0Y07ZZ
Brain Stem D0Y17ZZ
Breast
Left DMY07ZZ
Right DMY17ZZ
Bronchus DBY17ZZ
Cervix DUY17ZZ
Chest DWY27ZZ
Chest Wall DBY77ZZ
Colon DDY57ZZ
Diaphragm DBY87ZZ
Duodenum DDY27ZZ
Ear D9Y07ZZ
Esophagus DDY07ZZ
Eye D8Y07ZZ
Femur DPY97ZZ
Fibula DPYB7ZZ
Gallbladder DFY17ZZ
Gland
Adrenal DGY27ZZ
Parathyroid DGY47ZZ
Pituitary DGY07ZZ
Thyroid DGY57ZZ
Glands, Salivary D9Y67ZZ
Head and Neck DWY17ZZ
Hemibody DWY47ZZ
Humerus DPY67ZZ
Hypopharynx D9Y37ZZ
Ileum DDY47ZZ
Jejunum DDY37ZZ
Kidney DTY07ZZ
Larynx D9YB7ZZ
Liver DFY07ZZ
Lung DBY27ZZ
Mandible DPY37ZZ
Maxilla DPY27ZZ
Mediastinum DBY67ZZ
Mouth D9Y47ZZ
Nasopharynx D9YD7ZZ
Neck and Head DWY17ZZ
Nerve, Peripheral D0Y77ZZ
Nose D9Y17ZZ
Oropharynx D9YF7ZZ
Ovary DUY07ZZ
Palate
Hard D9Y87ZZ
Soft D9Y97ZZ
Pancreas DFY37ZZ
Parathyroid Gland DGY47ZZ
Pelvic Bones DPY87ZZ
Pelvic Region DWY67ZZ
Pineal Body DGY17ZZ
Pituitary Gland DGY07ZZ
Pleura DBY57ZZ
Prostate DVY07ZZ
Radius DPY77ZZ
Rectum DDY77ZZ
Rib DPY57ZZ
Sinuses D9Y77ZZ
Skin
Abdomen DHY87ZZ
Arm DHY47ZZ
Back DHY77ZZ
Buttock DHY97ZZ
Chest DHY67ZZ
Face DHY27ZZ
Leg DHYB7ZZ
Neck DHY37ZZ

Contact Radiation — continued
Skull DPY07ZZ
Spinal Cord D0Y67ZZ
Sternum DPY47ZZ
Stomach DDY17ZZ
Testis DVY17ZZ
Thyroid Gland DGY57ZZ
Tibia DPYB7ZZ
Tongue D9Y57ZZ
Trachea DBY07ZZ
Ulna DPY77ZZ
Ureter DTY17ZZ
Urethra DTY37ZZ
Uterus DUY27ZZ
Whole Body DWY57ZZ
CONTAK RENEWAL® 3 RF (HE) CRT-D
use Cardiac Resynchronization Defibrillator Pulse Generator in 0JH
Contegra® Pulmonary Valved Conduit
use Zooplastic Tissue in Heart and Great Vessels
Continuous Glucose Monitoring (CGM) device
use Monitoring Device
Continuous Negative Airway Pressure
24-96 Consecutive Hours, Ventilation 5A09459
Greater than 96 Consecutive Hours, Ventilation 5A09559
Less than 24 Consecutive Hours, Ventilation 5A09359
Continuous Positive Airway Pressure
24-96 Consecutive Hours, Ventilation 5A09457
Greater than 96 Consecutive Hours, Ventilation 5A09557
Less than 24 Consecutive Hours, Ventilation 5A09357
Continuous renal replacement therapy (CRRT) 5A1D90Z
Contraceptive Device
Change device in, Uterus and Cervix 0U2DXHZ
Insertion of device in
Cervix 0UHC
Subcutaneous Tissue and Fascia
Abdomen 0JH8
Chest 0JH6
Lower Arm
Left 0JHH
Right 0JHG
Lower Leg
Left 0JHP
Right 0JHN
Upper Arm
Left 0JHF
Right 0JHD
Upper Leg
Left 0JHM
Right 0JHL
Uterus 0UH9
Removal of device from
Subcutaneous Tissue and Fascia
Lower Extremity 0JPW
Trunk 0JPT
Upper Extremity 0JPV
Uterus and Cervix 0UPD
Revision of device in
Subcutaneous Tissue and Fascia
Lower Extremity 0JWW
Trunk 0JWT
Upper Extremity 0JWV
Uterus and Cervix 0UWD
Contractility Modulation Device
Abdomen 0JH8
Chest 0JH6

Control bleeding in
  Abdominal Wall 0W3F
  Ankle Region
    Left 0Y3L
    Right 0Y3K
  Arm
    Lower
      Left 0X3F
      Right 0X3D
    Upper
      Left 0X39
      Right 0X38
  Axilla
    Left 0X35
    Right 0X34
  Back
    Lower 0W3L
    Upper 0W3K
  Buttock
    Left 0Y31
    Right 0Y30
  Cavity, Cranial 0W31
  Chest Wall 0W38
  Elbow Region
    Left 0X3C
    Right 0X3B
  Extremity
    Lower
      Left 0Y3B
      Right 0Y39
    Upper
      Left 0X37
      Right 0X36
  Face 0W32
  Femoral Region
    Left 0Y38
    Right 0Y37
  Foot
    Left 0Y3N
    Right 0Y3M
  Gastrointestinal Tract 0W3P
  Genitourinary Tract 0W3R
  Hand
    Left 0X3K
    Right 0X3J
  Head 0W30
  Inguinal Region
    Left 0Y36
    Right 0Y35
  Jaw
    Lower 0W35
    Upper 0W34
  Knee Region
    Left 0Y3G
    Right 0Y3F
  Leg
    Lower
      Left 0Y3J
      Right 0Y3H
    Upper
      Left 0Y3D
      Right 0Y3C
  Mediastinum 0W3C
  Neck 0W36
  Oral Cavity and Throat 0W33
  Pelvic Cavity 0W3J
  Pericardial Cavity 0W3D
  Perineum
    Female 0W3N
    Male 0W3M
  Peritoneal Cavity 0W3G
  Pleural Cavity
    Left 0W3B
    Right 0W39
  Respiratory Tract 0W3Q
  Retroperitoneum 0W3H

Control bleeding in — *continued*
  Shoulder Region
    Left 0X33
    Right 0X32
  Wrist Region
    Left 0X3H
    Right 0X3G
Conus arteriosus
  use Ventricle, Right
Conus medullaris
  use Lumbar Spinal Cord
Conversion
  Cardiac rhythm 5A2204Z
  Gastrostomy to jejunostomy feeding
    device *see* Insertion of device in,
    Jejunum 0DHA
Cook Biodesign® Fistula Plug(s)
  use Nonautologous Tissue Substitute
Cook Biodesign® Hernia Graft(s)
  use Nonautologous Tissue Substitute
Cook Biodesign® Layered Graft(s)
  use Nonautologous Tissue Substitute
Cook Zenapro™ Layered Graft(s)
  use Nonautologous Tissue Substitute
Cook Zenith AAA Endovascular Graft
  use Intraluminal Device, Branched or
    Fenestrated, One or Two Arteries in 04V
  use Intraluminal Device, Branched or
    Fenestrated, Three or More Arteries in 04V
  use Intraluminal Device
Coracoacromial ligament
  use Shoulder Bursa and Ligament, Right
  use Shoulder Bursa and Ligament, Left
Coracobrachialis muscle
  use Upper Arm Muscle, Right
  use Upper Arm Muscle, Left
Coracoclavicular ligament
  use Shoulder Bursa and Ligament, Right
  use Shoulder Bursa and Ligament, Left
Coracohumeral ligament
  use Shoulder Bursa and Ligament, Right
  use Shoulder Bursa and Ligament, Left
Coracoid process
  use Scapula, Right
  use Scapula, Left
Cordotomy
  see Division, Central Nervous System and
    Cranial Nerves 008
Core needle biopsy
  see Excision with qualifier Diagnostic
CoreValve™ transcatheter aortic valve
  use Zooplastic Tissue in Heart and Great
    Vessels
Cormet™ Hip Resurfacing System
  use Resurfacing Device in Lower Joints
Corniculate cartilage
  use Larynx
CoRoent® XL
  use Interbody Fusion Device in Lower Joints
Coronary arteriography
  see Plain Radiography, Heart B20
  see Fluoroscopy, Heart B21
Corox® (OTW) Bipolar Lead
  use Cardiac Lead, Pacemaker in 02H
  use Cardiac Lead, Defibrillator in 02H
Corpus callosum
  use Brain
Corpus cavernosum
  use Penis
Corpus spongiosum
  use Penis
Corpus striatum
  use Basal Ganglia
Corrugator supercilii muscle
  use Facial Muscle
Cortical strip neurostimulator lead
  use Neurostimulator Lead in Central
    Nervous System and Cranial Nerves

Costatectomy
  see Excision, Upper Bones 0PB
  see Resection, Upper Bones 0PT
Costectomy
  see Excision, Upper Bones 0PB
  see Resection, Upper Bones 0PT
Costocervical trunk
  use Subclavian Artery, Right
  use Subclavian Artery, Left
Costochondrectomy
  see Excision, Upper Bones 0PB
  see Resection, Upper Bones 0PT
Costoclavicular ligament
  use Shoulder Bursa and Ligament, Right
  use Shoulder Bursa and Ligament, Left
Costosternoplasty
  see Repair, Upper Bones 0PQ
  see Replacement, Upper Bones 0PR
  see Supplement, Upper Bones 0PU
Costotomy
  see Division, Upper Bones 0P8
  see Drainage, Upper Bones 0P9
Costotransverse joint
  use Thoracic Vertebral Joint
Costotransverse ligament
  use Sternum Bursa and Ligament
  use Rib(s) Bursa and Ligament
Costovertebral joint
  use Thoracic Vertebral Joint
Costoxiphoid ligament
  use Sternum Bursa and Ligament
  use Rib(s) Bursa and Ligament
Counseling
  Family, for substance abuse, Other Family
    Counseling HZ63ZZZ
  Group
    12-Step HZ43ZZZ
    Behavioral HZ41ZZZ
    Cognitive HZ40ZZZ
    Cognitive-Behavioral HZ42ZZZ
    Confrontational HZ48ZZZ
    Continuing Care HZ49ZZZ
    Infectious Disease
      Post-Test HZ4CZZZ
      Pre-Test HZ4CZZZ
    Interpersonal HZ44ZZZ
    Motivational Enhancement HZ47ZZZ
    Psychoeducation HZ46ZZZ
    Spiritual HZ4BZZZ
    Vocational HZ45ZZZ
  Individual
    12-Step HZ33ZZZ
    Behavioral HZ31ZZZ
    Cognitive HZ30ZZZ
    Cognitive-Behavioral HZ32ZZZ
    Confrontational HZ38ZZZ
    Continuing Care HZ39ZZZ
    Infectious Disease
      Post-Test HZ3CZZZ
      Pre-Test HZ3CZZZ
    Interpersonal HZ34ZZZ
    Motivational Enhancement HZ37ZZZ
    Psychoeducation HZ36ZZZ
    Spiritual HZ3BZZZ
    Vocational HZ35ZZZ
  Mental Health Services
    Educational GZ60ZZZ
    Other Counseling GZ63ZZZ
    Vocational GZ61ZZZ
Countershock, cardiac 5A2204Z
Cowper's (bulbourethral) gland
  use Urethra
CPAP (continuous positive airway pressure)
  see Assistance, Respiratory 5A09
Craniectomy
  see Excision, Head and Facial Bones 0NB
  see Resection, Head and Facial Bones 0NT

Cranioplasty
see Repair, Head and Facial Bones 0NQ
see Replacement, Head and Facial Bones 0NR
see Supplement, Head and Facial Bones 0NU

Craniotomy
see Drainage, Central Nervous System and Cranial Nerves 009
see Division, Head and Facial Bones 0N8
see Drainage, Head and Facial Bones 0N9

Creation
Perineum
  Female 0W4N0
  Male 0W4M0
Valve
  Aortic 024F0
  Mitral 024G0
  Tricuspid 024J0

Cremaster muscle
use Perineum Muscle

Cribriform plate
use Ethmoid Bone, Right
use Ethmoid Bone, Left

Cricoid cartilage
use Trachea

Cricoidectomy
see Excision, Larynx 0CBS

Cricothyroid artery
use Thyroid Artery, Right
use Thyroid Artery, Left

Cricothyroid muscle
use Neck Muscle, Right
use Neck Muscle, Left

Crisis Intervention GZ2ZZZZ

CRRT (Continuous renal replacement therapy) 5A1D90Z

Crural fascia
use Subcutaneous Tissue and Fascia, Right Upper Leg
use Subcutaneous Tissue and Fascia, Left Upper Leg

Crushing, nerve
Cranial *see* Destruction, Central Nervous System and Cranial Nerves 005
Peripheral *see* Destruction, Peripheral Nervous System 015

Cryoablation
see Destruction

Cryotherapy
see Destruction

Cryptorchidectomy
see Excision, Male Reproductive System 0VB
see Resection, Male Reproductive System 0VT

Cryptorchiectomy
see Excision, Male Reproductive System 0VB
see Resection, Male Reproductive System 0VT

Cryptotomy
see Division, Gastrointestinal System 0D8
see Drainage, Gastrointestinal System 0D9

CT scan
see Computerized Tomography (CT Scan)

CT sialogram
see Computerized Tomography (CT Scan), Ear, Nose, Mouth and Throat B92

Cubital lymph node
use Lymphatic, Right Upper Extremity
use Lymphatic, Left Upper Extremity

Cubital nerve
use Ulnar Nerve

Cuboid bone
use Tarsal, Right
use Tarsal, Left

Cuboideonavicular joint
use Tarsal Joint, Right
use Tarsal Joint, Left

Culdocentesis
see Drainage, Cul-de-sac 0U9F

Culdoplasty
see Repair, Cul-de-sac 0UQF
see Supplement, Cul-de-sac 0UUF

Culdoscopy 0UJH8ZZ

Culdotomy
see Drainage, Cul-de-sac 0U9F

Culmen
use Cerebellum

Cultured epidermal cell autograft
use Autologous Tissue Substitute

Cuneiform cartilage
use Larynx

Cuneonavicular joint
use Tarsal Joint, Right
use Tarsal Joint, Left

Cuneonavicular ligament
use Foot Bursa and Ligament, Right
use Foot Bursa and Ligament, Left

Curettage
see Excision
see Extraction

Cutaneous (transverse) cervical nerve
use Cervical Plexus

CVP (central venous pressure)
see Measurement, Venous 4A04

Cyclodiathermy
see Destruction, Eye 085

Cyclophotocoagulation
see Destruction, Eye 085

CYPHER® Stent
use Intraluminal Device, Drug-eluting in Heart and Great Vessels

Cystectomy
see Excision, Bladder 0TBB
see Resection, Bladder 0TTB

Cystocele repair
see Repair, Subcutaneous Tissue and Fascia, Pelvic Region 0JQC

Cystography
see Plain Radiography, Urinary System BT0
see Fluoroscopy, Urinary System BT1

Cystolithotomy
see Extirpation, Bladder 0TCB

Cystopexy
see Repair, Bladder 0TQB
see Reposition, Bladder 0TSB

Cystoplasty
see Repair, Bladder 0TQB
see Replacement, Bladder 0TRB
see Supplement, Bladder 0TUB

Cystorrhaphy
see Repair, Bladder 0TQB

Cystoscopy 0TJB8ZZ

Cystostomy
see Bypass, Bladder 0T1B

Cystostomy tube
use Drainage Device

Cystotomy
see Drainage, Bladder 0T9B

Cystourethrography
see Plain Radiography, Urinary System BT0
see Fluoroscopy, Urinary System BT1

Cystourethroplasty
see Repair, Urinary System 0TQ
see Replacement, Urinary System 0TR
see Supplement, Urinary System 0TU

Cytarabine and Daunorubicin Liposome Antineoplastic XW0

D

DBS lead
use Neurostimulator Lead in Central Nervous System and Cranial Nerves

DeBakey Left Ventricular Assist Device
use Implantable Heart Assist System in Heart and Great Vessels

Debridement
Excisional *see* Excision
Non-excisional *see* Extraction

Decompression, Circulatory 6A15

Decortication, lung
see Extirpation, Respiratory System 0BC
see Release, Respiratory System 0BN

Deep brain neurostimulator lead
use Neurostimulator Lead in Central Nervous System and Cranial Nerves

Deep cervical fascia
use Subcutaneous Tissue and Fascia, Right Neck
use Subcutaneous Tissue and Fascia, Left Neck

Deep cervical vein
use Vertebral Vein, Right
use Vertebral Vein, Left

Deep circumflex iliac artery
use External Iliac Artery, Right
use External Iliac Artery, Left

Deep facial vein
use Face Vein, Right
use Face Vein, Left

Deep femoral (profunda femoris) vein
use Femoral Vein, Right
use Femoral Vein, Left

Deep femoral artery
use Femoral Artery, Right
use Femoral Artery, Left

Deep Inferior Epigastric Artery Perforator Flap
Replacement
  Bilateral 0HRV077
  Left 0HRU077
  Right 0HRT077
Transfer
  Left 0KXG
  Right 0KXF

Deep palmar arch
use Hand Artery, Right
use Hand Artery, Left

Deep transverse perineal muscle
use Perineum Muscle

Deferential artery
use Internal Iliac Artery, Right
use Internal Iliac Artery, Left

Defibrillator Generator
Abdomen 0JH8
Chest 0JH6

Defibrotide Sodium Anticoagulant XW0

Defitelio®
use Defibrotide Sodium Anticoagulant

Delivery
Cesarean *see* Extraction, Products of Conception 10D0
Forceps *see* Extraction, Products of Conception 10D0
Manually assisted 10E0XZZ
Products of Conception 10E0XZZ
Vacuum assisted *see* Extraction, Products of Conception 10D0

Delta frame external fixator
use External Fixation Device, Hybrid in 0PH
use External Fixation Device, Hybrid in 0PS
use External Fixation Device, Hybrid in 0QH
use External Fixation Device, Hybrid in 0QS

Delta III™ Reverse shoulder prosthesis
　use Synthetic Substitute, Reverse Ball and
　　Socket in 0RR
Deltoid fascia
　use Subcutaneous Tissue and Fascia, Right
　　Upper Arm
　use Subcutaneous Tissue and Fascia, Left
　　Upper Arm
Deltoid ligament
　use Ankle Bursa and Ligament, Right
　use Ankle Bursa and Ligament, Left
Deltoid muscle
　use Shoulder Muscle, Right
　use Shoulder Muscle, Left
Deltopectoral (infraclavicular) lymph node
　use Lymphatic, Right Upper Extremity
　use Lymphatic, Left Upper Extremity
Denervation
　Cranial nerve *see* Destruction, Central
　　Nervous System and Cranial Nerves 005
　Peripheral nerve *see* Destruction,
　　Peripheral Nervous System 015
Dens
　use Cervical Vertebra
Densitometry
　Plain Radiography
　　Femur
　　　Left BQ04ZZ1
　　　Right BQ03ZZ1
　　Hip
　　　Left BQ01ZZ1
　　　Right BQ00ZZ1
　　Spine
　　　Cervical BR00ZZ1
　　　Lumbar BR09ZZ1
　　　Thoracic BR07ZZ1
　　　Whole BR0GZZ1
　Ultrasonography
　　Elbow
　　　Left BP4HZZ1
　　　Right BP4GZZ1
　　Hand
　　　Left BP4PZZ1
　　　Right BP4NZZ1
　　Shoulder
　　　Left BP49ZZ1
　　　Right BP48ZZ1
　　Wrist
　　　Left BP4MZZ1
　　　Right BP4LZZ1
Denticulate (dentate) ligament
　use Spinal Meninges
Depressor anguli oris muscle
　use Facial Muscle
Depressor labii inferioris muscle
　use Facial Muscle
Depressor septi nasi muscle
　use Facial Muscle
Depressor supercilii muscle
　use Facial Muscle
Dermabrasion
　see Extraction, Skin and Breast 0HD
Dermis
　use Skin
Descending genicular artery
　use Femoral Artery, Right
　use Femoral Artery, Left
Destruction
　Acetabulum
　　Left 0Q55
　　Right 0Q54
　Adenoids 0C5Q
　Ampulla of Vater 0F5C
　Anal Sphincter 0D5R
　Anterior Chamber
　　Left 08533ZZ
　　Right 08523ZZ

Destruction — *continued*
　Anus 0D5Q
　Aorta
　　Abdominal 0450
　　Thoracic
　　　Ascending/Arch 025X
　　　Descending 025W
　Aortic Body 0G5D
　Appendix 0D5J
　Artery
　　Anterior Tibial
　　　Left 045Q
　　　Right 045P
　　Axillary
　　　Left 0356
　　　Right 0355
　　Brachial
　　　Left 0358
　　　Right 0357
　　Celiac 0451
　　Colic
　　　Left 0457
　　　Middle 0458
　　　Right 0456
　　Common Carotid
　　　Left 035J
　　　Right 035H
　　Common Iliac
　　　Left 045D
　　　Right 045C
　　External Carotid
　　　Left 035N
　　　Right 035M
　　External Iliac
　　　Left 045J
　　　Right 045H
　　Face 035R
　　Femoral
　　　Left 045L
　　　Right 045K
　　Foot
　　　Left 045W
　　　Right 045V
　　Gastric 0452
　　Hand
　　　Left 035F
　　　Right 035D
　　Hepatic 0453
　　Inferior Mesenteric 045B
　　Innominate 0352
　　Internal Carotid
　　　Left 035L
　　　Right 035K
　　Internal Iliac
　　　Left 045F
　　　Right 045E
　　Internal Mammary
　　　Left 0351
　　　Right 0350
　　Intracranial 035G
　　Lower 045Y
　　Peroneal
　　　Left 045U
　　　Right 045T
　　Popliteal
　　　Left 045N
　　　Right 045M
　　Posterior Tibial
　　　Left 045S
　　　Right 045R
　　Pulmonary
　　　Left 025R
　　　Right 025Q
　　Pulmonary Trunk 025P
　　Radial
　　　Left 035C

Destruction — *continued*
　Artery — *continued*
　　　Right 035B
　　Renal
　　　Left 045A
　　　Right 0459
　　Splenic 0454
　　Subclavian
　　　Left 0354
　　　Right 0353
　　Superior Mesenteric 0455
　　Temporal
　　　Left 035T
　　　Right 035S
　　Thyroid
　　　Left 035V
　　　Right 035U
　　Ulnar
　　　Left 035A
　　　Right 0359
　　Upper 035Y
　　Vertebral
　　　Left 035Q
　　　Right 035P
　Atrium
　　Left 0257
　　Right 0256
　Auditory Ossicle
　　Left 095A
　　Right 0959
　Basal Ganglia 0058
　Bladder 0T5B
　Bladder Neck 0T5C
　Bone
　　Ethmoid
　　　Left 0N5G
　　　Right 0N5F
　　Frontal 0N51
　　Hyoid 0N5X
　　Lacrimal
　　　Left 0N5J
　　　Right 0N5H
　　Nasal 0N5B
　　Occipital 0N57
　　Palatine
　　　Left 0N5L
　　　Right 0N5K
　　Parietal
　　　Left 0N54
　　　Right 0N53
　　Pelvic
　　　Left 0Q53
　　　Right 0Q52
　　Sphenoid 0N5C
　　Temporal
　　　Left 0N56
　　　Right 0N55
　　Zygomatic
　　　Left 0N5N
　　　Right 0N5M
　Brain 0050
　Breast
　　Bilateral 0H5V
　　Left 0H5U
　　Right 0H5T
　Bronchus
　　Lingula 0B59
　　Lower Lobe
　　　Left 0B5B
　　　Right 0B56
　　Main
　　　Left 0B57
　　　Right 0B53
　　Middle Lobe, Right 0B55
　　Upper Lobe
　　　Left 0B58
　　　Right 0B54

Destruction — *continued*
Buccal Mucosa 0C54
Bursa and Ligament
  Abdomen
    Left 0M5J
    Right 0M5H
  Ankle
    Left 0M5R
    Right 0M5Q
  Elbow
    Left 0M54
    Right 0M53
  Foot
    Left 0M5T
    Right 0M5S
  Hand
    Left 0M58
    Right 0M57
  Head and Neck 0M50
  Hip
    Left 0M5M
    Right 0M5L
  Knee
    Left 0M5P
    Right 0M5N
  Lower Extremity
    Left 0M5W
    Right 0M5V
  Perineum 0M5K
  Rib(s) 0M5G
  Shoulder
    Left 0M52
    Right 0M51
  Spine
    Lower 0M5D
    Upper 0M5C
  Sternum 0M5F
  Upper Extremity
    Left 0M5B
    Right 0M59
  Wrist
    Left 0M56
    Right 0M55
Carina 0B52
Carotid Bodies, Bilateral 0G58
Carotid Body
  Left 0G56
  Right 0G57
Carpal
  Left 0P5N
  Right 0P5M
Cecum 0D5H
Cerebellum 005C
Cerebral Hemisphere 0057
Cerebral Meninges 0051
Cerebral Ventricle 0056
Cervix 0U5C
Chordae Tendineae 0259
Choroid
  Left 085B
  Right 085A
Cisterna Chyli 075L
Clavicle
  Left 0P5B
  Right 0P59
Clitoris 0U5J
Coccygeal Glomus 0G5B
Coccyx 0Q5S
Colon
  Ascending 0D5K
  Descending 0D5M
  Sigmoid 0D5N
  Transverse 0D5L
Conduction Mechanism 0258
Conjunctiva
  Left 085TXZZ
  Right 085SXZZ

Destruction — *continued*
Cord
  Bilateral 0V5H
  Left 0V5G
  Right 0V5F
Cornea
  Left 0859XZZ
  Right 0858XZZ
Cul-de-sac 0U5F
Diaphragm 0B5T
Disc
  Cervical Vertebral 0R53
  Cervicothoracic Vertebral 0R55
  Lumbar Vertebral 0S52
  Lumbosacral 0S54
  Thoracic Vertebral 0R59
  Thoracolumbar Vertebral 0R5B
Duct
  Common Bile 0F59
  Cystic 0F58
  Hepatic
    Common 0F57
    Left 0F56
    Right 0F55
  Lacrimal
    Left 085Y
    Right 085X
  Pancreatic 0F5D
    Accessory 0F5F
  Parotid
    Left 0C5C
    Right 0C5B
Duodenum 0D59
Dura Mater 0052
Ear
  External
    Left 0951
    Right 0950
  External Auditory Canal
    Left 0954
    Right 0953
  Inner
    Left 095E
    Right 095D
  Middle
    Left 0956
    Right 0955
Endometrium 0U5B
Epididymis
  Bilateral 0V5L
  Left 0V5K
  Right 0V5J
Epiglottis 0C5R
Esophagogastric Junction 0D54
Esophagus 0D55
  Lower 0D53
  Middle 0D52
  Upper 0D51
Eustachian Tube
  Left 095G
  Right 095F
Eye
  Left 0851XZZ
  Right 0850XZZ
Eyelid
  Lower
    Left 085R
    Right 085Q
  Upper
    Left 085P
    Right 085N
Fallopian Tube
  Left 0U56
  Right 0U55
Fallopian Tubes, Bilateral 0U57
Femoral Shaft
  Left 0Q59
  Right 0Q58

Destruction — *continued*
Femur
  Lower
    Left 0Q5C
    Right 0Q5B
  Upper
    Left 0Q57
    Right 0Q56
Fibula
  Left 0Q5K
  Right 0Q5J
Finger Nail 0H5QXZZ
Gallbladder 0F54
Gingiva
  Lower 0C56
  Upper 0C55
Gland
  Adrenal
    Bilateral 0G54
    Left 0G52
    Right 0G53
  Lacrimal
    Left 085W
    Right 085V
  Minor Salivary 0C5J
  Parotid
    Left 0C59
    Right 0C58
  Pituitary 0G50
  Sublingual
    Left 0C5F
    Right 0C5D
  Submaxillary
    Left 0C5H
    Right 0C5G
  Vestibular 0U5L
Glenoid Cavity
  Left 0P58
  Right 0P57
Glomus Jugulare 0G5C
Humeral Head
  Left 0P5D
  Right 0P5C
Humeral Shaft
  Left 0P5G
  Right 0P5F
Hymen 0U5K
Hypothalamus 005A
Ileocecal Valve 0D5C
Ileum 0D5B
Intestine
  Large 0D5E
    Left 0D5G
    Right 0D5F
  Small 0D58
Iris
  Left 085D3ZZ
  Right 085C3ZZ
Jejunum 0D5A
Joint
  Acromioclavicular
    Left 0R5H
    Right 0R5G
  Ankle
    Left 0S5G
    Right 0S5F
  Carpal
    Left 0R5R
    Right 0R5Q
  Carpometacarpal
    Left 0R5T
    Right 0R5S
  Cervical Vertebral 0R51
  Cervicothoracic Vertebral 0R54
  Coccygeal 0S56
  Elbow
    Left 0R5M

Destruction — *continued*
Joint — *continued*
Right 0R5L
Finger Phalangeal
Left 0R5X
Right 0R5W
Hip
Left 0S5B
Right 0S59
Knee
Left 0S5D
Right 0S5C
Lumbar Vertebral 0S50
Lumbosacral 0S53
Metacarpophalangeal
Left 0R5V
Right 0R5U
Metatarsal-Phalangeal
Left 0S5N
Right 0S5M
Occipital-cervical 0R50
Sacrococcygeal 0S55
Sacroiliac
Left 0S58
Right 0S57
Shoulder
Left 0R5K
Right 0R5J
Sternoclavicular
Left 0R5F
Right 0R5E
Tarsal
Left 0S5J
Right 0S5H
Tarsometatarsal
Left 0S5L
Right 0S5K
Temporomandibular
Left 0R5D
Right 0R5C
Thoracic Vertebral 0R56
Thoracolumbar Vertebral 0R5A
Toe Phalangeal
Left 0S5Q
Right 0S5P
Wrist
Left 0R5P
Right 0R5N
Kidney
Left 0T51
Right 0T50
Kidney Pelvis
Left 0T54
Right 0T53
Larynx 0C5S
Lens
Left 085K3ZZ
Right 085J3ZZ
Lip
Lower 0C51
Upper 0C50
Liver 0F50
Left Lobe 0F52
Right Lobe 0F51
Lung
Bilateral 0B5M
Left 0B5L
Lower Lobe
Left 0B5J
Right 0B5F
Middle Lobe, Right 0B5D
Right 0B5K
Upper Lobe
Left 0B5G
Right 0B5C
Lung Lingula 0B5H

Destruction — *continued*
Lymphatic
Aortic 075D
Axillary
Left 0756
Right 0755
Head 0750
Inguinal
Left 075J
Right 075H
Internal Mammary
Left 0759
Right 0758
Lower Extremity
Left 075G
Right 075F
Mesenteric 075B
Neck
Left 0752
Right 0751
Pelvis 075C
Thoracic Duct 075K
Thorax 0757
Upper Extremity
Left 0754
Right 0753
Mandible
Left 0N5V
Right 0N5T
Maxilla 0N5R
Medulla Oblongata 005D
Mesentery 0D5V
Metacarpal
Left 0P5Q
Right 0P5P
Metatarsal
Left 0Q5P
Right 0Q5N
Muscle
Abdomen
Left 0K5L
Right 0K5K
Extraocular
Left 085M
Right 085L
Facial 0K51
Foot
Left 0K5W
Right 0K5V
Hand
Left 0K5D
Right 0K5C
Head 0K50
Hip
Left 0K5P
Right 0K5N
Lower Arm and Wrist
Left 0K5B
Right 0K59
Lower Leg
Left 0K5T
Right 0K5S
Neck
Left 0K53
Right 0K52
Papillary 025D
Perineum 0K5M
Shoulder
Left 0K56
Right 0K55
Thorax
Left 0K5J
Right 0K5H
Tongue, Palate, Pharynx 0K54
Trunk
Left 0K5G
Right 0K5F

Destruction — *continued*
Muscle — *continued*
Upper Arm
Left 0K58
Right 0K57
Upper Leg
Left 0K5R
Right 0K5Q
Nasal Mucosa and Soft Tissue 095K
Nasopharynx 095N
Nerve
Abdominal Sympathetic 015M
Abducens 005L
Accessory 005R
Acoustic 005N
Brachial Plexus 0153
Cervical 0151
Cervical Plexus 0150
Facial 005M
Femoral 015D
Glossopharyngeal 005P
Head and Neck Sympathetic 015K
Hypoglossal 005S
Lumbar 015B
Lumbar Plexus 0159
Lumbar Sympathetic 015N
Lumbosacral Plexus 015A
Median 0155
Oculomotor 005H
Olfactory 005F
Optic 005G
Peroneal 015H
Phrenic 0152
Pudendal 015C
Radial 0156
Sacral 015R
Sacral Plexus 015Q
Sacral Sympathetic 015P
Sciatic 015F
Thoracic 0158
Thoracic Sympathetic 015L
Tibial 015G
Trigeminal 005K
Trochlear 005J
Ulnar 0154
Vagus 005Q
Nipple
Left 0H5X
Right 0H5W
Omentum 0D5U
Orbit
Left 0N5Q
Right 0N5P
Ovary
Bilateral 0U52
Left 0U51
Right 0U50
Palate
Hard 0C52
Soft 0C53
Pancreas 0F5G
Para-aortic Body 0G59
Paraganglion Extremity 0G5F
Parathyroid Gland 0G5R
Inferior
Left 0G5P
Right 0G5N
Multiple 0G5Q
Superior
Left 0G5M
Right 0G5L
Patella
Left 0Q5F
Right 0Q5D
Penis 0V5S
Pericardium 025N
Peritoneum 0D5W

Destruction — *continued*
  Phalanx
    Finger
      Left 0P5V
      Right 0P5T
    Thumb
      Left 0P5S
      Right 0P5R
    Toe
      Left 0Q5R
      Right 0Q5Q
  Pharynx 0C5M
  Pineal Body 0G51
  Pleura
    Left 0B5P
    Right 0B5N
  Pons 005B
  Prepuce 0V5T
  Prostate 0V50
  Radius
    Left 0P5J
    Right 0P5H
  Rectum 0D5P
  Retina
    Left 085F3ZZ
    Right 085E3ZZ
  Retinal Vessel
    Left 085H3ZZ
    Right 085G3ZZ
  Ribs
    1 to 2 0P51
    3 or More 0P52
  Sacrum 0Q51
  Scapula
    Left 0P56
    Right 0P55
  Sclera
    Left 0857XZZ
    Right 0856XZZ
  Scrotum 0V55
  Septum
    Atrial 0255
    Nasal 095M
    Ventricular 025M
  Sinus
    Accessory 095P
    Ethmoid
      Left 095V
      Right 095U
    Frontal
      Left 095T
      Right 095S
    Mastoid
      Left 095C
      Right 095B
    Maxillary
      Left 095R
      Right 095Q
    Sphenoid
      Left 095X
      Right 095W
  Skin
    Abdomen 0H57XZ
    Back 0H56XZ
    Buttock 0H58XZ
    Chest 0H55XZ
    Ear
      Left 0H53XZ
      Right 0H52XZ
    Face 0H51XZ
    Foot
      Left 0H5NXZ
      Right 0H5MXZ
    Hand
      Left 0H5GXZ
      Right 0H5FXZ
    Inguinal 0H5AXZ

Destruction — *continued*
  Skin — *continued*
    Lower Arm
      Left 0H5EXZ
      Right 0H5DXZ
    Lower Leg
      Left 0H5LXZ
      Right 0H5KXZ
    Neck 0H54XZ
    Perineum 0H59XZ
    Scalp 0H50XZ
    Upper Arm
      Left 0H5CXZ
      Right 0H5BXZ
    Upper Leg
      Left 0H5JXZ
      Right 0H5HXZ
  Skull 0N50
  Spinal Cord
    Cervical 005W
    Lumbar 005Y
    Thoracic 005X
  Spinal Meninges 005T
  Spleen 075P
  Sternum 0P50
  Stomach 0D56
    Pylorus 0D57
  Subcutaneous Tissue and Fascia
    Abdomen 0J58
    Back 0J57
    Buttock 0J59
    Chest 0J56
    Face 0J51
    Foot
      Left 0J5R
      Right 0J5Q
    Hand
      Left 0J5K
      Right 0J5J
    Lower Arm
      Left 0J5H
      Right 0J5G
    Lower Leg
      Left 0J5P
      Right 0J5N
    Neck
      Left 0J55
      Right 0J54
    Pelvic Region 0J5C
    Perineum 0J5B
    Scalp 0J50
    Upper Arm
      Left 0J5F
      Right 0J5D
    Upper Leg
      Left 0J5M
      Right 0J5L
  Tarsal
    Left 0Q5M
    Right 0Q5L
  Tendon
    Abdomen
      Left 0L5G
      Right 0L5F
    Ankle
      Left 0L5T
      Right 0L5S
    Foot
      Left 0L5W
      Right 0L5V
    Hand
      Left 0L58
      Right 0L57
    Head and Neck 0L50
    Hip
      Left 0L5K
      Right 0L5J

Destruction — *continued*
  Tendon — *continued*
    Knee
      Left 0L5R
      Right 0L5Q
    Lower Arm and Wrist
      Left 0L56
      Right 0L55
    Lower Leg
      Left 0L5P
      Right 0L5N
    Perineum 0L5H
    Shoulder
      Left 0L52
      Right 0L51
    Thorax
      Left 0L5D
      Right 0L5C
    Trunk
      Left 0L5B
      Right 0L59
    Upper Arm
      Left 0L54
      Right 0L53
    Upper Leg
      Left 0L5M
      Right 0L5L
  Testis
    Bilateral 0V5C
    Left 0V5B
    Right 0V59
  Thalamus 0059
  Thymus 075M
  Thyroid Gland 0G5K
    Left Lobe 0G5G
    Right Lobe 0G5H
  Tibia
    Left 0Q5H
    Right 0Q5G
  Toe Nail 0H5RXZZ
  Tongue 0C57
  Tonsils 0C5P
  Tooth
    Lower 0C5X
    Upper 0C5W
  Trachea 0B51
  Tunica Vaginalis
    Left 0V57
    Right 0V56
  Turbinate, Nasal 095L
  Tympanic Membrane
    Left 0958
    Right 0957
  Ulna
    Left 0P5L
    Right 0P5K
  Ureter
    Left 0T57
    Right 0T56
  Urethra 0T5D
  Uterine Supporting Structure 0U54
  Uterus 0U59
  Uvula 0C5N
  Vagina 0U5G
  Valve
    Aortic 025F
    Mitral 025G
    Pulmonary 025H
    Tricuspid 025J
  Vas Deferens
    Bilateral 0V5Q
    Left 0V5P
    Right 0V5N
  Vein
    Axillary
      Left 0558
      Right 0557

Destruction — *continued*
  Vein — *continued*
    Azygos 0550
    Basilic
      Left 055C
      Right 055B
    Brachial
      Left 055A
      Right 0559
    Cephalic
      Left 055F
      Right 055D
    Colic 0657
    Common Iliac
      Left 065D
      Right 065C
    Coronary 0254
    Esophageal 0653
    External Iliac
      Left 065G
      Right 065F
    External Jugular
      Left 055Q
      Right 055P
    Face
      Left 055V
      Right 055T
    Femoral
      Left 065N
      Right 065M
    Foot
      Left 065V
      Right 065T
    Gastric 0652
    Hand
      Left 055H
      Right 055G
    Hemiazygos 0551
    Hepatic 0654
    Hypogastric
      Left 065J
      Right 065H
    Inferior Mesenteric 0656
    Innominate
      Left 0554
      Right 0553
    Internal Jugular
      Left 055N
      Right 055M
    Intracranial 055L
    Lower 065Y
    Portal 0658
    Pulmonary
      Left 025T
      Right 025S
    Renal
      Left 065B
      Right 0659
    Saphenous
      Left 065Q
      Right 065P
    Splenic 0651
    Subclavian
      Left 0556
      Right 0555
    Superior Mesenteric 0655
    Upper 055Y
    Vertebral
      Left 055S
      Right 055R
  Vena Cava
    Inferior 0650
    Superior 025V
  Ventricle
    Left 025L
    Right 025K

Destruction — *continued*
  Vertebra
    Cervical 0P53
    Lumbar 0Q50
    Thoracic 0P54
  Vesicle
    Bilateral 0V53
    Left 0V52
    Right 0V51
  Vitreous
    Left 08553ZZ
    Right 08543ZZ
  Vocal Cord
    Left 0C5V
    Right 0C5T
  Vulva 0U5M
Detachment
  Arm
    Lower
      Left 0X6F0Z
      Right 0X6D0Z
    Upper
      Left 0X690Z
      Right 0X680Z
  Elbow Region
    Left 0X6C0ZZ
    Right 0X6B0ZZ
  Femoral Region
    Left 0Y680ZZ
    Right 0Y670ZZ
  Finger
    Index
      Left 0X6P0Z
      Right 0X6N0Z
    Little
      Left 0X6W0Z
      Right 0X6V0Z
    Middle
      Left 0X6R0Z
      Right 0X6Q0Z
    Ring
      Left 0X6T0Z
      Right 0X6S0Z
  Foot
    Left 0Y6N0Z
    Right 0Y6M0Z
  Forequarter
    Left 0X610ZZ
    Right 0X600ZZ
  Hand
    Left 0X6K0Z
    Right 0X6J0Z
  Hindquarter
    Bilateral 0Y640ZZ
    Left 0Y630ZZ
    Right 0Y620ZZ
  Knee Region
    Left 0Y6G0ZZ
    Right 0Y6F0ZZ
  Leg
    Lower
      Left 0Y6J0Z
      Right 0Y6H0Z
    Upper
      Left 0Y6D0Z
      Right 0Y6C0Z
  Shoulder Region
    Left 0X630ZZ
    Right 0X620ZZ
  Thumb
    Left 0X6M0Z
    Right 0X6L0Z
  Toe
    1st
      Left 0Y6Q0Z
      Right 0Y6P0Z
    2nd

Detachment — *continued*
  Toe — *continued*
      Left 0Y6S0Z
      Right 0Y6R0Z
    3rd
      Left 0Y6U0Z
      Right 0Y6T0Z
    4th
      Left 0Y6W0Z
      Right 0Y6V0Z
    5th
      Left 0Y6Y0Z
      Right 0Y6X0Z
Determination, Mental status GZ14ZZZ
Detorsion
  see Release
  see Reposition
Detoxification Services, for substance abuse HZ2ZZZZ
Device Fitting F0DZ
Diagnostic Audiology
  see Audiology, Diagnostic
Diagnostic imaging
  see Imaging, Diagnostic
Diagnostic radiology
  see Imaging, Diagnostic
Dialysis
  Hemodialysis *see* Performance, Urinary 5A1D
  Peritoneal 3E1M39Z
Diaphragma sellae
  use Dura Mater
Diaphragmatic pacemaker generator
  use Stimulator Generator in Subcutaneous Tissue and Fascia
Diaphragmatic Pacemaker Lead
  Insertion of device in, Diaphragm 0BHT
  Removal of device from, Diaphragm 0BPT
  Revision of device in, Diaphragm 0BWT
Digital radiography, plain
  see Plain Radiography
Dilation
  Ampulla of Vater 0F7C
  Anus 0D7Q
  Aorta
    Abdominal 0470
    Thoracic
      Ascending/Arch 027X
      Descending 027W
  Artery
    Anterior Tibial
      Left 047Q
      Right 047P
    Axillary
      Left 0376
      Right 0375
    Brachial
      Left 0378
      Right 0377
    Celiac 0471
    Colic
      Left 0477
      Middle 0478
      Right 0476
    Common Carotid
      Left 037J
      Right 037H
    Common Iliac
      Left 047D
      Right 047C
    Coronary
      Four or More Arteries 0273
      One Artery 0270
      Three Arteries 0272
      Two Arteries 0271
    External Carotid
      Left 037N

Dilation — *continued*
  Artery — *continued*
    Right 037M
    External Iliac
      Left 047J
      Right 047H
    Face 037R
    Femoral
      Left 047L
      Right 047K
    Foot
      Left 047W
      Right 047V
    Gastric 0472
    Hand
      Left 037F
      Right 037D
    Hepatic 0473
    Inferior Mesenteric 047B
    Innominate 0372
    Internal Carotid
      Left 037L
      Right 037K
    Internal Iliac
      Left 047F
      Right 047E
    Internal Mammary
      Left 0371
      Right 0370
    Intracranial 037G
    Lower 047Y
    Peroneal
      Left 047U
      Right 047T
    Popliteal
      Left 047N
      Right 047M
    Posterior Tibial
      Left 047S
      Right 047R
    Pulmonary
      Left 027R
      Right 027Q
    Pulmonary Trunk 027P
    Radial
      Left 037C
      Right 037B
    Renal
      Left 047A
      Right 0479
    Splenic 0474
    Subclavian
      Left 0374
      Right 0373
    Superior Mesenteric 0475
    Temporal
      Left 037T
      Right 037S
    Thyroid
      Left 037V
      Right 037U
    Ulnar
      Left 037A
      Right 0379
    Upper 037Y
    Vertebral
      Left 037Q
      Right 037P
  Bladder 0T7B
  Bladder Neck 0T7C
  Bronchus
    Lingula 0B79
    Lower Lobe
      Left 0B7B
      Right 0B76
    Main
      Left 0B77

Dilation — *continued*
  Bronchus — *continued*
      Right 0B73
    Middle Lobe, Right 0B75
    Upper Lobe
      Left 0B78
      Right 0B74
  Carina 0B72
  Cecum 0D7H
  Cerebral Ventricle 0076
  Cervix 0U7C
  Colon
    Ascending 0D7K
    Descending 0D7M
    Sigmoid 0D7N
    Transverse 0D7L
  Duct
    Common Bile 0F79
    Cystic 0F78
    Hepatic
      Common 0F77
      Left 0F76
      Right 0F75
    Lacrimal
      Left 087Y
      Right 087X
    Pancreatic 0F7D
      Accessory 0F7F
    Parotid
      Left 0C7C
      Right 0C7B
  Duodenum 0D79
  Esophagogastric Junction 0D74
  Esophagus 0D75
    Lower 0D73
    Middle 0D72
    Upper 0D71
  Eustachian Tube
    Left 097G
    Right 097F
  Fallopian Tube
    Left 0U76
    Right 0U75
  Fallopian Tubes, Bilateral 0U77
  Hymen 0U7K
  Ileocecal Valve 0D7C
  Ileum 0D7B
  Intestine
    Large 0D7E
      Left 0D7G
      Right 0D7F
    Small 0D78
  Jejunum 0D7A
  Kidney Pelvis
    Left 0T74
    Right 0T73
  Larynx 0C7S
  Pharynx 0C7M
  Rectum 0D7P
  Stomach 0D76
    Pylorus 0D77
  Trachea 0B71
  Ureter
    Left 0T77
    Right 0T76
  Ureters, Bilateral 0T78
  Urethra 0T7D
  Uterus 0U79
  Vagina 0U7G
  Valve
    Aortic 027F
    Mitral 027G
    Pulmonary 027H
    Tricuspid 027J
  Vas Deferens
    Bilateral 0V7Q
    Left 0V7P

Dilation — *continued*
  Vas Deferens — *continued*
    Right 0V7N
  Vein
    Axillary
      Left 0578
      Right 0577
    Azygos 0570
    Basilic
      Left 057C
      Right 057B
    Brachial
      Left 057A
      Right 0579
    Cephalic
      Left 057F
      Right 057D
    Colic 0677
    Common Iliac
      Left 067D
      Right 067C
    Esophageal 0673
    External Iliac
      Left 067G
      Right 067F
    External Jugular
      Left 057Q
      Right 057P
    Face
      Left 057V
      Right 057T
    Femoral
      Left 067N
      Right 067M
    Foot
      Left 067V
      Right 067T
    Gastric 0672
    Hand
      Left 057H
      Right 057G
    Hemiazygos 0571
    Hepatic 0674
    Hypogastric
      Left 067J
      Right 067H
    Inferior Mesenteric 0676
    Innominate
      Left 0574
      Right 0573
    Internal Jugular
      Left 057N
      Right 057M
    Intracranial 057L
    Lower 067Y
    Portal 0678
    Pulmonary
      Left 027T
      Right 027S
    Renal
      Left 067B
      Right 0679
    Saphenous
      Left 067Q
      Right 067P
    Splenic 0671
    Subclavian
      Left 0576
      Right 0575
    Superior Mesenteric 0675
    Upper 057Y
    Vertebral
      Left 057S
      Right 057R
  Vena Cava
    Inferior 0670
    Superior 027V

Dilation — *continued*
  Ventricle
    Left 027L
    Right 027K
**Direct Lateral Interbody Fusion (DLIF)
  device**
  use Interbody Fusion Device in Lower
    Joints
Disarticulation
  see Detachment
Discectomy, diskectomy
  see Excision, Upper Joints 0RB
  see Resection, Upper Joints 0RT
  see Excision, Lower Joints 0SB
  see Resection, Lower Joints 0ST
Discography
  see Plain Radiography, Axial Skeleton,
    Except Skull and Facial Bones BR0
  see Fluoroscopy, Axial Skeleton, Except
    Skull and Facial Bones BR1
Distal humerus
  use Humeral Shaft, Right
  use Humeral Shaft, Left
Distal humerus, involving joint
  use Elbow Joint, Right
  use Elbow Joint, Left
Distal radioulnar joint
  use Wrist Joint, Right
  use Wrist Joint, Left
Diversion
  see Bypass
Diverticulectomy
  see Excision, Gastrointestinal System 0DB
Division
  Acetabulum
    Left 0Q85
    Right 0Q84
  Anal Sphincter 0D8R
  Basal Ganglia 0088
  Bladder Neck 0T8C
  Bone
    Ethmoid
      Left 0N8G
      Right 0N8F
    Frontal 0N81
    Hyoid 0N8X
    Lacrimal
      Left 0N8J
      Right 0N8H
    Nasal 0N8B
    Occipital 0N87
    Palatine
      Left 0N8L
      Right 0N8K
    Parietal
      Left 0N84
      Right 0N83
    Pelvic
      Left 0Q83
      Right 0Q82
    Sphenoid 0N8C
    Temporal
      Left 0N86
      Right 0N85
    Zygomatic
      Left 0N8N
      Right 0N8M
  Brain 0080
  Bursa and Ligament
    Abdomen
      Left 0M8J
      Right 0M8H
    Ankle
      Left 0M8R
      Right 0M8Q
    Elbow
      Left 0M84

Division — *continued*
  Bursa and Ligament — *continued*
    Right 0M83
    Foot
      Left 0M8T
      Right 0M8S
    Hand
      Left 0M88
      Right 0M87
    Head and Neck 0M80
    Hip
      Left 0M8M
      Right 0M8L
    Knee
      Left 0M8P
      Right 0M8N
    Lower Extremity
      Left 0M8W
      Right 0M8V
    Perineum 0M8K
    Rib(s) 0M8G
    Shoulder
      Left 0M82
      Right 0M81
    Spine
      Lower 0M8D
      Upper 0M8C
    Sternum 0M8F
    Upper Extremity
      Left 0M8B
      Right 0M89
    Wrist
      Left 0M86
      Right 0M85
  Carpal
    Left 0P8N
    Right 0P8M
  Cerebral Hemisphere 0087
  Chordae Tendineae 0289
  Clavicle
    Left 0P8B
    Right 0P89
  Coccyx 0Q8S
  Conduction Mechanism 0288
  Esophagogastric Junction 0D84
  Femoral Shaft
    Left 0Q89
    Right 0Q88
  Femur
    Lower
      Left 0Q8C
      Right 0Q8B
    Upper
      Left 0Q87
      Right 0Q86
  Fibula
    Left 0Q8K
    Right 0Q8J
  Gland, Pituitary 0G80
  Glenoid Cavity
    Left 0P88
    Right 0P87
  Humeral Head
    Left 0P8D
    Right 0P8C
  Humeral Shaft
    Left 0P8G
    Right 0P8F
  Hymen 0U8K
  Kidneys, Bilateral 0T82
  Mandible
    Left 0N8V
    Right 0N8T
  Maxilla 0N8R
  Metacarpal
    Left 0P8Q
    Right 0P8P

Division — *continued*
  Metatarsal
    Left 0Q8P
    Right 0Q8N
  Muscle
    Abdomen
      Left 0K8L
      Right 0K8K
    Facial 0K81
    Foot
      Left 0K8W
      Right 0K8V
    Hand
      Left 0K8D
      Right 0K8C
    Head 0K80
    Hip
      Left 0K8P
      Right 0K8N
    Lower Arm and Wrist
      Left 0K8B
      Right 0K89
    Lower Leg
      Left 0K8T
      Right 0K8S
    Neck
      Left 0K83
      Right 0K82
    Papillary 028D
    Perineum 0K8M
    Shoulder
      Left 0K86
      Right 0K85
    Thorax
      Left 0K8J
      Right 0K8H
    Tongue, Palate, Pharynx 0K84
    Trunk
      Left 0K8G
      Right 0K8F
    Upper Arm
      Left 0K88
      Right 0K87
    Upper Leg
      Left 0K8R
      Right 0K8Q
  Nerve
    Abdominal Sympathetic 018M
    Abducens 008L
    Accessory 008R
    Acoustic 008N
    Brachial Plexus 0183
    Cervical 0181
    Cervical Plexus 0180
    Facial 008M
    Femoral 018D
    Glossopharyngeal 008P
    Head and Neck Sympathetic 018K
    Hypoglossal 008S
    Lumbar 018B
    Lumbar Plexus 0189
    Lumbar Sympathetic 018N
    Lumbosacral Plexus 018A
    Median 0185
    Oculomotor 008H
    Olfactory 008F
    Optic 008G
    Peroneal 018H
    Phrenic 0182
    Pudendal 018C
    Radial 0186
    Sacral 018R
    Sacral Plexus 018Q
    Sacral Sympathetic 018P
    Sciatic 018F
    Thoracic 0188
    Thoracic Sympathetic 018L

Division — *continued*
  Nerve — *continued*
    Tibial 018G
    Trigeminal 008K
    Trochlear 008J
    Ulnar 0184
    Vagus 008Q
  Orbit
    Left 0N8Q
    Right 0N8P
  Ovary
    Bilateral 0U82
    Left 0U81
    Right 0U80
  Pancreas 0F8G
  Patella
    Left 0Q8F
    Right 0Q8D
  Perineum, Female 0W8NXZZ
  Phalanx
    Finger
      Left 0P8V
      Right 0P8T
    Thumb
      Left 0P8S
      Right 0P8R
    Toe
      Left 0Q8R
      Right 0Q8Q
  Radius
    Left 0P8J
    Right 0P8H
  Ribs
    1 to 2 0P81
    3 or More 0P82
  Sacrum 0Q81
  Scapula
    Left 0P86
    Right 0P85
  Skin
    Abdomen 0H87XZZ
    Back 0H86XZZ
    Buttock 0H88XZZ
    Chest 0H85XZZ
    Ear
      Left 0H83XZZ
      Right 0H82XZZ
    Face 0H81XZZ
    Foot
      Left 0H8NXZZ
      Right 0H8MXZZ
    Hand
      Left 0H8GXZZ
      Right 0H8FXZZ
    Inguinal 0H8AXZZ
    Lower Arm
      Left 0H8EXZZ
      Right 0H8DXZZ
    Lower Leg
      Left 0H8LXZZ
      Right 0H8KXZZ
    Neck 0H84XZZ
    Perineum 0H89XZZ
    Scalp 0H80XZZ
    Upper Arm
      Left 0H8CXZZ
      Right 0H8BXZZ
    Upper Leg
      Left 0H8JXZZ
      Right 0H8HXZZ
  Skull 0N80
  Spinal Cord
    Cervical 008W
    Lumbar 008Y
    Thoracic 008X
  Sternum 0P80
  Stomach, Pylorus 0D87

Division — *continued*
  Subcutaneous Tissue and Fascia
    Abdomen 0J88
    Back 0J87
    Buttock 0J89
    Chest 0J86
    Face 0J81
    Foot
      Left 0J8R
      Right 0J8Q
    Hand
      Left 0J8K
      Right 0J8J
    Head and Neck 0J8S
    Lower Arm
      Left 0J8H
      Right 0J8G
    Lower Extremity 0J8W
    Lower Leg
      Left 0J8P
      Right 0J8N
    Neck
      Left 0J85
      Right 0J84
    Pelvic Region 0J8C
    Perineum 0J8B
    Scalp 0J80
    Trunk 0J8T
    Upper Arm
      Left 0J8F
      Right 0J8D
    Upper Extremity 0J8V
    Upper Leg
      Left 0J8M
      Right 0J8L
  Tarsal
    Left 0Q8M
    Right 0Q8L
  Tendon
    Abdomen
      Left 0L8G
      Right 0L8F
    Ankle
      Left 0L8T
      Right 0L8S
    Foot
      Left 0L8W
      Right 0L8V
    Hand
      Left 0L88
      Right 0L87
    Head and Neck 0L80
    Hip
      Left 0L8K
      Right 0L8J
    Knee
      Left 0L8R
      Right 0L8Q
    Lower Arm and Wrist
      Left 0L86
      Right 0L85
    Lower Leg
      Left 0L8P
      Right 0L8N
    Perineum 0L8H
    Shoulder
      Left 0L82
      Right 0L81
    Thorax
      Left 0L8D
      Right 0L8C
    Trunk
      Left 0L8B
      Right 0L89
    Upper Arm
      Left 0L84
      Right 0L83

Division — *continued*
  Tendon — *continued*
    Upper Leg
      Left 0L8M
      Right 0L8L
  Thyroid Gland Isthmus 0G8J
  Tibia
    Left 0Q8H
    Right 0Q8G
  Turbinate, Nasal 098L
  Ulna
    Left 0P8L
    Right 0P8K
  Uterine Supporting Structure 0U84
  Vertebra
    Cervical 0P83
    Lumbar 0Q80
    Thoracic 0P84

Doppler study
  see Ultrasonography
Dorsal digital nerve
  use Radial Nerve
Dorsal metacarpal vein
  use Hand Vein, Right
  use Hand Vein, Left
Dorsal metatarsal artery
  use Foot Artery, Right
  use Foot Artery, Left
Dorsal metatarsal vein
  use Foot Vein, Right
  use Foot Vein, Left
Dorsal scapular artery
  use Subclavian Artery, Right
  use Subclavian Artery, Left
Dorsal scapular nerve
  use Brachial Plexus
Dorsal venous arch
  use Foot Vein, Right
  use Foot Vein, Left
Dorsalis pedis artery
  use Anterior Tibial Artery, Right
  use Anterior Tibial Artery, Left
Drainage
  Abdominal Wall 0W9F
  Acetabulum
    Left 0Q95
    Right 0Q94
  Adenoids 0C9Q
  Ampulla of Vater 0F9C
  Anal Sphincter 0D9R
  Ankle Region
    Left 0Y9L
    Right 0Y9K
  Anterior Chamber
    Left 0893
    Right 0892
  Anus 0D9Q
  Aorta, Abdominal 0490
  Aortic Body 0G9D
  Appendix 0D9J
  Arm
    Lower
      Left 0X9F
      Right 0X9D
    Upper
      Left 0X99
      Right 0X98
  Artery
    Anterior Tibial
      Left 049Q
      Right 049P
    Axillary
      Left 0396
      Right 0395
    Brachial
      Left 0398
      Right 0397

Drainage — *continued*
  Artery — *continued*
    Celiac 0491
    Colic
      Left 0497
      Middle 0498
      Right 0496
    Common Carotid
      Left 039J
      Right 039H
    Common Iliac
      Left 049D
      Right 049C
    External Carotid
      Left 039N
      Right 039M
    External Iliac
      Left 049J
      Right 049H
    Face 039R
    Femoral
      Left 049L
      Right 049K
    Foot
      Left 049W
      Right 049V
    Gastric 0492
    Hand
      Left 039F
      Right 039D
    Hepatic 0493
    Inferior Mesenteric 049B
    Innominate 0392
    Internal Carotid
      Left 039L
      Right 039K
    Internal Iliac
      Left 049F
      Right 049E
    Internal Mammary
      Left 0391
      Right 0390
    Intracranial 039G
    Lower 049Y
    Peroneal
      Left 049U
      Right 049T
    Popliteal
      Left 049N
      Right 049M
    Posterior Tibial
      Left 049S
      Right 049R
    Radial
      Left 039C
      Right 039B
    Renal
      Left 049A
      Right 0499
    Splenic 0494
    Subclavian
      Left 0394
      Right 0393
    Superior Mesenteric 0495
    Temporal
      Left 039T
      Right 039S
    Thyroid
      Left 039V
      Right 039U
    Ulnar
      Left 039A
      Right 0399
    Upper 039Y
    Vertebral
      Left 039Q
      Right 039P

Drainage — *continued*
  Auditory Ossicle
    Left 099A
    Right 0999
  Axilla
    Left 0X95
    Right 0X94
  Back
    Lower 0W9L
    Upper 0W9K
  Basal Ganglia 0098
  Bladder 0T9B
  Bladder Neck 0T9C
  Bone
    Ethmoid
      Left 0N9G
      Right 0N9F
    Frontal 0N91
    Hyoid 0N9X
    Lacrimal
      Left 0N9J
      Right 0N9H
    Nasal 0N9B
    Occipital 0N97
    Palatine
      Left 0N9L
      Right 0N9K
    Parietal
      Left 0N94
      Right 0N93
    Pelvic
      Left 0Q93
      Right 0Q92
    Sphenoid 0N9C
    Temporal
      Left 0N96
      Right 0N95
    Zygomatic
      Left 0N9N
      Right 0N9M
  Bone Marrow 079T
  Brain 0090
  Breast
    Bilateral 0H9V
    Left 0H9U
    Right 0H9T
  Bronchus
    Lingula 0B99
    Lower Lobe
      Left 0B9B
      Right 0B96
    Main
      Left 0B97
      Right 0B93
    Middle Lobe, Right 0B95
    Upper Lobe
      Left 0B98
      Right 0B94
  Buccal Mucosa 0C94
  Bursa and Ligament
    Abdomen
      Left 0M9J
      Right 0M9H
    Ankle
      Left 0M9R
      Right 0M9Q
    Elbow
      Left 0M94
      Right 0M93
    Foot
      Left 0M9T
      Right 0M9S
    Hand
      Left 0M98
      Right 0M97
    Head and Neck 0M90
    Hip

Drainage — *continued*
  Bursa and Ligament — *continued*
    Left 0M9M
    Right 0M9L
    Knee
      Left 0M9P
      Right 0M9N
    Lower Extremity
      Left 0M9W
      Right 0M9V
    Perineum 0M9K
    Rib(s) 0M9G
    Shoulder
      Left 0M92
      Right 0M91
    Spine
      Lower 0M9D
      Upper 0M9C
    Sternum 0M9F
    Upper Extremity
      Left 0M9B
      Right 0M99
    Wrist
      Left 0M96
      Right 0M95
  Buttock
    Left 0Y91
    Right 0Y90
  Carina 0B92
  Carotid Bodies, Bilateral 0G98
  Carotid Body
    Left 0G96
    Right 0G97
  Carpal
    Left 0P9N
    Right 0P9M
  Cavity, Cranial 0W91
  Cecum 0D9H
  Cerebellum 009C
  Cerebral Hemisphere 0097
  Cerebral Meninges 0091
  Cerebral Ventricle 0096
  Cervix 0U9C
  Chest Wall 0W98
  Choroid
    Left 089B
    Right 089A
  Cisterna Chyli 079L
  Clavicle
    Left 0P9B
    Right 0P99
  Clitoris 0U9J
  Coccygeal Glomus 0G9B
  Coccyx 0Q9S
  Colon
    Ascending 0D9K
    Descending 0D9M
    Sigmoid 0D9N
    Transverse 0D9L
  Conjunctiva
    Left 089T
    Right 089S
  Cord
    Bilateral 0V9H
    Left 0V9G
    Right 0V9F
  Cornea
    Left 0899
    Right 0898
  Cul-de-sac 0U9F
  Diaphragm 0B9T
  Disc
    Cervical Vertebral 0R93
    Cervicothoracic Vertebral 0R95
    Lumbar Vertebral 0S92
    Lumbosacral 0S94
    Thoracic Vertebral 0R99
    Thoracolumbar Vertebral 0R9B

Drainage — *continued*
- Duct
  - Common Bile 0F99
  - Cystic 0F98
  - Hepatic
    - Common 0F97
    - Left 0F96
    - Right 0F95
  - Lacrimal
    - Left 089Y
    - Right 089X
  - Pancreatic 0F9D
    - Accessory 0F9F
  - Parotid
    - Left 0C9C
    - Right 0C9B
- Duodenum 0D99
- Dura Mater 0092
- Ear
  - External
    - Left 0991
    - Right 0990
  - External Auditory Canal
    - Left 0994
    - Right 0993
  - Inner
    - Left 099E
    - Right 099D
  - Middle
    - Left 0996
    - Right 0995
- Elbow Region
  - Left 0X9C
  - Right 0X9B
- Epididymis
  - Bilateral 0V9L
  - Left 0V9K
  - Right 0V9J
- Epidural Space, Intracranial 0093
- Epiglottis 0C9R
- Esophagogastric Junction 0D94
- Esophagus 0D95
  - Lower 0D93
  - Middle 0D92
  - Upper 0D91
- Eustachian Tube
  - Left 099G
  - Right 099F
- Extremity
  - Lower
    - Left 0Y9B
    - Right 0Y99
  - Upper
    - Left 0X97
    - Right 0X96
- Eye
  - Left 0891
  - Right 0890
- Eyelid
  - Lower
    - Left 089R
    - Right 089Q
  - Upper
    - Left 089P
    - Right 089N
- Face 0W92
- Fallopian Tube
  - Left 0U96
  - Right 0U95
- Fallopian Tubes, Bilateral 0U97
- Femoral Region
  - Left 0Y98
  - Right 0Y97
- Femoral Shaft
  - Left 0Q99
  - Right 0Q98

Drainage — *continued*
- Femur
  - Lower
    - Left 0Q9C
    - Right 0Q9B
  - Upper
    - Left 0Q97
    - Right 0Q96
- Fibula
  - Left 0Q9K
  - Right 0Q9J
- Finger Nail 0H9Q
- Foot
  - Left 0Y9N
  - Right 0Y9M
- Gallbladder 0F94
- Gingiva
  - Lower 0C96
  - Upper 0C95
- Gland
  - Adrenal
    - Bilateral 0G94
    - Left 0G92
    - Right 0G93
  - Lacrimal
    - Left 089W
    - Right 089V
  - Minor Salivary 0C9J
  - Parotid
    - Left 0C99
    - Right 0C98
  - Pituitary 0G90
  - Sublingual
    - Left 0C9F
    - Right 0C9D
  - Submaxillary
    - Left 0C9H
    - Right 0C9G
  - Vestibular 0U9L
- Glenoid Cavity
  - Left 0P98
  - Right 0P97
- Glomus Jugulare 0G9C
- Hand
  - Left 0X9K
  - Right 0X9J
- Head 0W90
- Humeral Head
  - Left 0P9D
  - Right 0P9C
- Humeral Shaft
  - Left 0P9G
  - Right 0P9F
- Hymen 0U9K
- Hypothalamus 009A
- Ileocecal Valve 0D9C
- Ileum 0D9B
- Inguinal Region
  - Left 0Y96
  - Right 0Y95
- Intestine
  - Large 0D9E
    - Left 0D9G
    - Right 0D9F
  - Small 0D98
- Iris
  - Left 089D
  - Right 089C
- Jaw
  - Lower 0W95
  - Upper 0W94
- Jejunum 0D9A
- Joint
  - Acromioclavicular
    - Left 0R9H
    - Right 0R9G

Drainage — *continued*
- Joint — *continued*
  - Ankle
    - Left 0S9G
    - Right 0S9F
  - Carpal
    - Left 0R9R
    - Right 0R9Q
  - Carpometacarpal
    - Left 0R9T
    - Right 0R9S
  - Cervical Vertebral 0R91
  - Cervicothoracic Vertebral 0R94
  - Coccygeal 0S96
  - Elbow
    - Left 0R9M
    - Right 0R9L
  - Finger Phalangeal
    - Left 0R9X
    - Right 0R9W
  - Hip
    - Left 0S9B
    - Right 0S99
  - Knee
    - Left 0S9D
    - Right 0S9C
  - Lumbar Vertebral 0S90
  - Lumbosacral 0S93
  - Metacarpophalangeal
    - Left 0R9V
    - Right 0R9U
  - Metatarsal-Phalangeal
    - Left 0S9N
    - Right 0S9M
  - Occipital-cervical 0R90
  - Sacrococcygeal 0S95
  - Sacroiliac
    - Left 0S98
    - Right 0S97
  - Shoulder
    - Left 0R9K
    - Right 0R9J
  - Sternoclavicular
    - Left 0R9F
    - Right 0R9E
  - Tarsal
    - Left 0S9J
    - Right 0S9H
  - Tarsometatarsal
    - Left 0S9L
    - Right 0S9K
  - Temporomandibular
    - Left 0R9D
    - Right 0R9C
  - Thoracic Vertebral 0R96
  - Thoracolumbar Vertebral 0R9A
  - Toe Phalangeal
    - Left 0S9Q
    - Right 0S9P
  - Wrist
    - Left 0R9P
    - Right 0R9N
- Kidney
  - Left 0T91
  - Right 0T90
- Kidney Pelvis
  - Left 0T94
  - Right 0T93
- Knee Region
  - Left 0Y9G
  - Right 0Y9F
- Larynx 0C9S
- Leg
  - Lower
    - Left 0Y9J
    - Right 0Y9H
  - Upper

Drainage — *continued*
  Leg — *continued*
    Left 0Y9D
    Right 0Y9C
  Lens
    Left 089K
    Right 089J
  Lip
    Lower 0C91
    Upper 0C90
  Liver 0F90
    Left Lobe 0F92
    Right Lobe 0F91
  Lung
    Bilateral 0B9M
    Left 0B9L
    Lower Lobe
      Left 0B9J
      Right 0B9F
    Middle Lobe, Right 0B9D
    Right 0B9K
    Upper Lobe
      Left 0B9G
      Right 0B9C
  Lung Lingula 0B9H
  Lymphatic
    Aortic 079D
    Axillary
      Left 0796
      Right 0795
    Head 0790
    Inguinal
      Left 079J
      Right 079H
    Internal Mammary
      Left 0799
      Right 0798
    Lower Extremity
      Left 079G
      Right 079F
    Mesenteric 079B
    Neck
      Left 0792
      Right 0791
    Pelvis 079C
    Thoracic Duct 079K
    Thorax 0797
    Upper Extremity
      Left 0794
      Right 0793
  Mandible
    Left 0N9V
    Right 0N9T
  Maxilla 0N9R
  Mediastinum 0W9C
  Medulla Oblongata 009D
  Mesentery 0D9V
  Metacarpal
    Left 0P9Q
    Right 0P9P
  Metatarsal
    Left 0Q9P
    Right 0Q9N
  Muscle
    Abdomen
      Left 0K9L
      Right 0K9K
    Extraocular
      Left 089M
      Right 089L
    Facial 0K91
    Foot
      Left 0K9W
      Right 0K9V
    Hand
      Left 0K9D
      Right 0K9C

Drainage — *continued*
  Muscle — *continued*
    Head 0K90
    Hip
      Left 0K9P
      Right 0K9N
    Lower Arm and Wrist
      Left 0K9B
      Right 0K99
    Lower Leg
      Left 0K9T
      Right 0K9S
    Neck
      Left 0K93
      Right 0K92
    Perineum 0K9M
    Shoulder
      Left 0K96
      Right 0K95
    Thorax
      Left 0K9J
      Right 0K9H
    Tongue, Palate, Pharynx 0K94
    Trunk
      Left 0K9G
      Right 0K9F
    Upper Arm
      Left 0K98
      Right 0K97
    Upper Leg
      Left 0K9R
      Right 0K9Q
  Nasal Mucosa and Soft Tissue 099K
  Nasopharynx 099N
  Neck 0W96
  Nerve
    Abdominal Sympathetic 019M
    Abducens 009L
    Accessory 009R
    Acoustic 009N
    Brachial Plexus 0193
    Cervical 0191
    Cervical Plexus 0190
    Facial 009M
    Femoral 019D
    Glossopharyngeal 009P
    Head and Neck Sympathetic 019K
    Hypoglossal 009S
    Lumbar 019B
    Lumbar Plexus 0199
    Lumbar Sympathetic 019N
    Lumbosacral Plexus 019A
    Median 0195
    Oculomotor 009H
    Olfactory 009F
    Optic 009G
    Peroneal 019H
    Phrenic 0192
    Pudendal 019C
    Radial 0196
    Sacral 019R
    Sacral Plexus 019Q
    Sacral Sympathetic 019P
    Sciatic 019F
    Thoracic 0198
    Thoracic Sympathetic 019L
    Tibial 019G
    Trigeminal 009K
    Trochlear 009J
    Ulnar 0194
    Vagus 009Q
  Nipple
    Left 0H9X
    Right 0H9W
  Omentum 0D9U
  Oral Cavity and Throat 0W93

Drainage — *continued*
  Orbit
    Left 0N9Q
    Right 0N9P
  Ovary
    Bilateral 0U92
    Left 0U91
    Right 0U90
  Palate
    Hard 0C92
    Soft 0C93
  Pancreas 0F9G
  Para-aortic Body 0G99
  Paraganglion Extremity 0G9F
  Parathyroid Gland 0G9R
    Inferior
      Left 0G9P
      Right 0G9N
    Multiple 0G9Q
    Superior
      Left 0G9M
      Right 0G9L
  Patella
    Left 0Q9F
    Right 0Q9D
  Pelvic Cavity 0W9J
  Penis 0V9S
  Pericardial Cavity 0W9D
  Perineum
    Female 0W9N
    Male 0W9M
  Peritoneal Cavity 0W9G
  Peritoneum 0D9W
  Phalanx
    Finger
      Left 0P9V
      Right 0P9T
    Thumb
      Left 0P9S
      Right 0P9R
    Toe
      Left 0Q9R
      Right 0Q9Q
  Pharynx 0C9M
  Pineal Body 0G91
  Pleura
    Left 0B9P
    Right 0B9N
  Pleural Cavity
    Left 0W9B
    Right 0W99
  Pons 009B
  Prepuce 0V9T
  Products of Conception
    Amniotic Fluid
      Diagnostic 1090
      Therapeutic 1090
    Fetal Blood 1090
    Fetal Cerebrospinal Fluid 1090
    Fetal Fluid, Other 1090
    Fluid, Other 1090
  Prostate 0V90
  Radius
    Left 0P9J
    Right 0P9H
  Rectum 0D9P
  Retina
    Left 089F
    Right 089E
  Retinal Vessel
    Left 089H
    Right 089G
  Retroperitoneum 0W9H
  Ribs
    1 to 2 0P91
    3 or More 0P92
  Sacrum 0Q91

Drainage — *continued*
- Scapula
  - Left 0P96
  - Right 0P95
- Sclera
  - Left 0897
  - Right 0896
- Scrotum 0V95
- Septum, Nasal 099M
- Shoulder Region
  - Left 0X93
  - Right 0X92
- Sinus
  - Accessory 099P
  - Ethmoid
    - Left 099V
    - Right 099U
  - Frontal
    - Left 099T
    - Right 099S
  - Mastoid
    - Left 099C
    - Right 099B
  - Maxillary
    - Left 099R
    - Right 099Q
  - Sphenoid
    - Left 099X
    - Right 099W
- Skin
  - Abdomen 0H97
  - Back 0H96
  - Buttock 0H98
  - Chest 0H95
  - Ear
    - Left 0H93
    - Right 0H92
  - Face 0H91
  - Foot
    - Left 0H9N
    - Right 0H9M
  - Hand
    - Left 0H9G
    - Right 0H9F
  - Inguinal 0H9A
  - Lower Arm
    - Left 0H9E
    - Right 0H9D
  - Lower Leg
    - Left 0H9L
    - Right 0H9K
  - Neck 0H94
  - Perineum 0H99
  - Scalp 0H90
  - Upper Arm
    - Left 0H9C
    - Right 0H9B
  - Upper Leg
    - Left 0H9J
    - Right 0H9H
- Skull 0N90
- Spinal Canal 009U
- Spinal Cord
  - Cervical 009W
  - Lumbar 009Y
  - Thoracic 009X
- Spinal Meninges 009T
- Spleen 079P
- Sternum 0P90
- Stomach 0D96
  - Pylorus 0D97
- Subarachnoid Space, Intracranial 0095
- Subcutaneous Tissue and Fascia
  - Abdomen 0J98
  - Back 0J97
  - Buttock 0J99
  - Chest 0J96

Drainage — *continued*
- Subcutaneous Tissue and Fascia — *continued*
  - Face 0J91
  - Foot
    - Left 0J9R
    - Right 0J9Q
  - Hand
    - Left 0J9K
    - Right 0J9J
  - Lower Arm
    - Left 0J9H
    - Right 0J9G
  - Lower Leg
    - Left 0J9P
    - Right 0J9N
  - Neck
    - Left 0J95
    - Right 0J94
  - Pelvic Region 0J9C
  - Perineum 0J9B
  - Scalp 0J90
  - Upper Arm
    - Left 0J9F
    - Right 0J9D
  - Upper Leg
    - Left 0J9M
    - Right 0J9L
- Subdural Space, Intracranial 0094
- Tarsal
  - Left 0Q9M
  - Right 0Q9L
- Tendon
  - Abdomen
    - Left 0L9G
    - Right 0L9F
  - Ankle
    - Left 0L9T
    - Right 0L9S
  - Foot
    - Left 0L9W
    - Right 0L9V
  - Hand
    - Left 0L98
    - Right 0L97
  - Head and Neck 0L90
  - Hip
    - Left 0L9K
    - Right 0L9J
  - Knee
    - Left 0L9R
    - Right 0L9Q
  - Lower Arm and Wrist
    - Left 0L96
    - Right 0L95
  - Lower Leg
    - Left 0L9P
    - Right 0L9N
  - Perineum 0L9H
  - Shoulder
    - Left 0L92
    - Right 0L91
  - Thorax
    - Left 0L9D
    - Right 0L9C
  - Trunk
    - Left 0L9B
    - Right 0L99
  - Upper Arm
    - Left 0L94
    - Right 0L93
  - Upper Leg
    - Left 0L9M
    - Right 0L9L
- Testis
  - Bilateral 0V9C
  - Left 0V9B
  - Right 0V99

Drainage — *continued*
- Thalamus 0099
- Thymus 079M
- Thyroid Gland 0G9K
  - Left Lobe 0G9G
  - Right Lobe 0G9H
- Tibia
  - Left 0Q9H
  - Right 0Q9G
- Toe Nail 0H9R
- Tongue 0C97
- Tonsils 0C9P
- Tooth
  - Lower 0C9X
  - Upper 0C9W
- Trachea 0B91
- Tunica Vaginalis
  - Left 0V97
  - Right 0V96
- Turbinate, Nasal 099L
- Tympanic Membrane
  - Left 0998
  - Right 0997
- Ulna
  - Left 0P9L
  - Right 0P9K
- Ureter
  - Left 0T97
  - Right 0T96
- Ureters, Bilateral 0T98
- Urethra 0T9D
- Uterine Supporting Structure 0U94
- Uterus 0U99
- Uvula 0C9N
- Vagina 0U9G
- Vas Deferens
  - Bilateral 0V9Q
  - Left 0V9P
  - Right 0V9N
- Vein
  - Axillary
    - Left 0598
    - Right 0597
  - Azygos 0590
  - Basilic
    - Left 059C
    - Right 059B
  - Brachial
    - Left 059A
    - Right 0599
  - Cephalic
    - Left 059F
    - Right 059D
  - Colic 0697
  - Common Iliac
    - Left 069D
    - Right 069C
  - Esophageal 0693
  - External Iliac
    - Left 069G
    - Right 069F
  - External Jugular
    - Left 059Q
    - Right 059P
  - Face
    - Left 059V
    - Right 059T
  - Femoral
    - Left 069N
    - Right 069M
  - Foot
    - Left 069V
    - Right 069T
  - Gastric 0692
  - Hand
    - Left 059H
    - Right 059G

Drainage — *continued*
Vein — *continued*
Hemiazygos 0591
Hepatic 0694
Hypogastric
Left 069J
Right 069H
Inferior Mesenteric 0696
Innominate
Left 0594
Right 0593
Internal Jugular
Left 059N
Right 059M
Intracranial 059L
Lower 069Y
Portal 0698
Renal
Left 069B
Right 0699
Saphenous
Left 069Q
Right 069P
Splenic 0691
Subclavian
Left 0596
Right 0595
Superior Mesenteric 0695
Upper 059Y
Vertebral
Left 059S
Right 059R
Vena Cava, Inferior 0690
Vertebra
Cervical 0P93
Lumbar 0Q90
Thoracic 0P94
Vesicle
Bilateral 0V93
Left 0V92
Right 0V91
Vitreous
Left 0895
Right 0894
Vocal Cord
Left 0C9V
Right 0C9T
Vulva 0U9M
Wrist Region
Left 0X9H
Right 0X9G
Dressing
Abdominal Wall 2W23X4Z
Arm
Lower
Left 2W2DX4Z
Right 2W2CX4Z
Upper
Left 2W2BX4Z
Right 2W2AX4Z
Back 2W25X4Z
Chest Wall 2W24X4Z
Extremity
Lower
Left 2W2MX4Z
Right 2W2LX4Z
Upper
Left 2W29X4Z
Right 2W28X4Z
Face 2W21X4Z
Finger
Left 2W2KX4Z
Right 2W2JX4Z
Foot
Left 2W2TX4Z
Right 2W2SX4Z

Dressing — *continued*
Hand
Left 2W2FX4Z
Right 2W2EX4Z
Head 2W20X4Z
Inguinal Region
Left 2W27X4Z
Right 2W26X4Z
Leg
Lower
Left 2W2RX4Z
Right 2W2QX4Z
Upper
Left 2W2PX4Z
Right 2W2NX4Z
Neck 2W22X4Z
Thumb
Left 2W2HX4Z
Right 2W2GX4Z
Toe
Left 2W2VX4Z
Right 2W2UX4Z
Driver stent (RX) (OTW)
use Intraluminal Device
Drotrecogin alfa
see Introduction of Recombinant Human-activated Protein C
Duct of Santorini
use Pancreatic Duct, Accessory
Duct of Wirsung
use Pancreatic Duct
Ductogram, mammary
see Plain Radiography, Skin, Subcutaneous Tissue and Breast BH0
Ductography, mammary
see Plain Radiography, Skin, Subcutaneous Tissue and Breast BH0
Ductus deferens
use Vas Deferens, Right
use Vas Deferens, Left
use Vas Deferens, Bilateral
use Vas Deferens
Duodenal ampulla
use Ampulla of Vater
Duodenectomy
see Excision, Duodenum 0DB9
see Resection, Duodenum 0DT9
Duodenocholedochotomy
see Drainage, Gallbladder 0F94
Duodenocystostomy
see Bypass, Gallbladder 0F14
see Drainage, Gallbladder 0F94
Duodenoenterostomy
see Bypass, Gastrointestinal System 0D1
see Drainage, Gastrointestinal System 0D9
Duodenojejunal flexure
use Jejunum
Duodenolysis
see Release, Duodenum 0DN9
Duodenorrhaphy
see Repair, Duodenum 0DQ9
Duodenostomy
see Bypass, Duodenum 0D19
see Drainage, Duodenum 0D99
Duodenotomy
see Drainage, Duodenum 0D99
Dura mater, intracranial
use Dura Mater
Dura mater, spinal
use Spinal Meninges
DuraGraft® Endothelial Damage Inhibitor
use Endothelial Damage Inhibitor
DuraHeart® Left Ventricular Assist System
use Implantable Heart Assist System in Heart and Great Vessels
Dural venous sinus
use Intracranial Vein

Durata® Defibrillation Lead
use Cardiac Lead, Defibrillator in 02H
Dynesys® Dynamic Stabilization System
use Spinal Stabilization Device, Pedicle-Based in 0RH
use Spinal Stabilization Device, Pedicle-Based in 0SH

E

E-Luminexx™ (Biliary)(Vascular) Stent
use Intraluminal Device
Earlobe
use External Ear, Right
use External Ear, Left
use External Ear, Bilateral
ECCO2R (Extracorporeal Carbon Dioxide Removal) 5A0920Z
Echocardiogram
see Ultrasonography, Heart B24
Echography
see Ultrasonography
ECMO
see Performance, Circulatory 5A15
EDWARDS INTUITY Elite™ valve system
use Zooplastic Tissue, Rapid Deployment Technique in New Technology
EEG (electroencephalogram)
see Measurement, Central Nervous 4A00
EGD (esophagogastroduodenoscopy) 0DJ08ZZ
Eighth cranial nerve
use Acoustic Nerve
Ejaculatory duct
use Vas Deferens, Right
use Vas Deferens, Left
use Vas Deferens, Bilateral
use Vas Deferens
EKG (electrocardiogram)
see Measurement, Cardiac 4A02
Electrical bone growth stimulator (EBGS)
use Bone Growth Stimulator in Head and Facial Bones
use Bone Growth Stimulator in Upper Bones
use Bone Growth Stimulator in Lower Bones
Electrical muscle stimulation (EMS) lead
use Stimulator Lead in Muscles
Electrocautery
Destruction *see* Destruction
Repair *see* Repair
Electroconvulsive Therapy
Bilateral-Multiple Seizure GZB3ZZZ
Bilateral-Single Seizure GZB2ZZZ
Electroconvulsive Therapy, Other GZB4ZZZ
Unilateral-Multiple Seizure GZB1ZZZ
Unilateral-Single Seizure GZB0ZZZ
Electroencephalogram (EEG)
see Measurement, Central Nervous 4A00
Electromagnetic Therapy
Central Nervous 6A22
Urinary 6A21
Electronic muscle stimulator lead
use Stimulator Lead in Muscles
Electrophysiologic stimulation (EPS)
see Measurement, Cardiac 4A02
Electroshock therapy
see Electroconvulsive Therapy
Elevation, bone fragments, skull
see Reposition, Head and Facial Bones 0NS
Eleventh cranial nerve
use Accessory Nerve
Embolectomy
see Extirpation

Embolization
  see Occlusion
  see Restriction
Embolization coil(s)
  use Intraluminal Device
EMG (electromyogram)
  see Measurement, Musculoskeletal 4A0F
Encephalon
  use Brain
Endarterectomy
  see Extirpation, Upper Arteries 03C
  see Extirpation, Lower Arteries 04C
Endeavor® (III)(IV) (Sprint) Zotarolimus-eluting Coronary Stent System
  use Intraluminal Device, Drug-eluting in Heart and Great Vessels
Endologix AFX® Endovascular AAA System
  use Intraluminal Device
EndoSure® sensor
  use Monitoring Device, Pressure Sensor in 02H
ENDOTAK RELIANCE® (G) Defibrillation Lead
  use Cardiac Lead, Defibrillator in 02H
Endothelial damage inhibitor, applied to vein graft XY0VX83
Endotracheal tube (cuffed)(double-lumen)
  use Intraluminal Device, Endotracheal Airway in Respiratory System
Endurant® Endovascular Stent Graft
  use Intraluminal Device
Endurant® II AAA stent graft system
  use Intraluminal Device
Engineered Autologous Chimeric Antigen Receptor T-cell Immunotherapy XW0
Enlargement
  see Dilation
  see Repair
EnRhythm®
  use Pacemaker, Dual Chamber in 0JH
Enterorrhaphy
  see Repair, Gastrointestinal System 0DQ
Enterra® gastric neurostimulator
  use Stimulator Generator, Multiple Array in 0JH
Enucleation
  Eyeball *see* Resection, Eye 08T
  Eyeball with prosthetic implant *see* Replacement, Eye 08R
Ependyma
  use Cerebral Ventricle
Epic™ Stented Tissue Valve (aortic)
  use Zooplastic Tissue in Heart and Great Vessels
Epicel® cultured epidermal autograft
  use Autologous Tissue Substitute
Epidermis
  use Skin
Epididymectomy
  see Excision, Male Reproductive System 0VB
  see Resection, Male Reproductive System 0VT
Epididymoplasty
  see Repair, Male Reproductive System 0VQ
  see Supplement, Male Reproductive System 0VU
Epididymorrhaphy
  see Repair, Male Reproductive System 0VQ
Epididymotomy
  see Drainage, Male Reproductive System 0V9
Epidural space, spinal
  use Spinal Canal
Epiphysiodesis
  see Insertion of device in, Upper Bones 0PH

Epiphysiodesis — *continued*
  see Repair, Upper Bones 0PQ
  see Insertion of device in, Lower Bones 0QH
  see Repair, Lower Bones 0QQ
Epiploic foramen
  use Peritoneum
Epiretinal Visual Prosthesis
  Left 08H105Z
  Right 08H005Z
Episiorrhaphy
  see Repair, Perineum, Female 0WQN
Episiotomy
  see Division, Perineum, Female 0W8N
Epithalamus
  use Thalamus
Epitrochlear lymph node
  use Lymphatic, Right Upper Extremity
  use Lymphatic, Left Upper Extremity
EPS (electrophysiologic stimulation)
  see Measurement, Cardiac 4A02
Eptifibatide, infusion
  see Introduction of Platelet Inhibitor
ERCP (endoscopic retrograde cholangiopancreatography)
  see Fluoroscopy, Hepatobiliary System and Pancreas BF1
Erector spinae muscle
  use Trunk Muscle, Right
  use Trunk Muscle, Left
Esophageal artery
  use Upper Artery
Esophageal obturator airway (EOA)
  use Intraluminal Device, Airway in Gastrointestinal System
Esophageal plexus
  use Thoracic Sympathetic Nerve
Esophagectomy
  see Excision, Gastrointestinal System 0DB
  see Resection, Gastrointestinal System 0DT
Esophagocoloplasty
  see Repair, Gastrointestinal System 0DQ
  see Supplement, Gastrointestinal System 0DU
Esophagoenterostomy
  see Bypass, Gastrointestinal System 0D1
  see Drainage, Gastrointestinal System 0D9
Esophagoesophagostomy
  see Bypass, Gastrointestinal System 0D1
  see Drainage, Gastrointestinal System 0D9
Esophagogastrectomy
  see Excision, Gastrointestinal System 0DB
  see Resection, Gastrointestinal System 0DT
Esophagogastroduodenoscopy (EGD) 0DJ08ZZ
Esophagogastroplasty
  see Repair, Gastrointestinal System 0DQ
  see Supplement, Gastrointestinal System 0DU
Esophagogastroscopy 0DJ68ZZ
Esophagogastrostomy
  see Bypass, Gastrointestinal System 0D1
  see Drainage, Gastrointestinal System 0D9
Esophagojejunoplasty
  see Supplement, Gastrointestinal System 0DU
Esophagojejunostomy
  see Bypass, Gastrointestinal System 0D1
  see Drainage, Gastrointestinal System 0D9
Esophagomyotomy
  see Division, Esophagogastric Junction 0D84
Esophagoplasty
  see Repair, Gastrointestinal System 0DQ
  see Replacement, Esophagus 0DR5
  see Supplement, Gastrointestinal System 0DU

Esophagoplication
  see Restriction, Gastrointestinal System 0DV
Esophagorrhaphy
  see Repair, Gastrointestinal System 0DQ
Esophagoscopy 0DJ08ZZ
Esophagotomy
  see Drainage, Gastrointestinal System 0D9
Esteem® implantable hearing system
  use Hearing Device in Ear, Nose, Sinus
ESWL (extracorporeal shock wave lithotripsy)
  see Fragmentation
Ethmoidal air cell
  use Ethmoid Sinus, Right
  use Ethmoid Sinus, Left
Ethmoidectomy
  see Excision, Ear, Nose, Sinus 09B
  see Resection, Ear, Nose, Sinus 09T
  see Excision, Head and Facial Bones 0NB
  see Resection, Head and Facial Bones 0NT
Ethmoidotomy
  see Drainage, Ear, Nose, Sinus 099
Evacuation
  Hematoma *see* Extirpation
  Other Fluid *see* Drainage
Evera™ (XT)(S)(DR/VR)
  use Defibrillator Generator in 0JH
Everolimus-eluting coronary stent
  use Intraluminal Device, Drug-eluting in Heart and Great Vessels
Evisceration
  Eyeball *see* Resection, Eye 08T
  Eyeball with prosthetic implant *see* Replacement, Eye 08R
Ex-PRESS™ mini glaucoma shunt
  use Synthetic Substitute
Examination
  see Inspection
Exchange
  see Change device in
Excision
  Abdominal Wall 0WBF
  Acetabulum
    Left 0QB5
    Right 0QB4
  Adenoids 0CBQ
  Ampulla of Vater 0FBC
  Anal Sphincter 0DBR
  Ankle Region
    Left 0YBL
    Right 0YBK
  Anus 0DBQ
  Aorta
    Abdominal 04B0
    Thoracic
      Ascending/Arch 02BX
      Descending 02BW
  Aortic Body 0GBD
  Appendix 0DBJ
  Arm
    Lower
      Left 0XBF
      Right 0XBD
    Upper
      Left 0XB9
      Right 0XB8
  Artery
    Anterior Tibial
      Left 04BQ
      Right 04BP
    Axillary
      Left 03B6
      Right 03B5
    Brachial
      Left 03B8
      Right 03B7

Excision — continued
  Artery — continued
    Celiac 04B1
    Colic
      Left 04B7
      Middle 04B8
      Right 04B6
    Common Carotid
      Left 03BJ
      Right 03BH
    Common Iliac
      Left 04BD
      Right 04BC
    External Carotid
      Left 03BN
      Right 03BM
    External Iliac
      Left 04BJ
      Right 04BH
    Face 03BR
    Femoral
      Left 04BL
      Right 04BK
    Foot
      Left 04BW
      Right 04BV
    Gastric 04B2
    Hand
      Left 03BF
      Right 03BD
    Hepatic 04B3
    Inferior Mesenteric 04BB
    Innominate 03B2
    Internal Carotid
      Left 03BL
      Right 03BK
    Internal Iliac
      Left 04BF
      Right 04BE
    Internal Mammary
      Left 03B1
      Right 03B0
    Intracranial 03BG
    Lower 04BY
    Peroneal
      Left 04BU
      Right 04BT
    Popliteal
      Left 04BN
      Right 04BM
    Posterior Tibial
      Left 04BS
      Right 04BR
    Pulmonary
      Left 02BR
      Right 02BQ
    Pulmonary Trunk 02BP
    Radial
      Left 03BC
      Right 03BB
    Renal
      Left 04BA
      Right 04B9
    Splenic 04B4
    Subclavian
      Left 03B4
      Right 03B3
    Superior Mesenteric 04B5
    Temporal
      Left 03BT
      Right 03BS
    Thyroid
      Left 03BV
      Right 03BU
    Ulnar
      Left 03BA
      Right 03B9

Excision — continued
  Artery — continued
    Upper 03BY
    Vertebral
      Left 03BQ
      Right 03BP
  Atrium
    Left 02B7
    Right 02B6
  Auditory Ossicle
    Left 09BA
    Right 09B9
  Axilla
    Left 0XB5
    Right 0XB4
  Back
    Lower 0WBL
    Upper 0WBK
  Basal Ganglia 00B8
  Bladder 0TBB
  Bladder Neck 0TBC
  Bone
    Ethmoid
      Left 0NBG
      Right 0NBF
    Frontal 0NB1
    Hyoid 0NBX
    Lacrimal
      Left 0NBJ
      Right 0NBH
    Nasal 0NBB
    Occipital 0NB7
    Palatine
      Left 0NBL
      Right 0NBK
    Parietal
      Left 0NB4
      Right 0NB3
    Pelvic
      Left 0QB3
      Right 0QB2
    Sphenoid 0NBC
    Temporal
      Left 0NB6
      Right 0NB5
    Zygomatic
      Left 0NBN
      Right 0NBM
  Brain 00B0
  Breast
    Bilateral 0HBV
    Left 0HBU
    Right 0HBT
    Supernumerary 0HBY
  Bronchus
    Lingula 0BB9
    Lower Lobe
      Left 0BBB
      Right 0BB6
    Main
      Left 0BB7
      Right 0BB3
    Middle Lobe, Right 0BB5
    Upper Lobe
      Left 0BB8
      Right 0BB4
  Buccal Mucosa 0CB4
  Bursa and Ligament
    Abdomen
      Left 0MBJ
      Right 0MBH
    Ankle
      Left 0MBR
      Right 0MBQ
    Elbow
      Left 0MB4
      Right 0MB3

Excision — continued
  Bursa and Ligament — continued
    Foot
      Left 0MBT
      Right 0MBS
    Hand
      Left 0MB8
      Right 0MB7
    Head and Neck 0MB0
    Hip
      Left 0MBM
      Right 0MBL
    Knee
      Left 0MBP
      Right 0MBN
    Lower Extremity
      Left 0MBW
      Right 0MBV
    Perineum 0MBK
    Rib(s) 0MBG
    Shoulder
      Left 0MB2
      Right 0MB1
    Spine
      Lower 0MBD
      Upper 0MBC
    Sternum 0MBF
    Upper Extremity
      Left 0MBB
      Right 0MB9
    Wrist
      Left 0MB6
      Right 0MB5
  Buttock
    Left 0YB1
    Right 0YB0
  Carina 0BB2
  Carotid Bodies, Bilateral 0GB8
  Carotid Body
    Left 0GB6
    Right 0GB7
  Carpal
    Left 0PBN
    Right 0PBM
  Cecum 0DBH
  Cerebellum 00BC
  Cerebral Hemisphere 00B7
  Cerebral Meninges 00B1
  Cerebral Ventricle 00B6
  Cervix 0UBC
  Chest Wall 0WB8
  Chordae Tendineae 02B9
  Choroid
    Left 08BB
    Right 08BA
  Cisterna Chyli 07BL
  Clavicle
    Left 0PBB
    Right 0PB9
  Clitoris 0UBJ
  Coccygeal Glomus 0GBB
  Coccyx 0QBS
  Colon
    Ascending 0DBK
    Descending 0DBM
    Sigmoid 0DBN
    Transverse 0DBL
  Conduction Mechanism 02B8
  Conjunctiva
    Left 08BTXZ
    Right 08BSXZ
  Cord
    Bilateral 0VBH
    Left 0VBG
    Right 0VBF
  Cornea
    Left 08B9XZ
    Right 08B8XZ

Excision

ICD-10-PCS INDEX

Excision — *continued*
- Cul-de-sac 0UBF
- Diaphragm 0BBT
- Disc
  - Cervical Vertebral 0RB3
  - Cervicothoracic Vertebral 0RB5
  - Lumbar Vertebral 0SB2
  - Lumbosacral 0SB4
  - Thoracic Vertebral 0RB9
  - Thoracolumbar Vertebral 0RBB
- Duct
  - Common Bile 0FB9
  - Cystic 0FB8
  - Hepatic
    - Common 0FB7
    - Left 0FB6
    - Right 0FB5
  - Lacrimal
    - Left 08BY
    - Right 08BX
  - Pancreatic 0FBD
    - Accessory 0FBF
  - Parotid
    - Left 0CBC
    - Right 0CBB
- Duodenum 0DB9
- Dura Mater 00B2
- Ear
  - External
    - Left 09B1
    - Right 09B0
  - External Auditory Canal
    - Left 09B4
    - Right 09B3
  - Inner
    - Left 09BE
    - Right 09BD
  - Middle
    - Left 09B6
    - Right 09B5
- Elbow Region
  - Left 0XBC
  - Right 0XBB
- Epididymis
  - Bilateral 0VBL
  - Left 0VBK
  - Right 0VBJ
- Epiglottis 0CBR
- Esophagogastric Junction 0DB4
- Esophagus 0DB5
  - Lower 0DB3
  - Middle 0DB2
  - Upper 0DB1
- Eustachian Tube
  - Left 09BG
  - Right 09BF
- Extremity
  - Lower
    - Left 0YBB
    - Right 0YB9
  - Upper
    - Left 0XB7
    - Right 0XB6
- Eye
  - Left 08B1
  - Right 08B0
- Eyelid
  - Lower
    - Left 08BR
    - Right 08BQ
  - Upper
    - Left 08BP
    - Right 08BN
- Face 0WB2
- Fallopian Tube
  - Left 0UB6
  - Right 0UB5

Excision — *continued*
- Fallopian Tubes, Bilateral 0UB7
- Femoral Region
  - Left 0YB8
  - Right 0YB7
- Femoral Shaft
  - Left 0QB9
  - Right 0QB8
- Femur
  - Lower
    - Left 0QBC
    - Right 0QBB
  - Upper
    - Left 0QB7
    - Right 0QB6
- Fibula
  - Left 0QBK
  - Right 0QBJ
- Finger Nail 0HBQXZ
- Floor of mouth *see* Excision, Oral Cavity and Throat 0WB3
- Foot
  - Left 0YBN
  - Right 0YBM
- Gallbladder 0FB4
- Gingiva
  - Lower 0CB6
  - Upper 0CB5
- Gland
  - Adrenal
    - Bilateral 0GB4
    - Left 0GB2
    - Right 0GB3
  - Lacrimal
    - Left 08BW
    - Right 08BV
  - Minor Salivary 0CBJ
  - Parotid
    - Left 0CB9
    - Right 0CB8
  - Pituitary 0GB0
  - Sublingual
    - Left 0CBF
    - Right 0CBD
  - Submaxillary
    - Left 0CBH
    - Right 0CBG
  - Vestibular 0UBL
- Glenoid Cavity
  - Left 0PB8
  - Right 0PB7
- Glomus Jugulare 0GBC
- Hand
  - Left 0XBK
  - Right 0XBJ
- Head 0WB0
- Humeral Head
  - Left 0PBD
  - Right 0PBC
- Humeral Shaft
  - Left 0PBG
  - Right 0PBF
- Hymen 0UBK
- Hypothalamus 00BA
- Ileocecal Valve 0DBC
- Ileum 0DBB
- Inguinal Region
  - Left 0YB6
  - Right 0YB5
- Intestine
  - Large 0DBE
    - Left 0DBG
    - Right 0DBF
  - Small 0DB8
- Iris
  - Left 08BD3Z
  - Right 08BC3Z

Excision — *continued*
- Jaw
  - Lower 0WB5
  - Upper 0WB4
- Jejunum 0DBA
- Joint
  - Acromioclavicular
    - Left 0RBH
    - Right 0RBG
  - Ankle
    - Left 0SBG
    - Right 0SBF
  - Carpal
    - Left 0RBR
    - Right 0RBQ
  - Carpometacarpal
    - Left 0RBT
    - Right 0RBS
  - Cervical Vertebral 0RB1
  - Cervicothoracic Vertebral 0RB4
  - Coccygeal 0SB6
  - Elbow
    - Left 0RBM
    - Right 0RBL
  - Finger Phalangeal
    - Left 0RBX
    - Right 0RBW
  - Hip
    - Left 0SBB
    - Right 0SB9
  - Knee
    - Left 0SBD
    - Right 0SBC
  - Lumbar Vertebral 0SB0
  - Lumbosacral 0SB3
  - Metacarpophalangeal
    - Left 0RBV
    - Right 0RBU
  - Metatarsal-Phalangeal
    - Left 0SBN
    - Right 0SBM
  - Occipital-cervical 0RB0
  - Sacrococcygeal 0SB5
  - Sacroiliac
    - Left 0SB8
    - Right 0SB7
  - Shoulder
    - Left 0RBK
    - Right 0RBJ
  - Sternoclavicular
    - Left 0RBF
    - Right 0RBE
  - Tarsal
    - Left 0SBJ
    - Right 0SBH
  - Tarsometatarsal
    - Left 0SBL
    - Right 0SBK
  - Temporomandibular
    - Left 0RBD
    - Right 0RBC
  - Thoracic Vertebral 0RB6
  - Thoracolumbar Vertebral 0RBA
  - Toe Phalangeal
    - Left 0SBQ
    - Right 0SBP
  - Wrist
    - Left 0RBP
    - Right 0RBN
- Kidney
  - Left 0TB1
  - Right 0TB0
- Kidney Pelvis
  - Left 0TB4
  - Right 0TB3
- Knee Region
  - Left 0YBG
  - Right 0YBF

Excision — continued
Larynx 0CBS
Leg
  Lower
    Left 0YBJ
    Right 0YBH
  Upper
    Left 0YBD
    Right 0YBC
Lens
  Left 08BK3Z
  Right 08BJ3Z
Lip
  Lower 0CB1
  Upper 0CB0
Liver 0FB0
  Left Lobe 0FB2
  Right Lobe 0FB1
Lung
  Bilateral 0BBM
  Left 0BBL
  Lower Lobe
    Left 0BBJ
    Right 0BBF
  Middle Lobe, Right 0BBD
  Right 0BBK
  Upper Lobe
    Left 0BBG
    Right 0BBC
Lung Lingula 0BBH
Lymphatic
  Aortic 07BD
  Axillary
    Left 07B6
    Right 07B5
  Head 07B0
  Inguinal
    Left 07BJ
    Right 07BH
  Internal Mammary
    Left 07B9
    Right 07B8
  Lower Extremity
    Left 07BG
    Right 07BF
  Mesenteric 07BB
  Neck
    Left 07B2
    Right 07B1
  Pelvis 07BC
  Thoracic Duct 07BK
  Thorax 07B7
  Upper Extremity
    Left 07B4
    Right 07B3
Mandible
  Left 0NBV
  Right 0NBT
Maxilla 0NBR
Mediastinum 0WBC
Medulla Oblongata 00BD
Mesentery 0DBV
Metacarpal
  Left 0PBQ
  Right 0PBP
Metatarsal
  Left 0QBP
  Right 0QBN
Muscle
  Abdomen
    Left 0KBL
    Right 0KBK
  Extraocular
    Left 08BM
    Right 08BL
  Facial 0KB1
  Foot

Excision — continued
Muscle — continued
    Left 0KBW
    Right 0KBV
  Hand
    Left 0KBD
    Right 0KBC
  Head 0KB0
  Hip
    Left 0KBP
    Right 0KBN
  Lower Arm and Wrist
    Left 0KBB
    Right 0KB9
  Lower Leg
    Left 0KBT
    Right 0KBS
  Neck
    Left 0KB3
    Right 0KB2
  Papillary 02BD
  Perineum 0KBM
  Shoulder
    Left 0KB6
    Right 0KB5
  Thorax
    Left 0KBJ
    Right 0KBH
  Tongue, Palate, Pharynx 0KB4
  Trunk
    Left 0KBG
    Right 0KBF
  Upper Arm
    Left 0KB8
    Right 0KB7
  Upper Leg
    Left 0KBR
    Right 0KBQ
Nasal Mucosa and Soft Tissue 09BK
Nasopharynx 09BN
Neck 0WB6
Nerve
  Abdominal Sympathetic 01BM
  Abducens 00BL
  Accessory 00BR
  Acoustic 00BN
  Brachial Plexus 01B3
  Cervical 01B1
  Cervical Plexus 01B0
  Facial 00BM
  Femoral 01BD
  Glossopharyngeal 00BP
  Head and Neck Sympathetic 01BK
  Hypoglossal 00BS
  Lumbar 01BB
  Lumbar Plexus 01B9
  Lumbar Sympathetic 01BN
  Lumbosacral Plexus 01BA
  Median 01B5
  Oculomotor 00BH
  Olfactory 00BF
  Optic 00BG
  Peroneal 01BH
  Phrenic 01B2
  Pudendal 01BC
  Radial 01B6
  Sacral 01BR
  Sacral Plexus 01BQ
  Sacral Sympathetic 01BP
  Sciatic 01BF
  Thoracic 01B8
  Thoracic Sympathetic 01BL
  Tibial 01BG
  Trigeminal 00BK
  Trochlear 00BJ
  Ulnar 01B4
  Vagus 00BQ

Excision — continued
Nipple
  Left 0HBX
  Right 0HBW
Omentum 0DBU
Oral Cavity and Throat 0WB3
Orbit
  Left 0NBQ
  Right 0NBP
Ovary
  Bilateral 0UB2
  Left 0UB1
  Right 0UB0
Palate
  Hard 0CB2
  Soft 0CB3
Pancreas 0FBG
Para-aortic Body 0GB9
Paraganglion Extremity 0GBF
Parathyroid Gland 0GBR
  Inferior
    Left 0GBP
    Right 0GBN
  Multiple 0GBQ
  Superior
    Left 0GBM
    Right 0GBL
Patella
  Left 0QBF
  Right 0QBD
Penis 0VBS
Pericardium 02BN
Perineum
  Female 0WBN
  Male 0WBM
Peritoneum 0DBW
Phalanx
  Finger
    Left 0PBV
    Right 0PBT
  Thumb
    Left 0PBS
    Right 0PBR
  Toe
    Left 0QBR
    Right 0QBQ
Pharynx 0CBM
Pineal Body 0GB1
Pleura
  Left 0BBP
  Right 0BBN
Pons 00BB
Prepuce 0VBT
Prostate 0VB0
Radius
  Left 0PBJ
  Right 0PBH
Rectum 0DBP
Retina
  Left 08BF3Z
  Right 08BE3Z
Retroperitoneum 0WBH
Ribs
  1 to 2 0PB1
  3 or More 0PB2
Sacrum 0QB1
Scapula
  Left 0PB6
  Right 0PB5
Sclera
  Left 08B7XZ
  Right 08B6XZ
Scrotum 0VB5
Septum
  Atrial 02B5
  Nasal 09BM
  Ventricular 02BM

Excision — *continued*
- Shoulder Region
  - Left 0XB3
  - Right 0XB2
- Sinus
  - Accessory 09BP
  - Ethmoid
    - Left 09BV
    - Right 09BU
  - Frontal
    - Left 09BT
    - Right 09BS
  - Mastoid
    - Left 09BC
    - Right 09BB
  - Maxillary
    - Left 09BR
    - Right 09BQ
  - Sphenoid
    - Left 09BX
    - Right 09BW
- Skin
  - Abdomen 0HB7XZ
  - Back 0HB6XZ
  - Buttock 0HB8XZ
  - Chest 0HB5XZ
  - Ear
    - Left 0HB3XZ
    - Right 0HB2XZ
  - Face 0HB1XZ
  - Foot
    - Left 0HBNXZ
    - Right 0HBMXZ
  - Hand
    - Left 0HBGXZ
    - Right 0HBFXZ
  - Inguinal 0HBAXZ
  - Lower Arm
    - Left 0HBEXZ
    - Right 0HBDXZ
  - Lower Leg
    - Left 0HBLXZ
    - Right 0HBKXZ
  - Neck 0HB4XZ
  - Perineum 0HB9XZ
  - Scalp 0HB0XZ
  - Upper Arm
    - Left 0HBCXZ
    - Right 0HBBXZ
  - Upper Leg
    - Left 0HBJXZ
    - Right 0HBHXZ
- Skull 0NB0
- Spinal Cord
  - Cervical 00BW
  - Lumbar 00BY
  - Thoracic 00BX
- Spinal Meninges 00BT
- Spleen 07BP
- Sternum 0PB0
- Stomach 0DB6
  - Pylorus 0DB7
- Subcutaneous Tissue and Fascia
  - Abdomen 0JB8
  - Back 0JB7
  - Buttock 0JB9
  - Chest 0JB6
  - Face 0JB1
  - Foot
    - Left 0JBR
    - Right 0JBQ
  - Hand
    - Left 0JBK
    - Right 0JBJ
  - Lower Arm
    - Left 0JBH
    - Right 0JBG

Excision — *continued*
- Subcutaneous Tissue and Fascia — *continued*
  - Lower Leg
    - Left 0JBP
    - Right 0JBN
  - Neck
    - Left 0JB5
    - Right 0JB4
  - Pelvic Region 0JBC
  - Perineum 0JBB
  - Scalp 0JB0
  - Upper Arm
    - Left 0JBF
    - Right 0JBD
  - Upper Leg
    - Left 0JBM
    - Right 0JBL
- Tarsal
  - Left 0QBM
  - Right 0QBL
- Tendon
  - Abdomen
    - Left 0LBG
    - Right 0LBF
  - Ankle
    - Left 0LBT
    - Right 0LBS
  - Foot
    - Left 0LBW
    - Right 0LBV
  - Hand
    - Left 0LB8
    - Right 0LB7
  - Head and Neck 0LB0
  - Hip
    - Left 0LBK
    - Right 0LBJ
  - Knee
    - Left 0LBR
    - Right 0LBQ
  - Lower Arm and Wrist
    - Left 0LB6
    - Right 0LB5
  - Lower Leg
    - Left 0LBP
    - Right 0LBN
  - Perineum 0LBH
  - Shoulder
    - Left 0LB2
    - Right 0LB1
  - Thorax
    - Left 0LBD
    - Right 0LBC
  - Trunk
    - Left 0LBB
    - Right 0LB9
  - Upper Arm
    - Left 0LB4
    - Right 0LB3
  - Upper Leg
    - Left 0LBM
    - Right 0LBL
- Testis
  - Bilateral 0VBC
  - Left 0VBB
  - Right 0VB9
- Thalamus 00B9
- Thymus 07BM
- Thyroid Gland
  - Left Lobe 0GBG
  - Right Lobe 0GBH
- Thyroid Gland Isthmus 0GBJ
- Tibia
  - Left 0QBH
  - Right 0QBG
- Toe Nail 0HBRXZ

Excision — *continued*
- Tongue 0CB7
- Tonsils 0CBP
- Tooth
  - Lower 0CBX
  - Upper 0CBW
- Trachea 0BB1
- Tunica Vaginalis
  - Left 0VB7
  - Right 0VB6
- Turbinate, Nasal 09BL
- Tympanic Membrane
  - Left 09B8
  - Right 09B7
- Ulna
  - Left 0PBL
  - Right 0PBK
- Ureter
  - Left 0TB7
  - Right 0TB6
- Urethra 0TBD
- Uterine Supporting Structure 0UB4
- Uterus 0UB9
- Uvula 0CBN
- Vagina 0UBG
- Valve
  - Aortic 02BF
  - Mitral 02BG
  - Pulmonary 02BH
  - Tricuspid 02BJ
- Vas Deferens
  - Bilateral 0VBQ
  - Left 0VBP
  - Right 0VBN
- Vein
  - Axillary
    - Left 05B8
    - Right 05B7
  - Azygos 05B0
  - Basilic
    - Left 05BC
    - Right 05BB
  - Brachial
    - Left 05BA
    - Right 05B9
  - Cephalic
    - Left 05BF
    - Right 05BD
  - Colic 06B7
  - Common Iliac
    - Left 06BD
    - Right 06BC
  - Coronary 02B4
  - Esophageal 06B3
  - External Iliac
    - Left 06BG
    - Right 06BF
  - External Jugular
    - Left 05BQ
    - Right 05BP
  - Face
    - Left 05BV
    - Right 05BT
  - Femoral
    - Left 06BN
    - Right 06BM
  - Foot
    - Left 06BV
    - Right 06BT
  - Gastric 06B2
  - Hand
    - Left 05BH
    - Right 05BG
  - Hemiazygos 05B1
  - Hepatic 06B4
  - Hypogastric
    - Left 06BJ
    - Right 06BH

Excision — *continued*
  Vein — *continued*
    Inferior Mesenteric 06B6
    Innominate
      Left 05B4
      Right 05B3
    Internal Jugular
      Left 05BN
      Right 05BM
    Intracranial 05BL
    Lower 06BY
    Portal 06B8
    Pulmonary
      Left 02BT
      Right 02BS
    Renal
      Left 06BB
      Right 06B9
    Saphenous
      Left 06BQ
      Right 06BP
    Splenic 06B1
    Subclavian
      Left 05B6
      Right 05B5
    Superior Mesenteric 06B5
    Upper 05BY
    Vertebral
      Left 05BS
      Right 05BR
  Vena Cava
    Inferior 06B0
    Superior 02BV
  Ventricle
    Left 02BL
    Right 02BK
  Vertebra
    Cervical 0PB3
    Lumbar 0QB0
    Thoracic 0PB4
  Vesicle
    Bilateral 0VB3
    Left 0VB2
    Right 0VB1
  Vitreous
    Left 08B53Z
    Right 08B43Z
  Vocal Cord
    Left 0CBV
    Right 0CBT
  Vulva 0UBM
  Wrist Region
    Left 0XBH
    Right 0XBG
EXCLUDER® AAA Endoprosthesis
  use Intraluminal Device, Branched or
    Fenestrated, One or Two Arteries in 04V
  use Intraluminal Device, Branched or
    Fenestrated, Three or More Arteries in 04V
  use Intraluminal Device
EXCLUDER® IBE Endoprosthesis
  use Intraluminal Device, Branched or
    Fenestrated, One or Two Arteries in 04V
Exclusion, Left atrial appendage (LAA)
  see Occlusion, Atrium, Left 02L7
Exercise, rehabilitation
  see Motor Treatment, Rehabilitation F07
Exploration
  see Inspection
Express® (LD) Premounted Stent System
  use Intraluminal Device
Express® Biliary SD Monorail® Premounted Stent System
  use Intraluminal Device
Express® SD Renal Monorail® Premounted Stent System
  use Intraluminal Device

Extensor carpi radialis muscle
  use Lower Arm and Wrist Muscle, Right
  use Lower Arm and Wrist Muscle, Left
Extensor carpi ulnaris muscle
  use Lower Arm and Wrist Muscle, Right
  use Lower Arm and Wrist Muscle, Left
Extensor digitorum brevis muscle
  use Foot Muscle, Right
  use Foot Muscle, Left
Extensor digitorum longus muscle
  use Lower Leg Muscle, Right
  use Lower Leg Muscle, Left
Extensor hallucis brevis muscle
  use Foot Muscle, Right
  use Foot Muscle, Left
Extensor hallucis longus muscle
  use Lower Leg Muscle, Right
  use Lower Leg Muscle, Left
External anal sphincter
  use Anal Sphincter
External auditory meatus
  use External Auditory Canal, Right
  use External Auditory Canal, Left
External fixator
  use External Fixation Device in Head and Facial Bones
  use External Fixation Device in Upper Bones
  use External Fixation Device in Lower Bones
  use External Fixation Device in Upper Joints
  use External Fixation Device in Lower Joints
External maxillary artery
  use Face Artery
External naris
  use Nasal Mucosa and Soft Tissue
External oblique aponeurosis
  use Subcutaneous Tissue and Fascia, Trunk
External oblique muscle
  use Abdomen Muscle, Right
  use Abdomen Muscle, Left
External popliteal nerve
  use Peroneal Nerve
External pudendal artery
  use Femoral Artery, Right
  use Femoral Artery, Left
External pudendal vein
  use Saphenous Vein, Right
  use Saphenous Vein, Left
External urethral sphincter
  use Urethra
Extirpation
  Acetabulum
    Left 0QC5
    Right 0QC4
  Adenoids 0CCQ
  Ampulla of Vater 0FCC
  Anal Sphincter 0DCR
  Anterior Chamber
    Left 08C3
    Right 08C2
  Anus 0DCQ
  Aorta
    Abdominal 04C0
    Thoracic
      Ascending/Arch 02CX
      Descending 02CW
  Aortic Body 0GCD
  Appendix 0DCJ
  Artery
    Anterior Tibial
      Left 04CQ
      Right 04CP
    Axillary
      Left 03C6
      Right 03C5
    Brachial
      Left 03C8
      Right 03C7

Extirpation — *continued*
  Artery — *continued*
    Celiac 04C1
    Colic
      Left 04C7
      Middle 04C8
      Right 04C6
    Common Carotid
      Left 03CJ
      Right 03CH
    Common Iliac
      Left 04CD
      Right 04CC
    Coronary
      Four or More Arteries 02C3
      One Artery 02C0
      Three Arteries 02C2
      Two Arteries 02C1
    External Carotid
      Left 03CN
      Right 03CM
    External Iliac
      Left 04CJ
      Right 04CH
    Face 03CR
    Femoral
      Left 04CL
      Right 04CK
    Foot
      Left 04CW
      Right 04CV
    Gastric 04C2
    Hand
      Left 03CF
      Right 03CD
    Hepatic 04C3
    Inferior Mesenteric 04CB
    Innominate 03C2
    Internal Carotid
      Left 03CL
      Right 03CK
    Internal Iliac
      Left 04CF
      Right 04CE
    Internal Mammary
      Left 03C1
      Right 03C0
    Intracranial 03CG
    Lower 04CY
    Peroneal
      Left 04CU
      Right 04CT
    Popliteal
      Left 04CN
      Right 04CM
    Posterior Tibial
      Left 04CS
      Right 04CR
    Pulmonary
      Left 02CR
      Right 02CQ
    Pulmonary Trunk 02CP
    Radial
      Left 03CC
      Right 03CB
    Renal
      Left 04CA
      Right 04C9
    Splenic 04C4
    Subclavian
      Left 03C4
      Right 03C3
    Superior Mesenteric 04C5
    Temporal
      Left 03CT
      Right 03CS

Extirpation — *continued*
- Artery — *continued*
  - Thyroid
    - Left 03CV
    - Right 03CU
  - Ulnar
    - Left 03CA
    - Right 03C9
  - Upper 03CY
  - Vertebral
    - Left 03CQ
    - Right 03CP
- Atrium
  - Left 02C7
  - Right 02C6
- Auditory Ossicle
  - Left 09CA
  - Right 09C9
- Basal Ganglia 00C8
- Bladder 0TCB
- Bladder Neck 0TCC
- Bone
  - Ethmoid
    - Left 0NCG
    - Right 0NCF
  - Frontal 0NC1
  - Hyoid 0NCX
  - Lacrimal
    - Left 0NCJ
    - Right 0NCH
  - Nasal 0NCB
  - Occipital 0NC7
  - Palatine
    - Left 0NCL
    - Right 0NCK
  - Parietal
    - Left 0NC4
    - Right 0NC3
  - Pelvic
    - Left 0QC3
    - Right 0QC2
  - Sphenoid 0NCC
  - Temporal
    - Left 0NC6
    - Right 0NC5
  - Zygomatic
    - Left 0NCN
    - Right 0NCM
- Brain 00C0
- Breast
  - Bilateral 0HCV
  - Left 0HCU
  - Right 0HCT
- Bronchus
  - Lingula 0BC9
  - Lower Lobe
    - Left 0BCB
    - Right 0BC6
  - Main
    - Left 0BC7
    - Right 0BC3
  - Middle Lobe, Right 0BC5
  - Upper Lobe
    - Left 0BC8
    - Right 0BC4
- Buccal Mucosa 0CC4
- Bursa and Ligament
  - Abdomen
    - Left 0MCJ
    - Right 0MCH
  - Ankle
    - Left 0MCR
    - Right 0MCQ
  - Elbow
    - Left 0MC4
    - Right 0MC3
  - Foot

Extirpation — *continued*
- Bursa and Ligament — *continued*
  - Left 0MCT
  - Right 0MCS
  - Hand
    - Left 0MC8
    - Right 0MC7
  - Head and Neck 0MC0
  - Hip
    - Left 0MCM
    - Right 0MCL
  - Knee
    - Left 0MCP
    - Right 0MCN
  - Lower Extremity
    - Left 0MCW
    - Right 0MCV
  - Perineum 0MCK
  - Rib(s) 0MCG
  - Shoulder
    - Left 0MC2
    - Right 0MC1
  - Spine
    - Lower 0MCD
    - Upper 0MCC
  - Sternum 0MCF
  - Upper Extremity
    - Left 0MCB
    - Right 0MC9
  - Wrist
    - Left 0MC6
    - Right 0MC5
- Carina 0BC2
- Carotid Bodies, Bilateral 0GC8
- Carotid Body
  - Left 0GC6
  - Right 0GC7
- Carpal
  - Left 0PCN
  - Right 0PCM
- Cavity, Cranial 0WC1
- Cecum 0DCH
- Cerebellum 00CC
- Cerebral Hemisphere 00C7
- Cerebral Meninges 00C1
- Cerebral Ventricle 00C6
- Cervix 0UCC
- Chordae Tendineae 02C9
- Choroid
  - Left 08CB
  - Right 08CA
- Cisterna Chyli 07CL
- Clavicle
  - Left 0PCB
  - Right 0PC9
- Clitoris 0UCJ
- Coccygeal Glomus 0GCB
- Coccyx 0QCS
- Colon
  - Ascending 0DCK
  - Descending 0DCM
  - Sigmoid 0DCN
  - Transverse 0DCL
- Conduction Mechanism 02C8
- Conjunctiva
  - Left 08CTXZZ
  - Right 08CSXZZ
- Cord
  - Bilateral 0VCH
  - Left 0VCG
  - Right 0VCF
- Cornea
  - Left 08C9XZZ
  - Right 08C8XZZ
- Cul-de-sac 0UCF
- Diaphragm 0BCT

Extirpation — *continued*
- Disc
  - Cervical Vertebral 0RC3
  - Cervicothoracic Vertebral 0RC5
  - Lumbar Vertebral 0SC2
  - Lumbosacral 0SC4
  - Thoracic Vertebral 0RC9
  - Thoracolumbar Vertebral 0RCB
- Duct
  - Common Bile 0FC9
  - Cystic 0FC8
  - Hepatic
    - Common 0FC7
    - Left 0FC6
    - Right 0FC5
  - Lacrimal
    - Left 08CY
    - Right 08CX
  - Pancreatic 0FCD
    - Accessory 0FCF
  - Parotid
    - Left 0CCC
    - Right 0CCB
- Duodenum 0DC9
- Dura Mater 00C2
- Ear
  - External
    - Left 09C1
    - Right 09C0
  - External Auditory Canal
    - Left 09C4
    - Right 09C3
  - Inner
    - Left 09CE
    - Right 09CD
  - Middle
    - Left 09C6
    - Right 09C5
- Endometrium 0UCB
- Epididymis
  - Bilateral 0VCL
  - Left 0VCK
  - Right 0VCJ
- Epidural Space, Intracranial 00C3
- Epiglottis 0CCR
- Esophagogastric Junction 0DC4
- Esophagus 0DC5
  - Lower 0DC3
  - Middle 0DC2
  - Upper 0DC1
- Eustachian Tube
  - Left 09CG
  - Right 09CF
- Eye
  - Left 08C1XZZ
  - Right 08C0XZZ
- Eyelid
  - Lower
    - Left 08CR
    - Right 08CQ
  - Upper
    - Left 08CP
    - Right 08CN
- Fallopian Tube
  - Left 0UC6
  - Right 0UC5
- Fallopian Tubes, Bilateral 0UC7
- Femoral Shaft
  - Left 0QC9
  - Right 0QC8
- Femur
  - Lower
    - Left 0QCC
    - Right 0QCB
  - Upper
    - Left 0QC7
    - Right 0QC6

Extirpation — *continued*
Fibula
Left 0QCK
Right 0QCJ
Finger Nail 0HCQXZZ
Gallbladder 0FC4
Gastrointestinal Tract 0WCP
Genitourinary Tract 0WCR
Gingiva
Lower 0CC6
Upper 0CC5
Gland
Adrenal
Bilateral 0GC4
Left 0GC2
Right 0GC3
Lacrimal
Left 08CW
Right 08CV
Minor Salivary 0CCJ
Parotid
Left 0CC9
Right 0CC8
Pituitary 0GC0
Sublingual
Left 0CCF
Right 0CCD
Submaxillary
Left 0CCH
Right 0CCG
Vestibular 0UCL
Glenoid Cavity
Left 0PC8
Right 0PC7
Glomus Jugulare 0GCC
Humeral Head
Left 0PCD
Right 0PCC
Humeral Shaft
Left 0PCG
Right 0PCF
Hymen 0UCK
Hypothalamus 00CA
Ileocecal Valve 0DCC
Ileum 0DCB
Intestine
Large 0DCE
Left 0DCG
Right 0DCF
Small 0DC8
Iris
Left 08CD
Right 08CC
Jejunum 0DCA
Joint
Acromioclavicular
Left 0RCH
Right 0RCG
Ankle
Left 0SCG
Right 0SCF
Carpal
Left 0RCR
Right 0RCQ
Carpometacarpal
Left 0RCT
Right 0RCS
Cervical Vertebral 0RC1
Cervicothoracic Vertebral 0RC4
Coccygeal 0SC6
Elbow
Left 0RCM
Right 0RCL
Finger Phalangeal
Left 0RCX
Right 0RCW

Extirpation — *continued*
Joint — *continued*
Hip
Left 0SCB
Right 0SC9
Knee
Left 0SCD
Right 0SCC
Lumbar Vertebral 0SC0
Lumbosacral 0SC3
Metacarpophalangeal
Left 0RCV
Right 0RCU
Metatarsal-Phalangeal
Left 0SCN
Right 0SCM
Occipital-cervical 0RC0
Sacrococcygeal 0SC5
Sacroiliac
Left 0SC8
Right 0SC7
Shoulder
Left 0RCK
Right 0RCJ
Sternoclavicular
Left 0RCF
Right 0RCE
Tarsal
Left 0SCJ
Right 0SCH
Tarsometatarsal
Left 0SCL
Right 0SCK
Temporomandibular
Left 0RCD
Right 0RCC
Thoracic Vertebral 0RC6
Thoracolumbar Vertebral 0RCA
Toe Phalangeal
Left 0SCQ
Right 0SCP
Wrist
Left 0RCP
Right 0RCN
Kidney
Left 0TC1
Right 0TC0
Kidney Pelvis
Left 0TC4
Right 0TC3
Larynx 0CCS
Lens
Left 08CK
Right 08CJ
Lip
Lower 0CC1
Upper 0CC0
Liver 0FC0
Left Lobe 0FC2
Right Lobe 0FC1
Lung
Bilateral 0BCM
Left 0BCL
Lower Lobe
Left 0BCJ
Right 0BCF
Middle Lobe, Right 0BCD
Right 0BCK
Upper Lobe
Left 0BCG
Right 0BCC
Lung Lingula 0BCH
Lymphatic
Aortic 07CD
Axillary
Left 07C6
Right 07C5

Extirpation — *continued*
Lymphatic — *continued*
Head 07C0
Inguinal
Left 07CJ
Right 07CH
Internal Mammary
Left 07C9
Right 07C8
Lower Extremity
Left 07CG
Right 07CF
Mesenteric 07CB
Neck
Left 07C2
Right 07C1
Pelvis 07CC
Thoracic Duct 07CK
Thorax 07C7
Upper Extremity
Left 07C4
Right 07C3
Mandible
Left 0NCV
Right 0NCT
Maxilla 0NCR
Mediastinum 0WCC
Medulla Oblongata 00CD
Mesentery 0DCV
Metacarpal
Left 0PCQ
Right 0PCP
Metatarsal
Left 0QCP
Right 0QCN
Muscle
Abdomen
Left 0KCL
Right 0KCK
Extraocular
Left 08CM
Right 08CL
Facial 0KC1
Foot
Left 0KCW
Right 0KCV
Hand
Left 0KCD
Right 0KCC
Head 0KC0
Hip
Left 0KCP
Right 0KCN
Lower Arm and Wrist
Left 0KCB
Right 0KC9
Lower Leg
Left 0KCT
Right 0KCS
Neck
Left 0KC3
Right 0KC2
Papillary 02CD
Perineum 0KCM
Shoulder
Left 0KC6
Right 0KC5
Thorax
Left 0KCJ
Right 0KCH
Tongue, Palate, Pharynx 0KC4
Trunk
Left 0KCG
Right 0KCF
Upper Arm
Left 0KC8
Right 0KC7

Extirpation — *continued*
 Muscle — *continued*
  Upper Leg
   Left 0KCR
   Right 0KCQ
 Nasal Mucosa and Soft Tissue 09CK
 Nasopharynx 09CN
 Nerve
  Abdominal Sympathetic 01CM
  Abducens 00CL
  Accessory 00CR
  Acoustic 00CN
  Brachial Plexus 01C3
  Cervical 01C1
  Cervical Plexus 01C0
  Facial 00CM
  Femoral 01CD
  Glossopharyngeal 00CP
  Head and Neck Sympathetic 01CK
  Hypoglossal 00CS
  Lumbar 01CB
  Lumbar Plexus 01C9
  Lumbar Sympathetic 01CN
  Lumbosacral Plexus 01CA
  Median 01C5
  Oculomotor 00CH
  Olfactory 00CF
  Optic 00CG
  Peroneal 01CH
  Phrenic 01C2
  Pudendal 01CC
  Radial 01C6
  Sacral 01CR
  Sacral Plexus 01CQ
  Sacral Sympathetic 01CP
  Sciatic 01CF
  Thoracic 01C8
  Thoracic Sympathetic 01CL
  Tibial 01CG
  Trigeminal 00CK
  Trochlear 00CJ
  Ulnar 01C4
  Vagus 00CQ
 Nipple
  Left 0HCX
  Right 0HCW
 Omentum 0DCU
 Oral Cavity and Throat 0WC3
 Orbit
  Left 0NCQ
  Right 0NCP
 Orbital Atherectomy Technology X2C
 Ovary
  Bilateral 0UC2
  Left 0UC1
  Right 0UC0
 Palate
  Hard 0CC2
  Soft 0CC3
 Pancreas 0FCG
 Para-aortic Body 0GC9
 Paraganglion Extremity 0GCF
 Parathyroid Gland 0GCR
  Inferior
   Left 0GCP
   Right 0GCN
  Multiple 0GCQ
  Superior
   Left 0GCM
   Right 0GCL
 Patella
  Left 0QCF
  Right 0QCD
 Pelvic Cavity 0WCJ
 Penis 0VCS
 Pericardial Cavity 0WCD
 Pericardium 02CN

Extirpation — *continued*
 Peritoneal Cavity 0WCG
 Peritoneum 0DCW
 Phalanx
  Finger
   Left 0PCV
   Right 0PCT
  Thumb
   Left 0PCS
   Right 0PCR
  Toe
   Left 0QCR
   Right 0QCQ
 Pharynx 0CCM
 Pineal Body 0GC1
 Pleura
  Left 0BCP
  Right 0BCN
 Pleural Cavity
  Left 0WCB
  Right 0WC9
 Pons 00CB
 Prepuce 0VCT
 Prostate 0VC0
 Radius
  Left 0PCJ
  Right 0PCH
 Rectum 0DCP
 Respiratory Tract 0WCQ
 Retina
  Left 08CF
  Right 08CE
 Retinal Vessel
  Left 08CH
  Right 08CG
 Retroperitoneum 0WCH
 Ribs
  1 to 2 0PC1
  3 or More 0PC2
 Sacrum 0QC1
 Scapula
  Left 0PC6
  Right 0PC5
 Sclera
  Left 08C7XZZ
  Right 08C6XZZ
 Scrotum 0VC5
 Septum
  Atrial 02C5
  Nasal 09CM
  Ventricular 02CM
 Sinus
  Accessory 09CP
  Ethmoid
   Left 09CV
   Right 09CU
  Frontal
   Left 09CT
   Right 09CS
  Mastoid
   Left 09CC
   Right 09CB
  Maxillary
   Left 09CR
   Right 09CQ
  Sphenoid
   Left 09CX
   Right 09CW
 Skin
  Abdomen 0HC7XZZ
  Back 0HC6XZZ
  Buttock 0HC8XZZ
  Chest 0HC5XZZ
  Ear
   Left 0HC3XZZ
   Right 0HC2XZZ
  Face 0HC1XZZ

Extirpation — *continued*
 Skin — *continued*
  Foot
   Left 0HCNXZZ
   Right 0HCMXZZ
  Hand
   Left 0HCGXZZ
   Right 0HCFXZZ
  Inguinal 0HCAXZZ
  Lower Arm
   Left 0HCEXZZ
   Right 0HCDXZZ
  Lower Leg
   Left 0HCLXZZ
   Right 0HCKXZZ
  Neck 0HC4XZZ
  Perineum 0HC9XZZ
  Scalp 0HC0XZZ
  Upper Arm
   Left 0HCCXZZ
   Right 0HCBXZZ
  Upper Leg
   Left 0HCJXZZ
   Right 0HCHXZZ
 Spinal Canal 00CU
 Spinal Cord
  Cervical 00CW
  Lumbar 00CY
  Thoracic 00CX
 Spinal Meninges 00CT
 Spleen 07CP
 Sternum 0PC0
 Stomach 0DC6
  Pylorus 0DC7
 Subarachnoid Space, Intracranial 00C5
 Subcutaneous Tissue and Fascia
  Abdomen 0JC8
  Back 0JC7
  Buttock 0JC9
  Chest 0JC6
  Face 0JC1
  Foot
   Left 0JCR
   Right 0JCQ
  Hand
   Left 0JCK
   Right 0JCJ
  Lower Arm
   Left 0JCH
   Right 0JCG
  Lower Leg
   Left 0JCP
   Right 0JCN
  Neck
   Left 0JC5
   Right 0JC4
  Pelvic Region 0JCC
  Perineum 0JCB
  Scalp 0JC0
  Upper Arm
   Left 0JCF
   Right 0JCD
  Upper Leg
   Left 0JCM
   Right 0JCL
 Subdural Space, Intracranial 00C4
 Tarsal
  Left 0QCM
  Right 0QCL
 Tendon
  Abdomen
   Left 0LCG
   Right 0LCF
  Ankle
   Left 0LCT
   Right 0LCS

Extirpation — *continued*
Tendon — *continued*
Foot
Left 0LCW
Right 0LCV
Hand
Left 0LC8
Right 0LC7
Head and Neck 0LC0
Hip
Left 0LCK
Right 0LCJ
Knee
Left 0LCR
Right 0LCQ
Lower Arm and Wrist
Left 0LC6
Right 0LC5
Lower Leg
Left 0LCP
Right 0LCN
Perineum 0LCH
Shoulder
Left 0LC2
Right 0LC1
Thorax
Left 0LCD
Right 0LCC
Trunk
Left 0LCB
Right 0LC9
Upper Arm
Left 0LC4
Right 0LC3
Upper Leg
Left 0LCM
Right 0LCL
Testis
Bilateral 0VCC
Left 0VCB
Right 0VC9
Thalamus 00C9
Thymus 07CM
Thyroid Gland 0GCK
Left Lobe 0GCG
Right Lobe 0GCH
Tibia
Left 0QCH
Right 0QCG
Toe Nail 0HCRXZZ
Tongue 0CC7
Tonsils 0CCP
Tooth
Lower 0CCX
Upper 0CCW
Trachea 0BC1
Tunica Vaginalis
Left 0VC7
Right 0VC6
Turbinate, Nasal 09CL
Tympanic Membrane
Left 09C8
Right 09C7
Ulna
Left 0PCL
Right 0PCK
Ureter
Left 0TC7
Right 0TC6
Urethra 0TCD
Uterine Supporting Structure 0UC4
Uterus 0UC9
Uvula 0CCN
Vagina 0UCG
Valve
Aortic 02CF
Mitral 02CG

Extirpation — *continued*
Valve — *continued*
Pulmonary 02CH
Tricuspid 02CJ
Vas Deferens
Bilateral 0VCQ
Left 0VCP
Right 0VCN
Vein
Axillary
Left 05C8
Right 05C7
Azygos 05C0
Basilic
Left 05CC
Right 05CB
Brachial
Left 05CA
Right 05C9
Cephalic
Left 05CF
Right 05CD
Colic 06C7
Common Iliac
Left 06CD
Right 06CC
Coronary 02C4
Esophageal 06C3
External Iliac
Left 06CG
Right 06CF
External Jugular
Left 05CQ
Right 05CP
Face
Left 05CV
Right 05CT
Femoral
Left 06CN
Right 06CM
Foot
Left 06CV
Right 06CT
Gastric 06C2
Hand
Left 05CH
Right 05CG
Hemiazygos 05C1
Hepatic 06C4
Hypogastric
Left 06CJ
Right 06CH
Inferior Mesenteric 06C6
Innominate
Left 05C4
Right 05C3
Internal Jugular
Left 05CN
Right 05CM
Intracranial 05CL
Lower 06CY
Portal 06C8
Pulmonary
Left 02CT
Right 02CS
Renal
Left 06CB
Right 06C9
Saphenous
Left 06CQ
Right 06CP
Splenic 06C1
Subclavian
Left 05C6
Right 05C5
Superior Mesenteric 06C5
Upper 05CY

Extirpation — *continued*
Vein — *continued*
Vertebral
Left 05CS
Right 05CR
Vena Cava
Inferior 06C0
Superior 02CV
Ventricle
Left 02CL
Right 02CK
Vertebra
Cervical 0PC3
Lumbar 0QC0
Thoracic 0PC4
Vesicle
Bilateral 0VC3
Left 0VC2
Right 0VC1
Vitreous
Left 08C5
Right 08C4
Vocal Cord
Left 0CCV
Right 0CCT
Vulva 0UCM
Extracorporeal Carbon Dioxide Removal (ECCO2R) 5A0920Z
Extracorporeal shock wave lithotripsy
see Fragmentation
Extracranial-intracranial bypass (EC-IC)
see Bypass, Upper Arteries 031
Extraction
Acetabulum
Left 0QD50ZZ
Right 0QD40ZZ
Anus 0DDQ
Appendix 0DDJ
Auditory Ossicle
Left 09DA0ZZ
Right 09D90ZZ
Bone
Ethmoid
Left 0NDG0ZZ
Right 0NDF0ZZ
Frontal 0ND10ZZ
Hyoid 0NDX0ZZ
Lacrimal
Left 0NDJ0ZZ
Right 0NDH0ZZ
Nasal 0NDB0ZZ
Occipital 0ND70ZZ
Palatine
Left 0NDL0ZZ
Right 0NDK0ZZ
Parietal
Left 0ND40ZZ
Right 0ND30ZZ
Pelvic
Left 0QD30ZZ
Right 0QD20ZZ
Sphenoid 0NDC0ZZ
Temporal
Left 0ND60ZZ
Right 0ND50ZZ
Zygomatic
Left 0NDN0ZZ
Right 0NDM0ZZ
Bone Marrow
Iliac 07DR
Sternum 07DQ
Vertebral 07DS
Bronchus
Lingula 0BD9
Lower Lobe
Left 0BDB
Right 0BD6

Extraction — *continued*
  Bronchus — *continued*
    Main
      Left 0BD7
      Right 0BD3
    Middle Lobe, Right 0BD5
    Upper Lobe
      Left 0BD8
      Right 0BD4
  Bursa and Ligament
    Abdomen
      Left 0MDJ
      Right 0MDH
    Ankle
      Left 0MDR
      Right 0MDQ
    Elbow
      Left 0MD4
      Right 0MD3
    Foot
      Left 0MDT
      Right 0MDS
    Hand
      Left 0MD8
      Right 0MD7
    Head and Neck 0MD0
    Hip
      Left 0MDM
      Right 0MDL
    Knee
      Left 0MDP
      Right 0MDN
    Lower Extremity
      Left 0MDW
      Right 0MDV
    Perineum 0MDK
    Rib(s) 0MDG
    Shoulder
      Left 0MD2
      Right 0MD1
    Spine
      Lower 0MDD
      Upper 0MDC
    Sternum 0MDF
    Upper Extremity
      Left 0MDB
      Right 0MD9
    Wrist
      Left 0MD6
      Right 0MD5
  Carina 0BD2
  Carpal
    Left 0PDN0ZZ
    Right 0PDM0ZZ
  Cecum 0DDH
  Cerebral Meninges 00D1
  Cisterna Chyli 07DL
  Clavicle
    Left 0PDB0ZZ
    Right 0PD90ZZ
  Coccyx 0QDS0ZZ
  Colon
    Ascending 0DDK
    Descending 0DDM
    Sigmoid 0DDN
    Transverse 0DDL
  Cornea
    Left 08D9XZ
    Right 08D8XZ
  Duodenum 0DD9
  Dura Mater 00D2
  Endometrium 0UDB
  Esophagogastric Junction 0DD4
  Esophagus 0DD5
    Lower 0DD3
    Middle 0DD2
    Upper 0DD1

Extraction — *continued*
  Femoral Shaft
    Left 0QD90ZZ
    Right 0QD80ZZ
  Femur
    Lower
      Left 0QDC0ZZ
      Right 0QDB0ZZ
    Upper
      Left 0QD70ZZ
      Right 0QD60ZZ
  Fibula
    Left 0QDK0ZZ
    Right 0QDJ0ZZ
  Finger Nail 0HDQXZZ
  Glenoid Cavity
    Left 0PD80ZZ
    Right 0PD70ZZ
  Hair 0HDSXZZ
  Humeral Head
    Left 0PDD0ZZ
    Right 0PDC0ZZ
  Humeral Shaft
    Left 0PDG0ZZ
    Right 0PDF0ZZ
  Ileocecal Valve 0DDC
  Ileum 0DDB
  Intestine
    Large 0DDE
      Left 0DDG
      Right 0DDF
    Small 0DD8
  Jejunum 0DDA
  Kidney
    Left 0TD1
    Right 0TD0
  Lens
    Left 08DK3ZZ
    Right 08DJ3ZZ
  Lung
    Bilateral 0BDM
    Left 0BDL
    Lower Lobe
      Left 0BDJ
      Right 0BDF
    Middle Lobe, Right 0BDD
    Right 0BDK
    Upper Lobe
      Left 0BDG
      Right 0BDC
  Lung Lingula 0BDH
  Lymphatic
    Aortic 07DD
    Axillary
      Left 07D6
      Right 07D5
    Head 07D0
    Inguinal
      Left 07DJ
      Right 07DH
    Internal Mammary
      Left 07D9
      Right 07D8
    Lower Extremity
      Left 07DG
      Right 07DF
    Mesenteric 07DB
    Neck
      Left 07D2
      Right 07D1
    Pelvis 07DC
    Thoracic Duct 07DK
    Thorax 07D7
    Upper Extremity
      Left 07D4
      Right 07D3

Extraction — *continued*
  Mandible
    Left 0NDV0ZZ
    Right 0NDT0ZZ
  Maxilla 0NDR0ZZ
  Metacarpal
    Left 0PDQ0ZZ
    Right 0PDP0ZZ
  Metatarsal
    Left 0QDP0ZZ
    Right 0QDN0ZZ
  Muscle
    Abdomen
      Left 0KDL0ZZ
      Right 0KDK0ZZ
    Facial 0KD10ZZ
    Foot
      Left 0KDW0ZZ
      Right 0KDV0ZZ
    Hand
      Left 0KDD0ZZ
      Right 0KDC0ZZ
    Head 0KD00ZZ
    Hip
      Left 0KDP0ZZ
      Right 0KDN0ZZ
    Lower Arm and Wrist
      Left 0KDB0ZZ
      Right 0KD90ZZ
    Lower Leg
      Left 0KDT0ZZ
      Right 0KDS0ZZ
    Neck
      Left 0KD30ZZ
      Right 0KD20ZZ
    Perineum 0KDM0ZZ
    Shoulder
      Left 0KD60ZZ
      Right 0KD50ZZ
    Thorax
      Left 0KDJ0ZZ
      Right 0KDH0ZZ
    Tongue, Palate, Pharynx 0KD40ZZ
    Trunk
      Left 0KDG0ZZ
      Right 0KDF0ZZ
    Upper Arm
      Left 0KD80ZZ
      Right 0KD70ZZ
    Upper Leg
      Left 0KDR0ZZ
      Right 0KDQ0ZZ
  Nerve
    Abdominal Sympathetic 01DM
    Abducens 00DL
    Accessory 00DR
    Acoustic 00DN
    Brachial Plexus 01D3
    Cervical 01D1
    Cervical Plexus 01D0
    Facial 00DM
    Femoral 01DD
    Glossopharyngeal 00DP
    Head and Neck Sympathetic 01DK
    Hypoglossal 00DS
    Lumbar 01DB
    Lumbar Plexus 01D9
    Lumbar Sympathetic 01DN
    Lumbosacral Plexus 01DA
    Median 01D5
    Oculomotor 00DH
    Olfactory 00DF
    Optic 00DG
    Peroneal 01DH
    Phrenic 01D2
    Pudendal 01DC
    Radial 01D6

Extraction — *continued*
  Nerve — *continued*
    Sacral 01DR
    Sacral Plexus 01DQ
    Sacral Sympathetic 01DP
    Sciatic 01DF
    Thoracic 01D8
    Thoracic Sympathetic 01DL
    Tibial 01DG
    Trigeminal 00DK
    Trochlear 00DJ
    Ulnar 01D4
    Vagus 00DQ
  Orbit
    Left 0NDQ0ZZ
    Right 0NDP0ZZ
  Ova 0UDN
  Patella
    Left 0QDF0ZZ
    Right 0QDD0ZZ
  Phalanx
    Finger
      Left 0PDV0ZZ
      Right 0PDT0ZZ
    Thumb
      Left 0PDS0ZZ
      Right 0PDR0ZZ
    Toe
      Left 0QDR0ZZ
      Right 0QDQ0ZZ
  Pleura
    Left 0BDP
    Right 0BDN
  Products of Conception
    Classical 10D00Z0
    Ectopic 10D2
    Extraperitoneal 10D00Z2
    High Forceps 10D07Z5
    Internal Version 10D07Z7
    Low Cervical 10D00Z1
    Low Forceps 10D07Z3
    Mid Forceps 10D07Z4
    Other 10D07Z8
    Retained 10D1
    Vacuum 10D07Z6
  Radius
    Left 0PDJ0ZZ
    Right 0PDH0ZZ
  Rectum 0DDP
  Ribs
    1 to 2 0PD10ZZ
    3 or More 0PD20ZZ
  Sacrum 0QD10ZZ
  Scapula
    Left 0PD60ZZ
    Right 0PD50ZZ
  Septum, Nasal 09DM
  Sinus
    Accessory 09DP
    Ethmoid
      Left 09DV
      Right 09DU
    Frontal
      Left 09DT
      Right 09DS
    Mastoid
      Left 09DC
      Right 09DB
    Maxillary
      Left 09DR
      Right 09DQ
    Sphenoid
      Left 09DX
      Right 09DW
  Skin
    Abdomen 0HD7XZZ
    Back 0HD6XZZ

Extraction — *continued*
  Skin — *continued*
    Buttock 0HD8XZZ
    Chest 0HD5XZZ
    Ear
      Left 0HD3XZZ
      Right 0HD2XZZ
    Face 0HD1XZZ
    Foot
      Left 0HDNXZZ
      Right 0HDMXZZ
    Hand
      Left 0HDGXZZ
      Right 0HDFXZZ
    Inguinal 0HDAXZZ
    Lower Arm
      Left 0HDEXZZ
      Right 0HDDXZZ
    Lower Leg
      Left 0HDLXZZ
      Right 0HDKXZZ
    Neck 0HD4XZZ
    Perineum 0HD9XZZ
    Scalp 0HD0XZZ
    Upper Arm
      Left 0HDCXZZ
      Right 0HDBXZZ
    Upper Leg
      Left 0HDJXZZ
      Right 0HDHXZZ
  Skull 0ND00ZZ
  Spinal Meninges 00DT
  Spleen 07DP
  Sternum 0PD00ZZ
  Stomach 0DD6
    Pylorus 0DD7
  Subcutaneous Tissue and Fascia
    Abdomen 0JD8
    Back 0JD7
    Buttock 0JD9
    Chest 0JD6
    Face 0JD1
    Foot
      Left 0JDR
      Right 0JDQ
    Hand
      Left 0JDK
      Right 0JDJ
    Lower Arm
      Left 0JDH
      Right 0JDG
    Lower Leg
      Left 0JDP
      Right 0JDN
    Neck
      Left 0JD5
      Right 0JD4
    Pelvic Region 0JDC
    Perineum 0JDB
    Scalp 0JD0
    Upper Arm
      Left 0JDF
      Right 0JDD
    Upper Leg
      Left 0JDM
      Right 0JDL
  Tarsal
    Left 0QDM0ZZ
    Right 0QDL0ZZ
  Tendon
    Abdomen
      Left 0LDG0ZZ
      Right 0LDF0ZZ
    Ankle
      Left 0LDT0ZZ
      Right 0LDS0ZZ
    Foot

Extraction — *continued*
  Tendon — *continued*
      Left 0LDW0ZZ
      Right 0LDV0ZZ
    Hand
      Left 0LD80ZZ
      Right 0LD70ZZ
    Head and Neck 0LD00ZZ
    Hip
      Left 0LDK0ZZ
      Right 0LDJ0ZZ
    Knee
      Left 0LDR0ZZ
      Right 0LDQ0ZZ
    Lower Arm and Wrist
      Left 0LD60ZZ
      Right 0LD50ZZ
    Lower Leg
      Left 0LDP0ZZ
      Right 0LDN0ZZ
    Perineum 0LDH0ZZ
    Shoulder
      Left 0LD20ZZ
      Right 0LD10ZZ
    Thorax
      Left 0LDD0ZZ
      Right 0LDC0ZZ
    Trunk
      Left 0LDB0ZZ
      Right 0LD90ZZ
    Upper Arm
      Left 0LD40ZZ
      Right 0LD30ZZ
    Upper Leg
      Left 0LDM0ZZ
      Right 0LDL0ZZ
  Thymus 07DM
  Tibia
    Left 0QDH0ZZ
    Right 0QDG0ZZ
  Toe Nail 0HDRXZZ
  Tooth
    Lower 0CDXXZ
    Upper 0CDWXZ
  Trachea 0BD1
  Turbinate, Nasal 09DL
  Tympanic Membrane
    Left 09D8
    Right 09D7
  Ulna
    Left 0PDL0ZZ
    Right 0PDK0ZZ
  Vein
    Basilic
      Left 05DC
      Right 05DB
    Brachial
      Left 05DA
      Right 05D9
    Cephalic
      Left 05DF
      Right 05DD
    Femoral
      Left 06DN
      Right 06DM
    Foot
      Left 06DV
      Right 06DT
    Hand
      Left 05DH
      Right 05DG
    Lower 06DY
    Saphenous
      Left 06DQ
      Right 06DP
    Upper 05DY

Extraction — *continued*
Vertebra
Cervical 0PD30ZZ
Lumbar 0QD00ZZ
Thoracic 0PD40ZZ
Vocal Cord
Left 0CDV
Right 0CDT
Extradural space, intracranial
use Epidural Space, Intracranial
Extradural space, spinal
use Spinal Canal
Extreme Lateral Interbody Fusion (XLIF®) device
use Interbody Fusion Device in Lower Joints

F

Face lift
see Alteration, Face 0W02
Facet replacement spinal stabilization device
use Spinal Stabilization Device, Facet Replacement in 0RH
use Spinal Stabilization Device, Facet Replacement in 0SH
Facial artery
use Face Artery
Factor Xa Inhibitor Reversal Agent, Andexanet Alfa
use Andexanet Alfa, Factor Xa Inhibitor Reversal Agent
False vocal cord
use Larynx
Falx cerebri
use Dura Mater
Fascia lata
use Subcutaneous Tissue and Fascia, Right Upper Leg
use Subcutaneous Tissue and Fascia, Left Upper Leg
Fasciaplasty, fascioplasty
see Repair, Subcutaneous Tissue and Fascia 0JQ
see Replacement, Subcutaneous Tissue and Fascia 0JR
Fasciectomy
see Excision, Subcutaneous Tissue and Fascia 0JB
Fasciorrhaphy
see Repair, Subcutaneous Tissue and Fascia 0JQ
Fasciotomy
see Division, Subcutaneous Tissue and Fascia 0J8
see Drainage, Subcutaneous Tissue and Fascia 0J9
see Release
Feeding Device
Change device in
Lower 0D2DXUZ
Upper 0D20XUZ
Insertion of device in
Duodenum 0DH9
Esophagus 0DH5
Ileum 0DHB
Intestine, Small 0DH8
Jejunum 0DHA
Stomach 0DH6
Removal of device from
Esophagus 0DP5
Intestinal Tract
Lower 0DPD
Upper 0DP0
Stomach 0DP6

Feeding Device — *continued*
Revision of device in
Intestinal Tract
Lower 0DWD
Upper 0DW0
Stomach 0DW6
Femoral head
use Upper Femur, Right
use Upper Femur, Left
Femoral lymph node
use Lymphatic, Right Lower Extremity
use Lymphatic, Left Lower Extremity
Femoropatellar joint
use Knee Joint, Right
use Knee Joint, Left
use Knee Joint, Femoral Surface, Right
use Knee Joint, Femoral Surface, Left
Femorotibial joint
use Knee Joint, Right
use Knee Joint, Left
use Knee Joint, Tibial Surface, Right
use Knee Joint, Tibial Surface, Left
Fibular artery
use Peroneal Artery, Right
use Peroneal Artery, Left
Fibularis brevis muscle
use Lower Leg Muscle, Right
use Lower Leg Muscle, Left
Fibularis longus muscle
use Lower Leg Muscle, Right
use Lower Leg Muscle, Left
Fifth cranial nerve
use Trigeminal Nerve
Filum terminale
use Spinal Meninges
Fimbriectomy
see Excision, Female Reproductive System 0UB
see Resection, Female Reproductive System 0UT
Fine needle aspiration
Fluid or gas *see* Drainage
Tissue *see* Excision
First cranial nerve
use Olfactory Nerve
First intercostal nerve
use Brachial Plexus
Fistulization
see Bypass
see Drainage
see Repair
Fitting
Arch bars, for fracture reduction *see* Reposition, Mouth and Throat 0CS
Arch bars, for immobilization *see* Immobilization, Face 2W31
Artificial limb *see* Device Fitting, Rehabilitation F0D
Hearing aid *see* Device Fitting, Rehabilitation F0D
Ocular prosthesis F0DZ8UZ
Prosthesis, limb *see* Device Fitting, Rehabilitation F0D
Prosthesis, ocular F0DZ8UZ
Fixation, bone
External, with fracture reduction *see* Reposition
External, without fracture reduction *see* Insertion
Internal, with fracture reduction *see* Reposition
Internal, without fracture reduction *see* Insertion
FLAIR® Endovascular Stent Graft
use Intraluminal Device
Flexible Composite Mesh
use Synthetic Substitute

Flexor carpi radialis muscle
use Lower Arm and Wrist Muscle, Right
use Lower Arm and Wrist Muscle, Left
Flexor carpi ulnaris muscle
use Lower Arm and Wrist Muscle, Right
use Lower Arm and Wrist Muscle, Left
Flexor digitorum brevis muscle
use Foot Muscle, Right
use Foot Muscle, Left
Flexor digitorum longus muscle
use Lower Leg Muscle, Right
use Lower Leg Muscle, Left
Flexor hallucis brevis muscle
use Foot Muscle, Right
use Foot Muscle, Left
Flexor hallucis longus muscle
use Lower Leg Muscle, Right
use Lower Leg Muscle, Left
Flexor pollicis longus muscle
use Lower Arm and Wrist Muscle, Right
use Lower Arm and Wrist Muscle, Left
Fluoroscopy
Abdomen and Pelvis BW11
Airway, Upper BB1DZZZ
Ankle
Left BQ1H
Right BQ1G
Aorta
Abdominal B410
Laser, Intraoperative B410
Thoracic B310
Laser, Intraoperative B310
Thoraco-Abdominal B31P
Laser, Intraoperative B31P
Aorta and Bilateral Lower Extremity Arteries B41D
Laser, Intraoperative B41D
Arm
Left BP1FZZZ
Right BP1EZZZ
Artery
Brachiocephalic-Subclavian
Right B311
Laser, Intraoperative B311
Bronchial B31L
Laser, Intraoperative B31L
Bypass Graft, Other B21F
Cervico-Cerebral Arch B31Q
Laser, Intraoperative B31Q
Common Carotid
Bilateral B315
Laser, Intraoperative B315
Left B314
Laser, Intraoperative B314
Right B313
Laser, Intraoperative B313
Coronary
Bypass Graft
Multiple B213
Laser, Intraoperative B213
Single B212
Laser, Intraoperative B212
Multiple B211
Laser, Intraoperative B211
Single B210
Laser, Intraoperative B210
External Carotid
Bilateral B31C
Laser, Intraoperative B31C
Left B31B
Laser, Intraoperative B31B
Right B319
Laser, Intraoperative B319
Hepatic B412
Laser, Intraoperative B412
Inferior Mesenteric B415
Laser, Intraoperative B415

Fluoroscopy — *continued*
  Artery — *continued*
    Intercostal B31L
      Laser, Intraoperative B31L
    Internal Carotid
      Bilateral B318
        Laser, Intraoperative B318
      Left B317
        Laser, Intraoperative B317
      Right B316
        Laser, Intraoperative B316
    Internal Mammary Bypass Graft
      Left B218
      Right B217
    Intra-Abdominal
      Other B41B
      Laser, Intraoperative B41B
    Intracranial B31R
      Laser, Intraoperative B31R
    Lower
      Other B41J
      Laser, Intraoperative B41J
    Lower Extremity
      Bilateral and Aorta B41D
        Laser, Intraoperative B41D
      Left B41G
        Laser, Intraoperative B41G
      Right B41F
        Laser, Intraoperative B41F
    Lumbar B419
      Laser, Intraoperative B419
    Pelvic B41C
      Laser, Intraoperative B41C
    Pulmonary
      Left B31T
        Laser, Intraoperative B31T
      Right B31S
        Laser, Intraoperative B31S
    Pulmonary Trunk B31U
      Laser, Intraoperative B31U
    Renal
      Bilateral B418
        Laser, Intraoperative B418
      Left B417
        Laser, Intraoperative B417
      Right B416
        Laser, Intraoperative B416
    Spinal B31M
      Laser, Intraoperative B31M
    Splenic B413
      Laser, Intraoperative B413
    Subclavian
      Left B312
      Laser, Intraoperative B312
    Superior Mesenteric B414
      Laser, Intraoperative B414
    Upper
      Other B31N
      Laser, Intraoperative B31N
    Upper Extremity
      Bilateral B31K
        Laser, Intraoperative B31K
      Left B31J
        Laser, Intraoperative B31J
      Right B31H
        Laser, Intraoperative B31H
    Vertebral
      Bilateral B31G
        Laser, Intraoperative B31G
      Left B31F
        Laser, Intraoperative B31F
      Right B31D
        Laser, Intraoperative B31D
  Bile Duct BF10
    Pancreatic Duct and Gallbladder BF14
  Bile Duct and Gallbladder BF13

Fluoroscopy — *continued*
  Biliary Duct BF11
  Bladder BT10
    Kidney and Ureter BT14
      Left BT1F
      Right BT1D
  Bladder and Urethra BT1B
  Bowel, Small BD1
  Calcaneus
    Left BQ1KZZZ
    Right BQ1JZZZ
  Clavicle
    Left BP15ZZZ
    Right BP14ZZZ
  Coccyx BR1F
  Colon BD14
  Corpora Cavernosa BV10
  Dialysis Fistula B51W
  Dialysis Shunt B51W
  Diaphragm BB16ZZZ
  Disc
    Cervical BR11
    Lumbar BR13
    Thoracic BR12
  Duodenum BD19
  Elbow
    Left BP1H
    Right BP1G
  Epiglottis B91G
  Esophagus BD11
  Extremity
    Lower BW1C
    Upper BW1J
  Facet Joint
    Cervical BR14
    Lumbar BR16
    Thoracic BR15
  Fallopian Tube
    Bilateral BU12
    Left BU11
    Right BU10
  Fallopian Tube and Uterus BU18
  Femur
    Left BQ14ZZZ
    Right BQ13ZZZ
  Finger
    Left BP1SZZZ
    Right BP1RZZZ
  Foot
    Left BQ1MZZZ
    Right BQ1LZZZ
  Forearm
    Left BP1KZZZ
    Right BP1JZZZ
  Gallbladder BF12
    Bile Duct and Pancreatic Duct BF14
  Gallbladder and Bile Duct BF13
  Gastrointestinal, Upper BD1
  Hand
    Left BP1PZZZ
    Right BP1NZZZ
  Head and Neck BW19
  Heart
    Left B215
    Right B214
    Right and Left B216
  Hip
    Left BQ11
    Right BQ10
  Humerus
    Left BP1BZZZ
    Right BP1AZZZ
  Ileal Diversion Loop BT1C
  Ileal Loop, Ureters and Kidney BT1G
  Intracranial Sinus B512
  Joint
    Acromioclavicular, Bilateral BP13ZZZ

Fluoroscopy — *continued*
  Joint — *continued*
    Finger
      Left BP1D
      Right BP1C
    Foot
      Left BQ1Y
      Right BQ1X
    Hand
      Left BP1D
      Right BP1C
    Lumbosacral BR1B
    Sacroiliac BR1D
    Sternoclavicular
      Bilateral BP12ZZZ
      Left BP11ZZZ
      Right BP10ZZZ
    Temporomandibular
      Bilateral BN19
      Left BN18
      Right BN17
    Thoracolumbar BR18
    Toe
      Left BQ1Y
      Right BQ1X
  Kidney
    Bilateral BT13
    Ileal Loop and Ureter BT1G
    Left BT12
    Right BT11
    Ureter and Bladder BT14
      Left BT1F
      Right BT1D
  Knee
    Left BQ18
    Right BQ17
  Larynx B91J
  Leg
    Left BQ1FZZZ
    Right BQ1DZZZ
  Lung
    Bilateral BB14ZZZ
    Left BB13ZZZ
    Right BB12ZZZ
  Mediastinum BB1CZZZ
  Mouth BD1B
  Neck and Head BW19
  Oropharynx BD1B
  Pancreatic Duct BF1
    Gallbladder and Bile Buct BF14
  Patella
    Left BQ1WZZZ
    Right BQ1VZZZ
  Pelvis BR1C
  Pelvis and Abdomen BW11
  Pharynx B91G
  Ribs
    Left BP1YZZZ
    Right BP1XZZZ
  Sacrum BR1F
  Scapula
    Left BP17ZZZ
    Right BP16ZZZ
  Shoulder
    Left BP19
    Right BP18
  Sinus, Intracranial B512
  Spinal Cord B01B
  Spine
    Cervical BR10

Fluoroscopy — *continued*
  Spine — *continued*
    Lumbar BR19
    Thoracic BR17
    Whole BR1G
  Sternum BR1H
  Stomach BD12
  Toe
    Left BQ1QZZZ
    Right BQ1PZZZ
  Tracheobronchial Tree
    Bilateral BB19YZZ
    Left BB18YZZ
    Right BB17YZZ
  Ureter
    Ileal Loop and Kidney BT1G
    Kidney and Bladder BT14
      Left BT1F
      Right BT1D
    Left BT17
    Right BT16
  Urethra BT15
  Urethra and Bladder BT1B
  Uterus BU16
  Uterus and Fallopian Tube BU18
  Vagina BU19
  Vasa Vasorum BV18
  Vein
    Cerebellar B511
    Cerebral B511
    Epidural B510
    Jugular
      Bilateral B515
      Left B514
      Right B513
    Lower Extremity
      Bilateral B51D
      Left B51C
      Right B51B
    Other B51V
    Pelvic (Iliac)
      Left B51G
      Right B51F
    Pelvic (Iliac) Bilateral B51H
    Portal B51T
    Pulmonary
      Bilateral B51S
      Left B51R
      Right B51Q
    Renal
      Bilateral B51L
      Left B51K
      Right B51J
    Splanchnic B51T
    Subclavian
      Left B517
      Right B516
    Upper Extremity
      Bilateral B51P
      Left B51N
      Right B51M
  Vena Cava
    Inferior B519
    Superior B518
  Wrist
    Left BP1M
    Right BP1L
Fluoroscopy, laser intraoperative
  see Fluoroscopy, Heart B21
  see Fluoroscopy, Upper Arteries B31
  see Fluoroscopy, Lower Arteries B41
Flushing
  see Irrigation
Foley catheter
  use Drainage Device
Fontan completion procedure Stage II
  see Bypass, Vena Cava, Inferior 0610

Foramen magnum
  use Occipital Bone
Foramen of Monro (intraventricular)
  use Cerebral Ventricle
Foreskin
  use Prepuce
Formula™ Balloon-Expandable Renal Stent System
  use Intraluminal Device
Fossa of Rosenmuller
  use Nasopharynx
Fourth cranial nerve
  use Trochlear Nerve
Fourth ventricle
  use Cerebral Ventricle
Fovea
  use Retina, Right
  use Retina, Left
Fragmentation
  Ampulla of Vater 0FFC
  Anus 0DFQ
  Appendix 0DFJ
  Bladder 0TFB
  Bladder Neck 0TFC
  Bronchus
    Lingula 0BF9
    Lower Lobe
      Left 0BFB
      Right 0BF6
    Main
      Left 0BF7
      Right 0BF3
    Middle Lobe, Right 0BF5
    Upper Lobe
      Left 0BF8
      Right 0BF4
  Carina 0BF2
  Cavity, Cranial 0WF1
  Cecum 0DFH
  Cerebral Ventricle 00F6
  Colon
    Ascending 0DFK
    Descending 0DFM
    Sigmoid 0DFN
    Transverse 0DFL
  Duct
    Common Bile 0FF9
    Cystic 0FF8
    Hepatic
      Common 0FF7
      Left 0FF6
      Right 0FF5
    Pancreatic 0FFD
      Accessory 0FFF
    Parotid
      Left 0CFC
      Right 0CFB
  Duodenum 0DF9
  Epidural Space, Intracranial 00F3
  Esophagus 0DF5
  Fallopian Tube
    Left 0UF6
    Right 0UF5
  Fallopian Tubes, Bilateral 0UF7
  Gallbladder 0FF4
  Gastrointestinal Tract 0WFP
  Genitourinary Tract 0WFR
  Ileum 0DFB
  Intestine
    Large 0DFE
      Left 0DFG
      Right 0DFF
    Small 0DF8
  Jejunum 0DFA
  Kidney Pelvis
    Left 0TF4
    Right 0TF3

Fragmentation — *continued*
  Mediastinum 0WFC
  Oral Cavity and Throat 0WF3
  Pelvic Cavity 0WFJ
  Pericardial Cavity 0WFD
  Pericardium 02FN
  Peritoneal Cavity 0WFG
  Pleural Cavity
    Left 0WFB
    Right 0WF9
  Rectum 0DFP
  Respiratory Tract 0WFQ
  Spinal Canal 00FU
  Stomach 0DF6
  Subarachnoid Space, Intracranial 00F5
  Subdural Space, Intracranial 00F4
  Trachea 0BF1
  Ureter
    Left 0TF7
    Right 0TF6
  Urethra 0TFD
  Uterus 0UF9
  Vitreous
    Left 08F5
    Right 08F4
Freestyle (Stentless) Aortic Root Bioprosthesis
  use Zooplastic Tissue in Heart and Great Vessels
Frenectomy
  see Excision, Mouth and Throat 0CB
  see Resection, Mouth and Throat 0CT
Frenoplasty, frenuloplasty
  see Repair, Mouth and Throat 0CQ
  see Replacement, Mouth and Throat 0CR
  see Supplement, Mouth and Throat 0CU
Frenotomy
  see Drainage, Mouth and Throat 0C9
  see Release, Mouth and Throat 0CN
Frenulotomy
  see Drainage, Mouth and Throat 0C9
  see Release, Mouth and Throat 0CN
Frenulum labii inferioris
  use Lower Lip
Frenulum labii superioris
  use Upper Lip
Frenulum linguae
  use Tongue
Frenulumectomy
  see Excision, Mouth and Throat 0CB
  see Resection, Mouth and Throat 0CT
Frontal lobe
  use Cerebral Hemisphere
Frontal vein
  use Face Vein, Right
  use Face Vein, Left
Fulguration
  see Destruction
Fundoplication, gastroesophageal
  see Restriction, Esophagogastric Junction 0DV4
Fundus uteri
  use Uterus
Fusion
  Acromioclavicular
    Left 0RGH
    Right 0RGG
  Ankle
    Left 0SGG
    Right 0SGF
  Carpal
    Left 0RGR
    Right 0RGQ
  Carpometacarpal
    Left 0RGT
    Right 0RGS

Fusion — *continued*
  Cervical Vertebral 0RG1
    2 or more 0RG2
      Interbody Fusion Device
        Nanotextured Surface XRG2092
        Radiolucent Porous XRG20F3
      Interbody Fusion Device
        Nanotextured Surface XRG1092
        Radiolucent Porous XRG10F3
  Cervicothoracic Vertebral 0RG4
    Interbody Fusion Device
      Nanotextured Surface XRG4092
      Radiolucent Porous XRG40F3
  Coccygeal 0SG6
  Elbow
    Left 0RGM
    Right 0RGL
  Finger Phalangeal
    Left 0RGX
    Right 0RGW
  Hip
    Left 0SGB
    Right 0SG9
  Knee
    Left 0SGD
    Right 0SGC
  Lumbar Vertebral 0SG0
    2 or more 0SG1
      Interbody Fusion Device
        Nanotextured Surface XRGC092
        Radiolucent Porous XRGC0F3
      Interbody Fusion Device
        Nanotextured Surface XRGB092
        Radiolucent Porous XRGB0F3
  Lumbosacral 0SG3
    Interbody Fusion Device
      Nanotextured Surface XRGD092
      Radiolucent Porous XRGD0F3
  Metacarpophalangeal
    Left 0RGV
    Right 0RGU
  Metatarsal-Phalangeal
    Left 0SGN
    Right 0SGM
  Occipital-cervical 0RG0
    Interbody Fusion Device
      Nanotextured Surface XRG0092
      Radiolucent Porous XRG00F3
  Sacrococcygeal 0SG5
  Sacroiliac
    Left 0SG8
    Right 0SG7
  Shoulder
    Left 0RGK
    Right 0RGJ
  Sternoclavicular
    Left 0RGF
    Right 0RGE
  Tarsal
    Left 0SGJ
    Right 0SGH
  Tarsometatarsal
    Left 0SGL
    Right 0SGK
  Temporomandibular
    Left 0RGD
    Right 0RGC
  Thoracic Vertebral 0RG6
    2 to 7 0RG7
      Interbody Fusion Device
        Nanotextured Surface XRG7092
        Radiolucent Porous XRG70F3
    8 or more 0RG8
      Interbody Fusion Device
        Nanotextured Surface XRG8092
        Radiolucent Porous XRG80F3

Fusion — *continued*
  Thoracic Vertebral— *continued*
    Interbody Fusion Device
      Nanotextured Surface XRG6092
      Radiolucent Porous XRG60F3
  Thoracolumbar Vertebral 0RGA
    Interbody Fusion Device
      Nanotextured Surface XRGA092
      Radiolucent Porous XRGA0F3
  Toe Phalangeal
    Left 0SGQ
    Right 0SGP
  Wrist
    Left 0RGP
    Right 0RGN
Fusion screw (compression)(lag)(locking)
  use Internal Fixation Device in Upper Joints
  use Internal Fixation Device in Lower Joints

G

Gait training
  see Motor Treatment, Rehabilitation F07
Galea aponeurotica
  use Subcutaneous Tissue and Fascia, Scalp
GammaTile™
  use Radioactive Element, Cesium-131
    Collagen Implant in 00H
Ganglion impar (ganglion of Walther)
  use Sacral Sympathetic Nerve
Ganglionectomy
  Destruction of lesion *see* Destruction
  Excision of lesion *see* Excision
Gasserian ganglion
  use Trigeminal Nerve
Gastrectomy
  Partial *see* Excision, Stomach 0DB6
  Total *see* Resection, Stomach 0DT6
  Vertical (sleeve) *see* Excision, Stomach 0DB6
Gastric electrical stimulation (GES) lead
  use Stimulator Lead in Gastrointestinal
    System
Gastric lymph node
  use Lymphatic, Aortic
Gastric pacemaker lead
  use Stimulator Lead in Gastrointestinal System
Gastric plexus
  use Abdominal Sympathetic Nerve
Gastrocnemius muscle
  use Lower Leg Muscle, Right
  use Lower Leg Muscle, Left
Gastrocolic ligament
  use Omentum
Gastrocolic omentum
  use Omentum
Gastrocolostomy
  see Bypass, Gastrointestinal System 0D1
  see Drainage, Gastrointestinal System 0D9
Gastroduodenal artery
  use Hepatic Artery
Gastroduodenectomy
  see Excision, Gastrointestinal System 0DB
  see Resection, Gastrointestinal System 0DT
Gastroduodenoscopy 0DJ08ZZ
Gastroenteroplasty
  see Repair, Gastrointestinal System 0DQ
  see Supplement, Gastrointestinal
    System 0DU
Gastroenterostomy
  see Bypass, Gastrointestinal System 0D1
  see Drainage, Gastrointestinal System 0D9
Gastroesophageal (GE) junction
  use Esophagogastric Junction
Gastrogastrostomy
  see Bypass, Stomach 0D16
  see Drainage, Stomach 0D96

Gastrohepatic omentum
  use Omentum
Gastrojejunostomy
  see Bypass, Stomach 0D16
  see Drainage, Stomach 0D96
Gastrolysis
  see Release, Stomach 0DN6
Gastropexy
  see Repair, Stomach 0DQ6
  see Reposition, Stomach 0DS6
Gastrophrenic ligament
  use Omentum
Gastroplasty
  see Repair, Stomach 0DQ6
  see Supplement, Stomach 0DU6
Gastroplication
  see Restriction, Stomach 0DV6
Gastropylorectomy
  see Excision, Gastrointestinal System 0DB
Gastrorrhaphy
  see Repair, Stomach 0DQ6
Gastroscopy 0DJ68ZZ
Gastrosplenic ligament
  use Omentum
Gastrostomy
  see Bypass, Stomach 0D16
  see Drainage, Stomach 0D96
Gastrotomy
  see Drainage, Stomach 0D96
Gemellus muscle
  use Hip Muscle, Right
  use Hip Muscle, Left
Geniculate ganglion
  use Facial Nerve
Geniculate nucleus
  use Thalamus
Genioglossus muscle
  use Tongue, Palate, Pharynx Muscle
Genioplasty
  see Alteration, Jaw, Lower 0W05
Genitofemoral nerve
  use Lumbar Plexus
Gingivectomy
  see Excision, Mouth and Throat 0CB
Gingivoplasty
  see Repair, Mouth and Throat 0CQ
  see Replacement, Mouth and Throat 0CR
  see Supplement, Mouth and Throat 0CU
Glans penis
  use Prepuce
Glenohumeral joint
  use Shoulder Joint, Right
  use Shoulder Joint, Left
Glenohumeral ligament
  use Shoulder Bursa and Ligament, Right
  use Shoulder Bursa and Ligament, Left
Glenoid fossa (of scapula)
  use Glenoid Cavity, Right
  use Glenoid Cavity, Left
Glenoid ligament (labrum)
  use Shoulder Joint, Right
  use Shoulder Joint, Left
Globus pallidus
  use Basal Ganglia
Glomectomy
  see Excision, Endocrine System 0GB
  see Resection, Endocrine System 0GT
Glossectomy
  see Excision, Tongue 0CB7
  see Resection, Tongue 0CT7
Glossoepiglottic fold
  use Epiglottis
Glossopexy
  see Repair, Tongue 0CQ7
  see Reposition, Tongue 0CS7
Glossoplasty
  see Repair, Tongue 0CQ7

Glossoplasty — *continued*
  see Replacement, Tongue 0CR7
  see Supplement, Tongue 0CU7
Glossorrhaphy
  see Repair, Tongue 0CQ7
Glossotomy
  see Drainage, Tongue 0C97
Glottis
  use Larynx
Gluteal Artery Perforator Flap
  Replacement
    Bilateral 0HRV079
    Left 0HRU079
    Right 0HRT079
  Transfer
    Left 0KXG
    Right 0KXF
Gluteal lymph node
  use Lymphatic, Pelvis
Gluteal vein
  use Hypogastric Vein, Right
  use Hypogastric Vein, Left
Gluteus maximus muscle
  use Hip Muscle, Right
  use Hip Muscle, Left
Gluteus medius muscle
  use Hip Muscle, Right
  use Hip Muscle, Left
Gluteus minimus muscle
  use Hip Muscle, Right
  use Hip Muscle, Left
GORE EXCLUDER® AAA Endoprosthesis
  use Intraluminal Device, Branched or
    Fenestrated, One or Two Arteries in 04V
  use Intraluminal Device, Branched or
    Fenestrated, Three or More Arteries in 04V
  use Intraluminal Device
GORE EXCLUDER® IBE Endoprosthesis
  use Intraluminal Device, Branched or
    Fenestrated, One or Two Arteries in 04V
GORE TAG® Thoracic Endoprosthesis
  use Intraluminal Device
GORE® DUALMESH®
  use Synthetic Substitute
Gracilis muscle
  use Upper Leg Muscle, Right
  use Upper Leg Muscle, Left
Graft
  see Replacement
  see Supplement
Great auricular nerve
  use Cervical Plexus
Great cerebral vein
  use Intracranial Vein
Great(er) saphenous vein
  use Saphenous Vein, Right
  use Saphenous Vein, Left
Greater alar cartilage
  use Nasal Mucosa and Soft Tissue
Greater occipital nerve
  use Cervical Nerve
Greater Omentum
  use Omentum
Greater splanchnic nerve
  use Thoracic Sympathetic Nerve
Greater superficial petrosal nerve
  use Facial Nerve
Greater trochanter
  use Upper Femur, Right
  use Upper Femur, Left
Greater tuberosity
  use Humeral Head, Right
  use Humeral Head, Left
Greater vestibular (Bartholin's) gland
  use Vestibular Gland
Greater wing
  use Sphenoid Bone

Guedel airway
  use Intraluminal Device, Airway in Mouth
    and Throat
Guidance, catheter placement
  EKG *see* Measurement, Physiological
    Systems 4A0
  Fluoroscopy *see* Fluoroscopy, Veins B51
  Ultrasound *see* Ultrasonography, Veins B54

H

Hallux
  use 1st Toe, Right
  use 1st Toe, Left
Hamate bone
  use Carpal, Right
  use Carpal, Left
Hancock® Bioprosthesis (aortic) (mitral) valve
  use Zooplastic Tissue in Heart and Great
    Vessels
Hancock® Bioprosthetic Valved Conduit
  use Zooplastic Tissue in Heart and Great
    Vessels
Harvesting, stem cells
  see Pheresis, Circulatory 6A55
Head of fibula
  use Fibula, Right
  use Fibula, Left
Hearing Aid Assessment F14Z
Hearing Assessment F13Z
Hearing Device
  Bone Conduction
    Left 09HE
    Right 09HD
  Insertion of device in
    Left 0NH6
    Right 0NH5
  Multiple Channel Cochlear Prosthesis
    Left 09HE
    Right 09HD
  Removal of device from, Skull 0NP0
  Revision of device in, Skull 0NW0
  Single Channel Cochlear Prosthesis
    Left 09HE
    Right 09HD
Hearing Treatment F09Z
Heart Assist System
  Implantable
    Insertion of device in, Heart 02HA
    Removal of device from, Heart 02PA
    Revision of device in, Heart 02WA
  Short-term External
    Insertion of device in, Heart 02HA
    Removal of device from, Heart 02PA
    Revision of device in, Heart 02WA
HeartMate 3™ LVAS
  use Implantable Heart Assist System in
    Heart and Great Vessels
HeartMate II® Left Ventricular Assist Device (LVAD)
  use Implantable Heart Assist System in
    Heart and Great Vessels
HeartMate XVE® Left Ventricular Assist Device (LVAD)
  use Implantable Heart Assist System in
    Heart and Great Vessels
HeartMate® implantable heart assist system
  see Insertion of device in, Heart 02HA
Helix
  use External Ear, Right
  use External Ear, Left
  use External Ear, Bilateral
Hematopoietic cell transplant (HCT)
  see Transfusion, Circulatory 302

Hemicolectomy
  see Resection, Gastrointestinal System 0DT
Hemicystectomy
  see Excision, Urinary System 0TB
Hemigastrectomy
  see Excision, Gastrointestinal System 0DB
Hemiglossectomy
  see Excision, Mouth and Throat 0CB
Hemilaminectomy
  see Excision, Upper Bones 0PB
  see Excision, Lower Bones 0QB
Hemilaminotomy
  see Release, Central Nervous System and
    Cranial Nerves 00N
  see Release, Peripheral Nervous
    System 01N
  see Drainage, Upper Bones 0P9
  see Excision, Upper Bones 0PB
  see Release, Upper Bones 0PN
  see Drainage, Lower Bones 0Q9
  see Excision, Lower Bones 0QB
  see Release, Lower Bones 0QN
Hemilaryngectomy
  see Excision, Larynx 0CBS
Hemimandibulectomy
  see Excision, Head and Facial Bones 0NB
Hemimaxillectomy
  see Excision, Head and Facial Bones 0NB
Hemipylorectomy
  see Excision, Gastrointestinal System 0DB
Hemispherectomy
  see Excision, Central Nervous System and
    Cranial Nerves 00B
  see Resection, Central Nervous System and
    Cranial Nerves 00T
Hemithyroidectomy
  see Excision, Endocrine System 0GB
  see Resection, Endocrine System 0GT
Hemodialysis
  see Performance, Urinary 5A1D
Hemolung® Respiratory Assist System (RAS) 5A0920Z
Hepatectomy
  see Excision, Hepatobiliary System and
    Pancreas 0FB
  see Resection, Hepatobiliary System and
    Pancreas 0FT
Hepatic artery proper
  use Hepatic Artery
Hepatic flexure
  use Transverse Colon
Hepatic lymph node
  use Lymphatic, Aortic
Hepatic plexus
  use Abdominal Sympathetic Nerve
Hepatic portal vein
  use Portal Vein
Hepaticoduodenostomy
  see Bypass, Hepatobiliary System and
    Pancreas 0F1
  see Drainage, Hepatobiliary System and
    Pancreas 0F9
Hepaticotomy
  see Drainage, Hepatobiliary System and
    Pancreas 0F9
Hepatocholedochostomy
  see Drainage, Duct, Common Bile 0F99
Hepatogastric ligament
  use Omentum
Hepatopancreatic ampulla
  use Ampulla of Vater
Hepatopexy
  see Repair, Hepatobiliary System and
    Pancreas 0FQ
  see Reposition, Hepatobiliary System and
    Pancreas 0FS

Hepatorrhaphy
   see Repair, Hepatobiliary System and
   Pancreas 0FQ
Hepatotomy
   see Drainage, Hepatobiliary System and
   Pancreas 0F9
Herculink® (RX) Elite® Renal Stent System
   use Intraluminal Device
Herniorrhaphy
   see Repair, Anatomical Regions,
   General 0WQ
   see Repair, Anatomical Regions, Lower
   Extremities 0YQ
   with synthetic substitute
      see Supplement, Anatomical Regions,
      General 0WU
      see Supplement, Anatomical Regions,
      Lower Extremities 0YU
Hip (joint) liner
   use Liner in Lower Joints
Holter monitoring 4A12X45
Holter valve ventricular shunt
   use Synthetic Substitute
Humeroradial joint
   use Elbow Joint, Right
   use Elbow Joint, Left
Humeroulnar joint
   use Elbow Joint, Right
   use Elbow Joint, Left
Humerus, distal
   use Humeral Shaft, Right
   use Humeral Shaft, Left
Hydrocelectomy
   see Excision, Male Reproductive
   System 0VB
Hydrotherapy
   Assisted exercise in pool see Motor
   Treatment, Rehabilitation F07
   Whirlpool see Activities of Daily Living
   Treatment, Rehabilitation F08
Hymenectomy
   see Excision, Hymen 0UBK
   see Resection, Hymen 0UTK
Hymenoplasty
   see Repair, Hymen 0UQK
   see Supplement, Hymen 0UUK
Hymenorrhaphy
   see Repair, Hymen 0UQK
Hymenotomy
   see Division, Hymen 0U8K
   see Drainage, Hymen 0U9K
Hyoglossus muscle
   use Tongue, Palate, Pharynx Muscle
Hyoid artery
   use Thyroid Artery, Right
   use Thyroid Artery, Left
Hyperalimentation
   see Introduction of substance in or on
Hyperbaric oxygenation
   Decompression sickness treatment see
   Decompression, Circulatory 6A15
   Wound treatment see Assistance,
   Circulatory 5A05
Hyperthermia
   Radiation Therapy
      Abdomen DWY38ZZ
      Adrenal Gland DGY28ZZ
      Bile Ducts DFY28ZZ
      Bladder DTY28ZZ
      Bone, Other DPYC8ZZ
      Bone Marrow D7Y08ZZ
      Brain D0Y08ZZ
      Brain Stem D0Y18ZZ
      Breast
         Left DMY08ZZ
         Right DMY18ZZ
      Bronchus DBY18ZZ

Hyperthermia — continued
   Radiation Therapy — continued
      Cervix DUY18ZZ
      Chest DWY28ZZ
      Chest Wall DBY78ZZ
      Colon DDY58ZZ
      Diaphragm DBY88ZZ
      Duodenum DDY28ZZ
      Ear D9Y08ZZ
      Esophagus DDY08ZZ
      Eye D8Y08ZZ
      Femur DPY98ZZ
      Fibula DPYB8ZZ
      Gallbladder DFY18ZZ
      Gland
         Adrenal DGY28ZZ
         Parathyroid DGY48ZZ
         Pituitary DGY08ZZ
         Thyroid DGY58ZZ
      Glands, Salivary D9Y68ZZ
      Head and Neck DWY18ZZ
      Hemibody DWY48ZZ
      Humerus DPY68ZZ
      Hypopharynx D9Y38ZZ
      Ileum DDY48ZZ
      Jejunum DDY38ZZ
      Kidney DTY08ZZ
      Larynx D9YB8ZZ
      Liver DFY08ZZ
      Lung DBY28ZZ
      Lymphatics
         Abdomen D7Y68ZZ
         Axillary D7Y48ZZ
         Inguinal D7Y88ZZ
         Neck D7Y38ZZ
         Pelvis D7Y78ZZ
         Thorax D7Y58ZZ
      Mandible DPY38ZZ
      Maxilla DPY28ZZ
      Mediastinum DBY68ZZ
      Mouth D9Y48ZZ
      Nasopharynx D9YD8ZZ
      Neck and Head DWY18ZZ
      Nerve, Peripheral D0Y78ZZ
      Nose D9Y18ZZ
      Oropharynx D9YF8ZZ
      Ovary DUY08ZZ
      Palate
         Hard D9Y88ZZ
         Soft D9Y98ZZ
      Pancreas DFY38ZZ
      Parathyroid Gland DGY48ZZ
      Pelvic Bones DPY88ZZ
      Pelvic Region DWY68ZZ
      Pineal Body DGY18ZZ
      Pituitary Gland DGY08ZZ
      Pleura DBY58ZZ
      Prostate DVY08ZZ
      Radius DPY78ZZ
      Rectum DDY78ZZ
      Rib DPY58ZZ
      Sinuses D9Y78ZZ
      Skin
         Abdomen DHY88ZZ
         Arm DHY48ZZ
         Back DHY78ZZ
         Buttock DHY98ZZ
         Chest DHY68ZZ
         Face DHY28ZZ
         Leg DHYB8ZZ
         Neck DHY38ZZ
      Skull DPY08ZZ
      Spinal Cord D0Y68ZZ
      Spleen D7Y28ZZ
      Sternum DPY48ZZ
      Stomach DDY18ZZ
      Testis DVY18ZZ

Hyperthermia — continued
   Radiation Therapy — continued
      Thymus D7Y18ZZ
      Thyroid Gland DGY58ZZ
      Tibia DPYB8ZZ
      Tongue D9Y58ZZ
      Trachea DBY08ZZ
      Ulna DPY78ZZ
      Ureter DTY18ZZ
      Urethra DTY38ZZ
      Uterus DUY28ZZ
      Whole Body DWY58ZZ
      Whole Body 6A3Z
Hypnosis GZFZZZZ
Hypogastric artery
   use Internal Iliac Artery, Right
   use Internal Iliac Artery, Left
Hypopharynx
   use Pharynx
Hypophysectomy
   see Excision, Gland, Pituitary 0GB0
   see Resection, Gland, Pituitary 0GT0
Hypophysis
   use Pituitary Gland
Hypothalamotomy
   see Destruction, Thalamus 0059
Hypothenar muscle
   use Hand Muscle, Right
   use Hand Muscle, Left
Hypothermia, Whole Body 6A4Z
Hysterectomy
   Supracervical see Resection, Uterus 0UT9
   Total see Resection, Uterus 0UT9
Hysterolysis
   see Release, Uterus 0UN9
Hysteropexy
   see Repair, Uterus 0UQ9
   see Reposition, Uterus 0US9
Hysteroplasty
   see Repair, Uterus 0UQ9
Hysterorrhaphy
   see Repair, Uterus 0UQ9
Hysteroscopy 0UJD8ZZ
Hysterotomy
   see Drainage, Uterus 0U99
Hysterotrachelectomy
   see Resection, Uterus 0UT9
   see Resection, Cervix 0UTC
Hysterotracheloplasty
   see Repair, Uterus 0UQ9
Hysterotrachelorrhaphy
   see Repair, Uterus 0UQ9

I

IABP (Intra-aortic balloon pump)
   see Assistance, Cardiac 5A02
**IAEMT (Intraoperative anesthetic effect
   monitoring and titration)**
   see Monitoring, Central Nervous 4A10
**Idarucizumab, Dabigatran Reversal
   Agent** XW0
IHD (Intermittent hemodialysis) 5A1D70Z
Ileal artery
   use Superior Mesenteric Artery
Ileectomy
   see Excision, Ileum 0DBB
   see Resection, Ileum 0DTB
Ileocolic artery
   use Superior Mesenteric Artery
Ileocolic vein
   use Colic Vein
Ileopexy
   see Repair, Ileum 0DQB
   see Reposition, Ileum 0DSB

Ileorrhaphy
  see Repair, Ileum 0DQB
Ileoscopy 0DJD8ZZ
Ileostomy
  see Bypass, Ileum 0D1B
  see Drainage, Ileum 0D9B
Ileotomy
  see Drainage, Ileum 0D9B
Ileoureterostomy
  see Bypass, Urinary System 0T1
Iliac crest
  use Pelvic Bone, Right
  use Pelvic Bone, Left
Iliac fascia
  use Subcutaneous Tissue and Fascia, Right Upper Leg
  use Subcutaneous Tissue and Fascia, Left Upper Leg
Iliac lymph node
  use Lymphatic, Pelvis
Iliacus muscle
  use Hip Muscle, Right
  use Hip Muscle, Left
Iliofemoral ligament
  use Hip Bursa and Ligament, Right
  use Hip Bursa and Ligament, Left
Iliohypogastric nerve
  use Lumbar Plexus
Ilioinguinal nerve
  use Lumbar Plexus
Iliolumbar artery
  use Internal Iliac Artery, Right
  use Internal Iliac Artery, Left
Iliolumbar ligament
  use Lower Spine Bursa and Ligament
Iliotibial tract (band)
  use Subcutaneous Tissue and Fascia, Right Upper Leg
  use Subcutaneous Tissue and Fascia, Left Upper Leg
Ilium
  use Pelvic Bone, Right
  use Pelvic Bone, Left
Ilizarov external fixator
  use External Fixation Device, Ring in 0PH
  use External Fixation Device, Ring in 0PS
  use External Fixation Device, Ring in 0QH
  use External Fixation Device, Ring in 0QS
Ilizarov-Vecklich device
  use External Fixation Device, Limb Lengthening in 0PH
  use External Fixation Device, Limb Lengthening in 0QH
Imaging, diagnostic
  see Plain Radiography
  see Fluoroscopy
  see Computerized Tomography (CT Scan)
  see Magnetic Resonance Imaging (MRI)
  see Ultrasonography
Immobilization
  Abdominal Wall 2W33X
  Arm
    Lower
      Left 2W3DX
      Right 2W3CX
    Upper
      Left 2W3BX
      Right 2W3AX
  Back 2W35X
  Chest Wall 2W34X
  Extremity
    Lower
      Left 2W3MX
      Right 2W3LX
    Upper
      Left 2W39X
      Right 2W38X

Immobilization — *continued*
  Face 2W31X
  Finger
    Left 2W3KX
    Right 2W3JX
  Foot
    Left 2W3TX
    Right 2W3SX
  Hand
    Left 2W3FX
    Right 2W3EX
  Head 2W30X
  Inguinal Region
    Left 2W37X
    Right 2W36X
  Leg
    Lower
      Left 2W3RX
      Right 2W3QX
    Upper
      Left 2W3PX
      Right 2W3NX
  Neck 2W32X
  Thumb
    Left 2W3HX
    Right 2W3GX
  Toe
    Left 2W3VX
    Right 2W3UX
Immunization
  see Introduction of Serum, Toxoid, and Vaccine
Immunotherapy
  see Introduction of Immunotherapeutic Substance
Immunotherapy, antineoplastic
  Interferon *see* Introduction of Low-dose Interleukin-2
  Interleukin-2, high-dose *see* Introduction of High-dose Interleukin-2
  Interleukin-2, low-dose *see* Introduction of Low dose Interleukin-2
  Monoclonal antibody *see* Introduction of Monoclonal Antibody
  Proleukin, high-dose *see* Introduction of High-dose Interleukin-2
  Proleukin, low-dose *see* Introduction of Low-dose Interleukin-2
Impella® heart pump
  use Short-term External Heart Assist System in Heart and Great Vessels
Impeller Pump
  Continuous, Output 5A0221D
  Intermittent, Output 5A0211D
Implantable cardioverter-defibrillator (ICD)
  use Defibrillator Generator in 0JH
Implantable drug infusion pump (anti-spasmodic)(chemotherapy)(pain)
  use Infusion Device, Pump in Subcutaneous Tissue and Fascia
Implantable glucose monitoring device
  use Monitoring Device
Implantable hemodynamic monitor (IHM)
  use Monitoring Device, Hemodynamic in 0JH
Implantable hemodynamic monitoring system (IHMS)
  use Monitoring Device, Hemodynamic in 0JH
Implantable Miniature Telescope™ (IMT)
  use Synthetic Substitute, Intraocular Telescope in 08R
Implantation
  see Replacement
  see Insertion

Implanted (venous)(access) port
  use Vascular Access Device, Totally Implantable in Subcutaneous Tissue and Fascia
IMV (intermittent mandatory ventilation)
  see Assistance, Respiratory 5A09
In Vitro Fertilization 8E0ZXY1
Incision, abscess
  see Drainage
Incudectomy
  see Excision, Ear, Nose, Sinus 09B
  see Resection, Ear, Nose, Sinus 09T
Incudopexy
  see Repair, Ear, Nose, Sinus 09Q
  see Reposition, Ear, Nose, Sinus 09S
Incus
  use Auditory Ossicle, Right
  use Auditory Ossicle, Left
Induction of labor
  Artificial rupture of membranes *see* Drainage, Pregnancy 109
  Oxytocin *see* Introduction of Hormone
InDura®, intrathecal catheter (1P) (spinal)
  use Infusion Device
Inferior cardiac nerve
  use Thoracic Sympathetic Nerve
Inferior cerebellar vein
  use Intracranial Vein
Inferior cerebral vein
  use Intracranial Vein
Inferior epigastric artery
  use External Iliac Artery, Right
  use External Iliac Artery, Left
Inferior epigastric lymph node
  use Lymphatic, Pelvis
Inferior genicular artery
  use Popliteal Artery, Right
  use Popliteal Artery, Left
Inferior gluteal artery
  use Internal Iliac Artery, Right
  use Internal Iliac Artery, Left
Inferior gluteal nerve
  use Sacral Plexus
Inferior hypogastric plexus
  use Abdominal Sympathetic Nerve
Inferior labial artery
  use Face Artery
Inferior longitudinal muscle
  use Tongue, Palate, Pharynx Muscle
Inferior mesenteric ganglion
  use Abdominal Sympathetic Nerve
Inferior mesenteric lymph node
  use Lymphatic, Mesenteric
Inferior mesenteric plexus
  use Abdominal Sympathetic Nerve
Inferior oblique muscle
  use Extraocular Muscle, Right
  use Extraocular Muscle, Left
Inferior pancreaticoduodenal artery
  use Superior Mesenteric Artery
Inferior phrenic artery
  use Abdominal Aorta
Inferior rectus muscle
  use Extraocular Muscle, Right
  use Extraocular Muscle, Left
Inferior suprarenal artery
  use Renal Artery, Right
  use Renal Artery, Left
Inferior tarsal plate
  use Lower Eyelid, Right
  use Lower Eyelid, Left
Inferior thyroid vein
  use Innominate Vein, Right
  use Innominate Vein, Left
Inferior tibiofibular joint
  use Ankle Joint, Right
  use Ankle Joint, Left

Inferior turbinate
 use Nasal Turbinate
Inferior ulnar collateral artery
 use Brachial Artery, Right
 use Brachial Artery, Left
Inferior vesical artery
 use Internal Iliac Artery, Right
 use Internal Iliac Artery, Left
Infraauricular lymph node
 use Lymphatic, Head
Infraclavicular (deltopectoral) lymph node
 use Lymphatic, Right Upper Extremity
 use Lymphatic, Left Upper Extremity
Infrahyoid muscle
 use Neck Muscle, Right
 use Neck Muscle, Left
Infraparotid lymph node
 use Lymphatic, Head
Infraspinatus fascia
 use Subcutaneous Tissue and Fascia, Right
 Upper Arm
 use Subcutaneous Tissue and Fascia, Left
 Upper Arm
Infraspinatus muscle
 use Shoulder Muscle, Right
 use Shoulder Muscle, Left
Infundibulopelvic ligament
 use Uterine Supporting Structure
Infusion
 see Introduction of substance in or on
Infusion Device, Pump
 Insertion of device in
 Abdomen 0JH8
 Back 0JH7
 Chest 0JH6
 Lower Arm
 Left 0JHH
 Right 0JHG
 Lower Leg
 Left 0JHP
 Right 0JHN
 Trunk 0JHT
 Upper Arm
 Left 0JHF
 Right 0JHD
 Upper Leg
 Left 0JHM
 Right 0JHL
 Removal of device from
 Lower Extremity 0JPW
 Trunk 0JPT
 Upper Extremity 0JPV
 Revision of device in
 Lower Extremity 0JWW
 Trunk 0JWT
 Upper Extremity 0JWV
Infusion, glucarpidase
 Central vein 3E043GQ
 Peripheral vein 3E033GQ
Inguinal canal
 use Inguinal Region, Right
 use Inguinal Region, Left
 use Inguinal Region, Bilateral
Inguinal triangle
 use Inguinal Region, Right
 use Inguinal Region, Left
 use Inguinal Region, Bilateral
Injection
 see Introduction of substance in or on
Injection reservoir, port
 use Vascular Access Device, Totally
 Implantable in Subcutaneous Tissue and
 Fascia
Injection reservoir, pump
 use Infusion Device, Pump in Subcutaneous
 Tissue and Fascia

Injection, Concentrated Bone Marrow Aspirate (CBMA), intramuscular XK02303
Insemination, artificial 3E0P7LZ
Insertion
 Antimicrobial envelope *see* Introduction of Anti-infective
 Aqueous drainage shunt
 see Bypass, Eye 081
 see Drainage, Eye 089
 Products of Conception 10H0
 Spinal Stabilization Device
 see Insertion of device in, Upper
 Joints 0RH
 see Insertion of device in, Lower
 Joints 0SH
Insertion of device in
 Abdominal Wall 0WHF
 Acetabulum
 Left 0QH5
 Right 0QH4
 Anal Sphincter 0DHR
 Ankle Region
 Left 0YHL
 Right 0YHK
 Anus 0DHQ
 Aorta
 Abdominal 04H0
 Thoracic
 Ascending/Arch 02HX
 Descending 02HW
 Arm
 Lower
 Left 0XHF
 Right 0XHD
 Upper
 Left 0XH9
 Right 0XH8
 Artery
 Anterior Tibial
 Left 04HQ
 Right 04HP
 Axillary
 Left 03H6
 Right 03H5
 Brachial
 Left 03H8
 Right 03H7
 Celiac 04H1
 Colic
 Left 04H7
 Middle 04H8
 Right 04H6
 Common Carotid
 Left 03HJ
 Right 03HH
 Common Iliac
 Left 04HD
 Right 04HC
 External Carotid
 Left 03HN
 Right 03HM
 External Iliac
 Left 04HJ
 Right 04HH
 Face 03HR
 Femoral
 Left 04HL
 Right 04HK
 Foot
 Left 04HW
 Right 04HV
 Gastric 04H2
 Hand
 Left 03HF
 Right 03HD
 Hepatic 04H3
 Inferior Mesenteric 04HB

Insertion of device in — *continued*
 Artery — *continued*
 Innominate 03H2
 Internal Carotid
 Left 03HL
 Right 03HK
 Internal Iliac
 Left 04HF
 Right 04HE
 Internal Mammary
 Left 03H1
 Right 03H0
 Intracranial 03HG
 Lower 04HY
 Peroneal
 Left 04HU
 Right 04HT
 Popliteal
 Left 04HN
 Right 04HM
 Posterior Tibial
 Left 04HS
 Right 04HR
 Pulmonary
 Left 02HR
 Right 02HQ
 Pulmonary Trunk 02HP
 Radial
 Left 03HC
 Right 03HB
 Renal
 Left 04HA
 Right 04H9
 Splenic 04H4
 Subclavian
 Left 03H4
 Right 03H3
 Superior Mesenteric 04H5
 Temporal
 Left 03HT
 Right 03HS
 Thyroid
 Left 03HV
 Right 03HU
 Ulnar
 Left 03HA
 Right 03H9
 Upper 03HY
 Vertebral
 Left 03HQ
 Right 03HP
 Atrium
 Left 02H7
 Right 02H6
 Axilla
 Left 0XH5
 Right 0XH4
 Back
 Lower 0WHL
 Upper 0WHK
 Bladder 0THB
 Bladder Neck 0THC
 Bone
 Ethmoid
 Left 0NHG
 Right 0NHF
 Facial 0NHW
 Frontal 0NH1
 Hyoid 0NHX
 Lacrimal
 Left 0NHJ
 Right 0NHH
 Lower 0QHY
 Nasal 0NHB
 Occipital 0NH7
 Palatine
 Left 0NHL
 Right 0NHK

Insertion of device in — *continued*
- Bone — *continued*
  - Parietal
    - Left 0NH4
    - Right 0NH3
  - Pelvic
    - Left 0QH3
    - Right 0QH2
  - Sphenoid 0NHC
  - Temporal
    - Left 0NH6
    - Right 0NH5
  - Upper 0PHY
  - Zygomatic
    - Left 0NHN
    - Right 0NHM
- Brain 00H0
- Breast
  - Bilateral 0HHV
  - Left 0HHU
  - Right 0HHT
- Bronchus
  - Lingula 0BH9
  - Lower Lobe
    - Left 0BHB
    - Right 0BH6
  - Main
    - Left 0BH7
    - Right 0BH3
  - Middle Lobe, Right 0BH5
  - Upper Lobe
    - Left 0BH8
    - Right 0BH4
- Bursa and Ligament
  - Lower 0MHY
  - Upper 0MHX
- Buttock
  - Left 0YH1
  - Right 0YH0
- Carpal
  - Left 0PHN
  - Right 0PHM
- Cavity, Cranial 0WH1
- Cerebral Ventricle 00H6
- Cervix 0UHC
- Chest Wall 0WH8
- Cisterna Chyli 07HL
- Clavicle
  - Left 0PHB
  - Right 0PH9
- Coccyx 0QHS
- Cul-de-sac 0UHF
- Diaphragm 0BHT
- Disc
  - Cervical Vertebral 0RH3
  - Cervicothoracic Vertebral 0RH5
  - Lumbar Vertebral 0SH2
  - Lumbosacral 0SH4
  - Thoracic Vertebral 0RH9
  - Thoracolumbar Vertebral 0RHB
- Duct
  - Hepatobiliary 0FHB
  - Pancreatic 0FHD
- Duodenum 0DH9
- Ear
  - Inner
    - Left 09HE
    - Right 09HD
  - Left 09HJ
  - Right 09HH
- Elbow Region
  - Left 0XHC
  - Right 0XHB
- Epididymis and Spermatic Cord 0VHM
- Esophagus 0DH5
- Extremity
  - Lower

Insertion of device in — *continued*
- Extremity — *continued*
  - Left 0YHB
  - Right 0YH9
  - Upper
    - Left 0XH7
    - Right 0XH6
- Eye
  - Left 08H1
  - Right 08H0
- Face 0WH2
- Fallopian Tube 0UH8
- Femoral Region
  - Left 0YH8
  - Right 0YH7
- Femoral Shaft
  - Left 0QH9
  - Right 0QH8
- Femur
  - Lower
    - Left 0QHC
    - Right 0QHB
  - Upper
    - Left 0QH7
    - Right 0QH6
- Fibula
  - Left 0QHK
  - Right 0QHJ
- Foot
  - Left 0YHN
  - Right 0YHM
- Gallbladder 0FH4
- Gastrointestinal Tract 0WHP
- Genitourinary Tract 0WHR
- Gland
  - Endocrine 0GHS
  - Salivary 0CHA
- Glenoid Cavity
  - Left 0PH8
  - Right 0PH7
- Hand
  - Left 0XHK
  - Right 0XHJ
- Head 0WH0
- Heart 02HA
- Humeral Head
  - Left 0PHD
  - Right 0PHC
- Humeral Shaft
  - Left 0PHG
  - Right 0PHF
- Ileum 0DHB
- Inguinal Region
  - Left 0YH6
  - Right 0YH5
- Intestinal Tract
  - Lower 0DHD
  - Upper 0DH0
- Intestine
  - Large 0DHE
  - Small 0DH8
- Jaw
  - Lower 0WH5
  - Upper 0WH4
- Jejunum 0DHA
- Joint
  - Acromioclavicular
    - Left 0RHH
    - Right 0RHG
  - Ankle
    - Left 0SHG
    - Right 0SHF
  - Carpal
    - Left 0RHR
    - Right 0RHQ
  - Carpometacarpal
    - Left 0RHT

Insertion of device in — *continued*
- Joint — *continued*
  - Right 0RHS
  - Cervical Vertebral 0RH1
  - Cervicothoracic Vertebral 0RH4
  - Coccygeal 0SH6
  - Elbow
    - Left 0RHM
    - Right 0RHL
  - Finger Phalangeal
    - Left 0RHX
    - Right 0RHW
  - Hip
    - Left 0SHB
    - Right 0SH9
  - Knee
    - Left 0SHD
    - Right 0SHC
  - Lumbar Vertebral 0SH0
  - Lumbosacral 0SH3
  - Metacarpophalangeal
    - Left 0RHV
    - Right 0RHU
  - Metatarsal-Phalangeal
    - Left 0SHN
    - Right 0SHM
  - Occipital-cervical 0RH0
  - Sacrococcygeal 0SH5
  - Sacroiliac
    - Left 0SH8
    - Right 0SH7
  - Shoulder
    - Left 0RHK
    - Right 0RHJ
  - Sternoclavicular
    - Left 0RHF
    - Right 0RHE
  - Tarsal
    - Left 0SHJ
    - Right 0SHH
  - Tarsometatarsal
    - Left 0SHL
    - Right 0SHK
  - Temporomandibular
    - Left 0RHD
    - Right 0RHC
  - Thoracic Vertebral 0RH6
  - Thoracolumbar Vertebral 0RHA
  - Toe Phalangeal
    - Left 0SHQ
    - Right 0SHP
  - Wrist
    - Left 0RHP
    - Right 0RHN
- Kidney 0TH5
- Knee Region
  - Left 0YHG
  - Right 0YHF
- Larynx 0CHS
- Leg
  - Lower
    - Left 0YHJ
    - Right 0YHH
  - Upper
    - Left 0YHD
    - Right 0YHC
- Liver 0FH0
  - Left Lobe 0FH2
  - Right Lobe 0FH1
- Lung
  - Left 0BHL
  - Right 0BHK
- Lymphatic 07HN
  - Thoracic Duct 07HK
- Mandible
  - Left 0NHV
  - Right 0NHT

Insertion of device in — *continued*
Maxilla 0NHR
Mediastinum 0WHC
Metacarpal
  Left 0PHQ
  Right 0PHP
Metatarsal
  Left 0QHP
  Right 0QHN
Mouth and Throat 0CHY
Muscle
  Lower 0KHY
  Upper 0KHX
Nasal Mucosa and Soft Tissue 09HK
Nasopharynx 09HN
Neck 0WH6
Nerve
  Cranial 00HE
  Peripheral 01HY
Nipple
  Left 0HHX
  Right 0HHW
Oral Cavity and Throat 0WH3
Orbit
  Left 0NHQ
  Right 0NHP
Ovary 0UH3
Pancreas 0FHG
Patella
  Left 0QHF
  Right 0QHD
Pelvic Cavity 0WHJ
Penis 0VHS
Pericardial Cavity 0WHD
Pericardium 02HN
Perineum
  Female 0WHN
  Male 0WHM
Peritoneal Cavity 0WHG
Phalanx
  Finger
    Left 0PHV
    Right 0PHT
  Thumb
    Left 0PHS
    Right 0PHR
  Toe
    Left 0QHR
    Right 0QHQ
Pleura 0BHQ
Pleural Cavity
  Left 0WHB
  Right 0WH9
Prostate 0VH0
Prostate and Seminal Vesicles 0VH4
Radius
  Left 0PHJ
  Right 0PHH
Rectum 0DHP
Respiratory Tract 0WHQ
Retroperitoneum 0WHH
Ribs
  1 to 2 0PH1
  3 or More 0PH2
Sacrum 0QH1
Scapula
  Left 0PH6
  Right 0PH5
Scrotum and Tunica Vaginalis 0VH8
Shoulder Region
  Left 0XH3
  Right 0XH2
Sinus 09HY
Skin 0HHPXYZ
Skull 0NH0
Spinal Canal 00HU
Spinal Cord 00HV

Insertion of device in — *continued*
Spleen 07HP
Sternum 0PH0
Stomach 0DH6
Subcutaneous Tissue and Fascia
  Abdomen 0JH8
  Back 0JH7
  Buttock 0JH9
  Chest 0JH6
  Face 0JH1
  Foot
    Left 0JHR
    Right 0JHQ
  Hand
    Left 0JHK
    Right 0JHJ
  Head and Neck 0JHS
  Lower Arm
    Left 0JHH
    Right 0JHG
  Lower Extremity 0JHW
  Lower Leg
    Left 0JHP
    Right 0JHN
  Neck
    Left 0JH5
    Right 0JH4
  Pelvic Region 0JHC
  Perineum 0JHB
  Scalp 0JH0
  Trunk 0JHT
  Upper Arm
    Left 0JHF
    Right 0JHD
  Upper Extremity 0JHV
  Upper Leg
    Left 0JHM
    Right 0JHL
Tarsal
  Left 0QHM
  Right 0QHL
Tendon
  Lower 0LHY
  Upper 0LHX
Testis 0VHD
Thymus 07HM
Tibia
  Left 0QHH
  Right 0QHG
Tongue 0CH7
Trachea 0BH1
Tracheobronchial Tree 0BH0
Ulna
  Left 0PHL
  Right 0PHK
Ureter 0TH9
Urethra 0THD
Uterus 0UH9
Uterus and Cervix 0UHD
Vagina 0UHG
Vagina and Cul-de-sac 0UHH
Vas Deferens 0VHR
Vein
  Axillary
    Left 05H8
    Right 05H7
  Azygos 05H0
  Basilic
    Left 05HC
    Right 05HB
  Brachial
    Left 05HA
    Right 05H9
  Cephalic
    Left 05HF
    Right 05HD
  Colic 06H7

Insertion of device in — *continued*
Vein — *continued*
  Common Iliac
    Left 06HD
    Right 06HC
  Coronary 02H4
  Esophageal 06H3
  External Iliac
    Left 06HG
    Right 06HF
  External Jugular
    Left 05HQ
    Right 05HP
  Face
    Left 05HV
    Right 05HT
  Femoral
    Left 06HN
    Right 06HM
  Foot
    Left 06HV
    Right 06HT
  Gastric 06H2
  Hand
    Left 05HH
    Right 05HG
  Hemiazygos 05H1
  Hepatic 06H4
  Hypogastric
    Left 06HJ
    Right 06HH
  Inferior Mesenteric 06H6
  Innominate
    Left 05H4
    Right 05H3
  Internal Jugular
    Left 05HN
    Right 05HM
  Intracranial 05HL
  Lower 06HY
  Portal 06H8
  Pulmonary
    Left 02HT
    Right 02HS
  Renal
    Left 06HB
    Right 06H9
  Saphenous
    Left 06HQ
    Right 06HP
  Splenic 06H1
  Subclavian
    Left 05H6
    Right 05H5
  Superior Mesenteric 06H5
  Upper 05HY
  Vertebral
    Left 05HS
    Right 05HR
Vena Cava
  Inferior 06H0
  Superior 02HV
Ventricle
  Left 02HL
  Right 02HK
Vertebra
  Cervical 0PH3
  Lumbar 0QH0
  Thoracic 0PH4
Wrist Region
  Left 0XHH
  Right 0XHG
Inspection
  Abdominal Wall 0WJF
  Ankle Region
    Left 0YJL
    Right 0YJK

Inspection — *continued*

Arm
  Lower
    Left 0XJF
    Right 0XJD
  Upper
    Left 0XJ9
    Right 0XJ8
Artery
  Lower 04JY
  Upper 03JY
Axilla
  Left 0XJ5
  Right 0XJ4
Back
  Lower 0WJL
  Upper 0WJK
Bladder 0TJB
Bone
  Facial 0NJW
  Lower 0QJY
  Nasal 0NJB
  Upper 0PJY
Bone Marrow 07JT
Brain 00J0
Breast
  Left 0HJU
  Right 0HJT
Bursa and Ligament
  Lower 0MJY
  Upper 0MJX
Buttock
  Left 0YJ1
  Right 0YJ0
Cavity, Cranial 0WJ1
Chest Wall 0WJ8
Cisterna Chyli 07JL
Diaphragm 0BJT
Disc
  Cervical Vertebral 0RJ3
  Cervicothoracic Vertebral 0RJ5
  Lumbar Vertebral 0SJ2
  Lumbosacral 0SJ4
  Thoracic Vertebral 0RJ9
  Thoracolumbar Vertebral 0RJB
Duct
  Hepatobiliary 0FJB
  Pancreatic 0FJD
Ear
  Inner
    Left 09JE
    Right 09JD
  Left 09JJ
  Right 09JH
Elbow Region
  Left 0XJC
  Right 0XJB
Epididymis and Spermatic Cord 0VJM
Extremity
  Lower
    Left 0YJB
    Right 0YJ9
  Upper
    Left 0XJ7
    Right 0XJ6
Eye
  Left 08J1XZZ
  Right 08J0XZZ
Face 0WJ2
Fallopian Tube 0UJ8
Femoral Region
  Bilateral 0YJE
  Left 0YJ8
  Right 0YJ7
Finger Nail 0HJQXZZ
Foot
  Left 0YJN
  Right 0YJM

Inspection — *continued*

Gallbladder 0FJ4
Gastrointestinal Tract 0WJP
Genitourinary Tract 0WJR
Gland
  Adrenal 0GJ5
  Endocrine 0GJS
  Pituitary 0GJ0
  Salivary 0CJA
Great Vessel 02JY
Hand
  Left 0XJK
  Right 0XJJ
Head 0WJ0
Heart 02JA
Inguinal Region
  Bilateral 0YJA
  Left 0YJ6
  Right 0YJ5
Intestinal Tract
  Lower 0DJD
  Upper 0DJ0
Jaw
  Lower 0WJ5
  Upper 0WJ4
Joint
  Acromioclavicular
    Left 0RJH
    Right 0RJG
  Ankle
    Left 0SJG
    Right 0SJF
  Carpal
    Left 0RJR
    Right 0RJQ
  Carpometacarpal
    Left 0RJT
    Right 0RJS
  Cervical Vertebral 0RJ1
  Cervicothoracic Vertebral 0RJ4
  Coccygeal 0SJ6
  Elbow
    Left 0RJM
    Right 0RJL
  Finger Phalangeal
    Left 0RJX
    Right 0RJW
  Hip
    Left 0SJB
    Right 0SJ9
  Knee
    Left 0SJD
    Right 0SJC
  Lumbar Vertebral 0SJ0
  Lumbosacral 0SJ3
  Metacarpophalangeal
    Left 0RJV
    Right 0RJU
  Metatarsal-Phalangeal
    Left 0SJN
    Right 0SJM
  Occipital-cervical 0RJ0
  Sacrococcygeal 0SJ5
  Sacroiliac
    Left 0SJ8
    Right 0SJ7
  Shoulder
    Left 0RJK
    Right 0RJJ
  Sternoclavicular
    Left 0RJF
    Right 0RJE
  Tarsal
    Left 0SJJ
    Right 0SJH
  Tarsometatarsal
    Left 0SJL
    Right 0SJK

Inspection — *continued*

Joint — *continued*
  Temporomandibular
    Left 0RJD
    Right 0RJC
  Thoracic Vertebral 0RJ6
  Thoracolumbar Vertebral 0RJA
  Toe Phalangeal
    Left 0SJQ
    Right 0SJP
  Wrist
    Left 0RJP
    Right 0RJN
Kidney 0TJ5
Knee Region
  Left 0YJG
  Right 0YJF
Larynx 0CJS
Leg
  Lower
    Left 0YJJ
    Right 0YJH
  Upper
    Left 0YJD
    Right 0YJC
Lens
  Left 08JKXZZ
  Right 08JJXZZ
Liver 0FJ0
Lung
  Left 0BJL
  Right 0BJK
Lymphatic 07JN
  Thoracic Duct 07JK
Mediastinum 0WJC
Mesentery 0DJV
Mouth and Throat 0CJY
Muscle
  Extraocular
    Left 08JM
    Right 08JL
  Lower 0KJY
  Upper 0KJX
Nasal Mucosa and Soft Tissue 09JK
Neck 0WJ6
Nerve
  Cranial 00JE
  Peripheral 01JY
Omentum 0DJU
Oral Cavity and Throat 0WJ3
Ovary 0UJ3
Pancreas 0FJG
Parathyroid Gland 0GJR
Pelvic Cavity 0WJJ
Penis 0VJS
Pericardial Cavity 0WJD
Perineum
  Female 0WJN
  Male 0WJM
Peritoneal Cavity 0WJG
Peritoneum 0DJW
Pineal Body 0GJ1
Pleura 0BJQ
Pleural Cavity
  Left 0WJB
  Right 0WJ9
Products of Conception 10J0
  Ectopic 10J2
  Retained 10J1
Prostate and Seminal Vesicles 0VJ4
Respiratory Tract 0WJQ
Retroperitoneum 0WJH
Scrotum and Tunica Vaginalis 0VJ8
Shoulder Region
  Left 0XJ3
  Right 0XJ2
Sinus 09JY

Inspection — *continued*
  Skin 0HJPXZZ
  Skull 0NJ0
  Spinal Canal 00JU
  Spinal Cord 00JV
  Spleen 07JP
  Stomach 0DJ6
  Subcutaneous Tissue and Fascia
    Head and Neck 0JJS
    Lower Extremity 0JJW
    Trunk 0JJT
    Upper Extremity 0JJV
  Tendon
    Lower 0LJY
    Upper 0LJX
  Testis 0VJD
  Thymus 07JM
  Thyroid Gland 0GJK
  Toe Nail 0HJRXZZ
  Trachea 0BJ1
  Tracheobronchial Tree 0BJ0
  Tympanic Membrane
    Left 09J8
    Right 09J7
  Ureter 0TJ9
  Urethra 0TJD
  Uterus and Cervix 0UJD
  Vagina and Cul-de-sac 0UJH
  Vas Deferens 0VJR
  Vein
    Lower 06JY
    Upper 05JY
  Vulva 0UJM
  Wrist Region
    Left 0XJH
    Right 0XJG
Instillation
  see Introduction of substance in or on
Insufflation
  see Introduction of substance in or on
Interatrial septum
  use Atrial Septum
Interbody fusion (spine) cage
  use Interbody Fusion Device in Upper Joints
  use Interbody Fusion Device in Lower Joints
Interbody Fusion Device
  Nanotextured Surface
    Cervical Vertebral XRG1092
      2 or more XRG2092
    Cervicothoracic Vertebral XRG4092
    Lumbar Vertebral XRGB092
      2 or more XRGC092
    Lumbosacral XRGD092
    Occipital-cervical XRG0092
    Thoracic Vertebral XRG6092
      2 to 7 XRG7092
      8 or more XRG8092
    Thoracolumbar Vertebral XRGA092
  Radiolucent Porous
    Cervical Vertebral XRG10F3
      2 or more XRG20F3
    Cervicothoracic Vertebral XRG40F3
    Lumbar Vertebral XRGB0F3
      2 or more XRGC0F3
    Lumbosacral XRGD0F3
    Occipital-cervical XRG00F3
    Thoracic Vertebral XRG60F3
      2 to 7 XRG70F3
      8 or more XRG80F3
    Thoracolumbar Vertebral XRGA0F3
Intercarpal joint
  use Carpal Joint, Right
  use Carpal Joint, Left
Intercarpal ligament
  use Hand Bursa and Ligament, Right
  use Hand Bursa and Ligament, Left

Interclavicular ligament
  use Shoulder Bursa and Ligament, Right
  use Shoulder Bursa and Ligament, Left
Intercostal lymph node
  use Lymphatic, Thorax
Intercostal muscle
  use Thorax Muscle, Right
  use Thorax Muscle, Left
Intercostal nerve
  use Thoracic Nerve
Intercostobrachial nerve
  use Thoracic Nerve
Intercuneiform joint
  use Tarsal Joint, Right
  use Tarsal Joint, Left
Intercuneiform ligament
  use Foot Bursa and Ligament, Right
  use Foot Bursa and Ligament, Left
Intermediate bronchus
  use Main Bronchus, Right
Intermediate cuneiform bone
  use Tarsal, Right
  use Tarsal, Left
Intermittent hemodialysis (IHD) 5A1D70Z
Intermittent mandatory ventilation
  see Assistance, Respiratory 5A09
Intermittent Negative Airway Pressure
  24-96 Consecutive Hours, Ventilation 5A0945B
  Greater than 96 Consecutive Hours, Ventilation 5A0955B
  Less than 24 Consecutive Hours, Ventilation 5A0935B
Intermittent Positive Airway Pressure
  24-96 Consecutive Hours, Ventilation 5A09458
  Greater than 96 Consecutive Hours, Ventilation 5A09558
  Less than 24 Consecutive Hours, Ventilation 5A09358
Intermittent positive pressure breathing
  see Assistance, Respiratory 5A09
Internal (basal) cerebral vein
  use Intracranial Vein
Internal anal sphincter
  use Anal Sphincter
Internal carotid artery, intracranial portion
  use Intracranial Artery
Internal carotid plexus
  use Head and Neck Sympathetic Nerve
Internal iliac vein
  use Hypogastric Vein, Right
  use Hypogastric Vein, Left
Internal maxillary artery
  use External Carotid Artery, Right
  use External Carotid Artery, Left
Internal naris
  use Nasal Mucosa and Soft Tissue
Internal oblique muscle
  use Abdomen Muscle, Right
  use Abdomen Muscle, Left
Internal pudendal artery
  use Internal Iliac Artery, Right
  use Internal Iliac Artery, Left
Internal pudendal vein
  use Hypogastric Vein, Right
  use Hypogastric Vein, Left
Internal thoracic artery
  use Internal Mammary Artery, Right
  use Internal Mammary Artery, Left
  use Subclavian Artery, Right
  use Subclavian Artery, Left
Internal urethral sphincter
  use Urethra
Interphalangeal (IP) joint
  use Finger Phalangeal Joint, Right
  use Finger Phalangeal Joint, Left

Interphalangeal (IP) joint — *continued*
  use Toe Phalangeal Joint, Right
  use Toe Phalangeal Joint, Left
Interphalangeal ligament
  use Hand Bursa and Ligament, Right
  use Hand Bursa and Ligament, Left
  use Foot Bursa and Ligament, Right
  use Foot Bursa and Ligament, Left
Interrogation, cardiac rhythm related device
  Interrogation only *see* Measurement, Cardiac 4B02
  With cardiac function testing *see* Measurement, Cardiac 4A02
Interruption
  see Occlusion
Interspinalis muscle
  use Trunk Muscle, Right
  use Trunk Muscle, Left
Interspinous ligament
  use Head and Neck Bursa and Ligament
  use Upper Spine Bursa and Ligament
  use Lower Spine Bursa and Ligament
Interspinous process spinal stabilization device
  use Spinal Stabilization Device, Interspinous Process in 0RH
  use Spinal Stabilization Device, Interspinous Process in 0SH
InterStim® Therapy lead
  use Neurostimulator Lead in Peripheral Nervous System
InterStim® Therapy neurostimulator
  use Stimulator Generator, Single Array in 0JH
Intertransversarius muscle
  use Trunk Muscle, Right
  use Trunk Muscle, Left
Intertransverse ligament
  use Upper Spine Bursa and Ligament
  use Lower Spine Bursa and Ligament
Interventricular foramen (Monro)
  use Cerebral Ventricle
Interventricular septum
  use Ventricular Septum
Intestinal lymphatic trunk
  use Cisterna Chyli
Intraluminal Device
  Airway
    Esophagus 0DH5
    Mouth and Throat 0CHY
    Nasopharynx 09HN
  Bioactive
    Occlusion
      Common Carotid
        Left 03LJ
        Right 03LH
      External Carotid
        Left 03LN
        Right 03LM
      Internal Carotid
        Left 03LL
        Right 03LK
      Intracranial 03LG
      Vertebral
        Left 03LQ
        Right 03LP
    Restriction
      Common Carotid
        Left 03VJ
        Right 03VH
      External Carotid
        Left 03VN
        Right 03VM
      Internal Carotid
        Left 03VL
        Right 03VK

Intraluminal Device — *continued*
  Bioactive — *continued*
    Intracranial 03VG
    Vertebral
      Left 03VQ
      Right 03VP
  Endobronchial Valve
    Lingula 0BH9
    Lower Lobe
      Left 0BHB
      Right 0BH6
    Main
      Left 0BH7
      Right 0BH3
    Middle Lobe, Right 0BH5
    Upper Lobe
      Left 0BH8
      Right 0BH4
  Endotracheal Airway
    Change device in, Trachea 0B21XEZ
    Insertion of device in, Trachea 0BH1
  Pessary
    Change device in, Vagina and Cul-de-sac 0U2HXGZ
    Insertion of device in
      Cul-de-sac 0UHF
      Vagina 0UHG
Intramedullary (IM) rod (nail)
  use Internal Fixation Device, Intramedullary in Upper Bones
  use Internal Fixation Device, Intramedullary in Lower Bones
Intramedullary skeletal kinetic distractor (ISKD)
  use Internal Fixation Device, Intramedullary in Upper Bones
  use Internal Fixation Device, Intramedullary in Lower Bones
Intraocular Telescope
  Left 08RK30Z
  Right 08RJ30Z
Intraoperative Knee Replacement Sensor XR2
Intraoperative Radiation Therapy (IORT)
  Anus DDY8CZZ
  Bile Ducts DFY2CZZ
  Bladder DTY2CZZ
  Cervix DUY1CZZ
  Colon DDY5CZZ
  Duodenum DDY2CZZ
  Gallbladder DFY1CZZ
  Ileum DDY4CZZ
  Jejunum DDY3CZZ
  Kidney DTY0CZZ
  Larynx D9YBCZZ
  Liver DFY0CZZ
  Mouth D9Y4CZZ
  Nasopharynx D9YDCZZ
  Ovary DUY0CZZ
  Pancreas DFY3CZZ
  Pharynx D9YCCZZ
  Prostate DVY0CZZ
  Rectum DDY7CZZ
  Stomach DDY1CZZ
  Ureter DTY1CZZ
  Urethra DTY3CZZ
  Uterus DUY2CZZ
Intrauterine device (IUD)
  use Contraceptive Device in Female Reproductive System
Intravascular fluorescence angiography (IFA)
  see Monitoring, Physiological Systems 4A1
Introduction of substance in or on
  Artery
    Central 3E06
      Analgesics 3E06

Introduction of substance in or on — *continued*
  Artery — *continued*
    Anesthetic, Intracirculatory 3E06
    Anti-infective 3E06
    Anti-inflammatory 3E06
    Antiarrhythmic 3E06
    Antineoplastic 3E06
    Destructive Agent 3E06
    Diagnostic Substance, Other 3E06
    Electrolytic Substance 3E06
    Hormone 3E06
    Hypnotics 3E06
    Immunotherapeutic 3E06
    Nutritional Substance 3E06
    Platelet Inhibitor 3E06
    Radioactive Substance 3E06
    Sedatives 3E06
    Serum 3E06
    Thrombolytic 3E06
    Toxoid 3E06
    Vaccine 3E06
    Vasopressor 3E06
    Water Balance Substance 3E06
    Coronary 3E07
      Diagnostic Substance, Other 3E07
      Platelet Inhibitor 3E07
      Thrombolytic 3E07
    Peripheral 3E05
      Analgesics 3E05
      Anesthetic, Intracirculatory 3E05
      Anti-infective 3E05
      Anti-inflammatory 3E05
      Antiarrhythmic 3E05
      Antineoplastic 3E05
      Destructive Agent 3E05
      Diagnostic Substance, Other 3E05
      Electrolytic Substance 3E05
      Hormone 3E05
      Hypnotics 3E05
      Immunotherapeutic 3E05
      Nutritional Substance 3E05
      Platelet Inhibitor 3E05
      Radioactive Substance 3E05
      Sedatives 3E05
      Serum 3E05
      Thrombolytic 3E05
      Toxoid 3E05
      Vaccine 3E05
      Vasopressor 3E05
      Water Balance Substance 3E05
  Biliary Tract 3E0J
    Analgesics 3E0J
    Anesthetic Agent 3E0J
    Anti-infective 3E0J
    Anti-inflammatory 3E0J
    Antineoplastic 3E0J
    Destructive Agent 3E0J
    Diagnostic Substance, Other 3E0J
    Electrolytic Substance 3E0J
    Gas 3E0J
    Hypnotics 3E0J
    Islet Cells, Pancreatic 3E0J
    Nutritional Substance 3E0J
    Radioactive Substance 3E0J
    Sedatives 3E0J
    Water Balance Substance 3E0J
  Bone 3E0V
    Analgesics 3E0V3NZ
    Anesthetic Agent 3E0V3BZ
    Anti-infective 3E0V32
    Anti-inflammatory 3E0V33Z
    Antineoplastic 3E0V30
    Destructive Agent 3E0V3TZ
    Diagnostic Substance, Other 3E0V3KZ
    Electrolytic Substance 3E0V37Z
    Hypnotics 3E0V3NZ
    Nutritional Substance 3E0V36Z

Introduction of substance in or on — *continued*
  Bone — *continued*
    Radioactive Substance 3E0V3HZ
    Sedatives 3E0V3NZ
    Water Balance Substance 3E0V37Z
  Bone Marrow 3E0A3GC
    Antineoplastic 3E0A30
  Brain 3E0Q
    Analgesics 3E0Q
    Anesthetic Agent 3E0Q
    Anti-infective 3E0Q
    Anti-inflammatory 3E0Q
    Antineoplastic 3E0Q
    Destructive Agent 3E0Q
    Diagnostic Substance, Other 3E0Q
    Electrolytic Substance 3E0Q
    Gas 3E0Q
    Hypnotics 3E0Q
    Nutritional Substance 3E0Q
    Radioactive Substance 3E0Q
    Sedatives 3E0Q
    Stem Cells
      Embryonic 3E0Q
      Somatic 3E0Q
    Water Balance Substance 3E0Q
  Cranial Cavity 3E0Q
    Analgesics 3E0Q
    Anesthetic Agent 3E0Q
    Anti-infective 3E0Q
    Anti-inflammatory 3E0Q
    Antineoplastic 3E0Q
    Destructive Agent 3E0Q
    Diagnostic Substance, Other 3E0Q
    Electrolytic Substance 3E0Q
    Gas 3E0Q
    Hypnotics 3E0Q
    Nutritional Substance 3E0Q
    Radioactive Substance 3E0Q
    Sedatives 3E0Q
    Stem Cells
      Embryonic 3E0Q
      Somatic 3E0Q
    Water Balance Substance 3E0Q
  Ear 3E0B
    Analgesics 3E0B
    Anesthetic Agent 3E0B
    Anti-infective 3E0B
    Anti-inflammatory 3E0B
    Antineoplastic 3E0B
    Destructive Agent 3E0B
    Diagnostic Substance, Other 3E0B
    Hypnotics 3E0B
    Radioactive Substance 3E0B
    Sedatives 3E0B
  Epidural Space 3E0S3GC
    Analgesics 3E0S3NZ
    Anesthetic Agent 3E0S3BZ
    Anti-infective 3E0S32
    Anti-inflammatory 3E0S33Z
    Antineoplastic 3E0S30
    Destructive Agent 3E0S3TZ
    Diagnostic Substance, Other 3E0S3KZ
    Electrolytic Substance 3E0S37Z
    Gas 3E0S
    Hypnotics 3E0S3NZ
    Nutritional Substance 3E0S36Z
    Radioactive Substance 3E0S3HZ
    Sedatives 3E0S3NZ
    Water Balance Substance 3E0S37Z
  Eye 3E0C
    Analgesics 3E0C
    Anesthetic Agent 3E0C
    Anti-infective 3E0C
    Anti-inflammatory 3E0C
    Antineoplastic 3E0C
    Destructive Agent 3E0C
    Diagnostic Substance, Other 3E0C

Introduction of substance in or on — *continued*
  Eye — *continued*
    Gas 3E0C
    Hypnotics 3E0C
    Pigment 3E0C
    Radioactive Substance 3E0C
    Sedatives 3E0C
  Gastrointestinal Tract
    Lower 3E0H
      Analgesics 3E0H
      Anesthetic Agent 3E0H
      Anti-infective 3E0H
      Anti-inflammatory 3E0H
      Antineoplastic 3E0H
      Destructive Agent 3E0H
      Diagnostic Substance, Other 3E0H
      Electrolytic Substance 3E0H
      Gas 3E0H
      Hypnotics 3E0H
      Nutritional Substance 3E0H
      Radioactive Substance 3E0H
      Sedatives 3E0H
      Water Balance Substance 3E0H
    Upper 3E0G
      Analgesics 3E0G
      Anesthetic Agent 3E0G
      Anti-infective 3E0G
      Anti-inflammatory 3E0G
      Antineoplastic 3E0G
      Destructive Agent 3E0G
      Diagnostic Substance, Other 3E0G
      Electrolytic Substance 3E0G
      Gas 3E0G
      Hypnotics 3E0G
      Nutritional Substance 3E0G
      Radioactive Substance 3E0G
      Sedatives 3E0G
      Water Balance Substance 3E0G
  Genitourinary Tract 3E0K
    Analgesics 3E0K
    Anesthetic Agent 3E0K
    Anti-infective 3E0K
    Anti-inflammatory 3E0K
    Antineoplastic 3E0K
    Destructive Agent 3E0K
    Diagnostic Substance, Other 3E0K
    Electrolytic Substance 3E0K
    Gas 3E0K
    Hypnotics 3E0K
    Nutritional Substance 3E0K
    Radioactive Substance 3E0K
    Sedatives 3E0K
    Water Balance Substance 3E0K
  Heart 3E08
    Diagnostic Substance, Other 3E08
    Platelet Inhibitor 3E08
    Thrombolytic 3E08
  Joint 3E0U
    Analgesics 3E0U3NZ
    Anesthetic Agent 3E0U3BZ
    Anti-infective 3E0U
    Anti-inflammatory 3E0U33Z
    Antineoplastic 3E0U30
    Destructive Agent 3E0U3TZ
    Diagnostic Substance, Other 3E0U3KZ
    Electrolytic Substance 3E0U37Z
    Gas 3E0U3SF
    Hypnotics 3E0U3NZ
    Nutritional Substance 3E0U36Z
    Radioactive Substance 3E0U3HZ
    Sedatives 3E0U3NZ
    Water Balance Substance 3E0U37Z
  Lymphatic 3E0W3GC
    Analgesics 3E0W3NZ
    Anesthetic Agent 3E0W3BZ
    Anti-infective 3E0W32
    Anti-inflammatory 3E0W33Z

Introduction of substance in or on — *continued*
  Lymphatic — *continued*
    Antineoplastic 3E0W30
    Destructive Agent 3E0W3TZ
    Diagnostic Substance, Other 3E0W3KZ
    Electrolytic Substance 3E0W37Z
    Hypnotics 3E0W3NZ
    Nutritional Substance 3E0W36Z
    Radioactive Substance 3E0W3HZ
    Sedatives 3E0W3NZ
    Water Balance Substance 3E0W37Z
  Mouth 3E0D
    Analgesics 3E0D
    Anesthetic Agent 3E0D
    Anti-infective 3E0D
    Anti-inflammatory 3E0D
    Antiarrhythmic 3E0D
    Antineoplastic 3E0D
    Destructive Agent 3E0D
    Diagnostic Substance, Other 3E0D
    Electrolytic Substance 3E0D
    Hypnotics 3E0D
    Nutritional Substance 3E0D
    Radioactive Substance 3E0D
    Sedatives 3E0D
    Serum 3E0D
    Toxoid 3E0D
    Vaccine 3E0D
    Water Balance Substance 3E0D
  Mucous Membrane 3E00XGC
    Analgesics 3E00XNZ
    Anesthetic Agent 3E00XBZ
    Anti-infective 3E00X2
    Anti-inflammatory 3E00X3Z
    Antineoplastic 3E00X0
    Destructive Agent 3E00XTZ
    Diagnostic Substance, Other 3E00XKZ
    Hypnotics 3E00XNZ
    Pigment 3E00XMZ
    Sedatives 3E00XNZ
    Serum 3E00X4Z
    Toxoid 3E00X4Z
    Vaccine 3E00X4Z
  Muscle 3E023GC
    Analgesics 3E023NZ
    Anesthetic Agent 3E023BZ
    Anti-infective 3E0232
    Anti-inflammatory 3E0233Z
    Antineoplastic 3E0230
    Destructive Agent 3E023TZ
    Diagnostic Substance, Other 3E023KZ
    Electrolytic Substance 3E0237Z
    Hypnotics 3E023NZ
    Nutritional Substance 3E0236Z
    Radioactive Substance 3E023HZ
    Sedatives 3E023NZ
    Serum 3E0234Z
    Toxoid 3E0234Z
    Vaccine 3E0234Z
    Water Balance Substance 3E0237Z
  Nerve
    Cranial 3E0X3GC
      Anesthetic Agent 3E0X3BZ
      Anti-inflammatory 3E0X33Z
      Destructive Agent 3E0X3TZ
    Peripheral 3E0T3GC
      Anesthetic Agent 3E0T3BZ
      Anti-inflammatory 3E0T33Z
      Destructive Agent 3E0T3TZ
    Plexus 3E0T3GC
      Anesthetic Agent 3E0T3BZ
      Anti-inflammatory 3E0T33Z
      Destructive Agent 3E0T3TZ
  Nose 3E09
    Analgesics 3E09
    Anesthetic Agent 3E09
    Anti-infective 3E09

Introduction of substance in or on — *continued*
  Nose — *continued*
    Anti-inflammatory 3E09
    Antineoplastic 3E09
    Destructive Agent 3E09
    Diagnostic Substance, Other 3E09
    Hypnotics 3E09
    Radioactive Substance 3E09
    Sedatives 3E09
    Serum 3E09
    Toxoid 3E09
    Vaccine 3E09
  Pancreatic Tract 3E0J
    Analgesics 3E0J
    Anesthetic Agent 3E0J
    Anti-infective 3E0J
    Anti-inflammatory 3E0J
    Antineoplastic 3E0J
    Destructive Agent 3E0J
    Diagnostic Substance, Other 3E0J
    Electrolytic Substance 3E0J
    Gas 3E0J
    Hypnotics 3E0J
    Islet Cells, Pancreatic 3E0J
    Nutritional Substance 3E0J
    Radioactive Substance 3E0J
    Sedatives 3E0J
    Water Balance Substance 3E0J
  Pericardial Cavity 3E0Y
    Analgesics 3E0Y3NZ
    Anesthetic Agent 3E0Y3BZ
    Anti-infective 3E0Y32
    Anti-inflammatory 3E0Y33Z
    Antineoplastic 3E0Y
    Destructive Agent 3E0Y3TZ
    Diagnostic Substance, Other 3E0Y3KZ
    Electrolytic Substance 3E0Y37Z
    Gas 3E0Y
    Hypnotics 3E0Y3NZ
    Nutritional Substance 3E0Y36Z
    Radioactive Substance 3E0Y3HZ
    Sedatives 3E0Y3NZ
    Water Balance Substance 3E0Y37Z
  Peritoneal Cavity 3E0M
    Adhesion Barrier 3E0M
    Analgesics 3E0M3NZ
    Anesthetic Agent 3E0M3BZ
    Anti-infective 3E0M32
    Anti-inflammatory 3E0M33Z
    Antineoplastic 3E0M
    Destructive Agent 3E0M3TZ
    Diagnostic Substance, Other 3E0M3KZ
    Electrolytic Substance 3E0M37Z
    Gas 3E0M
    Hypnotics 3E0M3NZ
    Nutritional Substance 3E0M36Z
    Radioactive Substance 3E0M3HZ
    Sedatives 3E0M3NZ
    Water Balance Substance 3E0M37Z
  Pharynx 3E0D
    Analgesics 3E0D
    Anesthetic Agent 3E0D
    Anti-infective 3E0D
    Anti-inflammatory 3E0D
    Antiarrhythmic 3E0D
    Antineoplastic 3E0D
    Destructive Agent 3E0D
    Diagnostic Substance, Other 3E0D
    Electrolytic Substance 3E0D
    Hypnotics 3E0D
    Nutritional Substance 3E0D
    Radioactive Substance 3E0D
    Sedatives 3E0D
    Serum 3E0D
    Toxoid 3E0D
    Vaccine 3E0D
    Water Balance Substance 3E0D

Pleural Cavity 3E0L
  Adhesion Barrier 3E0L
  Analgesics 3E0L3NZ
  Anesthetic Agent 3E0L3BZ
  Anti-infective 3E0L32
  Anti-inflammatory 3E0L33Z
  Antineoplastic 3E0L
  Destructive Agent 3E0L3TZ
  Diagnostic Substance, Other 3E0L3KZ
  Electrolytic Substance 3E0L37Z
  Gas 3E0L
  Hypnotics 3E0L3NZ
  Nutritional Substance 3E0L36Z
  Radioactive Substance 3E0L3HZ
  Sedatives 3E0L3NZ
  Water Balance Substance 3E0L37Z
Products of Conception 3E0E
  Analgesics 3E0E
  Anesthetic Agent 3E0E
  Anti-infective 3E0E
  Anti-inflammatory 3E0E
  Antineoplastic 3E0E
  Destructive Agent 3E0E
  Diagnostic Substance, Other 3E0E
  Electrolytic Substance 3E0E
  Gas 3E0E
  Hypnotics 3E0E
  Nutritional Substance 3E0E
  Radioactive Substance 3E0E
  Sedatives 3E0E
  Water Balance Substance 3E0E
Reproductive
  Female 3E0P
    Adhesion Barrier 3E0P
    Analgesics 3E0P
    Anesthetic Agent 3E0P
    Anti-infective 3E0P
    Anti-inflammatory 3E0P
    Antineoplastic 3E0P
    Destructive Agent 3E0P
    Diagnostic Substance, Other 3E0P
    Electrolytic Substance 3E0P
    Gas 3E0P
    Hormone 3E0P
    Hypnotics 3E0P
    Nutritional Substance 3E0P
    Ovum, Fertilized 3E0P
    Radioactive Substance 3E0P
    Sedatives 3E0P
    Sperm 3E0P
    Water Balance Substance 3E0P
  Male 3E0N
    Analgesics 3E0N
    Anesthetic Agent 3E0N
    Anti-infective 3E0N
    Anti-inflammatory 3E0N
    Antineoplastic 3E0N
    Destructive Agent 3E0N
    Diagnostic Substance, Other 3E0N
    Electrolytic Substance 3E0N
    Gas 3E0N
    Hypnotics 3E0N
    Nutritional Substance 3E0N
    Radioactive Substance 3E0N
    Sedatives 3E0N
    Water Balance Substance 3E0N
Respiratory Tract 3E0F
  Analgesics 3E0F
  Anesthetic Agent 3E0F
  Anti-infective 3E0F
  Anti-inflammatory 3E0F
  Antineoplastic 3E0F
  Destructive Agent 3E0F
  Diagnostic Substance, Other 3E0F
  Electrolytic Substance 3E0F
  Gas 3E0F

Respiratory Tract — *continued*
  Hypnotics 3E0F
  Nutritional Substance 3E0F
  Radioactive Substance 3E0F
  Sedatives 3E0F
  Water Balance Substance 3E0F
Skin 3E00XGC
  Analgesics 3E00XNZ
  Anesthetic Agent 3E00XBZ
  Anti-infective 3E00X2
  Anti-inflammatory 3E00X3Z
  Antineoplastic 3E00X0
  Destructive Agent 3E00XTZ
  Diagnostic Substance, Other 3E00XKZ
  Hypnotics 3E00XNZ
  Pigment 3E00XMZ
  Sedatives 3E00XNZ
  Serum 3E00X4Z
  Toxoid 3E00X4Z
  Vaccine 3E00X4Z
Spinal Canal 3E0R3GC
  Analgesics 3E0R3NZ
  Anesthetic Agent 3E0R3BZ
  Anti-infective 3E0R32
  Anti-inflammatory 3E0R33Z
  Antineoplastic 3E0R30
  Destructive Agent 3E0R3TZ
  Diagnostic Substance, Other 3E0R3KZ
  Electrolytic Substance 3E0R37Z
  Gas 3E0R
  Hypnotics 3E0R3NZ
  Nutritional Substance 3E0R36Z
  Radioactive Substance 3E0R3HZ
  Sedatives 3E0R3NZ
  Stem Cells
    Embryonic 3E0R
    Somatic 3E0R
  Water Balance Substance 3E0R37Z
Subcutaneous Tissue 3E013GC
  Analgesics 3E013NZ
  Anesthetic Agent 3E013BZ
  Anti-infective 3E01
  Anti-inflammatory 3E0133Z
  Antineoplastic 3E0130
  Destructive Agent 3E013TZ
  Diagnostic Substance, Other 3E013KZ
  Electrolytic Substance 3E0137Z
  Hormone 3E013V
  Hypnotics 3E013NZ
  Nutritional Substance 3E0136Z
  Radioactive Substance 3E013HZ
  Sedatives 3E013NZ
  Serum 3E0134Z
  Toxoid 3E0134Z
  Vaccine 3E0134Z
  Water Balance Substance 3E0137Z
Vein
  Central 3E04
    Analgesics 3E04
    Anesthetic, Intracirculatory 3E04
    Anti-infective 3E04
    Anti-inflammatory 3E04
    Antiarrhythmic 3E04
    Antineoplastic 3E04
    Destructive Agent 3E04
    Diagnostic Substance, Other 3E04
    Electrolytic Substance 3E04
    Hormone 3E04
    Hypnotics 3E04
    Immunotherapeutic 3E04
    Nutritional Substance 3E04
    Platelet Inhibitor 3E04
    Radioactive Substance 3E04
    Sedatives 3E04
    Serum 3E04
    Thrombolytic 3E04

Vein — *continued*
    Toxoid 3E04
    Vaccine 3E04
    Vasopressor 3E04
    Water Balance Substance 3E04
  Peripheral 3E03
    Analgesics 3E03
    Anesthetic, Intracirculatory 3E03
    Anti-infective 3E03
    Anti-inflammatory 3E03
    Antiarrhythmic 3E03
    Antineoplastic 3E03
    Destructive Agent 3E03
    Diagnostic Substance, Other 3E03
    Electrolytic Substance 3E03
    Hormone 3E03
    Hypnotics 3E03
    Immunotherapeutic 3E03
    Islet Cells, Pancreatic 3E03
    Nutritional Substance 3E03
    Platelet Inhibitor 3E03
    Radioactive Substance 3E03
    Sedatives 3E03
    Serum 3E03
    Thrombolytic 3E03
    Toxoid 3E03
    Vaccine 3E03
    Vasopressor 3E03
    Water Balance Substance 3E03
Intubation
  Airway
    see Insertion of device in, Trachea 0BH1
    see Insertion of device in, Mouth and Throat 0CHY
    see Insertion of device in, Esophagus 0DH5
  Drainage device *see* Drainage
  Feeding Device *see* Insertion of device in, Gastrointestinal System 0DH
INTUITY Elite® valve system, EDWARDS
  use Zooplastic Tissue, Rapid Deployment Technique in New Technology
IPPB (intermittent positive pressure breathing)
  see Assistance, Respiratory 5A09
Iridectomy
  see Excision, Eye 08B
  see Resection, Eye 08T
Iridoplasty
  see Repair, Eye 08Q
  see Replacement, Eye 08R
  see Supplement, Eye 08U
Iridotomy
  see Drainage, Eye 089
Irrigation
  Biliary Tract, Irrigating Substance 3E1J
  Brain, Irrigating Substance 3E1Q38Z
  Cranial Cavity, Irrigating Substance 3E1Q38Z
  Ear, Irrigating Substance 3E1B
  Epidural Space, Irrigating Substance 3E1S38Z
  Eye, Irrigating Substance 3E1C
  Gastrointestinal Tract
    Lower, Irrigating Substance 3E1H
    Upper, Irrigating Substance 3E1G
  Genitourinary Tract, Irrigating Substance 3E1K
  Irrigating Substance 3C1ZX8Z
  Joint, Irrigating Substance 3E1U38Z
  Mucous Membrane, Irrigating Substance 3E10
  Nose, Irrigating Substance 3E19
  Pancreatic Tract, Irrigating Substance 3E1J
  Pericardial Cavity, Irrigating Substance 3E1Y38Z

Irrigation — *continued*
  Peritoneal Cavity
    Dialysate 3E1M39Z
    Irrigating Substance 3E1M38Z
  Pleural Cavity, Irrigating
    Substance 3E1L38Z
  Reproductive
    Female, Irrigating Substance 3E1P
    Male, Irrigating Substance 3E1N
  Respiratory Tract, Irrigating Substance 3E1F
  Skin, Irrigating Substance 3E10
  Spinal Canal, Irrigating Substance 3E1R38Z
Isavuconazole Anti-infective XW0
Ischiatic nerve
  use Sciatic Nerve
Ischiocavernosus muscle
  use Perineum Muscle
Ischiofemoral ligament
  use Hip Bursa and Ligament, Right
  use Hip Bursa and Ligament, Left
Ischium
  use Pelvic Bone, Right
  use Pelvic Bone, Left
Isolation 8E0ZXY6
Isotope Administration, Whole
  Body DWY5G
Itrel® (3)(4) neurostimulator
  use Stimulator Generator, Single Array
    in 0JH

J

Jejunal artery
  use Superior Mesenteric Artery
Jejunectomy
  see Excision, Jejunum 0DBA
  see Resection, Jejunum 0DTA
Jejunocolostomy
  see Bypass, Gastrointestinal System 0D1
  see Drainage, Gastrointestinal System 0D9
Jejunopexy
  see Repair, Jejunum 0DQA
  see Reposition, Jejunum 0DSA
Jejunostomy
  see Bypass, Jejunum 0D1A
  see Drainage, Jejunum 0D9A
Jejunotomy
  see Drainage, Jejunum 0D9A
Joint fixation plate
  use Internal Fixation Device in Upper Joints
  use Internal Fixation Device in Lower Joints
Joint liner (insert)
  use Liner in Lower Joints
Joint spacer (antibiotic)
  use Spacer in Upper Joints
  use Spacer in Lower Joints
Jugular body
  use Glomus Jugulare
Jugular lymph node
  use Lymphatic, Right Neck
  use Lymphatic, Left Neck

K

Kappa®
  use Pacemaker, Dual Chamber in 0JH
Kcentra®
  use 4-Factor Prothrombin Complex
    Concentrate
Keratectomy, kerectomy
  see Excision, Eye 08B
  see Resection, Eye 08T
Keratocentesis
  see Drainage, Eye 089

Keratoplasty
  see Repair, Eye 08Q
  see Replacement, Eye 08R
  see Supplement, Eye 08U
Keratotomy
  see Drainage, Eye 089
  see Repair, Eye 08Q
Kirschner wire (K-wire)
  use Internal Fixation Device in Head and
    Facial Bones
  use Internal Fixation Device in Upper Bones
  use Internal Fixation Device in Lower Bones
  use Internal Fixation Device in Upper Joints
  use Internal Fixation Device in Lower Joints
Knee (implant) insert
  use Liner in Lower Joints
KUB x-ray
  see Plain Radiography, Kidney, Ureter and
    Bladder BT04
Kuntscher nail
  use Internal Fixation Device, Intramedullary
    in Upper Bones
  use Internal Fixation Device, Intramedullary
    in Lower Bones

L

Labia majora
  use Vulva
Labia minora
  use Vulva
Labial gland
  use Upper Lip
  use Lower Lip
Labiectomy
  see Excision, Female Reproductive
    System 0UB
  see Resection, Female Reproductive
    System 0UT
Lacrimal canaliculus
  use Lacrimal Duct, Right
  use Lacrimal Duct, Left
Lacrimal punctum
  use Lacrimal Duct, Right
  use Lacrimal Duct, Left
Lacrimal sac
  use Lacrimal Duct, Right
  use Lacrimal Duct, Left
LAGB (laparoscopic adjustable gastric
  banding)
  Adjustment/revision 0DW64CZ
  Initial procedure 0DV64CZ
Laminectomy
  see Release, Central Nervous System and
    Cranial Nerves 00N
  see Release, Peripheral Nervous
    System 01N
  see Excision, Upper Bones 0PB
  see Excision, Lower Bones 0QB
Laminotomy
  see Release, Central Nervous System and
    Cranial Nerves 00N
  see Release, Peripheral Nervous
    System 01N
  see Drainage, Upper Bones 0P9
  see Excision, Upper Bones 0PB
  see Release, Upper Bones 0PN
  see Drainage, Lower Bones 0Q9
  see Excision, Lower Bones 0QB
  see Release, Lower Bones 0QN
LAP-BAND® adjustable gastric banding
  system
  use Extraluminal Device
Laparoscopic-assisted transanal pull-through
  see Excision, Gastrointestinal System 0DB
  see Resection, Gastrointestinal System 0DT

Laparoscopy
  see Inspection
Laparotomy
  Drainage *see* Drainage, Peritoneal
    Cavity 0W9G
  Exploratory *see* Inspection, Peritoneal
    Cavity 0WJG
Laryngectomy
  see Excision, Larynx 0CBS
  see Resection, Larynx 0CTS
Laryngocentesis
  see Drainage, Larynx 0C9S
Laryngogram
  see Fluoroscopy, Larynx B91J
Laryngopexy
  see Repair, Larynx 0CQS
Laryngopharynx
  use Pharynx
Laryngoplasty
  see Repair, Larynx 0CQS
  see Replacement, Larynx 0CRS
  see Supplement, Larynx 0CUS
Laryngorrhaphy
  see Repair, Larynx 0CQS
Laryngoscopy 0CJS8ZZ
Laryngotomy
  see Drainage, Larynx 0C9S
Laser Interstitial Thermal Therapy
  Adrenal Gland DGY2KZZ
  Anus DDY8KZZ
  Bile Ducts DFY2KZZ
  Brain D0Y0KZZ
  Brain Stem D0Y1KZZ
  Breast
    Left DMY0KZZ
    Right DMY1KZZ
  Bronchus DBY1KZZ
  Chest Wall DBY7KZZ
  Colon DDY5KZZ
  Diaphragm DBY8KZZ
  Duodenum DDY2KZZ
  Esophagus DDY0KZZ
  Gallbladder DFY1KZZ
  Gland
    Adrenal DGY2KZZ
    Parathyroid DGY4KZZ
    Pituitary DGY0KZZ
    Thyroid DGY5KZZ
  Ileum DDY4KZZ
  Jejunum DDY3KZZ
  Liver DFY0KZZ
  Lung DBY2KZZ
  Mediastinum DBY6KZZ
  Nerve, Peripheral D0Y7KZZ
  Pancreas DFY3KZZ
  Parathyroid Gland DGY4KZZ
  Pineal Body DGY1KZZ
  Pituitary Gland DGY0KZZ
  Pleura DBY5KZZ
  Prostate DVY0KZZ
  Rectum DDY7KZZ
  Spinal Cord D0Y6KZZ
  Stomach DDY1KZZ
  Thyroid Gland DGY5KZZ
  Trachea DBY0KZZ
Lateral (brachial) lymph node
  use Lymphatic, Right Axillary
  use Lymphatic, Left Axillary
Lateral canthus
  use Upper Eyelid, Right
  use Upper Eyelid, Left
Lateral collateral ligament (LCL)
  use Knee Bursa and Ligament, Right
  use Knee Bursa and Ligament, Left
Lateral condyle of femur
  use Lower Femur, Right
  use Lower Femur, Left

Lateral condyle of tibia
  use Tibia, Right
  use Tibia, Left
Lateral cuneiform bone
  use Tarsal, Right
  use Tarsal, Left
Lateral epicondyle of femur
  use Lower Femur, Right
  use Lower Femur, Left
Lateral epicondyle of humerus
  use Humeral Shaft, Right
  use Humeral Shaft, Left
Lateral femoral cutaneous nerve
  use Lumbar Plexus
Lateral malleolus
  use Fibula, Right
  use Fibula, Left
Lateral meniscus
  use Knee Joint, Right
  use Knee Joint, Left
Lateral nasal cartilage
  use Nasal Mucosa and Soft Tissue
Lateral plantar artery
  use Foot Artery, Right
  use Foot Artery, Left
Lateral plantar nerve
  use Tibial Nerve
Lateral rectus muscle
  use Extraocular Muscle, Right
  use Extraocular Muscle, Left
Lateral sacral artery
  use Internal Iliac Artery, Right
  use Internal Iliac Artery, Left
Lateral sacral vein
  use Hypogastric Vein, Right
  use Hypogastric Vein, Left
Lateral sural cutaneous nerve
  use Peroneal Nerve
Lateral tarsal artery
  use Foot Artery, Right
  use Foot Artery, Left
Lateral temporomandibular ligament
  use Head and Neck Bursa and Ligament
Lateral thoracic artery
  use Axillary Artery, Right
  use Axillary Artery, Left
Latissimus dorsi muscle
  use Trunk Muscle, Right
  use Trunk Muscle, Left
Latissimus Dorsi Myocutaneous Flap
  Replacement
    Bilateral 0HRV075
    Left 0HRU075
    Right 0HRT075
  Transfer
    Left 0KXG
    Right 0KXF
Lavage
  see Irrigation
  Bronchial alveolar, diagnostic *see* Drainage,
    Respiratory System 0B9
Least splanchnic nerve
  use Thoracic Sympathetic Nerve
Left ascending lumbar vein
  use Hemiazygos Vein
Left atrioventricular valve
  use Mitral Valve
Left auricular appendix
  use Atrium, Left
Left colic vein
  use Colic Vein
Left coronary sulcus
  use Heart, Left
Left gastric artery
  use Gastric Artery
Left gastroepiploic artery
  use Splenic Artery

Left gastroepiploic vein
  use Splenic Vein
Left inferior phrenic vein
  use Renal Vein, Left
Left inferior pulmonary vein
  use Pulmonary Vein, Left
Left jugular trunk
  use Thoracic Duct
Left lateral ventricle
  use Cerebral Ventricle
Left ovarian vein
  use Renal Vein, Left
Left second lumbar vein
  use Renal Vein, Left
Left subclavian trunk
  use Thoracic Duct
Left subcostal vein
  use Hemiazygos Vein
Left superior pulmonary vein
  use Pulmonary Vein, Left
Left suprarenal vein
  use Renal Vein, Left
Left testicular vein
  use Renal Vein, Left
Lengthening
  Bone, with device *see* Insertion of Limb
    Lengthening Device
  Muscle, by incision *see* Division,
    Muscles 0K8
  Tendon, by incision *see* Division,
    Tendons 0L8
Leptomeninges, intracranial
  use Cerebral Meninges
Leptomeninges, spinal
  use Spinal Meninges
Lesser alar cartilage
  use Nasal Mucosa and Soft Tissue
Lesser occipital nerve
  use Cervical Plexus
Lesser Omentum
  use Omentum
Lesser saphenous vein
  use Saphenous Vein, Right
  use Saphenous Vein, Left
Lesser splanchnic nerve
  use Thoracic Sympathetic Nerve
Lesser trochanter
  use Upper Femur, Right
  use Upper Femur, Left
Lesser tuberosity
  use Humeral Head, Right
  use Humeral Head, Left
Lesser wing
  use Sphenoid Bone
Leukopheresis, therapeutic
  see Pheresis, Circulatory 6A55
Levator anguli oris muscle
  use Facial Muscle
Levator ani muscle
  use Perineum Muscle
Levator labii superioris alaeque nasi muscle
  use Facial Muscle
Levator labii superioris muscle
  use Facial Muscle
Levator palpebrae superioris muscle
  use Upper Eyelid, Right
  use Upper Eyelid, Left
Levator scapulae muscle
  use Neck Muscle, Right
  use Neck Muscle, Left
Levator veli palatini muscle
  use Tongue, Palate, Pharynx Muscle
Levatores costarum muscle
  use Thorax Muscle, Right
  use Thorax Muscle, Left

LifeStent® (Flexstar)(XL) Vascular Stent System
  use Intraluminal Device
Ligament of head of fibula
  use Knee Bursa and Ligament, Right
  use Knee Bursa and Ligament, Left
Ligament of the lateral malleolus
  use Ankle Bursa and Ligament, Right
  use Ankle Bursa and Ligament, Left
Ligamentum flavum
  use Upper Spine Bursa and Ligament
  use Lower Spine Bursa and Ligament
Ligation
  see Occlusion
Ligation, hemorrhoid
  see Occlusion, Lower Veins, Hemorrhoidal
    Plexus
Light Therapy GZJZZZZ
Liner
  Removal of device from
    Hip
      Left 0SPB09Z
      Right 0SP909Z
    Knee
      Left 0SPD09Z
      Right 0SPC09Z
  Revision of device in
    Hip
      Left 0SWB09Z
      Right 0SW909Z
    Knee
      Left 0SWD09Z
      Right 0SWC09Z
  Supplement
    Hip
      Left 0SUB09Z
        Acetabular Surface 0SUE09Z
        Femoral Surface 0SUS09Z
      Right 0SU909Z
        Acetabular Surface 0SUA09Z
        Femoral Surface 0SUR09Z
    Knee
      Left 0SUD09
        Femoral Surface 0SUU09Z
        Tibial Surface 0SUW09Z
      Right 0SUC09
        Femoral Surface 0SUT09Z
        Tibial Surface 0SUV09Z
Lingual artery
  use External Carotid Artery, Right
  use External Carotid Artery, Left
Lingual tonsil
  use Pharynx
Lingulectomy, lung
  see Excision, Lung Lingula 0BBH
  see Resection, Lung Lingula 0BTH
Lithotripsy
  see Fragmentation
  with removal of fragments *see* Extirpation
LITT (laser interstitial thermal therapy)
  see Laser Interstitial Thermal Therapy
LIVIAN™ CRT-D
  use Cardiac Resynchronization Defibrillator
    Pulse Generator in 0JH
Lobectomy
  see Excision, Central Nervous System and
    Cranial Nerves 00B
  see Excision, Respiratory System 0BB
  see Resection, Respiratory System 0BT
  see Excision, Hepatobiliary System and
    Pancreas 0FB
  see Resection, Hepatobiliary System and
    Pancreas 0FT
  see Excision, Endocrine System 0GB
  see Resection, Endocrine System 0GT
Lobotomy
  see Division, Brain 0080

Localization
  see Map
  see Imaging
Locus ceruleus
  use Pons
Long thoracic nerve
  use Brachial Plexus
Loop ileostomy
  see Bypass, Ileum 0D1B
Loop recorder, implantable
  use Monitoring Device
Lower GI series
  see Fluoroscopy, Colon BD14
Lumbar artery
  use Abdominal Aorta
Lumbar facet joint
  use Lumbar Vertebral Joint
Lumbar ganglion
  use Lumbar Sympathetic Nerve
Lumbar lymph node
  use Lymphatic, Aortic
Lumbar lymphatic trunk
  use Cisterna Chyli
Lumbar splanchnic nerve
  use Lumbar Sympathetic Nerve
Lumbosacral facet joint
  use Lumbosacral Joint
Lumbosacral trunk
  use Lumbar Nerve
Lumpectomy
  see Excision
Lunate bone
  use Carpal, Right
  use Carpal, Left
Lunotriquetral ligament
  use Hand Bursa and Ligament, Right
  use Hand Bursa and Ligament, Left
Lymphadenectomy
  see Excision, Lymphatic and Hemic
    Systems 07B
  see Resection, Lymphatic and Hemic
    Systems 07T
Lymphadenotomy
  see Drainage, Lymphatic and Hemic
    Systems 079
Lymphangiectomy
  see Excision, Lymphatic and Hemic
    Systems 07B
  see Resection, Lymphatic and Hemic
    Systems 07T
Lymphangiogram
  see Plain Radiography, Lymphatic
    System B70
Lymphangioplasty
  see Repair, Lymphatic and Hemic
    Systems 07Q
  see Supplement, Lymphatic and Hemic
    Systems 07U
Lymphangiorrhaphy
  see Repair, Lymphatic and Hemic
    Systems 07Q
Lymphangiotomy
  see Drainage, Lymphatic and Hemic
    Systems 079
Lysis
  see Release

M

Macula
  use Retina, Right
  use Retina, Left
**MAGEC® Spinal Bracing and Distraction
  System**
  use Magnetically Controlled Growth Rod(s)
    in New Technology

Magnet extraction, ocular foreign body
  see Extirpation, Eye 08C
Magnetic Resonance Imaging (MRI)
  Abdomen BW30
  Ankle
    Left BQ3H
    Right BQ3G
  Aorta
    Abdominal B430
    Thoracic B330
  Arm
    Left BP3F
    Right BP3E
  Artery
    Celiac B431
    Cervico-Cerebral Arch B33Q
    Common Carotid, Bilateral B335
    Coronary
      Bypass Graft, Multiple B233
      Multiple B231
    Internal Carotid, Bilateral B338
    Intracranial B33R
    Lower Extremity
      Bilateral B43H
      Left B43G
      Right B43F
    Pelvic B43C
    Renal, Bilateral B438
    Spinal B33M
    Superior Mesenteric B434
    Upper Extremity
      Bilateral B33K
      Left B33J
      Right B33H
    Vertebral, Bilateral B33G
  Bladder BT30
  Brachial Plexus BW3P
  Brain B030
  Breast
    Bilateral BH32
    Left BH31
    Right BH30
  Calcaneus
    Left BQ3K
    Right BQ3J
  Chest BW33Y
  Coccyx BR3F
  Connective Tissue
    Lower Extremity BL31
    Upper Extremity BL30
  Corpora Cavernosa BV30
  Disc
    Cervical BR31
    Lumbar BR33
    Thoracic BR32
  Ear B930
  Elbow
    Left BP3H
    Right BP3G
  Eye
    Bilateral B837
    Left B836
    Right B835
  Femur
    Left BQ34
    Right BQ33
  Fetal Abdomen BY33
  Fetal Extremity BY35
  Fetal Head BY30
  Fetal Heart BY31
  Fetal Spine BY34
  Fetal Thorax BY32
  Fetus, Whole BY36
  Foot
    Left BQ3M
    Right BQ3L

Magnetic Resonance Imaging (MRI)
  — continued
  Forearm
    Left BP3K
    Right BP3J
  Gland
    Adrenal, Bilateral BG32
    Parathyroid BG33
    Parotid, Bilateral B936
    Salivary, Bilateral B93D
    Submandibular, Bilateral B939
    Thyroid BG34
  Head BW38
  Heart, Right and Left B236
  Hip
    Left BQ31
    Right BQ30
  Intracranial Sinus B532
  Joint
    Finger
      Left BP3D
      Right BP3C
    Hand
      Left BP3D
      Right BP3C
    Temporomandibular, Bilateral BN39
  Kidney
    Bilateral BT33
    Left BT32
    Right BT31
    Transplant BT39
  Knee
    Left BQ38
    Right BQ37
  Larynx B93J
  Leg
    Left BQ3F
    Right BQ3D
  Liver BF35
  Liver and Spleen BF36
  Lung Apices BB3G
  Nasopharynx B93F
  Neck BW3F
  Nerve
    Acoustic B03C
    Brachial Plexus BW3P
  Oropharynx B93F
  Ovary
    Bilateral BU35
    Left BU34
    Right BU33
  Ovary and Uterus BU3C
  Pancreas BF37
  Patella
    Left BQ3W
    Right BQ3V
  Pelvic Region BW3G
  Pelvis BR3C
  Pituitary Gland B039
  Plexus, Brachial BW3P
  Prostate BV33
  Retroperitoneum BW3H
  Sacrum BR3F
  Scrotum BV34
  Sella Turcica B039
  Shoulder
    Left BP39
    Right BP38
  Sinus
    Intracranial B532
    Paranasal B932
  Spinal Cord B03B
  Spine
    Cervical BR30
    Lumbar BR39
    Thoracic BR37
  Spleen and Liver BF36

Magnetic Resonance Imaging (MRI)
— continued
Subcutaneous Tissue
Abdomen BH3H
Extremity
Lower BH3J
Upper BH3F
Head BH3D
Neck BH3D
Pelvis BH3H
Thorax BH3G
Tendon
Lower Extremity BL33
Upper Extremity BL32
Testicle
Bilateral BV37
Left BV36
Right BV35
Toe
Left BQ3Q
Right BQ3P
Uterus BU36
Pregnant BU3B
Uterus and Ovary BU3C
Vagina BU39
Vein
Cerebellar B531
Cerebral B531
Jugular, Bilateral B535
Lower Extremity
Bilateral B53D
Left B53C
Right B53B
Other B53V
Pelvic (Iliac) Bilateral B53H
Portal B53T
Pulmonary, Bilateral B53S
Renal, Bilateral B53L
Splanchnic B53T
Upper Extremity
Bilateral B53P
Left B53N
Right B53M
Vena Cava
Inferior B539
Superior B538
Wrist
Left BP3M
Right BP3L
Magnetically Controlled Growth Rod(s)
Cervical XNS3
Lumbar XNS0
Thoracic XNS4
Malleotomy
see Drainage, Ear, Nose, Sinus 099
Malleus
use Auditory Ossicle, Right
use Auditory Ossicle, Left
Mammaplasty, mammoplasty
see Alteration, Skin and Breast 0H0
see Repair, Skin and Breast 0HQ
see Replacement, Skin and Breast 0HR
see Supplement, Skin and Breast 0HU
Mammary duct
use Breast, Right
use Breast, Left
use Breast, Bilateral
Mammary gland
use Breast, Right
use Breast, Left
use Breast, Bilateral
Mammectomy
see Excision, Skin and Breast 0HB
see Resection, Skin and Breast 0HT
Mammillary body
use Hypothalamus

Mammography
see Plain Radiography, Skin, Subcutaneous
Tissue and Breast BH0
Mammotomy
see Drainage, Skin and Breast 0H9
Mandibular nerve
use Trigeminal Nerve
Mandibular notch
use Mandible, Right
use Mandible, Left
Mandibulectomy
see Excision, Head and Facial Bones 0NB
see Resection, Head and Facial Bones 0NT
Manipulation
Adhesions see Release
Chiropractic see Chiropractic Manipulation
Manual removal, retained placenta
see Extraction, Products of Conception,
Retained 10D1
Manubrium
use Sternum
Map
Basal Ganglia 00K8
Brain 00K0
Cerebellum 00KC
Cerebral Hemisphere 00K7
Conduction Mechanism 02K8
Hypothalamus 00KA
Medulla Oblongata 00KD
Pons 00KB
Thalamus 00K9
Mapping
Doppler ultrasound see Ultrasonography
Electrocardiogram only see Measurement,
Cardiac 4A02
Mark IV™ Breathing Pacemaker System
use Stimulator Generator in Subcutaneous
Tissue and Fascia
Marsupialization
see Drainage
see Excision
Massage, cardiac
External 5A12012
Open 02QA0ZZ
Masseter muscle
use Head Muscle
Masseteric fascia
use Subcutaneous Tissue and Fascia, Face
Mastectomy
see Excision, Skin and Breast 0HB
see Resection, Skin and Breast 0HT
Mastoid (postauricular) lymph node
use Lymphatic, Right Neck
use Lymphatic, Left Neck
Mastoid air cells
use Mastoid Sinus, Right
use Mastoid Sinus, Left
Mastoid process
use Temporal Bone, Right
use Temporal Bone, Left
Mastoidectomy
see Excision, Ear, Nose, Sinus 09B
see Resection, Ear, Nose, Sinus 09T
Mastoidotomy
see Drainage, Ear, Nose, Sinus 099
Mastopexy
see Repair, Skin and Breast 0HQ
see Reposition, Skin and Breast 0HS
Mastorrhaphy
see Repair, Skin and Breast 0HQ
Mastotomy
see Drainage, Skin and Breast 0H9
Maxillary artery
use External Carotid Artery, Right
use External Carotid Artery, Left
Maxillary nerve
use Trigeminal Nerve

Maximo® II DR (VR)
use Defibrillator Generator in 0JH
Maximo® II DR CRT-D
use Cardiac Resynchronization Defibrillator
Pulse Generator in 0JH
Measurement
Arterial
Flow
Coronary 4A03
Peripheral 4A03
Pulmonary 4A03
Pressure
Coronary 4A03
Peripheral 4A03
Pulmonary 4A03
Thoracic, Other 4A03
Pulse
Coronary 4A03
Peripheral 4A03
Pulmonary 4A03
Saturation, Peripheral 4A03
Sound, Peripheral 4A03
Biliary
Flow 4A0C
Pressure 4A0C
Cardiac
Action Currents 4A02
Defibrillator 4B02XTZ
Electrical Activity 4A02
Guidance 4A02X4A
No Qualifier 4A02X4Z
Output 4A02
Pacemaker 4B02XSZ
Rate 4A02
Rhythm 4A02
Sampling and Pressure
Bilateral 4A02
Left Heart 4A02
Right Heart 4A02
Sound 4A02
Total Activity, Stress 4A02XM4
Central Nervous
Conductivity 4A00
Electrical Activity 4A00
Pressure 4A000BZ
Intracranial 4A00
Saturation, Intracranial 4A00
Stimulator 4B00XVZ
Temperature, Intracranial 4A00
Circulatory, Volume 4A05XLZ
Gastrointestinal
Motility 4A0B
Pressure 4A0B
Secretion 4A0B
Lymphatic
Flow 4A06
Pressure 4A06
Metabolism 4A0Z
Musculoskeletal
Contractility 4A0F
Stimulator 4B0FXVZ
Olfactory, Acuity 4A08X0Z
Peripheral Nervous
Conductivity
Motor 4A01
Sensory 4A01
Electrical Activity 4A01
Stimulator 4B01XVZ
Products of Conception
Cardiac
Electrical Activity 4A0H
Rate 4A0H
Rhythm 4A0H
Sound 4A0H
Nervous
Conductivity 4A0J
Electrical Activity 4A0J
Pressure 4A0J

Measurement — continued

Respiratory
  Capacity 4A09
  Flow 4A09
  Pacemaker 4B09XSZ
  Rate 4A09
  Resistance 4A09
  Total Activity 4A09
  Volume 4A09
Sleep 4A0ZXQZ
Temperature 4A0Z
Urinary
  Contractility 4A0D
  Flow 4A0D
  Pressure 4A0D
  Resistance 4A0D
  Volume 4A0D
Venous
  Flow
    Central 4A04
    Peripheral 4A04
    Portal 4A04
    Pulmonary 4A04
  Pressure
    Central 4A04
    Peripheral 4A04
    Portal 4A04
    Pulmonary 4A04
  Pulse
    Central 4A04
    Peripheral 4A04
    Portal 4A04
    Pulmonary 4A04
  Saturation, Peripheral 4A04
Visual
  Acuity 4A07X0Z
  Mobility 4A07X7Z
  Pressure 4A07XBZ

Meatoplasty, urethra
  see Repair, Urethra 0TQD
Meatotomy
  see Drainage, Urinary System 0T9
Mechanical ventilation
  see Performance, Respiratory 5A19
Medial canthus
  use Lower Eyelid, Right
  use Lower Eyelid, Left
Medial collateral ligament (MCL)
  use Knee Bursa and Ligament, Right
  use Knee Bursa and Ligament, Left
Medial condyle of femur
  use Lower Femur, Right
  use Lower Femur, Left
Medial condyle of tibia
  use Tibia, Right
  use Tibia, Left
Medial cuneiform bone
  use Tarsal, Right
  use Tarsal, Left
Medial epicondyle of femur
  use Lower Femur, Right
  use Lower Femur, Left
Medial epicondyle of humerus
  use Humeral Shaft, Right
  use Humeral Shaft, Left
Medial malleolus
  use Tibia, Right
  use Tibia, Left
Medial meniscus
  use Knee Joint, Right
  use Knee Joint, Left
Medial plantar artery
  use Foot Artery, Right
  use Foot Artery, Left
Medial plantar nerve
  use Tibial Nerve

Medial popliteal nerve
  use Tibial Nerve
Medial rectus muscle
  use Extraocular Muscle, Right
  use Extraocular Muscle, Left
Medial sural cutaneous nerve
  use Tibial Nerve
Median antebrachial vein
  use Basilic Vein, Right
  use Basilic Vein, Left
Median cubital vein
  use Basilic Vein, Right
  use Basilic Vein, Left
Median sacral artery
  use Abdominal Aorta
Mediastinal lymph node
  use Lymphatic, Thorax
Mediastinoscopy 0WJC4ZZ
Medication Management GZ3ZZZZ
  for substance abuse
    Antabuse HZ83ZZZ
    Bupropion HZ87ZZZ
    Clonidine HZ86ZZZ
    Levo-alpha-acetyl-methadol
      (LAAM) HZ82ZZZ
    Methadone Maintenance HZ81ZZZ
    Naloxone HZ85ZZZ
    Naltrexone HZ84ZZZ
    Nicotine Replacement HZ80ZZZ
    Other Replacement
      Medication HZ89ZZZ
    Psychiatric Medication HZ88ZZZ
Meditation 8E0ZXY5
**Medtronic Endurant® II AAA stent graft
system**
  use Intraluminal Device
Meissner's (submucous) plexus
  use Abdominal Sympathetic Nerve
Melody® transcatheter pulmonary valve
  use Zooplastic Tissue in Heart and Great
    Vessels
Membranous urethra
  use Urethra
Meningeorrhaphy
  see Repair, Cerebral Meninges 00Q1
  see Repair, Spinal Meninges 00QT
Meniscectomy, knee
  see Excision, Joint, Knee, Right 0SBC
  see Excision, Joint, Knee, Left 0SBD
Mental foramen
  use Mandible, Right
  use Mandible, Left
Mentalis muscle
  use Facial Muscle
Mentoplasty
  see Alteration, Jaw, Lower 0W05
Mesenterectomy
  see Excision, Mesentery 0DBV
Mesenteriorrhaphy, mesenterorrhaphy
  see Repair, Mesentery 0DQV
Mesenteriplication
  see Repair, Mesentery 0DQV
Mesoappendix
  use Mesentery
Mesocolon
  use Mesentery
Metacarpal ligament
  use Hand Bursa and Ligament, Right
  use Hand Bursa and Ligament, Left
Metacarpophalangeal ligament
  use Hand Bursa and Ligament, Right
  use Hand Bursa and Ligament, Left
Metal on metal bearing surface
  use Synthetic Substitute, Metal in 0SR
Metatarsal ligament
  use Foot Bursa and Ligament, Right
  use Foot Bursa and Ligament, Left

Metatarsectomy
  see Excision, Lower Bones 0QB
  see Resection, Lower Bones 0QT
Metatarsophalangeal (MTP) joint
  use Metatarsal-Phalangeal Joint, Right
  use Metatarsal-Phalangeal Joint, Left
Metatarsophalangeal ligament
  use Foot Bursa and Ligament, Right
  use Foot Bursa and Ligament, Left
Metathalamus
  use Thalamus
Micro-Driver® stent (RX) (OTW)
  use Intraluminal Device
MicroMed HeartAssist™
  use Implantable Heart Assist System in
    Heart and Great Vessels
Micrus CERECYTE® microcoil
  use Intraluminal Device, Bioactive in Upper
    Arteries
Midcarpal joint
  use Carpal Joint, Right
  use Carpal Joint, Left
Middle cardiac nerve
  use Thoracic Sympathetic Nerve
Middle cerebral artery
  use Intracranial Artery
Middle cerebral vein
  use Intracranial Vein
Middle colic vein
  use Colic Vein
Middle genicular artery
  use Popliteal Artery, Right
  use Popliteal Artery, Left
Middle hemorrhoidal vein
  use Hypogastric Vein, Right
  use Hypogastric Vein, Left
Middle rectal artery
  use Internal Iliac Artery, Right
  use Internal Iliac Artery, Left
Middle suprarenal artery
  use Abdominal Aorta
Middle temporal artery
  use Temporal Artery, Right
  use Temporal Artery, Left
Middle turbinate
  use Nasal Turbinate
MIRODERM™ Biologic Wound Matrix
  use Skin Substitute, Porcine Liver Derived
    in New Technology
MitraClip® valve repair system
  use Synthetic Substitute
Mitral annulus
  use Mitral Valve
Mitroflow® Aortic Pericardial Heart Valve
  use Zooplastic Tissue in Heart and Great
    Vessels
Mobilization, adhesions
  see Release
Molar gland
  use Buccal Mucosa
Monitoring
  Arterial
    Flow
      Coronary 4A13
      Peripheral 4A13
      Pulmonary 4A13
    Pressure
      Coronary 4A13
      Peripheral 4A13
      Pulmonary 4A13
    Pulse
      Coronary 4A13
      Peripheral 4A13
      Pulmonary 4A13
    Saturation, Peripheral 4A13
    Sound, Peripheral 4A13

Monitoring — *continued*
  Cardiac
    Electrical Activity 4A12
      Ambulatory 4A12X45
      No Qualifier 4A12X4Z
    Output 4A12
    Rate 4A12
    Rhythm 4A12
    Sound 4A12
    Total Activity, Stress 4A12XM4
    Vascular Perfusion, Indocyanine Green
      Dye 4A12XSH
  Central Nervous
    Conductivity 4A10
    Electrical Activity
      Intraoperative 4A10
      No Qualifier 4A10
    Pressure 4A100BZ
      Intracranial 4A10
    Saturation, Intracranial 4A10
    Temperature, Intracranial 4A10
  Gastrointestinal
    Motility 4A1B
    Pressure 4A1B
    Secretion 4A1B
    Vascular Perfusion, Indocyanine Green
      Dye 4A1BXSH
  Intraoperative Knee Replacement
  Sensor XR2
  Lymphatic
    Flow 4A16
    Pressure 4A16
  Peripheral Nervous
    Conductivity
      Motor 4A11
      Sensory 4A11
    Electrical Activity
      Intraoperative 4A11
      No Qualifier 4A11
  Products of Conception
    Cardiac
      Electrical Activity 4A1H
      Rate 4A1H
      Rhythm 4A1H
      Sound 4A1H
    Nervous
      Conductivity 4A1J
      Electrical Activity 4A1J
      Pressure 4A1J
  Respiratory
    Capacity 4A19
    Flow 4A19
    Rate 4A19
    Resistance 4A19
    Volume 4A19
  Skin and Breast, Vascular Perfusion,
  Indocyanine Green Dye 4A1GXSH
  Sleep 4A1ZXQZ
  Temperature 4A1Z
  Urinary
    Contractility 4A1D
    Flow 4A1D
    Pressure 4A1D
    Resistance 4A1D
    Volume 4A1D
  Venous
    Flow
      Central 4A14
      Peripheral 4A14
      Portal 4A14
      Pulmonary 4A14
    Pressure
      Central 4A14
      Peripheral 4A14
      Portal 4A14
      Pulmonary 4A14

Monitoring — *continued*
  Venous — *continued*
    Pulse
      Central 4A14
      Peripheral 4A14
      Portal 4A14
      Pulmonary 4A14
    Saturation
      Central 4A14
      Portal 4A14
      Pulmonary 4A14
Monitoring Device, Hemodynamic
  Abdomen 0JH8
  Chest 0JH6
Mosaic® Bioprosthesis (aortic) (mitral) valve
  use Zooplastic Tissue in Heart and Great
  Vessels
Motor Function Assessment F01
Motor Treatment F07
MR Angiography
  see Magnetic Resonance Imaging (MRI),
  Heart B23
  see Magnetic Resonance Imaging (MRI),
  Upper Arteries B33
  see Magnetic Resonance Imaging (MRI),
  Lower Arteries B43
MULTI-LINK (VISION®)(MINI-VISION®)
(ULTRA™) Coronary Stent System
  use Intraluminal Device
Multiple sleep latency test 4A0ZXQZ
Musculocutaneous nerve
  use Brachial Plexus
Musculopexy
  see Repair, Muscles 0KQ
  see Reposition, Muscles 0KS
Musculophrenic artery
  use Internal Mammary Artery, Right
  use Internal Mammary Artery, Left
Musculoplasty
  see Repair, Muscles 0KQ
  see Supplement, Muscles 0KU
Musculorrhaphy
  see Repair, Muscles 0KQ
Musculospiral nerve
  use Radial Nerve
Myectomy
  see Excision, Muscles 0KB
  see Resection, Muscles 0KT
Myelencephalon
  use Medulla Oblongata
Myelogram
  CT *see* Computerized Tomography (CT
  Scan), Central Nervous System B02
  MRI *see* Magnetic Resonance Imaging
  (MRI), Central Nervous System B03
Myenteric (Auerbach's) plexus
  use Abdominal Sympathetic Nerve
Myocardial Bridge Release
  see Release, Artery, Coronary
Myomectomy
  see Excision, Female Reproductive
  System 0UB
Myometrium
  use Uterus
Myopexy
  see Repair, Muscles 0KQ
  see Reposition, Muscles 0KS
Myoplasty
  see Repair, Muscles 0KQ
  see Supplement, Muscles 0KU
Myorrhaphy
  see Repair, Muscles 0KQ
Myoscopy
  see Inspection, Muscles 0KJ
Myotomy
  see Division, Muscles 0K8
  see Drainage, Muscles 0K9

Myringectomy
  see Excision, Ear, Nose, Sinus 09B
  see Resection, Ear, Nose, Sinus 09T
Myringoplasty
  see Repair, Ear, Nose, Sinus 09Q
  see Replacement, Ear, Nose, Sinus 09R
  see Supplement, Ear, Nose, Sinus 09U
Myringostomy
  see Drainage, Ear, Nose, Sinus 099
Myringotomy
  see Drainage, Ear, Nose, Sinus 099

N

Nail bed
  use Finger Nail
  use Toe Nail
Nail plate
  use Finger Nail
  use Toe Nail
nanoLOCK™ interbody fusion device
  use Interbody Fusion Device, Nanotextured
  Surface in New Technology
Narcosynthesis GZGZZZZ
Nasal cavity
  use Nasal Mucosa and Soft Tissue
Nasal concha
  use Nasal Turbinate
Nasalis muscle
  use Facial Muscle
Nasolacrimal duct
  use Lacrimal Duct, Right
  use Lacrimal Duct, Left
Nasopharyngeal airway (NPA)
  use Intraluminal Device, Airway in Ear,
  Nose, Sinus
Navicular bone
  use Tarsal, Right
  use Tarsal, Left
Near Infrared Spectroscopy, Circulatory
System 8E023DZ
Neck of femur
  use Upper Femur, Right
  use Upper Femur, Left
Neck of humerus (anatomical)(surgical)
  use Humeral Head, Right
  use Humeral Head, Left
Nephrectomy
  see Excision, Urinary System 0TB
  see Resection, Urinary System 0TT
Nephrolithotomy
  see Extirpation, Urinary System 0TC
Nephrolysis
  see Release, Urinary System 0TN
Nephropexy
  see Repair, Urinary System 0TQ
  see Reposition, Urinary System 0TS
Nephroplasty
  see Repair, Urinary System 0TQ
  see Supplement, Urinary System 0TU
Nephropyeloureterostomy
  see Bypass, Urinary System 0T1
  see Drainage, Urinary System 0T9
Nephrorrhaphy
  see Repair, Urinary System 0TQ
Nephroscopy, transurethral 0TJ58ZZ
Nephrostomy
  see Bypass, Urinary System 0T1
  see Drainage, Urinary System 0T9
Nephrotomography
  see Plain Radiography, Urinary System BT0
  see Fluoroscopy, Urinary System BT1
Nephrotomy
  see Division, Urinary System 0T8
  see Drainage, Urinary System 0T9

Nerve conduction study
  see Measurement, Central Nervous 4A00
  see Measurement, Peripheral Nervous 4A01
Nerve Function Assessment F01
Nerve to the stapedius
  use Facial Nerve
Nesiritide
  use Human B-type Natriuretic Peptide
Neurectomy
  see Excision, Central Nervous System and
    Cranial Nerves 00B
  see Excision, Peripheral Nervous
    System 01B
Neurexeresis
  see Extraction, Central Nervous System and
    Cranial Nerves 00D
  see Extraction, Peripheral Nervous
    System 01D
Neurohypophysis
  use Pituitary Gland
Neurolysis
  see Release, Central Nervous System and
    Cranial Nerves 00N
  see Release, Peripheral Nervous
    System 01N
Neuromuscular electrical stimulation
  (NEMS) lead
  use Stimulator Lead in Muscles
Neurophysiologic monitoring
  see Monitoring, Central Nervous 4A10
Neuroplasty
  see Repair, Central Nervous System and
    Cranial Nerves 00Q
  see Supplement, Central Nervous System
    and Cranial Nerves 00U
  see Repair, Peripheral Nervous System 01Q
  see Supplement, Peripheral Nervous
    System 01U
Neurorrhaphy
  see Repair, Central Nervous System and
    Cranial Nerves 00Q
  see Repair, Peripheral Nervous System 01Q
Neurostimulator Generator
  Insertion of device in, Skull 0NH00NZ
  Removal of device from, Skull 0NP00NZ
  Revision of device in, Skull 0NW00NZ
Neurostimulator generator, multiple
  channel
  use Stimulator Generator, Multiple Array
    in 0JH
Neurostimulator generator, multiple
  channel rechargeable
  use Stimulator Generator, Multiple Array
    Rechargeable in 0JH
Neurostimulator generator, single channel
  use Stimulator Generator, Single Array
    in 0JH
Neurostimulator generator, single channel
  rechargeable
  use Stimulator Generator, Single Array
    Rechargeable in 0JH
Neurostimulator Lead
  Insertion of device in
    Brain 00H0
    Cerebral Ventricle 00H6
    Nerve
      Cranial 00HE
      Peripheral 01HY
    Spinal Canal 00HU
    Spinal Cord 00HV
    Vein
      Azygos 05H0
      Innominate
        Left 05H4
        Right 05H3
  Removal of device from
    Brain 00P0

Neurostimulator Lead — continued
  Removal of device from — continued
    Cerebral Ventricle 00P6
    Nerve
      Cranial 00PE
      Peripheral 01PY
    Spinal Canal 00PU
    Spinal Cord 00PV
    Vein
      Azygos 05P0
      Innominate
        Left 05P4
        Right 05P3
  Revision of device in
    Brain 00W0
    Cerebral Ventricle 00W6
    Nerve
      Cranial 00WE
      Peripheral 01WY
    Spinal Canal 00WU
    Spinal Cord 00WV
    Vein
      Azygos 05W0
      Innominate
        Left 05W4
        Right 05W3
Neurotomy
  see Division, Central Nervous System and
    Cranial Nerves 008
  see Division, Peripheral Nervous
    System 018
Neurotripsy
  see Destruction, Central Nervous System
    and Cranial Nerves 005
  see Destruction, Peripheral Nervous
    System 015
Neutralization plate
  use Internal Fixation Device in Head and
    Facial Bones
  use Internal Fixation Device in Upper Bones
  use Internal Fixation Device in Lower Bones
New Technology
  Andexanet Alfa, Factor Xa Inhibitor
    Reversal Agent XW0
  Bezlotoxumab Monoclonal Antibody XW0
  Blinatumomab Antineoplastic
    Immunotherapy XW0
  Ceftazidime-Avibactam Anti-infective XW0
  Cerebral Embolic Filtration, Dual
    Filter X2A5312
  Concentrated Bone Marrow
    Aspirate XK02303
  Cytarabine and Daunorubicin Liposome
    Antineoplastic XW0
  Defibrotide Sodium Anticoagulant XW0
  Endothelial Damage Inhibitor XY0VX83
  Engineered Autologous Chimeric Antigen
    Receptor T-cell Immunotherapy XW0
  Fusion
    Cervical Vertebral
      2 or more
        Nanotextured Surface XRG2092
        Radiolucent Porous XRG20F3
      Interbody Fusion Device
        Nanotextured Surface XRG1092
        Radiolucent Porous XRG10F3
    Cervicothoracic Vertebral
      Nanotextured Surface XRG4092
      Radiolucent Porous XRG40F3
    Lumbar Vertebral
      2 or more
        Nanotextured Surface XRGC092
        Radiolucent Porous XRGC0F3
      Interbody Fusion Device
        Nanotextured Surface XRGB092
        Radiolucent Porous XRGB0F3

New Technology — continued
  Fusion — continued
    Lumbosacral
      Nanotextured Surface XRGD092
      Radiolucent Porous XRGD0F3
    Occipital-cervical
      Nanotextured Surface XRG0092
      Radiolucent Porous XRG00F3
    Thoracic Vertebral
      2 to 7
        Nanotextured Surface XRG7092
        Radiolucent Porous XRG70F3
      8 or more
        Nanotextured Surface XRG8092
        Radiolucent Porous XRG80F3
      Interbody Fusion Device
        Nanotextured Surface XRG6092
        Radiolucent Porous XRG60F3
    Thoracolumbar Vertebral
      Nanotextured Surface XRGA092
      Radiolucent Porous XRGA0F3
  Idarucizumab, Dabigatran Reversal
    Agent XW0
  Intraoperative Knee Replacement
    Sensor XR2
  Isavuconazole Anti-infective XW0
  Orbital Atherectomy Technology X2C
  Other New Technology Therapeutic
    Substance XW0
  Replacement
    Skin Substitute, Porcine Liver
      Derived XHRPXL2
    Zooplastic Tissue, Rapid Deployment
      Technique X2RF
  Reposition
    Cervical, Magnetically Controlled Growth
      Rod(s) XNS3
    Lumbar, Magnetically Controlled Growth
      Rod(s) XNS0
    Thoracic, Magnetically Controlled
      Growth Rod(s) XNS4
  Uridine Triacetate XW0DX82
Ninth cranial nerve
  use Glossopharyngeal Nerve
Nitinol framed polymer mesh
  use Synthetic Substitute
Non-tunneled central venous catheter
  use Infusion Device
Nonimaging Nuclear Medicine Assay
  Bladder, Kidneys and Ureters CT63
  Blood C763
  Kidneys, Ureters and Bladder CT63
  Lymphatics and Hematologic
    System C76YYZZ
  Ureters, Kidneys and Bladder CT63
  Urinary System CT6YYZZ
Nonimaging Nuclear Medicine Probe
  Abdomen CW50
  Abdomen and Chest CW54
  Abdomen and Pelvis CW51
  Brain C050
  Central Nervous System C05YYZZ
  Chest CW53
  Chest and Abdomen CW54
  Chest and Neck CW56
  Extremity
    Lower CP5PZZZ
    Upper CP5NZZZ
  Head and Neck CW5B
  Heart C25YYZZ
    Right and Left C256
  Lymphatics
    Head C75J
    Head and Neck C755
    Lower Extremity C75P
    Neck C75K
    Pelvic C75D

Nonimaging Nuclear Medicine Probe
— continued
Lymphatics — continued
Trunk C75M
Upper Chest C75L
Upper Extremity C75N
Lymphatics and Hematologic
System C75YYZZ
Musculoskeletal System, Other CP5YYZZ
Neck and Chest CW56
Neck and Head CW5B
Pelvic Region CW5J
Pelvis and Abdomen CW51
Spine CP55ZZZ
Nonimaging Nuclear Medicine Uptake
Endocrine System CG4YYZZ
Gland, Thyroid CG42
Nostril
use Nasal Mucosa and Soft Tissue
Novacor® Left Ventricular Assist Device
use Implantable Heart Assist System in
Heart and Great Vessels
**Novation® Ceramic AHS® (Articulation Hip
System)**
use Synthetic Substitute, Ceramic in 0SR
Nuclear medicine
see Planar Nuclear Medicine Imaging
see Tomographic (Tomo) Nuclear Medicine
Imaging
see Positron Emission Tomographic (PET)
Imaging
see Nonimaging Nuclear Medicine Uptake
see Nonimaging Nuclear Medicine Probe
see Nonimaging Nuclear Medicine Assay
see Systemic Nuclear Medicine Therapy
Nuclear scintigraphy
see Nuclear Medicine
Nutrition, concentrated substances
Enteral infusion 3E0G36Z
Parenteral (peripheral) infusion *see*
Introduction of Nutritional Substance

O

Obliteration
see Destruction
Obturator artery
use Internal Iliac Artery, Right
use Internal Iliac Artery, Left
Obturator lymph node
use Lymphatic, Pelvis
Obturator muscle
use Hip Muscle, Right
use Hip Muscle, Left
Obturator nerve
use Lumbar Plexus
Obturator vein
use Hypogastric Vein, Right
use Hypogastric Vein, Left
Obtuse margin
use Heart, Left
Occipital artery
use External Carotid Artery, Right
use External Carotid Artery, Left
Occipital lobe
use Cerebral Hemisphere
Occipital lymph node
use Lymphatic, Right Neck
use Lymphatic, Left Neck
Occipitofrontalis muscle
use Facial Muscle
Occlusion
Ampulla of Vater 0FLC
Anus 0DLQ

Occlusion — *continued*
Aorta
Abdominal 04L0
Thoracic, Descending 02LW3DJ
Artery
Anterior Tibial
Left 04LQ
Right 04LP
Axillary
Left 03L6
Right 03L5
Brachial
Left 03L8
Right 03L7
Celiac 04L1
Colic
Left 04L7
Middle 04L8
Right 04L6
Common Carotid
Left 03LJ
Right 03LH
Common Iliac
Left 04LD
Right 04LC
External Carotid
Left 03LN
Right 03LM
External Iliac
Left 04LJ
Right 04LH
Face 03LR
Femoral
Left 04LL
Right 04LK
Foot
Left 04LW
Right 04LV
Gastric 04L2
Hand
Left 03LF
Right 03LD
Hepatic 04L3
Inferior Mesenteric 04LB
Innominate 03L2
Internal Carotid
Left 03LL
Right 03LK
Internal Iliac
Left 04LF
Right 04LE
Internal Mammary
Left 03L1
Right 03L0
Intracranial 03LG
Lower 04LY
Peroneal
Left 04LU
Right 04LT
Popliteal
Left 04LN
Right 04LM
Posterior Tibial
Left 04LS
Right 04LR
Pulmonary
Left 02LR
Right 02LQ
Pulmonary Trunk 02LP
Radial
Left 03LC
Right 03LB
Renal
Left 04LA
Right 04L9
Splenic 04L4
Subclavian

Occlusion — *continued*
Artery — *continued*
Left 03L4
Right 03L3
Superior Mesenteric 04L5
Temporal
Left 03LT
Right 03LS
Thyroid
Left 03LV
Right 03LU
Ulnar
Left 03LA
Right 03L9
Upper 03LY
Vertebral
Left 03LQ
Right 03LP
Atrium, Left 02L7
Bladder 0TLB
Bladder Neck 0TLC
Bronchus
Lingula 0BL9
Lower Lobe
Left 0BLB
Right 0BL6
Main
Left 0BL7
Right 0BL3
Middle Lobe, Right 0BL5
Upper Lobe
Left 0BL8
Right 0BL4
Carina 0BL2
Cecum 0DLH
Cisterna Chyli 07LL
Colon
Ascending 0DLK
Descending 0DLM
Sigmoid 0DLN
Transverse 0DLL
Cord
Bilateral 0VLH
Left 0VLG
Right 0VLF
Cul-de-sac 0ULF
Duct
Common Bile 0FL9
Cystic 0FL8
Hepatic
Common 0FL7
Left 0FL6
Right 0FL5
Lacrimal
Left 08LY
Right 08LX
Pancreatic 0FLD
Accessory 0FLF
Parotid
Left 0CLC
Right 0CLB
Duodenum 0DL9
Esophagogastric Junction 0DL4
Esophagus 0DL5
Lower 0DL3
Middle 0DL2
Upper 0DL1
Fallopian Tube
Left 0UL6
Right 0UL5
Fallopian Tubes, Bilateral 0UL7
Ileocecal Valve 0DLC
Ileum 0DLB
Intestine
Large 0DLE
Left 0DLG
Right 0DLF
Small 0DL8

Occlusion — *continued*
Jejunum 0DLA
Kidney Pelvis
    Left 0TL4
    Right 0TL3
Left atrial appendage (LAA) *see* Occlusion, Atrium, Left 02L7
Lymphatic
    Aortic 07LD
    Axillary
        Left 07L6
        Right 07L5
    Head 07L0
    Inguinal
        Left 07LJ
        Right 07LH
    Internal Mammary
        Left 07L9
        Right 07L8
    Lower Extremity
        Left 07LG
        Right 07LF
    Mesenteric 07LB
    Neck
        Left 07L2
        Right 07L1
    Pelvis 07LC
    Thoracic Duct 07LK
    Thorax 07L7
    Upper Extremity
        Left 07L4
        Right 07L3
Rectum 0DLP
Stomach 0DL6
    Pylorus 0DL7
Trachea 0BL1
Ureter
    Left 0TL7
    Right 0TL6
Urethra 0TLD
Vagina 0ULG
Valve, Pulmonary 02LH
Vas Deferens
    Bilateral 0VLQ
    Left 0VLP
    Right 0VLN
Vein
    Axillary
        Left 05L8
        Right 05L7
    Azygos 05L0
    Basilic
        Left 05LC
        Right 05LB
    Brachial
        Left 05LA
        Right 05L9
    Cephalic
        Left 05LF
        Right 05LD
    Colic 06L7
    Common Iliac
        Left 06LD
        Right 06LC
    Esophageal 06L3
    External Iliac
        Left 06LG
        Right 06LF
    External Jugular
        Left 05LQ
        Right 05LP
    Face
        Left 05LV
        Right 05LT
    Femoral
        Left 06LN
        Right 06LM

Occlusion — *continued*
Vein — *continued*
    Foot
        Left 06LV
        Right 06LT
    Gastric 06L2
    Hand
        Left 05LH
        Right 05LG
    Hemiazygos 05L1
    Hepatic 06L4
    Hypogastric
        Left 06LJ
        Right 06LH
    Inferior Mesenteric 06L6
    Innominate
        Left 05L4
        Right 05L3
    Internal Jugular
        Left 05LN
        Right 05LM
    Intracranial 05LL
    Lower 06LY
    Portal 06L8
    Pulmonary
        Left 02LT
        Right 02LS
    Renal
        Left 06LB
        Right 06L9
    Saphenous
        Left 06LQ
        Right 06LP
    Splenic 06L1
    Subclavian
        Left 05L6
        Right 05L5
    Superior Mesenteric 06L5
    Upper 05LY
    Vertebral
        Left 05LS
        Right 05LR
    Vena Cava
        Inferior 06L0
        Superior 02LV
Occlusion, REBOA (resuscitative endovascular balloon occlusion of the aorta)
    02LW3DJ
    04L03DJ
Occupational therapy
    see Activities of Daily Living Treatment, Rehabilitation F08
Odentectomy
    see Excision, Mouth and Throat 0CB
    see Resection, Mouth and Throat 0CT
Odontoid process
    use Cervical Vertebra
Olecranon bursa
    use Elbow Bursa and Ligament, Right
    use Elbow Bursa and Ligament, Left
Olecranon process
    use Ulna, Right
    use Ulna, Left
Olfactory bulb
    use Olfactory Nerve
Omentectomy, omentumectomy
    see Excision, Gastrointestinal System 0DB
    see Resection, Gastrointestinal System 0DT
Omentofixation
    see Repair, Gastrointestinal System 0DQ
Omentoplasty
    see Repair, Gastrointestinal System 0DQ
    see Replacement, Gastrointestinal System 0DR
    see Supplement, Gastrointestinal System 0DU

Omentorrhaphy
    see Repair, Gastrointestinal System 0DQ
Omentotomy
    see Drainage, Gastrointestinal System 0D9
Omnilink Elite® Vascular Balloon Expandable Stent System
    use Intraluminal Device
Onychectomy
    see Excision, Skin and Breast 0HB
    see Resection, Skin and Breast 0HT
Onychoplasty
    see Repair, Skin and Breast 0HQ
    see Replacement, Skin and Breast 0HR
Onychotomy
    see Drainage, Skin and Breast 0H9
Oophorectomy
    see Excision, Female Reproductive System 0UB
    see Resection, Female Reproductive System 0UT
Oophoropexy
    see Repair, Female Reproductive System 0UQ
    see Reposition, Female Reproductive System 0US
Oophoroplasty
    see Repair, Female Reproductive System 0UQ
    see Supplement, Female Reproductive System 0UU
Oophororrhaphy
    see Repair, Female Reproductive System 0UQ
Oophorostomy
    see Drainage, Female Reproductive System 0U9
Oophorotomy
    see Division, Female Reproductive System 0U8
    see Drainage, Female Reproductive System 0U9
Oophorrhaphy
    see Repair, Female Reproductive System 0UQ
Open Pivot™ (mechanical) valve
    use Synthetic Substitute
Open Pivot™ Aortic Valve Graft (AVG)
    use Synthetic Substitute
Ophthalmic artery
    use Intracranial Artery
Ophthalmic nerve
    use Trigeminal Nerve
Ophthalmic vein
    use Intracranial Vein
Opponensplasty
    Tendon replacement *see* Replacement, Tendons 0LR
    Tendon transfer *see* Transfer, Tendons 0LX
Optic chiasma
    use Optic Nerve
Optic disc
    use Retina, Right
    use Retina, Left
Optic foramen
    use Sphenoid Bone
Optical coherence tomography, intravascular
    see Computerized Tomography (CT Scan)
Optimizer™ III implantable pulse generator
    use Contractility Modulation Device in 0JH
Orbicularis oculi muscle
    use Upper Eyelid, Right
    use Upper Eyelid, Left
Orbicularis oris muscle
    use Facial Muscle
Orbital Atherectomy Technology X2C

Orbital fascia
  use Subcutaneous Tissue and Fascia, Face
Orbital portion of ethmoid bone
  use Orbit, Right
  use Orbit, Left
Orbital portion of frontal bone
  use Orbit, Right
  use Orbit, Left
Orbital portion of lacrimal bone
  use Orbit, Right
  use Orbit, Left
Orbital portion of maxilla
  use Orbit, Right
  use Orbit, Left
Orbital portion of palatine bone
  use Orbit, Right
  use Orbit, Left
Orbital portion of sphenoid bone
  use Orbit, Right
  use Orbit, Left
Orbital portion of zygomatic bone
  use Orbit, Right
  use Orbit, Left
Orchectomy, orchidectomy, orchiectomy
  see Excision, Male Reproductive
    System 0VB
  see Resection, Male Reproductive
    System 0VT
Orchidoplasty, orchioplasty
  see Repair, Male Reproductive System 0VQ
  see Replacement, Male Reproductive
    System 0VR
  see Supplement, Male Reproductive
    System 0VU
Orchidorrhaphy, orchiorrhaphy
  see Repair, Male Reproductive System 0VQ
Orchidotomy, orchiotomy, orchotomy
  see Drainage, Male Reproductive
    System 0V9
Orchiopexy
  see Repair, Male Reproductive System 0VQ
  see Reposition, Male Reproductive
    System 0VS
Oropharyngeal airway (OPA)
  use Intraluminal Device, Airway in Mouth
    and Throat
Oropharynx
  use Pharynx
Ossiculectomy
  see Excision, Ear, Nose, Sinus 09B
  see Resection, Ear, Nose, Sinus 09T
Ossiculotomy
  see Drainage, Ear, Nose, Sinus 099
Ostectomy
  see Excision, Head and Facial Bones 0NB
  see Resection, Head and Facial Bones 0NT
  see Excision, Upper Bones 0PB
  see Resection, Upper Bones 0PT
  see Excision, Lower Bones 0QB
  see Resection, Lower Bones 0QT
Osteoclasis
  see Division, Head and Facial Bones 0N8
  see Division, Upper Bones 0P8
  see Division, Lower Bones 0Q8
Osteolysis
  see Release, Head and Facial Bones 0NN
  see Release, Upper Bones 0PN
  see Release, Lower Bones 0QN
Osteopathic Treatment
  Abdomen 7W09X
  Cervical 7W01X
  Extremity
    Lower 7W06X
    Upper 7W07X
  Head 7W00X
  Lumbar 7W03X

Osteopathic Treatment — *continued*
  Pelvis 7W05X
  Rib Cage 7W08X
  Sacrum 7W04X
  Thoracic 7W02X
Osteopexy
  see Repair, Head and Facial Bones 0NQ
  see Reposition, Head and Facial Bones 0NS
  see Repair, Upper Bones 0PQ
  see Reposition, Upper Bones 0PS
  see Repair, Lower Bones 0QQ
  see Reposition, Lower Bones 0QS
Osteoplasty
  see Repair, Head and Facial Bones 0NQ
  see Replacement, Head and Facial
    Bones 0NR
  see Supplement, Head and Facial
    Bones 0NU
  see Repair, Upper Bones 0PQ
  see Replacement, Upper Bones 0PR
  see Supplement, Upper Bones 0PU
  see Repair, Lower Bones 0QQ
  see Replacement, Lower Bones 0QR
  see Supplement, Lower Bones 0QU
Osteorrhaphy
  see Repair, Head and Facial Bones 0NQ
  see Repair, Upper Bones 0PQ
  see Repair, Lower Bones 0QQ
Osteotomy, ostotomy
  see Division, Head and Facial Bones 0N8
  see Drainage, Head and Facial Bones 0N9
  see Division, Upper Bones 0P8
  see Drainage, Upper Bones 0P9
  see Division, Lower Bones 0Q8
  see Drainage, Lower Bones 0Q9
Otic ganglion
  use Head and Neck Sympathetic Nerve
Otoplasty
  see Repair, Ear, Nose, Sinus 09Q
  see Replacement, Ear, Nose, Sinus 09R
  see Supplement, Ear, Nose, Sinus 09U
Otoscopy
  see Inspection, Ear, Nose, Sinus 09J
Oval window
  use Middle Ear, Right
  use Middle Ear, Left
Ovarian artery
  use Abdominal Aorta
Ovarian ligament
  use Uterine Supporting Structure
Ovariectomy
  see Excision, Female Reproductive
    System 0UB
  see Resection, Female Reproductive
    System 0UT
Ovariocentesis
  see Drainage, Female Reproductive
    System 0U9
Ovariopexy
  see Repair, Female Reproductive
    System 0UQ
  see Reposition, Female Reproductive
    System 0US
Ovariotomy
  see Division, Female Reproductive
    System 0U8
  see Drainage, Female Reproductive
    System 0U9
Ovatio™ CRT-D
  use Cardiac Resynchronization Defibrillator
    Pulse Generator in 0JH
Oversewing
  Gastrointestinal ulcer *see* Repair,
    Gastrointestinal System 0DQ
  Pleural bleb *see* Repair, Respiratory
    System 0BQ

Oviduct
  use Fallopian Tube, Right
  use Fallopian Tube, Left
Oximetry, Fetal pulse 10H073Z
OXINIUM™
  use Synthetic Substitute, Oxidized
    Zirconium on Polyethylene in 0SR
Oxygenation
  Extracorporeal membrane (ECMO) *see*
    Performance, Circulatory 5A15
  Hyperbaric *see* Assistance, Circulatory 5A05
  Supersaturated *see* Assistance,
    Circulatory 5A05

P

Pacemaker
  Dual Chamber
    Abdomen 0JH8
    Chest 0JH6
  Intracardiac
    Insertion of device in
      Atrium
        Left 02H7
        Right 02H6
      Vein, Coronary 02H4
      Ventricle
        Left 02HL
        Right 02HK
    Removal of device from, Heart 02PA
    Revision of device in, Heart 02WA
  Single Chamber
    Abdomen 0JH8
    Chest 0JH6
  Single Chamber Rate Responsive
    Abdomen 0JH8
    Chest 0JH6
Packing
  Abdominal Wall 2W43X5Z
  Anorectal 2Y43X5Z
  Arm
    Lower
      Left 2W4DX5Z
      Right 2W4CX5Z
    Upper
      Left 2W4BX5Z
      Right 2W4AX5Z
  Back 2W45X5Z
  Chest Wall 2W44X5Z
  Ear 2Y42X5Z
  Extremity
    Lower
      Left 2W4MX5Z
      Right 2W4LX5Z
    Upper
      Left 2W49X5Z
      Right 2W48X5Z
  Face 2W41X5Z
  Finger
    Left 2W4KX5Z
    Right 2W4JX5Z
  Foot
    Left 2W4TX5Z
    Right 2W4SX5Z
  Genital Tract, Female 2Y44X5Z
  Hand
    Left 2W4FX5Z
    Right 2W4EX5Z
  Head 2W40X5Z
  Inguinal Region
    Left 2W47X5Z
    Right 2W46X5Z
  Leg
    Lower
      Left 2W4RX5Z
      Right 2W4QX5Z

Packing — *continued*
  Leg — *continued*
    Upper
      Left 2W4PX5Z
      Right 2W4NX5Z
    Mouth and Pharynx 2Y40X5Z
    Nasal 2Y41X5Z
    Neck 2W42X5Z
    Thumb
      Left 2W4HX5Z
      Right 2W4GX5Z
    Toe
      Left 2W4VX5Z
      Right 2W4UX5Z
    Urethra 2Y45X5Z
Paclitaxel-eluting coronary stent
  use Intraluminal Device, Drug-eluting in
    Heart and Great Vessels
Paclitaxel-eluting peripheral stent
  use Intraluminal Device, Drug-eluting in
    Upper Arteries
  use Intraluminal Device, Drug-eluting in
    Lower Arteries
Palatine gland
  use Buccal Mucosa
Palatine tonsil
  use Tonsils
Palatine uvula
  use Uvula
Palatoglossal muscle
  use Tongue, Palate, Pharynx Muscle
Palatopharyngeal muscle
  use Tongue, Palate, Pharynx Muscle
Palatoplasty
  see Repair, Mouth and Throat 0CQ
  see Replacement, Mouth and Throat 0CR
  see Supplement, Mouth and Throat 0CU
Palatorrhaphy
  see Repair, Mouth and Throat 0CQ
Palmar (volar) digital vein
  use Hand Vein, Right
  use Hand Vein, Left
Palmar (volar) metacarpal vein
  use Hand Vein, Right
  use Hand Vein, Left
Palmar cutaneous nerve
  use Median Nerve
  use Radial Nerve
Palmar fascia (aponeurosis)
  use Subcutaneous Tissue and Fascia, Right
    Hand
  use Subcutaneous Tissue and Fascia, Left
    Hand
Palmar interosseous muscle
  use Hand Muscle, Right
  use Hand Muscle, Left
Palmar ulnocarpal ligament
  use Wrist Bursa and Ligament, Right
  use Wrist Bursa and Ligament, Left
Palmaris longus muscle
  use Lower Arm and Wrist Muscle, Right
  use Lower Arm and Wrist Muscle, Left
Pancreatectomy
  see Excision, Pancreas 0FBG
  see Resection, Pancreas 0FTG
Pancreatic artery
  use Splenic Artery
Pancreatic plexus
  use Abdominal Sympathetic Nerve
Pancreatic vein
  use Splenic Vein
Pancreaticoduodenostomy
  see Bypass, Hepatobiliary System and
    Pancreas 0F1
Pancreaticosplenic lymph node
  use Lymphatic, Aortic

Pancreatogram, endoscopic retrograde
  see Fluoroscopy, Pancreatic Duct BF18
Pancreatolithotomy
  see Extirpation, Pancreas 0FCG
Pancreatotomy
  see Division, Pancreas 0F8G
  see Drainage, Pancreas 0F9G
Panniculectomy
  see Excision, Skin, Abdomen 0HB7
  see Excision, Abdominal Wall 0WBF
Paraaortic lymph node
  use Lymphatic, Aortic
Paracentesis
  Eye *see* Drainage, Eye 089
  Peritoneal Cavity *see* Drainage, Peritoneal
    Cavity 0W9G
  Tympanum *see* Drainage, Ear, Nose,
    Sinus 099
Pararectal lymph node
  use Lymphatic, Mesenteric
Parasternal lymph node
  use Lymphatic, Thorax
Parathyroidectomy
  see Excision, Endocrine System 0GB
  see Resection, Endocrine System 0GT
Paratracheal lymph node
  use Lymphatic, Thorax
Paraurethral (Skene's) gland
  use Vestibular Gland
Parenteral nutrition, total
  see Introduction of Nutritional Substance
Parietal lobe
  use Cerebral Hemisphere
Parotid lymph node
  use Lymphatic, Head
Parotid plexus
  use Facial Nerve
Parotidectomy
  see Excision, Mouth and Throat 0CB
  see Resection, Mouth and Throat 0CT
Pars flaccida
  use Tympanic Membrane, Right
  use Tympanic Membrane, Left
Partial joint replacement
  Hip *see* Replacement, Lower Joints 0SR
  Knee *see* Replacement, Lower Joints 0SR
  Shoulder *see* Replacement, Upper Joints 0RR
Partially absorbable mesh
  use Synthetic Substitute
Patch, blood, spinal 3E0S3GC
Patellapexy
  see Repair, Lower Bones 0QQ
  see Reposition, Lower Bones 0QS
Patellaplasty
  see Repair, Lower Bones 0QQ
  see Replacement, Lower Bones 0QR
  see Supplement, Lower Bones 0QU
Patellar ligament
  use Knee Bursa and Ligament, Right
  use Knee Bursa and Ligament, Left
Patellar tendon
  use Knee Tendon, Right
  use Knee Tendon, Left
Patellectomy
  see Excision, Lower Bones 0QB
  see Resection, Lower Bones 0QT
Patellofemoral joint
  use Knee Joint, Right
  use Knee Joint, Left
  use Knee Joint, Femoral Surface, Right
  use Knee Joint, Femoral Surface, Left
Pectineus muscle
  use Upper Leg Muscle, Right
  use Upper Leg Muscle, Left
Pectoral (anterior) lymph node
  use Lymphatic, Right Axillary
  use Lymphatic, Left Axillary

Pectoral fascia
  use Subcutaneous Tissue and Fascia, Chest
Pectoralis major muscle
  use Thorax Muscle, Right
  use Thorax Muscle, Left
Pectoralis minor muscle
  use Thorax Muscle, Right
  use Thorax Muscle, Left
Pedicle-based dynamic stabilization device
  use Spinal Stabilization Device, Pedicle-
    Based in 0RH
  use Spinal Stabilization Device, Pedicle-
    Based in 0SH
PEEP (positive end expiratory pressure)
  see Assistance, Respiratory 5A09
**PEG (percutaneous endoscopic
  gastrostomy)** 0DH63UZ
**PEJ (percutaneous endoscopic
  jejunostomy)** 0DHA3UZ
Pelvic splanchnic nerve
  use Abdominal Sympathetic Nerve
  use Sacral Sympathetic Nerve
Penectomy
  see Excision, Male Reproductive
    System 0VB
  see Resection, Male Reproductive
    System 0VT
Penile urethra
  use Urethra
Perceval sutureless valve
  use Zooplastic Tissue, Rapid Deployment
    Technique in New Technology
**Percutaneous endoscopic
  gastrojejunostomy (PEG/J) tube**
  use Feeding Device in Gastrointestinal
    System
**Percutaneous endoscopic gastrostomy
  (PEG) tube**
  use Feeding Device in Gastrointestinal
    System
Percutaneous nephrostomy catheter
  use Drainage Device
**Percutaneous transluminal coronary
  angioplasty (PTCA)**
  see Dilation, Heart and Great Vessels 027
Performance
  Biliary
    Multiple, Filtration 5A1C60Z
    Single, Filtration 5A1C00Z
  Cardiac
    Continuous
      Output 5A1221Z
      Pacing 5A1223Z
    Intermittent, Pacing 5A1213Z
    Single, Output, Manual 5A12012
  Circulatory, Continuous, Oxygenation,
    Membrane 5A15223
  Respiratory
    24-96 Consecutive Hours,
      Ventilation 5A1945Z
    Greater than 96 Consecutive Hours,
      Ventilation 5A1955Z
    Less than 24 Consecutive Hours,
      Ventilation 5A1935Z
    Single, Ventilation,
      Nonmechanical 5A19054
  Urinary
    Continuous, Greater than 18 hours per
      day, Filtration 5A1D90Z
    Intermittent, Less than 6 Hours Per Day,
      Filtration 5A1D70Z
    Prolonged Intermittent, 6-18 hours per
      day, Filtration 5A1D80Z
Perfusion
  see Introduction of substance in or on
Perfusion, donor organ
  Heart 6AB50BZ

Perfusion, donor organ — *continued*
Kidney(s) 6ABT0BZ
Liver 6ABF0BZ
Lung(s) 6ABB0BZ
Pericardiectomy
see Excision, Pericardium 02BN
see Resection, Pericardium 02TN
Pericardiocentesis
see Drainage, Pericardial Cavity 0W9D
Pericardiolysis
see Release, Pericardium 02NN
Pericardiophrenic artery
use Internal Mammary Artery, Right
use Internal Mammary Artery, Left
Pericardioplasty
see Repair, Pericardium 02QN
see Replacement, Pericardium 02RN
see Supplement, Pericardium 02UN
Pericardiorrhaphy
see Repair, Pericardium 02QN
Pericardiostomy
see Drainage, Pericardial Cavity 0W9D
Pericardiotomy
see Drainage, Pericardial Cavity 0W9D
Perimetrium
use Uterus
Peripheral parenteral nutrition
see Introduction of Nutritional Substance
Peripherally inserted central catheter (PICC)
use Infusion Device
Peritoneal dialysis 3E1M39Z
Peritoneocentesis
see Drainage, Peritoneum 0D9W
see Drainage, Peritoneal Cavity 0W9G
Peritoneoplasty
see Repair, Peritoneum 0DQW
see Replacement, Peritoneum 0DRW
see Supplement, Peritoneum 0DUW
Peritoneoscopy 0DJW4ZZ
Peritoneotomy
see Drainage, Peritoneum 0D9W
Peritoneumectomy
see Excision, Peritoneum 0DBW
Peroneus brevis muscle
use Lower Leg Muscle, Right
use Lower Leg Muscle, Left
Peroneus longus muscle
use Lower Leg Muscle, Right
use Lower Leg Muscle, Left
Pessary ring
use Intraluminal Device, Pessary in Female Reproductive System
PET scan
see Positron Emission Tomographic (PET) Imaging
Petrous part of temporal bone
use Temporal Bone, Right
use Temporal Bone, Left
Phacoemulsification, lens
With IOL implant *see* Replacement, Eye 08R
Without IOL implant *see* Extraction, Eye 08D
Phalangectomy
see Excision, Upper Bones 0PB
see Resection, Upper Bones 0PT
see Excision, Lower Bones 0QB
see Resection, Lower Bones 0QT
Phallectomy
see Excision, Penis 0VBS
see Resection, Penis 0VTS
Phalloplasty
see Repair, Penis 0VQS
see Supplement, Penis 0VUS
Phallotomy
see Drainage, Penis 0V9S

Pharmacotherapy, for substance abuse
Antabuse HZ93ZZZ
Bupropion HZ97ZZZ
Clonidine HZ96ZZZ
Levo-alpha-acetyl-methadol (LAAM) HZ92ZZZ
Methadone Maintenance HZ91ZZZ
Naloxone HZ95ZZZ
Naltrexone HZ94ZZZ
Nicotine Replacement HZ90ZZZ
Psychiatric Medication HZ98ZZZ
Replacement Medication, Other HZ99ZZZ
Pharyngeal constrictor muscle
use Tongue, Palate, Pharynx Muscle
Pharyngeal plexus
use Vagus Nerve
Pharyngeal recess
use Nasopharynx
Pharyngeal tonsil
use Adenoids
Pharyngogram
see Fluoroscopy, Pharynx B91G
Pharyngoplasty
see Repair, Mouth and Throat 0CQ
see Replacement, Mouth and Throat 0CR
see Supplement, Mouth and Throat 0CU
Pharyngorrhaphy
see Repair, Mouth and Throat 0CQ
Pharyngotomy
see Drainage, Mouth and Throat 0C9
Pharyngotympanic tube
use Eustachian Tube, Right
use Eustachian Tube, Left
Pheresis
Erythrocytes 6A55
Leukocytes 6A55
Plasma 6A55
Platelets 6A55
Stem Cells
Cord Blood 6A55
Hematopoietic 6A55
Phlebectomy
see Excision, Upper Veins 05B
see Extraction, Upper Veins 05D
see Excision, Lower Veins 06B
see Extraction, Lower Veins 06D
Phlebography
see Plain Radiography, Veins B50
Impedance 4A04X51
Phleborrhaphy
see Repair, Upper Veins 05Q
see Repair, Lower Veins 06Q
Phlebotomy
see Drainage, Upper Veins 059
see Drainage, Lower Veins 069
Photocoagulation
for Destruction *see* Destruction
for Repair *see* Repair
Photopheresis, therapeutic
see Phototherapy, Circulatory 6A65
Phototherapy
Circulatory 6A65
Skin 6A60
Ultraviolet light *see* Ultraviolet Light Therapy, Physiological Systems 6A8
Phrenectomy, phrenoneurectomy
see Excision, Nerve, Phrenic 01B2
Phrenemphraxis
see Destruction, Nerve, Phrenic 0152
Phrenic nerve stimulator generator
use Stimulator Generator in Subcutaneous Tissue and Fascia
Phrenic nerve stimulator lead
use Diaphragmatic Pacemaker Lead in Respiratory System
Phreniclasis
see Destruction, Nerve, Phrenic 0152

Phrenicoexeresis
see Extraction, Nerve, Phrenic 01D2
Phrenicotomy
see Division, Nerve, Phrenic 0182
Phrenicotripsy
see Destruction, Nerve, Phrenic 0152
Phrenoplasty
see Repair, Respiratory System 0BQ
see Supplement, Respiratory System 0BU
Phrenotomy
see Drainage, Respiratory System 0B9
Physiatry
see Motor Treatment, Rehabilitation F07
Physical medicine
see Motor Treatment, Rehabilitation F07
Physical therapy
see Motor Treatment, Rehabilitation F07
PHYSIOMESH™ Flexible Composite Mesh
use Synthetic Substitute
Pia mater, intracranial
use Cerebral Meninges
Pia mater, spinal
use Spinal Meninges
Pinealectomy
see Excision, Pineal Body 0GB1
see Resection, Pineal Body 0GT1
Pinealoscopy 0GJ14ZZ
Pinealotomy
see Drainage, Pineal Body 0G91
Pinna
use External Ear, Right
use External Ear, Left
use External Ear, Bilateral
Pipeline™ Embolization device (PED)
use Intraluminal Device
Piriform recess (sinus)
use Pharynx
Piriformis muscle
use Hip Muscle, Right
use Hip Muscle, Left
PIRRT (Prolonged intermittent renal replacement therapy) 5A1D80Z
Pisiform bone
use Carpal, Right
use Carpal, Left
Pisohamate ligament
use Hand Bursa and Ligament, Right
use Hand Bursa and Ligament, Left
Pisometacarpal ligament
use Hand Bursa and Ligament, Right
use Hand Bursa and Ligament, Left
Pituitectomy
see Excision, Gland, Pituitary 0GB0
see Resection, Gland, Pituitary 0GT0
Plain film radiology
see Plain Radiography
Plain Radiography
Abdomen BW00ZZZ
Abdomen and Pelvis BW01ZZZ
Abdominal Lymphatic
Bilateral B701
Unilateral B700
Airway, Upper BB0DZZZ
Ankle
Left BQ0H
Right BQ0G
Aorta
Abdominal B400
Thoracic B300
Thoraco-Abdominal B30P
Aorta and Bilateral Lower Extremity Arteries B40D
Arch
Bilateral BN0DZZZ
Left BN0CZZZ
Right BN0BZZZ

Plain Radiography — *continued*
Arm
    Left BP0FZZZ
    Right BP0EZZZ
Artery
    Brachiocephalic-Subclavian, Right B301
    Bronchial B30L
    Bypass Graft, Other B20F
    Cervico-Cerebral Arch B30Q
    Common Carotid
        Bilateral B305
        Left B304
        Right B303
    Coronary
        Bypass Graft
            Multiple B203
            Single B202
        Multiple B201
        Single B200
    External Carotid
        Bilateral B30C
        Left B30B
        Right B309
    Hepatic B402
    Inferior Mesenteric B405
    Intercostal B30L
    Internal Carotid
        Bilateral B308
        Left B307
        Right B306
    Internal Mammary Bypass Graft
        Left B208
        Right B207
    Intra-Abdominal, Other B40B
    Intracranial B30R
    Lower, Other B40J
    Lower Extremity
        Bilateral and Aorta B40D
        Left B40G
        Right B40F
    Lumbar B409
    Pelvic B40C
    Pulmonary
        Left B30T
        Right B30S
    Renal
        Bilateral B408
        Left B407
        Right B406
        Transplant B40M
    Spinal B30M
    Splenic B403
    Subclavian, Left B302
    Superior Mesenteric B404
    Upper, Other B30N
    Upper Extremity
        Bilateral B30K
        Left B30J
        Right B30H
    Vertebral
        Bilateral B30G
        Left B30F
        Right B30D
Bile Duct BF00
Bile Duct and Gallbladder BF03
Bladder BT00
    Kidney and Ureter BT04
Bladder and Urethra BT0B
Bone
    Facial BN05ZZZ
    Nasal BN04ZZZ
Bones, Long, All BW0BZZZ
Breast
    Bilateral BH02ZZZ
    Left BH01ZZZ
    Right BH00ZZZ

Plain Radiography — *continued*
Calcaneus
    Left BQ0KZZZ
    Right BQ0JZZZ
Chest BW03ZZZ
Clavicle
    Left BP05ZZZ
    Right BP04ZZZ
Coccyx BR0FZZZ
Corpora Cavernosa BV00
Dialysis Fistula B50W
Dialysis Shunt B50W
Disc
    Cervical BR01
    Lumbar BR03
    Thoracic BR02
Duct
    Lacrimal
        Bilateral B802
        Left B801
        Right B800
    Mammary
        Multiple
            Left BH06
            Right BH05
        Single
            Left BH04
            Right BH03
Elbow
    Left BP0H
    Right BP0G
Epididymis
    Left BV02
    Right BV01
Extremity
    Lower BW0CZZZ
    Upper BW0JZZZ
Eye
    Bilateral B807ZZZ
    Left B806ZZZ
    Right B805ZZZ
Facet Joint
    Cervical BR04
    Lumbar BR06
    Thoracic BR05
Fallopian Tube
    Bilateral BU02
    Left BU01
    Right BU00
Fallopian Tube and Uterus BU08
Femur
    Left, Densitometry BQ04ZZ1
    Right, Densitometry BQ03ZZ1
Finger
    Left BP0SZZZ
    Right BP0RZZZ
Foot
    Left BQ0MZZZ
    Right BQ0LZZZ
Forearm
    Left BP0KZZZ
    Right BP0JZZZ
Gallbladder and Bile Duct BF03
Gland
    Parotid
        Bilateral B906
        Left B905
        Right B904
    Salivary
        Bilateral B90D
        Left B90C
        Right B90B
    Submandibular
        Bilateral B909
        Left B908
        Right B907

Plain Radiography — *continued*
Hand
    Left BP0PZZZ
    Right BP0NZZZ
Heart
    Left B205
    Right B204
    Right and Left B206
Hepatobiliary System, All BF0C
Hip
    Left BQ01
        Densitometry BQ01ZZ1
    Right BQ00
        Densitometry BQ00ZZ1
Humerus
    Left BP0BZZZ
    Right BP0AZZZ
Ileal Diversion Loop BT0C
Intracranial Sinus B502
Joint
    Acromioclavicular, Bilateral BP03ZZZ
    Finger
        Left BP0D
        Right BP0C
    Foot
        Left BQ0Y
        Right BQ0X
    Hand
        Left BP0D
        Right BP0C
    Lumbosacral BR0BZZZ
    Sacroiliac BR0D
    Sternoclavicular
        Bilateral BP02ZZZ
        Left BP01ZZZ
        Right BP00ZZZ
    Temporomandibular
        Bilateral BN09
        Left BN08
        Right BN07
    Thoracolumbar BR08ZZZ
    Toe
        Left BQ0Y
        Right BQ0X
Kidney
    Bilateral BT03
    Left BT02
    Right BT01
    Ureter and Bladder BT04
Knee
    Left BQ08
    Right BQ07
Leg
    Left BQ0FZZZ
    Right BQ0DZZZ
Lymphatic
    Head B704
    Lower Extremity
        Bilateral B70B
        Left B709
        Right B708
    Neck B704
    Pelvic B70C
    Upper Extremity
        Bilateral B707
        Left B706
        Right B705
Mandible BN06ZZZ
Mastoid B90HZZZ
Nasopharynx B90FZZZ
Optic Foramina
    Left B804ZZZ
    Right B803ZZZ
Orbit
    Bilateral BN03ZZZ
    Left BN02ZZZ
    Right BN01ZZZ

Plain Radiography — *continued*
Oropharynx B90FZZZ
Patella
  Left BQ0WZZZ
  Right BQ0VZZZ
Pelvis BR0CZZZ
Pelvis and Abdomen BW01ZZZ
Prostate BV03
Retroperitoneal Lymphatic
  Bilateral B701
  Unilateral B700
Ribs
  Left BP0YZZZ
  Right BP0XZZZ
Sacrum BR0FZZZ
Scapula
  Left BP07ZZZ
  Right BP06ZZZ
Shoulder
  Left BP09
  Right BP08
Sinus
  Intracranial B502
  Paranasal B902ZZZ
Skull BN00ZZZ
Spinal Cord B00B
Spine
  Cervical, Densitometry BR00ZZ1
  Lumbar, Densitometry BR09ZZ1
  Thoracic, Densitometry BR07ZZ1
  Whole, Densitometry BR0GZZ1
Sternum BR0HZZZ
Teeth
  All BN0JZZZ
  Multiple BN0HZZZ
Testicle
  Left BV06
  Right BV05
Toe
  Left BQ0QZZZ
  Right BQ0PZZZ
Tooth, Single BN0GZZZ
Tracheobronchial Tree
  Bilateral BB09YZZ
  Left BB08YZZ
  Right BB07YZZ
Ureter
  Bilateral BT08
  Kidney and Bladder BT04
  Left BT07
  Right BT06
Urethra BT05
Urethra and Bladder BT0B
Uterus BU06
Uterus and Fallopian Tube BU08
Vagina BU09
Vasa Vasorum BV08
Vein
  Cerebellar B501
  Cerebral B501
  Epidural B500
  Jugular
    Bilateral B505
    Left B504
    Right B503
  Lower Extremity
    Bilateral B50D
    Left B50C
    Right B50B
  Other B50V
  Pelvic (Iliac)
    Left B50G
    Right B50F
  Pelvic (Iliac) Bilateral B50H
  Portal B50T
  Pulmonary

Plain Radiography — *continued*
Vein — *continued*
  Bilateral B50S
  Left B50R
  Right B50Q
  Renal
    Bilateral B50L
    Left B50K
    Right B50J
  Splanchnic B50T
  Subclavian
    Left B507
    Right B506
  Upper Extremity
    Bilateral B50P
    Left B50N
    Right B50M
  Vena Cava
    Inferior B509
    Superior B508
  Whole Body BW0KZZZ
    Infant BW0MZZZ
  Whole Skeleton BW0LZZZ
  Wrist
    Left BP0M
    Right BP0L
Planar Nuclear Medicine Imaging
Abdomen CW10
Abdomen and Chest CW14
Abdomen and Pelvis CW11
Anatomical Region, Other CW1ZZZZ
Anatomical Regions, Multiple CW1YYZZ
Bladder, Kidneys and Ureters CT13
Bladder and Ureters CT1H
Blood C713
Bone Marrow C710
Brain C010
Breast CH1YYZZ
  Bilateral CH12
  Left CH11
  Right CH10
Bronchi and Lungs CB12
Central Nervous System C01YYZZ
Cerebrospinal Fluid C015
Chest CW13
Chest and Abdomen CW14
Chest and Neck CW16
Digestive System CD1YYZZ
Ducts, Lacrimal, Bilateral C819
Ear, Nose, Mouth and Throat C91YYZZ
Endocrine System CG1YYZZ
Extremity
  Lower CW1D
    Bilateral CP1F
    Left CP1D
    Right CP1C
  Upper CW1M
    Bilateral CP1B
    Left CP19
    Right CP18
Eye C81YYZZ
Gallbladder CF14
Gastrointestinal Tract CD17
  Upper CD15
Gland
  Adrenal, Bilateral CG14
  Parathyroid CG11
  Thyroid CG12
Glands, Salivary, Bilateral C91B
Head and Neck CW1B
Heart C21YYZZ
  Right and Left C216
Hepatobiliary System, All CF1C
Hepatobiliary System and
  Pancreas CF1YYZZ
Kidneys, Ureters and Bladder CT13
Liver CF15

Planar Nuclear Medicine Imaging — *continued*
Liver and Spleen CF16
Lungs and Bronchi CB12
Lymphatics
  Head C71J
  Head and Neck C715
  Lower Extremity C71P
  Neck C71K
  Pelvic C71D
  Trunk C71M
  Upper Chest C71L
  Upper Extremity C71N
Lymphatics and Hematologic
  System C71YYZZ
Musculoskeletal System
  All CP1Z
  Other CP1YYZZ
Myocardium C21G
Neck and Chest CW16
Neck and Head CW1B
Pancreas and Hepatobiliary
  System CF1YYZZ
Pelvic Region CW1J
Pelvis CP16
Pelvis and Abdomen CW11
Pelvis and Spine CP17
Reproductive System, Male CV1YYZZ
Respiratory System CB1YYZZ
Skin CH1YYZZ
Skull CP11
Spine CP15
Spine and Pelvis CP17
Spleen C712
Spleen and Liver CF16
Subcutaneous Tissue CH1YYZZ
Testicles, Bilateral CV19
Thorax CP14
Ureters, Kidneys and Bladder CT13
Ureters and Bladder CT1H
Urinary System CT1YYZZ
Veins C51YYZZ
  Central C51R
  Lower Extremity
    Bilateral C51D
    Left C51C
    Right C51B
  Upper Extremity
    Bilateral C51Q
    Left C51P
    Right C51N
Whole Body CW1N
Plantar digital vein
  use Foot Vein, Right
  use Foot Vein, Left
Plantar fascia (aponeurosis)
  use Subcutaneous Tissue and Fascia, Right
  Foot
  use Subcutaneous Tissue and Fascia, Left
  Foot
Plantar metatarsal vein
  use Foot Vein, Right
  use Foot Vein, Left
Plantar venous arch
  use Foot Vein, Right
  use Foot Vein, Left
Plaque Radiation
Abdomen DWY3FZZ
Adrenal Gland DGY2FZZ
Anus DDY8FZZ
Bile Ducts DFY2FZZ
Bladder DTY2FZZ
Bone, Other DPYCFZZ
Bone Marrow D7Y0FZZ
Brain D0Y0FZZ
Brain Stem D0Y1FZZ
Breast
  Left DMY0FZZ
  Right DMY1FZZ

Plaque Radiation — *continued*
Bronchus DBY1FZZ
Cervix DUY1FZZ
Chest DWY2FZZ
Chest Wall DBY7FZZ
Colon DDY5FZZ
Diaphragm DBY8FZZ
Duodenum DDY2FZZ
Ear D9Y0FZZ
Esophagus DDY0FZZ
Eye D8Y0FZZ
Femur DPY9FZZ
Fibula DPYBFZZ
Gallbladder DFY1FZZ
Gland
    Adrenal DGY2FZZ
    Parathyroid DGY4FZZ
    Pituitary DGY0FZZ
    Thyroid DGY5FZZ
Glands, Salivary D9Y6FZZ
Head and Neck DWY1FZZ
Hemibody DWY4FZZ
Humerus DPY6FZZ
Ileum DDY4FZZ
Jejunum DDY3FZZ
Kidney DTY0FZZ
Larynx D9YBFZZ
Liver DFY0FZZ
Lung DBY2FZZ
Lymphatics
    Abdomen D7Y6FZZ
    Axillary D7Y4FZZ
    Inguinal D7Y8FZZ
    Neck D7Y3FZZ
    Pelvis D7Y7FZZ
    Thorax D7Y5FZZ
Mandible DPY3FZZ
Maxilla DPY2FZZ
Mediastinum DBY6FZZ
Mouth D9Y4FZZ
Nasopharynx D9YDFZZ
Neck and Head DWY1FZZ
Nerve, Peripheral D0Y7FZZ
Nose D9Y1FZZ
Ovary DUY0FZZ
Palate
    Hard D9Y8FZZ
    Soft D9Y9FZZ
Pancreas DFY3FZZ
Parathyroid Gland DGY4FZZ
Pelvic Bones DPY8FZZ
Pelvic Region DWY6FZZ
Pharynx D9YCFZZ
Pineal Body DGY1FZZ
Pituitary Gland DGY0FZZ
Pleura DBY5FZZ
Prostate DVY0FZZ
Radius DPY7FZZ
Rectum DDY7FZZ
Rib DPY5FZZ
Sinuses D9Y7FZZ
Skin
    Abdomen DHY8FZZ
    Arm DHY4FZZ
    Back DHY7FZZ
    Buttock DHY9FZZ
    Chest DHY6FZZ
    Face DHY2FZZ
    Foot DHYCFZZ
    Hand DHY5FZZ
    Leg DHYBFZZ
    Neck DHY3FZZ
Skull DPY0FZZ
Spinal Cord D0Y6FZZ
Spleen D7Y2FZZ
Sternum DPY4FZZ
Stomach DDY1FZZ

Plaque Radiation — *continued*
Testis DVY1FZZ
Thymus D7Y1FZZ
Thyroid Gland DGY5FZZ
Tibia DPYBFZZ
Tongue D9Y5FZZ
Trachea DBY0FZZ
Ulna DPY7FZZ
Ureter DTY1FZZ
Urethra DTY3FZZ
Uterus DUY2FZZ
Whole Body DWY5FZZ
Plasmapheresis, therapeutic
    see Pheresis, Physiological Systems 6A5
Plateletpheresis, therapeutic
    see Pheresis, Physiological Systems 6A5
Platysma muscle
    use Neck Muscle, Right
    use Neck Muscle, Left
Pleurectomy
    see Excision, Respiratory System 0BB
    see Resection, Respiratory System 0BT
Pleurocentesis
    see Drainage, Anatomical Regions, General 0W9
Pleurodesis, pleurosclerosis
    Chemical injection *see* Introduction of substance in or on, Pleural Cavity 3E0L
    Surgical *see* Destruction, Respiratory System 0B5
Pleurolysis
    see Release, Respiratory System 0BN
Pleuroscopy 0BJQ4ZZ
Pleurotomy
    see Drainage, Respiratory System 0B9
Plica semilunaris
    use Conjunctiva, Right
    use Conjunctiva, Left
Plication
    see Restriction
Pneumectomy
    see Excision, Respiratory System 0BB
    see Resection, Respiratory System 0BT
Pneumocentesis
    see Drainage, Respiratory System 0B9
Pneumogastric nerve
    use Vagus Nerve
Pneumolysis
    see Release, Respiratory System 0BN
Pneumonectomy
    see Resection, Respiratory System 0BT
Pneumonolysis
    see Release, Respiratory System 0BN
Pneumonopexy
    see Repair, Respiratory System 0BQ
    see Reposition, Respiratory System 0BS
Pneumonorrhaphy
    see Repair, Respiratory System 0BQ
Pneumonotomy
    see Drainage, Respiratory System 0B9
Pneumotaxic center
    use Pons
Pneumotomy
    see Drainage, Respiratory System 0B9
Pollicization
    see Transfer, Anatomical Regions, Upper Extremities 0XX
Polyethylene socket
    use Synthetic Substitute, Polyethylene in 0SR
Polymethylmethacrylate (PMMA)
    use Synthetic Substitute
Polypectomy, gastrointestinal
    see Excision, Gastrointestinal System 0DB
Polypropylene mesh
    use Synthetic Substitute
Polysomnogram 4A1ZXQZ

Pontine tegmentum
    use Pons
Popliteal ligament
    use Knee Bursa and Ligament, Right
    use Knee Bursa and Ligament, Left
Popliteal lymph node
    use Lymphatic, Right Lower Extremity
    use Lymphatic, Left Lower Extremity
Popliteal vein
    use Femoral Vein, Right
    use Femoral Vein, Left
Popliteus muscle
    use Lower Leg Muscle, Right
    use Lower Leg Muscle, Left
Porcine (bioprosthetic) valve
    use Zooplastic Tissue in Heart and Great Vessels
Positive end expiratory pressure
    see Performance, Respiratory 5A19
Positron Emission Tomographic (PET) Imaging
    Brain C030
    Bronchi and Lungs CB32
    Central Nervous System C03YYZZ
    Heart C23YYZZ
    Lungs and Bronchi CB32
    Myocardium C23G
    Respiratory System CB3YYZZ
    Whole Body CW3NYZZ
Positron emission tomography
    see Positron Emission Tomographic (PET) Imaging
Postauricular (mastoid) lymph node
    use Lymphatic, Right Neck
    use Lymphatic, Left Neck
Postcava
    use Inferior Vena Cava
Posterior (subscapular) lymph node
    use Lymphatic, Right Axillary
    use Lymphatic, Left Axillary
Posterior auricular artery
    use External Carotid Artery, Right
    use External Carotid Artery, Left
Posterior auricular nerve
    use Facial Nerve
Posterior auricular vein
    use External Jugular Vein, Right
    use External Jugular Vein, Left
Posterior cerebral artery
    use Intracranial Artery
Posterior chamber
    use Eye, Right
    use Eye, Left
Posterior circumflex humeral artery
    use Axillary Artery, Right
    use Axillary Artery, Left
Posterior communicating artery
    use Intracranial Artery
Posterior cruciate ligament (PCL)
    use Knee Bursa and Ligament, Right
    use Knee Bursa and Ligament, Left
Posterior facial (retromandibular) vein
    use Face Vein, Right
    use Face Vein, Left
Posterior femoral cutaneous nerve
    use Sacral Plexus
Posterior inferior cerebellar artery (PICA)
    use Intracranial Artery
Posterior interosseous nerve
    use Radial Nerve
Posterior labial nerve
    use Pudendal Nerve
Posterior scrotal nerve
    use Pudendal Nerve
Posterior spinal artery
    use Vertebral Artery, Right
    use Vertebral Artery, Left

Posterior tibial recurrent artery
 use Anterior Tibial Artery, Right
 use Anterior Tibial Artery, Left
Posterior ulnar recurrent artery
 use Ulnar Artery, Right
 use Ulnar Artery, Left
Posterior vagal trunk
 use Vagus Nerve
PPN (peripheral parenteral nutrition)
 see Introduction of Nutritional Substance
Preauricular lymph node
 use Lymphatic, Head
Precava
 use Superior Vena Cava
Prepatellar bursa
 use Knee Bursa and Ligament, Right
 use Knee Bursa and Ligament, Left
Preputiotomy
 see Drainage, Male Reproductive
  System 0V9
Pressure support ventilation
 see Performance, Respiratory 5A19
PRESTIGE® Cervical Disc
 use Synthetic Substitute
Pretracheal fascia
 use Subcutaneous Tissue and Fascia, Right
  Neck
 use Subcutaneous Tissue and Fascia, Left
  Neck
Prevertebral fascia
 use Subcutaneous Tissue and Fascia, Right
  Neck
 use Subcutaneous Tissue and Fascia, Left
  Neck
**PrimeAdvanced™ neurostimulator
 (SureScan™)(MRI Safe)**
 use Stimulator Generator, Multiple Array
  in 0JH
Princeps pollicis artery
 use Hand Artery, Right
 use Hand Artery, Left
Probing, duct
 Diagnostic *see* Inspection
 Dilation *see* Dilation
PROCEED™ Ventral Patch
 use Synthetic Substitute
Procerus muscle
 use Facial Muscle
Proctectomy
 see Excision, Rectum 0DBP
 see Resection, Rectum 0DTP
Proctoclysis
 see Introduction of substance in or on,
  Gastrointestinal Tract, Lower 3E0H
Proctocolectomy
 see Excision, Gastrointestinal System 0DB
 see Resection, Gastrointestinal System 0DT
Proctocolpoplasty
 see Repair, Gastrointestinal System 0DQ
 see Supplement, Gastrointestinal
  System 0DU
Proctoperineoplasty
 see Repair, Gastrointestinal System 0DQ
 see Supplement, Gastrointestinal
  System 0DU
Proctoperineorrhaphy
 see Repair, Gastrointestinal System 0DQ
Proctopexy
 see Repair, Rectum 0DQP
 see Reposition, Rectum 0DSP
Proctoplasty
 see Repair, Rectum 0DQP
 see Supplement, Rectum 0DUP
Proctorrhaphy
 see Repair, Rectum 0DQP
Proctoscopy 0DJD8ZZ

Proctosigmoidectomy
 see Excision, Gastrointestinal System 0DB
 see Resection, Gastrointestinal System 0DT
Proctosigmoidoscopy 0DJD8ZZ
Proctostomy
 see Drainage, Rectum 0D9P
Proctotomy
 see Drainage, Rectum 0D9P
Prodisc®-C
 use Synthetic Substitute
Prodisc®-L
 use Synthetic Substitute
Production, atrial septal defect
 see Excision, Septum, Atrial 02B5
Profunda brachii
 use Brachial Artery, Right
 use Brachial Artery, Left
Profunda femoris (deep femoral) vein
 use Femoral Vein, Right
 use Femoral Vein, Left
**PROLENE® Polypropylene Hernia System
 (PHS)**
 use Synthetic Substitute
**Prolonged intermittent renal replacement
 therapy (PIRRT)** 5A1D80Z
Pronator quadratus muscle
 use Lower Arm and Wrist Muscle, Right
 use Lower Arm and Wrist Muscle, Left
Pronator teres muscle
 use Lower Arm and Wrist Muscle, Right
 use Lower Arm and Wrist Muscle, Left
Prostatectomy
 see Excision, Prostate 0VB0
 see Resection, Prostate 0VT0
Prostatic urethra
 use Urethra
Prostatomy, prostatotomy
 see Drainage, Prostate 0V90
Protecta™ XT CRT-D
 use Cardiac Resynchronization Defibrillator
  Pulse Generator in 0JH
Protecta XT™ DR (XT VR)
 use Defibrillator Generator in 0JH
Protege® RX Carotid Stent System
 use Intraluminal Device
Proximal radioulnar joint
 use Elbow Joint, Right
 use Elbow Joint, Left
Psoas muscle
 use Hip Muscle, Right
 use Hip Muscle, Left
PSV (pressure support ventilation)
 see Performance, Respiratory 5A19
Psychoanalysis GZ54ZZZ
Psychological Tests
 Cognitive Status GZ14ZZZ
 Developmental GZ10ZZZ
 Intellectual and
  Psychoeducational GZ12ZZZ
 Neurobehavioral Status GZ14ZZZ
 Neuropsychological GZ13ZZZ
 Personality and Behavioral GZ11ZZZ
Psychotherapy
 Family, Mental Health Services GZ72ZZZ
 Group
  GZHZZZZ
  Mental Health Services GZHZZZZ
 Individual
  see Psychotherapy, Individual, Mental
   Health Services
  for substance abuse
   12-Step HZ53ZZZ
   Behavioral HZ51ZZZ
   Cognitive HZ50ZZZ
   Cognitive-Behavioral HZ52ZZZ
   Confrontational HZ58ZZZ

Psychotherapy — *continued*
 Individual — *continued*
  Interactive HZ55ZZZ
  Interpersonal HZ54ZZZ
  Motivational Enhancement HZ57ZZZ
  Psychoanalysis HZ5BZZZ
  Psychodynamic HZ5CZZZ
  Psychoeducation HZ56ZZZ
  Psychophysiological HZ5DZZZ
  Supportive HZ59ZZZ
 Mental Health Services
  Behavioral GZ51ZZZ
  Cognitive GZ52ZZZ
  Cognitive-Behavioral GZ58ZZZ
  Interactive GZ50ZZZ
  Interpersonal GZ53ZZZ
  Psychoanalysis GZ54ZZZ
  Psychodynamic GZ55ZZZ
  Psychophysiological GZ59ZZZ
  Supportive GZ56ZZZ
**PTCA (percutaneous transluminal coronary
 angioplasty)**
 see Dilation, Heart and Great Vessels 027
Pterygoid muscle
 use Head Muscle
Pterygoid process
 use Sphenoid Bone
Pterygopalatine (sphenopalatine) ganglion
 use Head and Neck Sympathetic Nerve
Pubis
 use Pelvic Bone, Right
 use Pelvic Bone, Left
Pubofemoral ligament
 use Hip Bursa and Ligament, Right
 use Hip Bursa and Ligament, Left
Pudendal nerve
 use Sacral Plexus
**Pull-through, laparoscopic-assisted
 transanal**
 see Excision, Gastrointestinal System 0DB
 see Resection, Gastrointestinal System 0DT
Pull-through, rectal
 see Resection, Rectum 0DTP
Pulmoaortic canal
 use Pulmonary Artery, Left
Pulmonary annulus
 use Pulmonary Valve
Pulmonary artery wedge monitoring
 see Monitoring, Arterial 4A13
Pulmonary plexus
 use Vagus Nerve
 use Thoracic Sympathetic Nerve
Pulmonic valve
 use Pulmonary Valve
Pulpectomy
 see Excision, Mouth and Throat 0CB
Pulverization
 see Fragmentation
Pulvinar
 use Thalamus
Pump reservoir
 use Infusion Device, Pump in Subcutaneous
  Tissue and Fascia
Punch biopsy
 see Excision with qualifier Diagnostic
Puncture
 see Drainage
Puncture, lumbar
 see Drainage, Spinal Canal 009U
Pyelography
 see Plain Radiography, Urinary System BT0
 see Fluoroscopy, Urinary System BT1
Pyeloileostomy, urinary diversion
 see Bypass, Urinary System 0T1
Pyeloplasty
 see Repair, Urinary System 0TQ
 see Replacement, Urinary System 0TR
 see Supplement, Urinary System 0TU

Pyelorrhaphy
   see Repair, Urinary System 0TQ
Pyeloscopy 0TJ58ZZ
Pyelostomy
   see Bypass, Urinary System 0T1
   see Drainage, Urinary System 0T9
Pyelotomy
   see Drainage, Urinary System 0T9
Pylorectomy
   see Excision, Stomach, Pylorus 0DB7
   see Resection, Stomach, Pylorus 0DT7
Pyloric antrum
   use Stomach, Pylorus
Pyloric canal
   use Stomach, Pylorus
Pyloric sphincter
   use Stomach, Pylorus
Pylorodiosis
   see Dilation, Stomach, Pylorus 0D77
Pylorogastrectomy
   see Excision, Gastrointestinal System 0DB
   see Resection, Gastrointestinal System 0DT
Pyloroplasty
   see Repair, Stomach, Pylorus 0DQ7
   see Supplement, Stomach, Pylorus 0DU7
Pyloroscopy 0DJ68ZZ
Pylorotomy
   see Drainage, Stomach, Pylorus 0D97
Pyramidalis muscle
   use Abdomen Muscle, Right
   use Abdomen Muscle, Left

Q

Quadrangular cartilage
   use Nasal Septum
Quadrant resection of breast
   see Excision, Skin and Breast 0HB
Quadrate lobe
   use Liver
Quadratus femoris muscle
   use Hip Muscle, Right
   use Hip Muscle, Left
Quadratus lumborum muscle
   use Trunk Muscle, Right
   use Trunk Muscle, Left
Quadratus plantae muscle
   use Foot Muscle, Right
   use Foot Muscle, Left
Quadriceps (femoris)
   use Upper Leg Muscle, Right
   use Upper Leg Muscle, Left
Quarantine 8E0ZXY6

R

Radial collateral carpal ligament
   use Wrist Bursa and Ligament, Right
   use Wrist Bursa and Ligament, Left
Radial collateral ligament
   use Elbow Bursa and Ligament, Right
   use Elbow Bursa and Ligament, Left
Radial notch
   use Ulna, Right
   use Ulna, Left
Radial recurrent artery
   use Radial Artery, Right
   use Radial Artery, Left
Radial vein
   use Brachial Vein, Right
   use Brachial Vein, Left
Radialis indicis
   use Hand Artery, Right
   use Hand Artery, Left

Radiation Therapy
   see Beam Radiation
   see Brachytherapy
   see Stereotactic Radiosurgery
Radiation treatment
   see Radiation Therapy
Radiocarpal joint
   use Wrist Joint, Right
   use Wrist Joint, Left
Radiocarpal ligament
   use Wrist Bursa and Ligament, Right
   use Wrist Bursa and Ligament, Left
Radiography
   see Plain Radiography
Radiology, analog
   see Plain Radiography
Radiology, diagnostic
   see Imaging, Diagnostic
Radioulnar ligament
   use Wrist Bursa and Ligament, Right
   use Wrist Bursa and Ligament, Left
Range of motion testing
   see Motor Function Assessment,
   Rehabilitation F01
REALIZE® Adjustable Gastric Band
   use Extraluminal Device
Reattachment
   Abdominal Wall 0WMF0ZZ
   Ampulla of Vater 0FMC
   Ankle Region
      Left 0YML0ZZ
      Right 0YMK0ZZ
   Arm
      Lower
         Left 0XMF0ZZ
         Right 0XMD0ZZ
      Upper
         Left 0XM90ZZ
         Right 0XM80ZZ
   Axilla
      Left 0XM50ZZ
      Right 0XM40ZZ
   Back
      Lower 0WML0ZZ
      Upper 0WMK0ZZ
   Bladder 0TMB
   Bladder Neck 0TMC
   Breast
      Bilateral 0HMVXZZ
      Left 0HMUXZZ
      Right 0HMTXZZ
   Bronchus
      Lingula 0BM90ZZ
      Lower Lobe
         Left 0BMB0ZZ
         Right 0BM60ZZ
      Main
         Left 0BM70ZZ
         Right 0BM30ZZ
      Middle Lobe, Right 0BM50ZZ
      Upper Lobe
         Left 0BM80ZZ
         Right 0BM40ZZ
   Bursa and Ligament
      Abdomen
         Left 0MMJ
         Right 0MMH
      Ankle
         Left 0MMR
         Right 0MMQ
      Elbow
         Left 0MM4
         Right 0MM3
      Foot
         Left 0MMT
         Right 0MMS

Reattachment — *continued*
   Bursa and Ligament — *continued*
      Hand
         Left 0MM8
         Right 0MM7
      Head and Neck 0MM0
      Hip
         Left 0MMM
         Right 0MML
      Knee
         Left 0MMP
         Right 0MMN
      Lower Extremity
         Left 0MMW
         Right 0MMV
      Perineum 0MMK
      Rib(s) 0MMG
      Shoulder
         Left 0MM2
         Right 0MM1
      Spine
         Lower 0MMD
         Upper 0MMC
      Sternum 0MMF
      Upper Extremity
         Left 0MMB
         Right 0MM9
      Wrist
         Left 0MM6
         Right 0MM5
   Buttock
      Left 0YM10ZZ
      Right 0YM00ZZ
   Carina 0BM20ZZ
   Cecum 0DMH
   Cervix 0UMC
   Chest Wall 0WM80ZZ
   Clitoris 0UMJXZZ
   Colon
      Ascending 0DMK
      Descending 0DMM
      Sigmoid 0DMN
      Transverse 0DML
   Cord
      Bilateral 0VMH
      Left 0VMG
      Right 0VMF
   Cul-de-sac 0UMF
   Diaphragm 0BMT0ZZ
   Duct
      Common Bile 0FM9
      Cystic 0FM8
      Hepatic
         Common 0FM7
         Left 0FM6
         Right 0FM5
      Pancreatic 0FMD
         Accessory 0FMF
   Duodenum 0DM9
   Ear
      Left 09M1XZZ
      Right 09M0XZZ
   Elbow Region
      Left 0XMC0ZZ
      Right 0XMB0ZZ
   Esophagus 0DM5
   Extremity
      Lower
         Left 0YMB0ZZ
         Right 0YM90ZZ
      Upper
         Left 0XM70ZZ
         Right 0XM60ZZ
   Eyelid
      Lower
         Left 08MRXZZ
         Right 08MQXZZ

Reattachment — *continued*
  Eyelid — *continued*
    Upper
      Left 08MPXZZ
      Right 08MNXZZ
  Face 0WM20ZZ
  Fallopian Tube
    Left 0UM6
    Right 0UM5
  Fallopian Tubes, Bilateral 0UM7
  Femoral Region
    Left 0YM80ZZ
    Right 0YM70ZZ
  Finger
    Index
      Left 0XMP0ZZ
      Right 0XMN0ZZ
    Little
      Left 0XMW0ZZ
      Right 0XMV0ZZ
    Middle
      Left 0XMR0ZZ
      Right 0XMQ0ZZ
    Ring
      Left 0XMT0ZZ
      Right 0XMS0ZZ
  Foot
    Left 0YMN0ZZ
    Right 0YMM0ZZ
  Forequarter
    Left 0XM10ZZ
    Right 0XM00ZZ
  Gallbladder 0FM4
  Gland
    Left 0GM2
    Right 0GM3
  Hand
    Left 0XMK0ZZ
    Right 0XMJ0ZZ
  Hindquarter
    Bilateral 0YM40ZZ
    Left 0YM30ZZ
    Right 0YM20ZZ
  Hymen 0UMK
  Ileum 0DMB
  Inguinal Region
    Left 0YM60ZZ
    Right 0YM50ZZ
  Intestine
    Large 0DME
      Left 0DMG
      Right 0DMF
    Small 0DM8
  Jaw
    Lower 0WM50ZZ
    Upper 0WM40ZZ
  Jejunum 0DMA
  Kidney
    Left 0TM1
    Right 0TM0
  Kidney Pelvis
    Left 0TM4
    Right 0TM3
  Kidneys, Bilateral 0TM2
  Knee Region
    Left 0YMG0ZZ
    Right 0YMF0ZZ
  Leg
    Lower
      Left 0YMJ0ZZ
      Right 0YMH0ZZ
    Upper
      Left 0YMD0ZZ
      Right 0YMC0ZZ
  Lip
    Lower 0CM10ZZ
    Upper 0CM00ZZ

Reattachment — *continued*
  Liver 0FM0
    Left Lobe 0FM2
    Right Lobe 0FM1
  Lung
    Left 0BML0ZZ
    Lower Lobe
      Left 0BMJ0ZZ
      Right 0BMF0ZZ
    Middle Lobe, Right 0BMD0ZZ
    Right 0BMK0ZZ
    Upper Lobe
      Left 0BMG0ZZ
      Right 0BMC0ZZ
  Lung Lingula 0BMH0ZZ
  Muscle
    Abdomen
      Left 0KML
      Right 0KMK
    Facial 0KM1
    Foot
      Left 0KMW
      Right 0KMV
    Hand
      Left 0KMD
      Right 0KMC
    Head 0KM0
    Hip
      Left 0KMP
      Right 0KMN
    Lower Arm and Wrist
      Left 0KMB
      Right 0KM9
    Lower Leg
      Left 0KMT
      Right 0KMS
    Neck
      Left 0KM3
      Right 0KM2
    Perineum 0KMM
    Shoulder
      Left 0KM6
      Right 0KM5
    Thorax
      Left 0KMJ
      Right 0KMH
    Tongue, Palate, Pharynx 0KM4
    Trunk
      Left 0KMG
      Right 0KMF
    Upper Arm
      Left 0KM8
      Right 0KM7
    Upper Leg
      Left 0KMR
      Right 0KMQ
  Nasal Mucosa and Soft Tissue 09MKXZZ
  Neck 0WM60ZZ
  Nipple
    Left 0HMXXZZ
    Right 0HMWXZZ
  Ovary
    Bilateral 0UM2
    Left 0UM1
    Right 0UM0
  Palate, Soft 0CM30ZZ
  Pancreas 0FMG
  Parathyroid Gland 0GMR
    Inferior
      Left 0GMP
      Right 0GMN
    Multiple 0GMQ
    Superior
      Left 0GMM
      Right 0GML
  Penis 0VMSXZZ

Reattachment — *continued*
  Perineum
    Female 0WMN0ZZ
    Male 0WMM0ZZ
  Rectum 0DMP
  Scrotum 0VM5XZZ
  Shoulder Region
    Left 0XM30ZZ
    Right 0XM20ZZ
  Skin
    Abdomen 0HM7XZZ
    Back 0HM6XZZ
    Buttock 0HM8XZZ
    Chest 0HM5XZZ
    Ear
      Left 0HM3XZZ
      Right 0HM2XZZ
    Face 0HM1XZZ
    Foot
      Left 0HMNXZZ
      Right 0HMMXZZ
    Hand
      Left 0HMGXZZ
      Right 0HMFXZZ
    Inguinal 0HMAXZZ
    Lower Arm
      Left 0HMEXZZ
      Right 0HMDXZZ
    Lower Leg
      Left 0HMLXZZ
      Right 0HMKXZZ
    Neck 0HM4XZZ
    Perineum 0HM9XZZ
    Scalp 0HM0XZZ
    Upper Arm
      Left 0HMCXZZ
      Right 0HMBXZZ
    Upper Leg
      Left 0HMJXZZ
      Right 0HMHXZZ
  Stomach 0DM6
  Tendon
    Abdomen
      Left 0LMG
      Right 0LMF
    Ankle
      Left 0LMT
      Right 0LMS
    Foot
      Left 0LMW
      Right 0LMV
    Hand
      Left 0LM8
      Right 0LM7
    Head and Neck 0LM0
    Hip
      Left 0LMK
      Right 0LMJ
    Knee
      Left 0LMR
      Right 0LMQ
    Lower Arm and Wrist
      Left 0LM6
      Right 0LM5
    Lower Leg
      Left 0LMP
      Right 0LMN
    Perineum 0LMH
    Shoulder
      Left 0LM2
      Right 0LM1
    Thorax
      Left 0LMD
      Right 0LMC
    Trunk
      Left 0LMB
      Right 0LM9

Reattachment — *continued*
  Tendon — *continued*
    Upper Arm
      Left 0LM4
      Right 0LM3
    Upper Leg
      Left 0LMM
      Right 0LML
  Testis
    Bilateral 0VMC
    Left 0VMB
    Right 0VM9
  Thumb
    Left 0XMM0ZZ
    Right 0XML0ZZ
  Thyroid Gland
    Left Lobe 0GMG
    Right Lobe 0GMH
  Toe
    1st
      Left 0YMQ0ZZ
      Right 0YMP0ZZ
    2nd
      Left 0YMS0ZZ
      Right 0YMR0ZZ
    3rd
      Left 0YMU0ZZ
      Right 0YMT0ZZ
    4th
      Left 0YMW0ZZ
      Right 0YMV0ZZ
    5th
      Left 0YMY0ZZ
      Right 0YMX0ZZ
  Tongue 0CM70ZZ
  Tooth
    Lower 0CMX
    Upper 0CMW
  Trachea 0BM10ZZ
  Tunica Vaginalis
    Left 0VM7
    Right 0VM6
  Ureter
    Left 0TM7
    Right 0TM6
  Ureters, Bilateral 0TM8
  Urethra 0TMD
  Uterine Supporting Structure 0UM4
  Uterus 0UM9
  Uvula 0CMN0ZZ
  Vagina 0UMG
  Vulva 0UMMXZZ
  Wrist Region
    Left 0XMH0ZZ
    Right 0XMG0ZZ
REBOA (resuscitative endovascular balloon occlusion of the aorta)
  02LW3DJ
  04L03DJ
Rebound HRD® (Hernia Repair Device)
  use Synthetic Substitute
Recession
  see Repair
  see Reposition
Reclosure, disrupted abdominal wall
  0WQFXZZ
Reconstruction
  see Repair
  see Replacement
  see Supplement
Rectectomy
  see Excision, Rectum 0DBP
  see Resection, Rectum 0DTP
Rectocele repair
  see Repair, Subcutaneous Tissue and Fascia, Pelvic Region 0JQC

Rectopexy
  see Repair, Gastrointestinal System 0DQ
  see Reposition, Gastrointestinal System 0DS
Rectoplasty
  see Repair, Gastrointestinal System 0DQ
  see Supplement, Gastrointestinal System 0DU
Rectorrhaphy
  see Repair, Gastrointestinal System 0DQ
Rectoscopy 0DJD8ZZ
Rectosigmoid junction
  use Sigmoid Colon
Rectosigmoidectomy
  see Excision, Gastrointestinal System 0DB
  see Resection, Gastrointestinal System 0DT
Rectostomy
  see Drainage, Rectum 0D9P
Rectotomy
  see Drainage, Rectum 0D9P
Rectus abdominis muscle
  use Abdomen Muscle, Right
  use Abdomen Muscle, Left
Rectus femoris muscle
  use Upper Leg Muscle, Right
  use Upper Leg Muscle, Left
Recurrent laryngeal nerve
  use Vagus Nerve
Reduction
  Dislocation *see* Reposition
  Fracture *see* Reposition
  Intussusception, intestinal *see* Reposition, Gastrointestinal System 0DS
  Mammoplasty *see* Excision, Skin and Breast 0HB
  Prolapse *see* Reposition
  Torsion *see* Reposition
  Volvulus, gastrointestinal *see* Reposition, Gastrointestinal System 0DS
Refusion
  see Fusion
Rehabilitation
  see Speech Assessment, Rehabilitation F00
  see Motor Function Assessment, Rehabilitation F01
  see Activities of Daily Living Assessment, Rehabilitation F02
  see Speech Treatment, Rehabilitation F06
  see Motor Treatment, Rehabilitation F07
  see Activities of Daily Living Treatment, Rehabilitation F08
  see Hearing Treatment, Rehabilitation F09
  see Cochlear Implant Treatment, Rehabilitation F0B
  see Vestibular Treatment, Rehabilitation F0C
  see Device Fitting, Rehabilitation F0D
  see Caregiver Training, Rehabilitation F0F
Reimplantation
  see Reattachment
  see Reposition
  see Transfer
Reinforcement
  see Repair
  see Supplement
Relaxation, scar tissue
  see Release
Release
  Acetabulum
    Left 0QN5
    Right 0QN4
  Adenoids 0CNQ
  Ampulla of Vater 0FNC
  Anal Sphincter 0DNR
  Anterior Chamber
    Left 08N33ZZ
    Right 08N23ZZ
  Anus 0DNQ

Release — *continued*
  Aorta
    Abdominal 04N0
    Thoracic
      Ascending/Arch 02NX
      Descending 02NW
  Aortic Body 0GND
  Appendix 0DNJ
  Artery
    Anterior Tibial
      Left 04NQ
      Right 04NP
    Axillary
      Left 03N6
      Right 03N5
    Brachial
      Left 03N8
      Right 03N7
    Celiac 04N1
    Colic
      Left 04N7
      Middle 04N8
      Right 04N6
    Common Carotid
      Left 03NJ
      Right 03NH
    Common Iliac
      Left 04ND
      Right 04NC
    Coronary
      Four or More Arteries 02N3
      One Artery 02N0
      Three Arteries 02N2
      Two Arteries 02N1
    External Carotid
      Left 03NN
      Right 03NM
    External Iliac
      Left 04NJ
      Right 04NH
    Face 03NR
    Femoral
      Left 04NL
      Right 04NK
    Foot
      Left 04NW
      Right 04NV
    Gastric 04N2
    Hand
      Left 03NF
      Right 03ND
    Hepatic 04N3
    Inferior Mesenteric 04NB
    Innominate 03N2
    Internal Carotid
      Left 03NL
      Right 03NK
    Internal Iliac
      Left 04NF
      Right 04NE
    Internal Mammary
      Left 03N1
      Right 03N0
    Intracranial 03NG
    Lower 04NY
    Peroneal
      Left 04NU
      Right 04NT
    Popliteal
      Left 04NN
      Right 04NM
    Posterior Tibial
      Left 04NS
      Right 04NR
    Pulmonary
      Left 02NR
      Right 02NQ

Release — *continued*
  Artery — *continued*
    Pulmonary Trunk 02NP
    Radial
      Left 03NC
      Right 03NB
    Renal
      Left 04NA
      Right 04N9
    Splenic 04N4
    Subclavian
      Left 03N4
      Right 03N3
    Superior Mesenteric 04N5
    Temporal
      Left 03NT
      Right 03NS
    Thyroid
      Left 03NV
      Right 03NU
    Ulnar
      Left 03NA
      Right 03N9
    Upper 03NY
    Vertebral
      Left 03NQ
      Right 03NP
  Atrium
    Left 02N7
    Right 02N6
  Auditory Ossicle
    Left 09NA
    Right 09N9
  Basal Ganglia 00N8
  Bladder 0TNB
  Bladder Neck 0TNC
  Bone
    Ethmoid
      Left 0NNG
      Right 0NNF
    Frontal 0NN1
    Hyoid 0NNX
    Lacrimal
      Left 0NNJ
      Right 0NNH
    Nasal 0NNB
    Occipital 0NN7
    Palatine
      Left 0NNL
      Right 0NNK
    Parietal
      Left 0NN4
      Right 0NN3
    Pelvic
      Left 0QN3
      Right 0QN2
    Sphenoid 0NNC
    Temporal
      Left 0NN6
      Right 0NN5
    Zygomatic
      Left 0NNN
      Right 0NNM
  Brain 00N0
  Breast
    Bilateral 0HNV
    Left 0HNU
    Right 0HNT
  Bronchus
    Lingula 0BN9
    Lower Lobe
      Left 0BNB
      Right 0BN6
    Main
      Left 0BN7
      Right 0BN3
    Middle Lobe, Right 0BN5

Release — *continued*
  Bronchus — *continued*
    Upper Lobe
      Left 0BN8
      Right 0BN4
  Buccal Mucosa 0CN4
  Bursa and Ligament
    Abdomen
      Left 0MNJ
      Right 0MNH
    Ankle
      Left 0MNR
      Right 0MNQ
    Elbow
      Left 0MN4
      Right 0MN3
    Foot
      Left 0MNT
      Right 0MNS
    Hand
      Left 0MN8
      Right 0MN7
    Head and Neck 0MN0
    Hip
      Left 0MNM
      Right 0MNL
    Knee
      Left 0MNP
      Right 0MNN
    Lower Extremity
      Left 0MNW
      Right 0MNV
    Perineum 0MNK
    Rib(s) 0MNG
    Shoulder
      Left 0MN2
      Right 0MN1
    Spine
      Lower 0MND
      Upper 0MNC
    Sternum 0MNF
    Upper Extremity
      Left 0MNB
      Right 0MN9
    Wrist
      Left 0MN6
      Right 0MN5
  Carina 0BN2
  Carotid Bodies, Bilateral 0GN8
  Carotid Body
    Left 0GN6
    Right 0GN7
  Carpal
    Left 0PNN
    Right 0PNM
  Cecum 0DNH
  Cerebellum 00NC
  Cerebral Hemisphere 00N7
  Cerebral Meninges 00N1
  Cerebral Ventricle 00N6
  Cervix 0UNC
  Chordae Tendineae 02N9
  Choroid
    Left 08NB
    Right 08NA
  Cisterna Chyli 07NL
  Clavicle
    Left 0PNB
    Right 0PN9
  Clitoris 0UNJ
  Coccygeal Glomus 0GNB
  Coccyx 0QNS
  Colon
    Ascending 0DNK
    Descending 0DNM
    Sigmoid 0DNN
    Transverse 0DNL

Release — *continued*
  Conduction Mechanism 02N8
  Conjunctiva
    Left 08NTXZZ
    Right 08NSXZZ
  Cord
    Bilateral 0VNH
    Left 0VNG
    Right 0VNF
  Cornea
    Left 08N9XZZ
    Right 08N8XZZ
  Cul-de-sac 0UNF
  Diaphragm 0BNT
  Disc
    Cervical Vertebral 0RN3
    Cervicothoracic Vertebral 0RN5
    Lumbar Vertebral 0SN2
    Lumbosacral 0SN4
    Thoracic Vertebral 0RN9
    Thoracolumbar Vertebral 0RNB
  Duct
    Common Bile 0FN9
    Cystic 0FN8
    Hepatic
      Common 0FN7
      Left 0FN6
      Right 0FN5
    Lacrimal
      Left 08NY
      Right 08NX
    Pancreatic 0FND
      Accessory 0FNF
    Parotid
      Left 0CNC
      Right 0CNB
  Duodenum 0DN9
  Dura Mater 00N2
  Ear
    External
      Left 09N1
      Right 09N0
    External Auditory Canal
      Left 09N4
      Right 09N3
    Inner
      Left 09NE
      Right 09ND
    Middle
      Left 09N6
      Right 09N5
  Epididymis
    Bilateral 0VNL
    Left 0VNK
    Right 0VNJ
  Epiglottis 0CNR
  Esophagogastric Junction 0DN4
  Esophagus 0DN5
    Lower 0DN3
    Middle 0DN2
    Upper 0DN1
  Eustachian Tube
    Left 09NG
    Right 09NF
  Eye
    Left 08N1XZZ
    Right 08N0XZZ
  Eyelid
    Lower
      Left 08NR
      Right 08NQ
    Upper
      Left 08NP
      Right 08NN
  Fallopian Tube
    Left 0UN6
    Right 0UN5

Release — *continued*
  Fallopian Tubes, Bilateral 0UN7
  Femoral Shaft
    Left 0QN9
    Right 0QN8
  Femur
    Lower
      Left 0QNC
      Right 0QNB
    Upper
      Left 0QN7
      Right 0QN6
  Fibula
    Left 0QNK
    Right 0QNJ
  Finger Nail 0HNQXZZ
  Gallbladder 0FN4
  Gingiva
    Lower 0CN6
    Upper 0CN5
  Gland
    Adrenal
      Bilateral 0GN4
      Left 0GN2
      Right 0GN3
    Lacrimal
      Left 08NW
      Right 08NV
    Minor Salivary 0CNJ
    Parotid
      Left 0CN9
      Right 0CN8
    Pituitary 0GN0
    Sublingual
      Left 0CNF
      Right 0CND
    Submaxillary
      Left 0CNH
      Right 0CNG
    Vestibular 0UNL
  Glenoid Cavity
    Left 0PN8
    Right 0PN7
  Glomus Jugulare 0GNC
  Humeral Head
    Left 0PND
    Right 0PNC
  Humeral Shaft
    Left 0PNG
    Right 0PNF
  Hymen 0UNK
  Hypothalamus 00NA
  Ileocecal Valve 0DNC
  Ileum 0DNB
  Intestine
    Large 0DNE
      Left 0DNG
      Right 0DNF
    Small 0DN8
  Iris
    Left 08ND3ZZ
    Right 08NC3ZZ
  Jejunum 0DNA
  Joint
    Acromioclavicular
      Left 0RNH
      Right 0RNG
    Ankle
      Left 0SNG
      Right 0SNF
    Carpal
      Left 0RNR
      Right 0RNQ
    Carpometacarpal
      Left 0RNT
      Right 0RNS
    Cervical Vertebral 0RN1

Release — *continued*
  Joint — *continued*
    Cervicothoracic Vertebral 0RN4
    Coccygeal 0SN6
    Elbow
      Left 0RNM
      Right 0RNL
    Finger Phalangeal
      Left 0RNX
      Right 0RNW
    Hip
      Left 0SNB
      Right 0SN9
    Knee
      Left 0SND
      Right 0SNC
    Lumbar Vertebral 0SN0
    Lumbosacral 0SN3
    Metacarpophalangeal
      Left 0RNV
      Right 0RNU
    Metatarsal-Phalangeal
      Left 0SNN
      Right 0SNM
    Occipital-cervical 0RN0
    Sacrococcygeal 0SN5
    Sacroiliac
      Left 0SN8
      Right 0SN7
    Shoulder
      Left 0RNK
      Right 0RNJ
    Sternoclavicular
      Left 0RNF
      Right 0RNE
    Tarsal
      Left 0SNJ
      Right 0SNH
    Tarsometatarsal
      Left 0SNL
      Right 0SNK
    Temporomandibular
      Left 0RND
      Right 0RNC
    Thoracic Vertebral 0RN6
    Thoracolumbar Vertebral 0RNA
    Toe Phalangeal
      Left 0SNQ
      Right 0SNP
    Wrist
      Left 0RNP
      Right 0RNN
  Kidney
    Left 0TN1
    Right 0TN0
  Kidney Pelvis
    Left 0TN4
    Right 0TN3
  Larynx 0CNS
  Lens
    Left 08NK3ZZ
    Right 08NJ3ZZ
  Lip
    Lower 0CN1
    Upper 0CN0
  Liver 0FN0
    Left Lobe 0FN2
    Right Lobe 0FN1
  Lung
    Bilateral 0BNM
    Left 0BNL
    Lower Lobe
      Left 0BNJ
      Right 0BNF
    Middle Lobe, Right 0BND
    Right 0BNK
    Upper Lobe

Release — *continued*
  Lung — *continued*
    Left 0BNG
    Right 0BNC
  Lung Lingula 0BNH
  Lymphatic
    Aortic 07ND
    Axillary
      Left 07N6
      Right 07N5
    Head 07N0
    Inguinal
      Left 07NJ
      Right 07NH
    Internal Mammary
      Left 07N9
      Right 07N8
    Lower Extremity
      Left 07NG
      Right 07NF
    Mesenteric 07NB
    Neck
      Left 07N2
      Right 07N1
    Pelvis 07NC
    Thoracic Duct 07NK
    Thorax 07N7
    Upper Extremity
      Left 07N4
      Right 07N3
  Mandible
    Left 0NNV
    Right 0NNT
  Maxilla 0NNR
  Medulla Oblongata 00ND
  Mesentery 0DNV
  Metacarpal
    Left 0PNQ
    Right 0PNP
  Metatarsal
    Left 0QNP
    Right 0QNN
  Muscle
    Abdomen
      Left 0KNL
      Right 0KNK
    Extraocular
      Left 08NM
      Right 08NL
    Facial 0KN1
    Foot
      Left 0KNW
      Right 0KNV
    Hand
      Left 0KND
      Right 0KNC
    Head 0KN0
    Hip
      Left 0KNP
      Right 0KNN
    Lower Arm and Wrist
      Left 0KNB
      Right 0KN9
    Lower Leg
      Left 0KNT
      Right 0KNS
    Neck
      Left 0KN3
      Right 0KN2
    Papillary 02ND
    Perineum 0KNM
    Shoulder
      Left 0KN6
      Right 0KN5
    Thorax
      Left 0KNJ
      Right 0KNH

Release

Release — *continued*
  Muscle — *continued*
    Tongue, Palate, Pharynx 0KN4
    Trunk
      Left 0KNG
      Right 0KNF
    Upper Arm
      Left 0KN8
      Right 0KN7
    Upper Leg
      Left 0KNR
      Right 0KNQ
  Myocardial Bridge *see* Release, Artery, Coronary
  Nasal Mucosa and Soft Tissue 09NK
  Nasopharynx 09NN
  Nerve
    Abdominal Sympathetic 01NM
    Abducens 00NL
    Accessory 00NR
    Acoustic 00NN
    Brachial Plexus 01N3
    Cervical 01N1
    Cervical Plexus 01N0
    Facial 00NM
    Femoral 01ND
    Glossopharyngeal 00NP
    Head and Neck Sympathetic 01NK
    Hypoglossal 00NS
    Lumbar 01NB
    Lumbar Plexus 01N9
    Lumbar Sympathetic 01NN
    Lumbosacral Plexus 01NA
    Median 01N5
    Oculomotor 00NH
    Olfactory 00NF
    Optic 00NG
    Peroneal 01NH
    Phrenic 01N2
    Pudendal 01NC
    Radial 01N6
    Sacral 01NR
    Sacral Plexus 01NQ
    Sacral Sympathetic 01NP
    Sciatic 01NF
    Thoracic 01N8
    Thoracic Sympathetic 01NL
    Tibial 01NG
    Trigeminal 00NK
    Trochlear 00NJ
    Ulnar 01N4
    Vagus 00NQ
  Nipple
    Left 0HNX
    Right 0HNW
  Omentum 0DNU
  Orbit
    Left 0NNQ
    Right 0NNP
  Ovary
    Bilateral 0UN2
    Left 0UN1
    Right 0UN0
  Palate
    Hard 0CN2
    Soft 0CN3
  Pancreas 0FNG
  Para-aortic Body 0GN9
  Paraganglion Extremity 0GNF
  Parathyroid Gland 0GNR
    Inferior
      Left 0GNP
      Right 0GNN
    Multiple 0GNQ
    Superior
      Left 0GNM
      Right 0GNL

Release — *continued*
  Patella
    Left 0QNF
    Right 0QND
  Penis 0VNS
  Pericardium 02NN
  Peritoneum 0DNW
  Phalanx
    Finger
      Left 0PNV
      Right 0PNT
    Thumb
      Left 0PNS
      Right 0PNR
    Toe
      Left 0QNR
      Right 0QNQ
  Pharynx 0CNM
  Pineal Body 0GN1
  Pleura
    Left 0BNP
    Right 0BNN
  Pons 00NB
  Prepuce 0VNT
  Prostate 0VN0
  Radius
    Left 0PNJ
    Right 0PNH
  Rectum 0DNP
  Retina
    Left 08NF3ZZ
    Right 08NE3ZZ
  Retinal Vessel
    Left 08NH3ZZ
    Right 08NG3ZZ
  Ribs
    1 to 2 0PN1
    3 or More 0PN2
  Sacrum 0QN1
  Scapula
    Left 0PN6
    Right 0PN5
  Sclera
    Left 08N7XZZ
    Right 08N6XZZ
  Scrotum 0VN5
  Septum
    Atrial 02N5
    Nasal 09NM
    Ventricular 02NM
  Sinus
    Accessory 09NP
    Ethmoid
      Left 09NV
      Right 09NU
    Frontal
      Left 09NT
      Right 09NS
    Mastoid
      Left 09NC
      Right 09NB
    Maxillary
      Left 09NR
      Right 09NQ
    Sphenoid
      Left 09NX
      Right 09NW
  Skin
    Abdomen 0HN7XZZ
    Back 0HN6XZZ
    Buttock 0HN8XZZ
    Chest 0HN5XZZ
    Ear
      Left 0HN3XZZ
      Right 0HN2XZZ
    Face 0HN1XZZ
    Foot

Release — *continued*
  Skin — *continued*
      Left 0HNNXZZ
      Right 0HNMXZZ
    Hand
      Left 0HNGXZZ
      Right 0HNFXZZ
    Inguinal 0HNAXZZ
    Lower Arm
      Left 0HNEXZZ
      Right 0HNDXZZ
    Lower Leg
      Left 0HNLXZZ
      Right 0HNKXZZ
    Neck 0HN4XZZ
    Perineum 0HN9XZZ
    Scalp 0HN0XZZ
    Upper Arm
      Left 0HNCXZZ
      Right 0HNBXZZ
    Upper Leg
      Left 0HNJXZZ
      Right 0HNHXZZ
  Spinal Cord
    Cervical 00NW
    Lumbar 00NY
    Thoracic 00NX
  Spinal Meninges 00NT
  Spleen 07NP
  Sternum 0PN0
  Stomach 0DN6
    Pylorus 0DN7
  Subcutaneous Tissue and Fascia
    Abdomen 0JN8
    Back 0JN7
    Buttock 0JN9
    Chest 0JN6
    Face 0JN1
    Foot
      Left 0JNR
      Right 0JNQ
    Hand
      Left 0JNK
      Right 0JNJ
    Lower Arm
      Left 0JNH
      Right 0JNG
    Lower Leg
      Left 0JNP
      Right 0JNN
    Neck
      Left 0JN5
      Right 0JN4
    Pelvic Region 0JNC
    Perineum 0JNB
    Scalp 0JN0
    Upper Arm
      Left 0JNF
      Right 0JND
    Upper Leg
      Left 0JNM
      Right 0JNL
  Tarsal
    Left 0QNM
    Right 0QNL
  Tendon
    Abdomen
      Left 0LNG
      Right 0LNF
    Ankle
      Left 0LNT
      Right 0LNS
    Foot
      Left 0LNW
      Right 0LNV
    Hand
      Left 0LN8
      Right 0LN7

Release — *continued*
  Tendon — *continued*
    Head and Neck 0LN0
    Hip
      Left 0LNK
      Right 0LNJ
    Knee
      Left 0LNR
      Right 0LNQ
    Lower Arm and Wrist
      Left 0LN6
      Right 0LN5
    Lower Leg
      Left 0LNP
      Right 0LNN
    Perineum 0LNH
    Shoulder
      Left 0LN2
      Right 0LN1
    Thorax
      Left 0LND
      Right 0LNC
    Trunk
      Left 0LNB
      Right 0LN9
    Upper Arm
      Left 0LN4
      Right 0LN3
    Upper Leg
      Left 0LNM
      Right 0LNL
  Testis
    Bilateral 0VNC
    Left 0VNB
    Right 0VN9
  Thalamus 00N9
  Thymus 07NM
  Thyroid Gland 0GNK
    Left Lobe 0GNG
    Right Lobe 0GNH
  Tibia
    Left 0QNH
    Right 0QNG
  Toe Nail 0HNRXZZ
  Tongue 0CN7
  Tonsils 0CNP
  Tooth
    Lower 0CNX
    Upper 0CNW
  Trachea 0BN1
  Tunica Vaginalis
    Left 0VN7
    Right 0VN6
  Turbinate, Nasal 09NL
  Tympanic Membrane
    Left 09N8
    Right 09N7
  Ulna
    Left 0PNL
    Right 0PNK
  Ureter
    Left 0TN7
    Right 0TN6
  Urethra 0TND
  Uterine Supporting Structure 0UN4
  Uterus 0UN9
  Uvula 0CNN
  Vagina 0UNG
  Valve
    Aortic 02NF
    Mitral 02NG
    Pulmonary 02NH
    Tricuspid 02NJ
  Vas Deferens
    Bilateral 0VNQ
    Left 0VNP
    Right 0VNN

Release — *continued*
  Vein
    Axillary
      Left 05N8
      Right 05N7
    Azygos 05N0
    Basilic
      Left 05NC
      Right 05NB
    Brachial
      Left 05NA
      Right 05N9
    Cephalic
      Left 05NF
      Right 05ND
    Colic 06N7
    Common Iliac
      Left 06ND
      Right 06NC
    Coronary 02N4
    Esophageal 06N3
    External Iliac
      Left 06NG
      Right 06NF
    External Jugular
      Left 05NQ
      Right 05NP
    Face
      Left 05NV
      Right 05NT
    Femoral
      Left 06NN
      Right 06NM
    Foot
      Left 06NV
      Right 06NT
    Gastric 06N2
    Hand
      Left 05NH
      Right 05NG
    Hemiazygos 05N1
    Hepatic 06N4
    Hypogastric
      Left 06NJ
      Right 06NH
    Inferior Mesenteric 06N6
    Innominate
      Left 05N4
      Right 05N3
    Internal Jugular
      Left 05NN
      Right 05NM
    Intracranial 05NL
    Lower 06NY
    Portal 06N8
    Pulmonary
      Left 02NT
      Right 02NS
    Renal
      Left 06NB
      Right 06N9
    Saphenous
      Left 06NQ
      Right 06NP
    Splenic 06N1
    Subclavian
      Left 05N6
      Right 05N5
    Superior Mesenteric 06N5
    Upper 05NY
    Vertebral
      Left 05NS
      Right 05NR
  Vena Cava
    Inferior 06N0
    Superior 02NV

Release — *continued*
  Ventricle
    Left 02NL
    Right 02NK
  Vertebra
    Cervical 0PN3
    Lumbar 0QN0
    Thoracic 0PN4
  Vesicle
    Bilateral 0VN3
    Left 0VN2
    Right 0VN1
  Vitreous
    Left 08N53ZZ
    Right 08N43ZZ
  Vocal Cord
    Left 0CNV
    Right 0CNT
  Vulva 0UNM
Relocation
  see Reposition
Removal
  Abdominal Wall 2W53X
  Anorectal 2Y53X5Z
  Arm
    Lower
      Left 2W5DX
      Right 2W5CX
    Upper
      Left 2W5BX
      Right 2W5AX
  Back 2W55X
  Chest Wall 2W54X
  Ear 2Y52X5Z
  Extremity
    Lower
      Left 2W5MX
      Right 2W5LX
    Upper
      Left 2W59X
      Right 2W58X
  Face 2W51X
  Finger
    Left 2W5KX
    Right 2W5JX
  Foot
    Left 2W5TX
    Right 2W5SX
  Genital Tract, Female 2Y54X5Z
  Hand
    Left 2W5FX
    Right 2W5EX
  Head 2W50X
  Inguinal Region
    Left 2W57X
    Right 2W56X
  Leg
    Lower
      Left 2W5RX
      Right 2W5QX
    Upper
      Left 2W5PX
      Right 2W5NX
  Mouth and Pharynx 2Y50X5Z
  Nasal 2Y51X5Z
  Neck 2W52X
  Thumb
    Left 2W5HX
    Right 2W5GX
  Toe
    Left 2W5VX
    Right 2W5UX
  Urethra 2Y55X5Z
Removal of device from
  Abdominal Wall 0WPF
  Acetabulum
    Left 0QP5
    Right 0QP4

Removal of device from — *continued*
- Anal Sphincter 0DPR
- Anus 0DPQ
- Artery
  - Lower 04PY
  - Upper 03PY
- Back
  - Lower 0WPL
  - Upper 0WPK
- Bladder 0TPB
- Bone
  - Facial 0NPW
  - Lower 0QPY
  - Nasal 0NPB
  - Pelvic
    - Left 0QP3
    - Right 0QP2
  - Upper 0PPY
- Bone Marrow 07PT
- Brain 00P0
- Breast
  - Left 0HPU
  - Right 0HPT
- Bursa and Ligament
  - Lower 0MPY
  - Upper 0MPX
- Carpal
  - Left 0PPN
  - Right 0PPM
- Cavity, Cranial 0WP1
- Cerebral Ventricle 00P6
- Chest Wall 0WP8
- Cisterna Chyli 07PL
- Clavicle
  - Left 0PPB
  - Right 0PP9
- Coccyx 0QPS
- Diaphragm 0BPT
- Disc
  - Cervical Vertebral 0RP3
  - Cervicothoracic Vertebral 0RP5
  - Lumbar Vertebral 0SP2
  - Lumbosacral 0SP4
  - Thoracic Vertebral 0RP9
  - Thoracolumbar Vertebral 0RPB
- Duct
  - Hepatobiliary 0FPB
  - Pancreatic 0FPD
- Ear
  - Inner
    - Left 09PE
    - Right 09PD
  - Left 09PJ
  - Right 09PH
- Epididymis and Spermatic Cord 0VPM
- Esophagus 0DP5
- Extremity
  - Lower
    - Left 0YPB
    - Right 0YP9
  - Upper
    - Left 0XP7
    - Right 0XP6
- Eye
  - Left 08P1
  - Right 08P0
- Face 0WP2
- Fallopian Tube 0UP8
- Femoral Shaft
  - Left 0QP9
  - Right 0QP8
- Femur
  - Lower
    - Left 0QPC
    - Right 0QPB
  - Upper
    - Left 0QP7
    - Right 0QP6

Removal of device from — *continued*
- Fibula
  - Left 0QPK
  - Right 0QPJ
- Finger Nail 0HPQX
- Gallbladder 0FP4
- Gastrointestinal Tract 0WPP
- Genitourinary Tract 0WPR
- Gland
  - Adrenal 0GP5
  - Endocrine 0GPS
  - Pituitary 0GP0
  - Salivary 0CPA
- Glenoid Cavity
  - Left 0PP8
  - Right 0PP7
- Great Vessel 02PY
- Hair 0HPSX
- Head 0WP0
- Heart 02PA
- Humeral Head
  - Left 0PPD
  - Right 0PPC
- Humeral Shaft
  - Left 0PPG
  - Right 0PPF
- Intestinal Tract
  - Lower 0DPD
  - Upper 0DP0
- Jaw
  - Lower 0WP5
  - Upper 0WP4
- Joint
  - Acromioclavicular
    - Left 0RPH
    - Right 0RPG
  - Ankle
    - Left 0SPG
    - Right 0SPF
  - Carpal
    - Left 0RPR
    - Right 0RPQ
  - Carpometacarpal
    - Left 0RPT
    - Right 0RPS
  - Cervical Vertebral 0RP1
  - Cervicothoracic Vertebral 0RP4
  - Coccygeal 0SP6
  - Elbow
    - Left 0RPM
    - Right 0RPL
  - Finger Phalangeal
    - Left 0RPX
    - Right 0RPW
  - Hip
    - Left 0SPB
      - Acetabular Surface 0SPE
      - Femoral Surface 0SPS
    - Right 0SP9
      - Acetabular Surface 0SPA
      - Femoral Surface 0SPR
  - Knee
    - Left 0SPD
      - Femoral Surface 0SPU
      - Tibial Surface 0SPW
    - Right 0SPC
      - Femoral Surface 0SPT
      - Tibial Surface 0SPV
  - Lumbar Vertebral 0SP0
  - Lumbosacral 0SP3
  - Metacarpophalangeal
    - Left 0RPV
    - Right 0RPU
  - Metatarsal-Phalangeal
    - Left 0SPN
    - Right 0SPM
  - Occipital-cervical 0RP0

Removal of device from — *continued*
- Joint — *continued*
  - Sacrococcygeal 0SP5
  - Sacroiliac
    - Left 0SP8
    - Right 0SP7
  - Shoulder
    - Left 0RPK
    - Right 0RPJ
  - Sternoclavicular
    - Left 0RPF
    - Right 0RPE
  - Tarsal
    - Left 0SPJ
    - Right 0SPH
  - Tarsometatarsal
    - Left 0SPL
    - Right 0SPK
  - Temporomandibular
    - Left 0RPD
    - Right 0RPC
  - Thoracic Vertebral 0RP6
  - Thoracolumbar Vertebral 0RPA
  - Toe Phalangeal
    - Left 0SPQ
    - Right 0SPP
  - Wrist
    - Left 0RPP
    - Right 0RPN
- Kidney 0TP5
- Larynx 0CPS
- Lens
  - Left 08PK3
  - Right 08PJ3
- Liver 0FP0
- Lung
  - Left 0BPL
  - Right 0BPK
- Lymphatic 07PN
  - Thoracic Duct 07PK
- Mediastinum 0WPC
- Mesentery 0DPV
- Metacarpal
  - Left 0PPQ
  - Right 0PPP
- Metatarsal
  - Left 0QPP
  - Right 0QPN
- Mouth and Throat 0CPY
- Muscle
  - Extraocular
    - Left 08PM
    - Right 08PL
  - Lower 0KPY
  - Upper 0KPX
- Nasal Mucosa and Soft Tissue 09PK
- Neck 0WP6
- Nerve
  - Cranial 00PE
  - Peripheral 01PY
- Omentum 0DPU
- Ovary 0UP3
- Pancreas 0FPG
- Parathyroid Gland 0GPR
- Patella
  - Left 0QPF
  - Right 0QPD
- Pelvic Cavity 0WPJ
- Penis 0VPS
- Pericardial Cavity 0WPD
- Perineum
  - Female 0WPN
  - Male 0WPM
- Peritoneal Cavity 0WPG
- Peritoneum 0DPW
- Phalanx
  - Finger

Removal of device from — *continued*
  Phalanx — *continued*
    Left 0PPV
    Right 0PPT
  Thumb
    Left 0PPS
    Right 0PPR
  Toe
    Left 0QPR
    Right 0QPQ
  Pineal Body 0GP1
  Pleura 0BPQ
  Pleural Cavity
    Left 0WPB
    Right 0WP9
  Products of Conception 10P0
  Prostate and Seminal Vesicles 0VP4
  Radius
    Left 0PPJ
    Right 0PPH
  Rectum 0DPP
  Respiratory Tract 0WPQ
  Retroperitoneum 0WPH
  Ribs
    1 to 2 0PP1
    3 or More 0PP2
  Sacrum 0QP1
  Scapula
    Left 0PP6
    Right 0PP5
  Scrotum and Tunica Vaginalis 0VP8
  Sinus 09PY
  Skin 0HPPX
  Skull 0NP0
  Spinal Canal 00PU
  Spinal Cord 00PV
  Spleen 07PP
  Sternum 0PP0
  Stomach 0DP6
  Subcutaneous Tissue and Fascia
    Head and Neck 0JPS
    Lower Extremity 0JPW
    Trunk 0JPT
    Upper Extremity 0JPV
  Tarsal
    Left 0QPM
    Right 0QPL
  Tendon
    Lower 0LPY
    Upper 0LPX
  Testis 0VPD
  Thymus 07PM
  Thyroid Gland 0GPK
  Tibia
    Left 0QPH
    Right 0QPG
  Toe Nail 0HPRX
  Trachea 0BP1
  Tracheobronchial Tree 0BP0
  Tympanic Membrane
    Left 09P8
    Right 09P7
  Ulna
    Left 0PPL
    Right 0PPK
  Ureter 0TP9
  Urethra 0TPD
  Uterus and Cervix 0UPD
  Vagina and Cul-de-sac 0UPH
  Vas Deferens 0VPR
  Vein
    Azygos 05P0
    Innominate
      Left 05P4
      Right 05P3
    Lower 06PY
    Upper 05PY

Removal of device from — *continued*
  Vertebra
    Cervical 0PP3
    Lumbar 0QP0
    Thoracic 0PP4
  Vulva 0UPM
Renal calyx
  use Kidney, Right
  use Kidney, Left
  use Kidneys, Bilateral
  use Kidney
Renal capsule
  use Kidney, Right
  use Kidney, Left
  use Kidneys, Bilateral
  use Kidney
Renal cortex
  use Kidney, Right
  use Kidney, Left
  use Kidneys, Bilateral
  use Kidney
Renal dialysis
  see Performance, Urinary 5A1D
Renal plexus
  use Abdominal Sympathetic Nerve
Renal segment
  use Kidney, Right
  use Kidney, Left
  use Kidneys, Bilateral
  use Kidney
Renal segmental artery
  use Renal Artery, Right
  use Renal Artery, Left
Reopening, operative site
  Control of bleeding *see* Control bleeding in
  Inspection only *see* Inspection
Repair
  Abdominal Wall 0WQF
  Acetabulum
    Left 0QQ5
    Right 0QQ4
  Adenoids 0CQQ
  Ampulla of Vater 0FQC
  Anal Sphincter 0DQR
  Ankle Region
    Left 0YQL
    Right 0YQK
  Anterior Chamber
    Left 08Q33ZZ
    Right 08Q23ZZ
  Anus 0DQQ
  Aorta
    Abdominal 04Q0
    Thoracic
      Ascending/Arch 02QX
      Descending 02QW
  Aortic Body 0GQD
  Appendix 0DQJ
  Arm
    Lower
      Left 0XQF
      Right 0XQD
    Upper
      Left 0XQ9
      Right 0XQ8
  Artery
    Anterior Tibial
      Left 04QQ
      Right 04QP
    Axillary
      Left 03Q6
      Right 03Q5
    Brachial
      Left 03Q8
      Right 03Q7
    Celiac 04Q1
    Colic

Repair — *continued*
  Artery — *continued*
    Left 04Q7
    Middle 04Q8
    Right 04Q6
    Common Carotid
      Left 03QJ
      Right 03QH
    Common Iliac
      Left 04QD
      Right 04QC
    Coronary
      Four or More Arteries 02Q3
      One Artery 02Q0
      Three Arteries 02Q2
      Two Arteries 02Q1
    External Carotid
      Left 03QN
      Right 03QM
    External Iliac
      Left 04QJ
      Right 04QH
    Face 03QR
    Femoral
      Left 04QL
      Right 04QK
    Foot
      Left 04QW
      Right 04QV
    Gastric 04Q2
    Hand
      Left 03QF
      Right 03QD
    Hepatic 04Q3
    Inferior Mesenteric 04QB
    Innominate 03Q2
    Internal Carotid
      Left 03QL
      Right 03QK
    Internal Iliac
      Left 04QF
      Right 04QE
    Internal Mammary
      Left 03Q1
      Right 03Q0
    Intracranial 03QG
    Lower 04QY
    Peroneal
      Left 04QU
      Right 04QT
    Popliteal
      Left 04QN
      Right 04QM
    Posterior Tibial
      Left 04QS
      Right 04QR
    Pulmonary
      Left 02QR
      Right 02QQ
    Pulmonary Trunk 02QP
    Radial
      Left 03QC
      Right 03QB
    Renal
      Left 04QA
      Right 04Q9
    Splenic 04Q4
    Subclavian
      Left 03Q4
      Right 03Q3
    Superior Mesenteric 04Q5
    Temporal
      Left 03QT
      Right 03QS
    Thyroid
      Left 03QV
      Right 03QU

Repair — *continued*
  Artery — *continued*
    Ulnar
      Left 03QA
      Right 03Q9
    Upper 03QY
    Vertebral
      Left 03QQ
      Right 03QP
  Atrium
    Left 02Q7
    Right 02Q6
  Auditory Ossicle
    Left 09QA
    Right 09Q9
  Axilla
    Left 0XQ5
    Right 0XQ4
  Back
    Lower 0WQL
    Upper 0WQK
  Basal Ganglia 00Q8
  Bladder 0TQB
  Bladder Neck 0TQC
  Bone
    Ethmoid
      Left 0NQG
      Right 0NQF
    Frontal 0NQ1
    Hyoid 0NQX
    Lacrimal
      Left 0NQJ
      Right 0NQH
    Nasal 0NQB
    Occipital 0NQ7
    Palatine
      Left 0NQL
      Right 0NQK
    Parietal
      Left 0NQ4
      Right 0NQ3
    Pelvic
      Left 0QQ3
      Right 0QQ2
    Sphenoid 0NQC
    Temporal
      Left 0NQ6
      Right 0NQ5
    Zygomatic
      Left 0NQN
      Right 0NQM
  Brain 00Q0
  Breast
    Bilateral 0HQV
    Left 0HQU
    Right 0HQT
    Supernumerary 0HQY
  Bronchus
    Lingula 0BQ9
    Lower Lobe
      Left 0BQB
      Right 0BQ6
    Main
      Left 0BQ7
      Right 0BQ3
    Middle Lobe, Right 0BQ5
    Upper Lobe
      Left 0BQ8
      Right 0BQ4
  Buccal Mucosa 0CQ4
  Bursa and Ligament
    Abdomen
      Left 0MQJ
      Right 0MQH
    Ankle
      Left 0MQR
      Right 0MQQ

Repair — *continued*
  Bursa and Ligament — *continued*
    Elbow
      Left 0MQ4
      Right 0MQ3
    Foot
      Left 0MQT
      Right 0MQS
    Hand
      Left 0MQ8
      Right 0MQ7
    Head and Neck 0MQ0
    Hip
      Left 0MQM
      Right 0MQL
    Knee
      Left 0MQP
      Right 0MQN
    Lower Extremity
      Left 0MQW
      Right 0MQV
    Perineum 0MQK
    Rib(s) 0MQG
    Shoulder
      Left 0MQ2
      Right 0MQ1
    Spine
      Lower 0MQD
      Upper 0MQC
    Sternum 0MQF
    Upper Extremity
      Left 0MQB
      Right 0MQ9
    Wrist
      Left 0MQ6
      Right 0MQ5
  Buttock
    Left 0YQ1
    Right 0YQ0
  Carina 0BQ2
  Carotid Bodies, Bilateral 0GQ8
  Carotid Body
    Left 0GQ6
    Right 0GQ7
  Carpal
    Left 0PQN
    Right 0PQM
  Cecum 0DQH
  Cerebellum 00QC
  Cerebral Hemisphere 00Q7
  Cerebral Meninges 00Q1
  Cerebral Ventricle 00Q6
  Cervix 0UQC
  Chest Wall 0WQ8
  Chordae Tendineae 02Q9
  Choroid
    Left 08QB
    Right 08QA
  Cisterna Chyli 07QL
  Clavicle
    Left 0PQB
    Right 0PQ9
  Clitoris 0UQJ
  Coccygeal Glomus 0GQB
  Coccyx 0QQS
  Colon
    Ascending 0DQK
    Descending 0DQM
    Sigmoid 0DQN
    Transverse 0DQL
  Conduction Mechanism 02Q8
  Conjunctiva
    Left 08QTXZZ
    Right 08QSXZZ
  Cord
    Bilateral 0VQH
    Left 0VQG
    Right 0VQF

Repair — *continued*
  Cornea
    Left 08Q9XZZ
    Right 08Q8XZZ
  Cul-de-sac 0UQF
  Diaphragm 0BQT
  Disc
    Cervical Vertebral 0RQ3
    Cervicothoracic Vertebral 0RQ5
    Lumbar Vertebral 0SQ2
    Lumbosacral 0SQ4
    Thoracic Vertebral 0RQ9
    Thoracolumbar Vertebral 0RQB
  Duct
    Common Bile 0FQ9
    Cystic 0FQ8
    Hepatic
      Common 0FQ7
      Left 0FQ6
      Right 0FQ5
    Lacrimal
      Left 08QY
      Right 08QX
    Pancreatic 0FQD
      Accessory 0FQF
    Parotid
      Left 0CQC
      Right 0CQB
  Duodenum 0DQ9
  Dura Mater 00Q2
  Ear
    External
      Bilateral 09Q2
      Left 09Q1
      Right 09Q0
    External Auditory Canal
      Left 09Q4
      Right 09Q3
    Inner
      Left 09QE
      Right 09QD
    Middle
      Left 09Q6
      Right 09Q5
  Elbow Region
    Left 0XQC
    Right 0XQB
  Epididymis
    Bilateral 0VQL
    Left 0VQK
    Right 0VQJ
  Epiglottis 0CQR
  Esophagogastric Junction 0DQ4
  Esophagus 0DQ5
    Lower 0DQ3
    Middle 0DQ2
    Upper 0DQ1
  Eustachian Tube
    Left 09QG
    Right 09QF
  Extremity
    Lower
      Left 0YQB
      Right 0YQ9
    Upper
      Left 0XQ7
      Right 0XQ6
  Eye
    Left 08Q1XZZ
    Right 08Q0XZZ
  Eyelid
    Lower
      Left 08QR
      Right 08QQ
    Upper
      Left 08QP
      Right 08QN

Repair — *continued*
- Face 0WQ2
- Fallopian Tube
  - Left 0UQ6
  - Right 0UQ5
- Fallopian Tubes, Bilateral 0UQ7
- Femoral Region
  - Bilateral 0YQE
  - Left 0YQ8
  - Right 0YQ7
- Femoral Shaft
  - Left 0QQ9
  - Right 0QQ8
- Femur
  - Lower
    - Left 0QQC
    - Right 0QQB
  - Upper
    - Left 0QQ7
    - Right 0QQ6
- Fibula
  - Left 0QQK
  - Right 0QQJ
- Finger
  - Index
    - Left 0XQP
    - Right 0XQN
  - Little
    - Left 0XQW
    - Right 0XQV
  - Middle
    - Left 0XQR
    - Right 0XQQ
  - Ring
    - Left 0XQT
    - Right 0XQS
- Finger Nail 0HQQXZZ
- Floor of mouth *see* Repair, Oral Cavity and Throat 0WQ3
- Foot
  - Left 0YQN
  - Right 0YQM
- Gallbladder 0FQ4
- Gingiva
  - Lower 0CQ6
  - Upper 0CQ5
- Gland
  - Adrenal
    - Bilateral 0GQ4
    - Left 0GQ2
    - Right 0GQ3
  - Lacrimal
    - Left 08QW
    - Right 08QV
  - Minor Salivary 0CQJ
  - Parotid
    - Left 0CQ9
    - Right 0CQ8
  - Pituitary 0GQ0
  - Sublingual
    - Left 0CQF
    - Right 0CQD
  - Submaxillary
    - Left 0CQH
    - Right 0CQG
  - Vestibular 0UQL
- Glenoid Cavity
  - Left 0PQ8
  - Right 0PQ7
- Glomus Jugulare 0GQC
- Hand
  - Left 0XQK
  - Right 0XQJ
- Head 0WQ0
- Heart 02QA
  - Left 02QC
  - Right 02QB

Repair — *continued*
- Humeral Head
  - Left 0PQD
  - Right 0PQC
- Humeral Shaft
  - Left 0PQG
  - Right 0PQF
- Hymen 0UQK
- Hypothalamus 00QA
- Ileocecal Valve 0DQC
- Ileum 0DQB
- Inguinal Region
  - Bilateral 0YQA
  - Left 0YQ6
  - Right 0YQ5
- Intestine
  - Large 0DQE
    - Left 0DQG
    - Right 0DQF
  - Small 0DQ8
- Iris
  - Left 08QD3ZZ
  - Right 08QC3ZZ
- Jaw
  - Lower 0WQ5
  - Upper 0WQ4
- Jejunum 0DQA
- Joint
  - Acromioclavicular
    - Left 0RQH
    - Right 0RQG
  - Ankle
    - Left 0SQG
    - Right 0SQF
  - Carpal
    - Left 0RQR
    - Right 0RQQ
  - Carpometacarpal
    - Left 0RQT
    - Right 0RQS
  - Cervical Vertebral 0RQ1
  - Cervicothoracic Vertebral 0RQ4
  - Coccygeal 0SQ6
  - Elbow
    - Left 0RQM
    - Right 0RQL
  - Finger Phalangeal
    - Left 0RQX
    - Right 0RQW
  - Hip
    - Left 0SQB
    - Right 0SQ9
  - Knee
    - Left 0SQD
    - Right 0SQC
  - Lumbar Vertebral 0SQ0
  - Lumbosacral 0SQ3
  - Metacarpophalangeal
    - Left 0RQV
    - Right 0RQU
  - Metatarsal-Phalangeal
    - Left 0SQN
    - Right 0SQM
  - Occipital-cervical 0RQ0
  - Sacrococcygeal 0SQ5
  - Sacroiliac
    - Left 0SQ8
    - Right 0SQ7
  - Shoulder
    - Left 0RQK
    - Right 0RQJ
  - Sternoclavicular
    - Left 0RQF
    - Right 0RQE
  - Tarsal
    - Left 0SQJ
    - Right 0SQH

Repair — *continued*
- Joint — *continued*
  - Tarsometatarsal
    - Left 0SQL
    - Right 0SQK
  - Temporomandibular
    - Left 0RQD
    - Right 0RQC
  - Thoracic Vertebral 0RQ6
  - Thoracolumbar Vertebral 0RQA
  - Toe Phalangeal
    - Left 0SQQ
    - Right 0SQP
  - Wrist
    - Left 0RQP
    - Right 0RQN
- Kidney
  - Left 0TQ1
  - Right 0TQ0
- Kidney Pelvis
  - Left 0TQ4
  - Right 0TQ3
- Knee Region
  - Left 0YQG
  - Right 0YQF
- Larynx 0CQS
- Leg
  - Lower
    - Left 0YQJ
    - Right 0YQH
  - Upper
    - Left 0YQD
    - Right 0YQC
- Lens
  - Left 08QK3ZZ
  - Right 08QJ3ZZ
- Lip
  - Lower 0CQ1
  - Upper 0CQ0
- Liver 0FQ0
  - Left Lobe 0FQ2
  - Right Lobe 0FQ1
- Lung
  - Bilateral 0BQM
  - Left 0BQL
  - Lower Lobe
    - Left 0BQJ
    - Right 0BQF
  - Middle Lobe, Right 0BQD
  - Right 0BQK
  - Upper Lobe
    - Left 0BQG
    - Right 0BQC
- Lung Lingula 0BQH
- Lymphatic
  - Aortic 07QD
  - Axillary
    - Left 07Q6
    - Right 07Q5
  - Head 07Q0
  - Inguinal
    - Left 07QJ
    - Right 07QH
  - Internal Mammary
    - Left 07Q9
    - Right 07Q8
  - Lower Extremity
    - Left 07QG
    - Right 07QF
  - Mesenteric 07QB
  - Neck
    - Left 07Q2
    - Right 07Q1
  - Pelvis 07QC
  - Thoracic Duct 07QK
  - Thorax 07Q7
  - Upper Extremity

Repair — *continued*
Lymphatic — *continued*
Left 07Q4
Right 07Q3
Mandible
Left 0NQV
Right 0NQT
Maxilla 0NQR
Mediastinum 0WQC
Medulla Oblongata 00QD
Mesentery 0DQV
Metacarpal
Left 0PQQ
Right 0PQP
Metatarsal
Left 0QQP
Right 0QQN
Muscle
Abdomen
Left 0KQL
Right 0KQK
Extraocular
Left 08QM
Right 08QL
Facial 0KQ1
Foot
Left 0KQW
Right 0KQV
Hand
Left 0KQD
Right 0KQC
Head 0KQ0
Hip
Left 0KQP
Right 0KQN
Lower Arm and Wrist
Left 0KQB
Right 0KQ9
Lower Leg
Left 0KQT
Right 0KQS
Neck
Left 0KQ3
Right 0KQ2
Papillary 02QD
Perineum 0KQM
Shoulder
Left 0KQ6
Right 0KQ5
Thorax
Left 0KQJ
Right 0KQH
Tongue, Palate, Pharynx 0KQ4
Trunk
Left 0KQG
Right 0KQF
Upper Arm
Left 0KQ8
Right 0KQ7
Upper Leg
Left 0KQR
Right 0KQQ
Nasal Mucosa and Soft Tissue 09QK
Nasopharynx 09QN
Neck 0WQ6
Nerve
Abdominal Sympathetic 01QM
Abducens 00QL
Accessory 00QR
Acoustic 00QN
Brachial Plexus 01Q3
Cervical 01Q1
Cervical Plexus 01Q0
Facial 00QM
Femoral 01QD
Glossopharyngeal 00QP
Head and Neck Sympathetic 01QK

Repair — *continued*
Nerve — *continued*
Hypoglossal 00QS
Lumbar 01QB
Lumbar Plexus 01Q9
Lumbar Sympathetic 01QN
Lumbosacral Plexus 01QA
Median 01Q5
Oculomotor 00QH
Olfactory 00QF
Optic 00QG
Peroneal 01QH
Phrenic 01Q2
Pudendal 01QC
Radial 01Q6
Sacral 01QR
Sacral Plexus 01QQ
Sacral Sympathetic 01QP
Sciatic 01QF
Thoracic 01Q8
Thoracic Sympathetic 01QL
Tibial 01QG
Trigeminal 00QK
Trochlear 00QJ
Ulnar 01Q4
Vagus 00QQ
Nipple
Left 0HQX
Right 0HQW
Omentum 0DQU
Oral Cavity and Throat 0WQ3
Orbit
Left 0NQQ
Right 0NQP
Ovary
Bilateral 0UQ2
Left 0UQ1
Right 0UQ0
Palate
Hard 0CQ2
Soft 0CQ3
Pancreas 0FQG
Para-aortic Body 0GQ9
Paraganglion Extremity 0GQF
Parathyroid Gland 0GQR
Inferior
Left 0GQP
Right 0GQN
Multiple 0GQQ
Superior
Left 0GQM
Right 0GQL
Patella
Left 0QQF
Right 0QQD
Penis 0VQS
Pericardium 02QN
Perineum
Female 0WQN
Male 0WQM
Peritoneum 0DQW
Phalanx
Finger
Left 0PQV
Right 0PQT
Thumb
Left 0PQS
Right 0PQR
Toe
Left 0QQR
Right 0QQQ
Pharynx 0CQM
Pineal Body 0GQ1
Pleura
Left 0BQP
Right 0BQN
Pons 00QB

Repair — *continued*
Prepuce 0VQT
Products of Conception 10Q0
Prostate 0VQ0
Radius
Left 0PQJ
Right 0PQH
Rectum 0DQP
Retina
Left 08QF3ZZ
Right 08QE3ZZ
Retinal Vessel
Left 08QH3ZZ
Right 08QG3ZZ
Ribs
1 to 2 0PQ1
3 or More 0PQ2
Sacrum 0QQ1
Scapula
Left 0PQ6
Right 0PQ5
Sclera
Left 08Q7XZZ
Right 08Q6XZZ
Scrotum 0VQ5
Septum
Atrial 02Q5
Nasal 09QM
Ventricular 02QM
Shoulder Region
Left 0XQ3
Right 0XQ2
Sinus
Accessory 09QP
Ethmoid
Left 09QV
Right 09QU
Frontal
Left 09QT
Right 09QS
Mastoid
Left 09QC
Right 09QB
Maxillary
Left 09QR
Right 09QQ
Sphenoid
Left 09QX
Right 09QW
Skin
Abdomen 0HQ7XZZ
Back 0HQ6XZZ
Buttock 0HQ8XZZ
Chest 0HQ5XZZ
Ear
Left 0HQ3XZZ
Right 0HQ2XZZ
Face 0HQ1XZZ
Foot
Left 0HQNXZZ
Right 0HQMXZZ
Hand
Left 0HQGXZZ
Right 0HQFXZZ
Inguinal 0HQAXZZ
Lower Arm
Left 0HQEXZZ
Right 0HQDXZZ
Lower Leg
Left 0HQLXZZ
Right 0HQKXZZ
Neck 0HQ4XZZ
Perineum 0HQ9XZZ
Scalp 0HQ0XZZ
Upper Arm
Left 0HQCXZZ
Right 0HQBXZZ

Repair — *continued*
  Skin — *continued*
    Upper Leg
      Left 0HQJXZZ
      Right 0HQHXZZ
  Skull 0NQ0
  Spinal Cord
    Cervical 00QW
    Lumbar 00QY
    Thoracic 00QX
  Spinal Meninges 00QT
  Spleen 07QP
  Sternum 0PQ0
  Stomach 0DQ6
    Pylorus 0DQ7
  Subcutaneous Tissue and Fascia
    Abdomen 0JQ8
    Back 0JQ7
    Buttock 0JQ9
    Chest 0JQ6
    Face 0JQ1
    Foot
      Left 0JQR
      Right 0JQQ
    Hand
      Left 0JQK
      Right 0JQJ
    Lower Arm
      Left 0JQH
      Right 0JQG
    Lower Leg
      Left 0JQP
      Right 0JQN
    Neck
      Left 0JQ5
      Right 0JQ4
    Pelvic Region 0JQC
    Perineum 0JQB
    Scalp 0JQ0
    Upper Arm
      Left 0JQF
      Right 0JQD
    Upper Leg
      Left 0JQM
      Right 0JQL
  Tarsal
    Left 0QQM
    Right 0QQL
  Tendon
    Abdomen
      Left 0LQG
      Right 0LQF
    Ankle
      Left 0LQT
      Right 0LQS
    Foot
      Left 0LQW
      Right 0LQV
    Hand
      Left 0LQ8
      Right 0LQ7
    Head and Neck 0LQ0
    Hip
      Left 0LQK
      Right 0LQJ
    Knee
      Left 0LQR
      Right 0LQQ
    Lower Arm and Wrist
      Left 0LQ6
      Right 0LQ5
    Lower Leg
      Left 0LQP
      Right 0LQN
    Perineum 0LQH
    Shoulder
      Left 0LQ2

Repair — *continued*
  Tendon — *continued*
      Right 0LQ1
    Thorax
      Left 0LQD
      Right 0LQC
    Trunk
      Left 0LQB
      Right 0LQ9
    Upper Arm
      Left 0LQ4
      Right 0LQ3
    Upper Leg
      Left 0LQM
      Right 0LQL
  Testis
    Bilateral 0VQC
    Left 0VQB
    Right 0VQ9
  Thalamus 00Q9
  Thumb
    Left 0XQM
    Right 0XQL
  Thymus 07QM
  Thyroid Gland 0GQK
    Left Lobe 0GQG
    Right Lobe 0GQH
  Thyroid Gland Isthmus 0GQJ
  Tibia
    Left 0QQH
    Right 0QQG
  Toe
    1st
      Left 0YQQ
      Right 0YQP
    2nd
      Left 0YQS
      Right 0YQR
    3rd
      Left 0YQU
      Right 0YQT
    4th
      Left 0YQW
      Right 0YQV
    5th
      Left 0YQY
      Right 0YQX
  Toe Nail 0HQRXZZ
  Tongue 0CQ7
  Tonsils 0CQP
  Tooth
    Lower 0CQX
    Upper 0CQW
  Trachea 0BQ1
  Tunica Vaginalis
    Left 0VQ7
    Right 0VQ6
  Turbinate, Nasal 09QL
  Tympanic Membrane
    Left 09Q8
    Right 09Q7
  Ulna
    Left 0PQL
    Right 0PQK
  Ureter
    Left 0TQ7
    Right 0TQ6
  Urethra 0TQD
  Uterine Supporting Structure 0UQ4
  Uterus 0UQ9
  Uvula 0CQN
  Vagina 0UQG
  Valve
    Aortic 02QF
    Mitral 02QG
    Pulmonary 02QH
    Tricuspid 02QJ

Repair — *continued*
  Vas Deferens
    Bilateral 0VQQ
    Left 0VQP
    Right 0VQN
  Vein
    Axillary
      Left 05Q8
      Right 05Q7
    Azygos 05Q0
    Basilic
      Left 05QC
      Right 05QB
    Brachial
      Left 05QA
      Right 05Q9
    Cephalic
      Left 05QF
      Right 05QD
    Colic 06Q7
    Common Iliac
      Left 06QD
      Right 06QC
    Coronary 02Q4
    Esophageal 06Q3
    External Iliac
      Left 06QG
      Right 06QF
    External Jugular
      Left 05QQ
      Right 05QP
    Face
      Left 05QV
      Right 05QT
    Femoral
      Left 06QN
      Right 06QM
    Foot
      Left 06QV
      Right 06QT
    Gastric 06Q2
    Hand
      Left 05QH
      Right 05QG
    Hemiazygos 05Q1
    Hepatic 06Q4
    Hypogastric
      Left 06QJ
      Right 06QH
    Inferior Mesenteric 06Q6
    Innominate
      Left 05Q4
      Right 05Q3
    Internal Jugular
      Left 05QN
      Right 05QM
    Intracranial 05QL
    Lower 06QY
    Portal 06Q8
    Pulmonary
      Left 02QT
      Right 02QS
    Renal
      Left 06QB
      Right 06Q9
    Saphenous
      Left 06QQ
      Right 06QP
    Splenic 06Q1
    Subclavian
      Left 05Q6
      Right 05Q5
    Superior Mesenteric 06Q5
    Upper 05QY
    Vertebral
      Left 05QS
      Right 05QR

Repair — continued
Vena Cava
  Inferior 06Q0
  Superior 02QV
Ventricle
  Left 02QL
  Right 02QK
Vertebra
  Cervical 0PQ3
  Lumbar 0QQ0
  Thoracic 0PQ4
Vesicle
  Bilateral 0VQ3
  Left 0VQ2
  Right 0VQ1
Vitreous
  Left 08Q53ZZ
  Right 08Q43ZZ
Vocal Cord
  Left 0CQV
  Right 0CQT
Vulva 0UQM
Wrist Region
  Left 0XQH
  Right 0XQG

Repair, obstetric laceration, periurethral
0UQMXZZ

Replacement
Acetabulum
  Left 0QR5
  Right 0QR4
Ampulla of Vater 0FRC
Anal Sphincter 0DRR
Aorta
  Abdominal 04R0
  Thoracic
    Ascending/Arch 02RX
    Descending 02RW
Artery
  Anterior Tibial
    Left 04RQ
    Right 04RP
  Axillary
    Left 03R6
    Right 03R5
  Brachial
    Left 03R8
    Right 03R7
  Celiac 04R1
  Colic
    Left 04R7
    Middle 04R8
    Right 04R6
  Common Carotid
    Left 03RJ
    Right 03RH
  Common Iliac
    Left 04RD
    Right 04RC
  External Carotid
    Left 03RN
    Right 03RM
  External Iliac
    Left 04RJ
    Right 04RH
  Face 03RR
  Femoral
    Left 04RL
    Right 04RK
  Foot
    Left 04RW
    Right 04RV
  Gastric 04R2
  Hand
    Left 03RF
    Right 03RD
  Hepatic 04R3

Replacement — continued
Artery — continued
  Inferior Mesenteric 04RB
  Innominate 03R2
  Internal Carotid
    Left 03RL
    Right 03RK
  Internal Iliac
    Left 04RF
    Right 04RE
  Internal Mammary
    Left 03R1
    Right 03R0
  Intracranial 03RG
  Lower 04RY
  Peroneal
    Left 04RU
    Right 04RT
  Popliteal
    Left 04RN
    Right 04RM
  Posterior Tibial
    Left 04RS
    Right 04RR
  Pulmonary
    Left 02RR
    Right 02RQ
  Pulmonary Trunk 02RP
  Radial
    Left 03RC
    Right 03RB
  Renal
    Left 04RA
    Right 04R9
  Splenic 04R4
  Subclavian
    Left 03R4
    Right 03R3
  Superior Mesenteric 04R5
  Temporal
    Left 03RT
    Right 03RS
  Thyroid
    Left 03RV
    Right 03RU
  Ulnar
    Left 03RA
    Right 03R9
  Upper 03RY
  Vertebral
    Left 03RQ
    Right 03RP
Atrium
  Left 02R7
  Right 02R6
Auditory Ossicle
  Left 09RA0
  Right 09R90
Bladder 0TRB
Bladder Neck 0TRC
Bone
  Ethmoid
    Left 0NRG
    Right 0NRF
  Frontal 0NR1
  Hyoid 0NRX
  Lacrimal
    Left 0NRJ
    Right 0NRH
  Nasal 0NRB
  Occipital 0NR7
  Palatine
    Left 0NRL
    Right 0NRK
  Parietal
    Left 0NR4
    Right 0NR3

Replacement — continued
Bone — continued
  Pelvic
    Left 0QR3
    Right 0QR2
  Sphenoid 0NRC
  Temporal
    Left 0NR6
    Right 0NR5
  Zygomatic
    Left 0NRN
    Right 0NRM
Breast
  Bilateral 0HRV
  Left 0HRU
  Right 0HRT
Bronchus
  Lingula 0BR9
  Lower Lobe
    Left 0BRB
    Right 0BR6
  Main
    Left 0BR7
    Right 0BR3
  Middle Lobe, Right 0BR5
  Upper Lobe
    Left 0BR8
    Right 0BR4
Buccal Mucosa 0CR4
Bursa and Ligament
  Abdomen
    Left 0MRJ
    Right 0MRH
  Ankle
    Left 0MRR
    Right 0MRQ
  Elbow
    Left 0MR4
    Right 0MR3
  Foot
    Left 0MRT
    Right 0MRS
  Hand
    Left 0MR8
    Right 0MR7
  Head and Neck 0MR0
  Hip
    Left 0MRM
    Right 0MRL
  Knee
    Left 0MRP
    Right 0MRN
  Lower Extremity
    Left 0MRW
    Right 0MRV
  Perineum 0MRK
  Rib(s) 0MRG
  Shoulder
    Left 0MR2
    Right 0MR1
  Spine
    Lower 0MRD
    Upper 0MRC
  Sternum 0MRF
  Upper Extremity
    Left 0MRB
    Right 0MR9
  Wrist
    Left 0MR6
    Right 0MR5
Carina 0BR2
Carpal
  Left 0PRN
  Right 0PRM
Cerebral Meninges 00R1
Cerebral Ventricle 00R6
Chordae Tendineae 02R9

Replacement — *continued*
- Choroid
  - Left 08RB
  - Right 08RA
- Clavicle
  - Left 0PRB
  - Right 0PR9
- Coccyx 0QRS
- Conjunctiva
  - Left 08RTX
  - Right 08RSX
- Cornea
  - Left 08R9
  - Right 08R8
- Diaphragm 0BRT
- Disc
  - Cervical Vertebral 0RR30
  - Cervicothoracic Vertebral 0RR50
  - Lumbar Vertebral 0SR20
  - Lumbosacral 0SR40
  - Thoracic Vertebral 0RR90
  - Thoracolumbar Vertebral 0RRB0
- Duct
  - Common Bile 0FR9
  - Cystic 0FR8
  - Hepatic
    - Common 0FR7
    - Left 0FR6
    - Right 0FR5
  - Lacrimal
    - Left 08RY
    - Right 08RX
  - Pancreatic 0FRD
    - Accessory 0FRF
  - Parotid
    - Left 0CRC
    - Right 0CRB
- Dura Mater 00R2
- Ear
  - External
    - Bilateral 09R2
    - Left 09R1
    - Right 09R0
  - Inner
    - Left 09RE0
    - Right 09RD0
  - Middle
    - Left 09R60
    - Right 09R50
- Epiglottis 0CRR
- Esophagus 0DR5
- Eye
  - Left 08R1
  - Right 08R0
- Eyelid
  - Lower
    - Left 08RR
    - Right 08RQ
  - Upper
    - Left 08RP
    - Right 08RN
- Femoral Shaft
  - Left 0QR9
  - Right 0QR8
- Femur
  - Lower
    - Left 0QRC
    - Right 0QRB
  - Upper
    - Left 0QR7
    - Right 0QR6
- Fibula
  - Left 0QRK
  - Right 0QRJ
- Finger Nail 0HRQX
- Gingiva
  - Lower 0CR6
  - Upper 0CR5

Replacement — *continued*
- Glenoid Cavity
  - Left 0PR8
  - Right 0PR7
- Hair 0HRSX
- Humeral Head
  - Left 0PRD
  - Right 0PRC
- Humeral Shaft
  - Left 0PRG
  - Right 0PRF
- Iris
  - Left 08RD3
  - Right 08RC3
- Joint
  - Acromioclavicular
    - Left 0RRH0
    - Right 0RRG0
  - Ankle
    - Left 0SRG
    - Right 0SRF
  - Carpal
    - Left 0RRR0
    - Right 0RRQ0
  - Carpometacarpal
    - Left 0RRT0
    - Right 0RRS0
  - Cervical Vertebral 0RR10
  - Cervicothoracic Vertebral 0RR40
  - Coccygeal 0SR60
  - Elbow
    - Left 0RRM0
    - Right 0RRL0
  - Finger Phalangeal
    - Left 0RRX0
    - Right 0RRW0
  - Hip
    - Left 0SRB
      - Acetabular Surface 0SRE
      - Femoral Surface 0SRS
    - Right 0SR9
      - Acetabular Surface 0SRA
      - Femoral Surface 0SRR
  - Knee
    - Left 0SRD
      - Femoral Surface 0SRU
      - Tibial Surface 0SRW
    - Right 0SRC
      - Femoral Surface 0SRT
      - Tibial Surface 0SRV
  - Lumbar Vertebral 0SR00
  - Lumbosacral 0SR30
  - Metacarpophalangeal
    - Left 0RRV0
    - Right 0RRU0
  - Metatarsal-Phalangeal
    - Left 0SRN0
    - Right 0SRM0
  - Occipital-cervical 0RR00
  - Sacrococcygeal 0SR50
  - Sacroiliac
    - Left 0SR80
    - Right 0SR70
  - Shoulder
    - Left 0RRK
    - Right 0RRJ
  - Sternoclavicular
    - Left 0RRF0
    - Right 0RRE0
  - Tarsal
    - Left 0SRJ0
    - Right 0SRH0
  - Tarsometatarsal
    - Left 0SRL0
    - Right 0SRK0
  - Temporomandibular
    - Left 0RRD0
    - Right 0RRC0

Replacement — *continued*
- Joint — *continued*
  - Thoracic Vertebral 0RR60
  - Thoracolumbar Vertebral 0RRA0
  - Toe Phalangeal
    - Left 0SRQ0
    - Right 0SRP0
  - Wrist
    - Left 0RRP0
    - Right 0RRN0
- Kidney Pelvis
  - Left 0TR4
  - Right 0TR3
- Larynx 0CRS
- Lens
  - Left 08RK30Z
  - Right 08RJ30Z
- Lip
  - Lower 0CR1
  - Upper 0CR0
- Mandible
  - Left 0NRV
  - Right 0NRT
- Maxilla 0NRR
- Mesentery 0DRV
- Metacarpal
  - Left 0PRQ
  - Right 0PRP
- Metatarsal
  - Left 0QRP
  - Right 0QRN
- Muscle
  - Abdomen
    - Left 0KRL
    - Right 0KRK
  - Facial 0KR1
  - Foot
    - Left 0KRW
    - Right 0KRV
  - Hand
    - Left 0KRD
    - Right 0KRC
  - Head 0KR0
  - Hip
    - Left 0KRP
    - Right 0KRN
  - Lower Arm and Wrist
    - Left 0KRB
    - Right 0KR9
  - Lower Leg
    - Left 0KRT
    - Right 0KRS
  - Neck
    - Left 0KR3
    - Right 0KR2
  - Papillary 02RD
  - Perineum 0KRM
  - Shoulder
    - Left 0KR6
    - Right 0KR5
  - Thorax
    - Left 0KRJ
    - Right 0KRH
  - Tongue, Palate, Pharynx 0KR4
  - Trunk
    - Left 0KRG
    - Right 0KRF
  - Upper Arm
    - Left 0KR8
    - Right 0KR7
  - Upper Leg
    - Left 0KRR
    - Right 0KRQ
- Nasal Mucosa and Soft Tissue 09RK
- Nasopharynx 09RN
- Nerve
  - Abducens 00RL

Replacement — continued
  Nerve — continued
    Accessory 00RR
    Acoustic 00RN
    Cervical 01R1
    Facial 00RM
    Femoral 01RD
    Glossopharyngeal 00RP
    Hypoglossal 00RS
    Lumbar 01RB
    Median 01R5
    Oculomotor 00RH
    Olfactory 00RF
    Optic 00RG
    Peroneal 01RH
    Phrenic 01R2
    Pudendal 01RC
    Radial 01R6
    Sacral 01RR
    Sciatic 01RF
    Thoracic 01R8
    Tibial 01RG
    Trigeminal 00RK
    Trochlear 00RJ
    Ulnar 01R4
    Vagus 00RQ
  Nipple
    Left 0HRX
    Right 0HRW
  Omentum 0DRU
  Orbit
    Left 0NRQ
    Right 0NRP
  Palate
    Hard 0CR2
    Soft 0CR3
  Patella
    Left 0QRF
    Right 0QRD
  Pericardium 02RN
  Peritoneum 0DRW
  Phalanx
    Finger
      Left 0PRV
      Right 0PRT
    Thumb
      Left 0PRS
      Right 0PRR
    Toe
      Left 0QRR
      Right 0QRQ
  Pharynx 0CRM
  Radius
    Left 0PRJ
    Right 0PRH
  Retinal Vessel
    Left 08RH3
    Right 08RG3
  Ribs
    1 to 2 0PR1
    3 or More 0PR2
  Sacrum 0QR1
  Scapula
    Left 0PR6
    Right 0PR5
  Sclera
    Left 08R7X
    Right 08R6X
  Septum
    Atrial 02R5
    Nasal 09RM
    Ventricular 02RM
  Skin
    Abdomen 0HR7
    Back 0HR6
    Buttock 0HR8
    Chest 0HR5

Replacement — continued
  Skin — continued
    Ear
      Left 0HR3
      Right 0HR2
    Face 0HR1
    Foot
      Left 0HRN
      Right 0HRM
    Hand
      Left 0HRG
      Right 0HRF
    Inguinal 0HRA
    Lower Arm
      Left 0HRE
      Right 0HRD
    Lower Leg
      Left 0HRL
      Right 0HRK
    Neck 0HR4
    Perineum 0HR9
    Scalp 0HR0
    Upper Arm
      Left 0HRC
      Right 0HRB
    Upper Leg
      Left 0HRJ
      Right 0HRH
  Skin Substitute, Porcine Liver
    Derived XHRPXL2
  Skull 0NR0
  Spinal Meninges 00RT
  Sternum 0PR0
  Subcutaneous Tissue and Fascia
    Abdomen 0JR8
    Back 0JR7
    Buttock 0JR9
    Chest 0JR6
    Face 0JR1
    Foot
      Left 0JRR
      Right 0JRQ
    Hand
      Left 0JRK
      Right 0JRJ
    Lower Arm
      Left 0JRH
      Right 0JRG
    Lower Leg
      Left 0JRP
      Right 0JRN
    Neck
      Left 0JR5
      Right 0JR4
    Pelvic Region 0JRC
    Perineum 0JRB
    Scalp 0JR0
    Upper Arm
      Left 0JRF
      Right 0JRD
    Upper Leg
      Left 0JRM
      Right 0JRL
  Tarsal
    Left 0QRM
    Right 0QRL
  Tendon
    Abdomen
      Left 0LRG
      Right 0LRF
    Ankle
      Left 0LRT
      Right 0LRS
    Foot
      Left 0LRW
      Right 0LRV
    Hand

Replacement — continued
  Tendon — continued
    Left 0LR8
    Right 0LR7
    Head and Neck 0LR0
    Hip
      Left 0LRK
      Right 0LRJ
    Knee
      Left 0LRR
      Right 0LRQ
    Lower Arm and Wrist
      Left 0LR6
      Right 0LR5
    Lower Leg
      Left 0LRP
      Right 0LRN
    Perineum 0LRH
    Shoulder
      Left 0LR2
      Right 0LR1
    Thorax
      Left 0LRD
      Right 0LRC
    Trunk
      Left 0LRB
      Right 0LR9
    Upper Arm
      Left 0LR4
      Right 0LR3
    Upper Leg
      Left 0LRM
      Right 0LRL
  Testis
    Bilateral 0VRC0JZ
    Left 0VRB0JZ
    Right 0VR90JZ
  Thumb
    Left 0XRM
    Right 0XRL
  Tibia
    Left 0QRH
    Right 0QRG
  Toe Nail 0HRRX
  Tongue 0CR7
  Tooth
    Lower 0CRX
    Upper 0CRW
  Trachea 0BR1
  Turbinate, Nasal 09RL
  Tympanic Membrane
    Left 09R8
    Right 09R7
  Ulna
    Left 0PRL
    Right 0PRK
  Ureter
    Left 0TR7
    Right 0TR6
  Urethra 0TRD
  Uvula 0CRN
  Valve
    Aortic 02RF
    Mitral 02RG
    Pulmonary 02RH
    Tricuspid 02RJ
  Vein
    Axillary
      Left 05R8
      Right 05R7
    Azygos 05R0
    Basilic
      Left 05RC
      Right 05RB
    Brachial
      Left 05RA
      Right 05R9

Replacement — *continued*
Vein — *continued*
Cephalic
Left 05RF
Right 05RD
Colic 06R7
Common Iliac
Left 06RD
Right 06RC
Esophageal 06R3
External Iliac
Left 06RG
Right 06RF
External Jugular
Left 05RQ
Right 05RP
Face
Left 05RV
Right 05RT
Femoral
Left 06RN
Right 06RM
Foot
Left 06RV
Right 06RT
Gastric 06R2
Hand
Left 05RH
Right 05RG
Hemiazygos 05R1
Hepatic 06R4
Hypogastric
Left 06RJ
Right 06RH
Inferior Mesenteric 06R6
Innominate
Left 05R4
Right 05R3
Internal Jugular
Left 05RN
Right 05RM
Intracranial 05RL
Lower 06RY
Portal 06R8
Pulmonary
Left 02RT
Right 02RS
Renal
Left 06RB
Right 06R9
Saphenous
Left 06RQ
Right 06RP
Splenic 06R1
Subclavian
Left 05R6
Right 05R5
Superior Mesenteric 06R5
Upper 05RY
Vertebral
Left 05RS
Right 05RR
Vena Cava
Inferior 06R0
Superior 02RV
Ventricle
Left 02RL
Right 02RK
Vertebra
Cervical 0PR3
Lumbar 0QR0
Thoracic 0PR4
Vitreous
Left 08R53
Right 08R43
Vocal Cord
Left 0CRV
Right 0CRT

Replacement — *continued*
Zooplastic Tissue, Rapid Deployment
Technique X2RF
Replacement, hip
Partial or total *see* Replacement, Lower
Joints 0SR
Resurfacing only *see* Supplement, Lower
Joints 0SU
Replantation
see Reposition
Replantation, scalp
see Reattachment, Skin, Scalp 0HM0
Reposition
Acetabulum
Left 0QS5
Right 0QS4
Ampulla of Vater 0FSC
Anus 0DSQ
Aorta
Abdominal 04S0
Thoracic
Ascending/Arch 02SX0ZZ
Descending 02SW0ZZ
Artery
Anterior Tibial
Left 04SQ
Right 04SP
Axillary
Left 03S6
Right 03S5
Brachial
Left 03S8
Right 03S7
Celiac 04S1
Colic
Left 04S7
Middle 04S8
Right 04S6
Common Carotid
Left 03SJ
Right 03SH
Common Iliac
Left 04SD
Right 04SC
Coronary
One Artery 02S00ZZ
Two Arteries 02S10ZZ
External Carotid
Left 03SN
Right 03SM
External Iliac
Left 04SJ
Right 04SH
Face 03SR
Femoral
Left 04SL
Right 04SK
Foot
Left 04SW
Right 04SV
Gastric 04S2
Hand
Left 03SF
Right 03SD
Hepatic 04S3
Inferior Mesenteric 04SB
Innominate 03S2
Internal Carotid
Left 03SL
Right 03SK
Internal Iliac
Left 04SF
Right 04SE
Internal Mammary
Left 03S1
Right 03S0
Intracranial 03SG

Reposition — *continued*
Artery — *continued*
Lower 04SY
Peroneal
Left 04SU
Right 04ST
Popliteal
Left 04SN
Right 04SM
Posterior Tibial
Left 04SS
Right 04SR
Pulmonary
Left 02SR0ZZ
Right 02SQ0ZZ
Pulmonary Trunk 02SP0ZZ
Radial
Left 03SC
Right 03SB
Renal
Left 04SA
Right 04S9
Splenic 04S4
Subclavian
Left 03S4
Right 03S3
Superior Mesenteric 04S5
Temporal
Left 03ST
Right 03SS
Thyroid
Left 03SV
Right 03SU
Ulnar
Left 03SA
Right 03S9
Upper 03SY
Vertebral
Left 03SQ
Right 03SP
Auditory Ossicle
Left 09SA
Right 09S9
Bladder 0TSB
Bladder Neck 0TSC
Bone
Ethmoid
Left 0NSG
Right 0NSF
Frontal 0NS1
Hyoid 0NSX
Lacrimal
Left 0NSJ
Right 0NSH
Nasal 0NSB
Occipital 0NS7
Palatine
Left 0NSL
Right 0NSK
Parietal
Left 0NS4
Right 0NS3
Pelvic
Left 0QS3
Right 0QS2
Sphenoid 0NSC
Temporal
Left 0NS6
Right 0NS5
Zygomatic
Left 0NSN
Right 0NSM
Breast
Bilateral 0HSV0ZZ
Left 0HSU0ZZ
Right 0HST0ZZ

Reposition — continued
Bronchus
Lingula 0BS90ZZ
Lower Lobe
Left 0BSB0ZZ
Right 0BS60ZZ
Main
Left 0BS70ZZ
Right 0BS30ZZ
Middle Lobe, Right 0BS50ZZ
Upper Lobe
Left 0BS80ZZ
Right 0BS40ZZ
Bursa and Ligament
Abdomen
Left 0MSJ
Right 0MSH
Ankle
Left 0MSR
Right 0MSQ
Elbow
Left 0MS4
Right 0MS3
Foot
Left 0MST
Right 0MSS
Hand
Left 0MS8
Right 0MS7
Head and Neck 0MS0
Hip
Left 0MSM
Right 0MSL
Knee
Left 0MSP
Right 0MSN
Lower Extremity
Left 0MSW
Right 0MSV
Perineum 0MSK
Rib(s) 0MSG
Shoulder
Left 0MS2
Right 0MS1
Spine
Lower 0MSD
Upper 0MSC
Sternum 0MSF
Upper Extremity
Left 0MSB
Right 0MS9
Wrist
Left 0MS6
Right 0MS5
Carina 0BS20ZZ
Carpal
Left 0PSN
Right 0PSM
Cecum 0DSH
Cervix 0USC
Clavicle
Left 0PSB
Right 0PS9
Coccyx 0QSS
Colon
Ascending 0DSK
Descending 0DSM
Sigmoid 0DSN
Transverse 0DSL
Cord
Bilateral 0VSH
Left 0VSG
Right 0VSF
Cul-de-sac 0USF
Diaphragm 0BST0ZZ
Duct
Common Bile 0FS9

Reposition — continued
Duct — continued
Cystic 0FS8
Hepatic
Common 0FS7
Left 0FS6
Right 0FS5
Lacrimal
Left 08SY
Right 08SX
Pancreatic 0FSD
Accessory 0FSF
Parotid
Left 0CSC
Right 0CSB
Duodenum 0DS9
Ear
Bilateral 09S2
Left 09S1
Right 09S0
Epiglottis 0CSR
Esophagus 0DS5
Eustachian Tube
Left 09SG
Right 09SF
Eyelid
Lower
Left 08SR
Right 08SQ
Upper
Left 08SP
Right 08SN
Fallopian Tube
Left 0US6
Right 0US5
Fallopian Tubes, Bilateral 0US7
Femoral Shaft
Left 0QS9
Right 0QS8
Femur
Lower
Left 0QSC
Right 0QSB
Upper
Left 0QS7
Right 0QS6
Fibula
Left 0QSK
Right 0QSJ
Gallbladder 0FS4
Gland
Adrenal
Left 0GS2
Right 0GS3
Lacrimal
Left 08SW
Right 08SV
Glenoid Cavity
Left 0PS8
Right 0PS7
Hair 0HSSXZZ
Humeral Head
Left 0PSD
Right 0PSC
Humeral Shaft
Left 0PSG
Right 0PSF
Ileum 0DSB
Intestine
Large 0DSE
Small 0DS8
Iris
Left 08SD3ZZ
Right 08SC3ZZ
Jejunum 0DSA
Joint
Acromioclavicular

Reposition — continued
Joint — continued
Left 0RSH
Right 0RSG
Ankle
Left 0SSG
Right 0SSF
Carpal
Left 0RSR
Right 0RSQ
Carpometacarpal
Left 0RST
Right 0RSS
Cervical Vertebral 0RS1
Cervicothoracic Vertebral 0RS4
Coccygeal 0SS6
Elbow
Left 0RSM
Right 0RSL
Finger Phalangeal
Left 0RSX
Right 0RSW
Hip
Left 0SSB
Right 0SS9
Knee
Left 0SSD
Right 0SSC
Lumbar Vertebral 0SS0
Lumbosacral 0SS3
Metacarpophalangeal
Left 0RSV
Right 0RSU
Metatarsal-Phalangeal
Left 0SSN
Right 0SSM
Occipital-cervical 0RS0
Sacrococcygeal 0SS5
Sacroiliac
Left 0SS8
Right 0SS7
Shoulder
Left 0RSK
Right 0RSJ
Sternoclavicular
Left 0RSF
Right 0RSE
Tarsal
Left 0SSJ
Right 0SSH
Tarsometatarsal
Left 0SSL
Right 0SSK
Temporomandibular
Left 0RSD
Right 0RSC
Thoracic Vertebral 0RS6
Thoracolumbar Vertebral 0RSA
Toe Phalangeal
Left 0SSQ
Right 0SSP
Wrist
Left 0RSP
Right 0RSN
Kidney
Left 0TS1
Right 0TS0
Kidney Pelvis
Left 0TS4
Right 0TS3
Kidneys, Bilateral 0TS2
Lens
Left 08SK3ZZ
Right 08SJ3ZZ
Lip
Lower 0CS1
Upper 0CS0

Reposition — *continued*
Liver 0FS0
Lung
  Left 0BSL0ZZ
  Lower Lobe
    Left 0BSJ0ZZ
    Right 0BSF0ZZ
  Middle Lobe, Right 0BSD0ZZ
  Right 0BSK0ZZ
  Upper Lobe
    Left 0BSG0ZZ
    Right 0BSC0ZZ
Lung Lingula 0BSH0ZZ
Mandible
  Left 0NSV
  Right 0NST
Maxilla 0NSR
Metacarpal
  Left 0PSQ
  Right 0PSP
Metatarsal
  Left 0QSP
  Right 0QSN
Muscle
  Abdomen
    Left 0KSL
    Right 0KSK
  Extraocular
    Left 08SM
    Right 08SL
  Facial 0KS1
  Foot
    Left 0KSW
    Right 0KSV
  Hand
    Left 0KSD
    Right 0KSC
  Head 0KS0
  Hip
    Left 0KSP
    Right 0KSN
  Lower Arm and Wrist
    Left 0KSB
    Right 0KS9
  Lower Leg
    Left 0KST
    Right 0KSS
  Neck
    Left 0KS3
    Right 0KS2
  Perineum 0KSM
  Shoulder
    Left 0KS6
    Right 0KS5
  Thorax
    Left 0KSJ
    Right 0KSH
  Tongue, Palate, Pharynx 0KS4
  Trunk
    Left 0KSG
    Right 0KSF
  Upper Arm
    Left 0KS8
    Right 0KS7
  Upper Leg
    Left 0KSR
    Right 0KSQ
Nasal Mucosa and Soft Tissue 09SK
Nerve
  Abducens 00SL
  Accessory 00SR
  Acoustic 00SN
  Brachial Plexus 01S3
  Cervical 01S1
  Cervical Plexus 01S0
  Facial 00SM
  Femoral 01SD

Reposition — *continued*
Nerve — *continued*
  Glossopharyngeal 00SP
  Hypoglossal 00SS
  Lumbar 01SB
  Lumbar Plexus 01S9
  Lumbosacral Plexus 01SA
  Median 01S5
  Oculomotor 00SH
  Olfactory 00SF
  Optic 00SG
  Peroneal 01SH
  Phrenic 01S2
  Pudendal 01SC
  Radial 01S6
  Sacral 01SR
  Sacral Plexus 01SQ
  Sciatic 01SF
  Thoracic 01S8
  Tibial 01SG
  Trigeminal 00SK
  Trochlear 00SJ
  Ulnar 01S4
  Vagus 00SQ
Nipple
  Left 0HSXXZZ
  Right 0HSWXZZ
Orbit
  Left 0NSQ
  Right 0NSP
Ovary
  Bilateral 0US2
  Left 0US1
  Right 0US0
Palate
  Hard 0CS2
  Soft 0CS3
Pancreas 0FSG
Parathyroid Gland 0GSR
  Inferior
    Left 0GSP
    Right 0GSN
  Multiple 0GSQ
  Superior
    Left 0GSM
    Right 0GSL
Patella
  Left 0QSF
  Right 0QSD
Phalanx
  Finger
    Left 0PSV
    Right 0PST
  Thumb
    Left 0PSS
    Right 0PSR
  Toe
    Left 0QSR
    Right 0QSQ
Products of Conception 10S0
  Ectopic 10S2
Radius
  Left 0PSJ
  Right 0PSH
Rectum 0DSP
Retinal Vessel
  Left 08SH3ZZ
  Right 08SG3ZZ
Ribs
  1 to 2 0PS1
  3 or More 0PS2
Sacrum 0QS1
Scapula
  Left 0PS6
  Right 0PS5
Septum, Nasal 09SM

Reposition — *continued*
Sesamoid Bone(s) 1st Toe
  see Reposition, Metatarsal, Right 0QSN
  see Reposition, Metatarsal, Left 0QSP
Skull 0NS0
Spinal Cord
  Cervical 00SW
  Lumbar 00SY
  Thoracic 00SX
Spleen 07SP0ZZ
Sternum 0PS0
Stomach 0DS6
Tarsal
  Left 0QSM
  Right 0QSL
Tendon
  Abdomen
    Left 0LSG
    Right 0LSF
  Ankle
    Left 0LST
    Right 0LSS
  Foot
    Left 0LSW
    Right 0LSV
  Hand
    Left 0LS8
    Right 0LS7
  Head and Neck 0LS0
  Hip
    Left 0LSK
    Right 0LSJ
  Knee
    Left 0LSR
    Right 0LSQ
  Lower Arm and Wrist
    Left 0LS6
    Right 0LS5
  Lower Leg
    Left 0LSP
    Right 0LSN
  Perineum 0LSH
  Shoulder
    Left 0LS2
    Right 0LS1
  Thorax
    Left 0LSD
    Right 0LSC
  Trunk
    Left 0LSB
    Right 0LS9
  Upper Arm
    Left 0LS4
    Right 0LS3
  Upper Leg
    Left 0LSM
    Right 0LSL
Testis
  Bilateral 0VSC
  Left 0VSB
  Right 0VS9
Thymus 07SM0ZZ
Thyroid Gland
  Left Lobe 0GSG
  Right Lobe 0GSH
Tibia
  Left 0QSH
  Right 0QSG
Tongue 0CS7
Tooth
  Lower 0CSX
  Upper 0CSW
Trachea 0BS10ZZ
Turbinate, Nasal 09SL
Tympanic Membrane
  Left 09S8
  Right 09S7

Reposition — *continued*
- Ulna
  - Left 0PSL
  - Right 0PSK
- Ureter
  - Left 0TS7
  - Right 0TS6
- Ureters, Bilateral 0TS8
- Urethra 0TSD
- Uterine Supporting Structure 0US4
- Uterus 0US9
- Uvula 0CSN
- Vagina 0USG
- Vein
  - Axillary
    - Left 05S8
    - Right 05S7
  - Azygos 05S0
  - Basilic
    - Left 05SC
    - Right 05SB
  - Brachial
    - Left 05SA
    - Right 05S9
  - Cephalic
    - Left 05SF
    - Right 05SD
  - Colic 06S7
  - Common Iliac
    - Left 06SD
    - Right 06SC
  - Esophageal 06S3
  - External Iliac
    - Left 06SG
    - Right 06SF
  - External Jugular
    - Left 05SQ
    - Right 05SP
  - Face
    - Left 05SV
    - Right 05ST
  - Femoral
    - Left 06SN
    - Right 06SM
  - Foot
    - Left 06SV
    - Right 06ST
  - Gastric 06S2
  - Hand
    - Left 05SH
    - Right 05SG
  - Hemiazygos 05S1
  - Hepatic 06S4
  - Hypogastric
    - Left 06SJ
    - Right 06SH
  - Inferior Mesenteric 06S6
  - Innominate
    - Left 05S4
    - Right 05S3
  - Internal Jugular
    - Left 05SN
    - Right 05SM
  - Intracranial 05SL
  - Lower 06SY
  - Portal 06S8
  - Pulmonary
    - Left 02ST0ZZ
    - Right 02SS0ZZ
  - Renal
    - Left 06SB
    - Right 06S9
  - Saphenous
    - Left 06SQ
    - Right 06SP
  - Splenic 06S1
  - Subclavian

Reposition — *continued*
- Vein — *continued*
  - Left 05S6
  - Right 05S5
  - Superior Mesenteric 06S5
  - Upper 05SY
  - Vertebral
    - Left 05SS
    - Right 05SR
- Vena Cava
  - Inferior 06S0
  - Superior 02SV0ZZ
- Vertebra
  - Cervical 0PS3
    - Magnetically Controlled Growth Rod(s) XNS3
  - Lumbar 0QS0
    - Magnetically Controlled Growth Rod(s) XNS0
  - Thoracic 0PS4
    - Magnetically Controlled Growth Rod(s) XNS4
- Vocal Cord
  - Left 0CSV
  - Right 0CST

Resection
- Acetabulum
  - Left 0QT50ZZ
  - Right 0QT40ZZ
- Adenoids 0CTQ
- Ampulla of Vater 0FTC
- Anal Sphincter 0DTR
- Anus 0DTQ
- Aortic Body 0GTD
- Appendix 0DTJ
- Auditory Ossicle
  - Left 09TA
  - Right 09T9
- Bladder 0TTB
- Bladder Neck 0TTC
- Bone
  - Ethmoid
    - Left 0NTG0ZZ
    - Right 0NTF0ZZ
  - Frontal 0NT10ZZ
  - Hyoid 0NTX0ZZ
  - Lacrimal
    - Left 0NTJ0ZZ
    - Right 0NTH0ZZ
  - Nasal 0NTB0ZZ
  - Occipital 0NT70ZZ
  - Palatine
    - Left 0NTL0ZZ
    - Right 0NTK0ZZ
  - Parietal
    - Left 0NT40ZZ
    - Right 0NT30ZZ
  - Pelvic
    - Left 0QT30ZZ
    - Right 0QT20ZZ
  - Sphenoid 0NTC0ZZ
  - Temporal
    - Left 0NT60ZZ
    - Right 0NT50ZZ
  - Zygomatic
    - Left 0NTN0ZZ
    - Right 0NTM0ZZ
- Breast
  - Bilateral 0HTV0ZZ
  - Left 0HTU0ZZ
  - Right 0HTT0ZZ
  - Supernumerary 0HTY0ZZ
- Bronchus
  - Lingula 0BT9
  - Lower Lobe
    - Left 0BTB
    - Right 0BT6

Resection — *continued*
- Bronchus — *continued*
  - Main
    - Left 0BT7
    - Right 0BT3
  - Middle Lobe, Right 0BT5
  - Upper Lobe
    - Left 0BT8
    - Right 0BT4
- Bursa and Ligament
  - Abdomen
    - Left 0MTJ
    - Right 0MTH
  - Ankle
    - Left 0MTR
    - Right 0MTQ
  - Elbow
    - Left 0MT4
    - Right 0MT3
  - Foot
    - Left 0MTT
    - Right 0MTS
  - Hand
    - Left 0MT8
    - Right 0MT7
  - Head and Neck 0MT0
  - Hip
    - Left 0MTM
    - Right 0MTL
  - Knee
    - Left 0MTP
    - Right 0MTN
  - Lower Extremity
    - Left 0MTW
    - Right 0MTV
  - Perineum 0MTK
  - Rib(s) 0MTG
  - Shoulder
    - Left 0MT2
    - Right 0MT1
  - Spine
    - Lower 0MTD
    - Upper 0MTC
  - Sternum 0MTF
  - Upper Extremity
    - Left 0MTB
    - Right 0MT9
  - Wrist
    - Left 0MT6
    - Right 0MT5
- Carina 0BT2
- Carotid Bodies, Bilateral 0GT8
- Carotid Body
  - Left 0GT6
  - Right 0GT7
- Carpal
  - Left 0PTN0ZZ
  - Right 0PTM0ZZ
- Cecum 0DTH
- Cerebral Hemisphere 00T7
- Cervix 0UTC
- Chordae Tendineae 02T9
- Cisterna Chyli 07TL
- Clavicle
  - Left 0PTB0ZZ
  - Right 0PT90ZZ
- Clitoris 0UTJ
- Coccygeal Glomus 0GTB
- Coccyx 0QTS0ZZ
- Colon
  - Ascending 0DTK
  - Descending 0DTM
  - Sigmoid 0DTN
  - Transverse 0DTL
- Conduction Mechanism 02T8
- Cord
  - Bilateral 0VTH

Resection — *continued*
Cord — *continued*
  Left 0VTG
  Right 0VTF
Cornea
  Left 08T9XZZ
  Right 08T8XZZ
Cul-de-sac 0UTF
Diaphragm 0BTT
Disc
  Cervical Vertebral 0RT30ZZ
  Cervicothoracic Vertebral 0RT50ZZ
  Lumbar Vertebral 0ST20ZZ
  Lumbosacral 0ST40ZZ
  Thoracic Vertebral 0RT90ZZ
  Thoracolumbar Vertebral 0RTB0ZZ
Duct
  Common Bile 0FT9
  Cystic 0FT8
  Hepatic
    Common 0FT7
    Left 0FT6
    Right 0FT5
  Lacrimal
    Left 08TY
    Right 08TX
  Pancreatic 0FTD
    Accessory 0FTF
  Parotid
    Left 0CTC0ZZ
    Right 0CTB0ZZ
Duodenum 0DT9
Ear
  External
    Left 09T1
    Right 09T0
  Inner
    Left 09TE
    Right 09TD
  Middle
    Left 09T6
    Right 09T5
Epididymis
  Bilateral 0VTL
  Left 0VTK
  Right 0VTJ
Epiglottis 0CTR
Esophagogastric Junction 0DT4
Esophagus 0DT5
  Lower 0DT3
  Middle 0DT2
  Upper 0DT1
Eustachian Tube
  Left 09TG
  Right 09TF
Eye
  Left 08T1XZZ
  Right 08T0XZZ
Eyelid
  Lower
    Left 08TR
    Right 08TQ
  Upper
    Left 08TP
    Right 08TN
Fallopian Tube
  Left 0UT6
  Right 0UT5
Fallopian Tubes, Bilateral 0UT7
Femoral Shaft
  Left 0QT90ZZ
  Right 0QT80ZZ
Femur
  Lower
    Left 0QTC0ZZ
    Right 0QTB0ZZ
  Upper

Resection — *continued*
Femur — *continued*
    Left 0QT70ZZ
    Right 0QT60ZZ
Fibula
  Left 0QTK0ZZ
  Right 0QTJ0ZZ
Finger Nail 0HTQXZZ
Gallbladder 0FT4
Gland
  Adrenal
    Bilateral 0GT4
    Left 0GT2
    Right 0GT3
  Lacrimal
    Left 08TW
    Right 08TV
  Minor Salivary 0CTJ0ZZ
  Parotid
    Left 0CT90ZZ
    Right 0CT80ZZ
  Pituitary 0GT0
  Sublingual
    Left 0CTF0ZZ
    Right 0CTD0ZZ
  Submaxillary
    Left 0CTH0ZZ
    Right 0CTG0ZZ
  Vestibular 0UTL
Glenoid Cavity
  Left 0PT80ZZ
  Right 0PT70ZZ
Glomus Jugulare 0GTC
Humeral Head
  Left 0PTD0ZZ
  Right 0PTC0ZZ
Humeral Shaft
  Left 0PTG0ZZ
  Right 0PTF0ZZ
Hymen 0UTK
Ileocecal Valve 0DTC
Ileum 0DTB
Intestine
  Large 0DTE
    Left 0DTG
    Right 0DTF
  Small 0DT8
Iris
  Left 08TD3ZZ
  Right 08TC3ZZ
Jejunum 0DTA
Joint
  Acromioclavicular
    Left 0RTH0ZZ
    Right 0RTG0ZZ
  Ankle
    Left 0STG0ZZ
    Right 0STF0ZZ
  Carpal
    Left 0RTR0ZZ
    Right 0RTQ0ZZ
  Carpometacarpal
    Left 0RTT0ZZ
    Right 0RTS0ZZ
  Cervicothoracic Vertebral 0RT40ZZ
  Coccygeal 0ST60ZZ
  Elbow
    Left 0RTM0ZZ
    Right 0RTL0ZZ
  Finger Phalangeal
    Left 0RTX0ZZ
    Right 0RTW0ZZ
  Hip
    Left 0STB0ZZ
    Right 0ST90ZZ
  Knee
    Left 0STD0ZZ

Resection — *continued*
Joint — *continued*
    Right 0STC0ZZ
  Metacarpophalangeal
    Left 0RTV0ZZ
    Right 0RTU0ZZ
  Metatarsal-Phalangeal
    Left 0STN0ZZ
    Right 0STM0ZZ
  Sacrococcygeal 0ST50ZZ
  Sacroiliac
    Left 0ST80ZZ
    Right 0ST70ZZ
  Shoulder
    Left 0RTK0ZZ
    Right 0RTJ0ZZ
  Sternoclavicular
    Left 0RTF0ZZ
    Right 0RTE0ZZ
  Tarsal
    Left 0STJ0ZZ
    Right 0STH0ZZ
  Tarsometatarsal
    Left 0STL0ZZ
    Right 0STK0ZZ
  Temporomandibular
    Left 0RTD0ZZ
    Right 0RTC0ZZ
  Toe Phalangeal
    Left 0STQ0ZZ
    Right 0STP0ZZ
  Wrist
    Left 0RTP0ZZ
    Right 0RTN0ZZ
Kidney
  Left 0TT1
  Right 0TT0
Kidney Pelvis
  Left 0TT4
  Right 0TT3
Kidneys, Bilateral 0TT2
Larynx 0CTS
Lens
  Left 08TK3ZZ
  Right 08TJ3ZZ
Lip
  Lower 0CT1
  Upper 0CT0
Liver 0FT0
  Left Lobe 0FT2
  Right Lobe 0FT1
Lung
  Bilateral 0BTM
  Left 0BTL
  Lower Lobe
    Left 0BTJ
    Right 0BTF
  Middle Lobe, Right 0BTD
  Right 0BTK
  Upper Lobe
    Left 0BTG
    Right 0BTC
Lung Lingula 0BTH
Lymphatic
  Aortic 07TD
  Axillary
    Left 07T6
    Right 07T5
  Head 07T0
  Inguinal
    Left 07TJ
    Right 07TH
  Internal Mammary
    Left 07T9
    Right 07T8
  Lower Extremity
    Left 07TG

Resection — continued
Lymphatic — continued
Right 07TF
Mesenteric 07TB
Neck
Left 07T2
Right 07T1
Pelvis 07TC
Thoracic Duct 07TK
Thorax 07T7
Upper Extremity
Left 07T4
Right 07T3
Mandible
Left 0NTV0ZZ
Right 0NTT0ZZ
Maxilla 0NTR0ZZ
Metacarpal
Left 0PTQ0ZZ
Right 0PTP0ZZ
Metatarsal
Left 0QTP0ZZ
Right 0QTN0ZZ
Muscle
Abdomen
Left 0KTL
Right 0KTK
Extraocular
Left 08TM
Right 08TL
Facial 0KT1
Foot
Left 0KTW
Right 0KTV
Hand
Left 0KTD
Right 0KTC
Head 0KT0
Hip
Left 0KTP
Right 0KTN
Lower Arm and Wrist
Left 0KTB
Right 0KT9
Lower Leg
Left 0KTT
Right 0KTS
Neck
Left 0KT3
Right 0KT2
Papillary 02TD
Perineum 0KTM
Shoulder
Left 0KT6
Right 0KT5
Thorax
Left 0KTJ
Right 0KTH
Tongue, Palate, Pharynx 0KT4
Trunk
Left 0KTG
Right 0KTF
Upper Arm
Left 0KT8
Right 0KT7
Upper Leg
Left 0KTR
Right 0KTQ
Nasal Mucosa and Soft Tissue 09TK
Nasopharynx 09TN
Nipple
Left 0HTXXZZ
Right 0HTWXZZ
Omentum 0DTU
Orbit
Left 0NTQ0ZZ
Right 0NTP0ZZ

Resection — continued
Ovary
Bilateral 0UT2
Left 0UT1
Right 0UT0
Palate
Hard 0CT2
Soft 0CT3
Pancreas 0FTG
Para-aortic Body 0GT9
Paraganglion Extremity 0GTF
Parathyroid Gland 0GTR
Inferior
Left 0GTP
Right 0GTN
Multiple 0GTQ
Superior
Left 0GTM
Right 0GTL
Patella
Left 0QTF0ZZ
Right 0QTD0ZZ
Penis 0VTS
Pericardium 02TN
Phalanx
Finger
Left 0PTV0ZZ
Right 0PTT0ZZ
Thumb
Left 0PTS0ZZ
Right 0PTR0ZZ
Toe
Left 0QTR0ZZ
Right 0QTQ0ZZ
Pharynx 0CTM
Pineal Body 0GT1
Prepuce 0VTT
Products of Conception, Ectopic 10T2
Prostate 0VT0
Radius
Left 0PTJ0ZZ
Right 0PTH0ZZ
Rectum 0DTP
Ribs
1 to 2 0PT10ZZ
3 or More 0PT20ZZ
Scapula
Left 0PT60ZZ
Right 0PT50ZZ
Scrotum 0VT5
Septum
Atrial 02T5
Nasal 09TM
Ventricular 02TM
Sinus
Accessory 09TP
Ethmoid
Left 09TV
Right 09TU
Frontal
Left 09TT
Right 09TS
Mastoid
Left 09TC
Right 09TB
Maxillary
Left 09TR
Right 09TQ
Sphenoid
Left 09TX
Right 09TW
Spleen 07TP
Sternum 0PT00ZZ
Stomach 0DT6
Pylorus 0DT7
Tarsal
Left 0QTM0ZZ
Right 0QTL0ZZ

Resection — continued
Tendon
Abdomen
Left 0LTG
Right 0LTF
Ankle
Left 0LTT
Right 0LTS
Foot
Left 0LTW
Right 0LTV
Hand
Left 0LT8
Right 0LT7
Head and Neck 0LT0
Hip
Left 0LTK
Right 0LTJ
Knee
Left 0LTR
Right 0LTQ
Lower Arm and Wrist
Left 0LT6
Right 0LT5
Lower Leg
Left 0LTP
Right 0LTN
Perineum 0LTH
Shoulder
Left 0LT2
Right 0LT1
Thorax
Left 0LTD
Right 0LTC
Trunk
Left 0LTB
Right 0LT9
Upper Arm
Left 0LT4
Right 0LT3
Upper Leg
Left 0LTM
Right 0LTL
Testis
Bilateral 0VTC
Left 0VTB
Right 0VT9
Thymus 07TM
Thyroid Gland 0GTK
Left Lobe 0GTG
Right Lobe 0GTH
Thyroid Gland Isthmus 0GTJ
Tibia
Left 0QTH0ZZ
Right 0QTG0ZZ
Toe Nail 0HTRXZZ
Tongue 0CT7
Tonsils 0CTP
Tooth
Lower 0CTX0Z
Upper 0CTW0Z
Trachea 0BT1
Tunica Vaginalis
Left 0VT7
Right 0VT6
Turbinate, Nasal 09TL
Tympanic Membrane
Left 09T8
Right 09T7
Ulna
Left 0PTL0ZZ
Right 0PTK0ZZ
Ureter
Left 0TT7
Right 0TT6
Urethra 0TTD
Uterine Supporting Structure 0UT4

Resection — *continued*
Uterus 0UT9
Uvula 0CTN
Vagina 0UTG
Valve, Pulmonary 02TH
Vas Deferens
  Bilateral 0VTQ
  Left 0VTP
  Right 0VTN
Vesicle
  Bilateral 0VT3
  Left 0VT2
  Right 0VT1
Vitreous
  Left 08T53ZZ
  Right 08T43ZZ
Vocal Cord
  Left 0CTV
  Right 0CTT
Vulva 0UTM

Resection, Left ventricular outflow tract obstruction (LVOT)
see Dilation, Ventricle, Left 027L

Resection, Subaortic membrane (Left ventricular outflow tract obstruction)
see Dilation, Ventricle, Left 027L

Restoration, Cardiac, Single, Rhythm
5A2204Z

RestoreAdvanced® neurostimulator (SureScan®)(MRI Safe)
use Stimulator Generator, Multiple Array Rechargeable in 0JH

RestoreSensor® neurostimulator (SureScan®)(MRI Safe)
use Stimulator Generator, Multiple Array Rechargeable in 0JH

RestoreUltra® neurostimulator (SureScan®) (MRI Safe)
use Stimulator Generator, Multiple Array Rechargeable in 0JH

Restriction
Ampulla of Vater 0FVC
Anus 0DVQ
Aorta
  Abdominal 04V0
    Intraluminal Device, Branched or Fenestrated 04V0
  Thoracic
    Ascending/Arch, Intraluminal Device, Branched or Fenestrated 02VX
    Descending, Intraluminal Device, Branched or Fenestrated 02VW
Artery
  Anterior Tibial
    Left 04VQ
    Right 04VP
  Axillary
    Left 03V6
    Right 03V5
  Brachial
    Left 03V8
    Right 03V7
  Celiac 04V1
  Colic
    Left 04V7
    Middle 04V8
    Right 04V6
  Common Carotid
    Left 03VJ
    Right 03VH
  Common Iliac
    Left 04VD
    Right 04VC
  External Carotid
    Left 03VN
    Right 03VM
  External Iliac

Restriction — *continued*
Artery — *continued*
    Left 04VJ
    Right 04VH
  Face 03VR
  Femoral
    Left 04VL
    Right 04VK
  Foot
    Left 04VW
    Right 04VV
  Gastric 04V2
  Hand
    Left 03VF
    Right 03VD
  Hepatic 04V3
  Inferior Mesenteric 04VB
  Innominate 03V2
  Internal Carotid
    Left 03VL
    Right 03VK
  Internal Iliac
    Left 04VF
    Right 04VE
  Internal Mammary
    Left 03V1
    Right 03V0
  Intracranial 03VG
  Lower 04VY
  Peroneal
    Left 04VU
    Right 04VT
  Popliteal
    Left 04VN
    Right 04VM
  Posterior Tibial
    Left 04VS
    Right 04VR
  Pulmonary
    Left 02VR
    Right 02VQ
  Pulmonary Trunk 02VP
  Radial
    Left 03VC
    Right 03VB
  Renal
    Left 04VA
    Right 04V9
  Splenic 04V4
  Subclavian
    Left 03V4
    Right 03V3
  Superior Mesenteric 04V5
  Temporal
    Left 03VT
    Right 03VS
  Thyroid
    Left 03VV
    Right 03VU
  Ulnar
    Left 03VA
    Right 03V9
  Upper 03VY
  Vertebral
    Left 03VQ
    Right 03VP
Bladder 0TVB
Bladder Neck 0TVC
Bronchus
  Lingula 0BV9
  Lower Lobe
    Left 0BVB
    Right 0BV6
  Main
    Left 0BV7
    Right 0BV3
  Middle Lobe, Right 0BV5

Restriction — *continued*
Bronchus — *continued*
  Upper Lobe
    Left 0BV8
    Right 0BV4
Carina 0BV2
Cecum 0DVH
Cervix 0UVC
Cisterna Chyli 07VL
Colon
  Ascending 0DVK
  Descending 0DVM
  Sigmoid 0DVN
  Transverse 0DVL
Duct
  Common Bile 0FV9
  Cystic 0FV8
  Hepatic
    Common 0FV7
    Left 0FV6
    Right 0FV5
  Lacrimal
    Left 08VY
    Right 08VX
  Pancreatic 0FVD
    Accessory 0FVF
  Parotid
    Left 0CVC
    Right 0CVB
Duodenum 0DV9
Esophagogastric Junction 0DV4
Esophagus 0DV5
  Lower 0DV3
  Middle 0DV2
  Upper 0DV1
Heart 02VA
Ileocecal Valve 0DVC
Ileum 0DVB
Intestine
  Large 0DVE
    Left 0DVG
    Right 0DVF
  Small 0DV8
Jejunum 0DVA
Kidney Pelvis
  Left 0TV4
  Right 0TV3
Lymphatic
  Aortic 07VD
  Axillary
    Left 07V6
    Right 07V5
  Head 07V0
  Inguinal
    Left 07VJ
    Right 07VH
  Internal Mammary
    Left 07V9
    Right 07V8
  Lower Extremity
    Left 07VG
    Right 07VF
  Mesenteric 07VB
  Neck
    Left 07V2
    Right 07V1
  Pelvis 07VC
  Thoracic Duct 07VK
  Thorax 07V7
  Upper Extremity
    Left 07V4
    Right 07V3
Rectum 0DVP
Stomach 0DV6
  Pylorus 0DV7
Trachea 0BV1

Restriction — *continued*
Ureter
Left 0TV7
Right 0TV6
Urethra 0TVD
Valve, Mitral 02VG
Vein
Axillary
Left 05V8
Right 05V7
Azygos 05V0
Basilic
Left 05VC
Right 05VB
Brachial
Left 05VA
Right 05V9
Cephalic
Left 05VF
Right 05VD
Colic 06V7
Common Iliac
Left 06VD
Right 06VC
Esophageal 06V3
External Iliac
Left 06VG
Right 06VF
External Jugular
Left 05VQ
Right 05VP
Face
Left 05VV
Right 05VT
Femoral
Left 06VN
Right 06VM
Foot
Left 06VV
Right 06VT
Gastric 06V2
Hand
Left 05VH
Right 05VG
Hemiazygos 05V1
Hepatic 06V4
Hypogastric
Left 06VJ
Right 06VH
Inferior Mesenteric 06V6
Innominate
Left 05V4
Right 05V3
Internal Jugular
Left 05VN
Right 05VM
Intracranial 05VL
Lower 06VY
Portal 06V8
Pulmonary
Left 02VT
Right 02VS
Renal
Left 06VB
Right 06V9
Saphenous
Left 06VQ
Right 06VP
Splenic 06V1
Subclavian
Left 05V6
Right 05V5
Superior Mesenteric 06V5
Upper 05VY
Vertebral
Left 05VS
Right 05VR

Restriction — *continued*
Vena Cava
Inferior 06V0
Superior 02VV
Resurfacing Device
Removal of device from
Left 0SPB0BZ
Right 0SP90BZ
Revision of device in
Left 0SWB0BZ
Right 0SW90BZ
Supplement
Left 0SUB0BZ
Acetabular Surface 0SUE0BZ
Femoral Surface 0SUS0BZ
Right 0SU90BZ
Acetabular Surface 0SUA0BZ
Femoral Surface 0SUR0BZ
Resuscitation
Cardiopulmonary *see* Assistance,
Cardiac 5A02
Cardioversion 5A2204Z
Defibrillation 5A2204Z
Endotracheal intubation *see* Insertion of
device in, Trachea 0BH1
External chest compression 5A12012
Pulmonary 5A19054
**Resuscitative endovascular balloon
occlusion of the aorta (REBOA)**
02LW3DJ
04L03DJ
Resuture, Heart valve prosthesis
see Revision of device in, Heart and Great
Vessels 02W
Retained placenta, manual removal
see Extraction, Products of Conception,
Retained 10D1
Retraining
Cardiac *see* Motor Treatment,
Rehabilitation F07
Vocational *see* Activities of Daily Living
Treatment, Rehabilitation F08
Retrogasserian rhizotomy
see Division, Nerve, Trigeminal 008K
Retroperitoneal lymph node
use Lymphatic, Aortic
Retroperitoneal space
use Retroperitoneum
Retropharyngeal lymph node
use Lymphatic, Right Neck
use Lymphatic, Left Neck
Retropubic space
use Pelvic Cavity
Reveal® (DX)(XT)
use Monitoring Device
Reverse® total shoulder replacement
see Replacement, Upper Joints 0RR
Reverse® Shoulder Prosthesis
use Synthetic Substitute, Reverse Ball and
Socket in 0RR
Revision
Correcting a portion of existing device *see*
Revision of device in
Removal of device without replacement
see Removal of device from
Replacement of existing device
see Removal of device from
see Root operation to place new
device, e.g., Insertion, Replacement,
Supplement
Revision of device in
Abdominal Wall 0WWF
Acetabulum
Left 0QW5
Right 0QW4
Anal Sphincter 0DWR
Anus 0DWQ

Revision of device in — *continued*
Artery
Lower 04WY
Upper 03WY
Auditory Ossicle
Left 09WA
Right 09W9
Back
Lower 0WWL
Upper 0WWK
Bladder 0TWB
Bone
Facial 0NWW
Lower 0QWY
Nasal 0NWB
Pelvic
Left 0QW3
Right 0QW2
Upper 0PWY
Bone Marrow 07WT
Brain 00W0
Breast
Left 0HWU
Right 0HWT
Bursa and Ligament
Lower 0MWY
Upper 0MWX
Carpal
Left 0PWN
Right 0PWM
Cavity, Cranial 0WW1
Cerebral Ventricle 00W6
Chest Wall 0WW8
Cisterna Chyli 07WL
Clavicle
Left 0PWB
Right 0PW9
Coccyx 0QWS
Diaphragm 0BWT
Disc
Cervical Vertebral 0RW3
Cervicothoracic Vertebral 0RW5
Lumbar Vertebral 0SW2
Lumbosacral 0SW4
Thoracic Vertebral 0RW9
Thoracolumbar Vertebral 0RWB
Duct
Hepatobiliary 0FWB
Pancreatic 0FWD
Ear
Inner
Left 09WE
Right 09WD
Left 09WJ
Right 09WH
Epididymis and Spermatic Cord 0VWM
Esophagus 0DW5
Extremity
Lower
Left 0YWB
Right 0YW9
Upper
Left 0XW7
Right 0XW6
Eye
Left 08W1
Right 08W0
Face 0WW2
Fallopian Tube 0UW8
Femoral Shaft
Left 0QW9
Right 0QW8
Femur
Lower
Left 0QWC
Right 0QWB
Upper

Revision of device in — *continued*
  Femur — *continued*
    Left 0QW7
    Right 0QW6
  Fibula
    Left 0QWK
    Right 0QWJ
  Finger Nail 0HWQX
  Gallbladder 0FW4
  Gastrointestinal Tract 0WWP
  Genitourinary Tract 0WWR
  Gland
    Adrenal 0GW5
    Endocrine 0GWS
    Pituitary 0GW0
    Salivary 0CWA
  Glenoid Cavity
    Left 0PW8
    Right 0PW7
  Great Vessel 02WY
  Hair 0HWSX
  Head 0WW0
  Heart 02WA
  Humeral Head
    Left 0PWD
    Right 0PWC
  Humeral Shaft
    Left 0PWG
    Right 0PWF
  Intestinal Tract
    Lower 0DWD
    Upper 0DW0
  Intestine
    Large 0DWE
    Small 0DW8
  Jaw
    Lower 0WW5
    Upper 0WW4
  Joint
    Acromioclavicular
      Left 0RWH
      Right 0RWG
    Ankle
      Left 0SWG
      Right 0SWF
    Carpal
      Left 0RWR
      Right 0RWQ
    Carpometacarpal
      Left 0RWT
      Right 0RWS
    Cervical Vertebral 0RW1
    Cervicothoracic Vertebral 0RW4
    Coccygeal 0SW6
    Elbow
      Left 0RWM
      Right 0RWL
    Finger Phalangeal
      Left 0RWX
      Right 0RWW
    Hip
      Left 0SWB
        Acetabular Surface 0SWE
        Femoral Surface 0SWS
      Right 0SW9
        Acetabular Surface 0SWA
        Femoral Surface 0SWR
    Knee
      Left 0SWD
        Femoral Surface 0SWU
        Tibial Surface 0SWW
      Right 0SWC
        Femoral Surface 0SWT
        Tibial Surface 0SWV
    Lumbar Vertebral 0SW0
    Lumbosacral 0SW3
    Metacarpophalangeal

Revision of device in — *continued*
  Joint — *continued*
    Left 0RWV
    Right 0RWU
    Metatarsal-Phalangeal
      Left 0SWN
      Right 0SWM
    Occipital-cervical 0RW0
    Sacrococcygeal 0SW5
    Sacroiliac
      Left 0SW8
      Right 0SW7
    Shoulder
      Left 0RWK
      Right 0RWJ
    Sternoclavicular
      Left 0RWF
      Right 0RWE
    Tarsal
      Left 0SWJ
      Right 0SWH
    Tarsometatarsal
      Left 0SWL
      Right 0SWK
    Temporomandibular
      Left 0RWD
      Right 0RWC
    Thoracic Vertebral 0RW6
    Thoracolumbar Vertebral 0RWA
    Toe Phalangeal
      Left 0SWQ
      Right 0SWP
    Wrist
      Left 0RWP
      Right 0RWN
  Kidney 0TW5
  Larynx 0CWS
  Lens
    Left 08WK
    Right 08WJ
  Liver 0FW0
  Lung
    Left 0BWL
    Right 0BWK
  Lymphatic 07WN
    Thoracic Duct 07WK
  Mediastinum 0WWC
  Mesentery 0DWV
  Metacarpal
    Left 0PWQ
    Right 0PWP
  Metatarsal
    Left 0QWP
    Right 0QWN
  Mouth and Throat 0CWY
  Muscle
    Extraocular
      Left 08WM
      Right 08WL
    Lower 0KWY
    Upper 0KWX
  Nasal Mucosa and Soft Tissue 09WK
  Neck 0WW6
  Nerve
    Cranial 00WE
    Peripheral 01WY
  Omentum 0DWU
  Ovary 0UW3
  Pancreas 0FWG
  Parathyroid Gland 0GWR
  Patella
    Left 0QWF
    Right 0QWD
  Pelvic Cavity 0WWJ
  Penis 0VWS
  Pericardial Cavity 0WWD

Revision of device in — *continued*
  Perineum
    Female 0WWN
    Male 0WWM
  Peritoneal Cavity 0WWG
  Peritoneum 0DWW
  Phalanx
    Finger
      Left 0PWV
      Right 0PWT
    Thumb
      Left 0PWS
      Right 0PWR
    Toe
      Left 0QWR
      Right 0QWQ
  Pineal Body 0GW1
  Pleura 0BWQ
  Pleural Cavity
    Left 0WWB
    Right 0WW9
  Prostate and Seminal Vesicles 0VW4
  Radius
    Left 0PWJ
    Right 0PWH
  Respiratory Tract 0WWQ
  Retroperitoneum 0WWH
  Ribs
    1 to 2 0PW1
    3 or More 0PW2
  Sacrum 0QW1
  Scapula
    Left 0PW6
    Right 0PW5
  Scrotum and Tunica Vaginalis 0VW8
  Septum
    Atrial 02W5
    Ventricular 02WM
  Sinus 09WY
  Skin 0HWPX
  Skull 0NW0
  Spinal Canal 00WU
  Spinal Cord 00WV
  Spleen 07WP
  Sternum 0PW0
  Stomach 0DW6
  Subcutaneous Tissue and Fascia
    Head and Neck 0JWS
    Lower Extremity 0JWW
    Trunk 0JWT
    Upper Extremity 0JWV
  Tarsal
    Left 0QWM
    Right 0QWL
  Tendon
    Lower 0LWY
    Upper 0LWX
  Testis 0VWD
  Thymus 07WM
  Thyroid Gland 0GWK
  Tibia
    Left 0QWH
    Right 0QWG
  Toe Nail 0HWRX
  Trachea 0BW1
  Tracheobronchial Tree 0BW0
  Tympanic Membrane
    Left 09W8
    Right 09W7
  Ulna
    Left 0PWL
    Right 0PWK
  Ureter 0TW9
  Urethra 0TWD
  Uterus and Cervix 0UWD
  Vagina and Cul-de-sac 0UWH

Revision of device in — *continued*
Valve
Aortic 02WF
Mitral 02WG
Pulmonary 02WH
Tricuspid 02WJ
Vas Deferens 0VWR
Vein
Azygos 05W0
Innominate
Left 05W4
Right 05W3
Lower 06WY
Upper 05WY
Vertebra
Cervical 0PW3
Lumbar 0QW0
Thoracic 0PW4
Vulva 0UWM
Revo MRI™ SureScan® pacemaker
use Pacemaker, Dual Chamber in 0JH
rhBMP-2
use Recombinant Bone Morphogenetic
Protein
Rheos® System device
use Stimulator Generator in Subcutaneous
Tissue and Fascia
Rheos® System lead
use Stimulator Lead in Upper Arteries
Rhinopharynx
use Nasopharynx
Rhinoplasty
see Alteration, Nasal Mucosa and Soft
Tissue 090K
see Repair, Nasal Mucosa and Soft
Tissue 09QK
see Replacement, Nasal Mucosa and Soft
Tissue 09RK
see Supplement, Nasal Mucosa and Soft
Tissue 09UK
Rhinorrhaphy
see Repair, Nasal Mucosa and Soft
Tissue 09QK
Rhinoscopy 09JKXZZ
Rhizotomy
see Division, Central Nervous System and
Cranial Nerves 008
see Division, Peripheral Nervous
System 018
Rhomboid major muscle
use Trunk Muscle, Right
use Trunk Muscle, Left
Rhomboid minor muscle
use Trunk Muscle, Right
use Trunk Muscle, Left
Rhythm electrocardiogram
see Measurement, Cardiac 4A02
Rhytidectomy
see Face lift
Right ascending lumbar vein
use Azygos Vein
Right atrioventricular valve
use Tricuspid Valve
Right auricular appendix
use Atrium, Right
Right colic vein
use Colic Vein
Right coronary sulcus
use Heart, Right
Right gastric artery
use Gastric Artery
Right gastroepiploic vein
use Superior Mesenteric Vein
Right inferior phrenic vein
use Inferior Vena Cava
Right inferior pulmonary vein
use Pulmonary Vein, Right

Right jugular trunk
use Lymphatic, Right Neck
Right lateral ventricle
use Cerebral Ventricle
Right lymphatic duct
use Lymphatic, Right Neck
Right ovarian vein
use Inferior Vena Cava
Right second lumbar vein
use Inferior Vena Cava
Right subclavian trunk
use Lymphatic, Right Neck
Right subcostal vein
use Azygos Vein
Right superior pulmonary vein
use Pulmonary Vein, Right
Right suprarenal vein
use Inferior Vena Cava
Right testicular vein
use Inferior Vena Cava
Rima glottidis
use Larynx
Risorius muscle
use Facial Muscle
RNS® System lead
use Neurostimulator Lead in Central
Nervous System and Cranial Nerves
RNS® system neurostimulator generator
use Neurostimulator Generator in Head
and Facial Bones
Robotic Assisted Procedure
Extremity
Lower 8E0Y
Upper 8E0X
Head and Neck Region 8E09
Trunk Region 8E0W
Rotation of fetal head
Forceps 10S07ZZ
Manual 10S0XZZ
Round ligament of uterus
use Uterine Supporting Structure
Round window
use Inner Ear, Right
use Inner Ear, Left
Roux-en-Y operation
see Bypass, Gastrointestinal System 0D1
see Bypass, Hepatobiliary System and
Pancreas 0F1
Rupture
Adhesions *see* Release
Fluid collection *see* Drainage

S

Sacral ganglion
use Sacral Sympathetic Nerve
Sacral lymph node
use Lymphatic, Pelvis
Sacral nerve modulation (SNM) lead
use Stimulator Lead in Urinary System
Sacral neuromodulation lead
use Stimulator Lead in Urinary System
Sacral splanchnic nerve
use Sacral Sympathetic Nerve
Sacrectomy
see Excision, Lower Bones 0QB
Sacrococcygeal ligament
use Lower Spine Bursa and Ligament
Sacrococcygeal symphysis
use Sacrococcygeal Joint
Sacroiliac ligament
use Lower Spine Bursa and Ligament
Sacrospinous ligament
use Lower Spine Bursa and Ligament
Sacrotuberous ligament
use Lower Spine Bursa and Ligament

Salpingectomy
see Excision, Female Reproductive
System 0UB
see Resection, Female Reproductive
System 0UT
Salpingolysis
see Release, Female Reproductive
System 0UN
Salpingopexy
see Repair, Female Reproductive
System 0UQ
see Reposition, Female Reproductive
System 0US
Salpingopharyngeus muscle
use Tongue, Palate, Pharynx Muscle
Salpingoplasty
see Repair, Female Reproductive
System 0UQ
see Supplement, Female Reproductive
System 0UU
Salpingorrhaphy
see Repair, Female Reproductive
System 0UQ
Salpingoscopy 0UJ88ZZ
Salpingostomy
see Drainage, Female Reproductive
System 0U9
Salpingotomy
see Drainage, Female Reproductive
System 0U9
Salpinx
use Fallopian Tube, Right
use Fallopian Tube, Left
Saphenous nerve
use Femoral Nerve
SAPIEN® transcatheter aortic valve
use Zooplastic Tissue in Heart and Great
Vessels
Sartorius muscle
use Upper Leg Muscle, Right
use Upper Leg Muscle, Left
Scalene muscle
use Neck Muscle, Right
use Neck Muscle, Left
Scan
Computerized Tomography (CT) *see*
Computerized Tomography (CT Scan)
Radioisotope *see* Planar Nuclear Medicine
Imaging
Scaphoid bone
use Carpal, Right
use Carpal, Left
Scapholunate ligament
use Hand Bursa and Ligament, Right
use Hand Bursa and Ligament, Left
Scaphotrapezium ligament
use Hand Bursa and Ligament, Right
use Hand Bursa and Ligament, Left
Scapulectomy
see Excision, Upper Bones 0PB
see Resection, Upper Bones 0PT
Scapulopexy
see Repair, Upper Bones 0PQ
see Reposition, Upper Bones 0PS
Scarpa's (vestibular) ganglion
use Acoustic Nerve
Sclerectomy
see Excision, Eye 08B
Sclerotherapy, mechanical
see Destruction
Sclerotomy
see Drainage, Eye 089
Scrotectomy
see Excision, Male Reproductive System 0VB
see Resection, Male Reproductive
System 0VT

Scrotoplasty
see Repair, Male Reproductive System 0VQ
see Supplement, Male Reproductive System 0VU
Scrotorrhaphy
see Repair, Male Reproductive System 0VQ
Scrototomy
see Drainage, Male Reproductive System 0V9
Sebaceous gland
use Skin
Second cranial nerve
use Optic Nerve
Section, cesarean
see Extraction, Pregnancy 10D
Secura™ (DR) (VR)
use Defibrillator Generator in 0JH
Sella turcica
use Sphenoid Bone
Semicircular canal
use Inner Ear, Right
use Inner Ear, Left
Semimembranosus muscle
use Upper Leg Muscle, Right
use Upper Leg Muscle, Left
Semitendinosus muscle
use Upper Leg Muscle, Right
use Upper Leg Muscle, Left
Seprafilm®
use Adhesion Barrier
Septal cartilage
use Nasal Septum
Septectomy
see Excision, Heart and Great Vessels 02B
see Resection, Heart and Great Vessels 02T
see Excision, Ear, Nose, Sinus 09B
see Resection, Ear, Nose, Sinus 09T
Septoplasty
see Repair, Heart and Great Vessels 02Q
see Replacement, Heart and Great Vessels 02R
see Supplement, Heart and Great Vessels 02U
see Repair, Ear, Nose, Sinus 09Q
see Replacement, Ear, Nose, Sinus 09R
see Reposition, Ear, Nose, Sinus 09S
see Supplement, Ear, Nose, Sinus 09U
Septostomy, balloon atrial 02163Z7
Septotomy
see Drainage, Ear, Nose, Sinus 099
Sequestrectomy, bone
see Extirpation
Serratus anterior muscle
use Thorax Muscle, Right
use Thorax Muscle, Left
Serratus posterior muscle
use Trunk Muscle, Right
use Trunk Muscle, Left
Seventh cranial nerve
use Facial Nerve
Sheffield hybrid external fixator
use External Fixation Device, Hybrid in 0PH
use External Fixation Device, Hybrid in 0PS
use External Fixation Device, Hybrid in 0QH
use External Fixation Device, Hybrid in 0QS
Sheffield ring external fixator
use External Fixation Device, Ring in 0PH
use External Fixation Device, Ring in 0PS
use External Fixation Device, Ring in 0QH
use External Fixation Device, Ring in 0QS
Shirodkar cervical cerclage 0UVC7ZZ
Shock Wave Therapy, Musculoskeletal 6A93
Short gastric artery
use Splenic Artery
Shortening
see Excision
see Repair
see Reposition

Shunt creation
see Bypass
Sialoadenectomy
Complete *see* Resection, Mouth and Throat 0CT
Partial *see* Excision, Mouth and Throat 0CB
Sialodochoplasty
see Repair, Mouth and Throat 0CQ
see Replacement, Mouth and Throat 0CR
see Supplement, Mouth and Throat 0CU
Sialectomy
see Excision, Mouth and Throat 0CB
see Resection, Mouth and Throat 0CT
Sialography
see Plain Radiography, Ear, Nose, Mouth and Throat B90
Sialolithotomy
see Extirpation, Mouth and Throat 0CC
Sigmoid artery
use Inferior Mesenteric Artery
Sigmoid flexure
use Sigmoid Colon
Sigmoid vein
use Inferior Mesenteric Vein
Sigmoidectomy
see Excision, Gastrointestinal System 0DB
see Resection, Gastrointestinal System 0DT
Sigmoidorrhaphy
see Repair, Gastrointestinal System 0DQ
Sigmoidoscopy 0DJD8ZZ
Sigmoidotomy
see Drainage, Gastrointestinal System 0D9
Single lead pacemaker (atrium)(ventricle)
use Pacemaker, Single Chamber in 0JH
Single lead rate responsive pacemaker (atrium)(ventricle)
use Pacemaker, Single Chamber Rate Responsive in 0JH
Sinoatrial node
use Conduction Mechanism
Sinogram
Abdominal Wall *see* Fluoroscopy, Abdomen and Pelvis BW11
Chest Wall *see* Plain Radiography, Chest BW03
Retroperitoneum *see* Fluoroscopy, Abdomen and Pelvis BW11
Sinus venosus
use Atrium, Right
Sinusectomy
see Excision, Ear, Nose, Sinus 09B
see Resection, Ear, Nose, Sinus 09T
Sinusoscopy 09JY4ZZ
Sinusotomy
see Drainage, Ear, Nose, Sinus 099
Sirolimus-eluting coronary stent
use Intraluminal Device, Drug-eluting in Heart and Great Vessels
Sixth cranial nerve
use Abducens Nerve
Size reduction, breast
see Excision, Skin and Breast 0HB
SJM Biocor® Stented Valve System
use Zooplastic Tissue in Heart and Great Vessels
Skene's (paraurethral) gland
use Vestibular Gland
Skin Substitute, Porcine Liver Derived, Replacement XHRPXL2
Sling
Fascial, orbicularis muscle (mouth) *see* Supplement, Muscle, Facial 0KU1
Levator muscle, for urethral suspension *see* Reposition, Bladder Neck 0TSC
Pubococcygeal, for urethral suspension *see* Reposition, Bladder Neck 0TSC
Rectum *see* Reposition, Rectum 0DSP

Small bowel series
see Fluoroscopy, Bowel, Small BD13
Small saphenous vein
use Saphenous Vein, Right
use Saphenous Vein, Left
Snaring, polyp, colon
see Excision, Gastrointestinal System 0DB
Solar (celiac) plexus
use Abdominal Sympathetic Nerve
Soleus muscle
use Lower Leg Muscle, Right
use Lower Leg Muscle, Left
Spacer
Insertion of device in
Disc
Lumbar Vertebral 0SH2
Lumbosacral 0SH4
Joint
Acromioclavicular
Left 0RHH
Right 0RHG
Ankle
Left 0SHG
Right 0SHF
Carpal
Left 0RHR
Right 0RHQ
Carpometacarpal
Left 0RHT
Right 0RHS
Cervical Vertebral 0RH1
Cervicothoracic Vertebral 0RH4
Coccygeal 0SH6
Elbow
Left 0RHM
Right 0RHL
Finger Phalangeal
Left 0RHX
Right 0RHW
Hip
Left 0SHB
Right 0SH9
Knee
Left 0SHD
Right 0SHC
Lumbar Vertebral 0SH0
Lumbosacral 0SH3
Metacarpophalangeal
Left 0RHV
Right 0RHU
Metatarsal-Phalangeal
Left 0SHN
Right 0SHM
Occipital-cervical 0RH0
Sacrococcygeal 0SH5
Sacroiliac
Left 0SH8
Right 0SH7
Shoulder
Left 0RHK
Right 0RHJ
Sternoclavicular
Left 0RHF
Right 0RHE
Tarsal
Left 0SHJ
Right 0SHH
Tarsometatarsal
Left 0SHL
Right 0SHK
Temporomandibular
Left 0RHD
Right 0RHC
Thoracic Vertebral 0RH6
Thoracolumbar Vertebral 0RHA
Toe Phalangeal
Left 0SHQ

Spacer — *continued*
Insertion of device in — *continued*
Right 0SHP
Wrist
Left 0RHP
Right 0RHN
Removal of device from
Acromioclavicular
Left 0RPH
Right 0RPG
Ankle
Left 0SPG
Right 0SPF
Carpal
Left 0RPR
Right 0RPQ
Carpometacarpal
Left 0RPT
Right 0RPS
Cervical Vertebral 0RP1
Cervicothoracic Vertebral 0RP4
Coccygeal 0SP6
Elbow
Left 0RPM
Right 0RPL
Finger Phalangeal
Left 0RPX
Right 0RPW
Hip
Left 0SPB
Right 0SP9
Knee
Left 0SPD
Right 0SPC
Lumbar Vertebral 0SP0
Lumbosacral 0SP3
Metacarpophalangeal
Left 0RPV
Right 0RPU
Metatarsal-Phalangeal
Left 0SPN
Right 0SPM
Occipital-cervical 0RP0
Sacrococcygeal 0SP5
Sacroiliac
Left 0SP8
Right 0SP7
Shoulder
Left 0RPK
Right 0RPJ
Sternoclavicular
Left 0RPF
Right 0RPE
Tarsal
Left 0SPJ
Right 0SPH
Tarsometatarsal
Left 0SPL
Right 0SPK
Temporomandibular
Left 0RPD
Right 0RPC
Thoracic Vertebral 0RP6
Thoracolumbar Vertebral 0RPA
Toe Phalangeal
Left 0SPQ
Right 0SPP
Wrist
Left 0RPP
Right 0RPN
Revision of device in
Acromioclavicular
Left 0RWH
Right 0RWG
Ankle
Left 0SWG
Right 0SWF

Spacer — *continued*
Revision of device in — *continued*
Carpal
Left 0RWR
Right 0RWQ
Carpometacarpal
Left 0RWT
Right 0RWS
Cervical Vertebral 0RW1
Cervicothoracic Vertebral 0RW4
Coccygeal 0SW6
Elbow
Left 0RWM
Right 0RWL
Finger Phalangeal
Left 0RWX
Right 0RWW
Hip
Left 0SWB
Right 0SW9
Knee
Left 0SWD
Right 0SWC
Lumbar Vertebral 0SW0
Lumbosacral 0SW3
Metacarpophalangeal
Left 0RWV
Right 0RWU
Metatarsal-Phalangeal
Left 0SWN
Right 0SWM
Occipital-cervical 0RW0
Sacrococcygeal 0SW5
Sacroiliac
Left 0SW8
Right 0SW7
Shoulder
Left 0RWK
Right 0RWJ
Sternoclavicular
Left 0RWF
Right 0RWE
Tarsal
Left 0SWJ
Right 0SWH
Tarsometatarsal
Left 0SWL
Right 0SWK
Temporomandibular
Left 0RWD
Right 0RWC
Thoracic Vertebral 0RW6
Thoracolumbar Vertebral 0RWA
Toe Phalangeal
Left 0SWQ
Right 0SWP
Wrist
Left 0RWP
Right 0RWN
Spectroscopy
Intravascular 8E023DZ
Near infrared 8E023DZ
Speech Assessment F00
Speech therapy
see Speech Treatment, Rehabilitation F06
Speech Treatment F06
Sphenoidectomy
see Excision, Ear, Nose, Sinus 09B
see Resection, Ear, Nose, Sinus 09T
see Excision, Head and Facial Bones 0NB
see Resection, Head and Facial Bones 0NT
Sphenoidotomy
see Drainage, Ear, Nose, Sinus 099
Sphenomandibular ligament
use Head and Neck Bursa and Ligament
Sphenopalatine (pterygopalatine) ganglion
use Head and Neck Sympathetic Nerve

Sphincterorrhaphy, anal
see Repair, Anal Sphincter 0DQR
Sphincterotomy, anal
see Division, Anal Sphincter 0D8R
see Drainage, Anal Sphincter 0D9R
Spinal cord neurostimulator lead
use Neurostimulator Lead in Central Nervous System and Cranial Nerves
Spinal growth rods, magnetically controlled
use Magnetically Controlled Growth Rod(s) in New Technology
Spinal nerve, cervical
use Cervical Nerve
Spinal nerve, lumbar
use Lumbar Nerve
Spinal nerve, sacral
use Sacral Nerve
Spinal nerve, thoracic
use Thoracic Nerve
Spinal Stabilization Device
Facet Replacement
Cervical Vertebral 0RH1
Cervicothoracic Vertebral 0RH4
Lumbar Vertebral 0SH0
Lumbosacral 0SH3
Occipital-cervical 0RH0
Thoracic Vertebral 0RH6
Thoracolumbar Vertebral 0RHA
Interspinous Process
Cervical Vertebral 0RH1
Cervicothoracic Vertebral 0RH4
Lumbar Vertebral 0SH0
Lumbosacral 0SH3
Occipital-cervical 0RH0
Thoracic Vertebral 0RH6
Thoracolumbar Vertebral 0RHA
Pedicle-Based
Cervical Vertebral 0RH1
Cervicothoracic Vertebral 0RH4
Lumbar Vertebral 0SH0
Lumbosacral 0SH3
Occipital-cervical 0RH0
Thoracic Vertebral 0RH6
Thoracolumbar Vertebral 0RHA
Spinous process
use Cervical Vertebra
use Thoracic Vertebra
use Lumbar Vertebra
Spiral ganglion
use Acoustic Nerve
Spiration IBV™ Valve System
use Intraluminal Device, Endobronchial Valve in Respiratory System
Splenectomy
see Excision, Lymphatic and Hemic Systems 07B
see Resection, Lymphatic and Hemic Systems 07T
Splenic flexure
use Transverse Colon
Splenic plexus
use Abdominal Sympathetic Nerve
Splenius capitis muscle
use Head Muscle
Splenius cervicis muscle
use Neck Muscle, Right
use Neck Muscle, Left
Splenolysis
see Release, Lymphatic and Hemic Systems 07N
Splenopexy
see Repair, Lymphatic and Hemic Systems 07Q
see Reposition, Lymphatic and Hemic Systems 07S

Splenoplasty
  see Repair, Lymphatic and Hemic
    Systems 07Q
Splenorrhaphy
  see Repair, Lymphatic and Hemic
    Systems 07Q
Splenotomy
  see Drainage, Lymphatic and Hemic
    Systems 079
Splinting, musculoskeletal
  see Immobilization, Anatomical
    Regions 2W3
SPY system intravascular fluorescence
angiography
  see Monitoring, Physiological Systems 4A1
Stapedectomy
  see Excision, Ear, Nose, Sinus 09B
  see Resection, Ear, Nose, Sinus 09T
Stapediolysis
  see Release, Ear, Nose, Sinus 09N
Stapedioplasty
  see Repair, Ear, Nose, Sinus 09Q
  see Replacement, Ear, Nose, Sinus 09R
  see Supplement, Ear, Nose, Sinus 09U
Stapedotomy
  see Drainage, Ear, Nose, Sinus 099
Stapes
  use Auditory Ossicle, Right
  use Auditory Ossicle, Left
STELARA®
  use Other New Technology Therapeutic
    Substance
Stellate ganglion
  use Head and Neck Sympathetic Nerve
Stem cell transplant
  see Transfusion, Circulatory 302
Stensen's duct
  use Parotid Duct, Right
  use Parotid Duct, Left
Stent, intraluminal (cardiovascular)
(gastrointestinal)(hepatobiliary)(urinary)
  use Intraluminal Device
Stented tissue valve
  use Zooplastic Tissue in Heart and Great
    Vessels
Stereotactic Radiosurgery
  Abdomen DW23
  Adrenal Gland DG22
  Bile Ducts DF22
  Bladder DT22
  Bone Marrow D720
  Brain D020
  Brain Stem D021
  Breast
    Left DM20
    Right DM21
  Bronchus DB21
  Cervix DU21
  Chest DW22
  Chest Wall DB27
  Colon DD25
  Diaphragm DB28
  Duodenum DD22
  Ear D920
  Esophagus DD20
  Eye D820
  Gallbladder DF21
  Gamma Beam
    Abdomen DW23JZZ
    Adrenal Gland DG22JZZ
    Bile Ducts DF22JZZ
    Bladder DT22JZZ
    Bone Marrow D720JZZ
    Brain D020JZZ
    Brain Stem D021JZZ
    Breast
      Left DM20JZZ

Stereotactic Radiosurgery — *continued*
  Gamma Beam — *continued*
    Right DM21JZZ
    Bronchus DB21JZZ
    Cervix DU21JZZ
    Chest DW22JZZ
    Chest Wall DB27JZZ
    Colon DD25JZZ
    Diaphragm DB28JZZ
    Duodenum DD22JZZ
    Ear D920JZZ
    Esophagus DD20JZZ
    Eye D820JZZ
    Gallbladder DF21JZZ
    Gland
      Adrenal DG22JZZ
      Parathyroid DG24JZZ
      Pituitary DG20JZZ
      Thyroid DG25JZZ
    Glands, Salivary D926JZZ
    Head and Neck DW21JZZ
    Ileum DD24JZZ
    Jejunum DD23JZZ
    Kidney DT20JZZ
    Larynx D92BJZZ
    Liver DF20JZZ
    Lung DB22JZZ
    Lymphatics
      Abdomen D726JZZ
      Axillary D724JZZ
      Inguinal D728JZZ
      Neck D723JZZ
      Pelvis D727JZZ
      Thorax D725JZZ
    Mediastinum DB26JZZ
    Mouth D924JZZ
    Nasopharynx D92DJZZ
    Neck and Head DW21JZZ
    Nerve, Peripheral D027JZZ
    Nose D921JZZ
    Ovary DU20JZZ
    Palate
      Hard D928JZZ
      Soft D929JZZ
    Pancreas DF23JZZ
    Parathyroid Gland DG24JZZ
    Pelvic Region DW26JZZ
    Pharynx D92CJZZ
    Pineal Body DG21JZZ
    Pituitary Gland DG20JZZ
    Pleura DB25JZZ
    Prostate DV20JZZ
    Rectum DD27JZZ
    Sinuses D927JZZ
    Spinal Cord D026JZZ
    Spleen D722JZZ
    Stomach DD21JZZ
    Testis DV21JZZ
    Thymus D721JZZ
    Thyroid Gland DG25JZZ
    Tongue D925JZZ
    Trachea DB20JZZ
    Ureter DT21JZZ
    Urethra DT23JZZ
    Uterus DU22JZZ
  Gland
    Adrenal DG22
    Parathyroid DG24
    Pituitary DG20
    Thyroid DG25
  Glands, Salivary D926
  Head and Neck DW21
  Ileum DD24
  Jejunum DD23
  Kidney DT20
  Larynx D92B
  Liver DF20

Stereotactic Radiosurgery — *continued*
  Lung DB22
  Lymphatics
    Abdomen D726
    Axillary D724
    Inguinal D728
    Neck D723
    Pelvis D727
    Thorax D725
  Mediastinum DB26
  Mouth D924
  Nasopharynx D92D
  Neck and Head DW21
  Nerve, Peripheral D027
  Nose D921
  Other Photon
    Abdomen DW23DZZ
    Adrenal Gland DG22DZZ
    Bile Ducts DF22DZZ
    Bladder DT22DZZ
    Bone Marrow D720DZZ
    Brain D020DZZ
    Brain Stem D021DZZ
    Breast
      Left DM20DZZ
      Right DM21DZZ
    Bronchus DB21DZZ
    Cervix DU21DZZ
    Chest DW22DZZ
    Chest Wall DB27DZZ
    Colon DD25DZZ
    Diaphragm DB28DZZ
    Duodenum DD22DZZ
    Ear D920DZZ
    Esophagus DD20DZZ
    Eye D820DZZ
    Gallbladder DF21DZZ
    Gland
      Adrenal DG22DZZ
      Parathyroid DG24DZZ
      Pituitary DG20DZZ
      Thyroid DG25DZZ
    Glands, Salivary D926DZZ
    Head and Neck DW21DZZ
    Ileum DD24DZZ
    Jejunum DD23DZZ
    Kidney DT20DZZ
    Larynx D92BDZZ
    Liver DF20DZZ
    Lung DB22DZZ
    Lymphatics
      Abdomen D726DZZ
      Axillary D724DZZ
      Inguinal D728DZZ
      Neck D723DZZ
      Pelvis D727DZZ
      Thorax D725DZZ
    Mediastinum DB26DZZ
    Mouth D924DZZ
    Nasopharynx D92DDZZ
    Neck and Head DW21DZZ
    Nerve, Peripheral D027DZZ
    Nose D921DZZ
    Ovary DU20DZZ
    Palate
      Hard D928DZZ
      Soft D929DZZ
    Pancreas DF23DZZ
    Parathyroid Gland DG24DZZ
    Pelvic Region DW26DZZ
    Pharynx D92CDZZ
    Pineal Body DG21DZZ
    Pituitary Gland DG20DZZ
    Pleura DB25DZZ
    Prostate DV20DZZ
    Rectum DD27DZZ
    Sinuses D927DZZ

Stereotactic Radiosurgery — *continued*
  Other Photon — *continued*
    Spinal Cord D026DZZ
    Spleen D722DZZ
    Stomach DD21DZZ
    Testis DV21DZZ
    Thymus D721DZZ
    Thyroid Gland DG25DZZ
    Tongue D925DZZ
    Trachea DB20DZZ
    Ureter DT21DZZ
    Urethra DT23DZZ
    Uterus DU22DZZ
  Ovary DU20
  Palate
    Hard D928
    Soft D929
  Pancreas DF23
  Parathyroid Gland DG24
  Particulate
    Abdomen DW23HZZ
    Adrenal Gland DG22HZZ
    Bile Ducts DF22HZZ
    Bladder DT22HZZ
    Bone Marrow D720HZZ
    Brain D020HZZ
    Brain Stem D021HZZ
    Breast
      Left DM20HZZ
      Right DM21HZZ
    Bronchus DB21HZZ
    Cervix DU21HZZ
    Chest DW22HZZ
    Chest Wall DB27HZZ
    Colon DD25HZZ
    Diaphragm DB28HZZ
    Duodenum DD22HZZ
    Ear D920HZZ
    Esophagus DD20HZZ
    Eye D820HZZ
    Gallbladder DF21HZZ
    Gland
      Adrenal DG22HZZ
      Parathyroid DG24HZZ
      Pituitary DG20HZZ
      Thyroid DG25HZZ
    Glands, Salivary D926HZZ
    Head and Neck DW21HZZ
    Ileum DD24HZZ
    Jejunum DD23HZZ
    Kidney DT20HZZ
    Larynx D92BHZZ
    Liver DF20HZZ
    Lung DB22HZZ
    Lymphatics
      Abdomen D726HZZ
      Axillary D724HZZ
      Inguinal D728HZZ
      Neck D723HZZ
      Pelvis D727HZZ
      Thorax D725HZZ
    Mediastinum DB26HZZ
    Mouth D924HZZ
    Nasopharynx D92DHZZ
    Neck and Head DW21HZZ
    Nerve, Peripheral D027HZZ
    Nose D921HZZ
    Ovary DU20HZZ
    Palate
      Hard D928HZZ
      Soft D929HZZ
    Pancreas DF23HZZ
    Parathyroid Gland DG24HZZ
    Pelvic Region DW26HZZ
    Pharynx D92CHZZ
    Pineal Body DG21HZZ
    Pituitary Gland DG20HZZ

Stereotactic Radiosurgery — *continued*
  Particulate — *continued*
    Pleura DB25HZZ
    Prostate DV20HZZ
    Rectum DD27HZZ
    Sinuses D927HZZ
    Spinal Cord D026HZZ
    Spleen D722HZZ
    Stomach DD21HZZ
    Testis DV21HZZ
    Thymus D721HZZ
    Thyroid Gland DG25HZZ
    Tongue D925HZZ
    Trachea DB20HZZ
    Ureter DT21HZZ
    Urethra DT23HZZ
    Uterus DU22HZZ
  Pelvic Region DW26
  Pharynx D92C
  Pineal Body DG21
  Pituitary Gland DG20
  Pleura DB25
  Prostate DV20
  Rectum DD27
  Sinuses D927
  Spinal Cord D026
  Spleen D722
  Stomach DD21
  Testis DV21
  Thymus D721
  Thyroid Gland DG25
  Tongue D925
  Trachea DB20
  Ureter DT21
  Urethra DT23
  Uterus DU22
Sternoclavicular ligament
  use Shoulder Bursa and Ligament, Right
  use Shoulder Bursa and Ligament, Left
Sternocleidomastoid artery
  use Thyroid Artery, Right
  use Thyroid Artery, Left
Sternocleidomastoid muscle
  use Neck Muscle, Right
  use Neck Muscle, Left
Sternocostal ligament
  use Sternum Bursa and Ligament
  use Rib(s) Bursa and Ligament
Sternotomy
  see Division, Sternum 0P80
  see Drainage, Sternum 0P90
Stimulation, cardiac
  Cardioversion 5A2204Z
  Electrophysiologic testing *see*
    Measurement, Cardiac 4A02
Stimulator Generator
  Insertion of device in
    Abdomen 0JH8
    Back 0JH7
    Chest 0JH6
  Multiple Array
    Abdomen 0JH8
    Back 0JH7
    Chest 0JH6
  Multiple Array Rechargeable
    Abdomen 0JH8
    Back 0JH7
    Chest 0JH6
  Removal of device from, Subcutaneous
    Tissue and Fascia, Trunk 0JPT
  Revision of device in, Subcutaneous Tissue
    and Fascia, Trunk 0JWT
  Single Array
    Abdomen 0JH8
    Back 0JH7
    Chest 0JH6

Stimulator Generator — *continued*
  Single Array Rechargeable
    Abdomen 0JH8
    Back 0JH7
    Chest 0JH6
Stimulator Lead
  Insertion of device in
    Anal Sphincter 0DHR
    Artery
      Left 03HL
      Right 03HK
    Bladder 0THB
    Muscle
      Lower 0KHY
      Upper 0KHX
    Stomach 0DH6
    Ureter 0TH9
  Removal of device from
    Anal Sphincter 0DPR
    Artery, Upper 03PY
    Bladder 0TPB
    Muscle
      Lower 0KPY
      Upper 0KPX
    Stomach 0DP6
    Ureter 0TP9
  Revision of device in
    Anal Sphincter 0DWR
    Artery, Upper 03WY
    Bladder 0TWB
    Muscle
      Lower 0KWY
      Upper 0KWX
    Stomach 0DW6
    Ureter 0TW9
Stoma
  Excision
    Abdominal Wall 0WBFXZ2
    Neck 0WB6XZ2
  Repair
    Abdominal Wall 0WQFXZ2
    Neck 0WQ6XZ2
Stomatoplasty
  see Repair, Mouth and Throat 0CQ
  see Replacement, Mouth and Throat 0CR
  see Supplement, Mouth and Throat 0CU
Stomatorrhaphy
  see Repair, Mouth and Throat 0CQ
Stratos LV®
  use Cardiac Resynchronization Pacemaker
    Pulse Generator in 0JH
Stress test
  4A02XM4
  4A12XM4
Stripping
  see Extraction
Study
  Electrophysiologic stimulation, cardiac *see*
    Measurement, Cardiac 4A02
  Ocular motility 4A07X7Z
  Pulmonary airway flow measurement *see*
    Measurement, Respiratory 4A09
  Visual acuity 4A07X0Z
Styloglossus muscle
  use Tongue, Palate, Pharynx Muscle
Stylomandibular ligament
  use Head and Neck Bursa and Ligament
Stylopharyngeus muscle
  use Tongue, Palate, Pharynx Muscle
Subacromial bursa
  use Shoulder Bursa and Ligament, Right
  use Shoulder Bursa and Ligament, Left
Subaortic (common iliac) lymph node
  use Lymphatic, Pelvis
Subarachnoid space, spinal
  use Spinal Canal

Subclavicular (apical) lymph node
   use Lymphatic, Right Axillary
   use Lymphatic, Left Axillary
Subclavius muscle
   use Thorax Muscle, Right
   use Thorax Muscle, Left
Subclavius nerve
   use Brachial Plexus
Subcostal artery
   use Upper Artery
Subcostal muscle
   use Thorax Muscle, Right
   use Thorax Muscle, Left
Subcostal nerve
   use Thoracic Nerve
Subcutaneous injection reservoir, port
   use Vascular Access Device, Totally
      Implantable in Subcutaneous Tissue and
      Fascia
Subcutaneous injection reservoir, pump
   use Infusion Device, Pump in Subcutaneous
      Tissue and Fascia
Subdermal progesterone implant
   use Contraceptive Device in Subcutaneous
      Tissue and Fascia
Subdural space, spinal
   use Spinal Canal
Submandibular ganglion
   use Facial Nerve
   use Head and Neck Sympathetic Nerve
Submandibular gland
   use Submaxillary Gland, Right
   use Submaxillary Gland, Left
Submandibular lymph node
   use Lymphatic, Head
Submaxillary ganglion
   use Head and Neck Sympathetic Nerve
Submaxillary lymph node
   use Lymphatic, Head
Submental artery
   use Face Artery
Submental lymph node
   use Lymphatic, Head
Submucous (Meissner's) plexus
   use Abdominal Sympathetic Nerve
Suboccipital nerve
   use Cervical Nerve
Suboccipital venous plexus
   use Vertebral Vein, Right
   use Vertebral Vein, Left
Subparotid lymph node
   use Lymphatic, Head
Subscapular (posterior) lymph node
   use Lymphatic, Right Axillary
   use Lymphatic, Left Axillary
Subscapular aponeurosis
   use Subcutaneous Tissue and Fascia, Right
      Upper Arm
   use Subcutaneous Tissue and Fascia, Left
      Upper Arm
Subscapular artery
   use Axillary Artery, Right
   use Axillary Artery, Left
Subscapularis muscle
   use Shoulder Muscle, Right
   use Shoulder Muscle, Left
Substance Abuse Treatment
   Counseling
      Family, for substance abuse, Other
         Family Counseling HZ63ZZZ
      Group
         12-Step HZ43ZZZ
         Behavioral HZ41ZZZ
         Cognitive HZ40ZZZ
         Cognitive-Behavioral HZ42ZZZ
         Confrontational HZ48ZZZ
         Continuing Care HZ49ZZZ

Substance Abuse Treatment — *continued*
   Counseling — *continued*
      Infectious Disease
         Post-Test HZ4CZZZ
         Pre-Test HZ4CZZZ
      Interpersonal HZ44ZZZ
      Motivational Enhancement HZ47ZZZ
      Psychoeducation HZ46ZZZ
      Spiritual HZ4BZZZ
      Vocational HZ45ZZZ
   Individual
      12-Step HZ33ZZZ
      Behavioral HZ31ZZZ
      Cognitive HZ30ZZZ
      Cognitive-Behavioral HZ32ZZZ
      Confrontational HZ38ZZZ
      Continuing Care HZ39ZZZ
      Infectious Disease
         Post-Test HZ3CZZZ
         Pre-Test HZ3CZZZ
      Interpersonal HZ34ZZZ
      Motivational Enhancement HZ37ZZZ
      Psychoeducation HZ36ZZZ
      Spiritual HZ3BZZZ
      Vocational HZ35ZZZ
   Detoxification Services, for substance
      abuse HZ2ZZZZ
   Medication Management
      Antabuse HZ83ZZZ
      Bupropion HZ87ZZZ
      Clonidine HZ86ZZZ
      Levo-alpha-acetyl-methadol
         (LAAM) HZ82ZZZ
      Methadone Maintenance HZ81ZZZ
      Naloxone HZ85ZZZ
      Naltrexone HZ84ZZZ
      Nicotine Replacement HZ80ZZZ
      Other Replacement
         Medication HZ89ZZZ
      Psychiatric Medication HZ88ZZZ
   Pharmacotherapy
      Antabuse HZ93ZZZ
      Bupropion HZ97ZZZ
      Clonidine HZ96ZZZ
      Levo-alpha-acetyl-methadol
         (LAAM) HZ92ZZZ
      Methadone Maintenance HZ91ZZZ
      Naloxone HZ95ZZZ
      Naltrexone HZ94ZZZ
      Nicotine Replacement HZ90ZZZ
      Psychiatric Medication HZ98ZZZ
      Replacement Medication,
         Other HZ99ZZZ
   Psychotherapy
      12-Step HZ53ZZZ
      Behavioral HZ51ZZZ
      Cognitive HZ50ZZZ
      Cognitive-Behavioral HZ52ZZZ
      Confrontational HZ58ZZZ
      Interactive HZ55ZZZ
      Interpersonal HZ54ZZZ
      Motivational Enhancement HZ57ZZZ
      Psychoanalysis HZ5BZZZ
      Psychodynamic HZ5CZZZ
      Psychoeducation HZ56ZZZ
      Psychophysiological HZ5DZZZ
      Supportive HZ59ZZZ
Substantia nigra
   use Basal Ganglia
Subtalar (talocalcaneal) joint
   use Tarsal Joint, Right
   use Tarsal Joint, Left
Subtalar ligament
   use Foot Bursa and Ligament, Right
   use Foot Bursa and Ligament, Left
Subthalamic nucleus
   use Basal Ganglia

Suction curettage (D&C), nonobstetric
   see Extraction, Endometrium 0UDB
Suction curettage, obstetric post-delivery
   see Extraction, Products of Conception,
      Retained 10D1
Superficial circumflex iliac vein
   use Saphenous Vein, Right
   use Saphenous Vein, Left
Superficial epigastric artery
   use Femoral Artery, Right
   use Femoral Artery, Left
Superficial epigastric vein
   use Saphenous Vein, Right
   use Saphenous Vein, Left
Superficial Inferior Epigastric Artery Flap
   Replacement
      Bilateral 0HRV078
      Left 0HRU078
      Right 0HRT078
   Transfer
      Left 0KXG
      Right 0KXF
Superficial palmar arch
   use Hand Artery, Right
   use Hand Artery, Left
Superficial palmar venous arch
   use Hand Vein, Right
   use Hand Vein, Left
Superficial temporal artery
   use Temporal Artery, Right
   use Temporal Artery, Left
Superficial transverse perineal muscle
   use Perineum Muscle
Superior cardiac nerve
   use Thoracic Sympathetic Nerve
Superior cerebellar vein
   use Intracranial Vein
Superior cerebral vein
   use Intracranial Vein
Superior clunic (cluneal) nerve
   use Lumbar Nerve
Superior epigastric artery
   use Internal Mammary Artery, Right
   use Internal Mammary Artery, Left
Superior genicular artery
   use Popliteal Artery, Right
   use Popliteal Artery, Left
Superior gluteal artery
   use Internal Iliac Artery, Right
   use Internal Iliac Artery, Left
Superior gluteal nerve
   use Lumbar Plexus
Superior hypogastric plexus
   use Abdominal Sympathetic Nerve
Superior labial artery
   use Face Artery
Superior laryngeal artery
   use Thyroid Artery, Right
   use Thyroid Artery, Left
Superior laryngeal nerve
   use Vagus Nerve
Superior longitudinal muscle
   use Tongue, Palate, Pharynx Muscle
Superior mesenteric ganglion
   use Abdominal Sympathetic Nerve
Superior mesenteric lymph node
   use Lymphatic, Mesenteric
Superior mesenteric plexus
   use Abdominal Sympathetic Nerve
Superior oblique muscle
   use Extraocular Muscle, Right
   use Extraocular Muscle, Left
Superior olivary nucleus
   use Pons
Superior rectal artery
   use Inferior Mesenteric Artery

Superior rectal vein
  use Inferior Mesenteric Vein
Superior rectus muscle
  use Extraocular Muscle, Right
  use Extraocular Muscle, Left
Superior tarsal plate
  use Upper Eyelid, Right
  use Upper Eyelid, Left
Superior thoracic artery
  use Axillary Artery, Right
  use Axillary Artery, Left
Superior thyroid artery
  use External Carotid Artery, Right
  use External Carotid Artery, Left
  use Thyroid Artery, Right
  use Thyroid Artery, Left
Superior turbinate
  use Nasal Turbinate
Superior ulnar collateral artery
  use Brachial Artery, Right
  use Brachial Artery, Left
Supplement
  Abdominal Wall 0WUF
  Acetabulum
    Left 0QU5
    Right 0QU4
  Ampulla of Vater 0FUC
  Anal Sphincter 0DUR
  Ankle Region
    Left 0YUL
    Right 0YUK
  Anus 0DUQ
  Aorta
    Abdominal 04U0
    Thoracic
      Ascending/Arch 02UX
      Descending 02UW
  Arm
    Lower
      Left 0XUF
      Right 0XUD
    Upper
      Left 0XU9
      Right 0XU8
  Artery
    Anterior Tibial
      Left 04UQ
      Right 04UP
    Axillary
      Left 03U6
      Right 03U5
    Brachial
      Left 03U8
      Right 03U7
    Celiac 04U1
    Colic
      Left 04U7
      Middle 04U8
      Right 04U6
    Common Carotid
      Left 03UJ
      Right 03UH
    Common Iliac
      Left 04UD
      Right 04UC
    External Carotid
      Left 03UN
      Right 03UM
    External Iliac
      Left 04UJ
      Right 04UH
    Face 03UR
    Femoral
      Left 04UL
      Right 04UK
    Foot
      Left 04UW
      Right 04UV

Supplement — *continued*
  Artery — *continued*
    Gastric 04U2
    Hand
      Left 03UF
      Right 03UD
    Hepatic 04U3
    Inferior Mesenteric 04UB
    Innominate 03U2
    Internal Carotid
      Left 03UL
      Right 03UK
    Internal Iliac
      Left 04UF
      Right 04UE
    Internal Mammary
      Left 03U1
      Right 03U0
    Intracranial 03UG
    Lower 04UY
    Peroneal
      Left 04UU
      Right 04UT
    Popliteal
      Left 04UN
      Right 04UM
    Posterior Tibial
      Left 04US
      Right 04UR
    Pulmonary
      Left 02UR
      Right 02UQ
    Pulmonary Trunk 02UP
    Radial
      Left 03UC
      Right 03UB
    Renal
      Left 04UA
      Right 04U9
    Splenic 04U4
    Subclavian
      Left 03U4
      Right 03U3
    Superior Mesenteric 04U5
    Temporal
      Left 03UT
      Right 03US
    Thyroid
      Left 03UV
      Right 03UU
    Ulnar
      Left 03UA
      Right 03U9
    Upper 03UY
    Vertebral
      Left 03UQ
      Right 03UP
  Atrium
    Left 02U7
    Right 02U6
  Auditory Ossicle
    Left 09UA
    Right 09U9
  Axilla
    Left 0XU5
    Right 0XU4
  Back
    Lower 0WUL
    Upper 0WUK
  Bladder 0TUB
  Bladder Neck 0TUC
  Bone
    Ethmoid
      Left 0NUG
      Right 0NUF
    Frontal 0NU1
    Hyoid 0NUX

Supplement — *continued*
  Bone — *continued*
    Lacrimal
      Left 0NUJ
      Right 0NUH
    Nasal 0NUB
    Occipital 0NU7
    Palatine
      Left 0NUL
      Right 0NUK
    Parietal
      Left 0NU4
      Right 0NU3
    Pelvic
      Left 0QU3
      Right 0QU2
    Sphenoid 0NUC
    Temporal
      Left 0NU6
      Right 0NU5
    Zygomatic
      Left 0NUN
      Right 0NUM
  Breast
    Bilateral 0HUV
    Left 0HUU
    Right 0HUT
  Bronchus
    Lingula 0BU9
    Lower Lobe
      Left 0BUB
      Right 0BU6
    Main
      Left 0BU7
      Right 0BU3
    Middle Lobe, Right 0BU5
    Upper Lobe
      Left 0BU8
      Right 0BU4
  Buccal Mucosa 0CU4
  Bursa and Ligament
    Abdomen
      Left 0MUJ
      Right 0MUH
    Ankle
      Left 0MUR
      Right 0MUQ
    Elbow
      Left 0MU4
      Right 0MU3
    Foot
      Left 0MUT
      Right 0MUS
    Hand
      Left 0MU8
      Right 0MU7
    Head and Neck 0MU0
    Hip
      Left 0MUM
      Right 0MUL
    Knee
      Left 0MUP
      Right 0MUN
    Lower Extremity
      Left 0MUW
      Right 0MUV
    Perineum 0MUK
    Rib(s) 0MUG
    Shoulder
      Left 0MU2
      Right 0MU1
    Spine
      Lower 0MUD
      Upper 0MUC
    Sternum 0MUF
    Upper Extremity
      Left 0MUB
      Right 0MU9

Supplement — *continued*
  Bursa and Ligament — *continued*
    Wrist
      Left 0MU6
      Right 0MU5
  Buttock
    Left 0YU1
    Right 0YU0
  Carina 0BU2
  Carpal
    Left 0PUN
    Right 0PUM
  Cecum 0DUH
  Cerebral Meninges 00U1
  Cerebral Ventricle 00U6
  Chest Wall 0WU8
  Chordae Tendineae 02U9
  Cisterna Chyli 07UL
  Clavicle
    Left 0PUB
    Right 0PU9
  Clitoris 0UUJ
  Coccyx 0QUS
  Colon
    Ascending 0DUK
    Descending 0DUM
    Sigmoid 0DUN
    Transverse 0DUL
  Cord
    Bilateral 0VUH
    Left 0VUG
    Right 0VUF
  Cornea
    Left 08U9
    Right 08U8
  Cul-de-sac 0UUF
  Diaphragm 0BUT
  Disc
    Cervical Vertebral 0RU3
    Cervicothoracic Vertebral 0RU5
    Lumbar Vertebral 0SU2
    Lumbosacral 0SU4
    Thoracic Vertebral 0RU9
    Thoracolumbar Vertebral 0RUB
  Duct
    Common Bile 0FU9
    Cystic 0FU8
    Hepatic
      Common 0FU7
      Left 0FU6
      Right 0FU5
    Lacrimal
      Left 08UY
      Right 08UX
    Pancreatic 0FUD
      Accessory 0FUF
  Duodenum 0DU9
  Dura Mater 00U2
  Ear
    External
      Bilateral 09U2
      Left 09U1
      Right 09U0
    Inner
      Left 09UE
      Right 09UD
    Middle
      Left 09U6
      Right 09U5
  Elbow Region
    Left 0XUC
    Right 0XUB
  Epididymis
    Bilateral 0VUL
    Left 0VUK
    Right 0VUJ
  Epiglottis 0CUR

Supplement — *continued*
  Esophagogastric Junction 0DU4
  Esophagus 0DU5
    Lower 0DU3
    Middle 0DU2
    Upper 0DU1
  Extremity
    Lower
      Left 0YUB
      Right 0YU9
    Upper
      Left 0XU7
      Right 0XU6
  Eye
    Left 08U1
    Right 08U0
  Eyelid
    Lower
      Left 08UR
      Right 08UQ
    Upper
      Left 08UP
      Right 08UN
  Face 0WU2
  Fallopian Tube
    Left 0UU6
    Right 0UU5
  Fallopian Tubes, Bilateral 0UU7
  Femoral Region
    Bilateral 0YUE
    Left 0YU8
    Right 0YU7
  Femoral Shaft
    Left 0QU9
    Right 0QU8
  Femur
    Lower
      Left 0QUC
      Right 0QUB
    Upper
      Left 0QU7
      Right 0QU6
  Fibula
    Left 0QUK
    Right 0QUJ
  Finger
    Index
      Left 0XUP
      Right 0XUN
    Little
      Left 0XUW
      Right 0XUV
    Middle
      Left 0XUR
      Right 0XUQ
    Ring
      Left 0XUT
      Right 0XUS
  Foot
    Left 0YUN
    Right 0YUM
  Gingiva
    Lower 0CU6
    Upper 0CU5
  Glenoid Cavity
    Left 0PU8
    Right 0PU7
  Hand
    Left 0XUK
    Right 0XUJ
  Head 0WU0
  Heart 02UA
  Humeral Head
    Left 0PUD
    Right 0PUC
  Humeral Shaft
    Left 0PUG
    Right 0PUF

Supplement — *continued*
  Hymen 0UUK
  Ileocecal Valve 0DUC
  Ileum 0DUB
  Inguinal Region
    Bilateral 0YUA
    Left 0YU6
    Right 0YU5
  Intestine
    Large 0DUE
      Left 0DUG
      Right 0DUF
    Small 0DU8
  Iris
    Left 08UD
    Right 08UC
  Jaw
    Lower 0WU5
    Upper 0WU4
  Jejunum 0DUA
  Joint
    Acromioclavicular
      Left 0RUH
      Right 0RUG
    Ankle
      Left 0SUG
      Right 0SUF
    Carpal
      Left 0RUR
      Right 0RUQ
    Carpometacarpal
      Left 0RUT
      Right 0RUS
    Cervical Vertebral 0RU1
    Cervicothoracic Vertebral 0RU4
    Coccygeal 0SU6
    Elbow
      Left 0RUM
      Right 0RUL
    Finger Phalangeal
      Left 0RUX
      Right 0RUW
    Hip
      Left 0SUB
        Acetabular Surface 0SUE
        Femoral Surface 0SUS
      Right 0SU9
        Acetabular Surface 0SUA
        Femoral Surface 0SUR
    Knee
      Left 0SUD
        Femoral Surface 0SUU09Z
        Tibial Surface 0SUW09Z
      Right 0SUC
        Femoral Surface 0SUT09Z
        Tibial Surface 0SUV09Z
    Lumbar Vertebral 0SU0
    Lumbosacral 0SU3
    Metacarpophalangeal
      Left 0RUV
      Right 0RUU
    Metatarsal-Phalangeal
      Left 0SUN
      Right 0SUM
    Occipital-cervical 0RU0
    Sacrococcygeal 0SU5
    Sacroiliac
      Left 0SU8
      Right 0SU7
    Shoulder
      Left 0RUK
      Right 0RUJ
    Sternoclavicular
      Left 0RUF
      Right 0RUE
    Tarsal
      Left 0SUJ
      Right 0SUH

Supplement — *continued*
- Joint — *continued*
  - Tarsometatarsal
    - Left 0SUL
    - Right 0SUK
  - Temporomandibular
    - Left 0RUD
    - Right 0RUC
  - Thoracic Vertebral 0RU6
  - Thoracolumbar Vertebral 0RUA
  - Toe Phalangeal
    - Left 0SUQ
    - Right 0SUP
  - Wrist
    - Left 0RUP
    - Right 0RUN
- Kidney Pelvis
  - Left 0TU4
  - Right 0TU3
- Knee Region
  - Left 0YUG
  - Right 0YUF
- Larynx 0CUS
- Leg
  - Lower
    - Left 0YUJ
    - Right 0YUH
  - Upper
    - Left 0YUD
    - Right 0YUC
- Lip
  - Lower 0CU1
  - Upper 0CU0
- Lymphatic
  - Aortic 07UD
  - Axillary
    - Left 07U6
    - Right 07U5
  - Head 07U0
  - Inguinal
    - Left 07UJ
    - Right 07UH
  - Internal Mammary
    - Left 07U9
    - Right 07U8
  - Lower Extremity
    - Left 07UG
    - Right 07UF
  - Mesenteric 07UB
  - Neck
    - Left 07U2
    - Right 07U1
  - Pelvis 07UC
  - Thoracic Duct 07UK
  - Thorax 07U7
  - Upper Extremity
    - Left 07U4
    - Right 07U3
- Mandible
  - Left 0NUV
  - Right 0NUT
- Maxilla 0NUR
- Mediastinum 0WUC
- Mesentery 0DUV
- Metacarpal
  - Left 0PUQ
  - Right 0PUP
- Metatarsal
  - Left 0QUP
  - Right 0QUN
- Muscle
  - Abdomen
    - Left 0KUL
    - Right 0KUK
  - Extraocular
    - Left 08UM
    - Right 08UL

Supplement — *continued*
- Muscle — *continued*
  - Facial 0KU1
  - Foot
    - Left 0KUW
    - Right 0KUV
  - Hand
    - Left 0KUD
    - Right 0KUC
  - Head 0KU0
  - Hip
    - Left 0KUP
    - Right 0KUN
  - Lower Arm and Wrist
    - Left 0KUB
    - Right 0KU9
  - Lower Leg
    - Left 0KUT
    - Right 0KUS
  - Neck
    - Left 0KU3
    - Right 0KU2
  - Papillary 02UD
  - Perineum 0KUM
  - Shoulder
    - Left 0KU6
    - Right 0KU5
  - Thorax
    - Left 0KUJ
    - Right 0KUH
  - Tongue, Palate, Pharynx 0KU4
  - Trunk
    - Left 0KUG
    - Right 0KUF
  - Upper Arm
    - Left 0KU8
    - Right 0KU7
  - Upper Leg
    - Left 0KUR
    - Right 0KUQ
- Nasal Mucosa and Soft Tissue 09UK
- Nasopharynx 09UN
- Neck 0WU6
- Nerve
  - Abducens 00UL
  - Accessory 00UR
  - Acoustic 00UN
  - Cervical 01U1
  - Facial 00UM
  - Femoral 01UD
  - Glossopharyngeal 00UP
  - Hypoglossal 00US
  - Lumbar 01UB
  - Median 01U5
  - Oculomotor 00UH
  - Olfactory 00UF
  - Optic 00UG
  - Peroneal 01UH
  - Phrenic 01U2
  - Pudendal 01UC
  - Radial 01U6
  - Sacral 01UR
  - Sciatic 01UF
  - Thoracic 01U8
  - Tibial 01UG
  - Trigeminal 00UK
  - Trochlear 00UJ
  - Ulnar 01U4
  - Vagus 00UQ
- Nipple
  - Left 0HUX
  - Right 0HUW
- Omentum 0DUU
- Orbit
  - Left 0NUQ
  - Right 0NUP

Supplement — *continued*
- Palate
  - Hard 0CU2
  - Soft 0CU3
- Patella
  - Left 0QUF
  - Right 0QUD
- Penis 0VUS
- Pericardium 02UN
- Perineum
  - Female 0WUN
  - Male 0WUM
- Peritoneum 0DUW
- Phalanx
  - Finger
    - Left 0PUV
    - Right 0PUT
  - Thumb
    - Left 0PUS
    - Right 0PUR
  - Toe
    - Left 0QUR
    - Right 0QUQ
- Pharynx 0CUM
- Prepuce 0VUT
- Radius
  - Left 0PUJ
  - Right 0PUH
- Rectum 0DUP
- Retina
  - Left 08UF
  - Right 08UE
- Retinal Vessel
  - Left 08UH
  - Right 08UG
- Ribs
  - 1 to 2 0PU1
  - 3 or More 0PU2
- Sacrum 0QU1
- Scapula
  - Left 0PU6
  - Right 0PU5
- Scrotum 0VU5
- Septum
  - Atrial 02U5
  - Nasal 09UM
  - Ventricular 02UM
- Shoulder Region
  - Left 0XU3
  - Right 0XU2
- Skull 0NU0
- Spinal Meninges 00UT
- Sternum 0PU0
- Stomach 0DU6
  - Pylorus 0DU7
- Subcutaneous Tissue and Fascia
  - Abdomen 0JU8
  - Back 0JU7
  - Buttock 0JU9
  - Chest 0JU6
  - Face 0JU1
  - Foot
    - Left 0JUR
    - Right 0JUQ
  - Hand
    - Left 0JUK
    - Right 0JUJ
  - Lower Arm
    - Left 0JUH
    - Right 0JUG
  - Lower Leg
    - Left 0JUP
    - Right 0JUN
  - Neck
    - Left 0JU5
    - Right 0JU4
  - Pelvic Region 0JUC

Supplement — *continued*
  Subcutaneous Tissue and Fascia — *continued*
    Perineum 0JUB
    Scalp 0JU0
    Upper Arm
      Left 0JUF
      Right 0JUD
    Upper Leg
      Left 0JUM
      Right 0JUL
  Tarsal
    Left 0QUM
    Right 0QUL
  Tendon
    Abdomen
      Left 0LUG
      Right 0LUF
    Ankle
      Left 0LUT
      Right 0LUS
    Foot
      Left 0LUW
      Right 0LUV
    Hand
      Left 0LU8
      Right 0LU7
    Head and Neck 0LU0
    Hip
      Left 0LUK
      Right 0LUJ
    Knee
      Left 0LUR
      Right 0LUQ
    Lower Arm and Wrist
      Left 0LU6
      Right 0LU5
    Lower Leg
      Left 0LUP
      Right 0LUN
    Perineum 0LUH
    Shoulder
      Left 0LU2
      Right 0LU1
    Thorax
      Left 0LUD
      Right 0LUC
    Trunk
      Left 0LUB
      Right 0LU9
    Upper Arm
      Left 0LU4
      Right 0LU3
    Upper Leg
      Left 0LUM
      Right 0LUL
  Testis
    Bilateral 0VUC0
    Left 0VUB0
    Right 0VU90
  Thumb
    Left 0XUM
    Right 0XUL
  Tibia
    Left 0QUH
    Right 0QUG
  Toe
    1st
      Left 0YUQ
      Right 0YUP
    2nd
      Left 0YUS
      Right 0YUR
    3rd
      Left 0YUU
      Right 0YUT
    4th
      Left 0YUW

Supplement — *continued*
  Toe — *continued*
      Right 0YUV
    5th
      Left 0YUY
      Right 0YUX
  Tongue 0CU7
  Trachea 0BU1
  Tunica Vaginalis
    Left 0VU7
    Right 0VU6
  Turbinate, Nasal 09UL
  Tympanic Membrane
    Left 09U8
    Right 09U7
  Ulna
    Left 0PUL
    Right 0PUK
  Ureter
    Left 0TU7
    Right 0TU6
  Urethra 0TUD
  Uterine Supporting Structure 0UU4
  Uvula 0CUN
  Vagina 0UUG
  Valve
    Aortic 02UF
    Mitral 02UG
    Pulmonary 02UH
    Tricuspid 02UJ
  Vas Deferens
    Bilateral 0VUQ
    Left 0VUP
    Right 0VUN
  Vein
    Axillary
      Left 05U8
      Right 05U7
    Azygos 05U0
    Basilic
      Left 05UC
      Right 05UB
    Brachial
      Left 05UA
      Right 05U9
    Cephalic
      Left 05UF
      Right 05UD
    Colic 06U7
    Common Iliac
      Left 06UD
      Right 06UC
    Esophageal 06U3
    External Iliac
      Left 06UG
      Right 06UF
    External Jugular
      Left 05UQ
      Right 05UP
    Face
      Left 05UV
      Right 05UT
    Femoral
      Left 06UN
      Right 06UM
    Foot
      Left 06UV
      Right 06UT
    Gastric 06U2
    Hand
      Left 05UH
      Right 05UG
    Hemiazygos 05U1
    Hepatic 06U4
    Hypogastric
      Left 06UJ
      Right 06UH

Supplement — *continued*
  Vein — *continued*
    Inferior Mesenteric 06U6
    Innominate
      Left 05U4
      Right 05U3
    Internal Jugular
      Left 05UN
      Right 05UM
    Intracranial 05UL
    Lower 06UY
    Portal 06U8
    Pulmonary
      Left 02UT
      Right 02US
    Renal
      Left 06UB
      Right 06U9
    Saphenous
      Left 06UQ
      Right 06UP
    Splenic 06U1
    Subclavian
      Left 05U6
      Right 05U5
    Superior Mesenteric 06U5
    Upper 05UY
    Vertebral
      Left 05US
      Right 05UR
  Vena Cava
    Inferior 06U0
    Superior 02UV
  Ventricle
    Left 02UL
    Right 02UK
  Vertebra
    Cervical 0PU3
    Lumbar 0QU0
    Thoracic 0PU4
  Vesicle
    Bilateral 0VU3
    Left 0VU2
    Right 0VU1
  Vocal Cord
    Left 0CUV
    Right 0CUT
  Vulva 0UUM
  Wrist Region
    Left 0XUH
    Right 0XUG

Supraclavicular (Virchow's) lymph node
  use Lymphatic, Right Neck
  use Lymphatic, Left Neck
Supraclavicular nerve
  use Cervical Plexus
Suprahyoid lymph node
  use Lymphatic, Head
Suprahyoid muscle
  use Neck Muscle, Right
  use Neck Muscle, Left
Suprainguinal lymph node
  use Lymphatic, Pelvis
Supraorbital vein
  use Face Vein, Right
  use Face Vein, Left
Suprarenal gland
  use Adrenal Gland, Left
  use Adrenal Gland, Right
  use Adrenal Glands, Bilateral
  use Adrenal Gland
Suprarenal plexus
  use Abdominal Sympathetic Nerve
Suprascapular nerve
  use Brachial Plexus

Supraspinatus fascia
use Subcutaneous Tissue and Fascia, Right Upper Arm
use Subcutaneous Tissue and Fascia, Left Upper Arm
Supraspinatus muscle
use Shoulder Muscle, Right
use Shoulder Muscle, Left
Supraspinous ligament
use Upper Spine Bursa and Ligament
use Lower Spine Bursa and Ligament
Suprasternal notch
use Sternum
Supratrochlear lymph node
use Lymphatic, Right Upper Extremity
use Lymphatic, Left Upper Extremity
Sural artery
use Popliteal Artery, Right
use Popliteal Artery, Left
Suspension
Bladder Neck *see* Reposition, Bladder Neck 0TSC
Kidney *see* Reposition, Urinary System 0TS
Urethra *see* Reposition, Urinary System 0TS
Urethrovesical *see* Reposition, Bladder Neck 0TSC
Uterus *see* Reposition, Uterus 0US9
Vagina *see* Reposition, Vagina 0USG
Suture
Laceration repair *see* Repair
Ligation *see* Occlusion
Suture Removal
Extremity
Lower 8E0YXY8
Upper 8E0XXY8
Head and Neck Region 8E09XY8
Trunk Region 8E0WXY8
Sutureless valve, Perceval
use Zooplastic Tissue, Rapid Deployment Technique in New Technology
Sweat gland
use Skin
Sympathectomy
see Excision, Peripheral Nervous System 01B
SynCardia™ Total Artificial Heart
use Synthetic Substitute
Synchra™ CRT-P
use Cardiac Resynchronization Pacemaker Pulse Generator in 0JH
SynchroMed® pump
use Infusion Device, Pump in Subcutaneous Tissue and Fascia
Synechiotomy, iris
see Release, Eye 08N
Synovectomy
Lower joint *see* Excision, Lower Joints 0SB
Upper joint *see* Excision, Upper Joints 0RB
Systemic Nuclear Medicine Therapy
Abdomen CW70
Anatomical Regions, Multiple CW7YYZZ
Chest CW73
Thyroid CW7G
Whole Body CW7N

T

Takedown
Arteriovenous shunt *see* Removal of device from, Upper Arteries 03P
Arteriovenous shunt, with creation of new shunt *see* Bypass, Upper Arteries 031
Stoma
see Excision
see Reposition

Talent® Converter
use Intraluminal Device
Talent® Occluder
use Intraluminal Device
Talent® Stent Graft (abdominal)(thoracic)
use Intraluminal Device
Talocalcaneal (subtalar) joint
use Tarsal Joint, Right
use Tarsal Joint, Left
Talocalcaneal ligament
use Foot Bursa and Ligament, Right
use Foot Bursa and Ligament, Left
Talocalcaneonavicular joint
use Tarsal Joint, Right
use Tarsal Joint, Left
Talocalcaneonavicular ligament
use Foot Bursa and Ligament, Right
use Foot Bursa and Ligament, Left
Talocrural joint
use Ankle Joint, Right
use Ankle Joint, Left
Talofibular ligament
use Ankle Bursa and Ligament, Right
use Ankle Bursa and Ligament, Left
Talus bone
use Tarsal, Right
use Tarsal, Left
TandemHeart® System
use Short-term External Heart Assist System in Heart and Great Vessels
Tarsectomy
see Excision, Lower Bones 0QB
see Resection, Lower Bones 0QT
Tarsometatarsal ligament
use Foot Bursa and Ligament, Right
use Foot Bursa and Ligament, Left
Tarsorrhaphy
see Repair, Eye 08Q
Tattooing
Cornea 3E0CXMZ
Skin *see* Introduction of substance in or on, Skin 3E00
TAXUS® Liberte® Paclitaxel-eluting Coronary Stent System
use Intraluminal Device, Drug-eluting in Heart and Great Vessels
TBNA (transbronchial needle aspiration)
see Drainage, Respiratory System 0B9
Telemetry
4A12X4Z
Ambulatory 4A12X45
Temperature gradient study 4A0ZXKZ
Temporal lobe
use Cerebral Hemisphere
Temporalis muscle
use Head Muscle
Temporoparietalis muscle
use Head Muscle
Tendolysis
see Release, Tendons 0LN
Tendonectomy
see Excision, Tendons 0LB
see Resection, Tendons 0LT
Tendonoplasty, tenoplasty
see Repair, Tendons 0LQ
see Replacement, Tendons 0LR
see Supplement, Tendons 0LU
Tendorrhaphy
see Repair, Tendons 0LQ
Tendototomy
see Division, Tendons 0L8
see Drainage, Tendons 0L9
Tenectomy, tenonectomy
see Excision, Tendons 0LB
see Resection, Tendons 0LT
Tenolysis
see Release, Tendons 0LN

Tenontorrhaphy
see Repair, Tendons 0LQ
Tenontotomy
see Division, Tendons 0L8
see Drainage, Tendons 0L9
Tenorrhaphy
see Repair, Tendons 0LQ
Tenosynovectomy
see Excision, Tendons 0LB
see Resection, Tendons 0LT
Tenotomy
see Division, Tendons 0L8
see Drainage, Tendons 0L9
Tensor fasciae latae muscle
use Hip Muscle, Right
use Hip Muscle, Left
Tensor veli palatini muscle
use Tongue, Palate, Pharynx Muscle
Tenth cranial nerve
use Vagus Nerve
Tentorium cerebelli
use Dura Mater
Teres major muscle
use Shoulder Muscle, Right
use Shoulder Muscle, Left
Teres minor muscle
use Shoulder Muscle, Right
use Shoulder Muscle, Left
Termination of pregnancy
Aspiration curettage 10A07ZZ
Dilation and curettage 10A07ZZ
Hysterotomy 10A00ZZ
Intra-amniotic injection 10A03ZZ
Laminaria 10A07ZW
Vacuum 10A07Z6
Testectomy
see Excision, Male Reproductive System 0VB
see Resection, Male Reproductive System 0VT
Testicular artery
use Abdominal Aorta
Testing
Glaucoma 4A07XBZ
Hearing *see* Hearing Assessment, Diagnostic Audiology F13
Mental health *see* Psychological Tests
Muscle function, electromyography (EMG) *see* Measurement, Musculoskeletal 4A0F
Muscle function, manual *see* Motor Function Assessment, Rehabilitation F01
Neurophysiologic monitoring, intraoperative *see* Monitoring, Physiological Systems 4A1
Range of motion *see* Motor Function Assessment, Rehabilitation F01
Vestibular function *see* Vestibular Assessment, Diagnostic Audiology F15
Thalamectomy
see Excision, Thalamus 00B9
Thalamotomy
see Drainage, Thalamus 0099
Thenar muscle
use Hand Muscle, Right
use Hand Muscle, Left
Therapeutic Massage
Musculoskeletal System 8E0KX1Z
Reproductive System
Prostate 8E0VX1C
Rectum 8E0VX1D
Therapeutic occlusion coil(s)
use Intraluminal Device
Thermography 4A0ZXKZ
Thermotherapy, prostate
see Destruction, Prostate 0V50
Third cranial nerve
use Oculomotor Nerve

Third occipital nerve
  use Cervical Nerve

Third ventricle
  use Cerebral Ventricle

Thoracectomy
  see Excision, Anatomical Regions, General 0WB

Thoracentesis
  see Drainage, Anatomical Regions, General 0W9

Thoracic aortic plexus
  use Thoracic Sympathetic Nerve

Thoracic esophagus
  use Esophagus, Middle

Thoracic facet joint
  use Thoracic Vertebral Joint

Thoracic ganglion
  use Thoracic Sympathetic Nerve

Thoracoacromial artery
  use Axillary Artery, Right
  use Axillary Artery, Left

Thoracocentesis
  see Drainage, Anatomical Regions, General 0W9

Thoracolumbar facet joint
  use Thoracolumbar Vertebral Joint

Thoracoplasty
  see Repair, Anatomical Regions, General 0WQ
  see Supplement, Anatomical Regions, General 0WU

Thoracostomy tube
  use Drainage Device

Thoracostomy, for lung collapse
  see Drainage, Respiratory System 0B9

Thoracotomy
  see Drainage, Anatomical Regions, General 0W9

Thoratec® IVAD (Implantable Ventricular Assist Device)
  use Implantable Heart Assist System in Heart and Great Vessels

Thoratec Paracorporeal Ventricular Assist Device
  use Short-term External Heart Assist System in Heart and Great Vessels

Thrombectomy
  see Extirpation

Thymectomy
  see Excision, Lymphatic and Hemic Systems 07B
  see Resection, Lymphatic and Hemic Systems 07T

Thymopexy
  see Repair, Lymphatic and Hemic Systems 07Q
  see Reposition, Lymphatic and Hemic Systems 07S

Thymus gland
  use Thymus

Thyroarytenoid muscle
  use Neck Muscle, Right
  use Neck Muscle, Left

Thyrocervical trunk
  use Thyroid Artery, Right
  use Thyroid Artery, Left

Thyroid cartilage
  use Larynx

Thyroidectomy
  see Excision, Endocrine System 0GB
  see Resection, Endocrine System 0GT

Thyroidorrhaphy
  see Repair, Endocrine System 0GQ

Thyroidoscopy 0GJK4ZZ

Thyroidotomy
  see Drainage, Endocrine System 0G9

Tibial insert
  use Liner in Lower Joints

Tibialis anterior muscle
  use Lower Leg Muscle, Right
  use Lower Leg Muscle, Left

Tibialis posterior muscle
  use Lower Leg Muscle, Right
  use Lower Leg Muscle, Left

Tibiofemoral joint
  use Knee Joint, Right
  use Knee Joint, Left
  use Knee Joint, Tibial Surface, Right
  use Knee Joint, Tibial Surface, Left

Tissue bank graft
  use Nonautologous Tissue Substitute

Tissue Expander
  Insertion of device in
    Breast
      Bilateral 0HHV
      Left 0HHU
      Right 0HHT
    Nipple
      Left 0HHX
      Right 0HHW
    Subcutaneous Tissue and Fascia
      Abdomen 0JH8
      Back 0JH7
      Buttock 0JH9
      Chest 0JH6
      Face 0JH1
      Foot
        Left 0JHR
        Right 0JHQ
      Hand
        Left 0JHK
        Right 0JHJ
      Lower Arm
        Left 0JHH
        Right 0JHG
      Lower Leg
        Left 0JHP
        Right 0JHN
      Neck
        Left 0JH5
        Right 0JH4
      Pelvic Region 0JHC
      Perineum 0JHB
      Scalp 0JH0
      Upper Arm
        Left 0JHF
        Right 0JHD
      Upper Leg
        Left 0JHM
        Right 0JHL
  Removal of device from
    Breast
      Left 0HPU
      Right 0HPT
    Subcutaneous Tissue and Fascia
      Head and Neck 0JPS
      Lower Extremity 0JPW
      Trunk 0JPT
      Upper Extremity 0JPV
  Revision of device in
    Breast
      Left 0HWU
      Right 0HWT
    Subcutaneous Tissue and Fascia
      Head and Neck 0JWS
      Lower Extremity 0JWW
      Trunk 0JWT
      Upper Extremity 0JWV

Tissue expander (inflatable)(injectable)
  use Tissue Expander in Skin and Breast
  use Tissue Expander in Subcutaneous Tissue and Fascia

Tissue Plasminogen Activator (tPA)(r-tPA)
  use Other Thrombolytic

Titanium Sternal Fixation System (TSFS)
  use Internal Fixation Device, Rigid Plate in 0PH
  use Internal Fixation Device, Rigid Plate in 0PS

Tomographic (Tomo) Nuclear Medicine Imaging
  Abdomen CW20
  Abdomen and Chest CW24
  Abdomen and Pelvis CW21
  Anatomical Regions, Multiple CW2YYZZ
  Bladder, Kidneys and Ureters CT23
  Brain C020
  Breast CH2YYZZ
    Bilateral CH22
    Left CH21
    Right CH20
  Bronchi and Lungs CB22
  Central Nervous System C02YYZZ
  Cerebrospinal Fluid C025
  Chest CW23
  Chest and Abdomen CW24
  Chest and Neck CW26
  Digestive System CD2YYZZ
  Endocrine System CG2YYZZ
  Extremity
    Lower CW2D
      Bilateral CP2F
      Left CP2D
      Right CP2C
    Upper CW2M
      Bilateral CP2B
      Left CP29
      Right CP28
  Gallbladder CF24
  Gastrointestinal Tract CD27
  Gland, Parathyroid CG21
  Head and Neck CW2B
  Heart C22YYZZ
    Right and Left C226
  Hepatobiliary System and Pancreas CF2YYZZ
  Kidneys, Ureters and Bladder CT23
  Liver CF25
  Liver and Spleen CF26
  Lungs and Bronchi CB22
  Lymphatics and Hematologic System C72YYZZ
  Musculoskeletal System, Other CP2YYZZ
  Myocardium C22G
  Neck and Chest CW26
  Neck and Head CW2B
  Pancreas and Hepatobiliary System CF2YYZZ
  Pelvic Region CW2J
  Pelvis CP26
  Pelvis and Abdomen CW21
  Pelvis and Spine CP27
  Respiratory System CB2YYZZ
  Skin CH2YYZZ
  Skull CP21
  Skull and Cervical Spine CP23
  Spine
    Cervical CP22
    Cervical and Skull CP23
    Lumbar CP2H
    Thoracic CP2G
    Thoracolumbar CP2J
  Spine and Pelvis CP27
  Spleen C722
  Spleen and Liver CF26
  Subcutaneous Tissue CH2YYZZ
  Thorax CP24
  Ureters, Kidneys and Bladder CT23
  Urinary System CT2YYZZ

Tomography, computerized
  see Computerized Tomography (CT Scan)
Tongue, base of
  use Pharynx
Tonometry 4A07XBZ
Tonsillectomy
  see Excision, Mouth and Throat 0CB
  see Resection, Mouth and Throat 0CT
Tonsillotomy
  see Drainage, Mouth and Throat 0C9
Total Anomalous Pulmonary Venous Return (TAPVR) repair
  see Bypass, Atrium, Left 0217
  see Bypass, Vena Cava, Superior 021V
Total artificial (replacement) heart
  use Synthetic Substitute
Total parenteral nutrition (TPN)
  see Introduction of Nutritional Substance
Trachectomy
  see Excision, Trachea 0BB1
  see Resection, Trachea 0BT1
Trachelectomy
  see Excision, Cervix 0UBC
  see Resection, Cervix 0UTC
Trachelopexy
  see Repair, Cervix 0UQC
  see Reposition, Cervix 0USC
Tracheloplasty
  see Repair, Cervix 0UQC
Trachelorrhaphy
  see Repair, Cervix 0UQC
Trachelotomy
  see Drainage, Cervix 0U9C
Tracheobronchial lymph node
  use Lymphatic, Thorax
Tracheoesophageal fistulization 0B110D6
Tracheolysis
  see Release, Respiratory System 0BN
Tracheoplasty
  see Repair, Respiratory System 0BQ
  see Supplement, Respiratory System 0BU
Tracheorrhaphy
  see Repair, Respiratory System 0BQ
Tracheoscopy 0BJ18ZZ
Tracheostomy
  see Bypass, Respiratory System 0B1
Tracheostomy Device
  Bypass, Trachea 0B11
  Change device in, Trachea 0B21XFZ
  Removal of device from, Trachea 0BP1
  Revision of device in, Trachea 0BW1
Tracheostomy tube
  use Tracheostomy Device in Respiratory System
Tracheotomy
  see Drainage, Respiratory System 0B9
Traction
  Abdominal Wall 2W63X
  Arm
    Lower
      Left 2W6DX
      Right 2W6CX
    Upper
      Left 2W6BX
      Right 2W6AX
  Back 2W65X
  Chest Wall 2W64X
  Extremity
    Lower
      Left 2W6MX
      Right 2W6LX
    Upper
      Left 2W69X
      Right 2W68X
  Face 2W61X

Traction — *continued*
  Finger
    Left 2W6KX
    Right 2W6JX
  Foot
    Left 2W6TX
    Right 2W6SX
  Hand
    Left 2W6FX
    Right 2W6EX
  Head 2W60X
  Inguinal Region
    Left 2W67X
    Right 2W66X
  Leg
    Lower
      Left 2W6RX
      Right 2W6QX
    Upper
      Left 2W6PX
      Right 2W6NX
  Neck 2W62X
  Thumb
    Left 2W6HX
    Right 2W6GX
  Toe
    Left 2W6VX
    Right 2W6UX
Tractotomy
  see Division, Central Nervous System and Cranial Nerves 008
Tragus
  use External Ear, Right
  use External Ear, Left
  use External Ear, Bilateral
Training, caregiver
  see Caregiver Training
TRAM (transverse rectus abdominis myocutaneous) flap reconstruction
  Free *see* Replacement, Skin and Breast 0HR
  Pedicled *see* Transfer, Muscles 0KX
Transection
  see Division
Transfer
  Buccal Mucosa 0CX4
  Bursa and Ligament
    Abdomen
      Left 0MXJ
      Right 0MXH
    Ankle
      Left 0MXR
      Right 0MXQ
    Elbow
      Left 0MX4
      Right 0MX3
    Foot
      Left 0MXT
      Right 0MXS
    Hand
      Left 0MX8
      Right 0MX7
    Head and Neck 0MX0
    Hip
      Left 0MXM
      Right 0MXL
    Knee
      Left 0MXP
      Right 0MXN
    Lower Extremity
      Left 0MXW
      Right 0MXV
    Perineum 0MXK
    Rib(s) 0MXG
    Shoulder
      Left 0MX2
      Right 0MX1

Transfer — *continued*
  Bursa and Ligament — *continued*
    Spine
      Lower 0MXD
      Upper 0MXC
    Sternum 0MXF
    Upper Extremity
      Left 0MXB
      Right 0MX9
    Wrist
      Left 0MX6
      Right 0MX5
  Finger
    Left 0XXP0ZM
    Right 0XXN0ZL
  Gingiva
    Lower 0CX6
    Upper 0CX5
  Intestine
    Large 0DXE
    Small 0DX8
  Lip
    Lower 0CX1
    Upper 0CX0
  Muscle
    Abdomen
      Left 0KXL
      Right 0KXK
    Extraocular
      Left 08XM
      Right 08XL
    Facial 0KX1
    Foot
      Left 0KXW
      Right 0KXV
    Hand
      Left 0KXD
      Right 0KXC
    Head 0KX0
    Hip
      Left 0KXP
      Right 0KXN
    Lower Arm and Wrist
      Left 0KXB
      Right 0KX9
    Lower Leg
      Left 0KXT
      Right 0KXS
    Neck
      Left 0KX3
      Right 0KX2
    Perineum 0KXM
    Shoulder
      Left 0KX6
      Right 0KX5
    Thorax
      Left 0KXJ
      Right 0KXH
    Tongue, Palate, Pharynx 0KX4
    Trunk
      Left 0KXG
      Right 0KXF
    Upper Arm
      Left 0KX8
      Right 0KX7
    Upper Leg
      Left 0KXR
      Right 0KXQ
  Nerve
    Abducens 00XL
    Accessory 00XR
    Acoustic 00XN
    Cervical 01X1
    Facial 00XM
    Femoral 01XD
    Glossopharyngeal 00XP
    Hypoglossal 00XS

Transfer — *continued*
  Nerve — *continued*
    Lumbar 01XB
    Median 01X5
    Oculomotor 00XH
    Olfactory 00XF
    Optic 00XG
    Peroneal 01XH
    Phrenic 01X2
    Pudendal 01XC
    Radial 01X6
    Sciatic 01XF
    Thoracic 01X8
    Tibial 01XG
    Trigeminal 00XK
    Trochlear 00XJ
    Ulnar 01X4
    Vagus 00XQ
  Palate, Soft 0CX3
  Skin
    Abdomen 0HX7XZZ
    Back 0HX6XZZ
    Buttock 0HX8XZZ
    Chest 0HX5XZZ
    Ear
      Left 0HX3XZZ
      Right 0HX2XZZ
    Face 0HX1XZZ
    Foot
      Left 0HXNXZZ
      Right 0HXMXZZ
    Hand
      Left 0HXGXZZ
      Right 0HXFXZZ
    Inguinal 0HXAXZZ
    Lower Arm
      Left 0HXEXZZ
      Right 0HXDXZZ
    Lower Leg
      Left 0HXLXZZ
      Right 0HXKXZZ
    Neck 0HX4XZZ
    Perineum 0HX9XZZ
    Scalp 0HX0XZZ
    Upper Arm
      Left 0HXCXZZ
      Right 0HXBXZZ
    Upper Leg
      Left 0HXJXZZ
      Right 0HXHXZZ
  Stomach 0DX6
  Subcutaneous Tissue and Fascia
    Abdomen 0JX8
    Back 0JX7
    Buttock 0JX9
    Chest 0JX6
    Face 0JX1
    Foot
      Left 0JXR
      Right 0JXQ
    Hand
      Left 0JXK
      Right 0JXJ
    Lower Arm
      Left 0JXH
      Right 0JXG
    Lower Leg
      Left 0JXP
      Right 0JXN
    Neck
      Left 0JX5
      Right 0JX4
    Pelvic Region 0JXC
    Perineum 0JXB
    Scalp 0JX0
    Upper Arm
      Left 0JXF

Transfer — *continued*
  Subcutaneous Tissue and Fascia — *continued*
    Right 0JXD
    Upper Leg
      Left 0JXM
      Right 0JXL
  Tendon
    Abdomen
      Left 0LXG
      Right 0LXF
    Ankle
      Left 0LXT
      Right 0LXS
    Foot
      Left 0LXW
      Right 0LXV
    Hand
      Left 0LX8
      Right 0LX7
    Head and Neck 0LX0
    Hip
      Left 0LXK
      Right 0LXJ
    Knee
      Left 0LXR
      Right 0LXQ
    Lower Arm and Wrist
      Left 0LX6
      Right 0LX5
    Lower Leg
      Left 0LXP
      Right 0LXN
    Perineum 0LXH
    Shoulder
      Left 0LX2
      Right 0LX1
    Thorax
      Left 0LXD
      Right 0LXC
    Trunk
      Left 0LXB
      Right 0LX9
    Upper Arm
      Left 0LX4
      Right 0LX3
    Upper Leg
      Left 0LXM
      Right 0LXL
  Tongue 0CX7

Transfusion
  Artery
    Central
      Antihemophilic Factors 3026
      Blood
        Platelets 3026
        Red Cells 3026
          Frozen 3026
        White Cells 3026
        Whole 3026
      Bone Marrow 3026
      Factor IX 3026
      Fibrinogen 3026
      Globulin 3026
      Plasma
        Fresh 3026
        Frozen 3026
      Plasma Cryoprecipitate 3026
      Serum Albumin 3026
      Stem Cells
        Cord Blood 3026
        Hematopoietic 3026
    Peripheral
      Antihemophilic Factors 3025
      Blood
        Platelets 3025
        Red Cells 3025
          Frozen 3025

Transfusion — *continued*
  Artery — *continued*
        White Cells 3025
        Whole 3025
      Bone Marrow 3025
      Factor IX 3025
      Fibrinogen 3025
      Globulin 3025
      Plasma
        Fresh 3025
        Frozen 3025
      Plasma Cryoprecipitate 3025
      Serum Albumin 3025
      Stem Cells
        Cord Blood 3025
        Hematopoietic 3025
  Products of Conception
    Antihemophilic Factors 3027
    Blood
      Platelets 3027
      Red Cells 3027
        Frozen 3027
      White Cells 3027
      Whole 3027
    Factor IX 3027
    Fibrinogen 3027
    Globulin 3027
    Plasma
      Fresh 3027
      Frozen 3027
    Plasma Cryoprecipitate 3027
    Serum Albumin 3027
  Vein
    4-Factor Prothrombin Complex Concentrate 3028
    Central
      Antihemophilic Factors 3024
      Blood
        Platelets 3024
        Red Cells 3024
          Frozen 3024
        White Cells 3024
        Whole 3024
      Bone Marrow 3024
      Factor IX 3024
      Fibrinogen 3024
      Globulin 3024
      Plasma
        Fresh 3024
        Frozen 3024
      Plasma Cryoprecipitate 3024
      Serum Albumin 3024
      Stem Cells
        Cord Blood 3024
        Embryonic 3024
        Hematopoietic 3024
    Peripheral
      Antihemophilic Factors 3023
      Blood
        Platelets 3023
        Red Cells 3023
          Frozen 3023
        White Cells 3023
        Whole 3023
      Bone Marrow 3023
      Factor IX 3023
      Fibrinogen 3023
      Globulin 3023
      Plasma
        Fresh 3023
        Frozen 3023
      Plasma Cryoprecipitate 3023
      Serum Albumin 3023
      Stem Cells
        Cord Blood 3023
        Embryonic 3023
        Hematopoietic 3023

Transplant
  see Transplantation
Transplantation
  Bone marrow *see* Transfusion,
    Circulatory 302
  Esophagus 0DY50Z
  Face 0WY20Z
  Hand
    Left 0XYK0Z
    Right 0XYJ0Z
  Heart 02YA0Z
  Hematopoietic cell *see* Transfusion,
    Circulatory 302
  Intestine
    Large 0DYE0Z
    Small 0DY80Z
  Kidney
    Left 0TY10Z
    Right 0TY00Z
  Liver 0FY00Z
  Lung
    Bilateral 0BYM0Z
    Left 0BYL0Z
    Lower Lobe
      Left 0BYJ0Z
      Right 0BYF0Z
    Middle Lobe, Right 0BYD0Z
    Right 0BYK0Z
    Upper Lobe
      Left 0BYG0Z
      Right 0BYC0Z
  Lung Lingula 0BYH0Z
  Ovary
    Left 0UY10Z
    Right 0UY00Z
  Pancreas 0FYG0Z
  Products of Conception 10Y0
  Spleen 07YP0Z
  Stem cell *see* Transfusion, Circulatory 302
  Stomach 0DY60Z
  Thymus 07YM0Z
Transposition
  see Bypass
  see Reposition
  see Transfer
Transversalis fascia
  use Subcutaneous Tissue and Fascia, Trunk
Transverse (cutaneous) cervical nerve
  use Cervical Plexus
Transverse acetabular ligament
  use Hip Bursa and Ligament, Right
  use Hip Bursa and Ligament, Left
Transverse facial artery
  use Temporal Artery, Right
  use Temporal Artery, Left
Transverse foramen
  use Cervical Vertebra
Transverse humeral ligament
  use Shoulder Bursa and Ligament, Right
  use Shoulder Bursa and Ligament, Left
Transverse ligament of atlas
  use Head and Neck Bursa and Ligament
Transverse process
  use Cervical Vertebra
  use Thoracic Vertebra
  use Lumbar Vertebra
Transverse Rectus Abdominis
  Myocutaneous Flap
  Replacement
    Bilateral 0HRV076
    Left 0HRU076
    Right 0HRT076
  Transfer
    Left 0KXL
    Right 0KXK

Transverse scapular ligament
  use Shoulder Bursa and Ligament, Right
  use Shoulder Bursa and Ligament, Left
Transverse thoracis muscle
  use Thorax Muscle, Right
  use Thorax Muscle, Left
Transversospinalis muscle
  use Trunk Muscle, Right
  use Trunk Muscle, Left
Transversus abdominis muscle
  use Abdomen Muscle, Right
  use Abdomen Muscle, Left
Trapezium bone
  use Carpal, Right
  use Carpal, Left
Trapezius muscle
  use Trunk Muscle, Right
  use Trunk Muscle, Left
Trapezoid bone
  use Carpal, Right
  use Carpal, Left
Triceps brachii muscle
  use Upper Arm Muscle, Right
  use Upper Arm Muscle, Left
Tricuspid annulus
  use Tricuspid Valve
Trifacial nerve
  use Trigeminal Nerve
Trifecta™ Valve (aortic)
  use Zooplastic Tissue in Heart and Great
    Vessels
Trigone of bladder
  use Bladder
Trimming, excisional
  see Excision
Triquetral bone
  use Carpal, Right
  use Carpal, Left
Trochanteric bursa
  use Hip Bursa and Ligament, Right
  use Hip Bursa and Ligament, Left
TUMT (Transurethral microwave
  thermotherapy of prostate) 0V507ZZ
TUNA (transurethral needle ablation of
  prostate) 0V507ZZ
Tunneled central venous catheter
  use Vascular Access Device, Tunneled in
    Subcutaneous Tissue and Fascia
Tunneled spinal (intrathecal) catheter
  use Infusion Device
Turbinectomy
  see Excision, Ear, Nose, Sinus 09B
  see Resection, Ear, Nose, Sinus 09T
Turbinoplasty
  see Repair, Ear, Nose, Sinus 09Q
  see Replacement, Ear, Nose, Sinus 09R
  see Supplement, Ear, Nose, Sinus 09U
Turbinotomy
  see Division, Ear, Nose, Sinus 098
  see Drainage, Ear, Nose, Sinus 099
TURP (transurethral resection of prostate)
  see Excision, Prostate 0VB0
  see Resection, Prostate 0VT0
Twelfth cranial nerve
  use Hypoglossal Nerve
Two lead pacemaker
  use Pacemaker, Dual Chamber in 0JH
Tympanic cavity
  use Middle Ear, Right
  use Middle Ear, Left
Tympanic nerve
  use Glossopharyngeal Nerve
Tympanic part of temporal bone
  use Temporal Bone, Right
  use Temporal Bone, Left

Tympanogram
  see Hearing Assessment, Diagnostic
    Audiology F13
Tympanoplasty
  see Repair, Ear, Nose, Sinus 09Q
  see Replacement, Ear, Nose, Sinus 09R
  see Supplement, Ear, Nose, Sinus 09U
Tympanosympathectomy
  see Excision, Nerve, Head and Neck
    Sympathetic 01BK
Tympanotomy
  see Drainage, Ear, Nose, Sinus 099

U

Ulnar collateral carpal ligament
  use Wrist Bursa and Ligament, Right
  use Wrist Bursa and Ligament, Left
Ulnar collateral ligament
  use Elbow Bursa and Ligament, Right
  use Elbow Bursa and Ligament, Left
Ulnar notch
  use Radius, Right
  use Radius, Left
Ulnar vein
  use Brachial Vein, Right
  use Brachial Vein, Left
Ultrafiltration
  Hemodialysis *see* Performance,
    Urinary 5A1D
  Therapeutic plasmapheresis *see* Pheresis,
    Circulatory 6A55
Ultraflex™ Precision Colonic Stent System
  use Intraluminal Device
ULTRAPRO® Hernia System (UHS)
  use Synthetic Substitute
ULTRAPRO® Partially Absorbable
  Lightweight Mesh
  use Synthetic Substitute
ULTRAPRO® Plug
  use Synthetic Substitute
Ultrasonic osteogenic stimulator
  use Bone Growth Stimulator in Head and
    Facial Bones
  use Bone Growth Stimulator in Upper
    Bones
  use Bone Growth Stimulator in Lower
    Bones
Ultrasonography
  Abdomen BW40ZZZ
  Abdomen and Pelvis BW41ZZZ
  Abdominal Wall BH49ZZZ
  Aorta
    Abdominal, Intravascular B440ZZ3
    Thoracic, Intravascular B340ZZ3
  Appendix BD48ZZZ
  Artery
    Brachiocephalic-Subclavian, Right,
      Intravascular B341ZZ3
    Celiac and Mesenteric,
      Intravascular B44KZZ3
    Common Carotid
      Bilateral, Intravascular B345ZZ3
      Left, Intravascular B344ZZ3
      Right, Intravascular B343ZZ3
    Coronary
      Multiple B241YZZ
        Intravascular B241ZZ3
        Transesophageal B241ZZ4
      Single B240YZZ
        Intravascular B240ZZ3
        Transesophageal B240ZZ4
    Femoral, Intravascular B44LZZ3
    Inferior Mesenteric,
      Intravascular B445ZZ3

Ultrasonography — *continued*
 Artery — *continued*
  Internal Carotid
   Bilateral, Intravascular B348ZZ3
   Left, Intravascular B347ZZ3
   Right, Intravascular B346ZZ3
  Intra-Abdominal, Other,
   Intravascular B44BZZ3
  Intracranial, Intravascular B34RZZ3
  Lower Extremity
   Bilateral, Intravascular B44HZZ3
   Left, Intravascular B44GZZ3
   Right, Intravascular B44FZZ3
  Mesenteric and Celiac,
   Intravascular B44KZZ3
  Ophthalmic, Intravascular B34VZZ3
  Penile, Intravascular B44NZZ3
  Pulmonary
   Left, Intravascular B34TZZ3
   Right, Intravascular B34SZZ3
  Renal
   Bilateral, Intravascular B448ZZ3
   Left, Intravascular B447ZZ3
   Right, Intravascular B446ZZ3
  Subclavian, Left, Intravascular B342ZZ3
  Superior Mesenteric,
   Intravascular B444ZZ3
  Upper Extremity
   Bilateral, Intravascular B34KZZ3
   Left, Intravascular B34JZZ3
   Right, Intravascular B34HZZ3
 Bile Duct BF40ZZZ
 Bile Duct and Gallbladder BF43ZZZ
 Bladder BT40ZZZ
  and Kidney BT4JZZZ
 Brain B040ZZZ
 Breast
  Bilateral BH42ZZZ
  Left BH41ZZZ
  Right BH40ZZZ
 Chest Wall BH4BZZZ
 Coccyx BR4FZZZ
 Connective Tissue
  Lower Extremity BL41ZZZ
  Upper Extremity BL40ZZZ
 Duodenum BD49ZZZ
 Elbow
  Left, Densitometry BP4HZZ1
  Right, Densitometry BP4GZZ1
 Esophagus BD41ZZZ
 Extremity
  Lower BH48ZZZ
  Upper BH47ZZZ
 Eye
  Bilateral B847ZZZ
  Left B846ZZZ
  Right B845ZZZ
 Fallopian Tube
  Bilateral BU42
  Left BU41
  Right BU40
 Fetal Umbilical Cord BY47ZZZ
 Fetus
  First Trimester, Multiple
   Gestation BY4BZZZ
  Second Trimester, Multiple
   Gestation BY4DZZZ
  Single
   First Trimester BY49ZZZ
   Second Trimester BY4CZZZ
   Third Trimester BY4FZZZ
  Third Trimester, Multiple
   Gestation BY4GZZZ
 Gallbladder BF42ZZZ
 Gallbladder and Bile Duct BF43ZZZ
 Gastrointestinal Tract BD47ZZZ

Ultrasonography — *continued*
 Gland
  Adrenal
   Bilateral BG42ZZZ
   Left BG41ZZZ
   Right BG40ZZZ
  Parathyroid BG43ZZZ
  Thyroid BG44ZZZ
 Hand
  Left, Densitometry BP4PZZ1
  Right, Densitometry BP4NZZ1
 Head and Neck BH4CZZZ
 Heart
  Left B245YZZ
   Intravascular B245ZZ3
   Transesophageal B245ZZ4
  Pediatric B24DYZZ
   Intravascular B24DZZ3
   Transesophageal B24DZZ4
  Right B244YZZ
   Intravascular B244ZZ3
   Transesophageal B244ZZ4
  Right and Left B246YZZ
   Intravascular B246ZZ3
   Transesophageal B246ZZ4
 Heart with Aorta B24BYZZ
  Intravascular B24BZZ3
  Transesophageal B24BZZ4
 Hepatobiliary System, All BF4CZZZ
 Hip
  Bilateral BQ42ZZZ
  Left BQ41ZZZ
  Right BQ40ZZZ
 Kidney
  and Bladder BT4JZZZ
  Bilateral BT43ZZZ
  Left BT42ZZZ
  Right BT41ZZZ
  Transplant BT49ZZZ
 Knee
  Bilateral BQ49ZZZ
  Left BQ48ZZZ
  Right BQ47ZZZ
 Liver BF45ZZZ
 Liver and Spleen BF46ZZZ
 Mediastinum BB4CZZZ
 Neck BW4FZZZ
 Ovary
  Bilateral BU45
  Left BU44
  Right BU43
 Ovary and Uterus BU4C
 Pancreas BF47ZZZ
 Pelvic Region BW4GZZZ
 Pelvis and Abdomen BW41ZZZ
 Penis BV4BZZZ
 Pericardium B24CYZZ
  Intravascular B24CZZ3
  Transesophageal B24CZZ4
 Placenta BY48ZZZ
 Pleura BB4BZZZ
 Prostate and Seminal Vesicle BV49ZZZ
 Rectum BD4CZZZ
 Sacrum BR4FZZZ
 Scrotum BV44ZZZ
 Seminal Vesicle and Prostate BV49ZZZ
 Shoulder
  Left, Densitometry BP49ZZ1
  Right, Densitometry BP48ZZ1
 Spinal Cord B04BZZZ
 Spine
  Cervical BR40ZZZ
  Lumbar BR49ZZZ
  Thoracic BR47ZZZ
 Spleen and Liver BF46ZZZ
 Stomach BD42ZZZ

Ultrasonography — *continued*
 Tendon
  Lower Extremity BL43ZZZ
  Upper Extremity BL42ZZZ
 Ureter
  Bilateral BT48ZZZ
  Left BT47ZZZ
  Right BT46ZZZ
 Urethra BT45ZZZ
 Uterus BU46
 Uterus and Ovary BU4C
 Vein
  Jugular
   Left, Intravascular B544ZZ3
   Right, Intravascular B543ZZ3
  Lower Extremity
   Bilateral, Intravascular B54DZZ3
   Left, Intravascular B54CZZ3
   Right, Intravascular B54BZZ3
  Portal, Intravascular B54TZZ3
  Renal
   Bilateral, Intravascular B54LZZ3
   Left, Intravascular B54KZZ3
   Right, Intravascular B54JZZ3
  Splanchnic, Intravascular B54TZZ3
  Subclavian
   Left, Intravascular B547ZZ3
   Right, Intravascular B546ZZ3
  Upper Extremity
   Bilateral, Intravascular B54PZZ3
   Left, Intravascular B54NZZ3
   Right, Intravascular B54MZZ3
 Vena Cava
  Inferior, Intravascular B549ZZ3
  Superior, Intravascular B548ZZ3
 Wrist
  Left, Densitometry BP4MZZ1
  Right, Densitometry BP4LZZ1
Ultrasound bone healing system
 use Bone Growth Stimulator in Head and
  Facial Bones
 use Bone Growth Stimulator in Upper
  Bones
 use Bone Growth Stimulator in Lower
  Bones
Ultrasound Therapy
 Heart 6A75
 No Qualifier 6A75
 Vessels
  Head and Neck 6A75
  Other 6A75
  Peripheral 6A75
Ultraviolet Light Therapy, Skin 6A80
Umbilical artery
 use Internal Iliac Artery, Right
 use Internal Iliac Artery, Left
 use Lower Artery
Uniplanar external fixator
 use External Fixation Device, Monoplanar
  in 0PH
 use External Fixation Device, Monoplanar
  in 0PS
 use External Fixation Device, Monoplanar
  in 0QH
 use External Fixation Device, Monoplanar
  in 0QS
Upper GI series
 see Fluoroscopy, Gastrointestinal,
  Upper BD15
Ureteral orifice
 use Ureter, Right
 use Ureter, Left
 use Ureters, Bilateral
 use Ureter
Ureterectomy
 see Excision, Urinary System 0TB
 see Resection, Urinary System 0TT

Ureterocolostomy
  see Bypass, Urinary System 0T1
Ureterocystostomy
  see Bypass, Urinary System 0T1
Ureteroenterostomy
  see Bypass, Urinary System 0T1
Ureteroileostomy
  see Bypass, Urinary System 0T1
Ureterolithotomy
  see Extirpation, Urinary System 0TC
Ureterolysis
  see Release, Urinary System 0TN
Ureteroneocystostomy
  see Bypass, Urinary System 0T1
  see Reposition, Urinary System 0TS
Ureteropelvic junction (UPJ)
  use Kidney Pelvis, Right
  use Kidney Pelvis, Left
Ureteropexy
  see Repair, Urinary System 0TQ
  see Reposition, Urinary System 0TS
Ureteroplasty
  see Repair, Urinary System 0TQ
  see Replacement, Urinary System 0TR
  see Supplement, Urinary System 0TU
Ureteroplication
  see Restriction, Urinary System 0TV
Ureteropyelography
  see Fluoroscopy, Urinary System BT1
Ureterorrhaphy
  see Repair, Urinary System 0TQ
Ureteroscopy 0TJ98ZZ
Ureterostomy
  see Bypass, Urinary System 0T1
  see Drainage, Urinary System 0T9
Ureterotomy
  see Drainage, Urinary System 0T9
Ureteroureterostomy
  see Bypass, Urinary System 0T1
Ureterovesical orifice
  use Ureter, Right
  use Ureter, Left
  use Ureters, Bilateral
  use Ureter
Urethral catheterization, indwelling
  0T9B70Z
Urethrectomy
  see Excision, Urethra 0TBD
  see Resection, Urethra 0TTD
Urethrolithotomy
  see Extirpation, Urethra 0TCD
Urethrolysis
  see Release, Urethra 0TND
Urethropexy
  see Repair, Urethra 0TQD
  see Reposition, Urethra 0TSD
Urethroplasty
  see Repair, Urethra 0TQD
  see Replacement, Urethra 0TRD
  see Supplement, Urethra 0TUD
Urethrorrhaphy
  see Repair, Urethra 0TQD
Urethroscopy 0TJD8ZZ
Urethrotomy
  see Drainage, Urethra 0T9D
Uridine Triacetate XW0DX82
Urinary incontinence stimulator lead
  use Stimulator Lead in Urinary System
Urography
  see Fluoroscopy, Urinary System BT1
Ustekinumab
  use Other New Technology Therapeutic
  Substance
Uterine Artery
  use Internal Iliac Artery, Right
  use Internal Iliac Artery, Left

Uterine artery embolization (UAE)
  see Occlusion, Lower Arteries 04L
Uterine cornu
  use Uterus
Uterine tube
  use Fallopian Tube, Right
  use Fallopian Tube, Left
Uterine vein
  use Hypogastric Vein, Right
  use Hypogastric Vein, Left
Uvulectomy
  see Excision, Uvula 0CBN
  see Resection, Uvula 0CTN
Uvulorrhaphy
  see Repair, Uvula 0CQN
Uvulotomy
  see Drainage, Uvula 0C9N

V

Vaccination
  see Introduction of Serum, Toxoid, and
  Vaccine
Vacuum extraction, obstetric 10D07Z6
Vaginal artery
  use Internal Iliac Artery, Right
  use Internal Iliac Artery, Left
Vaginal pessary
  use Intraluminal Device, Pessary in Female
  Reproductive System
Vaginal vein
  use Hypogastric Vein, Right
  use Hypogastric Vein, Left
Vaginectomy
  see Excision, Vagina 0UBG
  see Resection, Vagina 0UTG
Vaginofixation
  see Repair, Vagina 0UQG
  see Reposition, Vagina 0USG
Vaginoplasty
  see Repair, Vagina 0UQG
  see Supplement, Vagina 0UUG
Vaginorrhaphy
  see Repair, Vagina 0UQG
Vaginoscopy 0UJH8ZZ
Vaginotomy
  see Drainage, Female Reproductive
  System 0U9
Vagotomy
  see Division, Nerve, Vagus 008Q
Valiant® Thoracic Stent Graft
  use Intraluminal Device
Valvotomy, valvulotomy
  see Division, Heart and Great Vessels 028
  see Release, Heart and Great Vessels 02N
Valvuloplasty
  see Repair, Heart and Great Vessels 02Q
  see Replacement, Heart and Great
  Vessels 02R
  see Supplement, Heart and Great
  Vessels 02U
Valvuloplasty, Alfieri Stitch
  see Restriction, Valve, Mitral 02VG
Vascular Access Device
  Totally Implantable
   Insertion of device in
    Abdomen 0JH8
    Chest 0JH6
    Lower Arm
     Left 0JHH
     Right 0JHG
    Lower Leg
     Left 0JHP
     Right 0JHN
    Upper Arm

Vascular Access Device — *continued*
  Totally Implantable — *continued*
     Left 0JHF
     Right 0JHD
    Upper Leg
     Left 0JHM
     Right 0JHL
   Removal of device from
    Lower Extremity 0JPW
    Trunk 0JPT
    Upper Extremity 0JPV
   Revision of device in
    Lower Extremity 0JWW
    Trunk 0JWT
    Upper Extremity 0JWV
  Tunneled
   Insertion of device in
    Abdomen 0JH8
    Chest 0JH6
    Lower Arm
     Left 0JHH
     Right 0JHG
    Lower Leg
     Left 0JHP
     Right 0JHN
    Upper Arm
     Left 0JHF
     Right 0JHD
    Upper Leg
     Left 0JHM
     Right 0JHL
   Removal of device from
    Lower Extremity 0JPW
    Trunk 0JPT
    Upper Extremity 0JPV
   Revision of device in
    Lower Extremity 0JWW
    Trunk 0JWT
    Upper Extremity 0JWV
Vasectomy
  see Excision, Male Reproductive System 0VB
Vasography
  see Plain Radiography, Male Reproductive
  System BV0
  see Fluoroscopy, Male Reproductive
  System BV1
Vasoligation
  see Occlusion, Male Reproductive
  System 0VL
Vasorrhaphy
  see Repair, Male Reproductive System 0VQ
Vasostomy
  see Bypass, Male Reproductive System 0V1
Vasotomy
  Drainage *see* Drainage, Male Reproductive
  System 0V9
  With ligation *see* Occlusion, Male
  Reproductive System 0VL
Vasovasostomy
  see Repair, Male Reproductive System 0VQ
Vastus intermedius muscle
  use Upper Leg Muscle, Right
  use Upper Leg Muscle, Left
Vastus lateralis muscle
  use Upper Leg Muscle, Right
  use Upper Leg Muscle, Left
Vastus medialis muscle
  use Upper Leg Muscle, Right
  use Upper Leg Muscle, Left
VCG (vectorcardiogram)
  see Measurement, Cardiac 4A02
Vectra® Vascular Access Graft
  use Vascular Access Device, Tunneled in
  Subcutaneous Tissue and Fascia
Venectomy
  see Excision, Upper Veins 05B
  see Excision, Lower Veins 06B

Venography
  see Plain Radiography, Veins B50
  see Fluoroscopy, Veins B51
Venorrhaphy
  see Repair, Upper Veins 05Q
  see Repair, Lower Veins 06Q
Venotripsy
  see Occlusion, Upper Veins 05L
  see Occlusion, Lower Veins 06L
Ventricular fold
  use Larynx
Ventriculoatriostomy
  see Bypass, Central Nervous System and
    Cranial Nerves 001
Ventriculocisternostomy
  see Bypass, Central Nervous System and
    Cranial Nerves 001
Ventriculogram, cardiac
  Combined left and right heart *see*
    Fluoroscopy, Heart, Right and Left B216
  Left ventricle *see* Fluoroscopy, Heart,
    Left B215
  Right ventricle *see* Fluoroscopy, Heart,
    Right B214
Ventriculopuncture, through previously
  implanted catheter 8C01X6J
Ventriculoscopy 00J04ZZ
Ventriculostomy
  External drainage *see* Drainage, Cerebral
    Ventricle 0096
  Internal shunt *see* Bypass, Cerebral
    Ventricle 0016
Ventriculovenostomy
  see Bypass, Cerebral Ventricle 0016
Ventrio™ Hernia Patch
  use Synthetic Substitute
VEP (visual evoked potential) 4A07X0Z
Vermiform appendix
  use Appendix
Vermilion border
  use Upper Lip
  use Lower Lip
Versa®
  use Pacemaker, Dual Chamber in 0JH
Version, obstetric
  External 10S0XZZ
  Internal 10S07ZZ
Vertebral arch
  use Cervical Vertebra
  use Thoracic Vertebra
  use Lumbar Vertebra
Vertebral body
  use Cervical Vertebra
  use Thoracic Vertebra
  use Lumbar Vertebra
Vertebral canal
  use Spinal Canal
Vertebral foramen
  use Cervical Vertebra
  use Thoracic Vertebra
  use Lumbar Vertebra
Vertebral lamina
  use Cervical Vertebra
  use Thoracic Vertebra
  use Lumbar Vertebra
Vertebral pedicle
  use Cervical Vertebra
  use Thoracic Vertebra
  use Lumbar Vertebra
Vesical vein
  use Hypogastric Vein, Right
  use Hypogastric Vein, Left
Vesicotomy
  see Drainage, Urinary System 0T9
Vesiculectomy
  see Excision, Male Reproductive
    System 0VB

Vesiculectomy — *continued*
  see Resection, Male Reproductive
    System 0VT
Vesiculogram, seminal
  see Plain Radiography, Male Reproductive
    System BV0
Vesiculotomy
  see Drainage, Male Reproductive
    System 0V9
Vestibular (Scarpa's) ganglion
  use Acoustic Nerve
Vestibular Assessment F15Z
Vestibular nerve
  use Acoustic Nerve
Vestibular Treatment F0C
Vestibulocochlear nerve
  use Acoustic Nerve
VH-IVUS (virtual histology intravascular ultrasound)
  see Ultrasonography, Heart B24
Virchow's (supraclavicular) lymph node
  use Lymphatic, Right Neck
  use Lymphatic, Left Neck
Virtuoso® (II) (DR) (VR)
  use Defibrillator Generator in 0JH
Vistogard®
  use Uridine Triacetate
Vitrectomy
  see Excision, Eye 08B
  see Resection, Eye 08T
Vitreous body
  use Vitreous, Right
  use Vitreous, Left
Viva™ (XT)(S)
  use Cardiac Resynchronization Defibrillator
    Pulse Generator in 0JH
Vocal fold
  use Vocal Cord, Right
  use Vocal Cord, Left
Vocational
  Assessment *see* Activities of Daily Living
    Assessment, Rehabilitation F02
  Retraining *see* Activities of Daily Living
    Treatment, Rehabilitation F08
Volar (palmar) digital vein
  use Hand Vein, Right
  use Hand Vein, Left
Volar (palmar) metacarpal vein
  use Hand Vein, Right
  use Hand Vein, Left
Vomer bone
  use Nasal Septum
Vomer of nasal septum
  use Nasal Bone
Voraxaze®
  use Glucarpidase
Vulvectomy
  see Excision, Female Reproductive
    System 0UB
  see Resection, Female Reproductive
    System 0UT
VYXEOS™
  use Cytarabine and Daunorubicin
    Liposome Antineoplastic

W

WALLSTENT® Endoprosthesis
  use Intraluminal Device
Washing
  see Irrigation
Wedge resection, pulmonary
  see Excision, Respiratory System 0BB
Window
  see Drainage
Wiring, dental 2W31X9Z

X

X-ray
  see Plain Radiography
X-STOP® Spacer
  use Spinal Stabilization Device,
    Interspinous Process in 0RH
  use Spinal Stabilization Device,
    Interspinous Process in 0SH
Xact® Carotid Stent System
  use Intraluminal Device
Xenograft
  use Zooplastic Tissue in Heart and Great
    Vessels
XIENCE™ Everolimus Eluting Coronary Stent System
  use Intraluminal Device, Drug-eluting in
    Heart and Great Vessels
Xiphoid process
  use Sternum
XLIF® System
  use Interbody Fusion Device in Lower
    Joints

Y

Yoga Therapy 8E0ZXY4

Z

Z-plasty, skin for scar contracture
  see Release, Skin and Breast 0HN
Zenith® AAA Endovascular Graft
  use Intraluminal Device, Branched or
    Fenestrated, One or Two Arteries in 04V
  use Intraluminal Device, Branched or
    Fenestrated, Three or More Arteries in 04V
  use Intraluminal Device
Zenith Flex® AAA Endovascular Graft
  use Intraluminal Device
Zenith TX2® TAA Endovascular Graft
  use Intraluminal Device
Zenith® Renu™ AAA Ancillary Graft
  use Intraluminal Device
Zilver® PTX® (paclitaxel) Drug-Eluting Peripheral Stent
  use Intraluminal Device, Drug-eluting in
    Upper Arteries
  use Intraluminal Device, Drug-eluting in
    Lower Arteries
Zimmer® NexGen® LPS Mobile Bearing Knee
  use Synthetic Substitute
Zimmer® NexGen® LPS-Flex Mobile Knee
  use Synthetic Substitute
ZINPLAVA™
  use Bezlotoxumab Monoclonal Antibody
Zonule of Zinn
  use Lens, Right
  use Lens, Left
Zooplastic Tissue, Rapid Deployment Technique, Replacement X2RF
Zotarolimus-eluting coronary stent
  use Intraluminal Device, Drug-eluting in
    Heart and Great Vessels
Zygomatic process of frontal bone
  use Frontal Bone
Zygomatic process of temporal bone
  use Temporal Bone, Right
  use Temporal Bone, Left
Zygomaticus muscle
  use Facial Muscle
Zyvox®
  use Oxazolidinones

This page intentionally left blank

ICD-10-PCS Tables

Medical and Surgical 001-0YW

Central Nervous System and Cranial Nerves 001-00X

0   **Medical and Surgical**
0   **Central Nervous System** and Cranial Nerves
1   **Bypass:** Altering the route of passage of the contents of a tubular body part

Body Part	Approach	Device	Qualifier
Character 4	Character 5	Character 6	Character 7
6 Cerebral Ventricle	**0** Open **3** Percutaneous **4** Percutaneous Endoscopic	**7** Autologous Tissue Substitute **J** Synthetic Substitute **K** Nonautologous Tissue Substitute	**0** Nasopharynx **1** Mastoid Sinus **2** Atrium **3** Blood Vessel **4** Pleural Cavity **5** Intestine **6** Peritoneal Cavity **7** Urinary Tract **8** Bone Marrow **B** Cerebral Cisterns
6 Cerebral Ventricle	**0** Open **3** Percutaneous **4** Percutaneous Endoscopic	**Z** No Device	**B** Cerebral Cisterns
U Spinal Canal	**0** Open **3** Percutaneous	**7** Autologous Tissue Substitute **J** Synthetic Substitute **K** Nonautologous Tissue Substitute	**4** Pleural Cavity **6** Peritoneal Cavity **7** Urinary Tract **9** Fallopian Tube

0   **Medical and Surgical**
0   **Central Nervous System** and Cranial Nerves
2   **Change:** Taking out or off a device from a body part and putting back an identical or similar device in or on the same body part without cutting or puncturing the skin or a mucous membrane

Body Part	Approach	Device	Qualifier
Character 4	Character 5	Character 6	Character 7
0 Brain **E** Cranial Nerve **U** Spinal Canal	**X** External	**0** Drainage Device **Y** Other Device	**Z** No Qualifier

LC Limited Coverage   **NC** Noncovered   **HAC** HAC-associated Procedure   **CC** Combination Cluster - See Appendix G for code lists
DRG Non-OR-Affecting MS-DRG Assignment   New/Revised Text in **Orange**   ♂ Male   ♀ Female

2018 ICD-10-PCS

159

CENTRAL NERVOUS SYSTEM AND CRANIAL NERVES 001-00X

0   Medical and Surgical
0   Central Nervous System and Cranial Nerves
5   Destruction: Physical eradication of all or a portion of a body part by the direct use of energy, force, or a destructive agent

Body Part	Approach	Device	Qualifier
Character 4	Character 5	Character 6	Character 7
0 Brain **1** Cerebral Meninges **2** Dura Mater **6** Cerebral Ventricle **7** Cerebral Hemisphere **8** Basal Ganglia **9** Thalamus **A** Hypothalamus **B** Pons **C** Cerebellum **D** Medulla Oblongata **F** Olfactory Nerve **G** Optic Nerve **H** Oculomotor Nerve **J** Trochlear Nerve **K** Trigeminal Nerve **L** Abducens Nerve **M** Facial Nerve **N** Acoustic Nerve **P** Glossopharyngeal Nerve **Q** Vagus Nerve **R** Accessory Nerve **S** Hypoglossal Nerve **T** Spinal Meninges **W** Cervical Spinal Cord **X** Thoracic Spinal Cord **Y** Lumbar Spinal Cord	**0** Open **3** Percutaneous **4** Percutaneous Endoscopic	**Z** No Device	**Z** No Qualifier

0   Medical and Surgical
0   Central Nervous System and Cranial Nerves
7   Change: Expanding an orifice or the lumen of a tubular body part

Body Part	Approach	Device	Qualifier
Character 4	Character 5	Character 6	Character 7
6 Cerebral Ventricle	**0** Open **3** Percutaneous **4** Percutaneous Endoscopic	Z No Device	Z No Qualifier

0   Medical and Surgical
0   Central Nervous System and Cranial Nerves
8   Division: Cutting into a body part, without draining fluids and/or gases from the body part, in order to separate or transect a body part

Body Part	Approach	Device	Qualifier
Character 4	Character 5	Character 6	Character 7
0 Brain **7** Cerebral Hemisphere **8** Basal Ganglia **F** Olfactory Nerve **G** Optic Nerve **H** Oculomotor Nerve **J** Trochlear Nerve **K** Trigeminal Nerve **L** Abducens Nerve **M** Facial Nerve **N** Acoustic Nerve **P** Glossopharyngeal Nerve **Q** Vagus Nerve **R** Accessory Nerve **S** Hypoglossal Nerve **W** Cervical Spinal Cord **X** Thoracic Spinal Cord **Y** Lumbar Spinal Cord	**0** Open **3** Percutaneous **4** Percutaneous Endoscopic	**Z** No Device	**Z** No Qualifier

LC Limited Coverage   **NC** Noncovered   **HAC** HAC-associated Procedure   **CC** Combination Cluster - See Appendix G for code lists
DRG Non-OR-Affecting MS-DRG Assignment   New/Revised Text in **Orange**   ♂ Male   ♀ Female

160   **2018 ICD-10-PCS**

0 Medical and Surgical
0 Central Nervous System and Cranial Nerves
9 Drainage: Taking or letting out fluids and/or gases from a body part

Body Part	Approach	Device	Qualifier
Character 4	Character 5	Character 6	Character 7
0 Brain **1** Cerebral Meninges **2** Dura Mater **3** Epidural Space, Intracranial **4** Subdural Space, Intracranial **5** Subarachnoid Space, Intracranial **6** Cerebral Ventricle **7** Cerebral Hemisphere **8** Basal Ganglia **9** Thalamus **A** Hypothalamus **B** Pons **C** Cerebellum **D** Medulla Oblongata **F** Olfactory Nerve **G** Optic Nerve **H** Oculomotor Nerve **J** Trochlear Nerve **K** Trigeminal Nerve **L** Abducens Nerve **M** Facial Nerve **N** Acoustic Nerve **P** Glossopharyngeal Nerve **Q** Vagus Nerve **R** Accessory Nerve **S** Hypoglossal Nerve **T** Spinal Meninges **U** Spinal Canal **W** Cervical Spinal Cord **X** Thoracic Spinal Cord **Y** Lumbar Spinal Cord	**0** Open **3** Percutaneous **4** Percutaneous Endoscopic	**0** Drainage Device	**Z** No Qualifier
0 Brain **1** Cerebral Meninges **2** Dura Mater **3** Epidural Space, Intracranial **4** Subdural Space, Intracranial **5** Subarachnoid Space, Intracranial **6** Cerebral Ventricle **7** Cerebral Hemisphere **8** Basal Ganglia **9** Thalamus **A** Hypothalamus **B** Pons **C** Cerebellum **D** Medulla Oblongata **F** Olfactory Nerve **G** Optic Nerve **H** Oculomotor Nerve **J** Trochlear Nerve **K** Trigeminal Nerve **L** Abducens Nerve **M** Facial Nerve **N** Acoustic Nerve **P** Glossopharyngeal Nerve **Q** Vagus Nerve **R** Accessory Nerve **S** Hypoglossal Nerve **T** Spinal Meninges **U** Spinal Canal **W** Cervical Spinal Cord **X** Thoracic Spinal Cord **Y** Lumbar Spinal Cord	**0** Open **3** Percutaneous **4** Percutaneous Endoscopic	**Z** No Device	**X** Diagnostic **Z** No Qualifier

LC Limited Coverage NC Noncovered HAC HAC-associated Procedure CC Combination Cluster - See Appendix G for code lists
DRG Non-OR-Affecting MS-DRG Assignment New/Revised Text in **Orange** ♂ Male ♀ Female

0 **Medical and Surgical**
0 **Central Nervous System** and Cranial Nerves
B **Excision:** Cutting out or off, without replacement, a portion of a body part

Body Part	Approach	Device	Qualifier
Character 4	Character 5	Character 6	Character 7
0 Brain 1 Cerebral Meninges 2 Dura Mater 6 Cerebral Ventricle 7 Cerebral Hemisphere 8 Basal Ganglia 9 Thalamus A Hypothalamus B Pons C Cerebellum D Medulla Oblongata F Olfactory Nerve G Optic Nerve H Oculomotor Nerve J Trochlear Nerve K Trigeminal Nerve L Abducens Nerve M Facial Nerve N Acoustic Nerve P Glossopharyngeal Nerve Q Vagus Nerve R Accessory Nerve S Hypoglossal Nerve T Spinal Meninges W Cervical Spinal Cord X Thoracic Spinal Cord Y Lumbar Spinal Cord	0 Open 3 Percutaneous 4 Percutaneous Endoscopic	Z No Device	X Diagnostic Z No Qualifier

LC Limited Coverage   **NC** Noncovered   **HAC** HAC-associated Procedure   **CC** Combination Cluster - See Appendix G for code lists
DRG Non-OR-Affecting MS-DRG Assignment   New/Revised Text in **Orange**   ♂ Male   ♀ Female

162

2018 ICD-10-PCS

CENTRAL NERVOUS SYSTEM AND CRANIAL NERVES 001-00X

0 **Medical and Surgical**
0 **Central Nervous System** and Cranial Nerves
C **Extirpation:** Taking or cutting out solid matter from a body part

Body Part	Approach	Device	Qualifier
Character 4	Character 5	Character 6	Character 7
0 Brain 1 Cerebral Meninges 2 Dura Mater 3 Epidural Space, Intracranial 4 Subdural Space, Intracranial 5 Subarachnoid Space, Intracranial 6 Cerebral Ventricle 7 Cerebral Hemisphere 8 Basal Ganglia 9 Thalamus A Hypothalamus B Pons C Cerebellum D Medulla Oblongata F Olfactory Nerve G Optic Nerve H Oculomotor Nerve J Trochlear Nerve K Trigeminal Nerve L Abducens Nerve M Facial Nerve N Acoustic Nerve P Glossopharyngeal Nerve Q Vagus Nerve R Accessory Nerve S Hypoglossal Nerve T Spinal Meninges U Spinal Canal W Cervical Spinal Cord X Thoracic Spinal Cord Y Lumbar Spinal Cord	0 Open 3 Percutaneous 4 Percutaneous Endoscopic	Z No Device	Z No Qualifier

0 **Medical and Surgical**
0 **Central Nervous System** and Cranial Nerves
D **Extraction:** Pulling or stripping out or off all or a portion of a body part by the use of force

Body Part	Approach	Device	Qualifier
Character 4	Character 5	Character 6	Character 7
1 Cerebral Meninges 2 Dura Mater F Olfactory Nerve G Optic Nerve H Oculomotor Nerve J Trochlear Nerve K Trigeminal Nerve L Abducens Nerve M Facial Nerve N Acoustic Nerve P Glossopharyngeal Nerve Q Vagus Nerve R Accessory Nerve S Hypoglossal Nerve T Spinal Meninges	0 Open 3 Percutaneous 4 Percutaneous Endoscopic	Z No Device	Z No Qualifier

0 **Medical and Surgical**
0 **Central Nervous System** and Cranial Nerves
F **Fragmentation:** Breaking solid matter in a body part into pieces

Body Part	Approach	Device	Qualifier
Character 4	Character 5	Character 6	Character 7
3 Epidural Space, Intracranial NC 4 Subdural Space, Intracranial NC 5 Subarachnoid Space, Intracranial NC 6 Cerebral Ventricle NC U Spinal Canal	0 Open 3 Percutaneous 4 Percutaneous Endoscopic X External	Z No Device	Z No Qualifier

NC 00F3XZZ   00F4XZZ   00F5XZZ   00F6XZZ

0 **Medical and Surgical**
0 **Central Nervous System** and Cranial Nerves
H **Insertion:** Putting in a nonbiological appliance that monitors, assists, performs, or prevents a physiological function but does not physically take the place of a body part

Body Part	Approach	Device	Qualifier
Character 4	Character 5	Character 6	Character 7
0 Brain CC	0 Open	2 Monitoring Device 3 Infusion Device 4 Radioactive Element, Cesium-131 Collagen Implant M Neurostimulator Lead Y Other Device	Z No Qualifier
0 Brain CC	3 Percutaneous 4 Percutaneous Endoscopic	2 Monitoring Device 3 Infusion Device M Neurostimulator Lead Y Other Device	Z No Qualifier
6 Cerebral Ventricle CC E Cranial Nerve CC U Spinal Canal CC V Spinal Cord CC	0 Open 3 Percutaneous 4 Percutaneous Endoscopic	2 Monitoring Device 3 Infusion Device M Neurostimulator Lead Y Other Device	Z No Qualifier

CC 00H00MZ   00H03MZ   00H04MZ   00H60MZ   00H63MZ   00H64MZ   00HE0MZ   00HE3MZ   00HE4MZ   00HU0MZ   00HU3MZ   00HU4MZ   00HV0MZ   00HV3MZ   00HV4MZ

0 **Medical and Surgical**
0 **Central Nervous System** and Cranial Nerves
J **Inspection:** Visually and/or manually exploring a body part

Body Part	Approach	Device	Qualifier
Character 4	Character 5	Character 6	Character 7
0 Brain ORG E Cranial Nerve U Spinal Canal ORG V Spinal Cord ORG	0 Open 3 Percutaneous 4 Percutaneous Endoscopic	Z No Device	Z No Qualifier

ORG 00J03ZZ   00JU3ZZ   00JV3ZZ

LC Limited Coverage   NC Noncovered   HAC HAC-associated Procedure   CC Combination Cluster - See Appendix G for code lists
ORG Non-OR-Affecting MS-DRG Assignment   New/Revised Text in **Orange**   ♂ Male   ♀ Female

164

2018 ICD-10-PCS

CENTRAL NERVOUS SYSTEM AND CRANIAL NERVES 001-00X

0 **Medical and Surgical**
0 **Central Nervous System** and Cranial Nerves
K **Map:** Locating the route of passage of electrical impulses and/or locating functional areas in a body part

Body Part	Approach	Device	Qualifier
Character 4	Character 5	Character 6	Character 7
0 Brain **7** Cerebral Hemisphere **8** Basal Ganglia **9** Thalamus **A** Hypothalamus **B** Pons **C** Cerebellum **D** Medulla Oblongata	**0** Open **3** Percutaneous **4** Percutaneous Endoscopic	**Z** No Device	**Z** No Qualifier

0 **Medical and Surgical**
0 **Central Nervous System** and Cranial Nerves
N **Release:** Freeing a body part from an abnormal physical constraint by cutting or by the use of force

Body Part	Approach	Device	Qualifier
Character 4	Character 5	Character 6	Character 7
0 Brain **1** Cerebral Meninges **2** Dura Mater **6** Cerebral Ventricle **7** Cerebral Hemisphere **8** Basal Ganglia **9** Thalamus **A** Hypothalamus **B** Pons **C** Cerebellum **D** Medulla Oblongata **F** Olfactory Nerve **G** Optic Nerve **H** Oculomotor Nerve **J** Trochlear Nerve **K** Trigeminal Nerve **L** Abducens Nerve **M** Facial Nerve **N** Acoustic Nerve **P** Glossopharyngeal Nerve **Q** Vagus Nerve **R** Accessory Nerve **S** Hypoglossal Nerve **T** Spinal Meninges **W** Cervical Spinal Cord **X** Thoracic Spinal Cord **Y** Lumbar Spinal Cord	**0** Open **3** Percutaneous **4** Percutaneous Endoscopic	**Z** No Device	**Z** No Qualifier

0 Medical and Surgical
0 Central Nervous System and Cranial Nerves
P Removal: Taking out or off a device from a body part

Body Part	Approach	Device	Qualifier
Character 4	**Character 5**	**Character 6**	**Character 7**
0 Brain **V** Spinal Cord	**0** Open **3** Percutaneous **4** Percutaneous Endoscopic	**0** Drainage Device **2** Monitoring Device **3** Infusion Device **7** Autologous Tissue Substitute **J** Synthetic Substitute **K** Nonautologous Tissue Substitute **M** Neurostimulator Lead **Y** Other Device	**Z** No Qualifier
0 Brain **V** Spinal Cord	**X** External	**0** Drainage Device **2** Monitoring Device **3** Infusion Device **M** Neurostimulator Lead	**Z** No Qualifier
6 Cerebral Ventricle **U** Spinal Canal	**0** Open **3** Percutaneous **4** Percutaneous Endoscopic	**0** Drainage Device **2** Monitoring Device **3** Infusion Device **J** Synthetic Substitute **M** Neurostimulator Lead **Y** Other Device	**Z** No Qualifier
6 Cerebral Ventricle **U** Spinal Canal	**X** External	**0** Drainage Device **2** Monitoring Device **3** Infusion Device **M** Neurostimulator Lead	**Z** No Qualifier
E Cranial Nerve	**0** Open **3** Percutaneous **4** Percutaneous Endoscopic	**0** Drainage Device **2** Monitoring Device **3** Infusion Device **7** Autologous Tissue Substitute **M** Neurostimulator Lead **Y** Other Device	**Z** No Qualifier
E Cranial Nerve	**X** External	**0** Drainage Device **2** Monitoring Device **3** Infusion Device **M** Neurostimulator Lead	**Z** No Qualifier

LC Limited Coverage NC Noncovered HAC HAC-associated Procedure CC Combination Cluster - See Appendix G for code lists
DRG Non-OR-Affecting MS-DRG Assignment New/Revised Text in **Orange** ♂ Male ♀ Female

166

2018 ICD-10-PCS

0   **Medical and Surgical**
0   **Central Nervous System** and Cranial Nerves
Q   **Repair:** Restoring, to the extent possible, a body part to its normal anatomic structure and function

Body Part	Approach	Device	Qualifier
Character 4	Character 5	Character 6	Character 7
0 Brain 1 Cerebral Meninges 2 Dura Mater 6 Cerebral Ventricle 7 Cerebral Hemisphere 8 Basal Ganglia 9 Thalamus A Hypothalamus B Pons C Cerebellum D Medulla Oblongata F Olfactory Nerve G Optic Nerve H Oculomotor Nerve J Trochlear Nerve K Trigeminal Nerve L Abducens Nerve M Facial Nerve N Acoustic Nerve P Glossopharyngeal Nerve Q Vagus Nerve R Accessory Nerve S Hypoglossal Nerve T Spinal Meninges W Cervical Spinal Cord X Thoracic Spinal Cord Y Lumbar Spinal Cord	0 Open 3 Percutaneous 4 Percutaneous Endoscopic	Z No Device	Z No Qualifier

0   **Medical and Surgical**
0   **Central Nervous System and Cranial Nerves**
R   **Replacement:** Putting in or on biological or synthetic material that physically takes the place and/or function of all or a portion of a body part

Body Part	Approach	Device	Qualifier
Character 4	Character 5	Character 6	Character 7
1 Cerebral Meninges 2 Dura Mater 6 Cerebral Ventricle F Olfactory Nerve G Optic Nerve H Oculomotor Nerve J Trochlear Nerve K Trigeminal Nerve L Abducens Nerve M Facial Nerve N Acoustic Nerve P Glossopharyngeal Nerve Q Vagus Nerve R Accessory Nerve S Hypoglossal Nerve T Spinal Meninges	0 Open 4 Percutaneous Endoscopic	7 Autologous Tissue Substitute J Synthetic Substitute K Nonautologous Tissue Substitute	Z No Qualifier

LC Limited Coverage   NC Noncovered   HAC HAC-associated Procedure   CC Combination Cluster - See Appendix G for code lists
DRG Non-OR-Affecting MS-DRG Assignment   New/Revised Text in **Orange**   ♂ Male   ♀ Female

2018 ICD-10-PCS

167

0 Medical and Surgical
0 Central Nervous System and Cranial Nerves
S Reposition: Moving to its normal location, or other suitable location, all or a portion of a body part

Body Part	Approach	Device	Qualifier
Character 4	Character 5	Character 6	Character 7
F Olfactory Nerve G Optic Nerve H Oculomotor Nerve J Trochlear Nerve K Trigeminal Nerve L Abducens Nerve M Facial Nerve N Acoustic Nerve P Glossopharyngeal Nerve Q Vagus Nerve R Accessory Nerve S Hypoglossal Nerve W Cervical Spinal Cord X Thoracic Spinal Cord Y Lumbar Spinal Cord	0 Open 3 Percutaneous 4 Percutaneous Endoscopic	Z No Device	Z No Qualifier

0 Medical and Surgical
0 Central Nervous System and Cranial Nerves
T Resection: Cutting out or off, without replacement, all of a body part

Body Part	Approach	Device	Qualifier
Character 4	Character 5	Character 6	Character 7
7 Cerebral Hemisphere	0 Open 3 Percutaneous 4 Percutaneous Endoscopic	Z No Device	Z No Qualifier

0 Medical and Surgical
0 Central Nervous System and Cranial Nerves
U Supplement: Putting in or on biological or synthetic material that physically reinforces and/or augments the function of a portion of a body part

Body Part	Approach	Device	Qualifier
Character 4	Character 5	Character 6	Character 7
1 Cerebral Meninges 2 Dura Mater 6 Cerebral Ventricle F Olfactory Nerve G Optic Nerve H Oculomotor Nerve J Trochlear Nerve K Trigeminal Nerve L Abducens Nerve M Facial Nerve N Acoustic Nerve P Glossopharyngeal Nerve Q Vagus Nerve R Accessory Nerve S Hypoglossal Nerve T Spinal Meninges	0 Open 3 Percutaneous 4 Percutaneous Endoscopic	7 Autologous Tissue Substitute J Synthetic Substitute K Nonautologous Tissue Substitute	Z No Qualifier

0 Medical and Surgical
0 Central Nervous System and Cranial Nerves
W Revision: Correcting, to the extent possible, a portion of a malfunctioning device or the position of a displaced device

Body Part	Approach	Device	Qualifier
Character 4	Character 5	Character 6	Character 7
0 Brain **V** Spinal Cord	**0** Open **3** Percutaneous **4** Percutaneous Endoscopic	**0** Drainage Device **2** Monitoring Device **3** Infusion Device **7** Autologous Tissue Substitute **J** Synthetic Substitute **K** Nonautologous Tissue Substitute **M** Neurostimulator Lead **Y** Other Device	**Z** No Qualifier
0 Brain **V** Spinal Cord	**X** External	**0** Drainage Device **2** Monitoring Device **3** Infusion Device **7** Autologous Tissue Substitute **J** Synthetic Substitute **K** Nonautologous Tissue Substitute **M** Neurostimulator Lead	**Z** No Qualifier
6 Cerebral Ventricle **U** Spinal Canal	**0** Open **3** Percutaneous **4** Percutaneous Endoscopic	**0** Drainage Device **2** Monitoring Device **3** Infusion Device **J** Synthetic Substitute **M** Neurostimulator Lead **Y** Other Device	**Z** No Qualifier
6 Cerebral Ventricle **U** Spinal Canal	**X** External	**0** Drainage Device **2** Monitoring Device **3** Infusion Device **J** Synthetic Substitute **M** Neurostimulator Lead	**Z** No Qualifier
E Cranial Nerve	**0** Open **3** Percutaneous **4** Percutaneous Endoscopic	**0** Drainage Device **2** Monitoring Device **3** Infusion Device **7** Autologous Tissue Substitute **M** Neurostimulator Lead **Y** Other Device	**Z** No Qualifier
E Cranial Nerve	**X** External	**0** Drainage Device **2** Monitoring Device **3** Infusion Device **7** Autologous Tissue Substitute **M** Neurostimulator Lead	**Z** No Qualifier

0 Medical and Surgical
0 Central Nervous System and Cranial Nerves
X Transfer: Moving, without taking out, all or a portion of a body part to another location to take over the function of all or a portion of a body part

Body Part	Approach	Device	Qualifier
Character 4	Character 5	Character 6	Character 7
F Olfactory Nerve **G** Optic Nerve **H** Oculomotor Nerve **J** Trochlear Nerve **K** Trigeminal Nerve **L** Abducens Nerve **M** Facial Nerve **N** Acoustic Nerve **P** Glossopharyngeal Nerve **Q** Vagus Nerve **R** Accessory Nerve **S** Hypoglossal Nerve	**0** Open **4** Percutaneous Endoscopic	**Z** No Device	**F** Olfactory Nerve **G** Optic Nerve **H** Oculomotor Nerve **J** Trochlear Nerve **K** Trigeminal Nerve **L** Abducens Nerve **M** Facial Nerve **N** Acoustic Nerve **P** Glossopharyngeal Nerve **Q** Vagus Nerve **R** Accessory Nerve **S** Hypoglossal Nerve

NOTES

Peripheral Nervous System 012-01X

0 **Medical and Surgical**
1 **Peripheral Nervous System**
2 **Change:** Taking out or off a device from a body part and putting back an identical or similar device in or on the same body part without cutting or puncturing the skin or a mucous membrane

Body Part	Approach	Device	Qualifier
Character 4	Character 5	Character 6	Character 7
Y Peripheral Nerve	**X** External	**0** Drainage Device **Y** Other Device	**Z** No Qualifier

0 **Medical and Surgical**
1 **Peripheral Nervous System**
5 **Destruction:** Physical eradication of all or a portion of a body part by the direct use of energy, force, or a destructive agent

Body Part	Approach	Device	Qualifier
Character 4	Character 5	Character 6	Character 7
0 Cervical Plexus **1** Cervical Nerve **2** Phrenic Nerve **3** Brachial Plexus **4** Ulnar Nerve **5** Median Nerve **6** Radial Nerve **8** Thoracic Nerve **9** Lumbar Plexus **A** Lumbosacral Plexus **B** Lumbar Nerve **C** Pudendal Nerve **D** Femoral Nerve **F** Sciatic Nerve **G** Tibial Nerve **H** Peroneal Nerve **K** Head and Neck Sympathetic Nerve **L** Thoracic Sympathetic Nerve **M** Abdominal Sympathetic Nerve **N** Lumbar Sympathetic Nerve **P** Sacral Sympathetic Nerve **Q** Sacral Plexus **R** Sacral Nerve	**0** Open **3** Percutaneous **4** Percutaneous Endoscopic	**Z** No Device	**Z** No Qualifier

---

0 **Medical and Surgical**
1 **Peripheral Nervous System**
8 **Division:** Cutting into a body part, without draining fluids and/or gases from the body part, in order to separate or transect a body part

Body Part	Approach	Device	Qualifier
Character 4	Character 5	Character 6	Character 7
0 Cervical Plexus **1** Cervical Nerve **2** Phrenic Nerve **3** Brachial Plexus **4** Ulnar Nerve **5** Median Nerve **6** Radial Nerve **8** Thoracic Nerve **9** Lumbar Plexus **A** Lumbosacral Plexus **B** Lumbar Nerve **C** Pudendal Nerve **D** Femoral Nerve **F** Sciatic Nerve **G** Tibial Nerve **H** Peroneal Nerve **K** Head and Neck Sympathetic Nerve **L** Thoracic Sympathetic Nerve **M** Abdominal Sympathetic Nerve **N** Lumbar Sympathetic Nerve **P** Sacral Sympathetic Nerve **Q** Sacral Plexus **R** Sacral Nerve	**0** Open **3** Percutaneous **4** Percutaneous Endoscopic	**Z** No Device	**Z** No Qualifier

0 **Medical and Surgical**
1 **Peripheral Nervous System**
9 **Drainage:** Taking or letting out fluids and/or gases from a body part

Body Part	Approach	Device	Qualifier
Character 4	Character 5	Character 6	Character 7
0 Cervical Plexus **1** Cervical Nerve **2** Phrenic Nerve **3** Brachial Plexus **4** Ulnar Nerve **5** Median Nerve **6** Radial Nerve **8** Thoracic Nerve **9** Lumbar Plexus **A** Lumbosacral Plexus **B** Lumbar Nerve **C** Pudendal Nerve **D** Femoral Nerve **F** Sciatic Nerve **G** Tibial Nerve **H** Peroneal Nerve **K** Head and Neck Sympathetic Nerve **L** Thoracic Sympathetic Nerve **M** Abdominal Sympathetic Nerve **N** Lumbar Sympathetic Nerve **P** Sacral Sympathetic Nerve **Q** Sacral Plexus **R** Sacral Nerve	**0** Open **3** Percutaneous **4** Percutaneous Endoscopic	**0** Drainage Device	**Z** No Qualifier

019 continued on next page

0   **Medical and Surgical**
1   **Peripheral Nervous System**
9   **Drainage:** Taking or letting out fluids and/or gases from a body part

019 continued from previous page

Body Part	Approach	Device	Qualifier
Character 4	Character 5	Character 6	Character 7
0 Cervical Plexus 1 Cervical Nerve 2 Phrenic Nerve 3 Brachial Plexus 4 Ulnar Nerve 5 Median Nerve 6 Radial Nerve 8 Thoracic Nerve 9 Lumbar Plexus A Lumbosacral Plexus B Lumbar Nerve C Pudendal Nerve D Femoral Nerve F Sciatic Nerve G Tibial Nerve H Peroneal Nerve K Head and Neck Sympathetic Nerve L Thoracic Sympathetic Nerve M Abdominal Sympathetic Nerve N Lumbar Sympathetic Nerve P Sacral Sympathetic Nerve Q Sacral Plexus R Sacral Nerve	0 Open 3 Percutaneous 4 Percutaneous Endoscopic	Z No Device	X Diagnostic Z No Qualifier

0   **Medical and Surgical**
1   **Peripheral Nervous System**
B   **Excision:** Cutting out or off, without replacement, a portion of a body part

Body Part	Approach	Device	Qualifier
Character 4	Character 5	Character 6	Character 7
0 Cervical Plexus 1 Cervical Nerve 2 Phrenic Nerve 3 Brachial Plexus 4 Ulnar Nerve 5 Median Nerve 6 Radial Nerve 8 Thoracic Nerve 9 Lumbar Plexus A Lumbosacral Plexus B Lumbar Nerve C Pudendal Nerve D Femoral Nerve F Sciatic Nerve G Tibial Nerve H Peroneal Nerve K Head and Neck Sympathetic Nerve L Thoracic Sympathetic Nerve M Abdominal Sympathetic Nerve N Lumbar Sympathetic Nerve P Sacral Sympathetic Nerve Q Sacral Plexus R Sacral Nerve	0 Open 3 Percutaneous 4 Percutaneous Endoscopic	Z No Device	X Diagnostic Z No Qualifier

LC Limited Coverage   NC Noncovered   HAC HAC-associated Procedure   CC Combination Cluster - See Appendix G for code lists
DRG Non-OR-Affecting MS-DRG Assignment   New/Revised Text in **Orange**   ♂ Male   ♀ Female

2018 ICD-10-PCS

173

PERIPHERAL NERVOUS SYSTEM 012-01X

0 **Medical and Surgical**
1 **Peripheral Nervous System**
C **Extirpation:** Taking or cutting out solid matter from a body part

Body Part	Approach	Device	Qualifier
Character 4	Character 5	Character 6	Character 7
0 Cervical Plexus **1** Cervical Nerve **2** Phrenic Nerve **3** Brachial Plexus **4** Ulnar Nerve **5** Median Nerve **6** Radial Nerve **8** Thoracic Nerve **9** Lumbar Plexus **A** Lumbosacral Plexus **B** Lumbar Nerve **C** Pudendal Nerve **D** Femoral Nerve **F** Sciatic Nerve **G** Tibial Nerve **H** Peroneal Nerve **K** Head and Neck Sympathetic Nerve **L** Thoracic Sympathetic Nerve **M** Abdominal Sympathetic Nerve **N** Lumbar Sympathetic Nerve **P** Sacral Sympathetic Nerve **Q** Sacral Plexus **R** Sacral Nerve	**0** Open **3** Percutaneous **4** Percutaneous Endoscopic	**Z** No Device	**Z** No Qualifier

0 **Medical and Surgical**
1 **Peripheral Nervous System**
D **Extraction:** Pulling or stripping out or off all or a portion of a body part by the use of force

Body Part	Approach	Device	Qualifier
Character 4	Character 5	Character 6	Character 7
0 Cervical Plexus **1** Cervical Nerve **2** Phrenic Nerve **3** Brachial Plexus **4** Ulnar Nerve **5** Median Nerve **6** Radial Nerve **8** Thoracic Nerve **9** Lumbar Plexus **A** Lumbosacral Plexus **B** Lumbar Nerve **C** Pudendal Nerve **D** Femoral Nerve **F** Sciatic Nerve **G** Tibial Nerve **H** Peroneal Nerve **K** Head and Neck Sympathetic Nerve **L** Thoracic Sympathetic Nerve **M** Abdominal Sympathetic Nerve **N** Lumbar Sympathetic Nerve **P** Sacral Sympathetic Nerve **Q** Sacral Plexus **R** Sacral Nerve	**0** Open **3** Percutaneous **4** Percutaneous Endoscopic	**Z** No Device	**Z** No Qualifier

LC Limited Coverage   NC Noncovered   HAC HAC-associated Procedure   CC Combination Cluster - See Appendix G for code lists
DRG Non-OR-Affecting MS-DRG Assignment   New/Revised Text in **Orange**   ♂ Male   ♀ Female

174

2018 ICD-10-PCS

0 Medical and Surgical
1 Peripheral Nervous System
H Insertion: Putting in a nonbiological appliance that monitors, assists, performs, or prevents a physiological function but does not physically take the place of a body part

Body Part	Approach	Device	Qualifier
Character 4	Character 5	Character 6	Character 7
Y Peripheral Nerve [CC]	0 Open 3 Percutaneous 4 Percutaneous Endoscopic	2 Monitoring Device M Neurostimulator Lead Y Other Device	Z No Qualifier

[CC] 01HY0MZ   01HY3MZ   01HY4MZ

0 Medical and Surgical
1 Peripheral Nervous System
J Inspection: Visually and/or manually exploring a body part

Body Part	Approach	Device	Qualifier
Character 4	Character 5	Character 6	Character 7
Y Peripheral Nerve	0 Open 3 Percutaneous 4 Percutaneous Endoscopic	Z No Device	Z No Qualifier

0 Medical and Surgical
1 Peripheral Nervous System
N Release: Freeing a body part from an abnormal physical constraint by cutting or by the use of force

Body Part	Approach	Device	Qualifier
Character 4	Character 5	Character 6	Character 7
0 Cervical Plexus 1 Cervical Nerve 2 Phrenic Nerve 3 Brachial Plexus 4 Ulnar Nerve 5 Median Nerve 6 Radial Nerve 8 Thoracic Nerve 9 Lumbar Plexus A Lumbosacral Plexus B Lumbar Nerve C Pudendal Nerve D Femoral Nerve F Sciatic Nerve G Tibial Nerve H Peroneal Nerve K Head and Neck Sympathetic Nerve L Thoracic Sympathetic Nerve M Abdominal Sympathetic Nerve N Lumbar Sympathetic Nerve P Sacral Sympathetic Nerve Q Sacral Plexus R Sacral Nerve	0 Open 3 Percutaneous 4 Percutaneous Endoscopic	Z No Device	Z No Qualifier

0 Medical and Surgical
1 Peripheral Nervous System
P Removal: Taking out or off a device from a body part

Body Part	Approach	Device	Qualifier
Character 4	Character 5	Character 6	Character 7
Y Peripheral Nerve	0 Open 3 Percutaneous 4 Percutaneous Endoscopic	0 Drainage Device 2 Monitoring Device 7 Autologous Tissue Substitute M Neurostimulator Lead Y Other Device	Z No Qualifier
Y Peripheral Nerve	X External	0 Drainage Device 2 Monitoring Device M Neurostimulator Lead	Z No Qualifier

---

[LC] Limited Coverage   [NC] Noncovered   [HAC] HAC-associated Procedure   [CC] Combination Cluster - See Appendix G for code lists
[DRG] Non-OR-Affecting MS-DRG Assignment   New/Revised Text in **Orange**   ♂ Male   ♀ Female

0 Medical and Surgical
1 Peripheral Nervous System
Q Repair: Restoring, to the extent possible, a body part to its normal anatomic structure and function

Body Part	Approach	Device	Qualifier
Character 4	Character 5	Character 6	Character 7
0 Cervical Plexus	0 Open	Z No Device	Z No Qualifier
1 Cervical Nerve	3 Percutaneous		
2 Phrenic Nerve	4 Percutaneous Endoscopic		
3 Brachial Plexus			
4 Ulnar Nerve			
5 Median Nerve			
6 Radial Nerve			
8 Thoracic Nerve			
9 Lumbar Plexus			
A Lumbosacral Plexus			
B Lumbar Nerve			
C Pudendal Nerve			
D Femoral Nerve			
F Sciatic Nerve			
G Tibial Nerve			
H Peroneal Nerve			
K Head and Neck Sympathetic Nerve			
L Thoracic Sympathetic Nerve			
M Abdominal Sympathetic Nerve			
N Lumbar Sympathetic Nerve			
P Sacral Sympathetic Nerve			
Q Sacral Plexus			
R Sacral Nerve			

0 Medical and Surgical
1 Peripheral Nervous System
R Replacement: Putting in or on biological or synthetic material that physically takes the place and/or function of all or a portion of a body part

Body Part	Approach	Device	Qualifier
Character 4	Character 5	Character 6	Character 7
1 Cervical Nerve	0 Open	7 Autologous Tissue Substitute	Z No Qualifier
2 Phrenic Nerve	4 Percutaneous Endoscopic	J Synthetic Substitute	
4 Ulnar Nerve		K Nonautologous Tissue Substitute	
5 Median Nerve			
6 Radial Nerve			
8 Thoracic Nerve			
B Lumbar Nerve			
C Pudendal Nerve			
D Femoral Nerve			
F Sciatic Nerve			
G Tibial Nerve			
H Peroneal Nerve			
R Sacral Nerve			

LC Limited Coverage   NC Noncovered   HAC HAC-associated Procedure   CC Combination Cluster - See Appendix G for code lists
DRG Non-OR-Affecting MS-DRG Assignment   New/Revised Text in Orange   ♂ Male   ♀ Female

176

2018 ICD-10-PCS

PERIPHERAL NERVOUS SYSTEM 012-01X

0 Medical and Surgical
1 Peripheral Nervous System
S Reposition: Moving to its normal location, or other suitable location, all or a portion of a body part

Body Part	Approach	Device	Qualifier
Character 4	Character 5	Character 6	Character 7
0 Cervical Plexus 1 Cervical Nerve 2 Phrenic Nerve 3 Brachial Plexus 4 Ulnar Nerve 5 Median Nerve 6 Radial Nerve 8 Thoracic Nerve 9 Lumbar Plexus A Lumbosacral Plexus B Lumbar Nerve C Pudendal Nerve D Femoral Nerve F Sciatic Nerve G Tibial Nerve H Peroneal Nerve Q Sacral Plexus R Sacral Nerve	0 Open 3 Percutaneous 4 Percutaneous Endoscopic	Z No Device	Z No Qualifier

0 Medical and Surgical
1 Peripheral Nervous System
U Supplement: Putting in or on biological or synthetic material that physically reinforces and/or augments the function of a portion of a body part

Body Part	Approach	Device	Qualifier
Character 4	Character 5	Character 6	Character 7
1 Cervical Nerve 2 Phrenic Nerve 4 Ulnar Nerve 5 Median Nerve 6 Radial Nerve 8 Thoracic Nerve B Lumbar Nerve C Pudendal Nerve D Femoral Nerve F Sciatic Nerve G Tibial Nerve H Peroneal Nerve R Sacral Nerve	0 Open 3 Percutaneous 4 Percutaneous Endoscopic	7 Autologous Tissue Substitute J Synthetic Substitute K Nonautologous Tissue Substitute	Z No Qualifier

0 Medical and Surgical
1 Peripheral Nervous System
W Revision: Correcting, to the extent possible, a portion of a malfunctioning device or the position of a displaced device

Body Part	Approach	Device	Qualifier
Character 4	Character 5	Character 6	Character 7
Y Peripheral Nerve	0 Open 3 Percutaneous 4 Percutaneous Endoscopic	0 Drainage Device 2 Monitoring Device 7 Autologous Tissue Substitute M Neurostimulator Lead Y Other Device	Z No Qualifier
Y Peripheral Nerve	X External	0 Drainage Device 2 Monitoring Device 7 Autologous Tissue Substitute M Neurostimulator Lead	Z No Qualifier

LC Limited Coverage   NC Noncovered   HAC HAC-associated Procedure   CC Combination Cluster - See Appendix G for code lists
DRG Non-OR-Affecting MS-DRG Assignment   New/Revised Text in Orange   ♂ Male   ♀ Female

2018 ICD-10-PCS

177

0 **Medical and Surgical**
1 **Peripheral Nervous System**
X **Transfer:** Moving, without taking out, all or a portion of a body part to another location to take over the function of all or a portion of a body part

Body Part	Approach	Device	Qualifier
Character 4	Character 5	Character 6	Character 7
1 Cervical Nerve 2 Phrenic Nerve	0 Open 4 Percutaneous Endoscopic	Z No Device	1 Cervical Nerve 2 Phrenic Nerve
4 Ulnar Nerve 5 Median Nerve 6 Radial Nerve	0 Open 4 Percutaneous Endoscopic	Z No Device	4 Ulnar Nerve 5 Median Nerve 6 Radial Nerve
8 Thoracic Nerve	0 Open 4 Percutaneous Endoscopic	Z No Device	8 Thoracic Nerve
B Lumbar Nerve C Pudendal Nerve	0 Open 4 Percutaneous Endoscopic	Z No Device	B Lumbar Nerve C Perineal Nerve
D Femoral Nerve F Sciatic Nerve G Tibial Nerve H Peroneal Nerve	0 Open 4 Percutaneous Endoscopic	Z No Device	D Femoral Nerve F Sciatic Nerve G Tibial Nerve H Peroneal Nerve

LC Limited Coverage   NC Noncovered   HAC HAC-associated Procedure   CC Combination Cluster - See Appendix G for code lists
DRG Non-OR-Affecting MS-DRG Assignment   New/Revised Text in **Orange**   ♂ Male   ♀ Female

NOTES

NOTES

Heart and Great Vessels 021-02Y

0 **Medical and Surgical**
2 **Heart and Great Vessels**
1 **Bypass:** Altering the route of passage of the contents of a tubular body part

Body Part	Approach	Device	Qualifier
Character 4	Character 5	Character 6	Character 7
0 Coronary Artery, One Artery HAC 1 Coronary Artery, Two Arteries HAC 2 Coronary Artery, Three Arteries HAC 3 Coronary Artery, Four or More Arteries HAC	0 Open	8 Zooplastic Tissue 9 Autologous Venous Tissue A Autologous Arterial Tissue J Synthetic Substitute K Nonautologous Tissue Substitute	3 Coronary Artery 8 Internal Mammary, Right 9 Internal Mammary, Left C Thoracic Artery F Abdominal Artery W Aorta
0 Coronary Artery, One Artery HAC 1 Coronary Artery, Two Arteries HAC 2 Coronary Artery, Three Arteries HAC 3 Coronary Artery, Four or More Arteries HAC	0 Open	Z No Device	3 Coronary Artery 8 Internal Mammary, Right 9 Internal Mammary, Left C Thoracic Artery F Abdominal Artery
0 Coronary Artery, One Artery 1 Coronary Artery, Two Arteries 2 Coronary Artery, Three Arteries 3 Coronary Artery, Four or More Arteries	3 Percutaneous	4 Intraluminal Device, Drug-eluting D Intraluminal Device	4 Coronary Vein
0 Coronary Artery, One Artery 1 Coronary Artery, Two Arteries 2 Coronary Artery, Three Arteries 3 Coronary Artery, Four or More Arteries	4 Percutaneous Endoscopic	4 Intraluminal Device, Drug-eluting D Intraluminal Device	4 Coronary Vein
0 Coronary Artery, One Artery HAC 1 Coronary Artery, Two Arteries HAC 2 Coronary Artery, Three Arteries HAC 3 Coronary Artery, Four or More Arteries HAC	4 Percutaneous Endoscopic	8 Zooplastic Tissue 9 Autologous Venous Tissue A Autologous Arterial Tissue J Synthetic Substitute K Nonautologous Tissue Substitute	3 Coronary Artery 8 Internal Mammary, Right 9 Internal Mammary, Left C Thoracic Artery F Abdominal Artery W Aorta
0 Coronary Artery, One Artery HAC 1 Coronary Artery, Two Arteries HAC 2 Coronary Artery, Three Arteries HAC 3 Coronary Artery, Four or More Arteries HAC	4 Percutaneous Endoscopic	Z No Device	3 Coronary Artery 8 Internal Mammary, Right 9 Internal Mammary, Left C Thoracic Artery F Abdominal Artery
6 Atrium, Right	0 Open 4 Percutaneous Endoscopic	8 Zooplastic Tissue 9 Autologous Venous Tissue A Autologous Arterial Tissue J Synthetic Substitute K Nonautologous Tissue Substitute	P Pulmonary Trunk Q Pulmonary Artery, Right R Pulmonary Artery, Left
6 Atrium, Right	0 Open 4 Percutaneous Endoscopic	Z No Device	7 Atrium, Left P Pulmonary Trunk Q Pulmonary Artery, Right R Pulmonary Artery, Left

021 continued on next page

LC Limited Coverage   NC Noncovered   HAC HAC-associated Procedure   CC Combination Cluster - See Appendix G for code lists
DRG Non-OR-Affecting MS-DRG Assignment   New/Revised Text in **Orange**   ♂ Male   ♀ Female

0 Medical and Surgical
2 Heart and Great Vessels
1 Bypass: Altering the route of passage of the contents of a tubular body part

021 continued from previous page

Body Part	Approach	Device	Qualifier
Character 4	Character 5	Character 6	Character 7
6 Atrium, Right	3 Percutaneous	Z No Device	7 Atrium, Left
7 Atrium, Left V Superior Vena Cava	0 Open 4 Percutaneous Endoscopic	8 Zooplastic Tissue 9 Autologous Venous Tissue A Autologous Arterial Tissue J Synthetic Substitute K Nonautologous Tissue Substitute Z No Device	P Pulmonary Trunk Q Pulmonary Artery, Right R Pulmonary Artery, Left S Pulmonary Vein, Right T Pulmonary Vein, Left U Pulmonary Vein, Confluence
K Ventricle, Right L Ventricle, Left	0 Open 4 Percutaneous Endoscopic	8 Zooplastic Tissue 9 Autologous Venous Tissue A Autologous Arterial Tissue J Synthetic Substitute K Nonautologous Tissue Substitute	P Pulmonary Trunk Q Pulmonary Artery, Right R Pulmonary Artery, Left
K Ventricle, Right L Ventricle, Left	0 Open 4 Percutaneous Endoscopic	Z No Device	5 Coronary Circulation 8 Internal Mammary, Right 9 Internal Mammary, Left C Thoracic Artery F Abdominal Artery P Pulmonary Trunk Q Pulmonary Artery, Right R Pulmonary Artery, Left W Aorta
P Pulmonary Trunk Q Pulmonary Artery, Right R Pulmonary Artery, Left	0 Open 4 Percutaneous Endoscopic	8 Zooplastic Tissue 9 Autologous Venous Tissue A Autologous Arterial Tissue J Synthetic Substitute K Nonautologous Tissue Substitute Z No Device	A Innominate Artery B Subclavian D Carotid
W Thoracic Aorta, Descending	0 Open	8 Zooplastic Tissue 9 Autologous Venous Tissue A Autologous Arterial Tissue Z No Device	B Subclavian D Carotid P Pulmonary Trunk Q Pulmonary Artery, Right R Pulmonary Artery, Left
W Thoracic Aorta, Descending	0 Open	J Synthetic Substitute K Nonautologous Tissue Substitute	B Subclavian D Carotid G Axillary Artery H Brachial Artery P Pulmonary Trunk Q Pulmonary Artery, Right R Pulmonary Artery, Left
W Thoracic Aorta, Descending	4 Percutaneous Endoscopic	8 Zooplastic Tissue 9 Autologous Venous Tissue A Autologous Arterial Tissue J Synthetic Substitute K Nonautologous Tissue Substitute Z No Device	B Subclavian D Carotid P Pulmonary Trunk Q Pulmonary Artery, Right R Pulmonary Artery, Left
X Thoracic Aorta, Ascending/Arch	0 Open 4 Percutaneous Endoscopic	8 Zooplastic Tissue 9 Autologous Venous Tissue A Autologous Arterial Tissue J Synthetic Substitute K Nonautologous Tissue Substitute Z No Device	B Subclavian D Carotid P Pulmonary Trunk Q Pulmonary Artery, Right R Pulmonary Artery, Left

021 continued on next page

LC Limited Coverage   NC Noncovered   HAC HAC-associated Procedure   CC Combination Cluster - See Appendix G for code lists
DRG Non-OR-Affecting MS-DRG Assignment   New/Revised Text in **Orange**   ♂ Male   ♀ Female

021 continued from previous page

HAC 0210083	0210088	0210089	021008C	021008F	021008W	0210093	0210098	0210099	021009C	021009F	021009W	02100A3
02100A8	02100A9	02100AC	02100AF	02100AW	02100J3	02100J8	02100J9	02100JC	02100JF	02100JW	02100K3	02100K8
02100K9	02100KC	02100KF	02100KW	02100Z3	02100Z8	02100Z9	02100ZC	02100ZF	0210483	0210488	0210489	021048C
021048F	021048W	0210493	0210498	0210499	021049C	021049F	021049W	02104A3	02104A8	02104A9	02104AC	02104AF
02104AW	02104J3	02104J8	02104J9	02104JC	02104JF	02104JW	02104K3	02104K8	02104K9	02104KC	02104KF	02104KW
02104Z3	02104Z8	02104Z9	02104ZC	02104ZF	0211083	0211088	0211089	021108C	021108F	021108W	0211093	0211098
0211099	021109C	021109F	021109W	02110A3	02110A8	02110A9	02110AC	02110AF	02110AW	02110J3	02110J8	02110J9
02110JC	02110JF	02110JW	02110K3	02110K8	02110K9	02110KC	02110KF	02110KW	02110Z3	02110Z8	02110Z9	02110ZC
02110ZF	0211483	0211488	0211489	021148C	021148F	021148W	0211493	0211498	0211499	021149C	021149F	021149W
02114A3	02114A8	02114A9	02114AC	02114AF	02114AW	02114J3	02114J8	02114J9	02114JC	02114JF	02114JW	02114K3
02114K8	02114K9	02114KC	02114KF	02114KW	02114Z3	02114Z8	02114Z9	02114ZC	02114ZF	0212083	0212088	0212089
021208C	021208F	021208W	0212093	0212098	0212099	021209C	021209F	021209W	02120A3	02120A8	02120A9	02120AC
02120AF	02120AW	02120J3	02120J8	02120J9	02120JC	02120JF	02120JW	02120K3	02120K8	02120K9	02120KC	02120KF
02120KW	02120Z3	02120Z8	02120Z9	02120ZC	02120ZF	0212483	0212488	0212489	021248C	021248F	021248W	0212493
0212498	0212499	021249C	021249F	021249W	02124A3	02124A8	02124A9	02124AC	02124AF	02124AW	02124J3	02124J8
02124J9	02124JC	02124JF	02124JW	02124K3	02124K8	02124K9	02124KC	02124KF	02124KW	02124Z3	02124Z8	02124Z9
02124ZC	02124ZF	0213083	0213088	0213089	021308C	021308F	021308W	0213093	0213098	0213099	021309C	021309F
021309W	02130A3	02130A8	02130A9	02130AC	02130AF	02130AW	02130J3	02130J8	02130J9	02130JC	02130JF	02130JW
02130K3	02130K8	02130K9	02130KC	02130KF	02130KW	02130Z3	02130Z8	02130Z9	02130ZC	02130ZF	0213483	0213488
0213489	021348C	021348F	021348W	0213493	0213498	0213499	021349C	021349F	021349W	02134A3	02134A8	02134A9
02134AC	02134AF	02134AW	02134J3	02134J8	02134J9	02134JC	02134JF	02134JW	02134K3	02134K8	02134K9	02134KC
02134KF	02134KW	02134Z3	02134Z8	02134Z9	02134ZC	02134ZF						

Surgical site infection, mediastinitis, following coronary artery bypass graft (CABG) and secondary diagnosis J98.51, J98.59.

0 Medical and Surgical
2 Heart and Great Vessels
4 Creation: Putting in or on biological or synthetic material to form a new body part that to the extent possible replicates the anatomic structure or function of an absent body part

Body Part	Approach	Device	Qualifier
Character 4	Character 5	Character 6	Character 7
F Aortic Valve	**0** Open	**7** Autologous Tissue Substitute **8** Zooplastic Tissue **J** Synthetic Substitute **K** Nonautologous Tissue Substitute	**J** Truncal Valve
G Mitral Valve **J** Tricuspid Valve	**0** Open	**7** Autologous Tissue Substitute **8** Zooplastic Tissue **J** Synthetic Substitute **K** Nonautologous Tissue Substitute	**2** Common Atrioventricular Valve

LC Limited Coverage   NC Noncovered   HAC HAC-associated Procedure   CC Combination Cluster - See Appendix G for code lists
DRG Non-OR-Affecting MS-DRG Assignment   New/Revised Text in **Orange**   ♂ Male   ♀ Female

2018 ICD-10-PCS

183

HEART AND GREAT VESSELS 021-02Y

0 Medical and Surgical
2 Heart and Great Vessels
5 Destruction: Physical eradication of all or a portion of a body part by the direct use of energy, force, or a destructive agent

Body Part	Approach	Device	Qualifier
Character 4	Character 5	Character 6	Character 7
4 Coronary Vein 5 Atrial Septum 6 Atrium, Right 8 Conduction Mechanism 9 Chordae Tendineae D Papillary Muscle F Aortic Valve G Mitral Valve H Pulmonary Valve J Tricuspid Valve K Ventricle, Right L Ventricle, Left M Ventricular Septum N Pericardium P Pulmonary Trunk Q Pulmonary Artery, Right R Pulmonary Artery, Left S Pulmonary Vein, Right T Pulmonary Vein, Left V Superior Vena Cava W Thoracic Aorta, Descending X Thoracic Aorta, Ascending/Arch	0 Open 3 Percutaneous 4 Percutaneous Endoscopic	Z No Device	Z No Qualifier
7 Atrium, Left ᴰᴿᴳ	0 Open 3 Percutaneous 4 Percutaneous Endoscopic	Z No Device	K Left Atrial Appendage Z No Qualifier

ᴰᴿᴳ 02570ZK   02573ZK   02574ZK

LC Limited Coverage   NC Noncovered   HAC HAC-associated Procedure   CC Combination Cluster - See Appendix G for code lists
ᴰᴿᴳ Non-OR-Affecting MS-DRG Assignment   New/Revised Text in **Orange**   ♂ Male   ♀ Female

184

2018 ICD-10-PCS

0   Medical and Surgical
2   Heart and Great Vessels
7   Dilation: Expanding an orifice or the lumen of a tubular body part

Body Part	Approach	Device	Qualifier
Character 4	Character 5	Character 6	Character 7
0 Coronary Artery, One Artery 1 Coronary Artery, Two Arteries 2 Coronary Artery, Three Arteries 3 Coronary Artery, Four or More Arteries	0 Open 3 Percutaneous 4 Percutaneous Endoscopic	4 Intraluminal Device, Drug-eluting 5 Intraluminal Device, Drug-eluting, Two 6 Intraluminal Device, Drug-eluting, Three 7 Intraluminal Device, Drug-eluting, Four or More D Intraluminal Device E Intraluminal Device, Two F Intraluminal Device, Three G Intraluminal Device, Four or More T Intraluminal Device, Radioactive Z No Device	6 Bifurcation Z No Qualifier
F Aortic Valve G Mitral Valve H Pulmonary Valve J Tricuspid Valve K Ventricle, Right L Ventricle, Left P Pulmonary Trunk Q Pulmonary Artery, Right S Pulmonary Vein, Right T Pulmonary Vein, Left V Superior Vena Cava W Thoracic Aorta, Descending X Thoracic Aorta, Ascending/Arch	0 Open 3 Percutaneous 4 Percutaneous Endoscopic	4 Intraluminal Device, Drug-eluting D Intraluminal Device Z No Device	Z No Qualifier
R Pulmonary Artery, Left	0 Open 3 Percutaneous 4 Percutaneous Endoscopic	4 Intraluminal Device, Drug-eluting D Intraluminal Device Z No Device	T Ductus Arteriosus Z No Qualifier

LC Limited Coverage   NC Noncovered   HAC HAC-associated Procedure   CC Combination Cluster - See Appendix G for code lists
DRG Non-OR-Affecting MS-DRG Assignment   New/Revised Text in **Orange**   ♂ Male   ♀ Female

2018 ICD-10-PCS

185

HEART AND GREAT VESSELS 021-02Y

0 Medical and Surgical
2 Heart and Great Vessels
8 Division: Cutting into a body part, without draining fluids and/or gases from the body part, in order to separate or transect a body part

Body Part	Approach	Device	Qualifier
Character 4	Character 5	Character 6	Character 7
8 Conduction Mechanism 9 Chordae Tendineae D Papillary Muscle	0 Open 3 Percutaneous 4 Percutaneous Endoscopic	Z No Device	Z No Qualifier

0 Medical and Surgical
2 Heart and Great Vessels
B Excision: Cutting out or off, without replacement, a portion of a body part

Body Part	Approach	Device	Qualifier
Character 4	Character 5	Character 6	Character 7
4 Coronary Vein 5 Atrial Septum 6 Atrium, Right 8 Conduction Mechanism 9 Chordae Tendineae D Papillary Muscle F Aortic Valve G Mitral Valve H Pulmonary Valve J Tricuspid Valve K Ventricle, Right 🅽🅲 L Ventricle, Left 🅽🅲 M Ventricular Septum N Pericardium P Pulmonary Trunk Q Pulmonary Artery, Right R Pulmonary Artery, Left S Pulmonary Vein, Right T Pulmonary Vein, Left V Superior Vena Cava W Thoracic Aorta, Descending X Thoracic Aorta, Ascending/Arch	0 Open 3 Percutaneous 4 Percutaneous Endoscopic	Z No Device	X Diagnostic Z No Qualifier
7 Atrium, Left	0 Open 3 Percutaneous 4 Percutaneous Endoscopic	Z No Device	K Left Atrial Appendage X Diagnostic Z No Qualifier

🅽🅲 02BK0ZZ   02BK3ZZ   02BK4ZZ   02BL0ZZ   02BL3ZZ   02BL4ZZ

0   Medical and Surgical
2   Heart and Great Vessels
C   Extirpation: Taking or cutting out solid matter from a body part

Body Part	Approach	Device	Qualifier
Character 4	Character 5	Character 6	Character 7
0 Coronary Artery, One Artery **1** Coronary Artery, Two Arteries **2** Coronary Artery, Three Arteries **3** Coronary Artery, Four or More Arteries	**0** Open **3** Percutaneous **4** Percutaneous Endoscopic	**Z** No Device	**6** Bifurcation **Z** No Qualifier
4 Coronary Vein **5** Atrial Septum **6** Atrium, Right **7** Atrium, Left **8** Conduction Mechanism **9** Chordae Tendineae **D** Papillary Muscle **F** Aortic Valve **G** Mitral Valve **H** Pulmonary Valve **J** Tricuspid Valve **K** Ventricle, Right **L** Ventricle, Left **M** Ventricular Septum **N** Pericardium **P** Pulmonary Trunk **Q** Pulmonary Artery, Right **R** Pulmonary Artery, Left **S** Pulmonary Vein, Right **T** Pulmonary Vein, Left **V** Superior Vena Cava **W** Thoracic Aorta, Descending **X** Thoracic Aorta, Ascending/Arch	**0** Open **3** Percutaneous **4** Percutaneous Endoscopic	**Z** No Device	**Z** No Qualifier

0   Medical and Surgical
2   Heart and Great Vessels
F   Fragmentation: Breaking solid matter in a body part into pieces

Body Part	Approach	Device	Qualifier
Character 4	Character 5	Character 6	Character 7
N Pericardium 🆖	**0** Open **3** Percutaneous **4** Percutaneous Endoscopic **X** External	**Z** No Device	**Z** No Qualifier

🆖 02FNXZZ

0 Medical and Surgical
2 Heart and Great Vessels
H Insertion: Putting in a nonbiological appliance that monitors, assists, performs, or prevents a physiological function but does not physically take the place of a body part

Body Part	Approach	Device	Qualifier
Character 4	Character 5	Character 6	Character 7
4 Coronary Vein CC DRG HAC 6 Atrium, Right CC DRG HAC 7 Atrium, Left CC DRG HAC K Ventricle, Right CC DRG HAC L Ventricle, Left CC DRG HAC	0 Open 3 Percutaneous 4 Percutaneous Endoscopic	0 Monitoring Device, Pressure Sensor 2 Monitoring Device 3 Infusion Device D Intraluminal Device J Cardiac Lead, Pacemaker K Cardiac Lead, Defibrillator M Cardiac Lead N Intracardiac Pacemaker Y Other Device	Z No Qualifier
A Heart NC LC	0 Open 3 Percutaneous 4 Percutaneous Endoscopic	Q Implantable Heart Assist System Y Other Device	Z No Qualifier
A Heart CC	0 Open 3 Percutaneous 4 Percutaneous Endoscopic	R Short term External Heart Assist System	J Intraoperative S Biventricular Z No Qualifier
N Pericardium CC HAC	0 Open 3 Percutaneous 4 Percutaneous Endoscopic	0 Monitoring Device, Pressure Sensor 2 Monitoring Device J Cardiac Lead, Pacemaker K Cardiac Lead, Defibrillator M Cardiac Lead Y Other Device	Z No Qualifier
P Pulmonary Trunk Q Pulmonary Artery, Right R Pulmonary Artery, Left S Pulmonary Vein, Right HAC T Pulmonary Vein, Left HAC V Superior Vena Cava HAC W Thoracic Aorta, Descending	0 Open 3 Percutaneous 4 Percutaneous Endoscopic	0 Monitoring Device, Pressure Sensor 2 Monitoring Device 3 Infusion Device D Intraluminal Device Y Other Device	Z No Qualifier
X Thoracic Aorta, Ascending/Arch	0 Open 3 Percutaneous 4 Percutaneous Endoscopic	0 Monitoring Device, Pressure Sensor 2 Monitoring Device 3 Infusion Device D Intraluminal Device	Z No Qualifier

LC 02HA0QZ

NC 02HA3QZ   02HA4QZ

HAC 02H633Z   02HK33Z   02HS33Z   02HS43Z   02HT33Z   02HT43Z   02HV33Z   02HV43Z

Iatrogenic pneumothorax w/ venous catheterization procedures and secondary diagnosis J95.811.

HAC 02H43JZ   02H43KZ   02H43MZ   02H63JZ   02H63MZ   02H73JZ   02H73MZ   02HK3JZ   02HL3JZ   02HN0JZ   02HN0MZ   02HN3JZ   02HN3MZ
02HN4JZ   02HN4MZ

Surgical site infection (SSI) following cardiac implantable electronic device (CIED) procedures and secondary diagnosis K68.11, T81.4XXA, T82.6XXA, T82.7XXA.

CC 02H40KZ   02H43JZ   02H43KZ   02H43MZ   02H44KZ   02H60KZ   02H63KZ   02H64KZ   02H70KZ   02H73KZ   02H74KZ   02HA0RS   02HA0RZ
02HA3RS   02HA4RS   02HA4RZ   02HK0KZ   02HK3KZ   02HK4KZ   02HL0KZ   02HL0MZ   02HL3KZ   02HL3MZ   02HL4KZ   02HL4MZ   02HN0JZ
02HN0KZ   02HN0MZ   02HN3JZ   02HN3KZ   02HN3MZ   02HN4JZ   02HN4KZ   02HN4MZ

DRG 02H40JZ   02H40MZ   02H44JZ   02H44MZ   02H60JZ   02H60MZ   02H63JZ   02H64JZ   02H64MZ   02H70JZ   02H70MZ   02H73JZ   02H74JZ
02H74MZ   02HK0JZ   02HK0MZ   02HK32Z   02HK3JZ   02HK3MZ   02HK4JZ   02HK4MZ   02HL0JZ

0 Medical and Surgical
2 Heart and Great Vessels
J Inspection: Visually and/or manually exploring a body part

Body Part	Approach	Device	Qualifier
Character 4	Character 5	Character 6	Character 7
A Heart Y Great Vessel	0 Open 3 Percutaneous 4 Percutaneous Endoscopic	Z No Device	Z No Qualifier

LC Limited Coverage   NC Noncovered   HAC HAC-associated Procedure   CC Combination Cluster - See Appendix G for code lists
DRG Non-OR-Affecting MS-DRG Assignment   New/Revised Text in **Orange**   ♂ Male   ♀ Female

0 Medical and Surgical
2 Heart and Great Vessels
K Map: Locating the route of passage of electrical impulses and/or locating functional areas in a body part

Body Part	Approach	Device	Qualifier
Character 4	**Character 5**	**Character 6**	**Character 7**
8 Conduction Mechanism	0 Open 3 Percutaneous 4 Percutaneous Endoscopic	Z No Device	Z No Qualifier

0 Medical and Surgical
2 Heart and Great Vessels
L Occlusion: Completely closing an orifice or the lumen of a tubular body part

Body Part	Approach	Device	Qualifier
Character 4	**Character 5**	**Character 6**	**Character 7**
7 Atrium, Left	0 Open 3 Percutaneous 4 Percutaneous Endoscopic	C Extraluminal Device D Intraluminal Device Z No Device	K Left Atrial Appendage
H Pulmonary Valve P Pulmonary Trunk Q Pulmonary Artery, Right S Pulmonary Vein, Right T Pulmonary Vein, Left V Superior Vena Cava	0 Open 3 Percutaneous 4 Percutaneous Endoscopic	C Extraluminal Device D Intraluminal Device Z No Device	Z No Qualifier
R Pulmonary Artery, Left	0 Open 3 Percutaneous 4 Percutaneous Endoscopic	C Extraluminal Device D Intraluminal Device Z No Device	T Ductus Arteriosus Z No Qualifier
W Thoracic Aorta, Descending	3 Percutaneous	D Intraluminal Device	J Temporary

0 Medical and Surgical
2 Heart and Great Vessels
N Release: Freeing a body part from an abnormal physical constraint by cutting or by the use of force

Body Part	Approach	Device	Qualifier
Character 4	**Character 5**	**Character 6**	**Character 7**
0 Coronary Artery, One Artery 1 Coronary Artery, Two Arteries 2 Coronary Artery, Three Arteries 3 Coronary Artery, Four or More Arteries 4 Coronary Vein 5 Atrial Septum 6 Atrium, Right 7 Atrium, Left 8 Conduction Mechanism 9 Chordae Tendineae D Papillary Muscle F Aortic Valve G Mitral Valve H Pulmonary Valve J Tricuspid Valve K Ventricle, Right L Ventricle, Left M Ventricular Septum N Pericardium P Pulmonary Trunk Q Pulmonary Artery, Right R Pulmonary Artery, Left S Pulmonary Vein, Right T Pulmonary Vein, Left V Superior Vena Cava W Thoracic Aorta, Descending X Thoracic Aorta, Ascending/Arch	0 Open 3 Percutaneous 4 Percutaneous Endoscopic	Z No Device	Z No Qualifier

LC Limited Coverage NC Noncovered HAC HAC-associated Procedure CC Combination Cluster - See Appendix G for code lists
DRG Non-OR-Affecting MS-DRG Assignment New/Revised Text in Orange ♂ Male ♀ Female

2018 ICD-10-PCS

189

0 Medical and Surgical
2 Heart and Great Vessels
P Removal: Taking out or off a device from a body part

Body Part	Approach	Device	Qualifier
Character 4	**Character 5**	**Character 6**	**Character 7**
A Heart HAC	**0** Open **3** Percutaneous **4** Percutaneous Endoscopic	**2** Monitoring Device **3** Infusion Device **7** Autologous Tissue Substitute **8** Zooplastic Tissue **C** Extraluminal Device **D** Intraluminal Device **J** Synthetic Substitute **K** Nonautologous Tissue Substitute **M** Cardiac Lead **N** Intracardiac Pacemaker **Q** Implantable Heart Assist System **Y** Other Device	**Z** No Qualifier
A Heart CC HAC	**0** Open **3** Percutaneous **4** Percutaneous Endoscopic	**R** Short-term External Heart Assist System	**S** Biventricular **Z** No Qualifier
A Heart HAC	**X** External	**2** Monitoring Device **3** Infusion Device **D** Intraluminal Device **M** Cardiac Lead	**Z** No Qualifier
Y Great Vessel	**0** Open **3** Percutaneous **4** Percutaneous Endoscopic	**2** Monitoring Device **3** Infusion Device **7** Autologous Tissue Substitute **8** Zooplastic Tissue **C** Extraluminal Device **D** Intraluminal Device **J** Synthetic Substitute **K** Nonautologous Tissue Substitute **Y** Other Device	**Z** No Qualifier
Y Great Vessel	**X** External	**2** Monitoring Device **3** Infusion Device **D** Intraluminal Device	**Z** No Qualifier

HAC 02PA0MZ   02PA3MZ   02PA4MZ   02PAXMZ
Surgical site infection (SSI) following cardiac implantable electronic device (CIED) procedures and secondary diagnosis K68.11, T81.4XXA, T82.6XXA, T82.7XXA.

CC 02PA0RZ   02PA3RZ   02PA4RZ

LC Limited Coverage   NC Noncovered   HAC HAC-associated Procedure   CC Combination Cluster - See Appendix G for code lists
DRG Non-OR-Affecting MS-DRG Assignment   New/Revised Text in **Orange**   ♂ Male   ♀ Female

190

2018 ICD-10-PCS

0 Medical and Surgical
2 Heart and Great Vessels
Q Repair: Restoring, to the extent possible, a body part to its normal anatomic structure and function

Body Part	Approach	Device	Qualifier
Character 4	Character 5	Character 6	Character 7
0 Coronary Artery, One Artery **1** Coronary Artery, Two Arteries **2** Coronary Artery, Three Arteries **3** Coronary Artery, Four or More Arteries **4** Coronary Vein **5** Atrial Septum **6** Atrium, Right **7** Atrium, Left **8** Conduction Mechanism **9** Chordae Tendineae **A** Heart **B** Heart, Right **C** Heart, Left **D** Papillary Muscle **H** Pulmonary Valve **K** Ventricle, Right **L** Ventricle, Left **M** Ventricular Septum **N** Pericardium **P** Pulmonary Trunk **Q** Pulmonary Artery, Right **R** Pulmonary Artery, Left **S** Pulmonary Vein, Right **T** Pulmonary Vein, Left **V** Superior Vena Cava **W** Thoracic Aorta, Descending **X** Thoracic Aorta, Ascending/Arch	**0** Open **3** Percutaneous **4** Percutaneous Endoscopic	**Z** No Device	**Z** No Qualifier
F Aortic Valve	**0** Open **3** Percutaneous **4** Percutaneous Endoscopic	**Z** No Device	**J** Truncal Valve **Z** No Qualifier
G Mitral Valve	**0** Open **3** Percutaneous **4** Percutaneous Endoscopic	**Z** No Device	**E** Atrioventricular Valve, Left **Z** No Qualifier
J Tricuspid Valve	**0** Open **3** Percutaneous **4** Percutaneous Endoscopic	**Z** No Device	**G** Atrioventricular Valve, Right **Z** No Qualifier

LC Limited Coverage   NC Noncovered   HAC HAC-associated Procedure   CC Combination Cluster - See Appendix G for code lists
DRG Non-OR-Affecting MS-DRG Assignment   New/Revised Text in Orange   ♂ Male   ♀ Female

2018 ICD-10-PCS

191

HEART AND GREAT VESSELS 021-02Y

0 Medical and Surgical
2 Heart and Great Vessels
R Replacement: Putting in or on biological or synthetic material that physically takes the place and/or function of all or a portion of a body part

Body Part	Approach	Device	Qualifier
Character 4	Character 5	Character 6	Character 7
5 Atrial Septum 6 Atrium, Right 7 Atrium, Left 9 Chordae Tendineae D Papillary Muscle K Ventricle, Right ᴺᶜ ᴸᶜ ᶜᶜ L Ventricle, Left ᴺᶜ ᴸᶜ ᶜᶜ M Ventricular Septum N Pericardium P Pulmonary Trunk Q Pulmonary Artery, Right R Pulmonary Artery, Left S Pulmonary Vein, Right T Pulmonary Vein, Left V Superior Vena Cava W Thoracic Aorta, Descending X Thoracic Aorta, Ascending/Arch	0 Open 4 Percutaneous Endoscopic	7 Autologous Tissue Substitute 8 Zooplastic Tissue J Synthetic Substitute K Nonautologous Tissue Substitute	Z No Qualifier
F Aortic Valve G Mitral Valve H Pulmonary Valve J Tricuspid Valve	0 Open 4 Percutaneous Endoscopic	7 Autologous Tissue Substitute 8 Zooplastic Tissue J Synthetic Substitute K Nonautologous Tissue Substitute	Z No Qualifier
F Aortic Valve G Mitral Valve H Pulmonary Valve J Tricuspid Valve	3 Percutaneous	7 Autologous Tissue Substitute 8 Zooplastic Tissue J Synthetic Substitute K Nonautologous Tissue Substitute	H Transapical Z No Qualifier

ᴸᶜ 02RK0JZ with 02RL0JZ
   Limited coverage when combined with diagnosis code Z00.6.
ᴺᶜ 02RK0JZ or 02RL0JZ with 02RL0JZ
   Noncovered except when combined with diagnosis code Z00.6.
ᶜᶜ 02RK0JZ   02RL0JZ

0 Medical and Surgical
2 Heart and Great Vessels
S Reposition: Moving to its normal location, or other suitable location, all or a portion of a body part

Body Part	Approach	Device	Qualifier
Character 4	Character 5	Character 6	Character 7
0 Coronary Artery, One Artery 1 Coronary Artery, Two Arteries P Pulmonary Trunk Q Pulmonary Artery, Right R Pulmonary Artery, Left S Pulmonary Vein, Right T Pulmonary Vein, Left V Superior Vena Cava W Thoracic Aorta, Descending X Thoracic Aorta, Ascending/Arch	0 Open	Z No Device	Z No Qualifier

ᴸᶜ Limited Coverage   ᴺᶜ Noncovered   ᴴᴬᶜ HAC-associated Procedure   ᶜᶜ Combination Cluster - See Appendix G for code lists
ᴰᴿᴳ Non-OR-Affecting MS-DRG Assignment   New/Revised Text in **Orange**   ♂ Male   ♀ Female

192   **2018 ICD-10-PCS**

0   Medical and Surgical
2   Heart and Great Vessels
T   Resection: Cutting out or off, without replacement, all of a body part

Body Part	Approach	Device	Qualifier
Character 4	Character 5	Character 6	Character 7
5 Atrial Septum 8 Conduction Mechanism 9 Chordae Tendineae D Papillary Muscle H Pulmonary Valve M Ventricular Septum N Pericardium	0 Open 3 Percutaneous 4 Percutaneous Endoscopic	Z No Device	Z No Qualifier

0   Medical and Surgical
2   Heart and Great Vessels
U   Supplement: Putting in or on biological or synthetic material that physically reinforces and/or augments the function of a portion of a body part

Body Part	Approach	Device	Qualifier
Character 4	Character 5	Character 6	Character 7
5 Atrial Septum 6 Atrium, Right 7 Atrium, Left 9 Chordae Tendineae A Heart D Papillary Muscle H Pulmonary Valve K Ventricle, Right L Ventricle, Left M Ventricular Septum N Pericardium P Pulmonary Trunk Q Pulmonary Artery, Right R Pulmonary Artery, Left S Pulmonary Vein, Right T Pulmonary Vein, Left V Superior Vena Cava W Thoracic Aorta, Descending X Thoracic Aorta, Ascending/Arch	0 Open 3 Percutaneous 4 Percutaneous Endoscopic	7 Autologous Tissue Substitute 8 Zooplastic Tissue J Synthetic Substitute K Nonautologous Tissue Substitute	Z No Qualifier
F Aortic Valve	0 Open 3 Percutaneous 4 Percutaneous Endoscopic	7 Autologous Tissue Substitute 8 Zooplastic Tissue J Synthetic Substitute K Nonautologous Tissue Substitute	J Truncal Valve Z No Qualifier
G Mitral Valve	0 Open 3 Percutaneous 4 Percutaneous Endoscopic	7 Autologous Tissue Substitute 8 Zooplastic Tissue J Synthetic Substitute K Nonautologous Tissue Substitute	E Atrioventricular Valve, Left Z No Qualifier
J Tricuspid Valve	0 Open 3 Percutaneous 4 Percutaneous Endoscopic	7 Autologous Tissue Substitute 8 Zooplastic Tissue J Synthetic Substitute K Nonautologous Tissue Substitute	G Atrioventricular Valve, Right Z No Qualifier

0 Medical and Surgical
2 Heart and Great Vessels
V Restriction: Partially closing an orifice or the lumen of a tubular body part

Body Part	Approach	Device	Qualifier
Character 4	**Character 5**	**Character 6**	**Character 7**
A Heart	0 Open 3 Percutaneous 4 Percutaneous Endoscopic	C Extraluminal Device Z No Device	Z No Qualifier
G Mitral Valve	0 Open 3 Percutaneous 4 Percutaneous Endoscopic	Z No Device	Z No Qualifier
P Pulmonary Trunk Q Pulmonary Artery, Right S Pulmonary Vein, Right T Pulmonary Vein, Left V Superior Vena Cava	0 Open 3 Percutaneous 4 Percutaneous Endoscopic	C Extraluminal Device D Intraluminal Device Z No Device	Z No Qualifier
R Pulmonary Artery, Left	0 Open 3 Percutaneous 4 Percutaneous Endoscopic	C Extraluminal Device D Intraluminal Device Z No Device	T Ductus Arteriosus Z No Qualifier
W Thoracic Aorta, Descending X Thoracic Aorta, Ascending/Arch	0 Open 3 Percutaneous 4 Percutaneous Endoscopic	C Extraluminal Device D Intraluminal Device E Intraluminal Device, Branched or Fenestrated, One or Two Arteries F Intraluminal Device, Branched or Fenestrated, Three or More Arteries Z No Device	Z No Qualifier

0 Medical and Surgical
2 Heart and Great Vessels
W Revision: Correcting, to the extent possible, a portion of a malfunctioning device or the position of a displaced device

Body Part	Approach	Device	Qualifier
Character 4	**Character 5**	**Character 6**	**Character 7**
5 Atrial Septum M Ventricular Septum	0 Open 4 Percutaneous Endoscopic	J Synthetic Substitute	Z No Qualifier
A Heart NC CC HAC LC	0 Open 3 Percutaneous 4 Percutaneous Endoscopic	2 Monitoring Device 3 Infusion Device 7 Autologous Tissue Substitute 8 Zooplastic Tissue C Extraluminal Device D Intraluminal Device J Synthetic Substitute K Nonautologous Tissue Substitute M Cardiac Lead N Intracardiac Pacemaker Q Implantable Heart Assist System Y Other Device	Z No Qualifier
A Heart	0 Open 3 Percutaneous 4 Percutaneous Endoscopic	R Short-term External Heart Assist System	S Biventricular Z No Qualifier
A Heart	X External	2 Monitoring Device 3 Infusion Device 7 Autologous Tissue Substitute 8 Zooplastic Tissue C Extraluminal Device D Intraluminal Device J Synthetic Substitute K Nonautologous Tissue Substitute M Cardiac Lead N Intracardiac Pacemaker Q Implantable Heart Assist System	Z No Qualifier

02W continued on next page

LC Limited Coverage   NC Noncovered   HAC HAC-associated Procedure   CC Combination Cluster - See Appendix G for code lists
DRG Non-OR-Affecting MS-DRG Assignment   New/Revised Text in **Orange**   ♂ Male   ♀ Female

0 Medical and Surgical
2 Heart and Great Vessels
W Revision: Correcting, to the extent possible, a portion of a malfunctioning device or the position of a displaced device

02W continued from previous page

Body Part	Approach	Device	Qualifier
Character 4	Character 5	Character 6	Character 7
A Heart	**X** External	**R** Short-term External Heart Assist System	**S** Biventricular **Z** No Qualifier
F Aortic Valve **G** Mitral Valve **H** Pulmonary Valve **J** Tricuspid Valve	**0** Open **3** Percutaneous **4** Percutaneous Endoscopic	**7** Autologous Tissue Substitute **8** Zooplastic Tissue **J** Synthetic Substitute **K** Nonautologous Tissue Substitute	**Z** No Qualifier
Y Great Vessel	**0** Open **3** Percutaneous **4** Percutaneous Endoscopic	**2** Monitoring Device **3** Infusion Device **7** Autologous Tissue Substitute **8** Zooplastic Tissue **C** Extraluminal Device **D** Intraluminal Device **J** Synthetic Substitute **K** Nonautologous Tissue Substitute **Y** Other Device	**Z** No Qualifier
Y Great Vessel	**X** External	**2** Monitoring Device **3** Infusion Device **7** Autologous Tissue Substitute **8** Zooplastic Tissue **C** Extraluminal Device **D** Intraluminal Device **J** Synthetic Substitute **K** Nonautologous Tissue Substitute	**Z** No Qualifier

LC 02WA0JZ 02WA0QZ

NC 02WA3QZ 02WA4QZ

HAC 02WA0MZ 02WA3MZ 02WA4MZ

Surgical site infection (SSI) following cardiac implantable electronic device (CIED) procedures and secondary diagnosis K68.11, T81.4XXA, T82.6XXA, T82.7XXA.

CC 02WA0QZ 02WA0RZ 02WA3QZ 02WA3RZ 02WA4QZ 02WA4RZ

0 Medical and Surgical
2 Heart and Great Vessels
Y Transplantation: Putting in or on all or a portion of a living body part taken from another individual or animal to physically take the place and/or function of all or a portion of a similar body part

Body Part	Approach	Device	Qualifier
Character 4	Character 5	Character 6	Character 7
A Heart LC	**0** Open	**Z** No Device	**0** Allogeneic **1** Syngeneic **2** Zooplastic

LC 02YA0Z0 02YA0Z1 02YA0Z2

NOTES

Upper Arteries 031-03W

0 Medical and Surgical
3 Upper Arteries
1 Bypass: Altering the route of passage of the contents of a tubular body part

Body Part	Approach	Device	Qualifier
Character 4	Character 5	Character 6	Character 7
2 Innominate Artery	0 Open	9 Autologous Venous Tissue A Autologous Arterial Tissue J Synthetic Substitute K Nonautologous Tissue Substitute Z No Device	0 Upper Arm Artery, Right 1 Upper Arm Artery, Left 2 Upper Arm Artery, Bilateral 3 Lower Arm Artery, Right 4 Lower Arm Artery, Left 5 Lower Arm Artery, Bilateral 6 Upper Leg Artery, Right 7 Upper Leg Artery, Left 8 Upper Leg Artery, Bilateral 9 Lower Leg Artery, Right B Lower Leg Artery, Left C Lower Leg Artery, Bilateral D Upper Arm Vein F Lower Arm Vein J Extracranial Artery, Right K Extracranial Artery, Left
3 Subclavian Artery, Right 4 Subclavian Artery, Left	0 Open	9 Autologous Venous Tissue A Autologous Arterial Tissue J Synthetic Substitute K Nonautologous Tissue Substitute Z No Device	0 Upper Arm Artery, Right 1 Upper Arm Artery, Left 2 Upper Arm Artery, Bilateral 3 Lower Arm Artery, Right 4 Lower Arm Artery, Left 5 Lower Arm Artery, Bilateral 6 Upper Leg Artery, Right 7 Upper Leg Artery, Left 8 Upper Leg Artery, Bilateral 9 Lower Leg Artery, Right B Lower Leg Artery, Left C Lower Leg Artery, Bilateral D Upper Arm Vein F Lower Arm Vein J Extracranial Artery, Right K Extracranial Artery, Left M Pulmonary Artery, Right N Pulmonary Artery, Left
5 Axillary Artery, Right 6 Axillary Artery, Left	0 Open	9 Autologous Venous Tissue A Autologous Arterial Tissue J Synthetic Substitute K Nonautologous Tissue Substitute Z No Device	0 Upper Arm Artery, Right 1 Upper Arm Artery, Left 2 Upper Arm Artery, Bilateral 3 Lower Arm Artery, Right 4 Lower Arm Artery, Left 5 Lower Arm Artery, Bilateral 6 Upper Leg Artery, Right 7 Upper Leg Artery, Left 8 Upper Leg Artery, Bilateral 9 Lower Leg Artery, Right B Lower Leg Artery, Left C Lower Leg Artery, Bilateral D Upper Arm Vein F Lower Arm Vein J Extracranial Artery, Right K Extracranial Artery, Left V Superior Vena Cava

031 continued on next page

031

0 **Medical and Surgical**
3 **Upper Arteries**
1 **Bypass:** Altering the route of passage of the contents of a tubular body part

031 continued from previous page

Body Part	Approach	Device	Qualifier
Character 4	**Character 5**	**Character 6**	**Character 7**
7 Brachial Artery, Right	0 Open	9 Autologous Venous Tissue A Autologous Arterial Tissue J Synthetic Substitute K Nonautologous Tissue Substitute Z No Device	0 Upper Arm Artery, Right 3 Lower Arm Artery, Right D Upper Arm Vein F Lower Arm Vein V Superior Vena Cava
8 Brachial Artery, Left	0 Open	9 Autologous Venous Tissue A Autologous Arterial Tissue J Synthetic Substitute K Nonautologous Tissue Substitute Z No Device	1 Upper Arm Artery, Left 4 Lower Arm Artery, Left D Upper Arm Vein F Lower Arm Vein V Superior Vena Cava
9 Ulnar Artery, Right B Radial Artery, Right	0 Open	9 Autologous Venous Tissue A Autologous Arterial Tissue J Synthetic Substitute K Nonautologous Tissue Substitute Z No Device	3 Lower Arm Artery, Right F Lower Arm Vein
A Ulnar Artery, Left C Radial Artery, Left	0 Open	9 Autologous Venous Tissue A Autologous Arterial Tissue J Synthetic Substitute K Nonautologous Tissue Substitute Z No Device	4 Lower Arm Artery, Left F Lower Arm Vein
G Intracranial Artery S Temporal Artery, Right NC T Temporal Artery, Left NC	0 Open	9 Autologous Venous Tissue A Autologous Arterial Tissue J Synthetic Substitute K Nonautologous Tissue Substitute Z No Device	G Intracranial Artery
H Common Carotid Artery, Right NC J Common Carotid Artery, Left NC	0 Open	9 Autologous Venous Tissue A Autologous Arterial Tissue J Synthetic Substitute K Nonautologous Tissue Substitute Z No Device	G Intracranial Artery J Extracranial Artery, Right K Extracranial Artery, Left
K Internal Carotid Artery, Right L Internal Carotid Artery, Left M External Carotid Artery, Right N External Carotid Artery, Left	0 Open	9 Autologous Venous Tissue A Autologous Arterial Tissue J Synthetic Substitute K Nonautologous Tissue Substitute Z No Device	J Extracranial Artery, Right K Extracranial Artery, Left

NC 031H09G 031H0AG 031H0JG 031H0KG 031H0ZG 031J09G 031J0AG 031J0JG 031J0KG 031J0ZG 031S09G 031S0AG 031S0JG
031S0KG 031S0ZG 031T09G 031T0AG 031T0JG 031T0KG 031T0ZG

LC Limited Coverage   NC Noncovered   HAC HAC-associated Procedure   CC Combination Cluster - See Appendix G for code lists
DRG Non-OR-Affecting MS-DRG Assignment   New/Revised Text in **Orange**   ♂ Male   ♀ Female

198

2018 ICD-10-PCS

0   Medical and Surgical
3   Upper Arteries
5   Destruction: Physical eradication of all or a portion of a body part by the direct use of energy, force, or a destructive agent

Body Part	Approach	Device	Qualifier
Character 4	Character 5	Character 6	Character 7
0 Internal Mammary Artery, Right 1 Internal Mammary Artery, Left 2 Innominate Artery 3 Subclavian Artery, Right 4 Subclavian Artery, Left 5 Axillary Artery, Right 6 Axillary Artery, Left 7 Brachial Artery, Right 8 Brachial Artery, Left 9 Ulnar Artery, Right A Ulnar Artery, Left B Radial Artery, Right C Radial Artery, Left D Hand Artery, Right F Hand Artery, Left G Intracranial Artery H Common Carotid Artery, Right J Common Carotid Artery, Left K Internal Carotid Artery, Right L Internal Carotid Artery, Left M External Carotid Artery, Right N External Carotid Artery, Left P Vertebral Artery, Right Q Vertebral Artery, Left R Face Artery S Temporal Artery, Right T Temporal Artery, Left U Thyroid Artery, Right V Thyroid Artery, Left Y Upper Artery	0 Open 3 Percutaneous 4 Percutaneous Endoscopic	Z No Device	Z No Qualifier

0   Medical and Surgical
3   Upper Arteries
7   Dilation: Expanding an orifice or the lumen of a tubular body part

Body Part	Approach	Device	Qualifier
Character 4	Character 5	Character 6	Character 7
0 Internal Mammary Artery, Right	0 Open	4 Intraluminal Device, Drug-eluting	6 Bifurcation
1 Internal Mammary Artery, Left	3 Percutaneous	5 Intraluminal Device, Drug-eluting, Two	Z No Qualifier
2 Innominate Artery	4 Percutaneous Endoscopic	6 Intraluminal Device, Drug-eluting, Three	
3 Subclavian Artery, Right		7 Intraluminal Device, Drug-eluting, Four or More	
4 Subclavian Artery, Left		D Intraluminal Device	
5 Axillary Artery, Right		E Intraluminal Device, Two	
6 Axillary Artery, Left		F Intraluminal Device, Three	
7 Brachial Artery, Right		G Intraluminal Device, Four or More	
8 Brachial Artery, Left		Z No Device	
9 Ulnar Artery, Right			
A Ulnar Artery, Left			
B Radial Artery, Right			
C Radial Artery, Left			
D Hand Artery, Right			
F Hand Artery, Left			
G Intracranial Artery 🅽🅲			
H Common Carotid Artery, Right			
J Common Carotid Artery, Left			
K Internal Carotid Artery, Right			
L Internal Carotid Artery, Left			
M External Carotid Artery, Right			
N External Carotid Artery, Left			
P Vertebral Artery, Right			
Q Vertebral Artery, Left			
R Face Artery			
S Temporal Artery, Right			
T Temporal Artery, Left			
U Thyroid Artery, Right			
V Thyroid Artery, Left			
Y Upper Artery			

🅽🅲   037G3Z6   037G3ZZ   037G4Z6   037G4ZZ

🅻🅲 Limited Coverage   🅽🅲 Noncovered   🅷🅰🅲 HAC-associated Procedure   🅲🅲 Combination Cluster - See Appendix G for code lists
🅳🆁🅶 Non-OR-Affecting MS-DRG Assignment   New/Revised Text in **Orange**   ♂ Male   ♀ Female

200

2018 ICD-10-PCS

0   Medical and Surgical
3   Upper Arteries
9   Drainage: Taking or letting out fluids and/or gases from a body part

Body Part	Approach	Device	Qualifier
Character 4	Character 5	Character 6	Character 7
0 Internal Mammary Artery, Right **1** Internal Mammary Artery, Left **2** Innominate Artery **3** Subclavian Artery, Right **4** Subclavian Artery, Left **5** Axillary Artery, Right **6** Axillary Artery, Left **7** Brachial Artery, Right **8** Brachial Artery, Left **9** Ulnar Artery, Right **A** Ulnar Artery, Left **B** Radial Artery, Right **C** Radial Artery, Left **D** Hand Artery, Right **F** Hand Artery, Left **G** Intracranial Artery **H** Common Carotid Artery, Right **J** Common Carotid Artery, Left **K** Internal Carotid Artery, Right **L** Internal Carotid Artery, Left **M** External Carotid Artery, Right **N** External Carotid Artery, Left **P** Vertebral Artery, Right **Q** Vertebral Artery, Left **R** Face Artery **S** Temporal Artery, Right **T** Temporal Artery, Left **U** Thyroid Artery, Right **V** Thyroid Artery, Left **Y** Upper Artery	**0** Open **3** Percutaneous **4** Percutaneous Endoscopic	**0** Drainage Device	**Z** No Qualifier
0 Internal Mammary Artery, Right **1** Internal Mammary Artery, Left **2** Innominate Artery **3** Subclavian Artery, Right **4** Subclavian Artery, Left **5** Axillary Artery, Right **6** Axillary Artery, Left **7** Brachial Artery, Right **8** Brachial Artery, Left **9** Ulnar Artery, Right **A** Ulnar Artery, Left **B** Radial Artery, Right **C** Radial Artery, Left **D** Hand Artery, Right **F** Hand Artery, Left **G** Intracranial Artery **H** Common Carotid Artery, Right **J** Common Carotid Artery, Left **K** Internal Carotid Artery, Right **L** Internal Carotid Artery, Left **M** External Carotid Artery, Right **N** External Carotid Artery, Left **P** Vertebral Artery, Right **Q** Vertebral Artery, Left **R** Face Artery **S** Temporal Artery, Right **T** Temporal Artery, Left **U** Thyroid Artery, Right **V** Thyroid Artery, Left **Y** Upper Artery	**0** Open **3** Percutaneous **4** Percutaneous Endoscopic	**Z** No Device	**X** Diagnostic **Z** No Qualifier

LC Limited Coverage   NC Noncovered   HAC HAC-associated Procedure   CC Combination Cluster - See Appendix G for code lists
DRG Non-OR-Affecting MS-DRG Assignment   New/Revised Text in **Orange**   ♂ Male   ♀ Female

2018 ICD-10-PCS

201

UPPER ARTERIES 031-03W

0 **Medical and Surgical**
3 **Upper Arteries**
B **Excision:** Cutting out or off, without replacement, a portion of a body part

Body Part	Approach	Device	Qualifier
Character 4	Character 5	Character 6	Character 7
0 Internal Mammary Artery, Right	**0** Open	**Z** No Device	**X** Diagnostic
1 Internal Mammary Artery, Left	**3** Percutaneous		**Z** No Qualifier
2 Innominate Artery	**4** Percutaneous Endoscopic		
3 Subclavian Artery, Right			
4 Subclavian Artery, Left			
5 Axillary Artery, Right			
6 Axillary Artery, Left			
7 Brachial Artery, Right			
8 Brachial Artery, Left			
9 Ulnar Artery, Right			
A Ulnar Artery, Left			
B Radial Artery, Right			
C Radial Artery, Left			
D Hand Artery, Right			
F Hand Artery, Left			
G Intracranial Artery			
H Common Carotid Artery, Right			
J Common Carotid Artery, Left			
K Internal Carotid Artery, Right			
L Internal Carotid Artery, Left			
M External Carotid Artery, Right			
N External Carotid Artery, Left			
P Vertebral Artery, Right			
Q Vertebral Artery, Left			
R Face Artery			
S Temporal Artery, Right			
T Temporal Artery, Left			
U Thyroid Artery, Right			
V Thyroid Artery, Left			
Y Upper Artery			

LC Limited Coverage   NC Noncovered   HAC HAC-associated Procedure   CC Combination Cluster - See Appendix G for code lists
DRG Non-OR-Affecting MS-DRG Assignment   New/Revised Text in Orange   ♂ Male   ♀ Female

202

2018 ICD-10-PCS

0 Medical and Surgical
3 Upper Arteries
C **Extirpation:** Taking or cutting out solid matter from a body part

Body Part	Approach	Device	Qualifier
Character 4	Character 5	Character 6	Character 7
0 Internal Mammary Artery, Right **1** Internal Mammary Artery, Left **2** Innominate Artery **3** Subclavian Artery, Right **4** Subclavian Artery, Left **5** Axillary Artery, Right **6** Axillary Artery, Left **7** Brachial Artery, Right **8** Brachial Artery, Left **9** Ulnar Artery, Right **A** Ulnar Artery, Left **B** Radial Artery, Right **C** Radial Artery, Left **D** Hand Artery, Right **F** Hand Artery, Left **G** Intracranial Artery **H** Common Carotid Artery, Right **J** Common Carotid Artery, Left **K** Internal Carotid Artery, Right **L** Internal Carotid Artery, Left **M** External Carotid Artery, Right **N** External Carotid Artery, Left **P** Vertebral Artery, Right **Q** Vertebral Artery, Left **R** Face Artery **S** Temporal Artery, Right **T** Temporal Artery, Left **U** Thyroid Artery, Right **V** Thyroid Artery, Left **Y** Upper Artery	**0** Open **3** Percutaneous **4** Percutaneous Endoscopic	**Z** No Device	**6** Bifurcation **Z** No Qualifier

0   Medical and Surgical
3   Upper Arteries
H   Insertion: Putting in a nonbiological appliance that monitors, assists, performs, or prevents a physiological function but does not physically take the place of a body part

Body Part	Approach	Device	Qualifier
Character 4	Character 5	Character 6	Character 7
0 Internal Mammary Artery, Right 1 Internal Mammary Artery, Left 2 Innominate Artery 3 Subclavian Artery, Right 4 Subclavian Artery, Left 5 Axillary Artery, Right 6 Axillary Artery, Left 7 Brachial Artery, Right 8 Brachial Artery, Left 9 Ulnar Artery, Right A Ulnar Artery, Left B Radial Artery, Right C Radial Artery, Left D Hand Artery, Right F Hand Artery, Left G Intracranial Artery H Common Carotid Artery, Right J Common Carotid Artery, Left M External Carotid Artery, Right N External Carotid Artery, Left P Vertebral Artery, Right Q Vertebral Artery, Left R Face Artery S Temporal Artery, Right T Temporal Artery, Left U Thyroid Artery, Right V Thyroid Artery, Left	0 Open 3 Percutaneous 4 Percutaneous Endoscopic	3 Infusion Device D Intraluminal Device	Z No Qualifier
K Internal Carotid Artery, Right L Internal Carotid Artery, Left	0 Open 3 Percutaneous 4 Percutaneous Endoscopic	3 Infusion Device D Intraluminal Device M Stimulator Lead	Z No Qualifier
Y Upper Artery	0 Open 3 Percutaneous 4 Percutaneous Endoscopic	2 Monitoring Device 3 Infusion Device D Intraluminal Device Y Other Device	Z No Qualifier

0   Medical and Surgical
3   Upper Arteries
J   Inspection: Visually and/or manually exploring a body part

Body Part	Approach	Device	Qualifier
Character 4	Character 5	Character 6	Character 7
Y Upper Artery	0 Open 3 Percutaneous 4 Percutaneous Endoscopic X External	Z No Device	Z No Qualifier

LC Limited Coverage   **NC** Noncovered   **HAC** HAC-associated Procedure   **CC** Combination Cluster - See Appendix G for code lists
DRG Non-OR-Affecting MS-DRG Assignment   New/Revised Text in **Orange**   ♂ Male   ♀ Female

204   2018 ICD-10-PCS

0   **Medical and Surgical**
3   **Upper Arteries**
L   **Occlusion:** Completely closing an orifice or the lumen of a tubular body part

Body Part	Approach	Device	Qualifier
Character 4	**Character 5**	**Character 6**	**Character 7**
0 Internal Mammary Artery, Right 1 Internal Mammary Artery, Left 2 Innominate Artery 3 Subclavian Artery, Right 4 Subclavian Artery, Left 5 Axillary Artery, Right 6 Axillary Artery, Left 7 Brachial Artery, Right 8 Brachial Artery, Left 9 Ulnar Artery, Right A Ulnar Artery, Left B Radial Artery, Right C Radial Artery, Left D Hand Artery, Right F Hand Artery, Left R Face Artery S Temporal Artery, Right T Temporal Artery, Left U Thyroid Artery, Right V Thyroid Artery, Left Y Upper Artery	0 Open 3 Percutaneous 4 Percutaneous Endoscopic	C Extraluminal Device D Intraluminal Device Z No Device	Z No Qualifier
G Intracranial Artery H Common Carotid Artery, Right J Common Carotid Artery, Left K Internal Carotid Artery, Right L Internal Carotid Artery, Left M External Carotid Artery, Right N External Carotid Artery, Left P Vertebral Artery, Right Q Vertebral Artery, Left	0 Open 3 Percutaneous 4 Percutaneous Endoscopic	B Intraluminal Device, Bioactive C Extraluminal Device D Intraluminal Device Z No Device	Z No Qualifier

LC Limited Coverage   NC Noncovered   HAC HAC-associated Procedure   CC Combination Cluster - See Appendix G for code lists
DRG Non-OR-Affecting MS-DRG Assignment   New/Revised Text in **Orange**   ♂ Male   ♀ Female

2018 ICD-10-PCS

205

UPPER ARTERIES 031-03W

0 **Medical and Surgical**
3 **Upper Arteries**
N **Release:** Freeing a body part from an abnormal physical constraint by cutting or by the use of force

Body Part	Approach	Device	Qualifier
Character 4	Character 5	Character 6	Character 7
0 Internal Mammary Artery, Right 1 Internal Mammary Artery, Left 2 Innominate Artery 3 Subclavian Artery, Right 4 Subclavian Artery, Left 5 Axillary Artery, Right 6 Axillary Artery, Left 7 Brachial Artery, Right 8 Brachial Artery, Left 9 Ulnar Artery, Right A Ulnar Artery, Left B Radial Artery, Right C Radial Artery, Left D Hand Artery, Right F Hand Artery, Left G Intracranial Artery H Common Carotid Artery, Right J Common Carotid Artery, Left K Internal Carotid Artery, Right L Internal Carotid Artery, Left M External Carotid Artery, Right N External Carotid Artery, Left P Vertebral Artery, Right Q Vertebral Artery, Left R Face Artery S Temporal Artery, Right T Temporal Artery, Left U Thyroid Artery, Right V Thyroid Artery, Left Y Upper Artery	0 Open 3 Percutaneous 4 Percutaneous Endoscopic	Z No Device	Z No Qualifier

0 **Medical and Surgical**
3 **Upper Arteries**
P **Removal:** Taking out or off a device from a body part

Body Part	Approach	Device	Qualifier
Character 4	Character 5	Character 6	Character 7
Y Upper Artery	0 Open 3 Percutaneous 4 Percutaneous Endoscopic	0 Drainage Device 2 Monitoring Device 3 Infusion Device 7 Autologous Tissue Substitute C Extraluminal Device D Intraluminal Device J Synthetic Substitute K Nonautologous Tissue Substitute M Stimulator Lead Y Other Device	Z No Qualifier
Y Upper Artery	X External	0 Drainage Device 2 Monitoring Device 3 Infusion Device D Intraluminal Device M Stimulator Lead	Z No Qualifier

0 **Medical and Surgical**
3 **Upper Arteries**
Q **Repair:** Restoring, to the extent possible, a body part to its normal anatomic structure and function

Body Part	Approach	Device	Qualifier
Character 4	Character 5	Character 6	Character 7
0 Internal Mammary Artery, Right	0 Open	Z No Device	Z No Qualifier
1 Internal Mammary Artery, Left	3 Percutaneous		
2 Innominate Artery	4 Percutaneous Endoscopic		
3 Subclavian Artery, Right			
4 Subclavian Artery, Left			
5 Axillary Artery, Right			
6 Axillary Artery, Left			
7 Brachial Artery, Right			
8 Brachial Artery, Left			
9 Ulnar Artery, Right			
A Ulnar Artery, Left			
B Radial Artery, Right			
C Radial Artery, Left			
D Hand Artery, Right			
F Hand Artery, Left			
G Intracranial Artery			
H Common Carotid Artery, Right			
J Common Carotid Artery, Left			
K Internal Carotid Artery, Right			
L Internal Carotid Artery, Left			
M External Carotid Artery, Right			
N External Carotid Artery, Left			
P Vertebral Artery, Right			
Q Vertebral Artery, Left			
R Face Artery			
S Temporal Artery, Right			
T Temporal Artery, Left			
U Thyroid Artery, Right			
V Thyroid Artery, Left			
Y Upper Artery			

0 **Medical and Surgical**
3 **Upper Arteries**
R **Replacement:** Putting in or on biological or synthetic material that physically takes the place and/or function of all or a portion of a body part

Body Part	Approach	Device	Qualifier
Character 4	Character 5	Character 6	Character 7
0 Internal Mammary Artery, Right 1 Internal Mammary Artery, Left 2 Innominate Artery 3 Subclavian Artery, Right 4 Subclavian Artery, Left 5 Axillary Artery, Right 6 Axillary Artery, Left 7 Brachial Artery, Right 8 Brachial Artery, Left 9 Ulnar Artery, Right A Ulnar Artery, Left B Radial Artery, Right C Radial Artery, Left D Hand Artery, Right F Hand Artery, Left G Intracranial Artery H Common Carotid Artery, Right J Common Carotid Artery, Left K Internal Carotid Artery, Right L Internal Carotid Artery, Left M External Carotid Artery, Right N External Carotid Artery, Left P Vertebral Artery, Right Q Vertebral Artery, Left R Face Artery S Temporal Artery, Right T Temporal Artery, Left U Thyroid Artery, Right V Thyroid Artery, Left Y Upper Artery	0 Open 4 Percutaneous Endoscopic	7 Autologous Tissue Substitute J Synthetic Substitute K Nonautologous Tissue Substitute	Z No Qualifier

LC Limited Coverage NC Noncovered HAC HAC-associated Procedure CC Combination Cluster - See Appendix G for code lists
DRG Non-OR-Affecting MS-DRG Assignment New/Revised Text in **Orange** ♂ Male ♀ Female

208

2018 ICD-10-PCS

0   **Medical and Surgical**
3   **Upper Arteries**
S   **Reposition:** Moving to its normal location, or other suitable location, all or a portion of a body part

Body Part	Approach	Device	Qualifier
Character 4	Character 5	Character 6	Character 7
0 Internal Mammary Artery, Right 1 Internal Mammary Artery, Left 2 Innominate Artery 3 Subclavian Artery, Right 4 Subclavian Artery, Left 5 Axillary Artery, Right 6 Axillary Artery, Left 7 Brachial Artery, Right 8 Brachial Artery, Left 9 Ulnar Artery, Right A Ulnar Artery, Left B Radial Artery, Right C Radial Artery, Left D Hand Artery, Right F Hand Artery, Left G Intracranial Artery H Common Carotid Artery, Right J Common Carotid Artery, Left K Internal Carotid Artery, Right L Internal Carotid Artery, Left M External Carotid Artery, Right N External Carotid Artery, Left P Vertebral Artery, Right Q Vertebral Artery, Left R Face Artery S Temporal Artery, Right T Temporal Artery, Left U Thyroid Artery, Right V Thyroid Artery, Left Y Upper Artery	0 Open 3 Percutaneous 4 Percutaneous Endoscopic	Z No Device	Z No Qualifier

LC Limited Coverage   NC Noncovered   HAC HAC-associated Procedure   CC Combination Cluster - See Appendix G for code lists
DRG Non-OR-Affecting MS-DRG Assignment   New/Revised Text in **Orange**   ♂ Male   ♀ Female

2018 ICD-10-PCS

209

UPPER ARTERIES 031-03W

0   **Medical and Surgical**
3   **Upper Arteries**
U   **Supplement:** Putting in or on biological or synthetic material that physically reinforces and/or augments the function of a portion of a body part

Body Part	Approach	Device	Qualifier
Character 4	Character 5	Character 6	Character 7
0 Internal Mammary Artery, Right 1 Internal Mammary Artery, Left 2 Innominate Artery 3 Subclavian Artery, Right 4 Subclavian Artery, Left 5 Axillary Artery, Right 6 Axillary Artery, Left 7 Brachial Artery, Right 8 Brachial Artery, Left 9 Ulnar Artery, Right A Ulnar Artery, Left B Radial Artery, Right C Radial Artery, Left D Hand Artery, Right F Hand Artery, Left G Intracranial Artery H Common Carotid Artery, Right J Common Carotid Artery, Left K Internal Carotid Artery, Right L Internal Carotid Artery, Left M External Carotid Artery, Right N External Carotid Artery, Left P Vertebral Artery, Right Q Vertebral Artery, Left R Face Artery S Temporal Artery, Right T Temporal Artery, Left U Thyroid Artery, Right V Thyroid Artery, Left Y Upper Artery	0 Open 3 Percutaneous 4 Percutaneous Endoscopic	7 Autologous Tissue Substitute J Synthetic Substitute K Nonautologous Tissue Substitute	Z No Qualifier

LC Limited Coverage   NC Noncovered   HAC HAC-associated Procedure   CC Combination Cluster - See Appendix G for code lists
DRG Non-OR-Affecting MS-DRG Assignment   New/Revised Text in **Orange**   ♂ Male   ♀ Female

210

2018 ICD-10-PCS

0   **Medical and Surgical**
3   **Upper Arteries**
V   **Restriction:** Partially closing an orifice or the lumen of a tubular body part

Body Part	Approach	Device	Qualifier
Character 4	Character 5	Character 6	Character 7
0 Internal Mammary Artery, Right 1 Internal Mammary Artery, Left 2 Innominate Artery 3 Subclavian Artery, Right 4 Subclavian Artery, Left 5 Axillary Artery, Right 6 Axillary Artery, Left 7 Brachial Artery, Right 8 Brachial Artery, Left 9 Ulnar Artery, Right A Ulnar Artery, Left B Radial Artery, Right C Radial Artery, Left D Hand Artery, Right F Hand Artery, Left R Face Artery S Temporal Artery, Right T Temporal Artery, Left U Thyroid Artery, Right V Thyroid Artery, Left Y Upper Artery	0 Open 3 Percutaneous 4 Percutaneous Endoscopic	C Extraluminal Device D Intraluminal Device Z No Device	Z No Qualifier
G Intracranial Artery H Common Carotid Artery, Right J Common Carotid Artery, Left K Internal Carotid Artery, Right L Internal Carotid Artery, Left M External Carotid Artery, Right N External Carotid Artery, Left P Vertebral Artery, Right Q Vertebral Artery, Left	0 Open 3 Percutaneous 4 Percutaneous Endoscopic	B Intraluminal Device, Bioactive C Extraluminal Device D Intraluminal Device Z No Device	Z No Qualifier

0   **Medical and Surgical**
3   **Upper Arteries**
W   **Revision:** Correcting, to the extent possible, a portion of a malfunctioning device or the position of a displaced device

Body Part	Approach	Device	Qualifier
Character 4	Character 5	Character 6	Character 7
Y Upper Artery	0 Open 3 Percutaneous 4 Percutaneous Endoscopic	0 Drainage Device 2 Monitoring Device 3 Infusion Device 7 Autologous Tissue Substitute C Extraluminal Device D Intraluminal Device J Synthetic Substitute K Nonautologous Tissue Substitute M Stimulator Lead Y Other Device	Z No Qualifier
Y Upper Artery	X External	0 Drainage Device 2 Monitoring Device 3 Infusion Device 7 Autologous Tissue Substitute C Extraluminal Device D Intraluminal Device J Synthetic Substitute K Nonautologous Tissue Substitute M Stimulator Lead	Z No Qualifier

NOTES

Lower Arteries 041-04W

0 Medical and Surgical
4 Lower Arteries
1 Bypass: Altering the route of passage of the contents of a tubular body part

Body Part	Approach	Device	Qualifier
Character 4	**Character 5**	**Character 6**	**Character 7**
0 Abdominal Aorta **C** Common Iliac Artery, Right **D** Common Iliac Artery, Left	**0** Open **4** Percutaneous Endoscopic	**9** Autologous Venous Tissue **A** Autologous Arterial Tissue **J** Synthetic Substitute **K** Nonautologous Tissue Substitute **Z** No Device	**0** Abdominal Aorta **1** Celiac Artery **2** Mesenteric Artery **3** Renal Artery, Right **4** Renal Artery, Left **5** Renal Artery, Bilateral **6** Common Iliac Artery, Right **7** Common Iliac Artery, Left **8** Common Iliac Arteries, Bilateral **9** Internal Iliac Artery, Right **B** Internal Iliac Artery, Left **C** Internal Iliac Arteries, Bilateral **D** External Iliac Artery, Right **F** External Iliac Artery, Left **G** External Iliac Arteries, Bilateral **H** Femoral Artery, Right **J** Femoral Artery, Left **K** Femoral Arteries, Bilateral **Q** Lower Extremity Artery **R** Lower Artery
3 Hepatic Artery **4** Splenic Artery	**0** Open **4** Percutaneous Endoscopic	**9** Autologous Venous Tissue **A** Autologous Arterial Tissue **J** Synthetic Substitute **K** Nonautologous Tissue Substitute **Z** No Device	**3** Renal Artery, Right **4** Renal Artery, Left **5** Renal Artery, Bilateral
E Internal Iliac Artery, Right **F** Internal Iliac Artery, Left **H** External Iliac Artery, Right **J** External Iliac Artery, Left	**0** Open **4** Percutaneous Endoscopic	**9** Autologous Venous Tissue **A** Autologous Arterial Tissue **J** Synthetic Substitute **K** Nonautologous Tissue Substitute **Z** No Device	**9** Internal Iliac Artery, Right **B** Internal Iliac Artery, Left **C** Internal Iliac Arteries, Bilateral **D** External Iliac Artery, Right **F** External Iliac Artery, Left **G** External Iliac Arteries, Bilateral **H** Femoral Artery, Right **J** Femoral Artery, Left **K** Femoral Arteries, Bilateral **P** Foot Artery **Q** Lower Extremity Artery
K Femoral Artery, Right **L** Femoral Artery, Left	**0** Open **4** Percutaneous Endoscopic	**9** Autologous Venous Tissue **A** Autologous Arterial Tissue **J** Synthetic Substitute **K** Nonautologous Tissue Substitute **Z** No Device	**H** Femoral Artery, Right **J** Femoral Artery, Left **K** Femoral Arteries, Bilateral **L** Popliteal Artery **M** Peroneal Artery **N** Posterior Tibial Artery **P** Foot Artery **Q** Lower Extremity Artery **S** Lower Extremity Vein
M Popliteal Artery, Right **N** Popliteal Artery, Left	**0** Open **4** Percutaneous Endoscopic	**9** Autologous Venous Tissue **A** Autologous Arterial Tissue **J** Synthetic Substitute **K** Nonautologous Tissue Substitute **Z** No Device	**L** Popliteal Artery **M** Peroneal Artery **P** Foot Artery **Q** Lower Extremity Artery **S** Lower Extremity Vein
T Peroneal Artery, Right **U** Peroneal Artery, Left **V** Foot Artery, Right **W** Foot Artery, Left	**0** Open **4** Percutaneous Endoscopic	**9** Autologous Venous Tissue **A** Autologous Arterial Tissue **J** Synthetic Substitute **K** Nonautologous Tissue Substitute **Z** No Device	**P** Foot Artery **Q** Lower Extremity Artery **S** Lower Extremity Vein

LC Limited Coverage **NC** Noncovered **HAC** HAC-associated Procedure **CC** Combination Cluster - See Appendix G for code lists
DRG Non-OR-Affecting MS-DRG Assignment New/Revised Text in **Orange** ♂ Male ♀ Female

2018 ICD-10-PCS

213

0   Medical and Surgical
4   Lower Arteries
5   Destruction: Physical eradication of all or a portion of a body part by the direct use of energy, force, or a destructive agent

Body Part	Approach	Device	Qualifier
Character 4	Character 5	Character 6	Character 7
0 Abdominal Aorta 1 Celiac Artery 2 Gastric Artery 3 Hepatic Artery 4 Splenic Artery 5 Superior Mesenteric Artery 6 Colic Artery, Right 7 Colic Artery, Left 8 Colic Artery, Middle 9 Renal Artery, Right A Renal Artery, Left B Inferior Mesenteric Artery C Common Iliac Artery, Right D Common Iliac Artery, Left E Internal Iliac Artery, Right F Internal Iliac Artery, Left H External Iliac Artery, Right J External Iliac Artery, Left K Femoral Artery, Right L Femoral Artery, Left M Popliteal Artery, Right N Popliteal Artery, Left P Anterior Tibial Artery, Right Q Anterior Tibial Artery, Left R Posterior Tibial Artery, Right S Posterior Tibial Artery, Left T Peroneal Artery, Right U Peroneal Artery, Left V Foot Artery, Right W Foot Artery, Left Y Lower Artery	0 Open 3 Percutaneous 4 Percutaneous Endoscopic	Z No Device	Z No Qualifier

0 Medical and Surgical
4 Lower Arteries
7 Dilation: Expanding an orifice or the lumen of a tubular body part

Body Part	Approach	Device	Qualifier
Character 4	Character 5	Character 6	Character 7
0 Abdominal Aorta 1 Celiac Artery 2 Gastric Artery 3 Hepatic Artery 4 Splenic Artery 5 Superior Mesenteric Artery 6 Colic Artery, Right 7 Colic Artery, Left 8 Colic Artery, Middle 9 Renal Artery, Right A Renal Artery, Left B Inferior Mesenteric Artery C Common Iliac Artery, Right D Common Iliac Artery, Left E Internal Iliac Artery, Right F Internal Iliac Artery, Left H External Iliac Artery, Right J External Iliac Artery, Left K Femoral Artery, Right L Femoral Artery, Left M Popliteal Artery, Right N Popliteal Artery, Left P Anterior Tibial Artery, Right Q Anterior Tibial Artery, Left R Posterior Tibial Artery, Right S Posterior Tibial Artery, Left T Peroneal Artery, Right U Peroneal Artery, Left V Foot Artery, Right W Foot Artery, Left Y Lower Artery	0 Open 3 Percutaneous 4 Percutaneous Endoscopic	4 Intraluminal Device, Drug-eluting D Intraluminal Device Z No Device	1 Drug-Coated Balloon 6 Bifurcation Z No Qualifier
0 Abdominal Aorta 1 Celiac Artery 2 Gastric Artery 3 Hepatic Artery 4 Splenic Artery 5 Superior Mesenteric Artery 6 Colic Artery, Right 7 Colic Artery, Left 8 Colic Artery, Middle 9 Renal Artery, Right A Renal Artery, Left B Inferior Mesenteric Artery C Common Iliac Artery, Right D Common Iliac Artery, Left E Internal Iliac Artery, Right F Internal Iliac Artery, Left H External Iliac Artery, Right J External Iliac Artery, Left K Femoral Artery, Right L Femoral Artery, Left M Popliteal Artery, Right N Popliteal Artery, Left P Anterior Tibial Artery, Right Q Anterior Tibial Artery, Left R Posterior Tibial Artery, Right S Posterior Tibial Artery, Left T Peroneal Artery, Right U Peroneal Artery, Left V Foot Artery, Right W Foot Artery, Left Y Lower Artery	0 Open 3 Percutaneous 4 Percutaneous Endoscopic	5 Intraluminal Device, Drug-eluting, Two 6 Intraluminal Device, Drug-eluting, Three 7 Intraluminal Device, Drug-eluting, Four or More E Intraluminal Device, Two F Intraluminal Device, Three G Intraluminal Device, Four or More	6 Bifurcation Z No Qualifier

0 **Medical and Surgical**
4 **Lower Arteries**
9 **Drainage:** Taking or letting out fluids and/or gases from a body part

Body Part	Approach	Device	Qualifier
Character 4	**Character 5**	**Character 6**	**Character 7**
0 Abdominal Aorta **1** Celiac Artery **2** Gastric Artery **3** Hepatic Artery **4** Splenic Artery **5** Superior Mesenteric Artery **6** Colic Artery, Right **7** Colic Artery, Left **8** Colic Artery, Middle **9** Renal Artery, Right **A** Renal Artery, Left **B** Inferior Mesenteric Artery **C** Common Iliac Artery, Right **D** Common Iliac Artery, Left **E** Internal Iliac Artery, Right **F** Internal Iliac Artery, Left **H** External Iliac Artery, Right **J** External Iliac Artery, Left **K** Femoral Artery, Right **L** Femoral Artery, Left **M** Popliteal Artery, Right **N** Popliteal Artery, Left **P** Anterior Tibial Artery, Right **Q** Anterior Tibial Artery, Left **R** Posterior Tibial Artery, Right **S** Posterior Tibial Artery, Left **T** Peroneal Artery, Right **U** Peroneal Artery, Left **V** Foot Artery, Right **W** Foot Artery, Left **Y** Lower Artery	**0** Open **3** Percutaneous **4** Percutaneous Endoscopic	**0** Drainage Device	**Z** No Qualifier
0 Abdominal Aorta **1** Celiac Artery **2** Gastric Artery **3** Hepatic Artery **4** Splenic Artery **5** Superior Mesenteric Artery **6** Colic Artery, Right **7** Colic Artery, Left **8** Colic Artery, Middle **9** Renal Artery, Right **A** Renal Artery, Left **B** Inferior Mesenteric Artery **C** Common Iliac Artery, Right **D** Common Iliac Artery, Left **E** Internal Iliac Artery, Right **F** Internal Iliac Artery, Left **H** External Iliac Artery, Right **J** External Iliac Artery, Left **K** Femoral Artery, Right **L** Femoral Artery, Left **M** Popliteal Artery, Right **N** Popliteal Artery, Left **P** Anterior Tibial Artery, Right **Q** Anterior Tibial Artery, Left **R** Posterior Tibial Artery, Right **S** Posterior Tibial Artery, Left **T** Peroneal Artery, Right **U** Peroneal Artery, Left **V** Foot Artery, Right **W** Foot Artery, Left **Y** Lower Artery	**0** Open **3** Percutaneous **4** Percutaneous Endoscopic	**Z** No Device	**X** Diagnostic **Z** No Qualifier

LC Limited Coverage   **NC** Noncovered   **HAC** HAC-associated Procedure   **CC** Combination Cluster - See Appendix G for code lists
DRG Non-OR-Affecting MS-DRG Assignment   New/Revised Text in **Orange**   ♂ Male   ♀ Female

216

2018 ICD-10-PCS

0 Medical and Surgical
4 Lower Arteries
B Excision: Cutting out or off, without replacement, a portion of a body part

Body Part	Approach	Device	Qualifier
Character 4	Character 5	Character 6	Character 7
0 Abdominal Aorta	0 Open	Z No Device	X Diagnostic
1 Celiac Artery	3 Percutaneous		Z No Qualifier
2 Gastric Artery	4 Percutaneous Endoscopic		
3 Hepatic Artery			
4 Splenic Artery			
5 Superior Mesenteric Artery			
6 Colic Artery, Right			
7 Colic Artery, Left			
8 Colic Artery, Middle			
9 Renal Artery, Right			
A Renal Artery, Left			
B Inferior Mesenteric Artery			
C Common Iliac Artery, Right			
D Common Iliac Artery, Left			
E Internal Iliac Artery, Right			
F Internal Iliac Artery, Left			
H External Iliac Artery, Right			
J External Iliac Artery, Left			
K Femoral Artery, Right			
L Femoral Artery, Left			
M Popliteal Artery, Right			
N Popliteal Artery, Left			
P Anterior Tibial Artery, Right			
Q Anterior Tibial Artery, Left			
R Posterior Tibial Artery, Right			
S Posterior Tibial Artery, Left			
T Peroneal Artery, Right			
U Peroneal Artery, Left			
V Foot Artery, Right			
W Foot Artery, Left			
Y Lower Artery			

LC Limited Coverage   NC Noncovered   HAC HAC-associated Procedure   CC Combination Cluster - See Appendix G for code lists
Non-OR-Affecting MS-DRG Assignment   New/Revised Text in **Orange**   ♂ Male   ♀ Female

2018 ICD-10-PCS

217

LOWER ARTERIES 041-04W

0 Medical and Surgical
4 Lower Arteries
C Extirpation: Taking or cutting out solid matter from a body part

Body Part		Approach		Device		Qualifier	
Character 4		**Character 5**		**Character 6**		**Character 7**	
0	Abdominal Aorta	0	Open	Z	No Device	6	Bifurcation
1	Celiac Artery	3	Percutaneous			Z	No Qualifier
2	Gastric Artery	4	Percutaneous Endoscopic				
3	Hepatic Artery						
4	Splenic Artery						
5	Superior Mesenteric Artery						
6	Colic Artery, Right						
7	Colic Artery, Left						
8	Colic Artery, Middle						
9	Renal Artery, Right						
A	Renal Artery, Left						
B	Inferior Mesenteric Artery						
C	Common Iliac Artery, Right						
D	Common Iliac Artery, Left						
E	Internal Iliac Artery, Right						
F	Internal Iliac Artery, Left						
H	External Iliac Artery, Right						
J	External Iliac Artery, Left						
K	Femoral Artery, Right						
L	Femoral Artery, Left						
M	Popliteal Artery, Right						
N	Popliteal Artery, Left						
P	Anterior Tibial Artery, Right						
Q	Anterior Tibial Artery, Left						
R	Posterior Tibial Artery, Right						
S	Posterior Tibial Artery, Left						
T	Peroneal Artery, Right						
U	Peroneal Artery, Left						
V	Foot Artery, Right						
W	Foot Artery, Left						
Y	Lower Artery						

LC Limited Coverage   NC Noncovered   HAC HAC-associated Procedure   CC Combination Cluster - See Appendix G for code lists
ÖÑÉ Non-OR-Affecting MS-DRG Assignment   New/Revised Text in **Orange**   ♂ Male   ♀ Female

218

2018 ICD-10-PCS

0 Medical and Surgical
4 Lower Arteries
H Insertion: Putting in a nonbiological appliance that monitors, assists, performs, or prevents a physiological function but does not physically take the place of a body part

Body Part	Approach	Device	Qualifier
Character 4	Character 5	Character 6	Character 7
0 Abdominal Aorta	**0** Open **3** Percutaneous **4** Percutaneous Endoscopic	**2** Monitoring Device **3** Infusion Device **D** Intraluminal Device	**Z** No Qualifier
1 Celiac Artery **2** Gastric Artery **3** Hepatic Artery **4** Splenic Artery **5** Superior Mesenteric Artery **6** Colic Artery, Right **7** Colic Artery, Left **8** Colic Artery, Middle **9** Renal Artery, Right **A** Renal Artery, Left **B** Inferior Mesenteric Artery **C** Common Iliac Artery, Right **D** Common Iliac Artery, Left **E** Internal Iliac Artery, Right **F** Internal Iliac Artery, Left **H** External Iliac Artery, Right **J** External Iliac Artery, Left **K** Femoral Artery, Right **L** Femoral Artery, Left **M** Popliteal Artery, Right **N** Popliteal Artery, Left **P** Anterior Tibial Artery, Right **Q** Anterior Tibial Artery, Left **R** Posterior Tibial Artery, Right **S** Posterior Tibial Artery, Left **T** Peroneal Artery, Right **U** Peroneal Artery, Left **V** Foot Artery, Right **W** Foot Artery, Left	**0** Open **3** Percutaneous **4** Percutaneous Endoscopic	**3** Infusion Device **D** Intraluminal Device	**Z** No Qualifier
Y Lower Artery	**0** Open **3** Percutaneous **4** Percutaneous Endoscopic	**2** Monitoring Device **3** Infusion Device **D** Intraluminal Device **Y** Other Device	**Z** No Qualifier

0 Medical and Surgical
4 Lower Arteries
J Inspection: Visually and/or manually exploring a body part

Body Part	Approach	Device	Qualifier
Character 4	Character 5	Character 6	Character 7
Y Lower Artery	**0** Open **3** Percutaneous **4** Percutaneous Endoscopic **X** External	**Z** No Device	**Z** No Qualifier

0   **Medical and Surgical**
4   **Lower Arteries**
L   **Occlusion:** Completely closing an orifice or the lumen of a tubular body part

Body Part	Approach	Device	Qualifier
Character 4	**Character 5**	**Character 6**	**Character 7**
0 Abdominal Aorta	0 Open 4 Percutaneous Endoscopic	C Extraluminal Device D Intraluminal Device Z No Device	Z No Qualifier
0 Abdominal Aorta	3 Percutaneous	C Extraluminal Device Z No Device	Z No Qualifier
0 Abdominal Aorta	3 Percutaneous	D Intraluminal Device	J Temporary Z No Qualifier
1 Celiac Artery 2 Gastric Artery 3 Hepatic Artery 4 Splenic Artery 5 Superior Mesenteric Artery 6 Colic Artery, Right 7 Colic Artery, Left 8 Colic Artery, Middle 9 Renal Artery, Right A Renal Artery, Left B Inferior Mesenteric Artery C Common Iliac Artery, Right D Common Iliac Artery, Left H External Iliac Artery, Right J External Iliac Artery, Left K Femoral Artery, Right L Femoral Artery, Left M Popliteal Artery, Right N Popliteal Artery, Left P Anterior Tibial Artery, Right Q Anterior Tibial Artery, Left R Posterior Tibial Artery, Right S Posterior Tibial Artery, Left T Peroneal Artery, Right U Peroneal Artery, Left V Foot Artery, Right W Foot Artery, Left Y Lower Artery	0 Open 3 Percutaneous 4 Percutaneous Endoscopic	C Extraluminal Device D Intraluminal Device Z No Device	Z No Qualifier
E Internal Iliac Artery, Right ♀	0 Open 3 Percutaneous 4 Percutaneous Endoscopic	C Extraluminal Device D Intraluminal Device Z No Device	T Uterine Artery, Right Z No Qualifier
F Internal Iliac Artery, Left ♀	0 Open 3 Percutaneous 4 Percutaneous Endoscopic	C Extraluminal Device D Intraluminal Device Z No Device	U Uterine Artery, Left Z No Qualifier

♀ 04LE0CT   04LE0DT   04LE0ZT   04LE3CT   04LE3DT   04LE3ZT   04LE4CT   04LE4DT   04LE4ZT   04LF0CU   04LF0DU   04LF0ZU   04LF3CU
04LF3DU   04LF3ZU   04LF4CU   04LF4DU   04LF4ZU

0 Medical and Surgical
4 Lower Arteries
N Release: Freeing a body part from an abnormal physical constraint by cutting or by the use of force

Body Part	Approach	Device	Qualifier
Character 4	Character 5	Character 6	Character 7
0 Abdominal Aorta **1** Celiac Artery **2** Gastric Artery **3** Hepatic Artery **4** Splenic Artery **5** Superior Mesenteric Artery **6** Colic Artery, Right **7** Colic Artery, Left **8** Colic Artery, Middle **9** Renal Artery, Right **A** Renal Artery, Left **B** Inferior Mesenteric Artery **C** Common Iliac Artery, Right **D** Common Iliac Artery, Left **E** Internal Iliac Artery, Right **F** Internal Iliac Artery, Left **H** External Iliac Artery, Right **J** External Iliac Artery, Left **K** Femoral Artery, Right **L** Femoral Artery, Left **M** Popliteal Artery, Right **N** Popliteal Artery, Left **P** Anterior Tibial Artery, Right **Q** Anterior Tibial Artery, Left **R** Posterior Tibial Artery, Right **S** Posterior Tibial Artery, Left **T** Peroneal Artery, Right **U** Peroneal Artery, Left **V** Foot Artery, Right **W** Foot Artery, Left **Y** Lower Artery	**0** Open **3** Percutaneous **4** Percutaneous Endoscopic	**Z** No Device	**Z** No Qualifier

0 Medical and Surgical
4 Lower Arteries
P Removal: Taking out or off a device from a body part

Body Part	Approach	Device	Qualifier
Character 4	Character 5	Character 6	Character 7
Y Lower Artery	**0** Open **3** Percutaneous **4** Percutaneous Endoscopic	**0** Drainage Device **2** Monitoring Device **3** Infusion Device **7** Autologous Tissue Substitute **C** Extraluminal Device **D** Intraluminal Device **J** Synthetic Substitute **K** Nonautologous Tissue Substitute **Y** Other Device	**Z** No Qualifier
Y Lower Artery	**X** External	**0** Drainage Device **1** Radioactive Element **2** Monitoring Device **3** Infusion Device **D** Intraluminal Device	**Z** No Qualifier

0   **Medical and Surgical**
4   **Lower Arteries**
Q   **Repair:** Restoring, to the extent possible, a body part to its normal anatomic structure and function

Body Part	Approach	Device	Qualifier
Character 4	Character 5	Character 6	Character 7
0 Abdominal Aorta	0 Open	Z No Device	Z No Qualifier
1 Celiac Artery	3 Percutaneous		
2 Gastric Artery	4 Percutaneous Endoscopic		
3 Hepatic Artery			
4 Splenic Artery			
5 Superior Mesenteric Artery			
6 Colic Artery, Right			
7 Colic Artery, Left			
8 Colic Artery, Middle			
9 Renal Artery, Right			
A Renal Artery, Left			
B Inferior Mesenteric Artery			
C Common Iliac Artery, Right			
D Common Iliac Artery, Left			
E Internal Iliac Artery, Right			
F Internal Iliac Artery, Left			
H External Iliac Artery, Right			
J External Iliac Artery, Left			
K Femoral Artery, Right			
L Femoral Artery, Left			
M Popliteal Artery, Right			
N Popliteal Artery, Left			
P Anterior Tibial Artery, Right			
Q Anterior Tibial Artery, Left			
R Posterior Tibial Artery, Right			
S Posterior Tibial Artery, Left			
T Peroneal Artery, Right			
U Peroneal Artery, Left			
V Foot Artery, Right			
W Foot Artery, Left			
Y Lower Artery			

LC Limited Coverage   NC Noncovered   HAC HAC-associated Procedure   CC Combination Cluster - See Appendix G for code lists
DRG Non-OR-Affecting MS-DRG Assignment   New/Revised Text in **Orange**   ♂ Male   ♀ Female

222

2018 ICD-10-PCS

0 Medical and Surgical
4 Lower Arteries
R Replacement: Putting in or on biological or synthetic material that physically takes the place and/or function of all or a portion of a body part

Body Part	Approach	Device	Qualifier
Character 4	Character 5	Character 6	Character 7
0 Abdominal Aorta **1** Celiac Artery **2** Gastric Artery **3** Hepatic Artery **4** Splenic Artery **5** Superior Mesenteric Artery **6** Colic Artery, Right **7** Colic Artery, Left **8** Colic Artery, Middle **9** Renal Artery, Right **A** Renal Artery, Left **B** Inferior Mesenteric Artery **C** Common Iliac Artery, Right **D** Common Iliac Artery, Left **E** Internal Iliac Artery, Right **F** Internal Iliac Artery, Left **H** External Iliac Artery, Right **J** External Iliac Artery, Left **K** Femoral Artery, Right **L** Femoral Artery, Left **M** Popliteal Artery, Right **N** Popliteal Artery, Left **P** Anterior Tibial Artery, Right **Q** Anterior Tibial Artery, Left **R** Posterior Tibial Artery, Right **S** Posterior Tibial Artery, Left **T** Peroneal Artery, Right **U** Peroneal Artery, Left **V** Foot Artery, Right **W** Foot Artery, Left **Y** Lower Artery	**0** Open **4** Percutaneous Endoscopic	**7** Autologous Tissue Substitute **J** Synthetic Substitute **K** Nonautologous Tissue Substitute	**Z** No Qualifier

0 **Medical and Surgical**
4 **Lower Arteries**
S **Reposition:** Moving to its normal location, or other suitable location, all or a portion of a body part

Body Part	Approach	Device	Qualifier
Character 4	Character 5	Character 6	Character 7
0 Abdominal Aorta	**0** Open	**Z** No Device	**Z** No Qualifier
1 Celiac Artery	**3** Percutaneous		
2 Gastric Artery	**4** Percutaneous Endoscopic		
3 Hepatic Artery			
4 Splenic Artery			
5 Superior Mesenteric Artery			
6 Colic Artery, Right			
7 Colic Artery, Left			
8 Colic Artery, Middle			
9 Renal Artery, Right			
A Renal Artery, Left			
B Inferior Mesenteric Artery			
C Common Iliac Artery, Right			
D Common Iliac Artery, Left			
E Internal Iliac Artery, Right			
F Internal Iliac Artery, Left			
H External Iliac Artery, Right			
J External Iliac Artery, Left			
K Femoral Artery, Right			
L Femoral Artery, Left			
M Popliteal Artery, Right			
N Popliteal Artery, Left			
P Anterior Tibial Artery, Right			
Q Anterior Tibial Artery, Left			
R Posterior Tibial Artery, Right			
S Posterior Tibial Artery, Left			
T Peroneal Artery, Right			
U Peroneal Artery, Left			
V Foot Artery, Right			
W Foot Artery, Left			
Y Lower Artery			

LC Limited Coverage   NC Noncovered   HAC HAC-associated Procedure   CC Combination Cluster - See Appendix G for code lists
DRG Non-OR-Affecting MS-DRG Assignment   New/Revised Text in Orange   ♂ Male   ♀ Female

224

2018 ICD-10-PCS

0 Medical and Surgical
4 Lower Arteries
U Supplement: Putting in or on biological or synthetic material that physically reinforces and/or augments the function of a portion of a body part

Body Part	Approach	Device	Qualifier
Character 4	Character 5	Character 6	Character 7
0 Abdominal Aorta 1 Celiac Artery 2 Gastric Artery 3 Hepatic Artery 4 Splenic Artery 5 Superior Mesenteric Artery 6 Colic Artery, Right 7 Colic Artery, Left 8 Colic Artery, Middle 9 Renal Artery, Right A Renal Artery, Left B Inferior Mesenteric Artery C Common Iliac Artery, Right D Common Iliac Artery, Left E Internal Iliac Artery, Right F Internal Iliac Artery, Left H External Iliac Artery, Right J External Iliac Artery, Left K Femoral Artery, Right L Femoral Artery, Left M Popliteal Artery, Right N Popliteal Artery, Left P Anterior Tibial Artery, Right Q Anterior Tibial Artery, Left R Posterior Tibial Artery, Right S Posterior Tibial Artery, Left T Peroneal Artery, Right U Peroneal Artery, Left V Foot Artery, Right W Foot Artery, Left Y Lower Artery	0 Open 3 Percutaneous 4 Percutaneous Endoscopic	7 Autologous Tissue Substitute J Synthetic Substitute K Nonautologous Tissue Substitute	Z No Qualifier

0   **Medical and Surgical**
4   **Lower Arteries**
V   **Restriction:** Partially closing an orifice or the lumen of a tubular body part

Body Part	Approach	Device	Qualifier
Character 4	Character 5	Character 6	Character 7
0 Abdominal Aorta	**0** Open **3** Percutaneous **4** Percutaneous Endoscopic	**C** Extraluminal Device **E** Intraluminal Device, Branched or Fenestrated, One or Two Arteries **F** Intraluminal Device, Branched or Fenestrated, Three or More Arteries **Z** No Device	**6** Bifurcation **Z** No Qualifier
0 Abdominal Aorta	**0** Open **3** Percutaneous **4** Percutaneous Endoscopic	**D** Intraluminal Device	**6** Bifurcation **J** Temporary **Z** No Qualifier
1 Celiac Artery **2** Gastric Artery **3** Hepatic Artery **4** Splenic Artery **5** Superior Mesenteric Artery **6** Colic Artery, Right **7** Colic Artery, Left **8** Colic Artery, Middle **9** Renal Artery, Right **A** Renal Artery, Left **B** Inferior Mesenteric Artery **E** Internal Iliac Artery, Right **F** Internal Iliac Artery, Left **H** External Iliac Artery, Right **J** External Iliac Artery, Left **K** Femoral Artery, Right **L** Femoral Artery, Left **M** Popliteal Artery, Right **N** Popliteal Artery, Left **P** Anterior Tibial Artery, Right **Q** Anterior Tibial Artery, Left **R** Posterior Tibial Artery, Right **S** Posterior Tibial Artery, Left **T** Peroneal Artery, Right **U** Peroneal Artery, Left **V** Foot Artery, Right **W** Foot Artery, Left **Y** Lower Artery	**0** Open **3** Percutaneous **4** Percutaneous Endoscopic	**C** Extraluminal Device **D** Intraluminal Device **Z** No Device	**Z** No Qualifier
C Common Iliac Artery, Right **D** Common Iliac Artery, Left	**0** Open **3** Percutaneous **4** Percutaneous Endoscopic	**C** Extraluminal Device **D** Intraluminal Device **E** Intraluminal Device, Branched or Fenestrated, One or Two Arteries **Z** No Device	**Z** No Qualifier

0 **Medical and Surgical**
4 **Lower Arteries**
W **Revision:** Correcting, to the extent possible, a portion of a malfunctioning device or the position of a displaced device

Body Part	Approach	Device	Qualifier
Character 4	Character 5	Character 6	Character 7
Y Lower Artery	**0** Open **3** Percutaneous **4** Percutaneous Endoscopic	**0** Drainage Device **2** Monitoring Device **3** Infusion Device **7** Autologous Tissue Substitute **C** Extraluminal Device **D** Intraluminal Device **J** Synthetic Substitute **K** Nonautologous Tissue Substitute **Y** Other Device	**Z** No Qualifier
Y Lower Artery	**X** External	**0** Drainage Device **2** Monitoring Device **3** Infusion Device **7** Autologous Tissue Substitute **C** Extraluminal Device **D** Intraluminal Device **J** Synthetic Substitute **K** Nonautologous Tissue Substitute	**Z** No Qualifier

NOTES

0   **Medical and Surgical**
5   **Upper Veins**
1   **Bypass:** Altering the route of passage of the contents of a tubular body part

Body Part	Approach	Device	Qualifier
Character 4	Character 5	Character 6	Character 7
0 Azygos Vein 1 Hemiazygos Vein 3 Innominate Vein, Right 4 Innominate Vein, Left 5 Subclavian Vein, Right 6 Subclavian Vein, Left 7 Axillary Vein, Right 8 Axillary Vein, Left 9 Brachial Vein, Right A Brachial Vein, Left B Basilic Vein, Right C Basilic Vein, Left D Cephalic Vein, Right F Cephalic Vein, Left G Hand Vein, Right H Hand Vein, Left L Intracranial Vein M Internal Jugular Vein, Right N Internal Jugular Vein, Left P External Jugular Vein, Right Q External Jugular Vein, Left R Vertebral Vein, Right S Vertebral Vein, Left T Face Vein, Right V Face Vein, Left	0 Open 4 Percutaneous Endoscopic	7 Autologous Tissue Substitute 9 Autologous Venous Tissue A Autologous Arterial Tissue J Synthetic Substitute K Nonautologous Tissue Substitute Z No Device	Y Upper Vein

LC Limited Coverage   NC Noncovered   HAC HAC-associated Procedure   CC Combination Cluster - See Appendix G for code lists
DRG Non-OR-Affecting MS-DRG Assignment   New/Revised Text in **Orange**   ♂ Male   ♀ Female

2018 ICD-10-PCS

229

UPPER VEINS 051-05W

0 Medical and Surgical
5 Upper Veins
5 Destruction: Physical eradication of all or a portion of a body part by the direct use of energy, force, or a destructive agent

Body Part	Approach	Device	Qualifier
Character 4	Character 5	Character 6	Character 7
0 Azygos Vein	**0** Open	**Z** No Device	**Z** No Qualifier
1 Hemiazygos Vein	**3** Percutaneous		
3 Innominate Vein, Right	**4** Percutaneous Endoscopic		
4 Innominate Vein, Left			
5 Subclavian Vein, Right			
6 Subclavian Vein, Left			
7 Axillary Vein, Right			
8 Axillary Vein, Left			
9 Brachial Vein, Right			
A Brachial Vein, Left			
B Basilic Vein, Right			
C Basilic Vein, Left			
D Cephalic Vein, Right			
F Cephalic Vein, Left			
G Hand Vein, Right			
H Hand Vein, Left			
L Intracranial Vein			
M Internal Jugular Vein, Right			
N Internal Jugular Vein, Left			
P External Jugular Vein, Right			
Q External Jugular Vein, Left			
R Vertebral Vein, Right			
S Vertebral Vein, Left			
T Face Vein, Right			
V Face Vein, Left			
Y Upper Vein			

0 Medical and Surgical
5 Upper Veins
7 Dilation: Expanding an orifice or the lumen of a tubular body part

Body Part	Approach	Device	Qualifier
Character 4	Character 5	Character 6	Character 7
0 Azygos Vein	**0** Open	**D** Intraluminal Device	**Z** No Qualifier
1 Hemiazygos Vein	**3** Percutaneous	**Z** No Device	
3 Innominate Vein, Right	**4** Percutaneous Endoscopic		
4 Innominate Vein, Left			
5 Subclavian Vein, Right			
6 Subclavian Vein, Left			
7 Axillary Vein, Right			
8 Axillary Vein, Left			
9 Brachial Vein, Right			
A Brachial Vein, Left			
B Basilic Vein, Right			
C Basilic Vein, Left			
D Cephalic Vein, Right			
F Cephalic Vein, Left			
G Hand Vein, Right			
H Hand Vein, Left			
L Intracranial Vein NC			
M Internal Jugular Vein, Right			
N Internal Jugular Vein, Left			
P External Jugular Vein, Right			
Q External Jugular Vein, Left			
R Vertebral Vein, Right			
S Vertebral Vein, Left			
T Face Vein, Right			
V Face Vein, Left			
Y Upper Vein			

NC 057L3ZZ   057L4ZZ

LC Limited Coverage   NC Noncovered   HAC HAC-associated Procedure   CC Combination Cluster - See Appendix G for code lists
DRG Non-OR-Affecting MS-DRG Assignment   New/Revised Text in **Orange**   ♂ Male   ♀ Female

0 Medical and Surgical

5 Upper Veins

9 Drainage: Taking or letting out fluids and/or gases from a body part

Body Part	Approach	Device	Qualifier
Character 4	Character 5	Character 6	Character 7
0 Azygos Vein **1** Hemiazygos Vein **3** Innominate Vein, Right **4** Innominate Vein, Left **5** Subclavian Vein, Right **6** Subclavian Vein, Left **7** Axillary Vein, Right **8** Axillary Vein, Left **9** Brachial Vein, Right **A** Brachial Vein, Left **B** Basilic Vein, Right **C** Basilic Vein, Left **D** Cephalic Vein, Right **F** Cephalic Vein, Left **G** Hand Vein, Right **H** Hand Vein, Left **L** Intracranial Vein **M** Internal Jugular Vein, Right **N** Internal Jugular Vein, Left **P** External Jugular Vein, Right **Q** External Jugular Vein, Left **R** Vertebral Vein, Right **S** Vertebral Vein, Left **T** Face Vein, Right **V** Face Vein, Left **Y** Upper Vein	**0** Open **3** Percutaneous **4** Percutaneous Endoscopic	**0** Drainage Device	**Z** No Qualifier
0 Azygos Vein **1** Hemiazygos Vein **3** Innominate Vein, Right **4** Innominate Vein, Left **5** Subclavian Vein, Right **6** Subclavian Vein, Left **7** Axillary Vein, Right **8** Axillary Vein, Left **9** Brachial Vein, Right **A** Brachial Vein, Left **B** Basilic Vein, Right **C** Basilic Vein, Left **D** Cephalic Vein, Right **F** Cephalic Vein, Left **G** Hand Vein, Right **H** Hand Vein, Left **L** Intracranial Vein **M** Internal Jugular Vein, Right **N** Internal Jugular Vein, Left **P** External Jugular Vein, Right **Q** External Jugular Vein, Left **R** Vertebral Vein, Right **S** Vertebral Vein, Left **T** Face Vein, Right **V** Face Vein, Left **Y** Upper Vein	**0** Open **3** Percutaneous **4** Percutaneous Endoscopic	**Z** No Device	**X** Diagnostic **Z** No Qualifier

LC Limited Coverage   **NC** Noncovered   **HAC** HAC-associated Procedure   **CC** Combination Cluster - See Appendix G for code lists

DRG Non-OR-Affecting MS-DRG Assignment   New/Revised Text in **Orange**   ♂ Male   ♀ Female

0 Medical and Surgical
5 Upper Veins
B Excision: Cutting out or off, without replacement, a portion of a body part

Body Part	Approach	Device	Qualifier
Character 4	Character 5	Character 6	Character 7
0 Azygos Vein	0 Open	Z No Device	X Diagnostic
1 Hemiazygos Vein	3 Percutaneous		Z No Qualifier
3 Innominate Vein, Right	4 Percutaneous Endoscopic		
4 Innominate Vein, Left			
5 Subclavian Vein, Right			
6 Subclavian Vein, Left			
7 Axillary Vein, Right			
8 Axillary Vein, Left			
9 Brachial Vein, Right			
A Brachial Vein, Left			
B Basilic Vein, Right			
C Basilic Vein, Left			
D Cephalic Vein, Right			
F Cephalic Vein, Left			
G Hand Vein, Right			
H Hand Vein, Left			
L Intracranial Vein			
M Internal Jugular Vein, Right			
N Internal Jugular Vein, Left			
P External Jugular Vein, Right			
Q External Jugular Vein, Left			
R Vertebral Vein, Right			
S Vertebral Vein, Left			
T Face Vein, Right			
V Face Vein, Left			
Y Upper Vein			

0 Medical and Surgical
5 Upper Veins
C Extirpation: Taking or cutting out solid matter from a body part

Body Part	Approach	Device	Qualifier
Character 4	Character 5	Character 6	Character 7
0 Azygos Vein	0 Open	Z No Device	Z No Qualifier
1 Hemiazygos Vein	3 Percutaneous		
3 Innominate Vein, Right	4 Percutaneous Endoscopic		
4 Innominate Vein, Left			
5 Subclavian Vein, Right			
6 Subclavian Vein, Left			
7 Axillary Vein, Right			
8 Axillary Vein, Left			
9 Brachial Vein, Right			
A Brachial Vein, Left			
B Basilic Vein, Right			
C Basilic Vein, Left			
D Cephalic Vein, Right			
F Cephalic Vein, Left			
G Hand Vein, Right			
H Hand Vein, Left			
L Intracranial Vein			
M Internal Jugular Vein, Right			
N Internal Jugular Vein, Left			
P External Jugular Vein, Right			
Q External Jugular Vein, Left			
R Vertebral Vein, Right			
S Vertebral Vein, Left			
T Face Vein, Right			
V Face Vein, Left			
Y Upper Vein			

LC Limited Coverage   NC Noncovered   HAC HAC-associated Procedure   CC Combination Cluster - See Appendix G for code lists
DRG Non-OR-Affecting MS-DRG Assignment   New/Revised Text in Orange   ♂ Male   ♀ Female

232

2018 ICD-10-PCS

0 Medical and Surgical
5 Upper Veins
D Extraction: Pulling or stripping out or off all or a portion of a body part by the use of force

Body Part	Approach	Device	Qualifier
Character 4	Character 5	Character 6	Character 7
9 Brachial Vein, Right A Brachial Vein, Left B Basilic Vein, Right C Basilic Vein, Left D Cephalic Vein, Right F Cephalic Vein, Left G Hand Vein, Right H Hand Vein, Left Y Upper Vein	0 Open 3 Percutaneous	Z No Device	Z No Qualifier

0 Medical and Surgical
5 Upper Veins
H Insertion: Putting in a nonbiological appliance that monitors, assists, performs, or prevents a physiological function but does not physically take the place of a body part

Body Part	Approach	Device	Qualifier
Character 4	Character 5	Character 6	Character 7
0 Azygos Vein 🅲🅲 🅷🅰🅲	0 Open 3 Percutaneous 4 Percutaneous Endoscopic	2 Monitoring Device 3 Infusion Device D Intraluminal Device M Neurostimulator Lead	Z No Qualifier
1 Hemiazygos Vein 🅷🅰🅲 5 Subclavian Vein, Right 🅷🅰🅲 6 Subclavian Vein, Left 🅷🅰🅲 7 Axillary Vein, Right 8 Axillary Vein, Left 9 Brachial Vein, Right A Brachial Vein, Left B Basilic Vein, Right C Basilic Vein, Left D Cephalic Vein, Right F Cephalic Vein, Left G Hand Vein, Right H Hand Vein, Left L Intracranial Vein M Internal Jugular Vein, Right 🅷🅰🅲 N Internal Jugular Vein, Left 🅷🅰🅲 P External Jugular Vein, Right 🅷🅰🅲 Q External Jugular Vein, Left 🅷🅰🅲 R Vertebral Vein, Right S Vertebral Vein, Left T Face Vein, Right V Face Vein, Left	0 Open 3 Percutaneous 4 Percutaneous Endoscopic	3 Infusion Device D Intraluminal Device	Z No Qualifier
3 Innominate Vein, Right 🅲🅲 🅷🅰🅲 4 Innominate Vein, Left 🅲🅲 🅷🅰🅲	0 Open 3 Percutaneous 4 Percutaneous Endoscopic	3 Infusion Device D Intraluminal Device M Neurostimulator Lead	Z No Qualifier
Y Upper Vein	0 Open 3 Percutaneous 4 Percutaneous Endoscopic	2 Monitoring Device 3 Infusion Device D Intraluminal Device Y Other Device	Z No Qualifier

🅷🅰🅲 05H033Z 05H043Z 05H133Z 05H143Z 05H333Z 05H343Z 05H433Z 05H443Z 05H533Z 05H543Z 05H633Z 05H643Z 05HM33Z
05HN33Z 05HP33Z 05HQ33Z
Iatrogenic pneumothorax w/ venous catheterization procedures and secondary diagnosis J95.811.
🅲🅲 05H00MZ 05H03MZ 05H04MZ 05H30MZ 05H33MZ 05H34MZ 05H40MZ 05H43MZ 05H44MZ

🅛🅒 Limited Coverage 🅝🅒 Noncovered 🅗🅐🅒 HAC-associated Procedure 🅒🅒 Combination Cluster - See Appendix G for code lists
🅓🅡🅖 Non-OR-Affecting MS-DRG Assignment New/Revised Text in **Orange** ♂ Male ♀ Female

0 Medical and Surgical
5 Upper Veins
J Inspection: Visually and/or manually exploring a body part

Body Part	Approach	Device	Qualifier
Character 4	Character 5	Character 6	Character 7
Y Upper Vein	0 Open 3 Percutaneous 4 Percutaneous Endoscopic X External	Z No Device	Z No Qualifier

0 Medical and Surgical
5 Upper Veins
L Occlusion: Completely closing an orifice or the lumen of a tubular body part

Body Part	Approach	Device	Qualifier
Character 4	Character 5	Character 6	Character 7
0 Azygos Vein 1 Hemiazygos Vein 3 Innominate Vein, Right 4 Innominate Vein, Left 5 Subclavian Vein, Right 6 Subclavian Vein, Left 7 Axillary Vein, Right 8 Axillary Vein, Left 9 Brachial Vein, Right A Brachial Vein, Left B Basilic Vein, Right C Basilic Vein, Left D Cephalic Vein, Right F Cephalic Vein, Left G Hand Vein, Right H Hand Vein, Left L Intracranial Vein M Internal Jugular Vein, Right N Internal Jugular Vein, Left P External Jugular Vein, Right Q External Jugular Vein, Left R Vertebral Vein, Right S Vertebral Vein, Left T Face Vein, Right V Face Vein, Left Y Upper Vein	0 Open 3 Percutaneous 4 Percutaneous Endoscopic	C Extraluminal Device D Intraluminal Device Z No Device	Z No Qualifier

0 Medical and Surgical
5 Upper Veins
N Release: Freeing a body part from an abnormal physical constraint by cutting or by the use of force

Body Part	Approach	Device	Qualifier
Character 4	Character 5	Character 6	Character 7
0 Azygos Vein 1 Hemiazygos Vein 3 Innominate Vein, Right 4 Innominate Vein, Left 5 Subclavian Vein, Right 6 Subclavian Vein, Left 7 Axillary Vein, Right 8 Axillary Vein, Left 9 Brachial Vein, Right A Brachial Vein, Left B Basilic Vein, Right C Basilic Vein, Left D Cephalic Vein, Right F Cephalic Vein, Left G Hand Vein, Right H Hand Vein, Left L Intracranial Vein M Internal Jugular Vein, Right N Internal Jugular Vein, Left P External Jugular Vein, Right Q External Jugular Vein, Left R Vertebral Vein, Right S Vertebral Vein, Left T Face Vein, Right V Face Vein, Left Y Upper Vein	0 Open 3 Percutaneous 4 Percutaneous Endoscopic	Z No Device	Z No Qualifier

0 Medical and Surgical
5 Upper Veins
P Removal: Taking out or off a device from a body part

Body Part	Approach	Device	Qualifier
Character 4	Character 5	Character 6	Character 7
0 Azygos Vein	0 Open 3 Percutaneous 4 Percutaneous Endoscopic X External	2 Monitoring Device M Neurostimulator Lead	Z No Qualifier
3 Innominate Vein, Right 4 Innominate Vein, Left	0 Open 3 Percutaneous 4 Percutaneous Endoscopic X External	M Neurostimulator Lead	Z No Qualifier
Y Upper Vein	0 Open 3 Percutaneous 4 Percutaneous Endoscopic	0 Drainage Device 2 Monitoring Device 3 Infusion Device 7 Autologous Tissue Substitute C Extraluminal Device D Intraluminal Device J Synthetic Substitute K Nonautologous Tissue Substitute Y Other Device	Z No Qualifier
Y Upper Vein	X External	0 Drainage Device 2 Monitoring Device 3 Infusion Device D Intraluminal Device	Z No Qualifier

LC Limited Coverage   NC Noncovered   HAC HAC-associated Procedure   CC Combination Cluster - See Appendix G for code lists
DRG Non-OR-Affecting MS-DRG Assignment   New/Revised Text in **Orange**   ♂ Male   ♀ Female

2018 ICD-10-PCS

235

UPPER VEINS 051-05W

0 Medical and Surgical
5 Upper Veins
Q Repair: Restoring, to the extent possible, a body part to its normal anatomic structure and function

Body Part	Approach	Device	Qualifier
Character 4	Character 5	Character 6	Character 7
0 Azygos Vein **1** Hemiazygos Vein **3** Innominate Vein, Right **4** Innominate Vein, Left **5** Subclavian Vein, Right **6** Subclavian Vein, Left **7** Axillary Vein, Right **8** Axillary Vein, Left **9** Brachial Vein, Right **A** Brachial Vein, Left **B** Basilic Vein, Right **C** Basilic Vein, Left **D** Cephalic Vein, Right **F** Cephalic Vein, Left **G** Hand Vein, Right **H** Hand Vein, Left **L** Intracranial Vein **M** Internal Jugular Vein, Right **N** Internal Jugular Vein, Left **P** External Jugular Vein, Right **Q** External Jugular Vein, Left **R** Vertebral Vein, Right **S** Vertebral Vein, Left **T** Face Vein, Right **V** Face Vein, Left **Y** Upper Vein	**0** Open **3** Percutaneous **4** Percutaneous Endoscopic	**Z** No Device	**Z** No Qualifier

0 Medical and Surgical
5 Upper Veins
R Replacement: Putting in or on biological or synthetic material that physically takes the place and/or function of all or a portion of a body part

Body Part	Approach	Device	Qualifier
Character 4	Character 5	Character 6	Character 7
0 Azygos Vein **1** Hemiazygos Vein **3** Innominate Vein, Right **4** Innominate Vein, Left **5** Subclavian Vein, Right **6** Subclavian Vein, Left **7** Axillary Vein, Right **8** Axillary Vein, Left **9** Brachial Vein, Right **A** Brachial Vein, Left **B** Basilic Vein, Right **C** Basilic Vein, Left **D** Cephalic Vein, Right **F** Cephalic Vein, Left **G** Hand Vein, Right **H** Hand Vein, Left **L** Intracranial Vein **M** Internal Jugular Vein, Right **N** Internal Jugular Vein, Left **P** External Jugular Vein, Right **Q** External Jugular Vein, Left **R** Vertebral Vein, Right **S** Vertebral Vein, Left **T** Face Vein, Right **V** Face Vein, Left **Y** Upper Vein	**0** Open **4** Percutaneous Endoscopic	**7** Autologous Tissue Substitute **J** Synthetic Substitute **K** Nonautologous Tissue Substitute	**Z** No Qualifier

LC Limited Coverage   NC Noncovered   HAC HAC-associated Procedure   CC Combination Cluster - See Appendix G for code lists
DRG Non-OR-Affecting MS-DRG Assignment   New/Revised Text in Orange   ♂ Male   ♀ Female

236

2018 ICD-10-PCS

0 **Medical and Surgical**
5 **Upper Veins**
S **Reposition:** Moving to its normal location, or other suitable location, all or a portion of a body part

Body Part	Approach	Device	Qualifier
Character 4	Character 5	Character 6	Character 7
0 Azygos Vein 1 Hemiazygos Vein 3 Innominate Vein, Right 4 Innominate Vein, Left 5 Subclavian Vein, Right 6 Subclavian Vein, Left 7 Axillary Vein, Right 8 Axillary Vein, Left 9 Brachial Vein, Right A Brachial Vein, Left B Basilic Vein, Right C Basilic Vein, Left D Cephalic Vein, Right F Cephalic Vein, Left G Hand Vein, Right H Hand Vein, Left L Intracranial Vein M Internal Jugular Vein, Right N Internal Jugular Vein, Left P External Jugular Vein, Right Q External Jugular Vein, Left R Vertebral Vein, Right S Vertebral Vein, Left T Face Vein, Right V Face Vein, Left Y Upper Vein	0 Open 3 Percutaneous 4 Percutaneous Endoscopic	Z No Device	Z No Qualifier

0 **Medical and Surgical**
5 **Upper Veins**
U **Supplement:** Putting in or on biological or synthetic material that physically reinforces and/or augments the function of a portion of a body part

Body Part	Approach	Device	Qualifier
Character 4	Character 5	Character 6	Character 7
0 Azygos Vein 1 Hemiazygos Vein 3 Innominate Vein, Right 4 Innominate Vein, Left 5 Subclavian Vein, Right 6 Subclavian Vein, Left 7 Axillary Vein, Right 8 Axillary Vein, Left 9 Brachial Vein, Right A Brachial Vein, Left B Basilic Vein, Right C Basilic Vein, Left D Cephalic Vein, Right F Cephalic Vein, Left G Hand Vein, Right H Hand Vein, Left L Intracranial Vein M Internal Jugular Vein, Right N Internal Jugular Vein, Left P External Jugular Vein, Right Q External Jugular Vein, Left R Vertebral Vein, Right S Vertebral Vein, Left T Face Vein, Right V Face Vein, Left Y Upper Vein	0 Open 3 Percutaneous 4 Percutaneous Endoscopic	7 Autologous Tissue Substitute J Synthetic Substitute K Nonautologous Tissue Substitute	Z No Qualifier

0   **Medical and Surgical**
5   **Upper Veins**
V   **Restriction:** Partially closing an orifice or the lumen of a tubular body part

Body Part	Approach	Device	Qualifier
Character 4	Character 5	Character 6	Character 7
0 Azygos Vein 1 Hemiazygos Vein 3 Innominate Vein, Right 4 Innominate Vein, Left 5 Subclavian Vein, Right 6 Subclavian Vein, Left 7 Axillary Vein, Right 8 Axillary Vein, Left 9 Brachial Vein, Right A Brachial Vein, Left B Basilic Vein, Right C Basilic Vein, Left D Cephalic Vein, Right F Cephalic Vein, Left G Hand Vein, Right H Hand Vein, Left L Intracranial Vein M Internal Jugular Vein, Right N Internal Jugular Vein, Left P External Jugular Vein, Right Q External Jugular Vein, Left R Vertebral Vein, Right S Vertebral Vein, Left T Face Vein, Right V Face Vein, Left Y Upper Vein	0 Open 3 Percutaneous 4 Percutaneous Endoscopic	C Extraluminal Device D Intraluminal Device Z No Device	Z No Qualifier

0   **Medical and Surgical**
5   **Upper Veins**
W   **Revision:** Correcting, to the extent possible, a portion of a malfunctioning device or the position of a displaced device

Body Part	Approach	Device	Qualifier
Character 4	Character 5	Character 6	Character 7
0 Azygos Vein	0 Open 3 Percutaneous 4 Percutaneous Endoscopic X External	2 Monitoring Device M Neurostimulator Lead	Z No Qualifier
3 Innominate Vein, Right 4 Innominate Vein, Left	0 Open 3 Percutaneous 4 Percutaneous Endoscopic X External	M Neurostimulator Lead	Z No Qualifier
Y Upper Vein	0 Open 3 Percutaneous 4 Percutaneous Endoscopic	0 Drainage Device 2 Monitoring Device 3 Infusion Device 7 Autologous Tissue Substitute C Extraluminal Device D Intraluminal Device J Synthetic Substitute K Nonautologous Tissue Substitute Y Other Device	Z No Qualifier
Y Upper Vein	X External	0 Drainage Device 2 Monitoring Device 3 Infusion Device 7 Autologous Tissue Substitute C Extraluminal Device D Intraluminal Device J Synthetic Substitute K Nonautologous Tissue Substitute	Z No Qualifier

Lower Veins 061-06W

0 **Medical and Surgical**
6 **Lower Veins**
1 **Bypass:** Altering the route of passage of the contents of a tubular body part

Body Part	Approach	Device	Qualifier
Character 4	Character 5	Character 6	Character 7
0 Inferior Vena Cava	**0** Open **4** Percutaneous Endoscopic	**7** Autologous Tissue Substitute **9** Autologous Venous Tissue **A** Autologous Arterial Tissue **J** Synthetic Substitute **K** Nonautologous Tissue Substitute **Z** No Device	**5** Superior Mesenteric Vein **6** Inferior Mesenteric Vein **P** Pulmonary Trunk **Q** Pulmonary Artery, Right **R** Pulmonary Artery, Left **Y** Lower Vein
1 Splenic Vein	**0** Open **4** Percutaneous Endoscopic	**7** Autologous Tissue Substitute **9** Autologous Venous Tissue **A** Autologous Arterial Tissue **J** Synthetic Substitute **K** Nonautologous Tissue Substitute **Z** No Device	**9** Renal Vein, Right **B** Renal Vein, Left **Y** Lower Vein
2 Gastric Vein **3** Esophageal Vein **4** Hepatic Vein **5** Superior Mesenteric Vein **6** Inferior Mesenteric Vein **7** Colic Vein **9** Renal Vein, Right **B** Renal Vein, Left **C** Common Iliac Vein, Right **D** Common Iliac Vein, Left **F** External Iliac Vein, Right **G** External Iliac Vein, Left **H** Hypogastric Vein, Right **J** Hypogastric Vein, Left **M** Femoral Vein, Right **N** Femoral Vein, Left **P** Saphenous Vein, Right **Q** Saphenous Vein, Left **T** Foot Vein, Right **V** Foot Vein, Left	**0** Open **4** Percutaneous Endoscopic	**7** Autologous Tissue Substitute **9** Autologous Venous Tissue **A** Autologous Arterial Tissue **J** Synthetic Substitute **K** Nonautologous Tissue Substitute **Z** No Device	**Y** Lower Vein
8 Portal Vein	**0** Open	**7** Autologous Tissue Substitute **9** Autologous Venous Tissue **A** Autologous Arterial Tissue **J** Synthetic Substitute **K** Nonautologous Tissue Substitute **Z** No Device	**9** Renal Vein, Right **B** Renal Vein, Left **Y** Lower Vein
8 Portal Vein	**3** Percutaneous	**J** Synthetic Substitute	**4** Hepatic Vein **Y** Lower Vein
8 Portal Vein	**4** Percutaneous Endoscopic	**7** Autologous Tissue Substitute **9** Autologous Venous Tissue **A** Autologous Arterial Tissue **K** Nonautologous Tissue Substitute **Z** No Device	**9** Renal Vein, Right **B** Renal Vein, Left **Y** Lower Vein
8 Portal Vein	**4** Percutaneous Endoscopic	**J** Synthetic Substitute	**4** Hepatic Vein **9** Renal Vein, Right **B** Renal Vein, Left **Y** Lower Vein

0 Medical and Surgical
6 Lower Veins
5 Destruction: Physical eradication of all or a portion of a body part by the direct use of energy, force, or a destructive agent

Body Part	Approach	Device	Qualifier
Character 4	Character 5	Character 6	Character 7
0 Inferior Vena Cava 1 Splenic Vein 2 Gastric Vein 3 Esophageal Vein 4 Hepatic Vein 5 Superior Mesenteric Vein 6 Inferior Mesenteric Vein 7 Colic Vein 8 Portal Vein 9 Renal Vein, Right B Renal Vein, Left C Common Iliac Vein, Right D Common Iliac Vein, Left F External Iliac Vein, Right G External Iliac Vein, Left H Hypogastric Vein, Right J Hypogastric Vein, Left M Femoral Vein, Right N Femoral Vein, Left P Saphenous Vein, Right Q Saphenous Vein, Left T Foot Vein, Right V Foot Vein, Left	0 Open 3 Percutaneous 4 Percutaneous Endoscopic	Z No Device	Z No Qualifier
Y Lower Vein	0 Open 3 Percutaneous 4 Percutaneous Endoscopic	Z No Device	C Hemorrhoidal Plexus Z No Qualifier

0 Medical and Surgical
6 Lower Veins
7 Dilation: Expanding an orifice or the lumen of a tubular body part

Body Part	Approach	Device	Qualifier
Character 4	Character 5	Character 6	Character 7
0 Inferior Vena Cava 1 Splenic Vein 2 Gastric Vein 3 Esophageal Vein 4 Hepatic Vein 5 Superior Mesenteric Vein 6 Inferior Mesenteric Vein 7 Colic Vein 8 Portal Vein 9 Renal Vein, Right B Renal Vein, Left C Common Iliac Vein, Right D Common Iliac Vein, Left F External Iliac Vein, Right G External Iliac Vein, Left H Hypogastric Vein, Right J Hypogastric Vein, Left M Femoral Vein, Right N Femoral Vein, Left P Saphenous Vein, Right Q Saphenous Vein, Left T Foot Vein, Right V Foot Vein, Left Y Lower Vein	0 Open 3 Percutaneous 4 Percutaneous Endoscopic	D Intraluminal Device Z No Device	Z No Qualifier

0 Medical and Surgical
6 Lower Veins
9 Drainage: Taking or letting out fluids and/or gases from a body part

Body Part	Approach	Device	Qualifier
Character 4	**Character 5**	**Character 6**	**Character 7**
0 Inferior Vena Cava **1** Splenic Vein **2** Gastric Vein **3** Esophageal Vein **4** Hepatic Vein **5** Superior Mesenteric Vein **6** Inferior Mesenteric Vein **7** Colic Vein **8** Portal Vein **9** Renal Vein, Right **B** Renal Vein, Left **C** Common Iliac Vein, Right **D** Common Iliac Vein, Left **F** External Iliac Vein, Right **G** External Iliac Vein, Left **H** Hypogastric Vein, Right **J** Hypogastric Vein, Left **M** Femoral Vein, Right **N** Femoral Vein, Left **P** Saphenous Vein, Right **Q** Saphenous Vein, Left **T** Foot Vein, Right **V** Foot Vein, Left **Y** Lower Vein	**0** Open **3** Percutaneous **4** Percutaneous Endoscopic	**0** Drainage Device	**Z** No Qualifier
0 Inferior Vena Cava **1** Splenic Vein **2** Gastric Vein **3** Esophageal Vein **4** Hepatic Vein **5** Superior Mesenteric Vein **6** Inferior Mesenteric Vein **7** Colic Vein **8** Portal Vein **9** Renal Vein, Right **B** Renal Vein, Left **C** Common Iliac Vein, Right **D** Common Iliac Vein, Left **F** External Iliac Vein, Right **G** External Iliac Vein, Left **H** Hypogastric Vein, Right **J** Hypogastric Vein, Left **M** Femoral Vein, Right **N** Femoral Vein, Left **P** Saphenous Vein, Right **Q** Saphenous Vein, Left **T** Foot Vein, Right **V** Foot Vein, Left **Y** Lower Vein	**0** Open **3** Percutaneous **4** Percutaneous Endoscopic	**Z** No Device	**X** Diagnostic **Z** No Qualifier

0 Medical and Surgical
6 Lower Veins
B Excision: Cutting out or off, without replacement, a portion of a body part

Body Part	Approach	Device	Qualifier
Character 4	Character 5	Character 6	Character 7
0 Inferior Vena Cava 1 Splenic Vein 2 Gastric Vein 3 Esophageal Vein 4 Hepatic Vein 5 Superior Mesenteric Vein 6 Inferior Mesenteric Vein 7 Colic Vein 8 Portal Vein 9 Renal Vein, Right B Renal Vein, Left C Common Iliac Vein, Right D Common Iliac Vein, Left F External Iliac Vein, Right G External Iliac Vein, Left H Hypogastric Vein, Right J Hypogastric Vein, Left M Femoral Vein, Right N Femoral Vein, Left P Saphenous Vein, Right Q Saphenous Vein, Left T Foot Vein, Right V Foot Vein, Left	0 Open 3 Percutaneous 4 Percutaneous Endoscopic	Z No Device	X Diagnostic Z No Qualifier
Y Lower Vein	0 Open 3 Percutaneous 4 Percutaneous Endoscopic	Z No Device	C Hemorrhoidal Plexus X Diagnostic Z No Qualifier

0 Medical and Surgical
6 Lower Veins
C Extirpation: Taking or cutting out solid matter from a body part

Body Part	Approach	Device	Qualifier
Character 4	Character 5	Character 6	Character 7
0 Inferior Vena Cava 1 Splenic Vein 2 Gastric Vein 3 Esophageal Vein 4 Hepatic Vein 5 Superior Mesenteric Vein 6 Inferior Mesenteric Vein 7 Colic Vein 8 Portal Vein 9 Renal Vein, Right B Renal Vein, Left C Common Iliac Vein, Right D Common Iliac Vein, Left F External Iliac Vein, Right G External Iliac Vein, Left H Hypogastric Vein, Right J Hypogastric Vein, Left M Femoral Vein, Right N Femoral Vein, Left P Saphenous Vein, Right Q Saphenous Vein, Left T Foot Vein, Right V Foot Vein, Left Y Lower Vein	0 Open 3 Percutaneous 4 Percutaneous Endoscopic	Z No Device	Z No Qualifier

0 Medical and Surgical
6 Lower Veins
D Extraction: Pulling or stripping out or off all or a portion of a body part by the use of force

Body Part	Approach	Device	Qualifier
Character 4	Character 5	Character 6	Character 7
M Femoral Vein, Right N Femoral Vein, Left P Saphenous Vein, Right Q Saphenous Vein, Left T Foot Vein, Right V Foot Vein, Left Y Lower Vein	0 Open 3 Percutaneous 4 Percutaneous Endoscopic	Z No Device	Z No Qualifier

0 Medical and Surgical
6 Lower Veins
H Insertion: Putting in a nonbiological appliance that monitors, assists, performs, or prevents a physiological function but does not physically take the place of a body part

Body Part	Approach	Device	Qualifier
Character 4	Character 5	Character 6	Character 7
0 Inferior Vena Cava	0 Open 3 Percutaneous	3 Infusion Device	T Via Umbilical Vein Z No Qualifier
0 Inferior Vena Cava	0 Open 3 Percutaneous	D Intraluminal Device	Z No Qualifier
0 Inferior Vena Cava	4 Percutaneous Endoscopic	3 Infusion Device D Intraluminal Device	Z No Qualifier
1 Splenic Vein 2 Gastric Vein 3 Esophageal Vein 4 Hepatic Vein 5 Superior Mesenteric Vein 6 Inferior Mesenteric Vein 7 Colic Vein 8 Portal Vein 9 Renal Vein, Right B Renal Vein, Left C Common Iliac Vein, Right D Common Iliac Vein, Left F External Iliac Vein, Right G External Iliac Vein, Left H Hypogastric Vein, Right J Hypogastric Vein, Left M Femoral Vein, Right N Femoral Vein, Left P Saphenous Vein, Right Q Saphenous Vein, Left T Foot Vein, Right V Foot Vein, Left	0 Open 3 Percutaneous 4 Percutaneous Endoscopic	3 Infusion Device D Intraluminal Device	Z No Qualifier
Y Lower Vein	0 Open 3 Percutaneous 4 Percutaneous Endoscopic	2 Monitoring Device 3 Infusion Device D Intraluminal Device Y Other Device	Z No Qualifier

LC Limited Coverage   NC Noncovered   HAC HAC-associated Procedure   CC Combination Cluster - See Appendix G for code lists
DRG Non-OR-Affecting MS-DRG Assignment   New/Revised Text in **Orange**   ♂ Male   ♀ Female

2018 ICD-10-PCS

245

LOWER VEINS 061-06W

0 **Medical and Surgical**
6 **Lower Veins**
J **Inspection:** Visually and/or manually exploring a body part

Body Part	Approach	Device	Qualifier
Character 4	Character 5	Character 6	Character 7
Y Lower Vein	0 Open 3 Percutaneous 4 Percutaneous Endoscopic X External	Z No Device	Z No Qualifier

0 **Medical and Surgical**
6 **Lower Veins**
L **Occlusion:** Completely closing an orifice or the lumen of a tubular body part

Body Part	Approach	Device	Qualifier
Character 4	Character 5	Character 6	Character 7
0 Inferior Vena Cava 1 Splenic Vein 2 Gastric Vein 4 Hepatic Vein 5 Superior Mesenteric Vein 6 Inferior Mesenteric Vein 7 Colic Vein 8 Portal Vein 9 Renal Vein, Right B Renal Vein, Left C Common Iliac Vein, Right D Common Iliac Vein, Left F External Iliac Vein, Right G External Iliac Vein, Left H Hypogastric Vein, Right J Hypogastric Vein, Left M Femoral Vein, Right N Femoral Vein, Left P Saphenous Vein, Right Q Saphenous Vein, Left T Foot Vein, Right V Foot Vein, Left	0 Open 3 Percutaneous 4 Percutaneous Endoscopic	C Extraluminal Device D Intraluminal Device Z No Device	Z No Qualifier
3 Esophageal Vein	0 Open 3 Percutaneous 4 Percutaneous Endoscopic 7 Via Natural or Artificial Opening 8 Via Natural or Artificial Opening Endoscopic	C Extraluminal Device D Intraluminal Device Z No Device	Z No Qualifier
Y Lower Vein	0 Open 3 Percutaneous 4 Percutaneous Endoscopic	C Extraluminal Device D Intraluminal Device Z No Device	C Hemorrhoidal Plexus Z No Qualifier

0 **Medical and Surgical**

6 **Lower Veins**

N **Release:** Freeing a body part from an abnormal physical constraint by cutting or by the use of force

Body Part	Approach	Device	Qualifier
Character 4	Character 5	Character 6	Character 7
0 Inferior Vena Cava 1 Splenic Vein 2 Gastric Vein 3 Esophageal Vein 4 Hepatic Vein 5 Superior Mesenteric Vein 6 Inferior Mesenteric Vein 7 Colic Vein 8 Portal Vein 9 Renal Vein, Right B Renal Vein, Left C Common Iliac Vein, Right D Common Iliac Vein, Left F External Iliac Vein, Right G External Iliac Vein, Left H Hypogastric Vein, Right J Hypogastric Vein, Left M Femoral Vein, Right N Femoral Vein, Left P Saphenous Vein, Right Q Saphenous Vein, Left T Foot Vein, Right V Foot Vein, Left Y Lower Vein	0 Open 3 Percutaneous 4 Percutaneous Endoscopic	Z No Device	Z No Qualifier

0 **Medical and Surgical**

6 **Lower Veins**

P **Removal:** Taking out or off a device from a body part

Body Part	Approach	Device	Qualifier
Character 4	Character 5	Character 6	Character 7
Y Lower Vein	0 Open 3 Percutaneous 4 Percutaneous Endoscopic	0 Drainage Device 2 Monitoring Device 3 Infusion Device 7 Autologous Tissue Substitute C Extraluminal Device D Intraluminal Device J Synthetic Substitute K Nonautologous Tissue Substitute Y Other Device	Z No Qualifier
Y Lower Vein	X External	0 Drainage Device 2 Monitoring Device 3 Infusion Device D Intraluminal Device	Z No Qualifier

06Q-06R

0   Medical and Surgical
6   Lower Veins
Q   Repair: Restoring, to the extent possible, a body part to its normal anatomic structure and function

Body Part	Approach	Device	Qualifier
Character 4	Character 5	Character 6	Character 7
0 Inferior Vena Cava 1 Splenic Vein 2 Gastric Vein 3 Esophageal Vein 4 Hepatic Vein 5 Superior Mesenteric Vein 6 Inferior Mesenteric Vein 7 Colic Vein 8 Portal Vein 9 Renal Vein, Right B Renal Vein, Left C Common Iliac Vein, Right D Common Iliac Vein, Left F External Iliac Vein, Right G External Iliac Vein, Left H Hypogastric Vein, Right J Hypogastric Vein, Left M Femoral Vein, Right N Femoral Vein, Left P Saphenous Vein, Right Q Saphenous Vein, Left T Foot Vein, Right V Foot Vein, Left Y Lower Vein	0 Open 3 Percutaneous 4 Percutaneous Endoscopic	Z No Device	Z No Qualifier

0   Medical and Surgical
6   Lower Veins
R   Replacement: Putting in or on biological or synthetic material that physically takes the place and/or function of all or a portion of a body part

Body Part	Approach	Device	Qualifier
Character 4	Character 5	Character 6	Character 7
0 Inferior Vena Cava 1 Splenic Vein 2 Gastric Vein 3 Esophageal Vein 4 Hepatic Vein 5 Superior Mesenteric Vein 6 Inferior Mesenteric Vein 7 Colic Vein 8 Portal Vein 9 Renal Vein, Right B Renal Vein, Left C Common Iliac Vein, Right D Common Iliac Vein, Left F External Iliac Vein, Right G External Iliac Vein, Left H Hypogastric Vein, Right J Hypogastric Vein, Left M Femoral Vein, Right N Femoral Vein, Left P Saphenous Vein, Right Q Saphenous Vein, Left T Foot Vein, Right V Foot Vein, Left Y Lower Vein	0 Open 4 Percutaneous Endoscopic	7 Autologous Tissue Substitute J Synthetic Substitute K Nonautologous Tissue Substitute	Z No Qualifier

LC Limited Coverage   NC Noncovered   HAC HAC-associated Procedure   CC Combination Cluster - See Appendix G for code lists
DRG Non-OR-Affecting MS-DRG Assignment   New/Revised Text in **Orange**   ♂ Male   ♀ Female

248

2018 ICD-10-PCS

0 **Medical and Surgical**

6 **Lower Veins**

S **Reposition:** Moving to its normal location, or other suitable location, all or a portion of a body part

Body Part	Approach	Device	Qualifier
Character 4	Character 5	Character 6	Character 7
0 Inferior Vena Cava 1 Splenic Vein 2 Gastric Vein 3 Esophageal Vein 4 Hepatic Vein 5 Superior Mesenteric Vein 6 Inferior Mesenteric Vein 7 Colic Vein 8 Portal Vein 9 Renal Vein, Right B Renal Vein, Left C Common Iliac Vein, Right D Common Iliac Vein, Left F External Iliac Vein, Right G External Iliac Vein, Left H Hypogastric Vein, Right J Hypogastric Vein, Left M Femoral Vein, Right N Femoral Vein, Left P Saphenous Vein, Right Q Saphenous Vein, Left T Foot Vein, Right V Foot Vein, Left Y Lower Vein	0 Open 3 Percutaneous 4 Percutaneous Endoscopic	Z No Device	Z No Qualifier

0 **Medical and Surgical**

6 **Lower Veins**

U **Supplement:** Putting in or on biological or synthetic material that physically reinforces and/or augments the function of a portion of a body part

Body Part	Approach	Device	Qualifier
Character 4	Character 5	Character 6	Character 7
0 Inferior Vena Cava 1 Splenic Vein 2 Gastric Vein 3 Esophageal Vein 4 Hepatic Vein 5 Superior Mesenteric Vein 6 Inferior Mesenteric Vein 7 Colic Vein 8 Portal Vein 9 Renal Vein, Right B Renal Vein, Left C Common Iliac Vein, Right D Common Iliac Vein, Left F External Iliac Vein, Right G External Iliac Vein, Left H Hypogastric Vein, Right J Hypogastric Vein, Left M Femoral Vein, Right N Femoral Vein, Left P Saphenous Vein, Right Q Saphenous Vein, Left T Foot Vein, Right V Foot Vein, Left Y Lower Vein	0 Open 3 Percutaneous 4 Percutaneous Endoscopic	7 Autologous Tissue Substitute J Synthetic Substitute K Nonautologous Tissue Substitute	Z No Qualifier

0   Medical and Surgical
6   Lower Veins
V   Restriction: Partially closing an orifice or the lumen of a tubular body part

Body Part	Approach	Device	Qualifier
Character 4	**Character 5**	**Character 6**	**Character 7**
0 Inferior Vena Cava 1 Splenic Vein 2 Gastric Vein 3 Esophageal Vein 4 Hepatic Vein 5 Superior Mesenteric Vein 6 Inferior Mesenteric Vein 7 Colic Vein 8 Portal Vein 9 Renal Vein, Right B Renal Vein, Left C Common Iliac Vein, Right D Common Iliac Vein, Left F External Iliac Vein, Right G External Iliac Vein, Left H Hypogastric Vein, Right J Hypogastric Vein, Left M Femoral Vein, Right N Femoral Vein, Left P Saphenous Vein, Right Q Saphenous Vein, Left T Foot Vein, Right V Foot Vein, Left Y Lower Vein	0 Open 3 Percutaneous 4 Percutaneous Endoscopic	C Extraluminal Device D Intraluminal Device Z No Device	Z No Qualifier

0   Medical and Surgical
6   Lower Veins
W   Revision: Correcting, to the extent possible, a portion of a malfunctioning device or the position of a displaced device

Body Part	Approach	Device	Qualifier
Character 4	**Character 5**	**Character 6**	**Character 7**
Y Lower Vein	0 Open 3 Percutaneous 4 Percutaneous Endoscopic	0 Drainage Device 2 Monitoring Device 3 Infusion Device 7 Autologous Tissue Substitute C Extraluminal Device D Intraluminal Device J Synthetic Substitute K Nonautologous Tissue Substitute Y Other Device	Z No Qualifier
Y Lower Vein	X External	0 Drainage Device 2 Monitoring Device 3 Infusion Device 7 Autologous Tissue Substitute C Extraluminal Device D Intraluminal Device J Synthetic Substitute K Nonautologous Tissue Substitute	Z No Qualifier

NOTES

NOTES

LYMPHATIC AND HEMIC SYSTEMS 072-07Y

Lymphatic and Hemic Systems 072-07Y

0 **Medical and Surgical**
7 **Lymphatic and Hemic Systems**
2 **Change:** Taking out or off a device from a body part and putting back an identical or similar device in or on the same body part without cutting or puncturing the skin or a mucous membrane

Body Part	Approach	Device	Qualifier
Character 4	Character 5	Character 6	Character 7
K Thoracic Duct **L** Cisterna Chyli **M** Thymus **N** Lymphatic **P** Spleen **T** Bone Marrow	**X** External	**0** Drainage Device **Y** Other Device	**Z** No Qualifier

0 **Medical and Surgical**
7 **Lymphatic and Hemic Systems**
5 **Destruction:** Physical eradication of all or a portion of a body part by the direct use of energy, force, or a destructive agent

Body Part	Approach	Device	Qualifier
Character 4	Character 5	Character 6	Character 7
0 Lymphatic, Head **1** Lymphatic, Right Neck **2** Lymphatic, Left Neck **3** Lymphatic, Right Upper Extremity **4** Lymphatic, Left Upper Extremity **5** Lymphatic, Right Axillary **6** Lymphatic, Left Axillary **7** Lymphatic, Thorax **8** Lymphatic, Internal Mammary, Right **9** Lymphatic, Internal Mammary, Left **B** Lymphatic, Mesenteric **C** Lymphatic, Pelvis **D** Lymphatic, Aortic **F** Lymphatic, Right Lower Extremity **G** Lymphatic, Left Lower Extremity **H** Lymphatic, Right Inguinal **J** Lymphatic, Left Inguinal **K** Thoracic Duct **L** Cisterna Chyli **M** Thymus **P** Spleen	**0** Open **3** Percutaneous **4** Percutaneous Endoscopic	**Z** No Device	**Z** No Qualifier

LC Limited Coverage   **NC** Noncovered   **HAC** HAC-associated Procedure   **CC** Combination Cluster - See Appendix G for code lists
DRG Non-OR-Affecting MS-DRG Assignment   New/Revised Text in **Orange**   ♂ Male   ♀ Female

253

0 Medical and Surgical
7 Lymphatic and Hemic Systems
9 Drainage: Taking or letting out fluids and/or gases from a body part

Body Part	Approach	Device	Qualifier
Character 4	Character 5	Character 6	Character 7
0 Lymphatic, Head 1 Lymphatic, Right Neck 2 Lymphatic, Left Neck 3 Lymphatic, Right Upper Extremity 4 Lymphatic, Left Upper Extremity 5 Lymphatic, Right Axillary 6 Lymphatic, Left Axillary 7 Lymphatic, Thorax 8 Lymphatic, Internal Mammary, Right 9 Lymphatic, Internal Mammary, Left B Lymphatic, Mesenteric C Lymphatic, Pelvis D Lymphatic, Aortic F Lymphatic, Right Lower Extremity G Lymphatic, Left Lower Extremity H Lymphatic, Right Inguinal J Lymphatic, Left Inguinal K Thoracic Duct L Cisterna Chyli	0 Open 3 Percutaneous 4 Percutaneous Endoscopic 8 Via Natural or Artificial Opening Endoscopic	0 Drainage Device	Z No Qualifier
0 Lymphatic, Head 1 Lymphatic, Right Neck 2 Lymphatic, Left Neck 3 Lymphatic, Right Upper Extremity 4 Lymphatic, Left Upper Extremity 5 Lymphatic, Right Axillary 6 Lymphatic, Left Axillary 7 Lymphatic, Thorax 8 Lymphatic, Internal Mammary, Right 9 Lymphatic, Internal Mammary, Left B Lymphatic, Mesenteric C Lymphatic, Pelvis D Lymphatic, Aortic F Lymphatic, Right Lower Extremity G Lymphatic, Left Lower Extremity H Lymphatic, Right Inguinal J Lymphatic, Left Inguinal K Thoracic Duct L Cisterna Chyli	0 Open 3 Percutaneous 4 Percutaneous Endoscopic 8 Via Natural or Artificial Opening Endoscopic	Z No Device	X Diagnostic Z No Qualifier
M Thymus ᴰᴿᴳ P Spleen T Bone Marrow	0 Open 3 Percutaneous 4 Percutaneous Endoscopic	0 Drainage Device	Z No Qualifier
M Thymus ᴰᴿᴳ P Spleen T Bone Marrow	0 Open 3 Percutaneous 4 Percutaneous Endoscopic	Z No Device	X Diagnostic Z No Qualifier

ᴰᴿᴳ 079M30Z 079M3ZZ

0 **Medical and Surgical**
7 **Lymphatic and Hemic Systems**
B **Excision:** Cutting out or off, without replacement, a portion of a body part

Body Part	Approach	Device	Qualifier
Character 4	Character 5	Character 6	Character 7

0 Lymphatic, Head
1 Lymphatic, Right Neck
2 Lymphatic, Left Neck
3 Lymphatic, Right Upper
   Extremity
4 Lymphatic, Left Upper Extremity
5 Lymphatic, Right Axillary
6 Lymphatic, Left Axillary
7 Lymphatic, Thorax
8 Lymphatic, Internal Mammary,
   Right
9 Lymphatic, Internal Mammary,
   Left
B Lymphatic, Mesenteric
C Lymphatic, Pelvis
D Lymphatic, Aortic
F Lymphatic, Right Lower
   Extremity
G Lymphatic, Left Lower Extremity
H Lymphatic, Right Inguinal CC
J Lymphatic, Left Inguinal CC
K Thoracic Duct
L Cisterna Chyli
M Thymus
P Spleen
	0 Open
	3 Percutaneous
	4 Percutaneous Endoscopic
		Z No Device	X Diagnostic
			Z No Qualifier

CC 07BH0ZZ   07BH4ZZ   07BJ0ZZ   07BJ4ZZ

0 **Medical and Surgical**
7 **Lymphatic and Hemic Systems**
C **Extirpation:** Taking or cutting out solid matter from a body part

Body Part	Approach	Device	Qualifier
Character 4	Character 5	Character 6	Character 7

0 Lymphatic, Head
1 Lymphatic, Right Neck
2 Lymphatic, Left Neck
3 Lymphatic, Right Upper
   Extremity
4 Lymphatic, Left Upper Extremity
5 Lymphatic, Right Axillary
6 Lymphatic, Left Axillary
7 Lymphatic, Thorax
8 Lymphatic, Internal Mammary,
   Right
9 Lymphatic, Internal Mammary,
   Left
B Lymphatic, Mesenteric
C Lymphatic, Pelvis
D Lymphatic, Aortic
F Lymphatic, Right Lower
   Extremity
G Lymphatic, Left Lower Extremity
H Lymphatic, Right Inguinal
J Lymphatic, Left Inguinal
K Thoracic Duct
L Cisterna Chyli
M Thymus
P Spleen
	0 Open
	3 Percutaneous
	4 Percutaneous Endoscopic
		Z No Device	Z No Qualifier

0 Medical and Surgical
7 Lymphatic and Hemic Systems
D Extraction: Pulling or stripping out or off all or a portion of a body part by the use of force

Body Part	Approach	Device	Qualifier
Character 4	Character 5	Character 6	Character 7
0 Lymphatic, Head 1 Lymphatic, Right Neck 2 Lymphatic, Left Neck 3 Lymphatic, Right Upper Extremity 4 Lymphatic, Left Upper Extremity 5 Lymphatic, Right Axillary 6 Lymphatic, Left Axillary 7 Lymphatic, Thorax 8 Lymphatic, Internal Mammary, Right 9 Lymphatic, Internal Mammary, Left B Lymphatic, Mesenteric C Lymphatic, Pelvis D Lymphatic, Aortic F Lymphatic, Right Lower Extremity G Lymphatic, Left Lower Extremity H Lymphatic, Right Inguinal J Lymphatic, Left Inguinal K Thoracic Duct L Cisterna Chyli	3 Percutaneous 4 Percutaneous Endoscopic 8 Via Natural or Artificial Opening Endoscopic	Z No Device	X Diagnostic
M Thymus P Spleen	3 Percutaneous 4 Percutaneous Endoscopic	Z No Device	X Diagnostic
Q Bone Marrow, Sternum R Bone Marrow, Iliac S Bone Marrow, Vertebral	0 Open 3 Percutaneous	Z No Device	X Diagnostic Z No Qualifier

0 Medical and Surgical
7 Lymphatic and Hemic Systems
H Insertion: Putting in a nonbiological appliance that monitors, assists, performs, or prevents a physiological function but does not physically take the place of a body part

Body Part	Approach	Device	Qualifier
Character 4	Character 5	Character 6	Character 7
K Thoracic Duct L Cisterna Chyli M Thymus N Lymphatic P Spleen	0 Open 3 Percutaneous 4 Percutaneous Endoscopic	3 Infusion Device Y Other Device	Z No Qualifier

0   **Medical and Surgical**
7   **Lymphatic and Hemic Systems**
J   **Inspection:** Visually and/or manually exploring a body part

Body Part	Approach	Device	Qualifier
Character 4	Character 5	Character 6	Character 7
K Thoracic Duct L Cisterna Chyli M Thymus T Bone Marrow	0 Open 3 Percutaneous 4 Percutaneous Endoscopic	Z No Device	Z No Qualifier
N Lymphatic	0 Open 3 Percutaneous 4 Percutaneous Endoscopic 8 Via Natural or Artificial Opening Endoscopic X External	Z No Device	Z No Qualifier
P Spleen	0 Open 3 Percutaneous 4 Percutaneous Endoscopic X External	Z No Device	Z No Qualifier

0   **Medical and Surgical**
7   **Lymphatic and Hemic Systems**
L   **Occlusion:** Completely closing an orifice or the lumen of a tubular body part

Body Part	Approach	Device	Qualifier
Character 4	Character 5	Character 6	Character 7
0 Lymphatic, Head 1 Lymphatic, Right Neck 2 Lymphatic, Left Neck 3 Lymphatic, Right Upper Extremity 4 Lymphatic, Left Upper Extremity 5 Lymphatic, Right Axillary 6 Lymphatic, Left Axillary 7 Lymphatic, Thorax 8 Lymphatic, Internal Mammary, Right 9 Lymphatic, Internal Mammary, Left B Lymphatic, Mesenteric C Lymphatic, Pelvis D Lymphatic, Aortic F Lymphatic, Right Lower Extremity G Lymphatic, Left Lower Extremity H Lymphatic, Right Inguinal J Lymphatic, Left Inguinal K Thoracic Duct L Cisterna Chyli	0 Open 3 Percutaneous 4 Percutaneous Endoscopic	C Extraluminal Device D Intraluminal Device Z No Device	Z No Qualifier

0 Medical and Surgical
7 Lymphatic and Hemic Systems
N Release: Freeing a body part from an abnormal physical constraint by cutting or by the use of force

Body Part	Approach	Device	Qualifier
Character 4	**Character 5**	**Character 6**	**Character 7**
0 Lymphatic, Head **1** Lymphatic, Right Neck **2** Lymphatic, Left Neck **3** Lymphatic, Right Upper Extremity **4** Lymphatic, Left Upper Extremity **5** Lymphatic, Right Axillary **6** Lymphatic, Left Axillary **7** Lymphatic, Thorax **8** Lymphatic, Internal Mammary, Right **9** Lymphatic, Internal Mammary, Left **B** Lymphatic, Mesenteric **C** Lymphatic, Pelvis **D** Lymphatic, Aortic **F** Lymphatic, Right Lower Extremity **G** Lymphatic, Left Lower Extremity **H** Lymphatic, Right Inguinal **J** Lymphatic, Left Inguinal **K** Thoracic Duct **L** Cisterna Chyli **M** Thymus **P** Spleen	**0** Open **3** Percutaneous **4** Percutaneous Endoscopic	**Z** No Device	**Z** No Qualifier

0 Medical and Surgical
7 Lymphatic and Hemic Systems
P Removal: Taking out or off a device from a body part

Body Part	Approach	Device	Qualifier
Character 4	**Character 5**	**Character 6**	**Character 7**
K Thoracic Duct **L** Cisterna Chyli **N** Lymphatic	**0** Open **3** Percutaneous **4** Percutaneous Endoscopic	**0** Drainage Device **3** Infusion Device **7** Autologous Tissue Substitute **C** Extraluminal Device **D** Intraluminal Device **J** Synthetic Substitute **K** Nonautologous Tissue Substitute **Y** Other Device	**Z** No Qualifier
K Thoracic Duct **L** Cisterna Chyli **N** Lymphatic	**X** External	**0** Drainage Device **3** Infusion Device **D** Intraluminal Device	**Z** No Qualifier
M Thymus **P** Spleen	**0** Open **3** Percutaneous **4** Percutaneous Endoscopic	**0** Drainage Device **3** Infusion Device **Y** Other Device	**Z** No Qualifier
M Thymus **P** Spleen	**X** External	**0** Drainage Device **3** Infusion Device	**Z** No Qualifier
T Bone Marrow	**0** Open **3** Percutaneous **4** Percutaneous Endoscopic **X** External	**0** Drainage Device	**Z** No Qualifier

LC Limited Coverage   NC Noncovered   HAC HAC-associated Procedure   CC Combination Cluster - See Appendix G for code lists
DRG Non-OR-Affecting MS-DRG Assignment   New/Revised Text in **Orange**   ♂ Male   ♀ Female

258   2018 ICD-10-PCS

0 Medical and Surgical

7 Lymphatic and Hemic Systems

Q Repair: Restoring, to the extent possible, a body part to its normal anatomic structure and function

Body Part	Approach	Device	Qualifier
Character 4	Character 5	Character 6	Character 7
0 Lymphatic, Head 1 Lymphatic, Right Neck 2 Lymphatic, Left Neck 3 Lymphatic, Right Upper Extremity 4 Lymphatic, Left Upper Extremity 5 Lymphatic, Right Axillary 6 Lymphatic, Left Axillary 7 Lymphatic, Thorax 8 Lymphatic, Internal Mammary, Right 9 Lymphatic, Internal Mammary, Left B Lymphatic, Mesenteric C Lymphatic, Pelvis D Lymphatic, Aortic F Lymphatic, Right Lower Extremity G Lymphatic, Left Lower Extremity H Lymphatic, Right Inguinal J Lymphatic, Left Inguinal K Thoracic Duct L Cisterna Chyli	0 Open 3 Percutaneous 4 Percutaneous Endoscopic 8 Via Natural or Artificial Opening Endoscopic	Z No Device	Z No Qualifier
M Thymus P Spleen	0 Open 3 Percutaneous 4 Percutaneous Endoscopic	Z No Device	Z No Qualifier

0 Medical and Surgical

7 Lymphatic and Hemic Systems

S Reposition: Moving to its normal location, or other suitable location, all or a portion of a body part

Body Part	Approach	Device	Qualifier
Character 4	Character 5	Character 6	Character 7
M Thymus P Spleen	0 Open	Z No Device	Z No Qualifier

LC Limited Coverage   NC Noncovered   HAC HAC-associated Procedure   CC Combination Cluster - See Appendix G for code lists
DRG Non-OR-Affecting MS-DRG Assignment   New/Revised Text in **Orange**   ♂ Male   ♀ Female

2018 ICD-10-PCS

259

LYMPHATIC AND HEMIC SYSTEMS 072-07Y

07Q-07S

0 Medical and Surgical
7 Lymphatic and Hemic Systems
T Resection: Cutting out or off, without replacement, all of a body part

Body Part	Approach	Device	Qualifier
Character 4	Character 5	Character 6	Character 7
0 Lymphatic, Head 1 Lymphatic, Right Neck 2 Lymphatic, Left Neck 3 Lymphatic, Right Upper Extremity 4 Lymphatic, Left Upper Extremity 5 Lymphatic, Right Axillary ⒸⒸ 6 Lymphatic, Left Axillary ⒸⒸ 7 Lymphatic, Thorax ⒸⒸ 8 Lymphatic, Internal Mammary, Right ⒸⒸ 9 Lymphatic, Internal Mammary, Left ⒸⒸ B Lymphatic, Mesenteric C Lymphatic, Pelvis D Lymphatic, Aortic F Lymphatic, Right Lower Extremity G Lymphatic, Left Lower Extremity H Lymphatic, Right Inguinal J Lymphatic, Left Inguinal K Thoracic Duct L Cisterna Chyli M Thymus P Spleen	0 Open 4 Percutaneous Endoscopic	Z No Device	Z No Qualifier

ⒸⒸ 07T50ZZ   07T60ZZ   07T70ZZ   07T80ZZ   07T90ZZ

0 Medical and Surgical
7 Lymphatic and Hemic Systems
U Supplement: Putting in or on biological or synthetic material that physically reinforces and/or augments the function of a portion of a body part

Body Part	Approach	Device	Qualifier
Character 4	Character 5	Character 6	Character 7
0 Lymphatic, Head 1 Lymphatic, Right Neck 2 Lymphatic, Left Neck 3 Lymphatic, Right Upper Extremity 4 Lymphatic, Left Upper Extremity 5 Lymphatic, Right Axillary 6 Lymphatic, Left Axillary 7 Lymphatic, Thorax 8 Lymphatic, Internal Mammary, Right 9 Lymphatic, Internal Mammary, Left B Lymphatic, Mesenteric C Lymphatic, Pelvis D Lymphatic, Aortic F Lymphatic, Right Lower Extremity G Lymphatic, Left Lower Extremity H Lymphatic, Right Inguinal J Lymphatic, Left Inguinal K Thoracic Duct L Cisterna Chyli	0 Open 4 Percutaneous Endoscopic	7 Autologous Tissue Substitute J Synthetic Substitute K Nonautologous Tissue Substitute	Z No Qualifier

ⒸⒸ Limited Coverage   ⓃⒸ Noncovered   ⒽⒶⒸ HAC-associated Procedure   ⒸⒸ Combination Cluster - See Appendix G for code lists
ⒹⓇⒼ Non-OR-Affecting MS-DRG Assignment   New/Revised Text in **Orange**   ♂ Male   ♀ Female

260

2018 ICD-10-PCS

0   **Medical and Surgical**
7   **Lymphatic and Hemic Systems**
V   **Restriction:** Partially closing an orifice or the lumen of a tubular body part

Body Part	Approach	Device	Qualifier
Character 4	Character 5	Character 6	Character 7
0 Lymphatic, Head 1 Lymphatic, Right Neck 2 Lymphatic, Left Neck 3 Lymphatic, Right Upper Extremity 4 Lymphatic, Left Upper Extremity 5 Lymphatic, Right Axillary 6 Lymphatic, Left Axillary 7 Lymphatic, Thorax 8 Lymphatic, Internal Mammary, Right 9 Lymphatic, Internal Mammary, Left B Lymphatic, Mesenteric C Lymphatic, Pelvis D Lymphatic, Aortic F Lymphatic, Right Lower Extremity G Lymphatic, Left Lower Extremity H Lymphatic, Right Inguinal J Lymphatic, Left Inguinal K Thoracic Duct L Cisterna Chyli	0 Open 3 Percutaneous 4 Percutaneous Endoscopic	C Extraluminal Device D Intraluminal Device Z No Device	Z No Qualifier

0   **Medical and Surgical**
7   **Lymphatic and Hemic Systems**
W   **Revision:** Correcting, to the extent possible, a portion of a malfunctioning device or the position of a displaced device

Body Part	Approach	Device	Qualifier
Character 4	Character 5	Character 6	Character 7
K Thoracic Duct L Cisterna Chyli N Lymphatic	0 Open 3 Percutaneous 4 Percutaneous Endoscopic	0 Drainage Device 3 Infusion Device 7 Autologous Tissue Substitute C Extraluminal Device D Intraluminal Device J Synthetic Substitute K Nonautologous Tissue Substitute Y Other Device	Z No Qualifier
K Thoracic Duct L Cisterna Chyli N Lymphatic	X External	0 Drainage Device 3 Infusion Device 7 Autologous Tissue Substitute C Extraluminal Device D Intraluminal Device J Synthetic Substitute K Nonautologous Tissue Substitute	Z No Qualifier
M Thymus P Spleen	0 Open 3 Percutaneous 4 Percutaneous Endoscopic	0 Drainage Device 3 Infusion Device Y Other Device	Z No Qualifier
M Thymus P Spleen	X External	0 Drainage Device 3 Infusion Device	Z No Qualifier
T Bone Marrow	0 Open 3 Percutaneous 4 Percutaneous Endoscopic X External	0 Drainage Device	Z No Qualifier

0 **Medical and Surgical**
7 **Lymphatic and Hemic Systems**
Y **Transplantation:** Putting in or on all or a portion of a living body part taken from another individual or animal to physically take the place and/or function of all or a portion of a similar body part

Body Part	Approach	Device	Qualifier
Character 4	Character 5	Character 6	Character 7
M Thymus **P** Spleen	**0** Open	**Z** No Device	**0** Allogeneic **1** Syngeneic **2** Zooplastic

LC Limited Coverage   **NC** Noncovered   **HAC** HAC-associated Procedure   **CC** Combination Cluster - See Appendix G for code lists
DRG Non-OR-Affecting MS-DRG Assignment   New/Revised Text in **Orange**   ♂ Male   ♀ Female

262

2018 ICD-10-PCS

NOTES

NOTES

Eye 080-08X

0   **Medical and Surgical**
8   **Eye**
0   **Alteration:** Modifying the anatomic structure of a body part without affecting the function of the body part

Body Part	Approach	Device	Qualifier
Character 4	Character 5	Character 6	Character 7
N Upper Eyelid, Right **P** Upper Eyelid, Left **Q** Lower Eyelid, Right **R** Lower Eyelid, Left	**0** Open **3** Percutaneous **X** External	**7** Autologous Tissue Substitute **J** Synthetic Substitute **K** Nonautologous Tissue Substitute **Z** No Device	**Z** No Qualifier

0   **Medical and Surgical**
8   **Eye**
1   **Bypass:** Altering the route of passage of the contents of a tubular body part

Body Part	Approach	Device	Qualifier
Character 4	Character 5	Character 6	Character 7
2 Anterior Chamber, Right **3** Anterior Chamber, Left	**3** Percutaneous	**J** Synthetic Substitute **K** Nonautologous Tissue Substitute **Z** No Device	**4** Sclera
X Lacrimal Duct, Right **Y** Lacrimal Duct, Left	**0** Open **3** Percutaneous	**J** Synthetic Substitute **K** Nonautologous Tissue Substitute **Z** No Device	**3** Nasal Cavity

0   **Medical and Surgical**
8   **Eye**
2   **Change:** Taking out or off a device from a body part and putting back an identical or similar device in or on the same body part without cutting or puncturing the skin or a mucous membrane

Body Part	Approach	Device	Qualifier
Character 4	Character 5	Character 6	Character 7
0 Eye, Right **1** Eye, Left	**X** External	**0** Drainage Device **Y** Other Device	**Z** No Qualifier

LC Limited Coverage   **NC** Noncovered   **HAC** HAC-associated Procedure   **CC** Combination Cluster - See Appendix G for code lists
DRG Non-OR-Affecting MS-DRG Assignment   New/Revised Text in **Orange**   ♂ Male   ♀ Female

2018 ICD-10-PCS

EYE 080-08X

265

0 Medical and Surgical
8 Eye
5 Destruction: Physical eradication of all or a portion of a body part by the direct use of energy, force, or a destructive agent

Body Part	Approach	Device	Qualifier
Character 4	Character 5	Character 6	Character 7
0 Eye, Right **1** Eye, Left **6** Sclera, Right **7** Sclera, Left **8** Cornea, Right **9** Cornea, Left **S** Conjunctiva, Right **T** Conjunctiva, Left	**X** External	**Z** No Device	**Z** No Qualifier
2 Anterior Chamber, Right **3** Anterior Chamber, Left **4** Vitreous, Right **5** Vitreous, Left **C** Iris, Right **D** Iris, Left **E** Retina, Right **F** Retina, Left **G** Retinal Vessel, Right **H** Retinal Vessel, Left **J** Lens, Right **K** Lens, Left	**3** Percutaneous	**Z** No Device	**Z** No Qualifier
A Choroid, Right **B** Choroid, Left **L** Extraocular Muscle, Right **M** Extraocular Muscle, Left **V** Lacrimal Gland, Right **W** Lacrimal Gland, Left	**0** Open **3** Percutaneous	**Z** No Device	**Z** No Qualifier
N Upper Eyelid, Right **P** Upper Eyelid, Left **Q** Lower Eyelid, Right **R** Lower Eyelid, Left	**0** Open **3** Percutaneous **X** External	**Z** No Device	**Z** No Qualifier
X Lacrimal Duct, Right **Y** Lacrimal Duct, Left	**0** Open **3** Percutaneous **7** Via Natural or Artificial Opening **8** Via Natural or Artificial Opening Endoscopic	**Z** No Device	**Z** No Qualifier

0 Medical and Surgical
8 Eye
7 Dilation: Expanding an orifice or the lumen of a tubular body part

Body Part	Approach	Device	Qualifier
Character 4	Character 5	Character 6	Character 7
X Lacrimal Duct, Right **Y** Lacrimal Duct, Left	**0** Open **3** Percutaneous **7** Via Natural or Artificial Opening **8** Via Natural or Artificial Opening Endoscopic	**D** Intraluminal Device **Z** No Device	**Z** No Qualifier

LC Limited Coverage   **NC** Noncovered   **HAC** HAC-associated Procedure   **CC** Combination Cluster - See Appendix G for code lists
DRG Non-OR-Affecting MS-DRG Assignment   New/Revised Text in **Orange**   ♂ Male   ♀ Female

266

EYE 080-08X

2018 ICD-10-PCS

0   Medical and Surgical
8   Eye
9   **Drainage:** Taking or letting out fluids and/or gases from a body part

Body Part	Approach	Device	Qualifier
Character 4	**Character 5**	**Character 6**	**Character 7**
0 Eye, Right **1** Eye, Left **6** Sclera, Right **7** Sclera, Left **8** Cornea, Right **9** Cornea, Left **S** Conjunctiva, Right **T** Conjunctiva, Left	**X** External	**0** Drainage Device	**Z** No Qualifier
0 Eye, Right **1** Eye, Left **6** Sclera, Right **7** Sclera, Left **8** Cornea, Right **9** Cornea, Left **S** Conjunctiva, Right **T** Conjunctiva, Left	**X** External	**Z** No Device	**X** Diagnostic **Z** No Qualifier
2 Anterior Chamber, Right **3** Anterior Chamber, Left **4** Vitreous, Right **5** Vitreous, Left **C** Iris, Right **D** Iris, Left **E** Retina, Right **F** Retina, Left **G** Retinal Vessel, Right **H** Retinal Vessel, Left **J** Lens, Right **K** Lens, Left	**3** Percutaneous	**0** Drainage Device	**Z** No Qualifier
2 Anterior Chamber, Right **3** Anterior Chamber, Left **4** Vitreous, Right **5** Vitreous, Left **C** Iris, Right **D** Iris, Left **E** Retina, Right **F** Retina, Left **G** Retinal Vessel, Right **H** Retinal Vessel, Left **J** Lens, Right **K** Lens, Left	**3** Percutaneous	**Z** No Device	**X** Diagnostic **Z** No Qualifier
A Choroid, Right **B** Choroid, Left **L** Extraocular Muscle, Right **M** Extraocular Muscle, Left **V** Lacrimal Gland, Right **W** Lacrimal Gland, Left	**0** Open **3** Percutaneous	**0** Drainage Device	**Z** No Qualifier
A Choroid, Right **B** Choroid, Left **L** Extraocular Muscle, Right **M** Extraocular Muscle, Left **V** Lacrimal Gland, Right **W** Lacrimal Gland, Left	**0** Open **3** Percutaneous	**Z** No Device	**X** Diagnostic **Z** No Qualifier
N Upper Eyelid, Right **P** Upper Eyelid, Left **Q** Lower Eyelid, Right **R** Lower Eyelid, Left	**0** Open **3** Percutaneous **X** External	**0** Drainage Device	**Z** No Qualifier

089 continued on next page

LC Limited Coverage   **NC** Noncovered   **HAC** HAC-associated Procedure   **CC** Combination Cluster - See Appendix G for code lists
DRG Non-OR-Affecting MS-DRG Assignment   New/Revised Text in **Orange**   ♂ Male   ♀ Female

0   Medical and Surgical
8   Eye
9   Drainage: Taking or letting out fluids and/or gases from a body part

089 continued from previous page

Body Part	Approach	Device	Qualifier
Character 4	Character 5	Character 6	Character 7
N Upper Eyelid, Right P Upper Eyelid, Left Q Lower Eyelid, Right R Lower Eyelid, Left	0 Open 3 Percutaneous X External	Z No Device	X Diagnostic Z No Qualifier
X Lacrimal Duct, Right Y Lacrimal Duct, Left	0 Open 3 Percutaneous 7 Via Natural or Artificial Opening 8 Via Natural or Artificial Opening Endoscopic	0 Drainage Device	Z No Qualifier
X Lacrimal Duct, Right Y Lacrimal Duct, Left	0 Open 3 Percutaneous 7 Via Natural or Artificial Opening 8 Via Natural or Artificial Opening Endoscopic	Z No Device	X Diagnostic Z No Qualifier

0   Medical and Surgical
8   Eye
B   Excision: Cutting out or off, without replacement, a portion of a body part

Body Part	Approach	Device	Qualifier
Character 4	Character 5	Character 6	Character 7
0 Eye, Right 1 Eye, Left N Upper Eyelid, Right P Upper Eyelid, Left Q Lower Eyelid, Right R Lower Eyelid, Left	0 Open 3 Percutaneous X External	Z No Device	X Diagnostic Z No Qualifier
4 Vitreous, Right 5 Vitreous, Left C Iris, Right D Iris, Left E Retina, Right F Retina, Left J Lens, Right K Lens, Left	3 Percutaneous	Z No Device	X Diagnostic Z No Qualifier
6 Sclera, Right 7 Sclera, Left 8 Cornea, Right 9 Cornea, Left S Conjunctiva, Right T Conjunctiva, Left	X External	Z No Device	X Diagnostic Z No Qualifier
A Choroid, Right B Choroid, Left L Extraocular Muscle, Right M Extraocular Muscle, Left V Lacrimal Gland, Right W Lacrimal Gland, Left	0 Open 3 Percutaneous	Z No Device	X Diagnostic Z No Qualifier
X Lacrimal Duct, Right Y Lacrimal Duct, Left	0 Open 3 Percutaneous 7 Via Natural or Artificial Opening 8 Via Natural or Artificial Opening Endoscopic	Z No Device	X Diagnostic Z No Qualifier

0   Medical and Surgical
8   Eye
C   Extirpation: Taking or cutting out solid matter from a body part

Body Part	Approach	Device	Qualifier
Character 4	Character 5	Character 6	Character 7
0 Eye, Right 1 Eye, Left 6 Sclera, Right 7 Sclera, Left 8 Cornea, Right 9 Cornea, Left S Conjunctiva, Right T Conjunctiva, Left	X External	Z No Device	Z No Qualifier
2 Anterior Chamber, Right 3 Anterior Chamber, Left 4 Vitreous, Right 5 Vitreous, Left C Iris, Right D Iris, Left E Retina, Right F Retina, Left G Retinal Vessel, Right H Retinal Vessel, Left J Lens, Right K Lens, Left	3 Percutaneous X External	Z No Device	Z No Qualifier
A Choroid, Right B Choroid, Left L Extraocular Muscle, Right M Extraocular Muscle, Left N Upper Eyelid, Right P Upper Eyelid, Left Q Lower Eyelid, Right R Lower Eyelid, Left V Lacrimal Gland, Right W Lacrimal Gland, Left	0 Open 3 Percutaneous X External	Z No Device	Z No Qualifier
X Lacrimal Duct, Right Y Lacrimal Duct, Left	0 Open 3 Percutaneous 7 Via Natural or Artificial Opening 8 Via Natural or Artificial Opening 　　Endoscopic	Z No Device	Z No Qualifier

0   Medical and Surgical
8   Eye
D   Extraction: Pulling or stripping out or off all or a portion of a body part by the use of force

Body Part	Approach	Device	Qualifier
Character 4	Character 5	Character 6	Character 7
8 Cornea, Right 9 Cornea, Left	X External	Z No Device	X Diagnostic Z No Qualifier
J Lens, Right K Lens, Left	3 Percutaneous	Z No Device	Z No Qualifier

0   Medical and Surgical
8   Eye
F   Fragmentation: Breaking solid matter in a body part into pieces

Body Part	Approach	Device	Qualifier
Character 4	Character 5	Character 6	Character 7
4 Vitreous, Right ⓃⒸ 5 Vitreous, Left ⓃⒸ	3 Percutaneous X External	Z No Device	Z No Qualifier

ⓃⒸ 08F4XZZ   08F5XZZ

ⓁⒸ Limited Coverage   ⓃⒸ Noncovered   ⒽⒶⒸ HAC-associated Procedure   ⒸⒸ Combination Cluster - See Appendix G for code lists
ᴰᴿᴳ Non-OR-Affecting MS-DRG Assignment   New/Revised Text in **Orange**   ♂ Male   ♀ Female

0 Medical and Surgical
8 Eye
H Insertion: Putting in a nonbiological appliance that monitors, assists, performs, or prevents a physiological function but does not physically take the place of a body part

Body Part	Approach	Device	Qualifier
Character 4	Character 5	Character 6	Character 7
0 Eye, Right 1 Eye, Left	0 Open	5 Epiretinal Visual Prosthesis Y Other Device	Z No Qualifier
0 Eye, Right 1 Eye, Left	3 Percutaneous	1 Radioactive Element 3 Infusion Device Y Other Device	Z No Qualifier
0 Eye, Right 1 Eye, Left	7 Via Natural or Artificial Opening 8 Via Natural or Artificial Opening Endoscopic	Y Other Device	Z No Qualifier
0 Eye, Right 1 Eye, Left	X External	1 Radioactive Element 3 Infusion Device	Z No Qualifier

0 Medical and Surgical
8 Eye
J Inspection: Visually and/or manually exploring a body part

Body Part	Approach	Device	Qualifier
Character 4	Character 5	Character 6	Character 7
0 Eye, Right 1 Eye, Left J Lens, Right K Lens, Left	X External	Z No Device	Z No Qualifier
L Extraocular Muscle, Right M Extraocular Muscle, Left	0 Open X External	Z No Device	Z No Qualifier

0 Medical and Surgical
8 Eye
L Occlusion: Completely closing an orifice or the lumen of a tubular body part

Body Part	Approach	Device	Qualifier
Character 4	Character 5	Character 6	Character 7
X Lacrimal Duct, Right Y Lacrimal Duct, Left	0 Open 3 Percutaneous	C Extraluminal Device D Intraluminal Device Z No Device	Z No Qualifier
X Lacrimal Duct, Right Y Lacrimal Duct, Left	7 Via Natural or Artificial Opening 8 Via Natural or Artificial Opening Endoscopic	D Intraluminal Device Z No Device	Z No Qualifier

0 Medical and Surgical
8 Eye
M Reattachment: Putting back in or on all or a portion of a separated body part to its normal location or other suitable location

Body Part	Approach	Device	Qualifier
Character 4	Character 5	Character 6	Character 7
N Upper Eyelid, Right P Upper Eyelid, Left Q Lower Eyelid, Right R Lower Eyelid, Left	X External	Z No Device	Z No Qualifier

LC Limited Coverage   NC Noncovered   HAC HAC-associated Procedure   CC Combination Cluster - See Appendix G for code lists
DRG Non-OR-Affecting MS-DRG Assignment   New/Revised Text in Orange   ♂ Male   ♀ Female
270   2018 ICD-10-PCS

0 **Medical and Surgical**
8 **Eye**
N **Release:** Freeing a body part from an abnormal physical constraint by cutting or by the use of force

Body Part	Approach	Device	Qualifier
Character 4	Character 5	Character 6	Character 7
0 Eye, Right 1 Eye, Left 6 Sclera, Right 7 Sclera, Left 8 Cornea, Right 9 Cornea, Left S Conjunctiva, Right T Conjunctiva, Left	X External	Z No Device	Z No Qualifier
2 Anterior Chamber, Right 3 Anterior Chamber, Left 4 Vitreous, Right 5 Vitreous, Left C Iris, Right D Iris, Left E Retina, Right F Retina, Left G Retinal Vessel, Right H Retinal Vessel, Left J Lens, Right K Lens, Left	3 Percutaneous	Z No Device	Z No Qualifier
A Choroid, Right B Choroid, Left L Extraocular Muscle, Right M Extraocular Muscle, Left V Lacrimal Gland, Right W Lacrimal Gland, Left	0 Open 3 Percutaneous	Z No Device	Z No Qualifier
N Upper Eyelid, Right P Upper Eyelid, Left Q Lower Eyelid, Right R Lower Eyelid, Left	0 Open 3 Percutaneous X External	Z No Device	Z No Qualifier
X Lacrimal Duct, Right Y Lacrimal Duct, Left	0 Open 3 Percutaneous 7 Via Natural or Artificial Opening 8 Via Natural or Artificial Opening Endoscopic	Z No Device	Z No Qualifier

0 Medical and Surgical
8 Eye
P Removal: Taking out or off a device from a body part

Body Part	Approach	Device	Qualifier
Character 4	Character 5	Character 6	Character 7
0 Eye, Right 1 Eye, Left	0 Open 3 Percutaneous 7 Via Natural or Artificial Opening 8 Via Natural or Artificial Opening Endoscopic	0 Drainage Device 1 Radioactive Element 3 Infusion Device 7 Autologous Tissue Substitute C Extraluminal Device D Intraluminal Device J Synthetic Substitute K Nonautologous Tissue Substitute Y Other Device	Z No Qualifier
0 Eye, Right 1 Eye, Left	X External	0 Drainage Device 1 Radioactive Element 3 Infusion Device 7 Autologous Tissue Substitute C Extraluminal Device D Intraluminal Device J Synthetic Substitute K Nonautologous Tissue Substitute	Z No Qualifier
J Lens, Right K Lens, Left	3 Percutaneous	J Synthetic Substitute Y Other Device	Z No Qualifier
L Extraocular Muscle, Right M Extraocular Muscle, Left	0 Open 3 Percutaneous	0 Drainage Device 7 Autologous Tissue Substitute J Synthetic Substitute K Nonautologous Tissue Substitute Y Other Device	Z No Qualifier

LC Limited Coverage   NC Noncovered   HAC HAC-associated Procedure   CC Combination Cluster - See Appendix G for code lists
DRG Non-OR-Affecting MS-DRG Assignment   New/Revised Text in Orange   ♂ Male   ♀ Female

272

2018 ICD-10-PCS

0 **Medical and Surgical**

8 **Eye**

Q **Repair:** Restoring, to the extent possible, a body part to its normal anatomic structure and function

Body Part	Approach	Device	Qualifier
Character 4	Character 5	Character 6	Character 7
0 Eye, Right 1 Eye, Left 6 Sclera, Right 7 Sclera, Left 8 Cornea, Right Ⓝ𝐂 9 Cornea, Left Ⓝ𝐂 S Conjunctiva, Right T Conjunctiva, Left	X External	Z No Device	Z No Qualifier
2 Anterior Chamber, Right 3 Anterior Chamber, Left 4 Vitreous, Right 5 Vitreous, Left C Iris, Right D Iris, Left E Retina, Right F Retina, Left G Retinal Vessel, Right H Retinal Vessel, Left J Lens, Right K Lens, Left	3 Percutaneous	Z No Device	Z No Qualifier
A Choroid, Right B Choroid, Left L Extraocular Muscle, Right M Extraocular Muscle, Left V Lacrimal Gland, Right W Lacrimal Gland, Left	0 Open 3 Percutaneous	Z No Device	Z No Qualifier
N Upper Eyelid, Right P Upper Eyelid, Left Q Lower Eyelid, Right R Lower Eyelid, Left	0 Open 3 Percutaneous X External	Z No Device	Z No Qualifier
X Lacrimal Duct, Right Y Lacrimal Duct, Left	0 Open 3 Percutaneous 7 Via Natural or Artificial Opening 8 Via Natural or Artificial Opening Endoscopic	Z No Device	Z No Qualifier

Ⓝ𝐂 08Q8XZZ   08Q9XZZ

0 Medical and Surgical
8 Eye
R Replacement: Putting in or on biological or synthetic material that physically takes the place and/or function of all or a portion of a body part

Body Part		Approach		Device		Qualifier	
Character 4		**Character 5**		**Character 6**		**Character 7**	
0 Eye, Right 1 Eye, Left A Choroid, Right B Choroid, Left		0 Open 3 Percutaneous		7 Autologous Tissue Substitute J Synthetic Substitute K Nonautologous Tissue Substitute		Z No Qualifier	
4 Vitreous, Right 5 Vitreous, Left C Iris, Right D Iris, Left G Retinal Vessel, Right H Retinal Vessel, Left		3 Percutaneous		7 Autologous Tissue Substitute J Synthetic Substitute K Nonautologous Tissue Substitute		Z No Qualifier	
6 Sclera, Right 7 Sclera, Left S Conjunctiva, Right T Conjunctiva, Left		X External		7 Autologous Tissue Substitute J Synthetic Substitute K Nonautologous Tissue Substitute		Z No Qualifier	
8 Cornea, Right 9 Cornea, Left		3 Percutaneous X External		7 Autologous Tissue Substitute J Synthetic Substitute K Nonautologous Tissue Substitute		Z No Qualifier	
J Lens, Right K Lens, Left		3 Percutaneous		0 Synthetic Substitute, Intraocular Telescope 7 Autologous Tissue Substitute J Synthetic Substitute K Nonautologous Tissue Substitute		Z No Qualifier	
N Upper Eyelid, Right P Upper Eyelid, Left Q Lower Eyelid, Right R Lower Eyelid, Left		0 Open 3 Percutaneous X External		7 Autologous Tissue Substitute J Synthetic Substitute K Nonautologous Tissue Substitute		Z No Qualifier	
X Lacrimal Duct, Right Y Lacrimal Duct, Left		0 Open 3 Percutaneous 7 Via Natural or Artificial Opening 8 Via Natural or Artificial Opening Endoscopic		7 Autologous Tissue Substitute J Synthetic Substitute K Nonautologous Tissue Substitute		Z No Qualifier	

LC Limited Coverage   NC Noncovered   HAC HAC-associated Procedure   CC Combination Cluster - See Appendix G for code lists
DRG Non-OR-Affecting MS-DRG Assignment   New/Revised Text in Orange   ♂ Male   ♀ Female

274

2018 ICD-10-PCS

0 **Medical and Surgical**
8 **Eye**
S **Reposition:** Moving to its normal location, or other suitable location, all or a portion of a body part

Body Part	Approach	Device	Qualifier
Character 4	Character 5	Character 6	Character 7
C Iris, Right D Iris, Left G Retinal Vessel, Right H Retinal Vessel, Left J Lens, Right K Lens, Left	3 Percutaneous	Z No Device	Z No Qualifier
L Extraocular Muscle, Right M Extraocular Muscle, Left V Lacrimal Gland, Right W Lacrimal Gland, Left	0 Open 3 Percutaneous	Z No Device	Z No Qualifier
N Upper Eyelid, Right P Upper Eyelid, Left Q Lower Eyelid, Right R Lower Eyelid, Left	0 Open 3 Percutaneous X External	Z No Device	Z No Qualifier
X Lacrimal Duct, Right Y Lacrimal Duct, Left	0 Open 3 Percutaneous 7 Via Natural or Artificial Opening 8 Via Natural or Artificial Opening Endoscopic	Z No Device	Z No Qualifier

0 **Medical and Surgical**
8 **Eye**
T **Resection:** Cutting out or off, without replacement, all of a body part

Body Part	Approach	Device	Qualifier
Character 4	Character 5	Character 6	Character 7
0 Eye, Right 1 Eye, Left 8 Cornea, Right 9 Cornea, Left	X External	Z No Device	Z No Qualifier
4 Vitreous, Right 5 Vitreous, Left C Iris, Right D Iris, Left J Lens, Right K Lens, Left	3 Percutaneous	Z No Device	Z No Qualifier
L Extraocular Muscle, Right M Extraocular Muscle, Left V Lacrimal Gland, Right W Lacrimal Gland, Left	0 Open 3 Percutaneous	Z No Device	Z No Qualifier
N Upper Eyelid, Right P Upper Eyelid, Left Q Lower Eyelid, Right R Lower Eyelid, Left	0 Open X External	Z No Device	Z No Qualifier
X Lacrimal Duct, Right Y Lacrimal Duct, Left	0 Open 3 Percutaneous 7 Via Natural or Artificial Opening 8 Via Natural or Artificial Opening Endoscopic	Z No Device	Z No Qualifier

0 **Medical and Surgical**
8 **Eye**
U **Supplement:** Putting in or on biological or synthetic material that physically reinforces and/or augments the function of a portion of a body part

Body Part	Approach	Device	Qualifier
Character 4	**Character 5**	**Character 6**	**Character 7**
0 Eye, Right 1 Eye, Left C Iris, Right D Iris, Left E Retina, Right F Retina, Left G Retinal Vessel, Right H Retinal Vessel, Left L Extraocular Muscle, Right M Extraocular Muscle, Left	0 Open 3 Percutaneous	7 Autologous Tissue Substitute J Synthetic Substitute K Nonautologous Tissue Substitute	Z No Qualifier
8 Cornea, Right ᴺᶜ 9 Cornea, Left ᴺᶜ N Upper Eyelid, Right P Upper Eyelid, Left Q Lower Eyelid, Right R Lower Eyelid, Left	0 Open 3 Percutaneous X External	7 Autologous Tissue Substitute J Synthetic Substitute K Nonautologous Tissue Substitute	Z No Qualifier
X Lacrimal Duct, Right Y Lacrimal Duct, Left	0 Open 3 Percutaneous 7 Via Natural or Artificial Opening 8 Via Natural or Artificial Opening Endoscopic	7 Autologous Tissue Substitute J Synthetic Substitute K Nonautologous Tissue Substitute	Z No Qualifier

ᴺᶜ 08U80KZ   08U83KZ   08U8XKZ   08U90KZ   08U93KZ   08U9XKZ

0 **Medical and Surgical**
8 **Eye**
V **Restriction:** Partially closing an orifice or the lumen of a tubular body part

Body Part	Approach	Device	Qualifier
Character 4	**Character 5**	**Character 6**	**Character 7**
X Lacrimal Duct, Right Y Lacrimal Duct, Left	0 Open 3 Percutaneous	C Extraluminal Device D Intraluminal Device Z No Device	Z No Qualifier
X Lacrimal Duct, Right Y Lacrimal Duct, Left	7 Via Natural or Artificial Opening 8 Via Natural or Artificial Opening Endoscopic	D Intraluminal Device Z No Device	Z No Qualifier

ᴸᶜ Limited Coverage   ᴺᶜ Noncovered   ᴴᴬᶜ HAC-associated Procedure   ᶜᶜ Combination Cluster - See Appendix G for code lists
⊗ Non-OR-Affecting MS-DRG Assignment   New/Revised Text in **Orange**   ♂ Male   ♀ Female

276

2018 ICD-10-PCS

0 Medical and Surgical
8 Eye
W Revision: Correcting, to the extent possible, a portion of a malfunctioning device or the position of a displaced device

Body Part	Approach	Device	Qualifier
Character 4	Character 5	Character 6	Character 7
0 Eye, Right **1** Eye, Left	**0** Open **3** Percutaneous **7** Via Natural or Artificial Opening **8** Via Natural or Artificial Opening Endoscopic	**0** Drainage Device **3** Infusion Device **7** Autologous Tissue Substitute **C** Extraluminal Device **D** Intraluminal Device **J** Synthetic Substitute **K** Nonautologous Tissue Substitute **Y** Other Device	**Z** No Qualifier
0 Eye, Right **1** Eye, Left	**X** External	**0** Drainage Device **3** Infusion Device **7** Autologous Tissue Substitute **C** Extraluminal Device **D** Intraluminal Device **J** Synthetic Substitute **K** Nonautologous Tissue Substitute	**Z** No Qualifier
J Lens, Right **K** Lens, Left	**3** Percutaneous	**J** Synthetic Substitute **Y** Other Device	**Z** No Qualifier
J Lens, Right **K** Lens, Left	**X** External	**J** Synthetic Substitute	**Z** No Qualifier
L Extraocular Muscle, Right **M** Extraocular Muscle, Left	**0** Open **3** Percutaneous	**0** Drainage Device **7** Autologous Tissue Substitute **J** Synthetic Substitute **K** Nonautologous Tissue Substitute **Y** Other Device	**Z** No Qualifier

0 Medical and Surgical
8 Eye
X Transfer: Moving, without taking out, all or a portion of a body part to another location to take over the function of all or a portion of a body part

Body Part	Approach	Device	Qualifier
Character 4	Character 5	Character 6	Character 7
L Extraocular Muscle, Right **M** Extraocular Muscle, Left	**0** Open **3** Percutaneous	**Z** No Device	**Z** No Qualifier

NOTES

Ear, Nose, Sinus 090-09W

0 Medical and Surgical
9 Ear, Nose, Sinus
0 Alteration: Modifying the anatomic structure of a body part without affecting the function of the body part

Body Part	Approach	Device	Qualifier
Character 4	Character 5	Character 6	Character 7
0 External Ear, Right **1** External Ear, Left **2** External Ear, Bilateral **K** Nasal Mucosa and Soft Tissue	**0** Open **3** Percutaneous **4** Percutaneous Endoscopic **X** External	**7** Autologous Tissue Substitute **J** Synthetic Substitute **K** Nonautologous Tissue Substitute **Z** No Device	**Z** No Qualifier

0 Medical and Surgical
9 Ear, Nose, Sinus
1 Bypass: Altering the route of passage of the contents of a tubular body part

Body Part	Approach	Device	Qualifier
Character 4	Character 5	Character 6	Character 7
D Inner Ear, Right **E** Inner Ear, Left	**0** Open	**7** Autologous Tissue Substitute **J** Synthetic Substitute **K** Nonautologous Tissue Substitute **Z** No Device	**0** Endolymphatic

0 Medical and Surgical
9 Ear, Nose, Sinus
2 Change: Taking out or off a device from a body part and putting back an identical or similar device in or on the same body part without cutting or puncturing the skin or a mucous membrane

Body Part	Approach	Device	Qualifier
Character 4	Character 5	Character 6	Character 7
H Ear, Right **J** Ear, Left **K** Nasal Mucosa and Soft Tissue **Y** Sinus	**X** External	**0** Drainage Device **Y** Other Device	**Z** No Qualifier

0 Medical and Surgical
9 Ear, Nose, Sinus
5 Destruction: Physical eradication of all or a portion of a body part by the direct use of energy, force, or a destructive agent

Body Part	Approach	Device	Qualifier
Character 4	Character 5	Character 6	Character 7
0 External Ear, Right **1** External Ear, Left	**0** Open **3** Percutaneous **4** Percutaneous Endoscopic **X** External	**Z** No Device	**Z** No Qualifier
3 External Auditory Canal, Right **4** External Auditory Canal, Left	**0** Open **3** Percutaneous **4** Percutaneous Endoscopic **7** Via Natural or Artificial Opening **8** Via Natural or Artificial Opening Endoscopic **X** External	**Z** No Device	**Z** No Qualifier
5 Middle Ear, Right **6** Middle Ear, Left **9** Auditory Ossicle, Right **A** Auditory Ossicle, Left **D** Inner Ear, Right **E** Inner Ear, Left	**0** Open **8** Via Natural or Artificial Opening Endoscopic	**Z** No Device	**Z** No Qualifier
7 Tympanic Membrane, Right **8** Tympanic Membrane, Left **F** Eustachian Tube, Right **G** Eustachian Tube, Left **L** Nasal Turbinate **N** Nasopharynx	**0** Open **3** Percutaneous **4** Percutaneous Endoscopic **7** Via Natural or Artificial Opening **8** Via Natural or Artificial Opening Endoscopic	**Z** No Device	**Z** No Qualifier
B Mastoid Sinus, Right **C** Mastoid Sinus, Left **M** Nasal Septum **P** Accessory Sinus **Q** Maxillary Sinus, Right **R** Maxillary Sinus, Left **S** Frontal Sinus, Right **T** Frontal Sinus, Left **U** Ethmoid Sinus, Right **V** Ethmoid Sinus, Left **W** Sphenoid Sinus, Right **X** Sphenoid Sinus, Left	**0** Open **3** Percutaneous **4** Percutaneous Endoscopic **8** Via Natural or Artificial Opening Endoscopic	**Z** No Device	**Z** No Qualifier
K Nasal Mucosa and Soft Tissue	**0** Open **3** Percutaneous **4** Percutaneous Endoscopic **8** Via Natural or Artificial Opening Endoscopic **X** External	**Z** No Device	**Z** No Qualifier

0 Medical and Surgical
9 Ear, Nose, Sinus
7 Dilation: Expanding an orifice or the lumen of a tubular body part

Body Part	Approach	Device	Qualifier
Character 4	Character 5	Character 6	Character 7
F Eustachian Tube, Right **G** Eustachian Tube, Left	**0** Open **7** Via Natural or Artificial Opening **8** Via Natural or Artificial Opening Endoscopic	**D** Intraluminal Device **Z** No Device	**Z** No Qualifier
F Eustachian Tube, Right **G** Eustachian Tube, Left	**3** Percutaneous **4** Percutaneous Endoscopic	**Z** No Device	**Z** No Qualifier

0 Medical and Surgical
9 Ear, Nose, Sinus
8 Division: Cutting into a body part, without draining fluids and/or gases from the body part, in order to separate or transect a body part

Body Part	Approach	Device	Qualifier
Character 4	Character 5	Character 6	Character 7
L Nasal Turbinate	**0** Open **3** Percutaneous **4** Percutaneous Endoscopic **7** Via Natural or Artificial Opening **8** Via Natural or Artificial Opening Endoscopic	**Z** No Device	**Z** No Qualifier

0 Medical and Surgical
9 Ear, Nose, Sinus
9 Drainage: Taking or letting out fluids and/or gases from a body part

Body Part	Approach	Device	Qualifier
Character 4	Character 5	Character 6	Character 7
0 External Ear, Right **1** External Ear, Left	**0** Open **3** Percutaneous **4** Percutaneous Endoscopic **X** External	**0** Drainage Device	**Z** No Qualifier
0 External Ear, Right **1** External Ear, Left	**0** Open **3** Percutaneous **4** Percutaneous Endoscopic **X** External	**Z** No Device	**X** Diagnostic **Z** No Qualifier
3 External Auditory Canal, Right **4** External Auditory Canal, Left **K** Nasal Mucosa and Soft Tissue	**0** Open **3** Percutaneous **4** Percutaneous Endoscopic **7** Via Natural or Artificial Opening **8** Via Natural or Artificial Opening Endoscopic **X** External	**0** Drainage Device	**Z** No Qualifier
3 External Auditory Canal, Right **4** External Auditory Canal, Left **K** Nasal Mucosa and Soft Tissue	**0** Open **3** Percutaneous **4** Percutaneous Endoscopic **7** Via Natural or Artificial Opening **8** Via Natural or Artificial Opening Endoscopic **X** External	**Z** No Device	**X** Diagnostic **Z** No Qualifier
5 Middle Ear, Right **6** Middle Ear, Left **9** Auditory Ossicle, Right **A** Auditory Ossicle, Left **D** Inner Ear, Right **E** Inner Ear, Left	**0** Open **7** Via Natural or Artificial Opening **8** Via Natural or Artificial Opening Endoscopic	**0** Drainage Device	**Z** No Qualifier
5 Middle Ear, Right **6** Middle Ear, Left **9** Auditory Ossicle, Right **A** Auditory Ossicle, Left **D** Inner Ear, Right **E** Inner Ear, Left	**0** Open **7** Via Natural or Artificial Opening **8** Via Natural or Artificial Opening Endoscopic	**Z** No Device	**X** Diagnostic **Z** No Qualifier

099 continued on next page

0 **Medical and Surgical**   099 continued from previous page
9 **Ear, Nose, Sinus**
9 **Drainage:** Taking or letting out fluids and/or gases from a body part

Body Part	Approach	Device	Qualifier
Character 4	Character 5	Character 6	Character 7
7 Tympanic Membrane, Right **8** Tympanic Membrane, Left **B** Mastoid Sinus, Right **C** Mastoid Sinus, Left **F** Eustachian Tube, Right **G** Eustachian Tube, Left **L** Nasal Turbinate **M** Nasal Septum **N** Nasopharynx **P** Accessory Sinus **Q** Maxillary Sinus, Right **R** Maxillary Sinus, Left **S** Frontal Sinus, Right **T** Frontal Sinus, Left **U** Ethmoid Sinus, Right **V** Ethmoid Sinus, Left **W** Sphenoid Sinus, Right **X** Sphenoid Sinus, Left	**0** Open **3** Percutaneous **4** Percutaneous Endoscopic **7** Via Natural or Artificial Opening **8** Via Natural or Artificial Opening Endoscopic	**0** Drainage Device	**Z** No Qualifier
7 Tympanic Membrane, Right **8** Tympanic Membrane, Left **B** Mastoid Sinus, Right **C** Mastoid Sinus, Left **F** Eustachian Tube, Right **G** Eustachian Tube, Left **L** Nasal Turbinate **M** Nasal Septum **N** Nasopharynx **P** Accessory Sinus **Q** Maxillary Sinus, Right **R** Maxillary Sinus, Left **S** Frontal Sinus, Right **T** Frontal Sinus, Left **U** Ethmoid Sinus, Right **V** Ethmoid Sinus, Left **W** Sphenoid Sinus, Right **X** Sphenoid Sinus, Left	**0** Open **3** Percutaneous **4** Percutaneous Endoscopic **7** Via Natural or Artificial Opening **8** Via Natural or Artificial Opening Endoscopic	**Z** No Device	**X** Diagnostic **Z** No Qualifier

LC Limited Coverage   NC Noncovered   HAC HAC-associated Procedure   CC Combination Cluster - See Appendix G for code lists
DRG Non-OR-Affecting MS-DRG Assignment   New/Revised Text in **Orange**   ♂ Male   ♀ Female

282

2018 ICD-10-PCS

0 **Medical and Surgical**
9 **Ear, Nose, Sinus**
B **Excision:** Cutting out or off, without replacement, a portion of a body part

Body Part	Approach	Device	Qualifier
Character 4	Character 5	Character 6	Character 7
0 External Ear, Right 1 External Ear, Left	0 Open 3 Percutaneous 4 Percutaneous Endoscopic X External	Z No Device	X Diagnostic Z No Qualifier
3 External Auditory Canal, Right 4 External Auditory Canal, Left	0 Open 3 Percutaneous 4 Percutaneous Endoscopic 7 Via Natural or Artificial Opening 8 Via Natural or Artificial Opening Endoscopic X External	Z No Device	X Diagnostic Z No Qualifier
5 Middle Ear, Right 6 Middle Ear, Left 9 Auditory Ossicle, Right A Auditory Ossicle, Left D Inner Ear, Right E Inner Ear, Left	0 Open 8 Via Natural or Artificial Opening Endoscopic	Z No Device	X Diagnostic Z No Qualifier
7 Tympanic Membrane, Right 8 Tympanic Membrane, Left F Eustachian Tube, Right G Eustachian Tube, Left L Nasal Turbinate N Nasopharynx	0 Open 3 Percutaneous 4 Percutaneous Endoscopic 7 Via Natural or Artificial Opening 8 Via Natural or Artificial Opening Endoscopic	Z No Device	X Diagnostic Z No Qualifier
B Mastoid Sinus, Right C Mastoid Sinus, Left M Nasal Septum P Accessory Sinus Q Maxillary Sinus, Right R Maxillary Sinus, Left S Frontal Sinus, Right T Frontal Sinus, Left U Ethmoid Sinus, Right V Ethmoid Sinus, Left W Sphenoid Sinus, Right X Sphenoid Sinus, Left	0 Open 3 Percutaneous 4 Percutaneous Endoscopic 8 Via Natural or Artificial Opening Endoscopic	Z No Device	X Diagnostic Z No Qualifier
K Nasal Mucosa and Soft Tissue	0 Open 3 Percutaneous 4 Percutaneous Endoscopic 8 Via Natural or Artificial Opening Endoscopic X External	Z No Device	X Diagnostic Z No Qualifier

LC Limited Coverage   NC Noncovered   HAC HAC-associated Procedure   CC Combination Cluster - See Appendix G for code lists
DRG Non-OR-Affecting MS-DRG Assignment   New/Revised Text in **Orange**   ♂ Male   ♀ Female

0 **Medical and Surgical**
9 **Ear, Nose, Sinus**
C **Extirpation:** Taking or cutting out solid matter from a body part

Body Part	Approach	Device	Qualifier
Character 4	Character 5	Character 6	Character 7
0 External Ear, Right 1 External Ear, Left	0 Open 3 Percutaneous 4 Percutaneous Endoscopic X External	Z No Device	Z No Qualifier
3 External Auditory Canal, Right 4 External Auditory Canal, Left	0 Open 3 Percutaneous 4 Percutaneous Endoscopic 7 Via Natural or Artificial Opening 8 Via Natural or Artificial Opening Endoscopic X External	Z No Device	Z No Qualifier
5 Middle Ear, Right 6 Middle Ear, Left 9 Auditory Ossicle, Right A Auditory Ossicle, Left D Inner Ear, Right E Inner Ear, Left	0 Open 8 Via Natural or Artificial Opening Endoscopic	Z No Device	Z No Qualifier
7 Tympanic Membrane, Right 8 Tympanic Membrane, Left F Eustachian Tube, Right G Eustachian Tube, Left L Nasal Turbinate N Nasopharynx	0 Open 3 Percutaneous 4 Percutaneous Endoscopic 7 Via Natural or Artificial Opening 8 Via Natural or Artificial Opening Endoscopic	Z No Device	Z No Qualifier
B Mastoid Sinus, Right C Mastoid Sinus, Left M Nasal Septum P Accessory Sinus Q Maxillary Sinus, Right R Maxillary Sinus, Left S Frontal Sinus, Right T Frontal Sinus, Left U Ethmoid Sinus, Right V Ethmoid Sinus, Left W Sphenoid Sinus, Right X Sphenoid Sinus, Left	0 Open 3 Percutaneous 4 Percutaneous Endoscopic 8 Via Natural or Artificial Opening Endoscopic	Z No Device	Z No Qualifier
K Nasal Mucosa and Soft Tissue	0 Open 3 Percutaneous 4 Percutaneous Endoscopic 8 Via Natural or Artificial Opening Endoscopic X External	Z No Device	Z No Qualifier

LC Limited Coverage   **NC** Noncovered   **HAC** HAC-associated Procedure   **CC** Combination Cluster - See Appendix G for code lists

DRG Non-OR-Affecting MS-DRG Assignment   New/Revised Text in **Orange**   ♂ Male   ♀ Female

284

2018 ICD-10-PCS

0 **Medical and Surgical**
9 **Ear, Nose, Sinus**
D **Extraction:** Pulling or stripping out or off all or a portion of a body part by the use of force

Body Part	Approach	Device	Qualifier
Character 4	**Character 5**	**Character 6**	**Character 7**
7 Tympanic Membrane, Right **8** Tympanic Membrane, Left **L** Nasal Turbinate	**0** Open **3** Percutaneous **4** Percutaneous Endoscopic **7** Via Natural or Artificial Opening **8** Via Natural or Artificial Opening Endoscopic	**Z** No Device	**Z** No Qualifier
9 Auditory Ossicle, Right **A** Auditory Ossicle, Left	**0** Open	**Z** No Device	**Z** No Qualifier
B Mastoid Sinus, Right **C** Mastoid Sinus, Left **M** Nasal Septum **P** Accessory Sinus **Q** Maxillary Sinus, Right **R** Maxillary Sinus, Left **S** Frontal Sinus, Right **T** Frontal Sinus, Left **U** Ethmoid Sinus, Right **V** Ethmoid Sinus, Left **W** Sphenoid Sinus, Right **X** Sphenoid Sinus, Left	**0** Open **3** Percutaneous **4** Percutaneous Endoscopic	**Z** No Device	**Z** No Qualifier

0 **Medical and Surgical**
9 **Ear, Nose, Sinus**
H **Insertion:** Putting in a nonbiological appliance that monitors, assists, performs, or prevents a physiological function but does not physically take the place of a body part

Body Part	Approach	Device	Qualifier
Character 4	**Character 5**	**Character 6**	**Character 7**

D Inner Ear, Right
E Inner Ear, Left
	0 Open
	3 Percutaneous
	4 Percutaneous Endoscopic
		4 Hearing Device, Bone Conduction
		5 Hearing Device, Single Channel
		   Cochlear Prosthesis
		6 Hearing Device, Multiple
		   Channel Cochlear Prosthesis
		S Hearing Device
			Z No Qualifier

H Ear, Right **J** Ear, Left **K** Nasal Mucosa and Soft Tissue **Y** Sinus	**0** Open **3** Percutaneous **4** Percutaneous Endoscopic **7** Via Natural or Artificial Opening **8** Via Natural or Artificial Opening Endoscopic	**Y** Other Device	**Z** No Qualifier
N Nasopharynx	**7** Via Natural or Artificial Opening **8** Via Natural or Artificial Opening Endoscopic	**B** Intraluminal Device, Airway	**Z** No Qualifier

0 **Medical and Surgical**
9 **Ear, Nose, Sinus**
J **Inspection:** Visually and/or manually exploring a body part

Body Part	Approach	Device	Qualifier
Character 4	**Character 5**	**Character 6**	**Character 7**
7 Tympanic Membrane, Right **8** Tympanic Membrane, Left **H** Ear, Right **J** Ear, Left	**0** Open **3** Percutaneous **4** Percutaneous Endoscopic **7** Via Natural or Artificial Opening **8** Via Natural or Artificial Opening Endoscopic **X** External	**Z** No Device	**Z** No Qualifier
D Inner Ear, Right **E** Inner Ear, Left **K** Nasal Mucosa and Soft tissue **Y** Sinus	**0** Open **3** Percutaneous **4** Percutaneous Endoscopic **8** Via Natural or Artificial Opening Endoscopic **X** External	**Z** No Device	**Z** No Qualifier

0 Medical and Surgical
9 Ear, Nose, Sinus
M Reattachment: Putting back in or on all or a portion of a separated body part to its normal location or other suitable location

Body Part	Approach	Device	Qualifier
Character 4	Character 5	Character 6	Character 7
0 External Ear, Right **1** External Ear, Left **K** Nasal Mucosa and Soft Tissue	**X** External	**Z** No Device	**Z** No Qualifier

0 Medical and Surgical
9 Ear, Nose, Sinus
N Release: Freeing a body part from an abnormal physical constraint by cutting or by the use of force

Body Part	Approach	Device	Qualifier
Character 4	Character 5	Character 6	Character 7
0 External Ear, Right **1** External Ear, Left	**0** Open **3** Percutaneous **4** Percutaneous Endoscopic **X** External	**Z** No Device	**Z** No Qualifier
3 External Auditory Canal, Right **4** External Auditory Canal, Left	**0** Open **3** Percutaneous **4** Percutaneous Endoscopic **7** Via Natural or Artificial Opening **8** Via Natural or Artificial Opening Endoscopic **X** External	**Z** No Device	**Z** No Qualifier
5 Middle Ear, Right **6** Middle Ear, Left **9** Auditory Ossicle, Right **A** Auditory Ossicle, Left **D** Inner Ear, Right **E** Inner Ear, Left	**0** Open **8** Via Natural or Artificial Opening Endoscopic	**Z** No Device	**Z** No Qualifier
7 Tympanic Membrane, Right **8** Tympanic Membrane, Left **F** Eustachian Tube, Right **G** Eustachian Tube, Left **L** Nasal Turbinate **N** Nasopharynx	**0** Open **3** Percutaneous **4** Percutaneous Endoscopic **7** Via Natural or Artificial Opening **8** Via Natural or Artificial Opening Endoscopic	**Z** No Device	**Z** No Qualifier
B Mastoid Sinus, Right **C** Mastoid Sinus, Left **M** Nasal Septum **P** Accessory Sinus **Q** Maxillary Sinus, Right **R** Maxillary Sinus, Left **S** Frontal Sinus, Right **T** Frontal Sinus, Left **U** Ethmoid Sinus, Right **V** Ethmoid Sinus, Left **W** Sphenoid Sinus, Right **X** Sphenoid Sinus, Left	**0** Open **3** Percutaneous **4** Percutaneous Endoscopic **8** Via Natural or Artificial Opening Endoscopic	**Z** No Device	**Z** No Qualifier
K Nasal Mucosa and Soft Tissue	**0** Open **3** Percutaneous **4** Percutaneous Endoscopic **8** Via Natural or Artificial Opening Endoscopic **X** External	**Z** No Device	**Z** No Qualifier

0 Medical and Surgical
9 Ear, Nose, Sinus
P Removal: Taking out or off a device from a body part

Body Part	Approach	Device	Qualifier
Character 4	Character 5	Character 6	Character 7
7 Tympanic Membrane, Right 8 Tympanic Membrane, Left	0 Open 7 Via Natural or Artificial Opening 8 Via Natural or Artificial Opening Endoscopic X External	0 Drainage Device	Z No Qualifier
D Inner Ear, Right E Inner Ear, Left	0 Open 7 Via Natural or Artificial Opening 8 Via Natural or Artificial Opening Endoscopic	S Hearing Device	Z No Qualifier
H Ear, Right J Ear, Left K Nasal Mucosa and Soft Tissue	0 Open 3 Percutaneous 4 Percutaneous Endoscopic 7 Via Natural or Artificial Opening 8 Via Natural or Artificial Opening Endoscopic	0 Drainage Device 7 Autologous Tissue Substitute D Intraluminal Device J Synthetic Substitute K Nonautologous Tissue Substitute Y Other Device	Z No Qualifier
H Ear, Right J Ear, Left K Nasal Mucosa and Soft Tissue	X External	0 Drainage Device 7 Autologous Tissue Substitute D Intraluminal Device J Synthetic Substitute K Nonautologous Tissue Substitute	Z No Qualifier
Y Sinus	0 Open 3 Percutaneous 4 Percutaneous Endoscopic	0 Drainage Device Y Other Device	Z No Qualifier
Y Sinus	7 Via Natural or Artificial Opening 8 Via Natural or Artificial Opening Endoscopic	Y Other Device	Z No Qualifier
Y Sinus	X External	0 Drainage Device	Z No Qualifier

0 Medical and Surgical
9 Ear, Nose, Sinus
Q Repair: Restoring, to the extent possible, a body part to its normal anatomic structure and function

Body Part	Approach	Device	Qualifier
Character 4	Character 5	Character 6	Character 7
0 External Ear, Right **1** External Ear, Left **2** External Ear, Bilateral	**0** Open **3** Percutaneous **4** Percutaneous Endoscopic **X** External	**Z** No Device	**Z** No Qualifier
3 External Auditory Canal, Right **4** External Auditory Canal, Left **F** Eustachian Tube, Right **G** Eustachian Tube, Left	**0** Open **3** Percutaneous **4** Percutaneous Endoscopic **7** Via Natural or Artificial Opening **8** Via Natural or Artificial Opening Endoscopic **X** External	**Z** No Device	**Z** No Qualifier
5 Middle Ear, Right **6** Middle Ear, Left **9** Auditory Ossicle, Right **A** Auditory Ossicle, Left **D** Inner Ear, Right **E** Inner Ear, Left	**0** Open **8** Via Natural or Artificial Opening Endoscopic	**Z** No Device	**Z** No Qualifier
7 Tympanic Membrane, Right **8** Tympanic Membrane, Left **L** Nasal Turbinate **N** Nasopharynx	**0** Open **3** Percutaneous **4** Percutaneous Endoscopic **7** Via Natural or Artificial Opening **8** Via Natural or Artificial Opening Endoscopic	**Z** No Device	**Z** No Qualifier
B Mastoid Sinus, Right **C** Mastoid Sinus, Left **M** Nasal Septum **P** Accessory Sinus **Q** Maxillary Sinus, Right **R** Maxillary Sinus, Left **S** Frontal Sinus, Right **T** Frontal Sinus, Left **U** Ethmoid Sinus, Right **V** Ethmoid Sinus, Left **W** Sphenoid Sinus, Right **X** Sphenoid Sinus, Left	**0** Open **3** Percutaneous **4** Percutaneous Endoscopic **8** Via Natural or Artificial Opening Endoscopic	**Z** No Device	**Z** No Qualifier
K Nasal Mucosa and Soft Tissue	**0** Open **3** Percutaneous **4** Percutaneous Endoscopic **8** Via Natural or Artificial Opening Endoscopic **X** External	**Z** No Device	**Z** No Qualifier

LC Limited Coverage   NC Noncovered   HAC HAC-associated Procedure   CC Combination Cluster - See Appendix G for code lists
DRG Non-OR-Affecting MS-DRG Assignment   New/Revised Text in **Orange**   ♂ Male   ♀ Female

288

2018 ICD-10-PCS

0 Medical and Surgical
9 Ear, Nose, Sinus
R Replacement: Putting in or on biological or synthetic material that physically takes the place and/or function of all or a portion of a body part

Body Part	Approach	Device	Qualifier
Character 4	Character 5	Character 6	Character 7
0 External Ear, Right 1 External Ear, Left 2 External Ear, Bilateral K Nasal Mucosa and Soft Tissue	0 Open X External	7 Autologous Tissue Substitute J Synthetic Substitute K Nonautologous Tissue Substitute	Z No Qualifier
5 Middle Ear, Right 6 Middle Ear, Left 9 Auditory Ossicle, Right A Auditory Ossicle, Left D Inner Ear, Right E Inner Ear, Left	0 Open	7 Autologous Tissue Substitute J Synthetic Substitute K Nonautologous Tissue Substitute	Z No Qualifier
7 Tympanic Membrane, Right 8 Tympanic Membrane, Left N Nasopharynx	0 Open 7 Via Natural or Artificial Opening 8 Via Natural or Artificial Opening Endoscopic	7 Autologous Tissue Substitute J Synthetic Substitute K Nonautologous Tissue Substitute	Z No Qualifier
L Nasal Turbinate	0 Open 3 Percutaneous 4 Percutaneous Endoscopic 7 Via Natural or Artificial Opening 8 Via Natural or Artificial Opening Endoscopic	7 Autologous Tissue Substitute J Synthetic Substitute K Nonautologous Tissue Substitute	Z No Qualifier
M Nasal Septum	0 Open 3 Percutaneous 4 Percutaneous Endoscopic	7 Autologous Tissue Substitute J Synthetic Substitute K Nonautologous Tissue Substitute	Z No Qualifier

0 Medical and Surgical
9 Ear, Nose, Sinus
S Reposition: Moving to its normal location, or other suitable location, all or a portion of a body part

Body Part	Approach	Device	Qualifier
Character 4	Character 5	Character 6	Character 7
0 External Ear, Right 1 External Ear, Left 2 External Ear, Bilateral K Nasal Mucosa and Soft Tissue	0 Open 4 Percutaneous Endoscopic X External	Z No Device	Z No Qualifier
7 Tympanic Membrane, Right 8 Tympanic Membrane, Left F Eustachian Tube, Right G Eustachian Tube, Left L Nasal Turbinate	0 Open 4 Percutaneous Endoscopic 7 Via Natural or Artificial Opening 8 Via Natural or Artificial Opening Endoscopic	Z No Device	Z No Qualifier
9 Auditory Ossicle, Right A Auditory Ossicle, Left M Nasal Septum	0 Open 4 Percutaneous Endoscopic	Z No Device	Z No Qualifier

0 **Medical and Surgical**
9 **Ear, Nose, Sinus**
T **Resection:** Cutting out or off, without replacement, all of a body part

Body Part	Approach	Device	Qualifier
Character 4	**Character 5**	**Character 6**	**Character 7**
0 External Ear, Right 1 External Ear, Left	0 Open 4 Percutaneous Endoscopic X External	Z No Device	Z No Qualifier
5 Middle Ear, Right 6 Middle Ear, Left 9 Auditory Ossicle, Right A Auditory Ossicle, Left D Inner Ear, Right E Inner Ear, Left	0 Open 8 Via Natural or Artificial Opening Endoscopic	Z No Device	Z No Qualifier
7 Tympanic Membrane, Right 8 Tympanic Membrane, Left F Eustachian Tube, Right G Eustachian Tube, Left L Nasal Turbinate N Nasopharynx	0 Open 4 Percutaneous Endoscopic 7 Via Natural or Artificial Opening 8 Via Natural or Artificial Opening Endoscopic	Z No Device	Z No Qualifier
B Mastoid Sinus, Right C Mastoid Sinus, Left M Nasal Septum P Accessory Sinus Q Maxillary Sinus, Right R Maxillary Sinus, Left S Frontal Sinus, Right T Frontal Sinus, Left U Ethmoid Sinus, Right V Ethmoid Sinus, Left W Sphenoid Sinus, Right X Sphenoid Sinus, Left	0 Open 4 Percutaneous Endoscopic 8 Via Natural or Artificial Opening Endoscopic	Z No Device	Z No Qualifier
K Nasal Mucosa and Soft Tissue	0 Open 4 Percutaneous Endoscopic 8 Via Natural or Artificial Opening Endoscopic X External	Z No Device	Z No Qualifier

LC Limited Coverage   NC Noncovered   HAC HAC-associated Procedure   CC Combination Cluster - See Appendix G for code lists
DRG Non-OR-Affecting MS-DRG Assignment   New/Revised Text in **Orange**   ♂ Male   ♀ Female

290

2018 ICD-10-PCS

0   **Medical and Surgical**
9   **Ear, Nose, Sinus**
U   **Supplement:** Putting in or on biological or synthetic material that physically reinforces and/or augments the function of a portion of a body part

Body Part	Approach	Device	Qualifier
Character 4	**Character 5**	**Character 6**	**Character 7**
0 External Ear, Right 1 External Ear, Left 2 External Ear, Bilateral	0 Open X External	7 Autologous Tissue Substitute J Synthetic Substitute K Nonautologous Tissue Substitute	Z No Qualifier
5 Middle Ear, Right 6 Middle Ear, Left 9 Auditory Ossicle, Right A Auditory Ossicle, Left D Inner Ear, Right E Inner Ear, Left	0 Open 8 Via Natural or Artificial Opening Endoscopic	7 Autologous Tissue Substitute J Synthetic Substitute K Nonautologous Tissue Substitute	Z No Qualifier
7 Tympanic Membrane, Right 8 Tympanic Membrane, Left N Nasopharynx	0 Open 7 Via Natural or Artificial Opening 8 Via Natural or Artificial Opening Endoscopic	7 Autologous Tissue Substitute J Synthetic Substitute K Nonautologous Tissue Substitute	Z No Qualifier
K Nasal Mucosa and Soft Tissue	0 Open 8 Via Natural or Artificial Opening Endoscopic X External	7 Autologous Tissue Substitute J Synthetic Substitute K Nonautologous Tissue Substitute	Z No Qualifier
L Nasal Turbinate	0 Open 3 Percutaneous 4 Percutaneous Endoscopic 7 Via Natural or Artificial Opening 8 Via Natural or Artificial Opening Endoscopic	7 Autologous Tissue Substitute J Synthetic Substitute K Nonautologous Tissue Substitute	Z No Qualifier
M Nasal Septum	0 Open 3 Percutaneous 4 Percutaneous Endoscopic 8 Via Natural or Artificial Opening Endoscopic	7 Autologous Tissue Substitute J Synthetic Substitute K Nonautologous Tissue Substitute	Z No Qualifier

LC Limited Coverage   NC Noncovered   HAC HAC-associated Procedure   CC Combination Cluster - See Appendix G for code lists
DRG Non-OR-Affecting MS-DRG Assignment   New/Revised Text in **Orange**   ♂ Male   ♀ Female

2018 ICD-10-PCS

291

EAR, NOSE, SINUS 090-09W

0 Medical and Surgical
9 Ear, Nose, Sinus
W Revision: Correcting, to the extent possible, a portion of a malfunctioning device or the position of a displaced device

Body Part		Approach		Device		Qualifier	
Character 4		**Character 5**		**Character 6**		**Character 7**	
7 Tympanic Membrane, Right 8 Tympanic Membrane, Left 9 Auditory Ossicle, Right A Auditory Ossicle, Left		0 Open 7 Via Natural or Artificial Opening 8 Via Natural or Artificial Opening Endoscopic		7 Autologous Tissue Substitute J Synthetic Substitute K Nonautologous Tissue Substitute		Z No Qualifier	
D Inner Ear, Right E Inner Ear, Left		0 Open 7 Via Natural or Artificial Opening 8 Via Natural or Artificial Opening Endoscopic		S Hearing Device		Z No Qualifier	
H Ear, Right J Ear, Left K Nasal Mucosa and Soft Tissue		0 Open 3 Percutaneous 4 Percutaneous Endoscopic 7 Via Natural or Artificial Opening 8 Via Natural or Artificial Opening Endoscopic		0 Drainage Device 7 Autologous Tissue Substitute D Intraluminal Device J Synthetic Substitute K Nonautologous Tissue Substitute Y Other Device		Z No Qualifier	
H Ear, Right J Ear, Left K Nasal Mucosa and Soft Tissue		X External		0 Drainage Device 7 Autologous Tissue Substitute D Intraluminal Device J Synthetic Substitute K Nonautologous Tissue Substitute		Z No Qualifier	
Y Sinus		0 Open 3 Percutaneous 4 Percutaneous Endoscopic		0 Drainage Device Y Other Device		Z No Qualifier	
Y Sinus		7 Via Natural or Artificial Opening 8 Via Natural or Artificial Opening Endoscopic		Y Other Device		Z No Qualifier	
Y Sinus		X External		0 Drainage Device		Z No Qualifier	

LC Limited Coverage   NC Noncovered   HAC HAC-associated Procedure   CC Combination Cluster - See Appendix G for code lists
DRG Non-OR-Affecting MS-DRG Assignment   New/Revised Text in **Orange**   ♂ Male   ♀ Female

292

2018 ICD-10-PCS

NOTES

NOTES

Respiratory System 0B1-0BY

0 Medical and Surgical
B Respiratory System
1 Bypass: Altering the route of passage of the contents of a tubular body part

Body Part	Approach	Device	Qualifier
Character 4	**Character 5**	**Character 6**	**Character 7**
1 Trachea	**0** Open	**D** Intraluminal Device	**6** Esophagus
1 Trachea	**0** Open	**F** Tracheostomy Device **Z** No Device	**4** Cutaneous
1 Trachea	**3** Percutaneous **4** Percutaneous Endoscopic	**F** Tracheostomy Device **Z** No Device	**4** Cutaneous

0 Medical and Surgical
B Respiratory System
2 Change: Taking out or off a device from a body part and putting back an identical or similar device in or on the same body part without cutting or puncturing the skin or a mucous membrane

Body Part	Approach	Device	Qualifier
Character 4	**Character 5**	**Character 6**	**Character 7**
0 Tracheobronchial Tree **K** Lung, Right **L** Lung, Left **Q** Pleura **T** Diaphragm	**X** External	**0** Drainage Device **Y** Other Device	**Z** No Qualifier
1 Trachea	**X** External	**0** Drainage Device **E** Intraluminal Device, Endotracheal Airway **F** Tracheostomy Device **Y** Other Device	**Z** No Qualifier

0 Medical and Surgical
B Respiratory System
5 Destruction: Physical eradication of all or a portion of a body part by the direct use of energy, force, or a destructive agent

Body Part	Approach	Device	Qualifier
Character 4	**Character 5**	**Character 6**	**Character 7**
1 Trachea **2** Carina **3** Main Bronchus, Right **4** Upper Lobe Bronchus, Right **5** Middle Lobe Bronchus, Right **6** Lower Lobe Bronchus, Right **7** Main Bronchus, Left **8** Upper Lobe Bronchus, Left **9** Lingula Bronchus **B** Lower Lobe Bronchus, Left **C** Upper Lung Lobe, Right **D** Middle Lung Lobe, Right **F** Lower Lung Lobe, Right **G** Upper Lung Lobe, Left **H** Lung Lingula **J** Lower Lung Lobe, Left **K** Lung, Right **L** Lung, Left **M** Lungs, Bilateral	**0** Open **3** Percutaneous **4** Percutaneous Endoscopic **7** Via Natural or Artificial Opening **8** Via Natural or Artificial Opening Endoscopic	**Z** No Device	**Z** No Qualifier
N Pleura, Right **P** Pleura, Left **T** Diaphragm	**0** Open **3** Percutaneous **4** Percutaneous Endoscopic	**Z** No Device	**Z** No Qualifier

---

0 **Medical and Surgical**
B **Respiratory System**
7 **Dilation:** Expanding an orifice or the lumen of a tubular body part

Body Part	Approach	Device	Qualifier
Character 4	Character 5	Character 6	Character 7
1 Trachea 2 Carina 3 Main Bronchus, Right 4 Upper Lobe Bronchus, Right 5 Middle Lobe Bronchus, Right 6 Lower Lobe Bronchus, Right 7 Main Bronchus, Left 8 Upper Lobe Bronchus, Left 9 Lingula Bronchus B Lower Lobe Bronchus, Left	0 Open 3 Percutaneous 4 Percutaneous Endoscopic 7 Via Natural or Artificial Opening 8 Via Natural or Artificial Opening Endoscopic	D Intraluminal Device Z No Device	Z No Qualifier

0 **Medical and Surgical**
B **Respiratory System**
9 **Drainage:** Taking or letting out fluids and/or gases from a body part

Body Part	Approach	Device	Qualifier
Character 4	Character 5	Character 6	Character 7
1 Trachea 2 Carina 3 Main Bronchus, Right 4 Upper Lobe Bronchus, Right 5 Middle Lobe Bronchus, Right 6 Lower Lobe Bronchus, Right 7 Main Bronchus, Left 8 Upper Lobe Bronchus, Left 9 Lingula Bronchus B Lower Lobe Bronchus, Left C Upper Lung Lobe, Right D Middle Lung Lobe, Right F Lower Lung Lobe, Right G Upper Lung Lobe, Left H Lung Lingula J Lower Lung Lobe, Left K Lung, Right L Lung, Left M Lungs, Bilateral	0 Open 3 Percutaneous 4 Percutaneous Endoscopic 7 Via Natural or Artificial Opening 8 Via Natural or Artificial Opening Endoscopic	0 Drainage Device	Z No Qualifier
1 Trachea 2 Carina 3 Main Bronchus, Right 4 Upper Lobe Bronchus, Right 5 Middle Lobe Bronchus, Right 6 Lower Lobe Bronchus, Right 7 Main Bronchus, Left 8 Upper Lobe Bronchus, Left 9 Lingula Bronchus B Lower Lobe Bronchus, Left C Upper Lung Lobe, Right D Middle Lung Lobe, Right F Lower Lung Lobe, Right G Upper Lung Lobe, Left H Lung Lingula J Lower Lung Lobe, Left K Lung, Right L Lung, Left M Lungs, Bilateral	0 Open 3 Percutaneous 4 Percutaneous Endoscopic 7 Via Natural or Artificial Opening 8 Via Natural or Artificial Opening Endoscopic	Z No Device	X Diagnostic Z No Qualifier

0B9 continued on next page

0 **Medical and Surgical**
B **Respiratory System**
9 **Drainage:** Taking or letting out fluids and/or gases from a body part

0B9 continued from previous page

Body Part	Approach	Device	Qualifier
Character 4	Character 5	Character 6	Character 7
N Pleura, Right P Pleura, Left	0 Open 3 Percutaneous 4 Percutaneous Endoscopic 8 Via Natural or Artificial Opening Endoscopic	0 Drainage Device	Z No Qualifier
N Pleura, Right P Pleura, Left	0 Open 3 Percutaneous 4 Percutaneous Endoscopic 8 Via Natural or Artificial Opening Endoscopic	Z No Device	X Diagnostic Z No Qualifier
T Diaphragm	0 Open 3 Percutaneous 4 Percutaneous Endoscopic	0 Drainage Device	Z No Qualifier
T Diaphragm	0 Open 3 Percutaneous 4 Percutaneous Endoscopic	Z No Device	X Diagnostic Z No Qualifier

0 **Medical and Surgical**
B **Respiratory System**
B **Excision:** Cutting out or off, without replacement, a portion of a body part

Body Part	Approach	Device	Qualifier
Character 4	Character 5	Character 6	Character 7
1 Trachea 2 Carina 3 Main Bronchus, Right 4 Upper Lobe Bronchus, Right 5 Middle Lobe Bronchus, Right 6 Lower Lobe Bronchus, Right 7 Main Bronchus, Left 8 Upper Lobe Bronchus, Left 9 Lingula Bronchus B Lower Lobe Bronchus, Left C Upper Lung Lobe, Right D Middle Lung Lobe, Right F Lower Lung Lobe, Right G Upper Lung Lobe, Left H Lung Lingula J Lower Lung Lobe, Left K Lung, Right L Lung, Left M Lungs, Bilateral	0 Open 3 Percutaneous 4 Percutaneous Endoscopic 7 Via Natural or Artificial Opening 8 Via Natural or Artificial Opening Endoscopic	Z No Device	X Diagnostic Z No Qualifier
N Pleura, Right P Pleura, Left	0 Open 3 Percutaneous 4 Percutaneous Endoscopic 8 Via Natural or Artificial Opening Endoscopic	Z No Device	X Diagnostic Z No Qualifier
T Diaphragm	0 Open 3 Percutaneous 4 Percutaneous Endoscopic	Z No Device	X Diagnostic Z No Qualifier

0   Medical and Surgical
B   Respiratory System
C   Extirpation: Taking or cutting out solid matter from a body part

Body Part	Approach	Device	Qualifier
Character 4	Character 5	Character 6	Character 7
1 Trachea 2 Carina 3 Main Bronchus, Right 4 Upper Lobe Bronchus, Right 5 Middle Lobe Bronchus, Right 6 Lower Lobe Bronchus, Right 7 Main Bronchus, Left 8 Upper Lobe Bronchus, Left 9 Lingula Bronchus B Lower Lobe Bronchus, Left C Upper Lung Lobe, Right D Middle Lung Lobe, Right F Lower Lung Lobe, Right G Upper Lung Lobe, Left H Lung Lingula J Lower Lung Lobe, Left K Lung, Right L Lung, Left M Lungs, Bilateral	0 Open 3 Percutaneous 4 Percutaneous Endoscopic 7 Via Natural or Artificial Opening 8 Via Natural or Artificial Opening Endoscopic	Z No Device	Z No Qualifier
N Pleura, Right P Pleura, Left T Diaphragm	0 Open 3 Percutaneous 4 Percutaneous Endoscopic	Z No Device	Z No Qualifier

0   Medical and Surgical
B   Respiratory System
D   Extraction: Pulling or stripping out or off all or a portion of a body part by the use of force

Body Part	Approach	Device	Qualifier
Character 4	Character 5	Character 6	Character 7
1 Trachea 2 Carina 3 Main Bronchus, Right 4 Upper Lobe Bronchus, Right 5 Middle Lobe Bronchus, Right 6 Lower Lobe Bronchus, Right 7 Main Bronchus, Left 8 Upper Lobe Bronchus, Left 9 Lingula Bronchus B Lower Lobe Bronchus, Left C Upper Lung Lobe, Right D Middle Lung Lobe, Right F Lower Lung Lobe, Right G Upper Lung Lobe, Left H Lung Lingula J Lower Lung Lobe, Left K Lung, Right L Lung, Left M Lungs, Bilateral	4 Percutaneous Endoscopic 8 Via Natural or Artificial Opening Endoscopic	Z No Device	X Diagnostic
N Pleura, Right P Pleura, Left	0 Open 3 Percutaneous 4 Percutaneous Endoscopic	Z No Device	X Diagnostic Z No Qualifier

0 Medical and Surgical
B Respiratory System
F Fragmentation: Breaking solid matter in a body part into pieces

Body Part	Approach	Device	Qualifier
Character 4	**Character 5**	**Character 6**	**Character 7**
1 Trachea NC 2 Carina NC 3 Main Bronchus, Right NC 4 Upper Lobe Bronchus, Right NC 5 Middle Lobe Bronchus, Right NC 6 Lower Lobe Bronchus, Right NC 7 Main Bronchus, Left NC 8 Upper Lobe Bronchus, Left NC 9 Lingula Bronchus NC B Lower Lobe Bronchus, Left NC	0 Open 3 Percutaneous 4 Percutaneous Endoscopic 7 Via Natural or Artificial Opening 8 Via Natural or Artificial Opening Endoscopic X External	Z No Device	Z No Qualifier

NC 0BF1XZZ   0BF2XZZ   0BF3XZZ   0BF4XZZ   0BF5XZZ   0BF6XZZ   0BF7XZZ   0BF8XZZ   0BF9XZZ   0BFBXZZ

0 Medical and Surgical
B Respiratory System
H Insertion: Putting in a nonbiological appliance that monitors, assists, performs, or prevents a physiological function but does not physically take the place of a body part

Body Part	Approach	Device	Qualifier
Character 4	**Character 5**	**Character 6**	**Character 7**
0 Tracheobronchial Tree	0 Open 3 Percutaneous 4 Percutaneous Endoscopic 7 Via Natural or Artificial Opening 8 Via Natural or Artificial Opening Endoscopic	1 Radioactive Element 2 Monitoring Device 3 Infusion Device D Intraluminal Device Y Other Device	Z No Qualifier
1 Trachea	0 Open	2 Monitoring Device D Intraluminal Device Y Other Device	Z No Qualifier
1 Trachea	3 Percutaneous	D Intraluminal Device E Intraluminal Device, Endotracheal Airway Y Other Device	Z No Qualifier
1 Trachea	4 Percutaneous Endoscopic	D Intraluminal Device Y Other Device	Z No Qualifier
1 Trachea	7 Via Natural or Artificial Opening 8 Via Natural or Artificial Opening Endoscopic	2 Monitoring Device D Intraluminal Device E Intraluminal Device, Endotracheal Airway Y Other Device	Z No Qualifier
3 Main Bronchus, Right 4 Upper Lobe Bronchus, Right 5 Middle Lobe Bronchus, Right 6 Lower Lobe Bronchus, Right 7 Main Bronchus, Left 8 Upper Lobe Bronchus, Left 9 Lingula Bronchus B Lower Lobe Bronchus, Left	0 Open 3 Percutaneous 4 Percutaneous Endoscopic 7 Via Natural or Artificial Opening 8 Via Natural or Artificial Opening Endoscopic	G Intraluminal Device, Endobronchial Valve	Z No Qualifier
K Lung, Right L Lung, Left	0 Open 3 Percutaneous 4 Percutaneous Endoscopic 7 Via Natural or Artificial Opening 8 Via Natural or Artificial Opening Endoscopic	1 Radioactive Element 2 Monitoring Device 3 Infusion Device Y Other Device	Z No Qualifier

0BH continued on next page

0 **Medical and Surgical**
B **Respiratory System**
H **Insertion:** Putting in a nonbiological appliance that monitors, assists, performs, or prevents a physiological function but does not physically take the place of a body part

Body Part	Approach	Device	Qualifier
Character 4	Character 5	Character 6	Character 7
Q Pleura	0 Open 3 Percutaneous 4 Percutaneous Endoscopic 7 Via Natural or Artificial Opening 8 Via Natural or Artificial Opening Endoscopic	Y Other Device	Z No Qualifier
T Diaphragm	0 Open 3 Percutaneous 4 Percutaneous Endoscopic	2 Monitoring Device M Diaphragmatic Pacemaker Lead Y Other Device	Z No Qualifier
T Diaphragm	7 Via Natural or Artificial Opening 8 Via Natural or Artificial Opening Endoscopic	Y Other Device	Z No Qualifier

0 **Medical and Surgical**
B **Respiratory System**
J **Inspection:** Visually and/or manually exploring a body part

Body Part	Approach	Device	Qualifier
Character 4	Character 5	Character 6	Character 7
0 Tracheobronchial Tree 1 Trachea K Lung, Right L Lung, Left Q Pleura T Diaphragm	0 Open 3 Percutaneous 4 Percutaneous Endoscopic 7 Via Natural or Artificial Opening 8 Via Natural or Artificial Opening Endoscopic X External	Z No Device	Z No Qualifier

0 **Medical and Surgical**
B **Respiratory System**
L **Occlusion:** Completely closing an orifice or the lumen of a tubular body part

Body Part	Approach	Device	Qualifier
Character 4	Character 5	Character 6	Character 7
1 Trachea 2 Carina 3 Main Bronchus, Right 4 Upper Lobe Bronchus, Right 5 Middle Lobe Bronchus, Right 6 Lower Lobe Bronchus, Right 7 Main Bronchus, Left 8 Upper Lobe Bronchus, Left 9 Lingula Bronchus B Lower Lobe Bronchus, Left	0 Open 3 Percutaneous 4 Percutaneous Endoscopic	C Extraluminal Device D Intraluminal Device Z No Device	Z No Qualifier
1 Trachea 2 Carina 3 Main Bronchus, Right 4 Upper Lobe Bronchus, Right 5 Middle Lobe Bronchus, Right 6 Lower Lobe Bronchus, Right 7 Main Bronchus, Left 8 Upper Lobe Bronchus, Left 9 Lingula Bronchus B Lower Lobe Bronchus, Left	7 Via Natural or Artificial Opening 8 Via Natural or Artificial Opening Endoscopic	D Intraluminal Device Z No Device	Z No Qualifier

LC Limited Coverage   NC Noncovered   HAC HAC-associated Procedure   CC Combination Cluster - See Appendix G for code lists
DRG Non-OR-Affecting MS-DRG Assignment   New/Revised Text in Orange   ♂ Male   ♀ Female

300

2018 ICD-10-PCS

0   **Medical and Surgical**
B   **Respiratory System**
M   **Reattachment:** Putting back in or on all or a portion of a separated body part to its normal location or other suitable location

Body Part	Approach	Device	Qualifier
Character 4	Character 5	Character 6	Character 7
1 Trachea 2 Carina 3 Main Bronchus, Right 4 Upper Lobe Bronchus, Right 5 Middle Lobe Bronchus, Right 6 Lower Lobe Bronchus, Right 7 Main Bronchus, Left 8 Upper Lobe Bronchus, Left 9 Lingula Bronchus B Lower Lobe Bronchus, Left C Upper Lung Lobe, Right D Middle Lung Lobe, Right F Lower Lung Lobe, Right G Upper Lung Lobe, Left H Lung Lingula J Lower Lung Lobe, Left K Lung, Right L Lung, Left T Diaphragm	0 Open	Z No Device	Z No Qualifier

0   **Medical and Surgical**
B   **Respiratory System**
N   **Release:** Freeing a body part from an abnormal physical constraint by cutting or by the use of force

Body Part	Approach	Device	Qualifier
Character 4	Character 5	Character 6	Character 7
1 Trachea 2 Carina 3 Main Bronchus, Right 4 Upper Lobe Bronchus, Right 5 Middle Lobe Bronchus, Right 6 Lower Lobe Bronchus, Right 7 Main Bronchus, Left 8 Upper Lobe Bronchus, Left 9 Lingula Bronchus B Lower Lobe Bronchus, Left C Upper Lung Lobe, Right D Middle Lung Lobe, Right F Lower Lung Lobe, Right G Upper Lung Lobe, Left H Lung Lingula J Lower Lung Lobe, Left K Lung, Right L Lung, Left M Lungs, Bilateral	0 Open 3 Percutaneous 4 Percutaneous Endoscopic 7 Via Natural or Artificial Opening 8 Via Natural or Artificial Opening Endoscopic	Z No Device	Z No Qualifier
N Pleura, Right P Pleura, Left T Diaphragm	0 Open 3 Percutaneous 4 Percutaneous Endoscopic	Z No Device	Z No Qualifier

LC Limited Coverage   NC Noncovered   HAC HAC-associated Procedure   CC Combination Cluster - See Appendix G for code lists
DRG Non-OR-Affecting MS-DRG Assignment   New/Revised Text in **Orange**   ♂ Male   ♀ Female

2018 ICD-10-PCS   **301**

0 **Medical and Surgical**
B **Respiratory System**
P **Removal:** Taking out or off a device from a body part

Body Part	Approach	Device	Qualifier
Character 4	**Character 5**	**Character 6**	**Character 7**
0 Tracheobronchial Tree	0 Open 3 Percutaneous 4 Percutaneous Endoscopic 7 Via Natural or Artificial Opening 8 Via Natural or Artificial Opening Endoscopic	0 Drainage Device 1 Radioactive Element 2 Monitoring Device 3 Infusion Device 7 Autologous Tissue Substitute C Extraluminal Device D Intraluminal Device J Synthetic Substitute K Nonautologous Tissue Substitute Y Other Device	Z No Qualifier
0 Tracheobronchial Tree	X External	0 Drainage Device 1 Radioactive Element 2 Monitoring Device 3 Infusion Device D Intraluminal Device	Z No Qualifier
1 Trachea	0 Open 3 Percutaneous 4 Percutaneous Endoscopic 7 Via Natural or Artificial Opening 8 Via Natural or Artificial Opening Endoscopic	0 Drainage Device 2 Monitoring Device 7 Autologous Tissue Substitute C Extraluminal Device D Intraluminal Device F Tracheostomy Device J Synthetic Substitute K Nonautologous Tissue Substitute	Z No Qualifier
1 Trachea	X External	0 Drainage Device 2 Monitoring Device D Intraluminal Device F Tracheostomy Device	Z No Qualifier
K Lung, Right L Lung, Left	0 Open 3 Percutaneous 4 Percutaneous Endoscopic 7 Via Natural or Artificial Opening 8 Via Natural or Artificial Opening Endoscopic	0 Drainage Device 1 Radioactive Element 2 Monitoring Device 3 Infusion Device Y Other Device	Z No Qualifier
K Lung, Right L Lung, Left	X External	0 Drainage Device 1 Radioactive Element 2 Monitoring Device 3 Infusion Device	Z No Qualifier
Q Pleura	0 Open 3 Percutaneous 4 Percutaneous Endoscopic 7 Via Natural or Artificial Opening 8 Via Natural or Artificial Opening Endoscopic	0 Drainage Device 1 Radioactive Element 2 Monitoring Device Y Other Device	Z No Qualifier
Q Pleura	X External	0 Drainage Device 1 Radioactive Element 2 Monitoring Device	Z No Qualifier
T Diaphragm	0 Open 3 Percutaneous 4 Percutaneous Endoscopic 7 Via Natural or Artificial Opening 8 Via Natural or Artificial Opening Endoscopic	0 Drainage Device 2 Monitoring Device 7 Autologous Tissue Substitute J Synthetic Substitute K Nonautologous Tissue Substitute M Diaphragmatic Pacemaker Lead Y Other Device	Z No Qualifier
T Diaphragm	X External	0 Drainage Device 2 Monitoring Device M Diaphragmatic Pacemaker Lead	Z No Qualifier

LC Limited Coverage   NC Noncovered   HAC HAC-associated Procedure   CC Combination Cluster - See Appendix G for code lists
Non-OR-Affecting MS-DRG Assignment   New/Revised Text in **Orange**   ♂ Male   ♀ Female

302

2018 ICD-10-PCS

0 Medical and Surgical
B Respiratory System
Q Repair: Restoring, to the extent possible, a body part to its normal anatomic structure and function

Body Part	Approach	Device	Qualifier
Character 4	Character 5	Character 6	Character 7
1 Trachea 2 Carina 3 Main Bronchus, Right 4 Upper Lobe Bronchus, Right 5 Middle Lobe Bronchus, Right 6 Lower Lobe Bronchus, Right 7 Main Bronchus, Left 8 Upper Lobe Bronchus, Left 9 Lingula Bronchus B Lower Lobe Bronchus, Left C Upper Lung Lobe, Right D Middle Lung Lobe, Right F Lower Lung Lobe, Right G Upper Lung Lobe, Left H Lung Lingula J Lower Lung Lobe, Left K Lung, Right L Lung, Left M Lungs, Bilateral	0 Open 3 Percutaneous 4 Percutaneous Endoscopic 7 Via Natural or Artificial Opening 8 Via Natural or Artificial Opening Endoscopic	Z No Device	Z No Qualifier
N Pleura, Right P Pleura, Left T Diaphragm	0 Open 3 Percutaneous 4 Percutaneous Endoscopic	Z No Device	Z No Qualifier

0 Medical and Surgical
B Respiratory System
R Replacement: Putting in or on biological or synthetic material that physically takes the place and/or function of all or a portion of a body part

Body Part	Approach	Device	Qualifier
Character 4	Character 5	Character 6	Character 7
1 Trachea 2 Carina 3 Main Bronchus, Right 4 Upper Lobe Bronchus, Right 5 Middle Lobe Bronchus, Right 6 Lower Lobe Bronchus, Right 7 Main Bronchus, Left 8 Upper Lobe Bronchus, Left 9 Lingula Bronchus B Lower Lobe Bronchus, Left T Diaphragm	0 Open 4 Percutaneous Endoscopic	7 Autologous Tissue Substitute J Synthetic Substitute K Nonautologous Tissue Substitute	Z No Qualifier

0 Medical and Surgical
B Respiratory System
S Reposition: Moving to its normal location, or other suitable location, all or a portion of a body part

Body Part	Approach	Device	Qualifier
Character 4	**Character 5**	**Character 6**	**Character 7**
1 Trachea 2 Carina 3 Main Bronchus, Right 4 Upper Lobe Bronchus, Right 5 Middle Lobe Bronchus, Right 6 Lower Lobe Bronchus, Right 7 Main Bronchus, Left 8 Upper Lobe Bronchus, Left 9 Lingula Bronchus B Lower Lobe Bronchus, Left C Upper Lung Lobe, Right D Middle Lung Lobe, Right F Lower Lung Lobe, Right G Upper Lung Lobe, Left H Lung Lingula J Lower Lung Lobe, Left K Lung, Right L Lung, Left T Diaphragm	0 Open	Z No Device	Z No Qualifier

0 Medical and Surgical
B Respiratory System
T Resection: Cutting out or off, without replacement, all of a body part

Body Part	Approach	Device	Qualifier
Character 4	**Character 5**	**Character 6**	**Character 7**
1 Trachea 2 Carina 3 Main Bronchus, Right 4 Upper Lobe Bronchus, Right 5 Middle Lobe Bronchus, Right 6 Lower Lobe Bronchus, Right 7 Main Bronchus, Left 8 Upper Lobe Bronchus, Left 9 Lingula Bronchus B Lower Lobe Bronchus, Left C Upper Lung Lobe, Right D Middle Lung Lobe, Right F Lower Lung Lobe, Right G Upper Lung Lobe, Left H Lung Lingula J Lower Lung Lobe, Left K Lung, Right L Lung, Left M Lungs, Bilateral T Diaphragm	0 Open 4 Percutaneous Endoscopic	Z No Device	Z No Qualifier

LC Limited Coverage   NC Noncovered   HAC HAC-associated Procedure   CC Combination Cluster - See Appendix G for code lists
DRG Non-OR-Affecting MS-DRG Assignment   New/Revised Text in **Orange**   ♂ Male   ♀ Female

304

2018 ICD-10-PCS

0 **Medical and Surgical**
B **Respiratory System**
U **Supplement:** Putting in or on biological or synthetic material that physically reinforces and/or augments the function of a portion of a body part

Body Part	Approach	Device	Qualifier
Character 4	Character 5	Character 6	Character 7
1 Trachea 2 Carina 3 Main Bronchus, Right 4 Upper Lobe Bronchus, Right 5 Middle Lobe Bronchus, Right 6 Lower Lobe Bronchus, Right 7 Main Bronchus, Left 8 Upper Lobe Bronchus, Left 9 Lingula Bronchus B Lower Lobe Bronchus, Left	0 Open 4 Percutaneous Endoscopic 8 Via Natural or Artificial Opening Endoscopic	7 Autologous Tissue Substitute J Synthetic Substitute K Nonautologous Tissue Substitute	Z No Qualifier
T Diaphragm	0 Open 4 Percutaneous Endoscopic	7 Autologous Tissue Substitute J Synthetic Substitute K Nonautologous Tissue Substitute	Z No Qualifier

0 **Medical and Surgical**
B **Respiratory System**
V **Restriction:** Partially closing an orifice or the lumen of a tubular body part

Body Part	Approach	Device	Qualifier
Character 4	Character 5	Character 6	Character 7
1 Trachea 2 Carina 3 Main Bronchus, Right 4 Upper Lobe Bronchus, Right 5 Middle Lobe Bronchus, Right 6 Lower Lobe Bronchus, Right 7 Main Bronchus, Left 8 Upper Lobe Bronchus, Left 9 Lingula Bronchus B Lower Lobe Bronchus, Left	0 Open 3 Percutaneous 4 Percutaneous Endoscopic	C Extraluminal Device D Intraluminal Device Z No Device	Z No Qualifier
1 Trachea 2 Carina 3 Main Bronchus, Right 4 Upper Lobe Bronchus, Right 5 Middle Lobe Bronchus, Right 6 Lower Lobe Bronchus, Right 7 Main Bronchus, Left 8 Upper Lobe Bronchus, Left 9 Lingula Bronchus B Lower Lobe Bronchus, Left	7 Via Natural or Artificial Opening 8 Via Natural or Artificial Opening Endoscopic	D Intraluminal Device Z No Device	Z No Qualifier

LC Limited Coverage   NC Noncovered   HAC HAC-associated Procedure   CC Combination Cluster - See Appendix G for code lists
DRG Non-OR-Affecting MS-DRG Assignment   New/Revised Text in **Orange**   ♂ Male   ♀ Female

2018 ICD-10-PCS

305

RESPIRATORY SYSTEM 0B1-0BY

0 **Medical and Surgical**
B **Respiratory System**
W **Revision:** Correcting, to the extent possible, a portion of a malfunctioning device or the position of a displaced device

Body Part	Approach	Device	Qualifier
Character 4	Character 5	Character 6	Character 7
0 Tracheobronchial Tree	**0** Open **3** Percutaneous **4** Percutaneous Endoscopic **7** Via Natural or Artificial Opening **8** Via Natural or Artificial Opening Endoscopic	**0** Drainage Device **2** Monitoring Device **3** Infusion Device **7** Autologous Tissue Substitute **C** Extraluminal Device **D** Intraluminal Device **J** Synthetic Substitute **K** Nonautologous Tissue Substitute **Y** Other Device	**Z** No Qualifier
0 Tracheobronchial Tree	**X** External	**0** Drainage Device **2** Monitoring Device **3** Infusion Device **7** Autologous Tissue Substitute **C** Extraluminal Device **D** Intraluminal Device **J** Synthetic Substitute **K** Nonautologous Tissue Substitute	**Z** No Qualifier
1 Trachea	**0** Open **3** Percutaneous **4** Percutaneous Endoscopic **7** Via Natural or Artificial Opening **8** Via Natural or Artificial Opening Endoscopic **X** External	**0** Drainage Device **2** Monitoring Device **7** Autologous Tissue Substitute **C** Extraluminal Device **D** Intraluminal Device **F** Tracheostomy Device **J** Synthetic Substitute **K** Nonautologous Tissue Substitute	**Z** No Qualifier
K Lung, Right **L** Lung, Left	**0** Open **3** Percutaneous **4** Percutaneous Endoscopic **7** Via Natural or Artificial Opening **8** Via Natural or Artificial Opening Endoscopic	**0** Drainage Device **2** Monitoring Device **3** Infusion Device **Y** Other Device	**Z** No Qualifier
K Lung, Right **L** Lung, Left	**X** External	**0** Drainage Device **2** Monitoring Device **3** Infusion Device	**Z** No Qualifier
Q Pleura	**0** Open **3** Percutaneous **4** Percutaneous Endoscopic **7** Via Natural or Artificial Opening **8** Via Natural or Artificial Opening Endoscopic	**0** Drainage Device **2** Monitoring Device **Y** Other Device	**Z** No Qualifier
Q Pleura	**X** External	**0** Drainage Device **2** Monitoring Device	**Z** No Qualifier
T Diaphragm	**0** Open **3** Percutaneous **4** Percutaneous Endoscopic **7** Via Natural or Artificial Opening **8** Via Natural or Artificial Opening Endoscopic	**0** Drainage Device **2** Monitoring Device **7** Autologous Tissue Substitute **J** Synthetic Substitute **K** Nonautologous Tissue Substitute **M** Diaphragmatic Pacemaker Lead **Y** Other Device	**Z** No Qualifier
T Diaphragm	**X** External	**0** Drainage Device **2** Monitoring Device **7** Autologous Tissue Substitute **J** Synthetic Substitute **K** Nonautologous Tissue Substitute **M** Diaphragmatic Pacemaker Lead	**Z** No Qualifier

LC Limited Coverage   **NC** Noncovered   **HAC** HAC-associated Procedure   **CC** Combination Cluster - See Appendix G for code lists
DRG Non-OR-Affecting MS-DRG Assignment   New/Revised Text in **Orange**   ♂ Male   ♀ Female

306

2018 ICD-10-PCS

0 **Medical and Surgical**
B **Respiratory System**
Y **Transplantation:** Putting in or on all or a portion of a living body part taken from another individual or animal to physically take the place and/or function of all or a portion of a similar body part

Body Part	Approach	Device	Qualifier
Character 4	Character 5	Character 6	Character 7
C Upper Lung Lobe, Right LC D Middle Lung Lobe, Right LC F Lower Lung Lobe, Right LC G Upper Lung Lobe, Left LC H Lung Lingula LC J Lower Lung Lobe, Left LC K Lung, Right LC L Lung, Left LC M Lungs, Bilateral LC	0 Open	Z No Device	0 Allogeneic 1 Syngeneic 2 Zooplastic

LC 0BYC0Z0   0BYC0Z1   0BYC0Z2   0BYD0Z0   0BYD0Z1   0BYD0Z2   0BYF0Z0   0BYF0Z1   0BYF0Z2   0BYG0Z0   0BYG0Z1   0BYG0Z2   0BYH0Z0
    0BYH0Z1   0BYH0Z2   0BYJ0Z0   0BYJ0Z1   0BYJ0Z2   0BYK0Z0   0BYK0Z1   0BYK0Z2   0BYL0Z0   0BYL0Z1   0BYL0Z2   0BYM0Z0   0BYM0Z1
    0BYM0Z2

LC Limited Coverage   NC Noncovered   HAC HAC-associated Procedure   CC Combination Cluster - See Appendix G for code lists
DRG Non-OR-Affecting MS-DRG Assignment   New/Revised Text in **Orange**   ♂ Male   ♀ Female

NOTES

Mouth and Throat 0C0-0CX

0 Medical and Surgical
C Mouth and Throat
0 Alteration: Modifying the anatomic structure of a body part without affecting the function of the body part

Body Part	Approach	Device	Qualifier
Character 4	**Character 5**	**Character 6**	**Character 7**
0 Upper Lip **1** Lower Lip	**X** External	**7** Autologous Tissue Substitute **J** Synthetic Substitute **K** Nonautologous Tissue Substitute **Z** No Device	**Z** No Qualifier

0 Medical and Surgical
C Mouth and Throat
2 Change: Taking out or off a device from a body part and putting back an identical or similar device in or on the same body part without cutting or puncturing the skin or a mucous membrane

Body Part	Approach	Device	Qualifier
Character 4	**Character 5**	**Character 6**	**Character 7**
A Salivary Gland **S** Larynx **Y** Mouth and Throat	**X** External	**0** Drainage Device **Y** Other Device	**Z** No Qualifier

0 Medical and Surgical
C Mouth and Throat
5 Destruction: Physical eradication of all or a portion of a body part by the direct use of energy, force, or a destructive agent

Body Part	Approach	Device	Qualifier
Character 4	**Character 5**	**Character 6**	**Character 7**
0 Upper Lip **1** Lower Lip **2** Hard Palate **3** Soft Palate **4** Buccal Mucosa **5** Upper Gingiva **6** Lower Gingiva **7** Tongue **N** Uvula **P** Tonsils **Q** Adenoids	**0** Open **3** Percutaneous **X** External	**Z** No Device	**Z** No Qualifier
8 Parotid Gland, Right **9** Parotid Gland, Left **B** Parotid Duct, Right **C** Parotid Duct, Left **D** Sublingual Gland, Right **F** Sublingual Gland, Left **G** Submaxillary Gland, Right **H** Submaxillary Gland, Left **J** Minor Salivary Gland	**0** Open **3** Percutaneous	**Z** No Device	**Z** No Qualifier
M Pharynx **R** Epiglottis **S** Larynx **T** Vocal Cord, Right **V** Vocal Cord, Left	**0** Open **3** Percutaneous **4** Percutaneous Endoscopic **7** Via Natural or Artificial Opening **8** Via Natural or Artificial Opening Endoscopic	**Z** No Device	**Z** No Qualifier
W Upper Tooth **X** Lower Tooth	**0** Open **X** External	**Z** No Device	**0** Single **1** Multiple **2** All

0 Medical and Surgical
C Mouth and Throat
7 Dilation: Expanding an orifice or the lumen of a tubular body part

Body Part	Approach	Device	Qualifier
Character 4	Character 5	Character 6	Character 7
B Parotid Duct, Right C Parotid Duct, Left	0 Open 3 Percutaneous 7 Via Natural or Artificial Opening	D Intraluminal Device Z No Device	Z No Qualifier
M Pharynx	7 Via Natural or Artificial Opening 8 Via Natural or Artificial Opening Endoscopic	D Intraluminal Device Z No Device	Z No Qualifier
S Larynx	0 Open 3 Percutaneous 4 Percutaneous Endoscopic 7 Via Natural or Artificial Opening 8 Via Natural or Artificial Opening Endoscopic	D Intraluminal Device Z No Device	Z No Qualifier

0 Medical and Surgical
C Mouth and Throat
9 Drainage: Taking or letting out fluids and/or gases from a body part

Body Part	Approach	Device	Qualifier
Character 4	Character 5	Character 6	Character 7
0 Upper Lip 1 Lower Lip 2 Hard Palate 3 Soft Palate 4 Buccal Mucosa 5 Upper Gingiva 6 Lower Gingiva 7 Tongue N Uvula P Tonsils Q Adenoids	0 Open 3 Percutaneous X External	0 Drainage Device	Z No Qualifier
0 Upper Lip 1 Lower Lip 2 Hard Palate 3 Soft Palate 4 Buccal Mucosa 5 Upper Gingiva 6 Lower Gingiva 7 Tongue N Uvula P Tonsils Q Adenoids	0 Open 3 Percutaneous X External	Z No Device	X Diagnostic Z No Qualifier
8 Parotid Gland, Right 9 Parotid Gland, Left B Parotid Duct, Right C Parotid Duct, Left D Sublingual Gland, Right F Sublingual Gland, Left G Submaxillary Gland, Right H Submaxillary Gland, Left J Minor Salivary Gland	0 Open 3 Percutaneous	0 Drainage Device	Z No Qualifier

0C9 continued on next page

LC Limited Coverage   NC Noncovered   HAC HAC-associated Procedure   CC Combination Cluster - See Appendix G for code lists
DRG Non-OR-Affecting MS-DRG Assignment   New/Revised Text in **Orange**   ♂ Male   ♀ Female

0 **Medical and Surgical**
C **Mouth and Throat**
9 **Drainage:** Taking or letting out fluids and/or gases from a body part

0C9 continued from previous page

Body Part	Approach	Device	Qualifier
Character 4	**Character 5**	**Character 6**	**Character 7**
8 Parotid Gland, Right 9 Parotid Gland, Left B Parotid Duct, Right C Parotid Duct, Left D Sublingual Gland, Right F Sublingual Gland, Left G Submaxillary Gland, Right H Submaxillary Gland, Left J Minor Salivary Gland	0 Open 3 Percutaneous	Z No Device	X Diagnostic Z No Qualifier
M Pharynx R Epiglottis S Larynx T Vocal Cord, Right V Vocal Cord, Left	0 Open 3 Percutaneous 4 Percutaneous Endoscopic 7 Via Natural or Artificial Opening 8 Via Natural or Artificial Opening Endoscopic	0 Drainage Device	Z No Qualifier
M Pharynx R Epiglottis S Larynx T Vocal Cord, Right V Vocal Cord, Left	0 Open 3 Percutaneous 4 Percutaneous Endoscopic 7 Via Natural or Artificial Opening 8 Via Natural or Artificial Opening Endoscopic	Z No Device	X Diagnostic Z No Qualifier
W Upper Tooth X Lower Tooth	0 Open X External	0 Drainage Device Z No Device	0 Single 1 Multiple 2 All

0 **Medical and Surgical**
C **Mouth and Throat**
B **Excision:** Cutting out or off, without replacement, a portion of a body part

Body Part	Approach	Device	Qualifier
Character 4	**Character 5**	**Character 6**	**Character 7**
0 Upper Lip 1 Lower Lip 2 Hard Palate 3 Soft Palate 4 Buccal Mucosa 5 Upper Gingiva 6 Lower Gingiva 7 Tongue N Uvula P Tonsils Q Adenoids	0 Open 3 Percutaneous X External	Z No Device	X Diagnostic Z No Qualifier
8 Parotid Gland, Right 9 Parotid Gland, Left B Parotid Duct, Right C Parotid Duct, Left D Sublingual Gland, Right F Sublingual Gland, Left G Submaxillary Gland, Right H Submaxillary Gland, Left J Minor Salivary Gland	0 Open 3 Percutaneous	Z No Device	X Diagnostic Z No Qualifier
M Pharynx R Epiglottis S Larynx T Vocal Cord, Right V Vocal Cord, Left	0 Open 3 Percutaneous 4 Percutaneous Endoscopic 7 Via Natural or Artificial Opening 8 Via Natural or Artificial Opening Endoscopic	Z No Device	X Diagnostic Z No Qualifier
W Upper Tooth X Lower Tooth	0 Open X External	Z No Device	0 Single 1 Multiple 2 All

0 Medical and Surgical
C Mouth and Throat
C Extirpation: Taking or cutting out solid matter from a body part

Body Part	Approach	Device	Qualifier
Character 4	Character 5	Character 6	Character 7
0 Upper Lip 1 Lower Lip 2 Hard Palate 3 Soft Palate 4 Buccal Mucosa 5 Upper Gingiva 6 Lower Gingiva 7 Tongue N Uvula P Tonsils Q Adenoids	0 Open 3 Percutaneous X External	Z No Device	Z No Qualifier
8 Parotid Gland, Right 9 Parotid Gland, Left B Parotid Duct, Right C Parotid Duct, Left D Sublingual Gland, Right F Sublingual Gland, Left G Submaxillary Gland, Right H Submaxillary Gland, Left J Minor Salivary Gland	0 Open 3 Percutaneous	Z No Device	Z No Qualifier
M Pharynx R Epiglottis S Larynx T Vocal Cord, Right V Vocal Cord, Left	0 Open 3 Percutaneous 4 Percutaneous Endoscopic 7 Via Natural or Artificial Opening 8 Via Natural or Artificial Opening Endoscopic	Z No Device	Z No Qualifier
W Upper Tooth X Lower Tooth	0 Open X External	Z No Device	0 Single 1 Multiple 2 All

0 Medical and Surgical
C Mouth and Throat
D Extraction: Pulling or stripping out or off all or a portion of a body part by the use of force

Body Part	Approach	Device	Qualifier
Character 4	Character 5	Character 6	Character 7
T Vocal Cord, Right V Vocal Cord, Left	0 Open 3 Percutaneous 4 Percutaneous Endoscopic 7 Via Natural or Artificial Opening 8 Via Natural or Artificial Opening Endoscopic	Z No Device	Z No Qualifier
W Upper Tooth X Lower Tooth	X External	Z No Device	0 Single 1 Multiple 2 All

0 Medical and Surgical
C Mouth and Throat
F Fragmentation: Breaking solid matter in a body part into pieces

Body Part	Approach	Device	Qualifier
Character 4	Character 5	Character 6	Character 7
B Parotid Duct, Right NC C Parotid Duct, Left NC	0 Open 3 Percutaneous 7 Via Natural or Artificial Opening X External	Z No Device	Z No Qualifier

NC 0CFBXZZ   0CFCXZZ

LC Limited Coverage   NC Noncovered   HAC HAC-associated Procedure   CC Combination Cluster - See Appendix G for code lists
DRG Non-OR-Affecting MS-DRG Assignment   New/Revised Text in **Orange**   ♂ Male   ♀ Female

312

2018 ICD-10-PCS

MOUTH AND THROAT 0C0-0CX

0 Medical and Surgical
C Mouth and Throat
H Insertion: Putting in a nonbiological appliance that monitors, assists, performs, or prevents a physiological function but does not physically take the place of a body part

Body Part	Approach	Device	Qualifier
Character 4	Character 5	Character 6	Character 7
7 Tongue	0 Open 3 Percutaneous X External	1 Radioactive Element	Z No Qualifier
A Salivary Gland S Larynx	0 Open 3 Percutaneous 7 Via Natural or Artificial Opening 8 Via Natural or Artificial Opening Endoscopic	Y Other Device	Z No Qualifier
Y Mouth and Throat	0 Open 3 Percutaneous	Y Other Device	Z No Qualifier
Y Mouth and Throat	7 Via Natural or Artificial Opening 8 Via Natural or Artificial Opening Endoscopic	B Intraluminal Device, Airway Y Other Device	Z No Qualifier

0 Medical and Surgical
C Mouth and Throat
J Inspection: Visually and/or manually exploring a body part

Body Part	Approach	Device	Qualifier
Character 4	Character 5	Character 6	Character 7
A Salivary Gland	0 Open 3 Percutaneous X External	Z No Device	Z No Qualifier
S Larynx Y Mouth and Throat	0 Open 3 Percutaneous 4 Percutaneous Endoscopic 7 Via Natural or Artificial Opening 8 Via Natural or Artificial Opening Endoscopic X External	Z No Device	Z No Qualifier

0 Medical and Surgical
C Mouth and Throat
L Occlusion: Completely closing an orifice or the lumen of a tubular body part

Body Part	Approach	Device	Qualifier
Character 4	Character 5	Character 6	Character 7
B Parotid Duct, Right C Parotid Duct, Left	0 Open 3 Percutaneous 4 Percutaneous Endoscopic	C Extraluminal Device D Intraluminal Device Z No Device	Z No Qualifier
B Parotid Duct, Right C Parotid Duct, Left	7 Via Natural or Artificial Opening 8 Via Natural or Artificial Opening Endoscopic	D Intraluminal Device Z No Device	Z No Qualifier

0 Medical and Surgical
C Mouth and Throat
M Reattachment: Putting back in or on all or a portion of a separated body part to its normal location or other suitable location

Body Part	Approach	Device	Qualifier
Character 4	Character 5	Character 6	Character 7
0 Upper Lip 1 Lower Lip 3 Soft Palate 7 Tongue N Uvula	0 Open	Z No Device	Z No Qualifier
W Upper Tooth X Lower Tooth	0 Open X External	Z No Device	0 Single 1 Multiple 2 All

LC Limited Coverage NC Noncovered HAC HAC-associated Procedure CC Combination Cluster - See Appendix G for code lists
DRG Non-OR-Affecting MS-DRG Assignment New/Revised Text in **Orange** ♂ Male ♀ Female

2018 ICD-10-PCS 313

0   Medical and Surgical
C   Mouth and Throat
N   Release: Freeing a body part from an abnormal physical constraint by cutting or by the use of force

Body Part	Approach	Device	Qualifier
Character 4	**Character 5**	**Character 6**	**Character 7**
0 Upper Lip 1 Lower Lip 2 Hard Palate 3 Soft Palate 4 Buccal Mucosa 5 Upper Gingiva 6 Lower Gingiva 7 Tongue N Uvula P Tonsils Q Adenoids	0 Open 3 Percutaneous X External	Z No Device	Z No Qualifier
8 Parotid Gland, Right 9 Parotid Gland, Left B Parotid Duct, Right C Parotid Duct, Left D Sublingual Gland, Right F Sublingual Gland, Left G Submaxillary Gland, Right H Submaxillary Gland, Left J Minor Salivary Gland	0 Open 3 Percutaneous	Z No Device	Z No Qualifier
M Pharynx R Epiglottis S Larynx T Vocal Cord, Right V Vocal Cord, Left	0 Open 3 Percutaneous 4 Percutaneous Endoscopic 7 Via Natural or Artificial Opening 8 Via Natural or Artificial Opening Endoscopic	Z No Device	Z No Qualifier
W Upper Tooth X Lower Tooth	0 Open X External	Z No Device	0 Single 1 Multiple 2 All

0   Medical and Surgical
C   Mouth and Throat
P   Removal: Taking out or off a device from a body part

Body Part	Approach	Device	Qualifier
Character 4	**Character 5**	**Character 6**	**Character 7**
A Salivary Gland	0 Open 3 Percutaneous	0 Drainage Device C Extraluminal Device Y Other Device	Z No Qualifier
A Salivary Gland	7 Via Natural or Artificial Opening 8 Via Natural or Artificial Opening Endoscopic	Y Other Device	Z No Qualifier
S Larynx	0 Open 3 Percutaneous 7 Via Natural or Artificial Opening 8 Via Natural or Artificial Opening Endoscopic	0 Drainage Device 7 Autologous Tissue Substitute D Intraluminal Device J Synthetic Substitute K Nonautologous Tissue Substitute Y Other Device	Z No Qualifier
S Larynx	X External	0 Drainage Device 7 Autologous Tissue Substitute D Intraluminal Device J Synthetic Substitute K Nonautologous Tissue Substitute	Z No Qualifier

0CP continued on next page

LC Limited Coverage   NC Noncovered   HAC HAC-associated Procedure   CC Combination Cluster - See Appendix G for code lists
DRG Non-OR-Affecting MS-DRG Assignment   New/Revised Text in **Orange**   ♂ Male   ♀ Female

314

2018 ICD-10-PCS

0 Medical and Surgical
C Mouth and Throat
P Removal: Taking out or off a device from a body part

0CP continued from previous page

Body Part	Approach	Device	Qualifier
Character 4	**Character 5**	**Character 6**	**Character 7**
Y Mouth and Throat	**0** Open **3** Percutaneous **7** Via Natural or Artificial Opening **8** Via Natural or Artificial Opening Endoscopic	**0** Drainage Device **1** Radioactive Element **7** Autologous Tissue Substitute **D** Intraluminal Device **J** Synthetic Substitute **K** Nonautologous Tissue Substitute **Y** Other Device	**Z** No Qualifier
Y Mouth and Throat	**X** External	**0** Drainage Device **1** Radioactive Element **7** Autologous Tissue Substitute **D** Intraluminal Device **J** Synthetic Substitute **K** Nonautologous Tissue Substitute	**Z** No Qualifier

0 Medical and Surgical
C Mouth and Throat
Q Repair: Restoring, to the extent possible, a body part to its normal anatomic structure and function

Body Part	Approach	Device	Qualifier
Character 4	**Character 5**	**Character 6**	**Character 7**
0 Upper Lip **1** Lower Lip **2** Hard Palate **3** Soft Palate **4** Buccal Mucosa **5** Upper Gingiva **6** Lower Gingiva **7** Tongue **N** Uvula **P** Tonsils **Q** Adenoids	**0** Open **3** Percutaneous **X** External	**Z** No Device	**Z** No Qualifier
8 Parotid Gland, Right **9** Parotid Gland, Left **B** Parotid Duct, Right **C** Parotid Duct, Left **D** Sublingual Gland, Right **F** Sublingual Gland, Left **G** Submaxillary Gland, Right **H** Submaxillary Gland, Left **J** Minor Salivary Gland	**0** Open **3** Percutaneous	**Z** No Device	**Z** No Qualifier
M Pharynx **R** Epiglottis **S** Larynx **T** Vocal Cord, Right **V** Vocal Cord, Left	**0** Open **3** Percutaneous **4** Percutaneous Endoscopic **7** Via Natural or Artificial Opening **8** Via Natural or Artificial Opening Endoscopic	**Z** No Device	**Z** No Qualifier
W Upper Tooth **X** Lower Tooth	**0** Open **X** External	**Z** No Device	**0** Single **1** Multiple **2** All

LC Limited Coverage   NC Noncovered   HAC HAC-associated Procedure   CC Combination Cluster - See Appendix G for code lists
DRG Non-OR-Affecting MS-DRG Assignment   New/Revised Text in **Orange**   ♂ Male   ♀ Female

0 Medical and Surgical
C Mouth and Throat
R Replacement: Putting in or on biological or synthetic material that physically takes the place and/or function of all or a portion of a body part

Body Part	Approach	Device	Qualifier
Character 4	Character 5	Character 6	Character 7
0 Upper Lip 1 Lower Lip 2 Hard Palate 3 Soft Palate 4 Buccal Mucosa 5 Upper Gingiva 6 Lower Gingiva 7 Tongue N Uvula	0 Open 3 Percutaneous X External	7 Autologous Tissue Substitute J Synthetic Substitute K Nonautologous Tissue Substitute	Z No Qualifier
B Parotid Duct, Right C Parotid Duct, Left	0 Open 3 Percutaneous	7 Autologous Tissue Substitute J Synthetic Substitute K Nonautologous Tissue Substitute	Z No Qualifier
M Pharynx R Epiglottis S Larynx T Vocal Cord, Right V Vocal Cord, Left	0 Open 7 Via Natural or Artificial Opening 8 Via Natural or Artificial Opening Endoscopic	7 Autologous Tissue Substitute J Synthetic Substitute K Nonautologous Tissue Substitute	Z No Qualifier
W Upper Tooth X Lower Tooth	0 Open X External	7 Autologous Tissue Substitute J Synthetic Substitute K Nonautologous Tissue Substitute	0 Single 1 Multiple 2 All

0 Medical and Surgical
C Mouth and Throat
S Reposition: Moving to its normal location, or other suitable location, all or a portion of a body part

Body Part	Approach	Device	Qualifier
Character 4	Character 5	Character 6	Character 7
0 Upper Lip 1 Lower Lip 2 Hard Palate 3 Soft Palate 7 Tongue N Uvula	0 Open X External	Z No Device	Z No Qualifier
B Parotid Duct, Right C Parotid Duct, Left	0 Open 3 Percutaneous	Z No Device	Z No Qualifier
R Epiglottis T Vocal Cord, Right V Vocal Cord, Left	0 Open 7 Via Natural or Artificial Opening 8 Via Natural or Artificial Opening Endoscopic	Z No Device	Z No Qualifier
W Upper Tooth X Lower Tooth	0 Open X External	5 External Fixation Device Z No Device	0 Single 1 Multiple 2 All

LC Limited Coverage   NC Noncovered   HAC HAC-associated Procedure   CC Combination Cluster - See Appendix G for code lists
DRG Non-OR-Affecting MS-DRG Assignment   New/Revised Text in Orange   ♂ Male   ♀ Female

316

2018 ICD-10-PCS

MOUTH AND THROAT 0C0-0CX

0 **Medical and Surgical**
C **Mouth and Throat**
T **Resection:** Cutting out or off, without replacement, all of a body part

Body Part	Approach	Device	Qualifier
Character 4	Character 5	Character 6	Character 7
0 Upper Lip 1 Lower Lip 2 Hard Palate 3 Soft Palate 7 Tongue N Uvula P Tonsils Q Adenoids	0 Open X External	Z No Device	Z No Qualifier
8 Parotid Gland, Right 9 Parotid Gland, Left B Parotid Duct, Right C Parotid Duct, Left D Sublingual Gland, Right F Sublingual Gland, Left G Submaxillary Gland, Right H Submaxillary Gland, Left J Minor Salivary Gland	0 Open	Z No Device	Z No Qualifier
M Pharynx R Epiglottis S Larynx T Vocal Cord, Right V Vocal Cord, Left	0 Open 4 Percutaneous Endoscopic 7 Via Natural or Artificial Opening 8 Via Natural or Artificial Opening Endoscopic	Z No Device	Z No Qualifier
W Upper Tooth X Lower Tooth	0 Open	Z No Device	0 Single 1 Multiple 2 All

0 **Medical and Surgical**
C **Mouth and Throat**
U **Supplement:** Putting in or on biological or synthetic material that physically reinforces and/or augments the function of a portion of a body part

Body Part	Approach	Device	Qualifier
Character 4	Character 5	Character 6	Character 7
0 Upper Lip 1 Lower Lip 2 Hard Palate 3 Soft Palate 4 Buccal Mucosa 5 Upper Gingiva 6 Lower Gingiva 7 Tongue N Uvula	0 Open 3 Percutaneous X External	7 Autologous Tissue Substitute J Synthetic Substitute K Nonautologous Tissue Substitute	Z No Qualifier
M Pharynx R Epiglottis S Larynx T Vocal Cord, Right V Vocal Cord, Left	0 Open 7 Via Natural or Artificial Opening 8 Via Natural or Artificial Opening Endoscopic	7 Autologous Tissue Substitute J Synthetic Substitute K Nonautologous Tissue Substitute	Z No Qualifier

0 **Medical and Surgical**
C **Mouth and Throat**
V **Restriction:** Partially closing an orifice or the lumen of a tubular body part

Body Part	Approach	Device	Qualifier
Character 4	**Character 5**	**Character 6**	**Character 7**
B Parotid Duct, Right **C** Parotid Duct, Left	**0** Open **3** Percutaneous	**C** Extraluminal Device **D** Intraluminal Device **Z** No Device	**Z** No Qualifier
B Parotid Duct, Right **C** Parotid Duct, Left	**7** Via Natural or Artificial Opening **8** Via Natural or Artificial Opening Endoscopic	**D** Intraluminal Device **Z** No Device	**Z** No Qualifier

0 **Medical and Surgical**
C **Mouth and Throat**
W **Revision:** Correcting, to the extent possible, a portion of a malfunctioning device or the position of a displaced device

Body Part	Approach	Device	Qualifier
Character 4	**Character 5**	**Character 6**	**Character 7**
A Salivary Gland	**0** Open **3** Percutaneous	**0** Drainage Device **C** Extraluminal Device **Y** Other Device	**Z** No Qualifier
A Salivary Gland	**7** Via Natural or Artificial Opening **8** Via Natural or Artificial Opening Endoscopic	**Y** Other Device	**Z** No Qualifier
A Salivary Gland	**X** External	**0** Drainage Device **C** Extraluminal Device	**Z** No Qualifier
S Larynx	**0** Open **3** Percutaneous **7** Via Natural or Artificial Opening **8** Via Natural or Artificial Opening Endoscopic	**0** Drainage Device **7** Autologous Tissue Substitute **D** Intraluminal Device **J** Synthetic Substitute **K** Nonautologous Tissue Substitute **Y** Other Device	**Z** No Qualifier
S Larynx	**X** External	**0** Drainage Device **7** Autologous Tissue Substitute **D** Intraluminal Device **J** Synthetic Substitute **K** Nonautologous Tissue Substitute	**Z** No Qualifier
Y Mouth and Throat	**0** Open **3** Percutaneous **7** Via Natural or Artificial Opening **8** Via Natural or Artificial Opening Endoscopic	**0** Drainage Device **1** Radioactive Element **7** Autologous Tissue Substitute **D** Intraluminal Device **J** Synthetic Substitute **K** Nonautologous Tissue Substitute **Y** Other Device	**Z** No Qualifier
Y Mouth and Throat	**X** External	**0** Drainage Device **1** Radioactive Element **7** Autologous Tissue Substitute **D** Intraluminal Device **J** Synthetic Substitute **K** Nonautologous Tissue Substitute	**Z** No Qualifier

0 **Medical and Surgical**
C **Mouth and Throat**
X **Transfer:** Moving, without taking out, all or a portion of a body part to another location to take over the function of all or a portion of a body part

Body Part	Approach	Device	Qualifier
Character 4	**Character 5**	**Character 6**	**Character 7**
0 Upper Lip **1** Lower Lip **3** Soft Palate **4** Buccal Mucosa **5** Upper Gingiva **6** Lower Gingiva **7** Tongue	**0** Open **X** External	**Z** No Device	**Z** No Qualifier

NOTES

NOTES

Gastrointestinal System 0D1-0DY

0 **Medical and Surgical**
D **Gastrointestinal System**
1 **Bypass:** Altering the route of passage of the contents of a tubular body part

Body Part	Approach	Device	Qualifier
Character 4	Character 5	Character 6	Character 7
1 Esophagus, Upper 2 Esophagus, Middle 3 Esophagus, Lower 5 Esophagus	0 Open 4 Percutaneous Endoscopic 8 Via Natural or Artificial Opening Endoscopic	7 Autologous Tissue Substitute J Synthetic Substitute K Nonautologous Tissue Substitute Z No Device	4 Cutaneous 6 Stomach 9 Duodenum A Jejunum B Ileum
1 Esophagus, Upper 2 Esophagus, Middle 3 Esophagus, Lower 5 Esophagus	3 Percutaneous	J Synthetic Substitute	4 Cutaneous
6 Stomach ᴴᴬᶜ 9 Duodenum	0 Open 4 Percutaneous Endoscopic 8 Via Natural or Artificial Opening Endoscopic	7 Autologous Tissue Substitute J Synthetic Substitute K Nonautologous Tissue Substitute Z No Device	4 Cutaneous 9 Duodenum A Jejunum B Ileum L Transverse Colon
6 Stomach 9 Duodenum	3 Percutaneous	J Synthetic Substitute	4 Cutaneous
A Jejunum	0 Open 4 Percutaneous Endoscopic 8 Via Natural or Artificial Opening Endoscopic	7 Autologous Tissue Substitute J Synthetic Substitute K Nonautologous Tissue Substitute Z No Device	4 Cutaneous A Jejunum B Ileum H Cecum K Ascending Colon L Transverse Colon M Descending Colon N Sigmoid Colon P Rectum Q Anus
A Jejunum	3 Percutaneous	J Synthetic Substitute	4 Cutaneous
B Ileum	0 Open 4 Percutaneous Endoscopic 8 Via Natural or Artificial Opening Endoscopic	7 Autologous Tissue Substitute J Synthetic Substitute K Nonautologous Tissue Substitute Z No Device	4 Cutaneous B Ileum H Cecum K Ascending Colon L Transverse Colon M Descending Colon N Sigmoid Colon P Rectum Q Anus
B Ileum	3 Percutaneous	J Synthetic Substitute	4 Cutaneous
H Cecum	0 Open 4 Percutaneous Endoscopic 8 Via Natural or Artificial Opening Endoscopic	7 Autologous Tissue Substitute J Synthetic Substitute K Nonautologous Tissue Substitute Z No Device	4 Cutaneous H Cecum K Ascending Colon L Transverse Colon M Descending Colon N Sigmoid Colon P Rectum
H Cecum	3 Percutaneous	J Synthetic Substitute	4 Cutaneous
K Ascending Colon	0 Open 4 Percutaneous Endoscopic 8 Via Natural or Artificial Opening Endoscopic	7 Autologous Tissue Substitute J Synthetic Substitute K Nonautologous Tissue Substitute Z No Device	4 Cutaneous K Ascending Colon L Transverse Colon M Descending Colon N Sigmoid Colon P Rectum
K Ascending Colon	3 Percutaneous	J Synthetic Substitute	4 Cutaneous

0D1 continued on next page

ᴸᶜ Limited Coverage ᴺᶜ Noncovered ᴴᴬᶜ HAC-associated Procedure ᶜᶜ Combination Cluster - See Appendix G for code lists
ᴰᴿᴳ Non-OR-Affecting MS-DRG Assignment New/Revised Text in **Orange** ♂ Male ♀ Female

0 **Medical and Surgical**
D **Gastrointestinal System**
1 **Bypass:** Altering the route of passage of the contents of a tubular body part

0D1 continued from previous page

Body Part	Approach	Device	Qualifier
Character 4	Character 5	Character 6	Character 7
L Transverse Colon	0 Open 4 Percutaneous Endoscopic 8 Via Natural or Artificial Opening Endoscopic	7 Autologous Tissue Substitute J Synthetic Substitute K Nonautologous Tissue Substitute Z No Device	4 Cutaneous L Transverse Colon M Descending Colon N Sigmoid Colon P Rectum
L Transverse Colon	3 Percutaneous	J Synthetic Substitute	4 Cutaneous
M Descending Colon	0 Open 4 Percutaneous Endoscopic 8 Via Natural or Artificial Opening Endoscopic	7 Autologous Tissue Substitute J Synthetic Substitute K Nonautologous Tissue Substitute Z No Device	4 Cutaneous M Descending Colon N Sigmoid Colon P Rectum
M Descending Colon	3 Percutaneous	J Synthetic Substitute	4 Cutaneous
N Sigmoid Colon	0 Open 4 Percutaneous Endoscopic 8 Via Natural or Artificial Opening Endoscopic	7 Autologous Tissue Substitute J Synthetic Substitute K Nonautologous Tissue Substitute Z No Device	4 Cutaneous N Sigmoid Colon P Rectum
N Sigmoid Colon	3 Percutaneous	J Synthetic Substitute	4 Cutaneous

HAC 0D16079   0D1607A   0D1607B   0D1607L   0D160J9   0D160JA   0D160JB   0D160JL   0D160K9   0D160KA   0D160KB   0D160KL   0D160Z9
0D160ZA   0D160ZB   0D160ZL   0D16479   0D1647A   0D1647B   0D1647L   0D164J9   0D164JA   0D164JB   0D164JL   0D164K9   0D164KA
0D164KB   0D164KL   0D164Z9   0D164ZA   0D164ZB   0D164ZL   0D16879   0D1687A   0D1687B   0D1687L   0D168J9   0D168JA   0D168JB
0D168JL   0D168K9   0D168KA   0D168KB   0D168KL   0D168Z9   0D168ZA   0D168ZB   0D168ZL
Surgical site infection following bariatric surgery procedures and principal diagnoses E66.01 and secondary diagnoses K68.11, K95.01, K95.81, T81.4XXA.

0 **Medical and Surgical**
D **Gastrointestinal System**
2 **Change:** Taking out or off a device from a body part and putting back an identical or similar device in or on the same body part without cutting or puncturing the skin or a mucous membrane

Body Part	Approach	Device	Qualifier
Character 4	Character 5	Character 6	Character 7
0 Upper Intestinal Tract D Lower Intestinal Tract	X External	0 Drainage Device U Feeding Device Y Other Device	Z No Qualifier
U Omentum V Mesentery W Peritoneum	X External	0 Drainage Device Y Other Device	Z No Qualifier

LC Limited Coverage   NC Noncovered   HAC HAC-associated Procedure   CC Combination Cluster - See Appendix G for code lists
DRG Non-OR-Affecting MS-DRG Assignment   New/Revised Text in **Orange**   ♂ Male   ♀ Female

322

2018 ICD-10-PCS

0 **Medical and Surgical**
D **Gastrointestinal System**
5 **Destruction:** Physical eradication of all or a portion of a body part by the direct use of energy, force, or a destructive agent

Body Part	Approach	Device	Qualifier
Character 4	**Character 5**	**Character 6**	**Character 7**
1 Esophagus, Upper 2 Esophagus, Middle 3 Esophagus, Lower 4 Esophagogastric Junction 5 Esophagus 6 Stomach 7 Stomach, Pylorus 8 Small Intestine 9 Duodenum A Jejunum B Ileum C Ileocecal Valve E Large Intestine F Large Intestine, Right G Large Intestine, Left H Cecum J Appendix K Ascending Colon L Transverse Colon M Descending Colon N Sigmoid Colon P Rectum	0 Open 3 Percutaneous 4 Percutaneous Endoscopic 7 Via Natural or Artificial Opening 8 Via Natural or Artificial Opening Endoscopic	Z No Device	Z No Qualifier
Q Anus	0 Open 3 Percutaneous 4 Percutaneous Endoscopic 7 Via Natural or Artificial Opening 8 Via Natural or Artificial Opening Endoscopic X External	Z No Device	Z No Qualifier
R Anal Sphincter U Omentum V Mesentery W Peritoneum	0 Open 3 Percutaneous 4 Percutaneous Endoscopic	Z No Device	Z No Qualifier

LC Limited Coverage   NC Noncovered   HAC HAC-associated Procedure   CC Combination Cluster - See Appendix G for code lists
DRG Non-OR-Affecting MS-DRG Assignment   New/Revised Text in **Orange**   ♂ Male   ♀ Female

2018 ICD-10-PCS

323

0 **Medical and Surgical**
D **Gastrointestinal System**
7 **Dilation:** Expanding an orifice or the lumen of a tubular body part

Body Part	Approach	Device	Qualifier
Character 4	Character 5	Character 6	Character 7
1 Esophagus, Upper 2 Esophagus, Middle 3 Esophagus, Lower 4 Esophagogastric Junction 5 Esophagus 6 Stomach 7 Stomach, Pylorus 8 Small Intestine 9 Duodenum A Jejunum B Ileum C Ileocecal Valve E Large Intestine F Large Intestine, Right G Large Intestine, Left H Cecum K Ascending Colon L Transverse Colon M Descending Colon N Sigmoid Colon P Rectum Q Anus	0 Open 3 Percutaneous 4 Percutaneous Endoscopic 7 Via Natural or Artificial Opening 8 Via Natural or Artificial Opening Endoscopic	D Intraluminal Device Z No Device	Z No Qualifier

0 **Medical and Surgical**
D **Gastrointestinal System**
8 **Division:** Cutting into a body part, without draining fluids and/or gases from the body part, in order to separate or transect a body part

Body Part	Approach	Device	Qualifier
Character 4	Character 5	Character 6	Character 7
4 Esophagogastric Junction 7 Stomach, Pylorus	0 Open 3 Percutaneous 4 Percutaneous Endoscopic 7 Via Natural or Artificial Opening 8 Via Natural or Artificial Opening Endoscopic	Z No Device	Z No Qualifier
R Anal Sphincter	0 Open 3 Percutaneous	Z No Device	Z No Qualifier

LC Limited Coverage   NC Noncovered   HAC HAC-associated Procedure   CC Combination Cluster - See Appendix G for code lists
DRG Non-OR-Affecting MS-DRG Assignment   New/Revised Text in **Orange**   ♂ Male   ♀ Female

324

2018 ICD-10-PCS

0 **Medical and Surgical**
D **Gastrointestinal System**
9 **Drainage:** Taking or letting out fluids and/or gases from a body part

Body Part Character 4	Approach Character 5	Device Character 6	Qualifier Character 7
1 Esophagus, Upper 2 Esophagus, Middle 3 Esophagus, Lower 4 Esophagogastric Junction 5 Esophagus 6 Stomach 7 Stomach, Pylorus 8 Small Intestine 9 Duodenum A Jejunum B Ileum C Ileocecal Valve E Large Intestine F Large Intestine, Right G Large Intestine, Left H Cecum J Appendix K Ascending Colon L Transverse Colon M Descending Colon N Sigmoid Colon P Rectum	0 Open 3 Percutaneous 4 Percutaneous Endoscopic 7 Via Natural or Artificial Opening 8 Via Natural or Artificial Opening Endoscopic	0 Drainage Device	Z No Qualifier
1 Esophagus, Upper 2 Esophagus, Middle 3 Esophagus, Lower 4 Esophagogastric Junction 5 Esophagus 6 Stomach 7 Stomach, Pylorus 8 Small Intestine 9 Duodenum A Jejunum B Ileum C Ileocecal Valve E Large Intestine F Large Intestine, Right G Large Intestine, Left H Cecum J Appendix K Ascending Colon L Transverse Colon M Descending Colon N Sigmoid Colon P Rectum	0 Open 3 Percutaneous 4 Percutaneous Endoscopic 7 Via Natural or Artificial Opening 8 Via Natural or Artificial Opening Endoscopic	Z No Device	X Diagnostic Z No Qualifier
Q Anus	0 Open 3 Percutaneous 4 Percutaneous Endoscopic 7 Via Natural or Artificial Opening 8 Via Natural or Artificial Opening Endoscopic X External	0 Drainage Device	Z No Qualifier
Q Anus	0 Open 3 Percutaneous 4 Percutaneous Endoscopic 7 Via Natural or Artificial Opening 8 Via Natural or Artificial Opening Endoscopic X External	Z No Device	X Diagnostic Z No Qualifier

0D9 continued on next page

LC Limited Coverage   NC Noncovered   HAC HAC-associated Procedure   CC Combination Cluster - See Appendix G for code lists
DRG Non-OR-Affecting MS-DRG Assignment   New/Revised Text in **Orange**   ♂ Male   ♀ Female

0 Medical and Surgical
D Gastrointestinal System
9 Drainage: Taking or letting out fluids and/or gases from a body part

0D9 continued from previous page

Body Part	Approach	Device	Qualifier
Character 4	**Character 5**	**Character 6**	**Character 7**
R Anal Sphincter **U** Omentum **V** Mesentery **W** Peritoneum	**0** Open **3** Percutaneous **4** Percutaneous Endoscopic	**0** Drainage Device	**Z** No Qualifier
R Anal Sphincter **U** Omentum **V** Mesentery **W** Peritoneum	**0** Open **3** Percutaneous **4** Percutaneous Endoscopic	**Z** No Device	**X** Diagnostic **Z** No Qualifier

0 Medical and Surgical
D Gastrointestinal System
B Excision: Cutting out or off, without replacement, a portion of a body part

Body Part	Approach	Device	Qualifier
Character 4	**Character 5**	**Character 6**	**Character 7**
1 Esophagus, Upper **2** Esophagus, Middle **3** Esophagus, Lower **4** Esophagogastric Junction **5** Esophagus **7** Stomach, Pylorus **8** Small Intestine **9** Duodenum **A** Jejunum **B** Ileum **C** Ileocecal Valve **E** Large Intestine **F** Large Intestine, Right **H** Cecum **J** Appendix **K** Ascending Colon **P** Rectum	**0** Open **3** Percutaneous **4** Percutaneous Endoscopic **7** Via Natural or Artificial Opening **8** Via Natural or Artificial Opening Endoscopic	**Z** No Device	**X** Diagnostic **Z** No Qualifier
6 Stomach	**0** Open **3** Percutaneous **4** Percutaneous Endoscopic **7** Via Natural or Artificial Opening **8** Via Natural or Artificial Opening Endoscopic	**Z** No Device	**3** Vertical **X** Diagnostic **Z** No Qualifier
G Large Intestine, Left **L** Transverse Colon **M** Descending Colon **N** Sigmoid Colon	**0** Open **3** Percutaneous **4** Percutaneous Endoscopic **7** Via Natural or Artificial Opening **8** Via Natural or Artificial Opening Endoscopic	**Z** No Device	**X** Diagnostic **Z** No Qualifier
G Large Intestine, Left **L** Transverse Colon **M** Descending Colon **N** Sigmoid Colon	**F** Via Natural or Artificial Opening With Percutaneous Endoscopic Assistance	**Z** No Device	**Z** No Qualifier
Q Anus	**0** Open **3** Percutaneous **4** Percutaneous Endoscopic **7** Via Natural or Artificial Opening **8** Via Natural or Artificial Opening Endoscopic **X** External	**Z** No Device	**X** Diagnostic **Z** No Qualifier

0DB continued on next page

LC Limited Coverage   **NC** Noncovered   **HAC** HAC-associated Procedure   **CC** Combination Cluster - See Appendix G for code lists
DRG Non-OR-Affecting MS-DRG Assignment   New/Revised Text in **Orange**   ♂ Male   ♀ Female

326

2018 ICD-10-PCS

0DB continued from previous page

0 Medical and Surgical
D Gastrointestinal System
B **Excision:** Cutting out or off, without replacement, a portion of a body part

Body Part	Approach	Device	Qualifier
Character 4	Character 5	Character 6	Character 7
R Anal Sphincter **U** Omentum **V** Mesentery **W** Peritoneum	**0** Open **3** Percutaneous **4** Percutaneous Endoscopic	**Z** No Device	**X** Diagnostic **Z** No Qualifier

0 Medical and Surgical
D Gastrointestinal System
C **Extirpation:** Taking or cutting out solid matter from a body part

Body Part	Approach	Device	Qualifier
Character 4	Character 5	Character 6	Character 7
1 Esophagus, Upper **2** Esophagus, Middle **3** Esophagus, Lower **4** Esophagogastric Junction **5** Esophagus **6** Stomach **7** Stomach, Pylorus **8** Small Intestine **9** Duodenum **A** Jejunum **B** Ileum **C** Ileocecal Valve **E** Large Intestine **F** Large Intestine, Right **G** Large Intestine, Left **H** Cecum **J** Appendix **K** Ascending Colon **L** Transverse Colon **M** Descending Colon **N** Sigmoid Colon **P** Rectum	**0** Open **3** Percutaneous **4** Percutaneous Endoscopic **7** Via Natural or Artificial Opening **8** Via Natural or Artificial Opening Endoscopic	**Z** No Device	**Z** No Qualifier
Q Anus	**0** Open **3** Percutaneous **4** Percutaneous Endoscopic **7** Via Natural or Artificial Opening **8** Via Natural or Artificial Opening Endoscopic **X** External	**Z** No Device	**Z** No Qualifier
R Anal Sphincter **U** Omentum **V** Mesentery **W** Peritoneum	**0** Open **3** Percutaneous **4** Percutaneous Endoscopic	**Z** No Device	**Z** No Qualifier

IC Limited Coverage **NC** Noncovered **HAC** HAC-associated Procedure **CC** Combination Cluster - See Appendix G for code lists
DRG Non-OR-Affecting MS-DRG Assignment New/Revised Text in **Orange** ♂ Male ♀ Female

2018 ICD-10-PCS

327

GASTROINTESTINAL SYSTEM 0D1-0DY

0DB-0DC

0 Medical and Surgical
D Gastrointestinal System
D Extraction: Pulling or stripping out or off all or a portion of a body part by the use of force

Body Part	Approach	Device	Qualifier
Character 4	Character 5	Character 6	Character 7
1 Esophagus, Upper 2 Esophagus, Middle 3 Esophagus, Lower 4 Esophagogastric Junction 5 Esophagus 6 Stomach 7 Stomach, Pylorus 8 Small Intestine 9 Duodenum A Jejunum B Ileum C Ileocecal Valve E Large Intestine F Large Intestine, Right G Large Intestine, Left H Cecum J Appendix K Ascending Colon L Transverse Colon M Descending Colon N Sigmoid Colon P Rectum	3 Percutaneous 4 Percutaneous Endoscopic 8 Via Natural or Artificial Opening Endoscopic	Z No Device	X Diagnostic
Q Anus	3 Percutaneous 4 Percutaneous Endoscopic 8 Via Natural or Artificial Opening Endoscopic X External	Z No Device	X Diagnostic

0 Medical and Surgical
D Gastrointestinal System
F Fragmentation: Breaking solid matter in a body part into pieces

Body Part	Approach	Device	Qualifier
Character 4	Character 5	Character 6	Character 7
5 Esophagus NC 6 Stomach NC 8 Small Intestine NC 9 Duodenum NC A Jejunum NC B Ileum NC E Large Intestine NC F Large Intestine, Right NC G Large Intestine, Left NC H Cecum NC J Appendix NC K Ascending Colon NC L Transverse Colon NC M Descending Colon NC N Sigmoid Colon NC P Rectum NC Q Anus NC	0 Open 3 Percutaneous 4 Percutaneous Endoscopic 7 Via Natural or Artificial Opening 8 Via Natural or Artificial Opening Endoscopic X External	Z No Device	Z No Qualifier

NC 0DF5XZZ   0DF6XZZ   0DF8XZZ   0DF9XZZ   0DFAXZZ   0DFBXZZ   0DFEXZZ   0DFFXZZ   0DFGXZZ   0DFHXZZ   0DFJXZZ   0DFKXZZ   0DFLXZZ
0DFMXZZ   0DFNXZZ   0DFPXZZ   0DFQXZZ

0   Medical and Surgical
D   Gastrointestinal System
H   Insertion: Putting in a nonbiological appliance that monitors, assists, performs, or prevents a physiological function but does not physically take the place of a body part

Body Part	Approach	Device	Qualifier
Character 4	Character 5	Character 6	Character 7
0 Upper Intestinal Tract D Lower Intestinal Tract	0 Open 3 Percutaneous 4 Percutaneous Endoscopic 7 Via Natural or Artificial Opening 8 Via Natural or Artificial Opening Endoscopic	Y Other Device	Z No Qualifier
5 Esophagus	0 Open 3 Percutaneous 4 Percutaneous Endoscopic	1 Radioactive Element 2 Monitoring Device 3 Infusion Device D Intraluminal Device U Feeding Device Y Other Device	Z No Qualifier
5 Esophagus	7 Via Natural or Artificial Opening 8 Via Natural or Artificial Opening Endoscopic	1 Radioactive Element 2 Monitoring Device 3 Infusion Device B Intraluminal Device, Airway D Intraluminal Device U Feeding Device Y Other Device	Z No Qualifier
6 Stomach ☒	0 Open 3 Percutaneous 4 Percutaneous Endoscopic	2 Monitoring Device 3 Infusion Device D Intraluminal Device M Stimulator Lead U Feeding Device Y Other Device	Z No Qualifier
6 Stomach	7 Via Natural or Artificial Opening 8 Via Natural or Artificial Opening Endoscopic	2 Monitoring Device 3 Infusion Device D Intraluminal Device U Feeding Device Y Other Device	Z No Qualifier
8 Small Intestine 9 Duodenum A Jejunum B Ileum	0 Open 3 Percutaneous 4 Percutaneous Endoscopic 7 Via Natural or Artificial Opening 8 Via Natural or Artificial Opening Endoscopic	2 Monitoring Device 3 Infusion Device D Intraluminal Device U Feeding Device	Z No Qualifier
E Large Intestine	0 Open 3 Percutaneous 4 Percutaneous Endoscopic 7 Via Natural or Artificial Opening 8 Via Natural or Artificial Opening Endoscopic	D Intraluminal Device	Z No Qualifier
P Rectum	0 Open 3 Percutaneous 4 Percutaneous Endoscopic 7 Via Natural or Artificial Opening 8 Via Natural or Artificial Opening Endoscopic	1 Radioactive Element D Intraluminal Device	Z No Qualifier
Q Anus	0 Open 3 Percutaneous 4 Percutaneous Endoscopic	D Intraluminal Device L Artificial Sphincter	Z No Qualifier
Q Anus	7 Via Natural or Artificial Opening 8 Via Natural or Artificial Opening Endoscopic	D Intraluminal Device	Z No Qualifier
R Anal Sphincter	0 Open 3 Percutaneous 4 Percutaneous Endoscopic	M Stimulator Lead	Z No Qualifier

☒ 0DH60MZ   0DH63MZ   0DH64MZ

☒ Limited Coverage   ☒ Noncovered   ☒ HAC-associated Procedure   ☒ Combination Cluster - See Appendix G for code lists
☒ Non-OR-Affecting MS-DRG Assignment   New/Revised Text in **Orange**   ♂ Male   ♀ Female

0 **Medical and Surgical**
D **Gastrointestinal System**
J **Inspection:** Visually and/or manually exploring a body part

Body Part	Approach	Device	Qualifier
Character 4	Character 5	Character 6	Character 7
0 Upper Intestinal Tract **6** Stomach **D** Lower Intestinal Tract	**0** Open **3** Percutaneous **4** Percutaneous Endoscopic **7** Via Natural or Artificial Opening **8** Via Natural or Artificial Opening Endoscopic **X** External	**Z** No Device	**Z** No Qualifier
U Omentum **V** Mesentery **W** Peritoneum	**0** Open **3** Percutaneous **4** Percutaneous Endoscopic **X** External	**Z** No Device	**Z** No Qualifier

0 **Medical and Surgical**
D **Gastrointestinal System**
L **Occlusion:** Completely closing an orifice or the lumen of a tubular body part

Body Part	Approach	Device	Qualifier
Character 4	Character 5	Character 6	Character 7
1 Esophagus, Upper **2** Esophagus, Middle **3** Esophagus, Lower **4** Esophagogastric Junction **5** Esophagus **6** Stomach **7** Stomach, Pylorus **8** Small Intestine **9** Duodenum **A** Jejunum **B** Ileum **C** Ileocecal Valve **E** Large Intestine **F** Large Intestine, Right **G** Large Intestine, Left **H** Cecum **K** Ascending Colon **L** Transverse Colon **M** Descending Colon **N** Sigmoid Colon **P** Rectum	**0** Open **3** Percutaneous **4** Percutaneous Endoscopic	**C** Extraluminal Device **D** Intraluminal Device **Z** No Device	**Z** No Qualifier
1 Esophagus, Upper **2** Esophagus, Middle **3** Esophagus, Lower **4** Esophagogastric Junction **5** Esophagus **6** Stomach **7** Stomach, Pylorus **8** Small Intestine **9** Duodenum **A** Jejunum **B** Ileum **C** Ileocecal Valve **E** Large Intestine **F** Large Intestine, Right **G** Large Intestine, Left **H** Cecum **K** Ascending Colon **L** Transverse Colon **M** Descending Colon **N** Sigmoid Colon **P** Rectum	**7** Via Natural or Artificial Opening **8** Via Natural or Artificial Opening Endoscopic	**D** Intraluminal Device **Z** No Device	**Z** No Qualifier

0DL continued on next page

LC Limited Coverage **NC** Noncovered **HAC** HAC-associated Procedure **CC** Combination Cluster - See Appendix G for code lists
DRG Non-OR-Affecting MS-DRG Assignment   New/Revised Text in **Orange**   ♂ Male   ♀ Female

330

2018 ICD-10-PCS

0 Medical and Surgical
D Gastrointestinal System
L Occlusion: Completely closing an orifice or the lumen of a tubular body part

0DL continued from previous page

Body Part	Approach	Device	Qualifier
Character 4	**Character 5**	**Character 6**	**Character 7**
Q Anus	**0** Open **3** Percutaneous **4** Percutaneous Endoscopic **X** External	**C** Extraluminal Device **D** Intraluminal Device **Z** No Device	**Z** No Qualifier
Q Anus	**7** Via Natural or Artificial Opening **8** Via Natural or Artificial Opening Endoscopic	**D** Intraluminal Device **Z** No Device	**Z** No Qualifier

0 Medical and Surgical
D Gastrointestinal System
M Reattachment: Putting back in or on all or a portion of a separated body part to its normal location or other suitable location

Body Part	Approach	Device	Qualifier
Character 4	**Character 5**	**Character 6**	**Character 7**
5 Esophagus **6** Stomach **8** Small Intestine **9** Duodenum **A** Jejunum **B** Ileum **E** Large Intestine **F** Large Intestine, Right **G** Large Intestine, Left **H** Cecum **K** Ascending Colon **L** Transverse Colon **M** Descending Colon **N** Sigmoid Colon **P** Rectum	**0** Open **4** Percutaneous Endoscopic	**Z** No Device	**Z** No Qualifier

0 Medical and Surgical
D Gastrointestinal System
N Release: Freeing a body part from an abnormal physical constraint by cutting or by the use of force

Body Part	Approach	Device	Qualifier
Character 4	**Character 5**	**Character 6**	**Character 7**
1 Esophagus, Upper **2** Esophagus, Middle **3** Esophagus, Lower **4** Esophagogastric Junction **5** Esophagus **6** Stomach **7** Stomach, Pylorus **8** Small Intestine **9** Duodenum **A** Jejunum **B** Ileum **C** Ileocecal Valve **E** Large Intestine **F** Large Intestine, Right **G** Large Intestine, Left **H** Cecum **J** Appendix **K** Ascending Colon **L** Transverse Colon **M** Descending Colon **N** Sigmoid Colon **P** Rectum	**0** Open **3** Percutaneous **4** Percutaneous Endoscopic **7** Via Natural or Artificial Opening **8** Via Natural or Artificial Opening Endoscopic	**Z** No Device	**Z** No Qualifier

0DN continued on next page

LC Limited Coverage   NC Noncovered   HAC HAC-associated Procedure   CC Combination Cluster - See Appendix G for code lists
DRG Non-OR-Affecting MS-DRG Assignment   New/Revised Text in **Orange**   ♂ Male   ♀ Female

0 Medical and Surgical
D Gastrointestinal System
N Release: Freeing a body part from an abnormal physical constraint by cutting or by the use of force

ODN continued from previous page

Body Part	Approach	Device	Qualifier
Character 4	Character 5	Character 6	Character 7
Q Anus	**0** Open **3** Percutaneous **4** Percutaneous Endoscopic **7** Via Natural or Artificial Opening **8** Via Natural or Artificial Opening Endoscopic **X** External	**Z** No Device	**Z** No Qualifier
R Anal Sphincter **U** Omentum **V** Mesentery **W** Peritoneum	**0** Open **3** Percutaneous **4** Percutaneous Endoscopic	**Z** No Device	**Z** No Qualifier

0 Medical and Surgical
D Gastrointestinal System
P Removal: Taking out or off a device from a body part

Body Part	Approach	Device	Qualifier
Character 4	Character 5	Character 6	Character 7
0 Upper Intestinal Tract **D** Lower Intestinal Tract	**0** Open **3** Percutaneous **4** Percutaneous Endoscopic **7** Via Natural or Artificial Opening **8** Via Natural or Artificial Opening Endoscopic	**0** Drainage Device **2** Monitoring Device **3** Infusion Device **7** Autologous Tissue Substitute **C** Extraluminal Device **D** Intraluminal Device **J** Synthetic Substitute **K** Nonautologous Tissue Substitute **U** Feeding Device **Y** Other Device	**Z** No Qualifier
0 Upper Intestinal Tract **D** Lower Intestinal Tract	**X** External	**0** Drainage Device **2** Monitoring Device **3** Infusion Device **D** Intraluminal Device **U** Feeding Device	**Z** No Qualifier
5 Esophagus	**0** Open **3** Percutaneous **4** Percutaneous Endoscopic	**1** Radioactive Element **2** Monitoring Device **3** Infusion Device **U** Feeding Device **Y** Other Device	**Z** No Qualifier
5 Esophagus	**7** Via Natural or Artificial Opening **8** Via Natural or Artificial Opening Endoscopic	**1** Radioactive Element **D** Intraluminal Device **Y** Other Device	**Z** No Qualifier
5 Esophagus	**X** External	**1** Radioactive Element **2** Monitoring Device **3** Infusion Device **D** Intraluminal Device **U** Feeding Device	**Z** No Qualifier
6 Stomach	**0** Open **3** Percutaneous **4** Percutaneous Endoscopic	**0** Drainage Device **2** Monitoring Device **3** Infusion Device **7** Autologous Tissue Substitute **C** Extraluminal Device **D** Intraluminal Device **J** Synthetic Substitute **K** Nonautologous Tissue Substitute **M** Stimulator Lead **U** Feeding Device **Y** Other Device	**Z** No Qualifier

ODP continued on next page

0 **Medical and Surgical**

0DP continued from previous page

D **Gastrointestinal System**
P **Removal:** Taking out or off a device from a body part

Body Part	Approach	Device	Qualifier
Character 4	Character 5	Character 6	Character 7
6 Stomach	7 Via Natural or Artificial Opening 8 Via Natural or Artificial Opening Endoscopic	0 Drainage Device 2 Monitoring Device 3 Infusion Device 7 Autologous Tissue Substitute C Extraluminal Device D Intraluminal Device J Synthetic Substitute K Nonautologous Tissue Substitute U Feeding Device Y Other Device	Z No Qualifier
6 Stomach	X External	0 Drainage Device 2 Monitoring Device 3 Infusion Device D Intraluminal Device U Feeding Device	Z No Qualifier
P Rectum	0 Open 3 Percutaneous 4 Percutaneous Endoscopic 7 Via Natural or Artificial Opening 8 Via Natural or Artificial Opening Endoscopic X External	1 Radioactive Element	Z No Qualifier
Q Anus	0 Open 3 Percutaneous 4 Percutaneous Endoscopic 7 Via Natural or Artificial Opening 8 Via Natural or Artificial Opening Endoscopic	L Artificial Sphincter	Z No Qualifier
R Anal Sphincter	0 Open 3 Percutaneous 4 Percutaneous Endoscopic	M Stimulator Lead	Z No Qualifier
U Omentum V Mesentery W Peritoneum	0 Open 3 Percutaneous 4 Percutaneous Endoscopic	0 Drainage Device 1 Radioactive Element 7 Autologous Tissue Substitute J Synthetic Substitute K Nonautologous Tissue Substitute	Z No Qualifier

LC Limited Coverage   NC Noncovered   HAC HAC-associated Procedure   CC Combination Cluster - See Appendix G for code lists
DRG Non-OR-Affecting MS-DRG Assignment   New/Revised Text in **Orange**   ♂ Male   ♀ Female

2018 ICD-10-PCS   333

0 **Medical and Surgical**
D **Gastrointestinal System**
Q **Repair:** Restoring, to the extent possible, a body part to its normal anatomic structure and function

Body Part	Approach	Device	Qualifier
Character 4	Character 5	Character 6	Character 7
1 Esophagus, Upper 2 Esophagus, Middle 3 Esophagus, Lower 4 Esophagogastric Junction 5 Esophagus 6 Stomach 7 Stomach, Pylorus 8 Small Intestine CC 9 Duodenum CC A Jejunum CC B Ileum CC C Ileocecal Valve E Large Intestine CC F Large Intestine, Right CC G Large Intestine, Left CC H Cecum CC J Appendix K Ascending Colon CC L Transverse Colon CC M Descending Colon CC N Sigmoid Colon CC P Rectum	0 Open 3 Percutaneous 4 Percutaneous Endoscopic 7 Via Natural or Artificial Opening 8 Via Natural or Artificial Opening Endoscopic	**Z** No Device	**Z** No Qualifier
Q Anus	0 Open 3 Percutaneous 4 Percutaneous Endoscopic 7 Via Natural or Artificial Opening 8 Via Natural or Artificial Opening Endoscopic X External	**Z** No Device	**Z** No Qualifier
R Anal Sphincter U Omentum V Mesentery W Peritoneum	0 Open 3 Percutaneous 4 Percutaneous Endoscopic	**Z** No Device	**Z** No Qualifier

CC 0DQ80ZZ   0DQ90ZZ   0DQA0ZZ   0DQB0ZZ   0DQE0ZZ   0DQF0ZZ   0DQG0ZZ   0DQH0ZZ   0DQK0ZZ   0DQL0ZZ   0DQM0ZZ   0DQN0ZZ

0 **Medical and Surgical**
D **Gastrointestinal System**
R **Replacement:** Putting in or on biological or synthetic material that physically takes the place and/or function of all or a portion of a body part

Body Part	Approach	Device	Qualifier
Character 4	Character 5	Character 6	Character 7
5 Esophagus	0 Open 4 Percutaneous Endoscopic 7 Via Natural or Artificial Opening 8 Via Natural or Artificial Opening Endoscopic	7 Autologous Tissue Substitute J Synthetic Substitute K Nonautologous Tissue Substitute	**Z** No Qualifier
R Anal Sphincter U Omentum V Mesentery W Peritoneum	0 Open 4 Percutaneous Endoscopic	7 Autologous Tissue Substitute J Synthetic Substitute K Nonautologous Tissue Substitute	**Z** No Qualifier

CC Limited Coverage   NC Noncovered   HAC HAC-associated Procedure   CC Combination Cluster - See Appendix G for code lists
⊕ Non-OR-Affecting MS-DRG Assignment   New/Revised Text in **Orange**   ♂ Male   ♀ Female

334

2018 ICD-10-PCS

0 Medical and Surgical
D Gastrointestinal System
S Reposition: Moving to its normal location, or other suitable location, all or a portion of a body part

Body Part	Approach	Device	Qualifier
Character 4	Character 5	Character 6	Character 7
5 Esophagus 6 Stomach 9 Duodenum A Jejunum B Ileum H Cecum K Ascending Colon L Transverse Colon M Descending Colon N Sigmoid Colon P Rectum Q Anus	0 Open 4 Percutaneous Endoscopic 7 Via Natural or Artificial Opening 8 Via Natural or Artificial Opening Endoscopic X External	Z No Device	Z No Qualifier
8 Small Intestine E Large Intestine	0 Open 4 Percutaneous Endoscopic 7 Via Natural or Artificial Opening 8 Via Natural or Artificial Opening Endoscopic	Z No Device	Z No Qualifier

0 Medical and Surgical
D Gastrointestinal System
T Resection: Cutting out or off, without replacement, all of a body part

Body Part	Approach	Device	Qualifier
Character 4	Character 5	Character 6	Character 7
1 Esophagus, Upper 2 Esophagus, Middle 3 Esophagus, Lower 4 Esophagogastric Junction 5 Esophagus 6 Stomach 7 Stomach, Pylorus 8 Small Intestine 9 Duodenum **CC** A Jejunum B Ileum C Ileocecal Valve E Large Intestine F Large Intestine, Right H Cecum J Appendix K Ascending Colon P Rectum Q Anus	0 Open 4 Percutaneous Endoscopic 7 Via Natural or Artificial Opening 8 Via Natural or Artificial Opening Endoscopic	Z No Device	Z No Qualifier
G Large Intestine, Left L Transverse Colon M Descending Colon N Sigmoid Colon	0 Open 4 Percutaneous Endoscopic 7 Via Natural or Artificial Opening 8 Via Natural or Artificial Opening Endoscopic F Via Natural or Artificial Opening With Percutaneous Endoscopic Assistance	Z No Device	Z No Qualifier
R Anal Sphincter U Omentum	0 Open 4 Percutaneous Endoscopic	Z No Device	Z No Qualifier

CC 0DT90ZZ

0 **Medical and Surgical**
D **Gastrointestinal System**
U **Supplement:** Putting in or on biological or synthetic material that physically reinforces and/or augments the function of a portion of a body part

Body Part	Approach	Device	Qualifier
Character 4	**Character 5**	**Character 6**	**Character 7**
1 Esophagus, Upper 2 Esophagus, Middle 3 Esophagus, Lower 4 Esophagogastric Junction 5 Esophagus 6 Stomach 7 Stomach, Pylorus 8 Small Intestine 9 Duodenum A Jejunum B Ileum C Ileocecal Valve E Large Intestine F Large Intestine, Right G Large Intestine, Left H Cecum K Ascending Colon L Transverse Colon M Descending Colon N Sigmoid Colon P Rectum	0 Open 4 Percutaneous Endoscopic 7 Via Natural or Artificial Opening 8 Via Natural or Artificial Opening Endoscopic	7 Autologous Tissue Substitute J Synthetic Substitute K Nonautologous Tissue Substitute	Z No Qualifier
Q Anus	0 Open 4 Percutaneous Endoscopic 7 Via Natural or Artificial Opening 8 Via Natural or Artificial Opening Endoscopic X External	7 Autologous Tissue Substitute J Synthetic Substitute K Nonautologous Tissue Substitute	Z No Qualifier
R Anal Sphincter U Omentum V Mesentery W Peritoneum	0 Open 4 Percutaneous Endoscopic	7 Autologous Tissue Substitute J Synthetic Substitute K Nonautologous Tissue Substitute	Z No Qualifier

0 **Medical and Surgical**
D **Gastrointestinal System**
V **Restriction:** Partially closing an orifice or the lumen of a tubular body part

Body Part	Approach	Device	Qualifier
Character 4	**Character 5**	**Character 6**	**Character 7**
1 Esophagus, Upper 2 Esophagus, Middle 3 Esophagus, Lower 4 Esophagogastric Junction 5 Esophagus 6 Stomach HAC 7 Stomach, Pylorus 8 Small Intestine 9 Duodenum A Jejunum B Ileum C Ileocecal Valve E Large Intestine F Large Intestine, Right G Large Intestine, Left H Cecum K Ascending Colon L Transverse Colon M Descending Colon N Sigmoid Colon P Rectum	0 Open 3 Percutaneous 4 Percutaneous Endoscopic	C Extraluminal Device D Intraluminal Device Z No Device	Z No Qualifier

0DV continued on next page

LC Limited Coverage NC Noncovered HAC HAC-associated Procedure CC Combination Cluster - See Appendix G for code lists
Non-OR-Affecting MS-DRG Assignment New/Revised Text in **Orange** ♂ Male ♀ Female

336   **2018 ICD-10-PCS**

0 **Medical and Surgical**
D **Gastrointestinal System**
V **Restriction:** Partially closing an orifice or the lumen of a tubular body part

0DV continued from previous page

Body Part	Approach	Device	Qualifier
Character 4	Character 5	Character 6	Character 7
1 Esophagus, Upper 2 Esophagus, Middle 3 Esophagus, Lower 4 Esophagogastric Junction 5 Esophagus 6 Stomach NC 7 Stomach, Pylorus 8 Small Intestine 9 Duodenum A Jejunum B Ileum C Ileocecal Valve E Large Intestine F Large Intestine, Right G Large Intestine, Left H Cecum K Ascending Colon L Transverse Colon M Descending Colon N Sigmoid Colon P Rectum	7 Via Natural or Artificial Opening 8 Via Natural or Artificial Opening Endoscopic	D Intraluminal Device Z No Device	Z No Qualifier
Q Anus	0 Open 3 Percutaneous 4 Percutaneous Endoscopic X External	C Extraluminal Device D Intraluminal Device Z No Device	Z No Qualifier
Q Anus	7 Via Natural or Artificial Opening 8 Via Natural or Artificial Opening Endoscopic	D Intraluminal Device Z No Device	Z No Qualifier

NC 0DV67DZ   0DV68DZ
HAC 0DV64CZ
  Surgical A1:E1309 infection following bariatric surgery procedures and principal diagnoses E66.01 and secondary diagnoses K68.11, K95.01, K95.81, T81.4XXA.

0 **Medical and Surgical**
D **Gastrointestinal System**
W **Revision:** Correcting, to the extent possible, a portion of a malfunctioning device or the position of a displaced device

Body Part	Approach	Device	Qualifier
Character 4	Character 5	Character 6	Character 7
0 Upper Intestinal Tract D Lower Intestinal Tract	0 Open 3 Percutaneous 4 Percutaneous Endoscopic 7 Via Natural or Artificial Opening 8 Via Natural or Artificial Opening Endoscopic	0 Drainage Device 2 Monitoring Device 3 Infusion Device 7 Autologous Tissue Substitute C Extraluminal Device D Intraluminal Device J Synthetic Substitute K Nonautologous Tissue Substitute U Feeding Device Y Other Device	Z No Qualifier
0 Upper Intestinal Tract D Lower Intestinal Tract	X External	0 Drainage Device 2 Monitoring Device 3 Infusion Device 7 Autologous Tissue Substitute C Extraluminal Device D Intraluminal Device J Synthetic Substitute K Nonautologous Tissue Substitute U Feeding Device	Z No Qualifier

0DW continued on next page

0 Medical and Surgical
D Gastrointestinal System

0DW continued from previous page

W Revision: Correcting, to the extent possible, a portion of a malfunctioning device or the position of a displaced device

Body Part	Approach	Device	Qualifier
Character 4	Character 5	Character 6	Character 7
5 Esophagus	0 Open 3 Percutaneous 4 Percutaneous Endoscopic	Y Other Device	Z No Qualifier
5 Esophagus	7 Via Natural or Artificial Opening 8 Via Natural or Artificial Opening Endoscopic	D Intraluminal Device Y Other Device	Z No Qualifier
5 Esophagus	X External	D Intraluminal Device	Z No Qualifier
6 Stomach	0 Open 3 Percutaneous 4 Percutaneous Endoscopic	0 Drainage Device 2 Monitoring Device 3 Infusion Device 7 Autologous Tissue Substitute C Extraluminal Device D Intraluminal Device J Synthetic Substitute K Nonautologous Tissue Substitute M Stimulator Lead U Feeding Device Y Other Device	Z No Qualifier
6 Stomach	7 Via Natural or Artificial Opening 8 Via Natural or Artificial Opening Endoscopic	0 Drainage Device 2 Monitoring Device 3 Infusion Device 7 Autologous Tissue Substitute C Extraluminal Device D Intraluminal Device J Synthetic Substitute K Nonautologous Tissue Substitute U Feeding Device Y Other Device	Z No Qualifier
6 Stomach	X External	0 Drainage Device 2 Monitoring Device 3 Infusion Device 7 Autologous Tissue Substitute C Extraluminal Device D Intraluminal Device J Synthetic Substitute K Nonautologous Tissue Substitute U Feeding Device	Z No Qualifier
8 Small Intestine E Large Intestine	0 Open 4 Percutaneous Endoscopic 7 Via Natural or Artificial Opening 8 Via Natural or Artificial Opening Endoscopic	7 Autologous Tissue Substitute J Synthetic Substitute K Nonautologous Tissue Substitute	Z No Qualifier
Q Anus	0 Open 3 Percutaneous 4 Percutaneous Endoscopic 7 Via Natural or Artificial Opening 8 Via Natural or Artificial Opening Endoscopic	L Artificial Sphincter	Z No Qualifier
R Anal Sphincter	0 Open 3 Percutaneous 4 Percutaneous Endoscopic	M Stimulator Lead	Z No Qualifier
U Omentum V Mesentery W Peritoneum	0 Open 3 Percutaneous 4 Percutaneous Endoscopic	0 Drainage Device 7 Autologous Tissue Substitute J Synthetic Substitute K Nonautologous Tissue Substitute	Z No Qualifier

LC Limited Coverage   NC Noncovered   HAC HAC-associated Procedure   CC Combination Cluster - See Appendix G for code lists

⚕ Non-OR-Affecting MS-DRG Assignment   New/Revised Text in **Orange**   ♂ Male   ♀ Female

0 Medical and Surgical
D Gastrointestinal System
X Transfer: Moving, without taking out, all or a portion of a body part to another location to take over the function of all or a portion of a body part

Body Part	Approach	Device	Qualifier
Character 4	Character 5	Character 6	Character 7
6 Stomach **8** Small Intestine **E** Large Intestine	**0** Open **4** Percutaneous Endoscopic	**Z** No Device	**5** Esophagus

0 Medical and Surgical
D Gastrointestinal System
Y Transplantation: Putting in or on all or a portion of a living body part taken from another individual or animal to physically take the place and/or function of all or a portion of a similar body part

Body Part	Approach	Device	Qualifier
Character 4	Character 5	Character 6	Character 7
5 Esophagus **6** Stomach **8** Small Intestine LC **E** Large Intestine LC	**0** Open	**Z** No Device	**0** Allogeneic **1** Syngeneic **2** Zooplastic

LC 0DY80Z0   0DY80Z1   0DY80Z2   0DYE0Z0   0DYE0Z1   0DYE0Z2

LC Limited Coverage   NC Noncovered   HAC HAC-associated Procedure   CC Combination Cluster - See Appendix G for code lists
DRG Non-OR-Affecting MS-DRG Assignment   New/Revised Text in **Orange**   ♂ Male   ♀ Female

2018 ICD-10-PCS

339

0DX-0DY

GASTROINTESTINAL SYSTEM 0D1-0DY

NOTES

Hepatobiliary System and Pancreas 0F1-0FY

0   Medical and Surgical
F   Hepatobiliary System and Pancreas
1   Bypass: Altering the route of passage of the contents of a tubular body part

Body Part	Approach	Device	Qualifier
Character 4	Character 5	Character 6	Character 7
4 Gallbladder **5** Hepatic Duct, Right **6** Hepatic Duct, Left **7** Hepatic Duct, Common **8** Cystic Duct **9** Common Bile Duct	**0** Open **4** Percutaneous Endoscopic	**D** Intraluminal Device **Z** No Device	**3** Duodenum **4** Stomach **5** Hepatic Duct, Right **6** Hepatic Duct, Left **7** Hepatic Duct, Caudate **8** Cystic Duct **9** Common Bile Duct **B** Small Intestine
D Pancreatic Duct **F** Pancreatic Duct, Accessory **G** Pancreas	**0** Open **4** Percutaneous Endoscopic	**D** Intraluminal Device **Z** No Device	**3** Duodenum **B** Small Intestine **C** Large Intestine

0   Medical and Surgical
F   Hepatobiliary System and Pancreas
2   Change: Taking out or off a device from a body part and putting back an identical or similar device in or on the same body part without cutting or puncturing the skin or a mucous membrane

Body Part	Approach	Device	Qualifier
Character 4	Character 5	Character 6	Character 7
0 Liver **4** Gallbladder **B** Hepatobiliary Duct **D** Pancreatic Duct **G** Pancreas	**X** External	**0** Drainage Device **Y** Other Device	**Z** No Qualifier

0   Medical and Surgical
F   Hepatobiliary System and Pancreas
5   Destruction: Physical eradication of all or a portion of a body part by the direct use of energy, force, or a destructive agent

Body Part	Approach	Device	Qualifier
Character 4	Character 5	Character 6	Character 7
0 Liver **1** Liver, Right Lobe **2** Liver, Left Lobe	**0** Open **3** Percutaneous **4** Percutaneous Endoscopic	**Z** No Device	**Z** No Qualifier
4 Gallbladder **G** Pancreas	**0** Open **3** Percutaneous **4** Percutaneous Endoscopic **8** Via Natural or Artificial Opening Endoscopic	**Z** No Device	**Z** No Qualifier
5 Hepatic Duct, Right **6** Hepatic Duct, Left **7** Hepatic Duct, Common **8** Cystic Duct **9** Common Bile Duct **C** Ampulla of Vater **D** Pancreatic Duct **F** Pancreatic Duct, Accessory	**0** Open **3** Percutaneous **4** Percutaneous Endoscopic **7** Via Natural or Artificial Opening **8** Via Natural or Artificial Opening Endoscopic	**Z** No Device	**Z** No Qualifier

Limited Coverage **Noncovered** **HAC-associated Procedure** **Combination Cluster - See Appendix G for code lists**
Non-OR-Affecting MS-DRG Assignment   New/Revised Text in Orange   ♂ Male   ♀ Female

2018 ICD-10-PCS

341

0 **Medical and Surgical**
F **Hepatobiliary System and Pancreas**
7 **Dilation:** Expanding an orifice or the lumen of a tubular body part

Body Part	Approach	Device	Qualifier
Character 4	Character 5	Character 6	Character 7
5 Hepatic Duct, Right 6 Hepatic Duct, Left 7 Hepatic Duct, Common 8 Cystic Duct 9 Common Bile Duct C Ampulla of Vater D Pancreatic Duct F Pancreatic Duct, Accessory	0 Open 3 Percutaneous 4 Percutaneous Endoscopic 7 Via Natural or Artificial Opening 8 Via Natural or Artificial Opening Endoscopic	D Intraluminal Device Z No Device	Z No Qualifier

0 **Medical and Surgical**
F **Hepatobiliary System and Pancreas**
8 **Division:** Cutting into a body part, without draining fluids and/or gases from the body part, in order to separate or transect a body part

Body Part	Approach	Device	Qualifier
Character 4	Character 5	Character 6	Character 7
G Pancreas	0 Open 3 Percutaneous 4 Percutaneous Endoscopic	Z No Device	Z No Qualifier

0 **Medical and Surgical**
F **Hepatobiliary System and Pancreas**
9 **Drainage:** Taking or letting out fluids and/or gases from a body part

Body Part	Approach	Device	Qualifier
Character 4	Character 5	Character 6	Character 7
0 Liver 1 Liver, Right Lobe 2 Liver, Left Lobe	0 Open 3 Percutaneous 4 Percutaneous Endoscopic	0 Drainage Device	Z No Qualifier
0 Liver 1 Liver, Right Lobe 2 Liver, Left Lobe	0 Open 3 Percutaneous 4 Percutaneous Endoscopic	Z No Device	X Diagnostic Z No Qualifier
4 Gallbladder G Pancreas	0 Open 3 Percutaneous 4 Percutaneous Endoscopic 8 Via Natural or Artificial Opening Endoscopic	0 Drainage Device	Z No Qualifier
4 Gallbladder G Pancreas	0 Open 3 Percutaneous 4 Percutaneous Endoscopic 8 Via Natural or Artificial Opening Endoscopic	Z No Device	X Diagnostic Z No Qualifier
5 Hepatic Duct, Right 6 Hepatic Duct, Left 7 Hepatic Duct, Common 8 Cystic Duct 9 Common Bile Duct C Ampulla of Vater D Pancreatic Duct F Pancreatic Duct, Accessory	0 Open 3 Percutaneous 4 Percutaneous Endoscopic 7 Via Natural or Artificial Opening 8 Via Natural or Artificial Opening Endoscopic	0 Drainage Device	Z No Qualifier
5 Hepatic Duct, Right 6 Hepatic Duct, Left 7 Hepatic Duct, Common 8 Cystic Duct 9 Common Bile Duct C Ampulla of Vater D Pancreatic Duct F Pancreatic Duct, Accessory	0 Open 3 Percutaneous 4 Percutaneous Endoscopic 7 Via Natural or Artificial Opening 8 Via Natural or Artificial Opening Endoscopic	Z No Device	X Diagnostic Z No Qualifier

LC Limited Coverage   NC Noncovered   HAC HAC-associated Procedure   CC Combination Cluster - See Appendix G for code lists
DRG Non-OR-Affecting MS-DRG Assignment   New/Revised Text in **Orange**   ♂ Male   ♀ Female

342   2018 ICD-10-PCS

0 **Medical and Surgical**
F **Hepatobiliary System and Pancreas**
B **Excision:** Cutting out or off, without replacement, a portion of a body part

Body Part	Approach	Device	Qualifier
Character 4	Character 5	Character 6	Character 7
0 Liver 1 Liver, Right Lobe 2 Liver, Left Lobe	0 Open 3 Percutaneous 4 Percutaneous Endoscopic	Z No Device	X Diagnostic Z No Qualifier
4 Gallbladder G Pancreas	0 Open 3 Percutaneous 4 Percutaneous Endoscopic 8 Via Natural or Artificial Opening Endoscopic	Z No Device	X Diagnostic Z No Qualifier
5 Hepatic Duct, Right 6 Hepatic Duct, Left 7 Hepatic Duct, Common 8 Cystic Duct 9 Common Bile Duct C Ampulla of Vater D Pancreatic Duct F Pancreatic Duct, Accessory	0 Open 3 Percutaneous 4 Percutaneous Endoscopic 7 Via Natural or Artificial Opening 8 Via Natural or Artificial Opening Endoscopic	Z No Device	X Diagnostic Z No Qualifier

0 **Medical and Surgical**
F **Hepatobiliary System and Pancreas**
C **Extirpation:** Taking or cutting out solid matter from a body part

Body Part	Approach	Device	Qualifier
Character 4	Character 5	Character 6	Character 7
0 Liver 1 Liver, Right Lobe 2 Liver, Left Lobe	0 Open 3 Percutaneous 4 Percutaneous Endoscopic	Z No Device	Z No Qualifier
4 Gallbladder G Pancreas	0 Open 3 Percutaneous 4 Percutaneous Endoscopic 8 Via Natural or Artificial Opening Endoscopic	Z No Device	Z No Qualifier
5 Hepatic Duct, Right 6 Hepatic Duct, Left 7 Hepatic Duct, Common 8 Cystic Duct 9 Common Bile Duct C Ampulla of Vater D Pancreatic Duct F Pancreatic Duct, Accessory	0 Open 3 Percutaneous 4 Percutaneous Endoscopic 7 Via Natural or Artificial Opening 8 Via Natural or Artificial Opening Endoscopic	Z No Device	Z No Qualifier

0 **Medical and Surgical**
F **Hepatobiliary System and Pancreas**
F **Fragmentation:** Breaking solid matter in a body part into pieces

Body Part	Approach	Device	Qualifier
Character 4	Character 5	Character 6	Character 7
4 Gallbladder NC 5 Hepatic Duct, Right NC 6 Hepatic Duct, Left NC 7 Hepatic Duct, Common 8 Cystic Duct NC 9 Common Bile Duct NC C Ampulla of Vater NC D Pancreatic Duct NC F Pancreatic Duct, Accessory NC	0 Open 3 Percutaneous 4 Percutaneous Endoscopic 7 Via Natural or Artificial Opening 8 Via Natural or Artificial Opening Endoscopic X External	Z No Device	Z No Qualifier

NC 0FF4XZZ   0FF5XZZ   0FF6XZZ   0FF8XZZ   0FF9XZZ   0FFCXZZ   0FFDXZZ   0FFFXZZ

LC Limited Coverage   NC Noncovered   HAC HAC-associated Procedure   CC Combination Cluster - See Appendix G for code lists
DRG Non-OR-Affecting MS-DRG Assignment   New/Revised Text in **Orange**   ♂ Male   ♀ Female

2018 ICD-10-PCS

343

HEPATOBILIARY SYSTEM AND PANCREAS 0F1-0FY

0   Medical and Surgical
F   Hepatobiliary System and Pancreas
H   Insertion: Putting in a nonbiological appliance that monitors, assists, performs, or prevents a physiological function but does not physically take the place of a body part

Body Part	Approach	Device	Qualifier
Character 4	**Character 5**	**Character 6**	**Character 7**
0 Liver **4** Gallbladder **G** Pancreas	**0** Open **3** Percutaneous **4** Percutaneous Endoscopic	**2** Monitoring Device **3** Infusion Device **Y** Other Device	**Z** No Qualifier
1 Liver, Right Lobe **2** Liver, Left Lobe	**0** Open **3** Percutaneous **4** Percutaneous Endoscopic	**2** Monitoring Device **3** Infusion Device	**Z** No Qualifier
B Hepatobiliary Duct **D** Pancreatic Duct	**0** Open **3** Percutaneous **4** Percutaneous Endoscopic **7** Via Natural or Artificial Opening **8** Via Natural or Artificial Opening Endoscopic	**1** Radioactive Element **2** Monitoring Device **3** Infusion Device **D** Intraluminal Device **Y** Other Device	**Z** No Qualifier

0   Medical and Surgical
F   Hepatobiliary System and Pancreas
J   Inspection: Visually and/or manually exploring a body part

Body Part	Approach	Device	Qualifier
Character 4	**Character 5**	**Character 6**	**Character 7**
0 Liver ᴰᴿᴳ	**0** Open **3** Percutaneous **4** Percutaneous Endoscopic **X** External	**Z** No Device	**Z** No Qualifier
4 Gallbladder **G** Pancreas	**0** Open **3** Percutaneous **4** Percutaneous Endoscopic **8** Via Natural or Artificial Opening Endoscopic **X** External	**Z** No Device	**Z** No Qualifier
B Hepatobiliary Duct **D** Pancreatic Duct	**0** Open **3** Percutaneous **4** Percutaneous Endoscopic **7** Via Natural or Artificial Opening **8** Via Natural or Artificial Opening Endoscopic	**Z** No Device	**Z** No Qualifier

ᴰᴿᴳ 0FJ03ZZ

🅛🅒 Limited Coverage   🅝🅒 Noncovered   🅗🅐🅒 HAC-associated Procedure   🅒🅒 Combination Cluster - See Appendix G for code lists
ᴰᴿᴳ Non-OR-Affecting MS-DRG Assignment   New/Revised Text in **Orange**   ♂ Male   ♀ Female

344   **2018 ICD-10-PCS**

0 Medical and Surgical
F Hepatobiliary System and Pancreas
L Occlusion: Completely closing an orifice or the lumen of a tubular body part

Body Part	Approach	Device	Qualifier
Character 4	Character 5	Character 6	Character 7
5 Hepatic Duct, Right 6 Hepatic Duct, Left 7 Hepatic Duct, Common 8 Cystic Duct 9 Common Bile Duct C Ampulla of Vater D Pancreatic Duct F Pancreatic Duct, Accessory	0 Open 3 Percutaneous 4 Percutaneous Endoscopic	C Extraluminal Device D Intraluminal Device Z No Device	Z No Qualifier
5 Hepatic Duct, Right 6 Hepatic Duct, Left 7 Hepatic Duct, Common 8 Cystic Duct 9 Common Bile Duct C Ampulla of Vater D Pancreatic Duct F Pancreatic Duct, Accessory	7 Via Natural or Artificial Opening 8 Via Natural or Artificial Opening Endoscopic	D Intraluminal Device Z No Device	Z No Qualifier

0 Medical and Surgical
F Hepatobiliary System and Pancreas
M Reattachment: Putting back in or on all or a portion of a separated body part to its normal location or other suitable location

Body Part	Approach	Device	Qualifier
Character 4	Character 5	Character 6	Character 7
0 Liver 1 Liver, Right Lobe 2 Liver, Left Lobe 4 Gallbladder 5 Hepatic Duct, Right 6 Hepatic Duct, Left 7 Hepatic Duct, Common 8 Cystic Duct 9 Common Bile Duct C Ampulla of Vater D Pancreatic Duct F Pancreatic Duct, Accessory G Pancreas	0 Open 4 Percutaneous Endoscopic	Z No Device	Z No Qualifier

0 Medical and Surgical
F Hepatobiliary System and Pancreas
N Release: Freeing a body part from an abnormal physical constraint by cutting or by the use of force

Body Part	Approach	Device	Qualifier
Character 4	Character 5	Character 6	Character 7
0 Liver 1 Liver, Right Lobe 2 Liver, Left Lobe	0 Open 3 Percutaneous 4 Percutaneous Endoscopic	Z No Device	Z No Qualifier
4 Gallbladder G Pancreas	0 Open 3 Percutaneous 4 Percutaneous Endoscopic 8 Via Natural or Artificial Opening Endoscopic	Z No Device	Z No Qualifier
5 Hepatic Duct, Right 6 Hepatic Duct, Left 7 Hepatic Duct, Common 8 Cystic Duct 9 Common Bile Duct C Ampulla of Vater D Pancreatic Duct F Pancreatic Duct, Accessory	0 Open 3 Percutaneous 4 Percutaneous Endoscopic 7 Via Natural or Artificial Opening 8 Via Natural or Artificial Opening Endoscopic	Z No Device	Z No Qualifier

0   Medical and Surgical
F   Hepatobiliary System and Pancreas
P   Removal: Taking out or off a device from a body part

Body Part	Approach	Device	Qualifier
Character 4	Character 5	Character 6	Character 7
0 Liver	**0** Open **3** Percutaneous **4** Percutaneous Endoscopic	**0** Drainage Device **2** Monitoring Device **3** Infusion Device **Y** Other Device	**Z** No Qualifier
0 Liver	**X** External	**0** Drainage Device **2** Monitoring Device **3** Infusion Device	**Z** No Qualifier
4 Gallbladder **G** Pancreas	**0** Open **3** Percutaneous **4** Percutaneous Endoscopic	**0** Drainage Device **2** Monitoring Device **3** Infusion Device **D** Intraluminal Device **Y** Other Device	**Z** No Qualifier
4 Gallbladder **G** Pancreas	**X** External	**0** Drainage Device **2** Monitoring Device **3** Infusion Device **D** Intraluminal Device	**Z** No Qualifier
B Hepatobiliary Duct **D** Pancreatic Duct	**0** Open **3** Percutaneous **4** Percutaneous Endoscopic **7** Via Natural or Artificial Opening **8** Via Natural or Artificial Opening Endoscopic	**0** Drainage Device **1** Radioactive Element **2** Monitoring Device **3** Infusion Device **7** Autologous Tissue Substitute **C** Extraluminal Device **D** Intraluminal Device **J** Synthetic Substitute **K** Nonautologous Tissue Substitute **Y** Other Device	**Z** No Qualifier
B Hepatobiliary Duct **D** Pancreatic Duct	**X** External	**0** Drainage Device **1** Radioactive Element **2** Monitoring Device **3** Infusion Device **D** Intraluminal Device	**Z** No Qualifier

0   Medical and Surgical
F   Hepatobiliary System and Pancreas
Q   Repair: Restoring, to the extent possible, a body part to its normal anatomic structure and function

Body Part	Approach	Device	Qualifier
Character 4	Character 5	Character 6	Character 7
0 Liver **1** Liver, Right Lobe **2** Liver, Left Lobe	**0** Open **3** Percutaneous **4** Percutaneous Endoscopic	**Z** No Device	**Z** No Qualifier
4 Gallbladder **G** Pancreas	**0** Open **3** Percutaneous **4** Percutaneous Endoscopic **8** Via Natural or Artificial Opening Endoscopic	**Z** No Device	**Z** No Qualifier
5 Hepatic Duct, Right **6** Hepatic Duct, Left **7** Hepatic Duct, Common **8** Cystic Duct **9** Common Bile Duct **C** Ampulla of Vater **D** Pancreatic Duct **F** Pancreatic Duct, Accessory	**0** Open **3** Percutaneous **4** Percutaneous Endoscopic **7** Via Natural or Artificial Opening **8** Via Natural or Artificial Opening Endoscopic	**Z** No Device	**Z** No Qualifier

LC Limited Coverage   NC Noncovered   HAC HAC-associated Procedure   CC Combination Cluster - See Appendix G for code lists
DRG Non-OR-Affecting MS-DRG Assignment   New/Revised Text in **Orange**   ♂ Male   ♀ Female

346

2018 ICD-10-PCS

0   Medical and Surgical
F   Hepatobiliary System and Pancreas
R   Replacement: Putting in or on biological or synthetic material that physically takes the place and/or function of all or a portion of a body part

Body Part	Approach	Device	Qualifier
Character 4	Character 5	Character 6	Character 7
5 Hepatic Duct, Right 6 Hepatic Duct, Left 7 Hepatic Duct, Common 8 Cystic Duct 9 Common Bile Duct C Ampulla of Vater D Pancreatic Duct F Pancreatic Duct, Accessory	0 Open 4 Percutaneous Endoscopic 8 Via Natural or Artificial Opening Endoscopic	7 Autologous Tissue Substitute J Synthetic Substitute K Nonautologous Tissue Substitute	Z No Qualifier

0   Medical and Surgical
F   Hepatobiliary System and Pancreas
S   Reposition: Moving to its normal location, or other suitable location, all or a portion of a body part

Body Part	Approach	Device	Qualifier
Character 4	Character 5	Character 6	Character 7
0 Liver 4 Gallbladder 5 Hepatic Duct, Right 6 Hepatic Duct, Left 7 Hepatic Duct, Common 8 Cystic Duct 9 Common Bile Duct C Ampulla of Vater D Pancreatic Duct F Pancreatic Duct, Accessory G Pancreas	0 Open 4 Percutaneous Endoscopic	Z No Device	Z No Qualifier

0   Medical and Surgical
F   Hepatobiliary System and Pancreas
T   Resection: Cutting out or off, without replacement, all of a body part

Body Part	Approach	Device	Qualifier
Character 4	Character 5	Character 6	Character 7
0 Liver 1 Liver, Right Lobe 2 Liver, Left Lobe 4 Gallbladder G Pancreas **CC**	0 Open 4 Percutaneous Endoscopic	Z No Device	Z No Qualifier
5 Hepatic Duct, Right 6 Hepatic Duct, Left 7 Hepatic Duct, Common 8 Cystic Duct 9 Common Bile Duct C Ampulla of Vater D Pancreatic Duct F Pancreatic Duct, Accessory	0 Open 4 Percutaneous Endoscopic 7 Via Natural or Artificial Opening 8 Via Natural or Artificial Opening Endoscopic	Z No Device	Z No Qualifier

CC 0FTG0ZZ

CC Limited Coverage   **NC** Noncovered   **HAC** HAC-associated Procedure   **CC** Combination Cluster - See Appendix G for code lists
096 Non-OR-Affecting MS-DRG Assignment   New/Revised Text in **Orange**   ♂ Male   ♀ Female

2018 ICD-10-PCS   **347**

0 Medical and Surgical
F Hepatobiliary System and Pancreas
U Supplement: Putting in or on biological or synthetic material that physically reinforces and/or augments the function of a portion of a body part

Body Part	Approach	Device	Qualifier
Character 4	Character 5	Character 6	Character 7
5 Hepatic Duct, Right 6 Hepatic Duct, Left 7 Hepatic Duct, Common 8 Cystic Duct 9 Common Bile Duct C Ampulla of Vater D Pancreatic Duct F Pancreatic Duct, Accessory	0 Open 3 Percutaneous 4 Percutaneous Endoscopic 8 Via Natural or Artificial Opening Endoscopic	7 Autologous Tissue Substitute J Synthetic Substitute K Nonautologous Tissue Substitute	Z No Qualifier

0 Medical and Surgical
F Hepatobiliary System and Pancreas
V Restriction: Partially closing an orifice or the lumen of a tubular body part

Body Part	Approach	Device	Qualifier
Character 4	Character 5	Character 6	Character 7
5 Hepatic Duct, Right 6 Hepatic Duct, Left 7 Hepatic Duct, Common 8 Cystic Duct 9 Common Bile Duct C Ampulla of Vater D Pancreatic Duct F Pancreatic Duct, Accessory	0 Open 3 Percutaneous 4 Percutaneous Endoscopic	C Extraluminal Device D Intraluminal Device Z No Device	Z No Qualifier
5 Hepatic Duct, Right 6 Hepatic Duct, Left 7 Hepatic Duct, Common 8 Cystic Duct 9 Common Bile Duct C Ampulla of Vater D Pancreatic Duct F Pancreatic Duct, Accessory	7 Via Natural or Artificial Opening 8 Via Natural or Artificial Opening Endoscopic	D Intraluminal Device Z No Device	Z No Qualifier

0 Medical and Surgical
F Hepatobiliary System and Pancreas
W Revision: Correcting, to the extent possible, a portion of a malfunctioning device or the position of a displaced device

Body Part	Approach	Device	Qualifier
Character 4	Character 5	Character 6	Character 7
0 Liver	0 Open 3 Percutaneous 4 Percutaneous Endoscopic	0 Drainage Device 2 Monitoring Device 3 Infusion Device Y Other Device	Z No Qualifier
0 Liver	X External	0 Drainage Device 2 Monitoring Device 3 Infusion Device	Z No Qualifier
4 Gallbladder G Pancreas	0 Open 3 Percutaneous 4 Percutaneous Endoscopic	0 Drainage Device 2 Monitoring Device 3 Infusion Device D Intraluminal Device Y Other Device	Z No Qualifier
4 Gallbladder G Pancreas	X External	0 Drainage Device 2 Monitoring Device 3 Infusion Device D Intraluminal Device	Z No Qualifier

0FW continued on next page

0   **Medical and Surgical**
F   **Hepatobiliary System and Pancreas**
W   **Revision:** Correcting, to the extent possible, a portion of a malfunctioning device or the position of a displaced device

0FW continued from previous page

Body Part	Approach	Device	Qualifier
Character 4	Character 5	Character 6	Character 7
B Hepatobiliary Duct **D** Pancreatic Duct	**0** Open **3** Percutaneous **4** Percutaneous Endoscopic **7** Via Natural or Artificial Opening **8** Via Natural or Artificial Opening Endoscopic	**0** Drainage Device **2** Monitoring Device **3** Infusion Device **7** Autologous Tissue Substitute **C** Extraluminal Device **D** Intraluminal Device **J** Synthetic Substitute **K** Nonautologous Tissue Substitute **Y** Other Device	**Z** No Qualifier
B Hepatobiliary Duct **D** Pancreatic Duct	**X** External	**0** Drainage Device **2** Monitoring Device **3** Infusion Device **7** Autologous Tissue Substitute **C** Extraluminal Device **D** Intraluminal Device **J** Synthetic Substitute **K** Nonautologous Tissue Substitute	**Z** No Qualifier

0   **Medical and Surgical**
F   **Hepatobiliary System and Pancreas**
Y   **Transplantation:** Putting in or on all or a portion of a living body part taken from another individual or animal to physically take the place and/or function of all or a portion of a similar body part

Body Part	Approach	Device	Qualifier
Character 4	Character 5	Character 6	Character 7
0 Liver 𝐋𝐂 **G** Pancreas 𝐍𝐂 𝐋𝐂 𝐂𝐂	**0** Open	**Z** No Device	**0** Allogeneic **1** Syngeneic **2** Zooplastic

𝐋𝐂   0FY00Z0   0FY00Z1   0FY00Z2   0FYG0Z0   0FYG0Z1

𝐍𝐂   0FYG0Z2

𝐍𝐂   0FYG0Z0   0FYG0Z1

The procedure idenitified is a noncovered procedure except when combined with procedures codes 0TY00Z0, 0TY00Z1, 0TY00Z2, 0TY10Z0, 0TY10Z1, 0TY10Z2 and with diagnosis codes: E10.10, E10.11, E10.21, E10.22, E10.29, E10.311, E10.319, E10.3211, E10.3212, E10.3213, E10.3219, E10.3291, E10.3292, E10.3293, E10.3299, E10.3311, E10.3312, E10.3313, E10.3319, E10.3391, E10.3392, E10.3393, E10.3399, E10.3411, E10.3412, E10.3413, E10.3419, E10.3491, E10.3492, E10.3493, E10.3499, E10.3511, E10.3512, E10.3513, E10.3519, E10.3521, E10.3522, E10.3523, E10.3529, E10.3531, E10.3532, E10.3533, E10.3539, E10.3541, E10.3542, E10.3543, E10.3549, E10.3551, E10.3552, E10.3553, E10.3559, E10.3591, E10.3592, E10.3593, E10.3599, E10.36, E10.37X1, E10.37X2, E10.37X3, E10.37X9, E10.39, E10.40, E10.41, E10.42, E10.43, E10.44, E10.49, E10.51, E10.52, E10.59, E10.610, E10.618, E10.620, E10.621, E10.622, E10.628, E10.630, E10.638, E10.641, E10.649, E10.65, E10.69, E10.8, E10.9, E89.1 .

𝐂𝐂   0FYG0Z0   0FYG0Z1   0FYG0Z2

𝐋𝐂 Limited Coverage   𝐍𝐂 Noncovered   𝐇𝐀𝐂 HAC-associated Procedure   𝐂𝐂 Combination Cluster - See Appendix G for code lists
𝐃𝐑𝐆 Non-OR-Affecting MS-DRG Assignment   New/Revised Text in **Orange**   ♂ Male   ♀ Female

2018 ICD-10-PCS

349

NOTES

Endocrine System 0G2-0GW

0 Medical and Surgical
G Endocrine System
2 Change: Taking out or off a device from a body part and putting back an identical or similar device in or on the same body part without cutting or puncturing the skin or a mucous membrane

Body Part	Approach	Device	Qualifier
Character 4	Character 5	Character 6	Character 7
0 Pituitary Gland **1** Pineal Body **5** Adrenal Gland **K** Thyroid Gland **R** Parathyroid Gland **S** Endocrine Gland	**X** External	**0** Drainage Device **Y** Other Device	**Z** No Qualifier

0 Medical and Surgical
G Endocrine System
5 Destruction: Physical eradication of all or a portion of a body part by the direct use of energy, force, or a destructive agent

Body Part	Approach	Device	Qualifier
Character 4	Character 5	Character 6	Character 7
0 Pituitary Gland **1** Pineal Body **2** Adrenal Gland, Left **3** Adrenal Gland, Right **4** Adrenal Glands, Bilateral **6** Carotid Body, Left **7** Carotid Body, Right **8** Carotid Bodies, Bilateral **9** Para-aortic Body **B** Coccygeal Glomus **C** Glomus Jugulare **D** Aortic Body **F** Paraganglion Extremity **G** Thyroid Gland Lobe, Left **H** Thyroid Gland Lobe, Right **K** Thyroid Gland **L** Superior Parathyroid Gland, Right **M** Superior Parathyroid Gland, Left **N** Inferior Parathyroid Gland, Right **P** Inferior Parathyroid Gland, Left **Q** Parathyroid Glands, Multiple **R** Parathyroid Gland	**0** Open **3** Percutaneous **4** Percutaneous Endoscopic	**Z** No Device	**Z** No Qualifier

0 Medical and Surgical
G Endocrine System
8 Division: Cutting into a body part, without draining fluids and/or gases from the body part, in order to separate or transect a body part

Body Part	Approach	Device	Qualifier
Character 4	Character 5	Character 6	Character 7
0 Pituitary Gland **J** Thyroid Gland Isthmus	**0** Open **3** Percutaneous **4** Percutaneous Endoscopic	**Z** No Device	**Z** No Qualifier

LC Limited Coverage   NC Noncovered   HAC HAC-associated Procedure   CC Combination Cluster - See Appendix G for code lists
DRG Non-OR-Affecting MS-DRG Assignment   New/Revised Text in **Orange**   ♂ Male   ♀ Female

2018 ICD-10-PCS

351

0   **Medical and Surgical**
G   **Endocrine System**
9   **Drainage:** Taking or letting out fluids and/or gases from a body part

Body Part	Approach	Device	Qualifier
Character 4	Character 5	Character 6	Character 7
0 Pituitary Gland 1 Pineal Body 2 Adrenal Gland, Left 3 Adrenal Gland, Right 4 Adrenal Glands, Bilateral 6 Carotid Body, Left 7 Carotid Body, Right 8 Carotid Bodies, Bilateral 9 Para-aortic Body B Coccygeal Glomus C Glomus Jugulare D Aortic Body F Paraganglion Extremity G Thyroid Gland Lobe, Left H Thyroid Gland Lobe, Right K Thyroid Gland L Superior Parathyroid Gland, Right M Superior Parathyroid Gland, Left N Inferior Parathyroid Gland, Right P Inferior Parathyroid Gland, Left Q Parathyroid Glands, Multiple R Parathyroid Gland	0 Open 3 Percutaneous 4 Percutaneous Endoscopic	0 Drainage Device	Z No Qualifier
0 Pituitary Gland 1 Pineal Body 2 Adrenal Gland, Left 3 Adrenal Gland, Right 4 Adrenal Glands, Bilateral 6 Carotid Body, Left 7 Carotid Body, Right 8 Carotid Bodies, Bilateral 9 Para-aortic Body B Coccygeal Glomus C Glomus Jugulare D Aortic Body F Paraganglion Extremity G Thyroid Gland Lobe, Left H Thyroid Gland Lobe, Right K Thyroid Gland L Superior Parathyroid Gland, Right M Superior Parathyroid Gland, Left N Inferior Parathyroid Gland, Right P Inferior Parathyroid Gland, Left Q Parathyroid Glands, Multiple R Parathyroid Gland	0 Open 3 Percutaneous 4 Percutaneous Endoscopic	Z No Device	X Diagnostic Z No Qualifier

0 **Medical and Surgical**
G **Endocrine System**
B **Excision:** Cutting out or off, without replacement, a portion of a body part

Body Part	Approach	Device	Qualifier
Character 4	Character 5	Character 6	Character 7
0 Pituitary Gland **1** Pineal Body **2** Adrenal Gland, Left **3** Adrenal Gland, Right **4** Adrenal Glands, Bilateral **6** Carotid Body, Left **7** Carotid Body, Right **8** Carotid Bodies, Bilateral **9** Para-aortic Body **B** Coccygeal Glomus **C** Glomus Jugulare **D** Aortic Body **F** Paraganglion Extremity **G** Thyroid Gland Lobe, Left **H** Thyroid Gland Lobe, Right **J** Thyroid Gland Isthmus **L** Superior Parathyroid Gland, Right **M** Superior Parathyroid Gland, Left **N** Inferior Parathyroid Gland, Right **P** Inferior Parathyroid Gland, Left **Q** Parathyroid Glands, Multiple **R** Parathyroid Gland	**0** Open **3** Percutaneous **4** Percutaneous Endoscopic	**Z** No Device	**X** Diagnostic **Z** No Qualifier

0 **Medical and Surgical**
G **Endocrine System**
C **Extirpation:** Taking or cutting out solid matter from a body part

Body Part	Approach	Device	Qualifier
Character 4	Character 5	Character 6	Character 7
0 Pituitary Gland **1** Pineal Body **2** Adrenal Gland, Left **3** Adrenal Gland, Right **4** Adrenal Glands, Bilateral **6** Carotid Body, Left **7** Carotid Body, Right **8** Carotid Bodies, Bilateral **9** Para-aortic Body **B** Coccygeal Glomus **C** Glomus Jugulare **D** Aortic Body **F** Paraganglion Extremity **G** Thyroid Gland Lobe, Left **H** Thyroid Gland Lobe, Right **K** Thyroid Gland **L** Superior Parathyroid Gland, Right **M** Superior Parathyroid Gland, Left **N** Inferior Parathyroid Gland, Right **P** Inferior Parathyroid Gland, Left **Q** Parathyroid Glands, Multiple **R** Parathyroid Gland	**0** Open **3** Percutaneous **4** Percutaneous Endoscopic	**Z** No Device	**Z** No Qualifier

LC Limited Coverage   **NC** Noncovered   **HAC** HAC-associated Procedure   **CC** Combination Cluster - See Appendix G for code lists
DRG Non-OR-Affecting MS-DRG Assignment   New/Revised Text in **Orange**   ♂ Male   ♀ Female

2018 ICD-10-PCS

353

ENDOCRINE SYSTEM 0G2-0GW

0   Medical and Surgical

G   Endocrine System

H   Insertion: Putting in a nonbiological appliance that monitors, assists, performs, or prevents a physiological function but does not physically take the place of a body part

Body Part	Approach	Device	Qualifier
Character 4	Character 5	Character 6	Character 7
S Endocrine Gland	**0** Open **3** Percutaneous **4** Percutaneous Endoscopic	**2** Monitoring Device **3** Infusion Device **Y** Other Device	**Z** No Qualifier

0   Medical and Surgical

G   Endocrine System

J   Inspection: Visually and/or manually exploring a body part

Body Part	Approach	Device	Qualifier
Character 4	Character 5	Character 6	Character 7
0 Pituitary Gland **1** Pineal Body **5** Adrenal Gland **K** Thyroid Gland **R** Parathyroid Gland **S** Endocrine Gland	**0** Open **3** Percutaneous **4** Percutaneous Endoscopic	**Z** No Device	**Z** No Qualifier

0   Medical and Surgical

G   Endocrine System

M   Reattachment: Putting back in or on all or a portion of a separated body part to its normal location or other suitable location

Body Part	Approach	Device	Qualifier
Character 4	Character 5	Character 6	Character 7
2 Adrenal Gland, Left **3** Adrenal Gland, Right **G** Thyroid Gland Lobe, Left **H** Thyroid Gland Lobe, Right **L** Superior Parathyroid Gland, Right **M** Superior Parathyroid Gland, Left **N** Inferior Parathyroid Gland, Right **P** Inferior Parathyroid Gland, Left **Q** Parathyroid Glands, Multiple **R** Parathyroid Gland	**0** Open **4** Percutaneous Endoscopic	**Z** No Device	**Z** No Qualifier

0 Medical and Surgical
G Endocrine System
N Release: Freeing a body part from an abnormal physical constraint by cutting or by the use of force

Body Part	Approach	Device	Qualifier
Character 4	Character 5	Character 6	Character 7
0 Pituitary Gland 1 Pineal Body 2 Adrenal Gland, Left 3 Adrenal Gland, Right 4 Adrenal Glands, Bilateral 6 Carotid Body, Left 7 Carotid Body, Right 8 Carotid Bodies, Bilateral 9 Para-aortic Body B Coccygeal Glomus C Glomus Jugulare D Aortic Body F Paraganglion Extremity G Thyroid Gland Lobe, Left H Thyroid Gland Lobe, Right K Thyroid Gland L Superior Parathyroid Gland, Right M Superior Parathyroid Gland, Left N Inferior Parathyroid Gland, Right P Inferior Parathyroid Gland, Left Q Parathyroid Glands, Multiple R Parathyroid Gland	0 Open 3 Percutaneous 4 Percutaneous Endoscopic	Z No Device	Z No Qualifier

0 Medical and Surgical
G Endocrine System
P Removal: Taking out or off a device from a body part

Body Part	Approach	Device	Qualifier
Character 4	Character 5	Character 6	Character 7
0 Pituitary Gland 1 Pineal Body 5 Adrenal Gland K Thyroid Gland R Parathyroid Gland	0 Open 3 Percutaneous 4 Percutaneous Endoscopic X External	0 Drainage Device	Z No Qualifier
S Endocrine Gland	0 Open 3 Percutaneous 4 Percutaneous Endoscopic	0 Drainage Device 2 Monitoring Device 3 Infusion Device Y Other Device	Z No Qualifier
S Endocrine Gland	X External	0 Drainage Device 2 Monitoring Device 3 Infusion Device	Z No Qualifier

LC Limited Coverage   NC Noncovered   HAC HAC-associated Procedure   CC Combination Cluster - See Appendix G for code lists
DRG Non-OR-Affecting MS-DRG Assignment   New/Revised Text in **Orange**   ♂ Male   ♀ Female

2018 ICD-10-PCS

355

0 Medical and Surgical
G Endocrine System
Q Repair: Restoring, to the extent possible, a body part to its normal anatomic structure and function

Body Part	Approach	Device	Qualifier
Character 4	Character 5	Character 6	Character 7
0 Pituitary Gland 1 Pineal Body 2 Adrenal Gland, Left 3 Adrenal Gland, Right 4 Adrenal Glands, Bilateral 6 Carotid Body, Left 7 Carotid Body, Right 8 Carotid Bodies, Bilateral 9 Para-aortic Body B Coccygeal Glomus C Glomus Jugulare D Aortic Body F Paraganglion Extremity G Thyroid Gland Lobe, Left H Thyroid Gland Lobe, Right J Thyroid Gland Isthmus K Thyroid Gland L Superior Parathyroid Gland, Right M Superior Parathyroid Gland, Left N Inferior Parathyroid Gland, Right P Inferior Parathyroid Gland, Left Q Parathyroid Glands, Multiple R Parathyroid Gland	0 Open 3 Percutaneous 4 Percutaneous Endoscopic	Z No Device	Z No Qualifier

0 Medical and Surgical
G Endocrine System
S Reposition: Moving to its normal location, or other suitable location, all or a portion of a body part

Body Part	Approach	Device	Qualifier
Character 4	Character 5	Character 6	Character 7
2 Adrenal Gland, Left 3 Adrenal Gland, Right G Thyroid Gland Lobe, Left H Thyroid Gland Lobe, Right L Superior Parathyroid Gland, Right M Superior Parathyroid Gland, Left N Inferior Parathyroid Gland, Right P Inferior Parathyroid Gland, Left Q Parathyroid Glands, Multiple R Parathyroid Gland	0 Open 4 Percutaneous Endoscopic	Z No Device	Z No Qualifier

0 **Medical and Surgical**
G **Endocrine System**
T **Resection:** Cutting out or off, without replacement, all of a body part

Body Part	Approach	Device	Qualifier
Character 4	Character 5	Character 6	Character 7
0 Pituitary Gland 1 Pineal Body 2 Adrenal Gland, Left 3 Adrenal Gland, Right 4 Adrenal Glands, Bilateral 6 Carotid Body, Left 7 Carotid Body, Right 8 Carotid Bodies, Bilateral 9 Para-aortic Body B Coccygeal Glomus C Glomus Jugulare D Aortic Body F Paraganglion Extremity G Thyroid Gland Lobe, Left H Thyroid Gland Lobe, Right J Thyroid Gland Isthmus K Thyroid Gland L Superior Parathyroid Gland, Right M Superior Parathyroid Gland, Left N Inferior Parathyroid Gland, Right P Inferior Parathyroid Gland, Left Q Parathyroid Glands, Multiple R Parathyroid Gland	0 Open 4 Percutaneous Endoscopic	Z No Device	Z No Qualifier

0 **Medical and Surgical**
G **Endocrine System**
W **Revision:** Correcting, to the extent possible, a portion of a malfunctioning device or the position of a displaced device

Body Part	Approach	Device	Qualifier
Character 4	Character 5	Character 6	Character 7
0 Pituitary Gland 1 Pineal Body 5 Adrenal Gland K Thyroid Gland R Parathyroid Gland	0 Open 3 Percutaneous 4 Percutaneous Endoscopic X External	0 Drainage Device	Z No Qualifier
S Endocrine Gland	0 Open 3 Percutaneous 4 Percutaneous Endoscopic	0 Drainage Device 2 Monitoring Device 3 Infusion Device Y Other Device	Z No Qualifier
S Endocrine Gland	X External	0 Drainage Device 2 Monitoring Device 3 Infusion Device	Z No Qualifier

LC Limited Coverage   **NC** Noncovered   **HAC** HAC-associated Procedure   **CC** Combination Cluster - See Appendix G for code lists
DRG Non-OR-Affecting MS-DRG Assignment   New/Revised Text in **Orange**   ♂ Male   ♀ Female

2018 ICD-10-PCS

357

NOTES

Skin and Breast 0H0-0HX

0 Medical and Surgical
H Skin and Breast
0 Alteration: Modifying the anatomic structure of a body part without affecting the function of the body part

Body Part	Approach	Device	Qualifier
Character 4	Character 5	Character 6	Character 7
T Breast, Right **U** Breast, Left **V** Breast, Bilateral	**0** Open **3** Percutaneous **X** External	**7** Autologous Tissue Substitute **J** Synthetic Substitute **K** Nonautologous Tissue Substitute **Z** No Device	**Z** No Qualifier

0 Medical and Surgical
H Skin and Breast
2 Change: Taking out or off a device from a body part and putting back an identical or similar device in or on the same body part without cutting or puncturing the skin or a mucous membrane

Body Part	Approach	Device	Qualifier
Character 4	Character 5	Character 6	Character 7
P Skin **T** Breast, Right **U** Breast, Left	**X** External	**0** Drainage Device **Y** Other Device	**Z** No Qualifier

0 Medical and Surgical
H Skin and Breast
5 Destruction: Physical eradication of all or a portion of a body part by the direct use of energy, force, or a destructive agent

Body Part	Approach	Device	Qualifier
Character 4	Character 5	Character 6	Character 7
0 Skin, Scalp **1** Skin, Face **2** Skin, Right Ear **3** Skin, Left Ear **4** Skin, Neck **5** Skin, Chest **6** Skin, Back **7** Skin, Abdomen **8** Skin, Buttock **9** Skin, Perineum **A** Skin, Inguinal **B** Skin, Right Upper Arm **C** Skin, Left Upper Arm **D** Skin, Right Lower Arm **E** Skin, Left Lower Arm **F** Skin, Right Hand **G** Skin, Left Hand **H** Skin, Right Upper Leg **J** Skin, Left Upper Leg **K** Skin, Right Lower Leg **L** Skin, Left Lower Leg **M** Skin, Right Foot **N** Skin, Left Foot	**X** External	**Z** No Device	**D** Multiple **Z** No Qualifier
Q Finger Nail **R** Toe Nail	**X** External	**Z** No Device	**Z** No Qualifier
T Breast, Right **U** Breast, Left **V** Breast, Bilateral **W** Nipple, Right **X** Nipple, Left	**0** Open **3** Percutaneous **7** Via Natural or Artificial Opening **8** Via Natural or Artificial Opening Endoscopic **X** External	**Z** No Device	**Z** No Qualifier

LC Limited Coverage   **NC** Noncovered   **HAC** HAC-associated Procedure   **CC** Combination Cluster - See Appendix G for code lists
DRG Non-OR-Affecting MS-DRG Assignment   New/Revised Text in **Orange**   ♂ Male   ♀ Female

0 **Medical and Surgical**
H **Skin and Breast**
8 **Division:** Cutting into a body part, without draining fluids and/or gases from the body part, in order to separate or transect a body part

Body Part	Approach	Device	Qualifier
Character 4	Character 5	Character 6	Character 7
0 Skin, Scalp	X External	Z No Device	Z No Qualifier
1 Skin, Face			
2 Skin, Right Ear			
3 Skin, Left Ear			
4 Skin, Neck			
5 Skin, Chest			
6 Skin, Back			
7 Skin, Abdomen			
8 Skin, Buttock			
9 Skin, Perineum			
A Skin, Inguinal			
B Skin, Right Upper Arm			
C Skin, Left Upper Arm			
D Skin, Right Lower Arm			
E Skin, Left Lower Arm			
F Skin, Right Hand			
G Skin, Left Hand			
H Skin, Right Upper Leg			
J Skin, Left Upper Leg			
K Skin, Right Lower Leg			
L Skin, Left Lower Leg			
M Skin, Right Foot			
N Skin, Left Foot			

0 **Medical and Surgical**
H **Skin and Breast**
9 **Drainage:** Taking or letting out fluids and/or gases from a body part

Body Part	Approach	Device	Qualifier
Character 4	Character 5	Character 6	Character 7
0 Skin, Scalp	X External	0 Drainage Device	Z No Qualifier
1 Skin, Face			
2 Skin, Right Ear			
3 Skin, Left Ear			
4 Skin, Neck			
5 Skin, Chest			
6 Skin, Back			
7 Skin, Abdomen			
8 Skin, Buttock			
9 Skin, Perineum			
A Skin, Inguinal			
B Skin, Right Upper Arm			
C Skin, Left Upper Arm			
D Skin, Right Lower Arm			
E Skin, Left Lower Arm			
F Skin, Right Hand			
G Skin, Left Hand			
H Skin, Right Upper Leg			
J Skin, Left Upper Leg			
K Skin, Right Lower Leg			
L Skin, Left Lower Leg			
M Skin, Right Foot			
N Skin, Left Foot			
Q Finger Nail			
R Toe Nail			

0H9 continued on next page

0 **Medical and Surgical**
H **Skin and Breast**
9 **Drainage:** Taking or letting out fluids and/or gases from a body part

Body Part	Approach	Device	Qualifier
Character 4	Character 5	Character 6	Character 7
0 Skin, Scalp 1 Skin, Face 2 Skin, Right Ear 3 Skin, Left Ear 4 Skin, Neck 5 Skin, Chest 6 Skin, Back 7 Skin, Abdomen 8 Skin, Buttock 9 Skin, Perineum A Skin, Inguinal B Skin, Right Upper Arm C Skin, Left Upper Arm D Skin, Right Lower Arm E Skin, Left Lower Arm F Skin, Right Hand G Skin, Left Hand H Skin, Right Upper Leg J Skin, Left Upper Leg K Skin, Right Lower Leg L Skin, Left Lower Leg M Skin, Right Foot N Skin, Left Foot Q Finger Nail R Toe Nail	X External	Z No Device	X Diagnostic Z No Qualifier
T Breast, Right U Breast, Left V Breast, Bilateral W Nipple, Right X Nipple, Left	0 Open 3 Percutaneous 7 Via Natural or Artificial Opening 8 Via Natural or Artificial Opening Endoscopic X External	0 Drainage Device	Z No Qualifier
T Breast, Right U Breast, Left V Breast, Bilateral W Nipple, Right X Nipple, Left	0 Open 3 Percutaneous 7 Via Natural or Artificial Opening 8 Via Natural or Artificial Opening Endoscopic X External	Z No Device	X Diagnostic Z No Qualifier

LC Limited Coverage   NC Noncovered   HAC HAC-associated Procedure   CC Combination Cluster - See Appendix G for code lists
DRG Non-OR-Affecting MS-DRG Assignment   New/Revised Text in **Orange**   ♂ Male   ♀ Female

2018 ICD-10-PCS

361

SKIN AND BREAST 0H0-0HX

0   Medical and Surgical
H   Skin and Breast
B   Excision: Cutting out or off, without replacement, a portion of a body part

Body Part	Approach	Device	Qualifier
Character 4	**Character 5**	**Character 6**	**Character 7**
0 Skin, Scalp	**X** External	**Z** No Device	**X** Diagnostic
1 Skin, Face			**Z** No Qualifier
2 Skin, Right Ear			
3 Skin, Left Ear			
4 Skin, Neck			
5 Skin, Chest			
6 Skin, Back			
7 Skin, Abdomen			
8 Skin, Buttock			
9 Skin, Perineum ⓓⓡⓖ			
A Skin, Inguinal			
B Skin, Right Upper Arm			
C Skin, Left Upper Arm			
D Skin, Right Lower Arm			
E Skin, Left Lower Arm			
F Skin, Right Hand			
G Skin, Left Hand			
H Skin, Right Upper Leg			
J Skin, Left Upper Leg			
K Skin, Right Lower Leg			
L Skin, Left Lower Leg			
M Skin, Right Foot			
N Skin, Left Foot			
Q Finger Nail			
R Toe Nail			
T Breast, Right	**0** Open	**Z** No Device	**X** Diagnostic
U Breast, Left	**3** Percutaneous		**Z** No Qualifier
V Breast, Bilateral	**7** Via Natural or Artificial Opening		
W Nipple, Right	**8** Via Natural or Artificial Opening Endoscopic		
X Nipple, Left			
Y Supernumerary Breast	**X** External		

ⓓⓡⓖ 0HB9XZZ

ⓁⒸ Limited Coverage   ⓃⒸ Noncovered   ⒽⒶⒸ HAC-associated Procedure   ⒸⒸ Combination Cluster - See Appendix G for code lists
ⓓⓡⓖ Non-OR-Affecting MS-DRG Assignment   New/Revised Text in **Orange**   ♂ Male   ♀ Female

362

2018 ICD-10-PCS

0 Medical and Surgical
H Skin and Breast
C Extirpation: Taking or cutting out solid matter from a body part

Body Part	Approach	Device	Qualifier
Character 4	Character 5	Character 6	Character 7
0 Skin, Scalp **1** Skin, Face **2** Skin, Right Ear **3** Skin, Left Ear **4** Skin, Neck **5** Skin, Chest **6** Skin, Back **7** Skin, Abdomen **8** Skin, Buttock **9** Skin, Perineum **A** Skin, Inguinal **B** Skin, Right Upper Arm **C** Skin, Left Upper Arm **D** Skin, Right Lower Arm **E** Skin, Left Lower Arm **F** Skin, Right Hand **G** Skin, Left Hand **H** Skin, Right Upper Leg **J** Skin, Left Upper Leg **K** Skin, Right Lower Leg **L** Skin, Left Lower Leg **M** Skin, Right Foot **N** Skin, Left Foot **Q** Finger Nail **R** Toe Nail	**X** External	**Z** No Device	**Z** No Qualifier
T Breast, Right **U** Breast, Left **V** Breast, Bilateral **W** Nipple, Right **X** Nipple, Left	**0** Open **3** Percutaneous **7** Via Natural or Artificial Opening **8** Via Natural or Artificial Opening Endoscopic **X** External	**Z** No Device	**Z** No Qualifier

LC Limited Coverage   NC Noncovered   HAC HAC-associated Procedure   CC Combination Cluster - See Appendix G for code lists
DRG Non-OR-Affecting MS-DRG Assignment   New/Revised Text in **Orange**   ♂ Male   ♀ Female

2018 ICD-10-PCS

363

0   Medical and Surgical
H   Skin and Breast
D   Extraction: Pulling or stripping out or off all or a portion of a body part by the use of force

Body Part	Approach	Device	Qualifier
Character 4	Character 5	Character 6	Character 7
0 Skin, Scalp	**X** External	**Z** No Device	**Z** No Qualifier
1 Skin, Face			
2 Skin, Right Ear			
3 Skin, Left Ear			
4 Skin, Neck			
5 Skin, Chest			
6 Skin, Back			
7 Skin, Abdomen			
8 Skin, Buttock			
9 Skin, Perineum			
A Skin, Inguinal			
B Skin, Right Upper Arm			
C Skin, Left Upper Arm			
D Skin, Right Lower Arm			
E Skin, Left Lower Arm			
F Skin, Right Hand			
G Skin, Left Hand			
H Skin, Right Upper Leg			
J Skin, Left Upper Leg			
K Skin, Right Lower Leg			
L Skin, Left Lower Leg			
M Skin, Right Foot			
N Skin, Left Foot			
Q Finger Nail			
R Toe Nail			
S Hair			

0   Medical and Surgical
H   Skin and Breast
H   Insertion: Putting in a nonbiological appliance that monitors, assists, performs, or prevents a physiological function but does not physically take the place of a body part

Body Part	Approach	Device	Qualifier
Character 4	Character 5	Character 6	Character 7
P Skin	**X** External	**Y** Other Device	**Z** No Qualifier
T Breast, Right **U** Breast, Left	**0** Open **3** Percutaneous **7** Via Natural or Artificial Opening **8** Via Natural or Artificial Opening Endoscopic	**1** Radioactive Element **N** Tissue Expander **Y** Other Device	**Z** No Qualifier
T Breast, Right **U** Breast, Left	**X** External	**1** Radioactive Element	**Z** No Qualifier
V Breast, Bilateral **W** Nipple, Right **X** Nipple, Left	**0** Open **3** Percutaneous **7** Via Natural or Artificial Opening **8** Via Natural or Artificial Opening Endoscopic	**1** Radioactive Element **N** Tissue Expander	**Z** No Qualifier
V Breast, Bilateral **W** Nipple, Right **X** Nipple, Left	**X** External	**1** Radioactive Element	**Z** No Qualifier

LC Limited Coverage   NC Noncovered   HAC HAC-associated Procedure   CC Combination Cluster - See Appendix G for code lists
DRG Non-OR-Affecting MS-DRG Assignment   New/Revised Text in **Orange**   ♂ Male   ♀ Female

364

2018 ICD-10-PCS

0 **Medical and Surgical**
H **Skin and Breast**
J **Inspection:** Visually and/or manually exploring a body part

Body Part	Approach	Device	Qualifier
Character 4	**Character 5**	**Character 6**	**Character 7**
P Skin **Q** Finger Nail **R** Toe Nail	**X** External	**Z** No Device	**Z** No Qualifier
T Breast, Right **U** Breast, Left	**0** Open **3** Percutaneous **7** Via Natural or Artificial Opening **8** Via Natural or Artificial Opening Endoscopic **X** External	**Z** No Device	**Z** No Qualifier

0 **Medical and Surgical**
H **Skin and Breast**
M **Reattachment:** Putting back in or on all or a portion of a separated body part to its normal location or other suitable location

Body Part	Approach	Device	Qualifier
Character 4	**Character 5**	**Character 6**	**Character 7**
0 Skin, Scalp **1** Skin, Face **2** Skin, Right Ear **3** Skin, Left Ear **4** Skin, Neck **5** Skin, Chest **6** Skin, Back **7** Skin, Abdomen **8** Skin, Buttock **9** Skin, Perineum **A** Skin, Inguinal **B** Skin, Right Upper Arm **C** Skin, Left Upper Arm **D** Skin, Right Lower Arm **E** Skin, Left Lower Arm **F** Skin, Right Hand **G** Skin, Left Hand **H** Skin, Right Upper Leg **J** Skin, Left Upper Leg **K** Skin, Right Lower Leg **L** Skin, Left Lower Leg **M** Skin, Right Foot **N** Skin, Left Foot **T** Breast, Right **U** Breast, Left **V** Breast, Bilateral **W** Nipple, Right **X** Nipple, Left	**X** External	**Z** No Device	**Z** No Qualifier

0 Medical and Surgical
H Skin and Breast
N Release: Freeing a body part from an abnormal physical constraint by cutting or by the use of force

Body Part	Approach	Device	Qualifier
Character 4	Character 5	Character 6	Character 7
0 Skin, Scalp 1 Skin, Face 2 Skin, Right Ear 3 Skin, Left Ear 4 Skin, Neck 5 Skin, Chest 6 Skin, Back 7 Skin, Abdomen 8 Skin, Buttock 9 Skin, Perineum A Skin, Inguinal B Skin, Right Upper Arm C Skin, Left Upper Arm D Skin, Right Lower Arm E Skin, Left Lower Arm F Skin, Right Hand G Skin, Left Hand H Skin, Right Upper Leg J Skin, Left Upper Leg K Skin, Right Lower Leg L Skin, Left Lower Leg M Skin, Right Foot N Skin, Left Foot Q Finger Nail R Toe Nail	X External	Z No Device	Z No Qualifier
T Breast, Right U Breast, Left V Breast, Bilateral W Nipple, Right X Nipple, Left	0 Open 3 Percutaneous 7 Via Natural or Artificial Opening 8 Via Natural or Artificial Opening Endoscopic X External	Z No Device	Z No Qualifier

0 Medical and Surgical
H Skin and Breast
P Removal: Taking out or off a device from a body part

Body Part	Approach	Device	Qualifier
Character 4	Character 5	Character 6	Character 7
P Skin	X External	0 Drainage Device 7 Autologous Tissue Substitute J Synthetic Substitute K Nonautologous Tissue Substitute Y Other Device	Z No Qualifier
Q Finger Nail R Toe Nail	X External	0 Drainage Device 7 Autologous Tissue Substitute J Synthetic Substitute K Nonautologous Tissue Substitute	Z No Qualifier
S Hair	X External	7 Autologous Tissue Substitute J Synthetic Substitute K Nonautologous Tissue Substitute	Z No Qualifier
T Breast, Right U Breast, Left	0 Open 3 Percutaneous 7 Via Natural or Artificial Opening 8 Via Natural or Artificial Opening Endoscopic	0 Drainage Device 1 Radioactive Element 7 Autologous Tissue Substitute J Synthetic Substitute K Nonautologous Tissue Substitute N Tissue Expander Y Other Device	Z No Qualifier

0HP continued on next page

0 **Medical and Surgical**
H **Skin and Breast**
P **Removal:** Taking out or off a device from a body part

0HP continued from previous page

Body Part	Approach	Device	Qualifier
Character 4	Character 5	Character 6	Character 7
T Breast, Right **U** Breast, Left	**X** External	**0** Drainage Device **1** Radioactive Element **7** Autologous Tissue Substitute **J** Synthetic Substitute **K** Nonautologous Tissue Substitute	**Z** No Qualifier

0 **Medical and Surgical**
H **Skin and Breast**
Q **Repair:** Restoring, to the extent possible, a body part to its normal anatomic structure and function

Body Part	Approach	Device	Qualifier
Character 4	Character 5	Character 6	Character 7
0 Skin, Scalp **1** Skin, Face **2** Skin, Right Ear **3** Skin, Left Ear **4** Skin, Neck **5** Skin, Chest **6** Skin, Back **7** Skin, Abdomen **8** Skin, Buttock **9** Skin, Perineum **A** Skin, Inguinal **B** Skin, Right Upper Arm **C** Skin, Left Upper Arm **D** Skin, Right Lower Arm **E** Skin, Left Lower Arm **F** Skin, Right Hand **G** Skin, Left Hand **H** Skin, Right Upper Leg **J** Skin, Left Upper Leg **K** Skin, Right Lower Leg **L** Skin, Left Lower Leg **M** Skin, Right Foot **N** Skin, Left Foot **Q** Finger Nail **R** Toe Nail	**X** External	**Z** No Device	**Z** No Qualifier
T Breast, Right **U** Breast, Left **V** Breast, Bilateral **W** Nipple, Right **X** Nipple, Left **Y** Supernumerary Breast	**0** Open **3** Percutaneous **7** Via Natural or Artificial Opening **8** Via Natural or Artificial Opening Endoscopic **X** External	**Z** No Device	**Z** No Qualifier

LC Limited Coverage   **NC** Noncovered   **HAC** HAC-associated Procedure   **CC** Combination Cluster - See Appendix G for code lists
🚺 Non-OR-Affecting MS-DRG Assignment   New/Revised Text in **Orange**   ♂ Male   ♀ Female

2018 ICD-10-PCS

367

SKIN AND BREAST 0H0-0HX

0 Medical and Surgical
H Skin and Breast
R Replacement: Putting in or on biological or synthetic material that physically takes the place and/or function of all or a portion of a body part

Body Part	Approach	Device	Qualifier
Character 4	Character 5	Character 6	Character 7
0 Skin, Scalp 1 Skin, Face 2 Skin, Right Ear 3 Skin, Left Ear 4 Skin, Neck 5 Skin, Chest 6 Skin, Back 7 Skin, Abdomen 8 Skin, Buttock 9 Skin, Perineum A Skin, Inguinal B Skin, Right Upper Arm C Skin, Left Upper Arm D Skin, Right Lower Arm E Skin, Left Lower Arm F Skin, Right Hand G Skin, Left Hand H Skin, Right Upper Leg J Skin, Left Upper Leg K Skin, Right Lower Leg L Skin, Left Lower Leg M Skin, Right Foot N Skin, Left Foot	X External	7 Autologous Tissue Substitute K Nonautologous Tissue Substitute	3 Full Thickness 4 Partial Thickness
0 Skin, Scalp 1 Skin, Face 2 Skin, Right Ear 3 Skin, Left Ear 4 Skin, Neck 5 Skin, Chest 6 Skin, Back 7 Skin, Abdomen 8 Skin, Buttock 9 Skin, Perineum A Skin, Inguinal B Skin, Right Upper Arm C Skin, Left Upper Arm D Skin, Right Lower Arm E Skin, Left Lower Arm F Skin, Right Hand G Skin, Left Hand H Skin, Right Upper Leg J Skin, Left Upper Leg K Skin, Right Lower Leg L Skin, Left Lower Leg M Skin, Right Foot N Skin, Left Foot	X External	J Synthetic Substitute	3 Full Thickness 4 Partial Thickness Z No Qualifier
Q Finger Nail R Toe Nail S Hair	X External	7 Autologous Tissue Substitute J Synthetic Substitute K Nonautologous Tissue Substitute	Z No Qualifier
T Breast, Right U Breast, Left V Breast, Bilateral	0 Open	7 Autologous Tissue Substitute	5 Latissimus Dorsi Myocutaneous Flap 6 Transverse Rectus Abdominis Myocutaneous Flap 7 Deep Inferior Epigastric Artery Perforator Flap 8 Superficial Inferior Epigastric Artery Flap 9 Gluteal Artery Perforator Flap Z No Qualifier

0HR continued on next page

LC Limited Coverage NC Noncovered HAC HAC-associated Procedure CC Combination Cluster - See Appendix G for code lists
DRG Non-OR-Affecting MS-DRG Assignment New/Revised Text in Orange ♂ Male ♀ Female

0 Medical and Surgical
H Skin and Breast
R Replacement: Putting in or on biological or synthetic material that physically takes the place and/or function of all or a portion of a body part

0HR continued from previous page

Body Part	Approach	Device	Qualifier
Character 4	Character 5	Character 6	Character 7
T Breast, Right U Breast, Left V Breast, Bilateral	0 Open	J Synthetic Substitute K Nonautologous Tissue Substitute	Z No Qualifier
T Breast, Right CC U Breast, Left CC V Breast, Bilateral CC	3 Percutaneous X External	7 Autologous Tissue Substitute J Synthetic Substitute K Nonautologous Tissue Substitute	Z No Qualifier
W Nipple, Right X Nipple, Left	0 Open 3 Percutaneous X External	7 Autologous Tissue Substitute J Synthetic Substitute K Nonautologous Tissue Substitute	Z No Qualifier

CC 0HRT37Z   0HRU37Z   0HRV37Z

0 Medical and Surgical
H Skin and Breast
S Reposition: Moving to its normal location, or other suitable location, all or a portion of a body part

Body Part	Approach	Device	Qualifier
Character 4	Character 5	Character 6	Character 7
S Hair W Nipple, Right X Nipple, Left	X External	Z No Device	Z No Qualifier
T Breast, Right U Breast, Left V Breast, Bilateral	0 Open	Z No Device	Z No Qualifier

0 Medical and Surgical
H Skin and Breast
T Resection: Cutting out or off, without replacement, all of a body part

Body Part	Approach	Device	Qualifier
Character 4	Character 5	Character 6	Character 7
Q Finger Nail R Toe Nail W Nipple, Right X Nipple, Left	X External	Z No Device	Z No Qualifier
T Breast, Right CC U Breast, Left CC V Breast, Bilateral CC Y Supernumerary Breast	0 Open	Z No Device	Z No Qualifier

CC 0HTT0ZZ   0HTU0ZZ   0HTV0ZZ

LC Limited Coverage   NC Noncovered   HAC HAC-associated Procedure   CC Combination Cluster - See Appendix G for code lists
DRG Non-OR-Affecting MS-DRG Assignment   New/Revised Text in Orange   ♂ Male   ♀ Female

2018 ICD-10-PCS

369

0 **Medical and Surgical**
H **Skin and Breast**
U **Supplement:** Putting in or on biological or synthetic material that physically reinforces and/or augments the function of a portion of a body part

Body Part	Approach	Device	Qualifier
Character 4	Character 5	Character 6	Character 7
T Breast, Right **U** Breast, Left **V** Breast, Bilateral **W** Nipple, Right **X** Nipple, Left	**0** Open **3** Percutaneous **7** Via Natural or Artificial Opening **8** Via Natural or Artificial Opening Endoscopic **X** External	**7** Autologous Tissue Substitute **J** Synthetic Substitute **K** Nonautologous Tissue Substitute	**Z** No Qualifier

0 **Medical and Surgical**
H **Skin and Breast**
W **Revision:** Correcting, to the extent possible, a portion of a malfunctioning device or the position of a displaced device

Body Part	Approach	Device	Qualifier
Character 4	Character 5	Character 6	Character 7
P Skin	**X** External	**0** Drainage Device **7** Autologous Tissue Substitute **J** Synthetic Substitute **K** Nonautologous Tissue Substitute **Y** Other Device	**Z** No Qualifier
Q Finger Nail **R** Toe Nail	**X** External	**0** Drainage Device **7** Autologous Tissue Substitute **J** Synthetic Substitute **K** Nonautologous Tissue Substitute	**Z** No Qualifier
S Hair	**X** External	**7** Autologous Tissue Substitute **J** Synthetic Substitute **K** Nonautologous Tissue Substitute	**Z** No Qualifier
T Breast, Right **U** Breast, Left	**0** Open **3** Percutaneous **7** Via Natural or Artificial Opening **8** Via Natural or Artificial Opening Endoscopic	**0** Drainage Device **7** Autologous Tissue Substitute **J** Synthetic Substitute **K** Nonautologous Tissue Substitute **N** Tissue Expander **Y** Other Device	**Z** No Qualifier
T Breast, Right **U** Breast, Left	**X** External	**0** Drainage Device **7** Autologous Tissue Substitute **J** Synthetic Substitute **K** Nonautologous Tissue Substitute	**Z** No Qualifier

LC Limited Coverage   **NC** Noncovered   **HAC** HAC-associated Procedure   **CC** Combination Cluster - See Appendix G for code lists
DRG Non-OR-Affecting MS-DRG Assignment   New/Revised Text in **Orange**   ♂ Male   ♀ Female

370

2018 ICD-10-PCS

0 Medical and Surgical
H Skin and Breast
X Transfer: Moving, without taking out, all or a portion of a body part to another location to take over the function of all or a portion of a body part

Body Part	Approach	Device	Qualifier
Character 4	Character 5	Character 6	Character 7
0 Skin, Scalp	**X** External	**Z** No Device	**Z** No Qualifier
1 Skin, Face			
2 Skin, Right Ear			
3 Skin, Left Ear			
4 Skin, Neck			
5 Skin, Chest			
6 Skin, Back			
7 Skin, Abdomen			
8 Skin, Buttock			
9 Skin, Perineum			
A Skin, Inguinal			
B Skin, Right Upper Arm			
C Skin, Left Upper Arm			
D Skin, Right Lower Arm			
E Skin, Left Lower Arm			
F Skin, Right Hand			
G Skin, Left Hand			
H Skin, Right Upper Leg			
J Skin, Left Upper Leg			
K Skin, Right Lower Leg			
L Skin, Left Lower Leg			
M Skin, Right Foot			
N Skin, Left Foot			

LC Limited Coverage   NC Noncovered   HAC HAC-associated Procedure   CC Combination Cluster - See Appendix G for code lists
DRG Non-OR-Affecting MS-DRG Assignment   New/Revised Text in **Orange**   ♂ Male   ♀ Female

2018 ICD-10-PCS   371

SKIN AND BREAST 0H0-0HX

NOTES

Subcutaneous Tissue and Fascia 0J0-0JX

0 **Medical and Surgical**
J **Subcutaneous Tissue and Fascia**
0 **Alteration:** Modifying the anatomic structure of a body part without affecting the function of the body part

Body Part	Approach	Device	Qualifier
Character 4	Character 5	Character 6	Character 7
1 Subcutaneous Tissue and Fascia, Face **4** Subcutaneous Tissue and Fascia, Right Neck **5** Subcutaneous Tissue and Fascia, Left Neck **6** Subcutaneous Tissue and Fascia, Chest **7** Subcutaneous Tissue and Fascia, Back **8** Subcutaneous Tissue and Fascia, Abdomen **9** Subcutaneous Tissue and Fascia, Buttock **D** Subcutaneous Tissue and Fascia, Right Upper Arm **F** Subcutaneous Tissue and Fascia, Left Upper Arm **G** Subcutaneous Tissue and Fascia, Right Lower Arm **H** Subcutaneous Tissue and Fascia, Left Lower Arm **L** Subcutaneous Tissue and Fascia, Right Upper Leg **M** Subcutaneous Tissue and Fascia, Left Upper Leg **N** Subcutaneous Tissue and Fascia, Right Lower Leg **P** Subcutaneous Tissue and Fascia, Left Lower Leg	**0** Open **3** Percutaneous	**Z** No Device	**Z** No Qualifier

0 **Medical and Surgical**
J **Subcutaneous Tissue and Fascia**
2 **Change:** Taking out or off a device from a body part and putting back an identical or similar device in or on the same body part without cutting or puncturing the skin or a mucous membrane

Body Part	Approach	Device	Qualifier
Character 4	Character 5	Character 6	Character 7
S Subcutaneous Tissue and Fascia, Head and Neck **T** Subcutaneous Tissue and Fascia, Trunk **V** Subcutaneous Tissue and Fascia, Upper Extremity **W** Subcutaneous Tissue and Fascia, Lower Extremity	**X** External	**0** Drainage Device **Y** Other Device	**Z** No Qualifier

LC Limited Coverage   NC Noncovered   HAC HAC-associated Procedure   CC Combination Cluster - See Appendix G for code lists
DRG Non-OR-Affecting MS-DRG Assignment   New/Revised Text in **Orange**   ♂ Male   ♀ Female

2018 ICD-10-PCS
373

0 **Medical and Surgical**
J **Subcutaneous Tissue and Fascia**
5 **Destruction:** Physical eradication of all or a portion of a body part by the direct use of energy, force, or a destructive agent

Body Part	Approach	Device	Qualifier
Character 4	Character 5	Character 6	Character 7
0 Subcutaneous Tissue and Fascia, Scalp	0 Open	Z No Device	Z No Qualifier
1 Subcutaneous Tissue and Fascia, Face	3 Percutaneous		
4 Subcutaneous Tissue and Fascia, Right Neck			
5 Subcutaneous Tissue and Fascia, Left Neck			
6 Subcutaneous Tissue and Fascia, Chest			
7 Subcutaneous Tissue and Fascia, Back			
8 Subcutaneous Tissue and Fascia, Abdomen			
9 Subcutaneous Tissue and Fascia, Buttock			
B Subcutaneous Tissue and Fascia, Perineum			
C Subcutaneous Tissue and Fascia, Pelvic Region			
D Subcutaneous Tissue and Fascia, Right Upper Arm			
F Subcutaneous Tissue and Fascia, Left Upper Arm			
G Subcutaneous Tissue and Fascia, Right Lower Arm			
H Subcutaneous Tissue and Fascia, Left Lower Arm			
J Subcutaneous Tissue and Fascia, Right Hand			
K Subcutaneous Tissue and Fascia, Left Hand			
L Subcutaneous Tissue and Fascia, Right Upper Leg			
M Subcutaneous Tissue and Fascia, Left Upper Leg			
N Subcutaneous Tissue and Fascia, Right Lower Leg			
P Subcutaneous Tissue and Fascia, Left Lower Leg			
Q Subcutaneous Tissue and Fascia, Right Foot			
R Subcutaneous Tissue and Fascia, Left Foot			

LC Limited Coverage   NC Noncovered   HAC HAC-associated Procedure   CC Combination Cluster - See Appendix G for code lists
DRG Non-OR-Affecting MS-DRG Assignment   New/Revised Text in **Orange**   ♂ Male   ♀ Female

0 **Medical and Surgical**
J **Subcutaneous Tissue and Fascia**
8 **Division:** Cutting into a body part, without draining fluids and/or gases from the body part, in order to separate or transect a body part

Body Part	Approach	Device	Qualifier
Character 4	Character 5	Character 6	Character 7
0 Subcutaneous Tissue and Fascia, Scalp	**0** Open	**Z** No Device	**Z** No Qualifier
1 Subcutaneous Tissue and Fascia, Face	**3** Percutaneous		
4 Subcutaneous Tissue and Fascia, Right Neck			
5 Subcutaneous Tissue and Fascia, Left Neck			
6 Subcutaneous Tissue and Fascia, Chest			
7 Subcutaneous Tissue and Fascia, Back			
8 Subcutaneous Tissue and Fascia, Abdomen			
9 Subcutaneous Tissue and Fascia, Buttock			
B Subcutaneous Tissue and Fascia, Perineum			
C Subcutaneous Tissue and Fascia, Pelvic Region			
D Subcutaneous Tissue and Fascia, Right Upper Arm			
F Subcutaneous Tissue and Fascia, Left Upper Arm			
G Subcutaneous Tissue and Fascia, Right Lower Arm			
H Subcutaneous Tissue and Fascia, Left Lower Arm			
J Subcutaneous Tissue and Fascia, Right Hand			
K Subcutaneous Tissue and Fascia, Left Hand			
L Subcutaneous Tissue and Fascia, Right Upper Leg			
M Subcutaneous Tissue and Fascia, Left Upper Leg			
N Subcutaneous Tissue and Fascia, Right Lower Leg			
P Subcutaneous Tissue and Fascia, Left Lower Leg			
Q Subcutaneous Tissue and Fascia, Right Foot			
R Subcutaneous Tissue and Fascia, Left Foot			
S Subcutaneous Tissue and Fascia, Head and Neck			
T Subcutaneous Tissue and Fascia, Trunk			
V Subcutaneous Tissue and Fascia, Upper Extremity			
W Subcutaneous Tissue and Fascia, Lower Extremity			

LC Limited Coverage   NC Noncovered   HAC HAC-associated Procedure   CC Combination Cluster - See Appendix G for code lists
DRG Non-OR-Affecting MS-DRG Assignment   New/Revised Text in Orange   ♂ Male   ♀ Female

2018 ICD-10-PCS

375

0 **Medical and Surgical**
J **Subcutaneous Tissue and Fascia**
9 **Drainage:** Taking or letting out fluids and/or gases from a body part

Body Part	Approach	Device	Qualifier
Character 4	Character 5	Character 6	Character 7
0 Subcutaneous Tissue and Fascia, Scalp	0 Open	0 Drainage Device	Z No Qualifier
1 Subcutaneous Tissue and Fascia, Face	3 Percutaneous		
4 Subcutaneous Tissue and Fascia, Right Neck			
5 Subcutaneous Tissue and Fascia, Left Neck			
6 Subcutaneous Tissue and Fascia, Chest			
7 Subcutaneous Tissue and Fascia, Back			
8 Subcutaneous Tissue and Fascia, Abdomen			
9 Subcutaneous Tissue and Fascia, Buttock			
B Subcutaneous Tissue and Fascia, Perineum			
C Subcutaneous Tissue and Fascia, Pelvic Region			
D Subcutaneous Tissue and Fascia, Right Upper Arm			
F Subcutaneous Tissue and Fascia, Left Upper Arm			
G Subcutaneous Tissue and Fascia, Right Lower Arm			
H Subcutaneous Tissue and Fascia, Left Lower Arm			
J Subcutaneous Tissue and Fascia, Right Hand			
K Subcutaneous Tissue and Fascia, Left Hand			
L Subcutaneous Tissue and Fascia, Right Upper Leg			
M Subcutaneous Tissue and Fascia, Left Upper Leg			
N Subcutaneous Tissue and Fascia, Right Lower Leg			
P Subcutaneous Tissue and Fascia, Left Lower Leg			
Q Subcutaneous Tissue and Fascia, Right Foot			
R Subcutaneous Tissue and Fascia, Left Foot			

0J9 continued on next page

0 **Medical and Surgical**
J **Subcutaneous Tissue and Fascia**
9 **Drainage:** Taking or letting out fluids and/or gases from a body part

0J9 continued from previous page

Body Part	Approach	Device	Qualifier
Character 4	Character 5	Character 6	Character 7
0 Subcutaneous Tissue and Fascia, Scalp	0 Open	Z No Device	X Diagnostic
1 Subcutaneous Tissue and Fascia, Face	3 Percutaneous		Z No Qualifier
4 Subcutaneous Tissue and Fascia, Right Neck			
5 Subcutaneous Tissue and Fascia, Left Neck			
6 Subcutaneous Tissue and Fascia, Chest			
7 Subcutaneous Tissue and Fascia, Back			
8 Subcutaneous Tissue and Fascia, Abdomen			
9 Subcutaneous Tissue and Fascia, Buttock			
B Subcutaneous Tissue and Fascia, Perineum			
C Subcutaneous Tissue and Fascia, Pelvic Region			
D Subcutaneous Tissue and Fascia, Right Upper Arm			
F Subcutaneous Tissue and Fascia, Left Upper Arm			
G Subcutaneous Tissue and Fascia, Right Lower Arm			
H Subcutaneous Tissue and Fascia, Left Lower Arm			
J Subcutaneous Tissue and Fascia, Right Hand			
K Subcutaneous Tissue and Fascia, Left Hand			
L Subcutaneous Tissue and Fascia, Right Upper Leg			
M Subcutaneous Tissue and Fascia, Left Upper Leg			
N Subcutaneous Tissue and Fascia, Right Lower Leg			
P Subcutaneous Tissue and Fascia, Left Lower Leg			
Q Subcutaneous Tissue and Fascia, Right Foot			
R Subcutaneous Tissue and Fascia, Left Foot			

0 Medical and Surgical
J Subcutaneous Tissue and Fascia
B Excision: Cutting out or off, without replacement, a portion of a body part

Body Part	Approach	Device	Qualifier
Character 4	Character 5	Character 6	Character 7
0 Subcutaneous Tissue and Fascia, Scalp	**0** Open	**Z** No Device	**X** Diagnostic
1 Subcutaneous Tissue and Fascia, Face	**3** Percutaneous		**Z** No Qualifier
4 Subcutaneous Tissue and Fascia, Right Neck ᴅᴿᴳ			
5 Subcutaneous Tissue and Fascia, Left Neck ᴅᴿᴳ			
6 Subcutaneous Tissue and Fascia, Chest ᴅᴿᴳ			
7 Subcutaneous Tissue and Fascia, Back ᴅᴿᴳ			
8 Subcutaneous Tissue and Fascia, Abdomen ᴅᴿᴳ			
9 Subcutaneous Tissue and Fascia, Buttock ᴅᴿᴳ			
B Subcutaneous Tissue and Fascia, Perineum ᴅᴿᴳ			
C Subcutaneous Tissue and Fascia, Pelvic Region ᴅᴿᴳ			
D Subcutaneous Tissue and Fascia, Right Upper Arm ᴅᴿᴳ			
F Subcutaneous Tissue and Fascia, Left Upper Arm ᴅᴿᴳ			
G Subcutaneous Tissue and Fascia, Right Lower Arm ᴅᴿᴳ			
H Subcutaneous Tissue and Fascia, Left Lower Arm ᴅᴿᴳ			
J Subcutaneous Tissue and Fascia, Right Hand			
K Subcutaneous Tissue and Fascia, Left Hand			
L Subcutaneous Tissue and Fascia, Right Upper Leg ᴅᴿᴳ			
M Subcutaneous Tissue and Fascia, Left Upper Leg ᴅᴿᴳ			
N Subcutaneous Tissue and Fascia, Right Lower Leg ᴅᴿᴳ			
P Subcutaneous Tissue and Fascia, Left Lower Leg ᴅᴿᴳ			
Q Subcutaneous Tissue and Fascia, Right Foot ᴅᴿᴳ			
R Subcutaneous Tissue and Fascia, Left Foot ᴅᴿᴳ			

ᴅᴿᴳ 0JB43ZZ 0JB53ZZ 0JB63ZZ 0JB73ZZ 0JB83ZZ 0JB93ZZ 0JBB3ZZ 0JBC3ZZ 0JBD3ZZ 0JBF3ZZ 0JBG3ZZ 0JBH3ZZ 0JBL3ZZ
0JBM3ZZ 0JBN3ZZ 0JBP3ZZ 0JBQ3ZZ 0JBR3ZZ

LC Limited Coverage **NC** Noncovered **HAC** HAC-associated Procedure **CC** Combination Cluster - See Appendix G for code lists
ᴅᴿᴳ Non-OR-Affecting MS-DRG Assignment New/Revised Text in **Orange** ♂ Male ♀ Female

378

2018 ICD-10-PCS

0 Medical and Surgical
J Subcutaneous Tissue and Fascia
C Extirpation: Taking or cutting out solid matter from a body part

Body Part	Approach	Device	Qualifier
Character 4	Character 5	Character 6	Character 7
0 Subcutaneous Tissue and Fascia, Scalp	**0** Open	**Z** No Device	**Z** No Qualifier
1 Subcutaneous Tissue and Fascia, Face	**3** Percutaneous		
4 Subcutaneous Tissue and Fascia, Right Neck			
5 Subcutaneous Tissue and Fascia, Left Neck			
6 Subcutaneous Tissue and Fascia, Chest			
7 Subcutaneous Tissue and Fascia, Back			
8 Subcutaneous Tissue and Fascia, Abdomen			
9 Subcutaneous Tissue and Fascia, Buttock			
B Subcutaneous Tissue and Fascia, Perineum			
C Subcutaneous Tissue and Fascia, Pelvic Region			
D Subcutaneous Tissue and Fascia, Right Upper Arm			
F Subcutaneous Tissue and Fascia, Left Upper Arm			
G Subcutaneous Tissue and Fascia, Right Lower Arm			
H Subcutaneous Tissue and Fascia, Left Lower Arm			
J Subcutaneous Tissue and Fascia, Right Hand			
K Subcutaneous Tissue and Fascia, Left Hand			
L Subcutaneous Tissue and Fascia, Right Upper Leg			
M Subcutaneous Tissue and Fascia, Left Upper Leg			
N Subcutaneous Tissue and Fascia, Right Lower Leg			
P Subcutaneous Tissue and Fascia, Left Lower Leg			
Q Subcutaneous Tissue and Fascia, Right Foot			
R Subcutaneous Tissue and Fascia, Left Foot			

0   Medical and Surgical
J   Subcutaneous Tissue and Fascia
D   Extraction: Pulling or stripping out or off all or a portion of a body part by the use of force

Body Part	Approach	Device	Qualifier
Character 4	Character 5	Character 6	Character 7
0 Subcutaneous Tissue and Fascia, Scalp	**0** Open	**Z** No Device	**Z** No Qualifier
1 Subcutaneous Tissue and Fascia, Face	**3** Percutaneous		
4 Subcutaneous Tissue and Fascia, Right Neck			
5 Subcutaneous Tissue and Fascia, Left Neck			
6 Subcutaneous Tissue and Fascia, Chest ⫏			
7 Subcutaneous Tissue and Fascia, Back ⫏			
8 Subcutaneous Tissue and Fascia, Abdomen ⫏			
9 Subcutaneous Tissue and Fascia, Buttock ⫏			
B Subcutaneous Tissue and Fascia, Perineum			
C Subcutaneous Tissue and Fascia, Pelvic Region			
D Subcutaneous Tissue and Fascia, Right Upper Arm			
F Subcutaneous Tissue and Fascia, Left Upper Arm			
G Subcutaneous Tissue and Fascia, Right Lower Arm			
H Subcutaneous Tissue and Fascia, Left Lower Arm			
J Subcutaneous Tissue and Fascia, Right Hand			
K Subcutaneous Tissue and Fascia, Left Hand			
L Subcutaneous Tissue and Fascia, Right Upper Leg ⫏			
M Subcutaneous Tissue and Fascia, Left Upper Leg ⫏			
N Subcutaneous Tissue and Fascia, Right Lower Leg			
P Subcutaneous Tissue and Fascia, Left Lower Leg			
Q Subcutaneous Tissue and Fascia, Right Foot			
R Subcutaneous Tissue and Fascia, Left Foot			

⫏ 0JD63ZZ   0JD73ZZ   0JD83ZZ   0JD93ZZ   0JDL3ZZ   0JDM3ZZ

LC Limited Coverage   **NC** Noncovered   **HAC** HAC-associated Procedure   **CC** Combination Cluster - See Appendix G for code lists
DRG Non-OR-Affecting MS-DRG Assignment   New/Revised Text in **Orange**   ♂ Male   ♀ Female

380

2018 ICD-10-PCS

SUBCUTANEOUS TISSUE AND FASCIA 0J0-0JX

0 **Medical and Surgical**
J **Subcutaneous Tissue and Fascia**
H **Insertion:** Putting in a nonbiological appliance that monitors, assists, performs, or prevents a physiological function but does not physically take the place of a body part

Body Part	Approach	Device	Qualifier
Character 4	Character 5	Character 6	Character 7
0 Subcutaneous Tissue and Fascia, Scalp **1** Subcutaneous Tissue and Fascia, Face **4** Subcutaneous Tissue and Fascia, Right Neck **5** Subcutaneous Tissue and Fascia, Left Neck **9** Subcutaneous Tissue and Fascia, Buttock **B** Subcutaneous Tissue and Fascia, Perineum **C** Subcutaneous Tissue and Fascia, Pelvic Region **J** Subcutaneous Tissue and Fascia, Right Hand **K** Subcutaneous Tissue and Fascia, Left Hand **Q** Subcutaneous Tissue and Fascia, Right Foot **R** Subcutaneous Tissue and Fascia, Left Foot	**0** Open **3** Percutaneous	**N** Tissue Expander	**Z** No Qualifier
6 Subcutaneous Tissue and Fascia, Chest CC HAC **8** Subcutaneous Tissue and Fascia, Abdomen NC CC HAC	**0** Open **3** Percutaneous	**0** Monitoring Device, Hemodynamic **2** Monitoring Device **4** Pacemaker, Single Chamber **5** Pacemaker, Single Chamber Rate Responsive **6** Pacemaker, Dual Chamber **7** Cardiac Resynchronization Pacemaker Pulse Generator **8** Defibrillator Generator **9** Cardiac Resynchronization Defibrillator Pulse Generator **A** Contractility Modulation Device **B** Stimulator Generator, Single Array **C** Stimulator Generator, Single Array Rechargeable **D** Stimulator Generator, Multiple Array **E** Stimulator Generator, Multiple Array Rechargeable **H** Contraceptive Device **M** Stimulator Generator **N** Tissue Expander **P** Cardiac Rhythm Related Device **V** Infusion Device, Pump **W** Vascular Access Device, Totally Implantable **X** Vascular Access Device, Tunneled	**Z** No Qualifier

0JH continued on next page

0 Medical and Surgical
J Subcutaneous Tissue and Fascia

0JH continued from previous page

H Insertion: Putting in a nonbiological appliance that monitors, assists, performs, or prevents a physiological function but does not physically take the place of a body part

Body Part	Approach	Device	Qualifier
Character 4	Character 5	Character 6	Character 7
7 Subcutaneous Tissue and Fascia, Back NC CC	0 Open 3 Percutaneous	B Stimulator Generator, Single Array C Stimulator Generator, Single Array Rechargeable D Stimulator Generator, Multiple Array E Stimulator Generator, Multiple Array Rechargeable M Stimulator Generator N Tissue Expander V Infusion Device, Pump	Z No Qualifier
D Subcutaneous Tissue and Fascia, Right Upper Arm F Subcutaneous Tissue and Fascia, Left Upper Arm G Subcutaneous Tissue and Fascia, Right Lower Arm H Subcutaneous Tissue and Fascia, Left Lower Arm L Subcutaneous Tissue and Fascia, Right Upper Leg DRG M Subcutaneous Tissue and Fascia, Left Upper Leg DRG N Subcutaneous Tissue and Fascia, Right Lower Leg DRG P Subcutaneous Tissue and Fascia, Left Lower Leg DRG	0 Open 3 Percutaneous	H Contraceptive Device N Tissue Expander V Infusion Device, Pump W Vascular Access Device, Totally Implantable X Vascular Access Device, Tunneled	Z No Qualifier
S Subcutaneous Tissue and Fascia, Head and Neck V Subcutaneous Tissue and Fascia, Upper Extremity W Subcutaneous Tissue and Fascia, Lower Extremity	0 Open 3 Percutaneous	1 Radioactive Element 3 Infusion Device Y Other Device	Z No Qualifier
T Subcutaneous Tissue and Fascia, Trunk	0 Open 3 Percutaneous	1 Radioactive Element 3 Infusion Device V Infusion Device, Pump Y Other Device	Z No Qualifier

NC 0JH70MZ   0JH73MZ   0JH80MZ   0JH83MZ

CC 0JH608Z   0JH609Z   0JH60AZ   0JH60BZ   0JH60CZ   0JH60DZ   0JH60EZ   0JH638Z   0JH639Z   0JH63AZ   0JH63BZ   0JH63CZ   0JH63DZ
0JH63EZ   0JH70BZ   0JH70CZ   0JH70DZ   0JH70EZ   0JH73BZ   0JH73CZ   0JH73DZ   0JH73EZ   0JH808Z   0JH809Z   0JH80AZ   0JH80BZ
0JH80CZ   0JH80DZ   0JH80EZ   0JH838Z   0JH839Z   0JH83AZ   0JH83BZ   0JH83CZ   0JH83DZ   0JH83EZ

HAC 0JH604Z   0JH605Z   0JH606Z   0JH607Z   0JH608Z   0JH609Z   0JH60PZ   0JH634Z   0JH635Z   0JH636Z   0JH637Z   0JH638Z   0JH639Z
0JH63PZ   0JH804Z   0JH805Z   0JH806Z   0JH807Z   0JH808Z   0JH809Z   0JH80PZ   0JH834Z   0JH835Z   0JH836Z   0JH837Z   0JH838Z
0JH839Z   0JH83PZ

Surgical site infection (SSI) following cardiac implantable electronic device (CIED) procedures and secondary diagnosis K68.11, T81.4XXA, T82.6XXA, T82.7XXA.

HAC 0JH63XZ

Iatrogenic pneumothorax w/ venous catheterization procedures and secondary diagnosis J95.811.

DRG 0JHL0WZ   0JHL0XZ   0JHL3WZ   0JHL3XZ   0JHM0WZ   0JHM0XZ   0JHM3WZ   0JHM3XZ   0JHN0WZ   0JHN0XZ   0JHN3HZ   0JHN3WZ   0JHN3XZ
0JHP0HZ   0JHP0WZ   0JHP0XZ   0JHP3HZ   0JHP3WZ   0JHP3XZ

LC Limited Coverage   NC Noncovered   HAC HAC-associated Procedure   CC Combination Cluster - See Appendix G for code lists
DRG Non-OR-Affecting MS-DRG Assignment   New/Revised Text in Orange   ♂ Male   ♀ Female

382

2018 ICD-10-PCS

0 Medical and Surgical
J Subcutaneous Tissue and Fascia
J Inspection: Visually and/or manually exploring a body part

Body Part	Approach	Device	Qualifier
Character 4	Character 5	Character 6	Character 7
S Subcutaneous Tissue and Fascia, Head and Neck **T** Subcutaneous Tissue and Fascia, Trunk **V** Subcutaneous Tissue and Fascia, Upper Extremity **W** Subcutaneous Tissue and Fascia, Lower Extremity	**0** Open **3** Percutaneous **X** External	**Z** No Device	**Z** No Qualifier

0 Medical and Surgical
J Subcutaneous Tissue and Fascia
N Release: Freeing a body part from an abnormal physical constraint by cutting or by the use of force

Body Part	Approach	Device	Qualifier
Character 4	Character 5	Character 6	Character 7
0 Subcutaneous Tissue and Fascia, Scalp **1** Subcutaneous Tissue and Fascia, Face **4** Subcutaneous Tissue and Fascia, Right Neck **5** Subcutaneous Tissue and Fascia, Left Neck **6** Subcutaneous Tissue and Fascia, Chest **7** Subcutaneous Tissue and Fascia, Back **8** Subcutaneous Tissue and Fascia, Abdomen **9** Subcutaneous Tissue and Fascia, Buttock **B** Subcutaneous Tissue and Fascia, Perineum **C** Subcutaneous Tissue and Fascia, Pelvic Region **D** Subcutaneous Tissue and Fascia, Right Upper Arm **F** Subcutaneous Tissue and Fascia, Left Upper Arm **G** Subcutaneous Tissue and Fascia, Right Lower Arm **H** Subcutaneous Tissue and Fascia, Left Lower Arm **J** Subcutaneous Tissue and Fascia, Right Hand **K** Subcutaneous Tissue and Fascia, Left Hand **L** Subcutaneous Tissue and Fascia, Right Upper Leg **M** Subcutaneous Tissue and Fascia, Left Upper Leg **N** Subcutaneous Tissue and Fascia, Right Lower Leg **P** Subcutaneous Tissue and Fascia, Left Lower Leg **Q** Subcutaneous Tissue and Fascia, Right Foot **R** Subcutaneous Tissue and Fascia, Left Foot	**0** Open **3** Percutaneous **X** External	**Z** No Device	**Z** No Qualifier

0 **Medical and Surgical**
J **Subcutaneous Tissue and Fascia**
P **Removal:** Taking out or off a device from a body part

Body Part	Approach	Device	Qualifier
Character 4	**Character 5**	**Character 6**	**Character 7**
S Subcutaneous Tissue and Fascia, Head and Neck	0 Open 3 Percutaneous	0 Drainage Device 1 Radioactive Element 3 Infusion Device 7 Autologous Tissue Substitute J Synthetic Substitute K Nonautologous Tissue Substitute N Tissue Expander Y Other Device	Z No Qualifier
S Subcutaneous Tissue and Fascia, Head and Neck	X External	0 Drainage Device 1 Radioactive Element 3 Infusion Device	Z No Qualifier
T Subcutaneous Tissue and Fascia, Trunk ᴴᴬᶜ	0 Open 3 Percutaneous	0 Drainage Device 1 Radioactive Element 2 Monitoring Device 3 Infusion Device 7 Autologous Tissue Substitute H Contraceptive Device J Synthetic Substitute K Nonautologous Tissue Substitute M Stimulator Generator N Tissue Expander P Cardiac Rhythm Related Device V Infusion Device, Pump W Vascular Access Device, Totally Implantable X Vascular Access Device, Tunneled Y Other Device	Z No Qualifier
T Subcutaneous Tissue and Fascia, Trunk	X External	0 Drainage Device 1 Radioactive Element 2 Monitoring Device 3 Infusion Device H Contraceptive Device V Infusion Device, Pump X Vascular Access Device, Tunneled	Z No Qualifier
V Subcutaneous Tissue and Fascia, Upper Extremity W Subcutaneous Tissue and Fascia, Lower Extremity	0 Open 3 Percutaneous	0 Drainage Device 1 Radioactive Element 3 Infusion Device 7 Autologous Tissue Substitute H Contraceptive Device J Synthetic Substitute K Nonautologous Tissue Substitute N Tissue Expander V Infusion Device, Pump W Vascular Access Device, Totally Implantable X Vascular Access Device, Tunneled Y Other Device	Z No Qualifier
V Subcutaneous Tissue and Fascia, Upper Extremity W Subcutaneous Tissue and Fascia, Lower Extremity	X External	0 Drainage Device 1 Radioactive Element 3 Infusion Device H Contraceptive Device V Infusion Device, Pump X Vascular Access Device, Tunneled	Z No Qualifier

ᴴᴬᶜ 0JPT0PZ   0JPT3PZ

Surgical site infection (SSI) following cardiac implantable electronic device (CIED) procedures and secondary diagnosis K68.11, T81.4XXA, T82.6XXA, T82.7XXA.

0 Medical and Surgical
J Subcutaneous Tissue and Fascia
Q Repair: Restoring, to the extent possible, a body part to its normal anatomic structure and function

Body Part	Approach	Device	Qualifier
Character 4	Character 5	Character 6	Character 7
0 Subcutaneous Tissue and Fascia, Scalp **1** Subcutaneous Tissue and Fascia, Face **4** Subcutaneous Tissue and Fascia, Right Neck **5** Subcutaneous Tissue and Fascia, Left Neck **6** Subcutaneous Tissue and Fascia, Chest **7** Subcutaneous Tissue and Fascia, Back **8** Subcutaneous Tissue and Fascia, Abdomen **9** Subcutaneous Tissue and Fascia, Buttock **B** Subcutaneous Tissue and Fascia, Perineum **C** Subcutaneous Tissue and Fascia, Pelvic Region **D** Subcutaneous Tissue and Fascia, Right Upper Arm **F** Subcutaneous Tissue and Fascia, Left Upper Arm **G** Subcutaneous Tissue and Fascia, Right Lower Arm **H** Subcutaneous Tissue and Fascia, Left Lower Arm **J** Subcutaneous Tissue and Fascia, Right Hand **K** Subcutaneous Tissue and Fascia, Left Hand **L** Subcutaneous Tissue and Fascia, Right Upper Leg **M** Subcutaneous Tissue and Fascia, Left Upper Leg **N** Subcutaneous Tissue and Fascia, Right Lower Leg **P** Subcutaneous Tissue and Fascia, Left Lower Leg **Q** Subcutaneous Tissue and Fascia, Right Foot **R** Subcutaneous Tissue and Fascia, Left Foot	**0** Open **3** Percutaneous	**Z** No Device	**Z** No Qualifier

0 Medical and Surgical
J Subcutaneous Tissue and Fascia
R Replacement: Putting in or on biological or synthetic material that physically takes the place and/or function of all or a portion of a body part

Body Part	Approach	Device	Qualifier
Character 4	Character 5	Character 6	Character 7
0 Subcutaneous Tissue and Fascia, Scalp 1 Subcutaneous Tissue and Fascia, Face 4 Subcutaneous Tissue and Fascia, Right Neck 5 Subcutaneous Tissue and Fascia, Left Neck 6 Subcutaneous Tissue and Fascia, Chest 7 Subcutaneous Tissue and Fascia, Back 8 Subcutaneous Tissue and Fascia, Abdomen 9 Subcutaneous Tissue and Fascia, Buttock B Subcutaneous Tissue and Fascia, Perineum C Subcutaneous Tissue and Fascia, Pelvic Region D Subcutaneous Tissue and Fascia, Right Upper Arm F Subcutaneous Tissue and Fascia, Left Upper Arm G Subcutaneous Tissue and Fascia, Right Lower Arm H Subcutaneous Tissue and Fascia, Left Lower Arm J Subcutaneous Tissue and Fascia, Right Hand K Subcutaneous Tissue and Fascia, Left Hand L Subcutaneous Tissue and Fascia, Right Upper Leg M Subcutaneous Tissue and Fascia, Left Upper Leg N Subcutaneous Tissue and Fascia, Right Lower Leg P Subcutaneous Tissue and Fascia, Left Lower Leg Q Subcutaneous Tissue and Fascia, Right Foot R Subcutaneous Tissue and Fascia, Left Foot	0 Open 3 Percutaneous	7 Autologous Tissue Substitute J Synthetic Substitute K Nonautologous Tissue Substitute	Z No Qualifier

0   **Medical and Surgical**
J   **Subcutaneous Tissue and Fascia**
U   **Supplement:** Putting in or on biological or synthetic material that physically reinforces and/or augments the function of a portion of a body part

Body Part	Approach	Device	Qualifier
Character 4	Character 5	Character 6	Character 7
0 Subcutaneous Tissue and Fascia, Scalp **1** Subcutaneous Tissue and Fascia, Face **4** Subcutaneous Tissue and Fascia, Right Neck **5** Subcutaneous Tissue and Fascia, Left Neck **6** Subcutaneous Tissue and Fascia, Chest **7** Subcutaneous Tissue and Fascia, Back **8** Subcutaneous Tissue and Fascia, Abdomen **9** Subcutaneous Tissue and Fascia, Buttock **B** Subcutaneous Tissue and Fascia, Perineum **C** Subcutaneous Tissue and Fascia, Pelvic Region **D** Subcutaneous Tissue and Fascia, Right Upper Arm **F** Subcutaneous Tissue and Fascia, Left Upper Arm **G** Subcutaneous Tissue and Fascia, Right Lower Arm **H** Subcutaneous Tissue and Fascia, Left Lower Arm **J** Subcutaneous Tissue and Fascia, Right Hand **K** Subcutaneous Tissue and Fascia, Left Hand **L** Subcutaneous Tissue and Fascia, Right Upper Leg **M** Subcutaneous Tissue and Fascia, Left Upper Leg **N** Subcutaneous Tissue and Fascia, Right Lower Leg **P** Subcutaneous Tissue and Fascia, Left Lower Leg **Q** Subcutaneous Tissue and Fascia, Right Foot **R** Subcutaneous Tissue and Fascia, Left Foot	**0** Open **3** Percutaneous	**7** Autologous Tissue Substitute **J** Synthetic Substitute **K** Nonautologous Tissue Substitute	**Z** No Qualifier

0   **Medical and Surgical**
J   **Subcutaneous Tissue and Fascia**
W   **Revision:** Correcting, to the extent possible, a portion of a malfunctioning device or the position of a displaced device

Body Part	Approach	Device	Qualifier
Character 4	Character 5	Character 6	Character 7
S Subcutaneous Tissue and Fascia, Head and Neck 🏷	**0** Open **3** Percutaneous	**0** Drainage Device **3** Infusion Device **7** Autologous Tissue Substitute **J** Synthetic Substitute **K** Nonautologous Tissue Substitute **N** Tissue Expander **Y** Other Device	**Z** No Qualifier

0JW continued on next page

0 Medical and Surgical
J Subcutaneous Tissue and Fascia

OJW continued from previous page

W Revision: Correcting, to the extent possible, a portion of a malfunctioning device or the position of a displaced device

Body Part	Approach	Device	Qualifier
Character 4	Character 5	Character 6	Character 7
S Subcutaneous Tissue and Fascia, Head and Neck	**X** External	**0** Drainage Device **3** Infusion Device **7** Autologous Tissue Substitute **J** Synthetic Substitute **K** Nonautologous Tissue Substitute **N** Tissue Expander	**Z** No Qualifier
T Subcutaneous Tissue and Fascia, Trunk ⬛DRG	**0** Open **3** Percutaneous	**0** Drainage Device **2** Monitoring Device **3** Infusion Device **7** Autologous Tissue Substitute **H** Contraceptive Device **J** Synthetic Substitute **K** Nonautologous Tissue Substitute **M** Stimulator Generator **N** Tissue Expander **P** Cardiac Rhythm Related Device **V** Infusion Device, Pump **W** Vascular Access Device, Totally Implantable **X** Vascular Access Device, Tunneled **Y** Other Device	**Z** No Qualifier
T Subcutaneous Tissue and Fascia, Trunk	**X** External	**0** Drainage Device **2** Monitoring Device **3** Infusion Device **7** Autologous Tissue Substitute **H** Contraceptive Device **J** Synthetic Substitute **K** Nonautologous Tissue Substitute **M** Stimulator Generator **N** Tissue Expander **P** Cardiac Rhythm Related Device **V** Infusion Device, Pump **W** Vascular Access Device, Totally Implantable **X** Vascular Access Device, Tunneled	**Z** No Qualifier
V Subcutaneous Tissue and Fascia, Upper Extremity DRG **W** Subcutaneous Tissue and Fascia, Lower Extremity DRG	**0** Open **3** Percutaneous	**0** Drainage Device **3** Infusion Device **7** Autologous Tissue Substitute **H** Contraceptive Device **J** Synthetic Substitute **K** Nonautologous Tissue Substitute **N** Tissue Expander **V** Infusion Device, Pump **W** Vascular Access Device, Totally Implantable **X** Vascular Access Device, Tunneled **Y** Other Device	**Z** No Qualifier
V Subcutaneous Tissue and Fascia, Upper Extremity **W** Subcutaneous Tissue and Fascia, Lower Extremity	**X** External	**0** Drainage Device **3** Infusion Device **7** Autologous Tissue Substitute **H** Contraceptive Device **J** Synthetic Substitute **K** Nonautologous Tissue Substitute **N** Tissue Expander **V** Infusion Device, Pump **W** Vascular Access Device, Totally Implantable **X** Vascular Access Device, Tunneled	**Z** No Qualifier

OJW continued on next page

LC Limited Coverage   NC Noncovered   HAC HAC-associated Procedure   CC Combination Cluster - See Appendix G for code lists
DRG Non-OR-Affecting MS-DRG Assignment   New/Revised Text in **Orange**   ♂ Male   ♀ Female

0JW continued from previous page

HAC 0JWT0PZ   0JWT3PZ

Surgical site infection (SSI) following cardiac implantable electronic device (CIED) procedures and secondary diagnosis K68.11, T81.4XXA, T82.6XXA, T82.7XXA.

DRG 0JWS00Z 0JWS03Z 0JWS07Z 0JWS0JZ 0JWS0KZ 0JWS0NZ 0JWS30Z 0JWS33Z 0JWS37Z 0JWS3JZ 0JWS3KZ 0JWS3NZ 0JWT00Z
0JWT03Z 0JWT07Z 0JWT0HZ 0JWT0JZ 0JWT0KZ 0JWT0NZ 0JWT0VZ 0JWT0WZ 0JWT0XZ 0JWT30Z 0JWT33Z 0JWT37Z 0JWT3HZ
0JWT3JZ 0JWT3KZ 0JWT3NZ 0JWT3VZ 0JWT3WZ 0JWT3XZ 0JWV00Z 0JWV03Z 0JWV07Z 0JWV0HZ 0JWV0JZ 0JWV0KZ 0JWV0NZ
0JWV0VZ 0JWV0WZ 0JWV0XZ 0JWV30Z 0JWV33Z 0JWV37Z 0JWV3HZ 0JWV3JZ 0JWV3KZ 0JWV3NZ 0JWV3VZ 0JWV3WZ 0JWV3XZ
0JWW00Z 0JWW03Z 0JWW07Z 0JWW0HZ 0JWW0JZ 0JWW0KZ 0JWW0NZ 0JWW0VZ 0JWW0WZ 0JWW0XZ 0JWW30Z 0JWW33Z 0JWW37Z
0JWW3HZ 0JWW3JZ 0JWW3KZ 0JWW3NZ 0JWW3VZ 0JWW3WZ 0JWW3XZ

0 **Medical and Surgical**
J **Subcutaneous Tissue and Fascia**
X **Transfer:** Moving, without taking out, all or a portion of a body part to another location to take over the function of all or a portion of a body part

Body Part	Approach	Device	Qualifier
Character 4	Character 5	Character 6	Character 7
0 Subcutaneous Tissue and Fascia, Scalp **1** Subcutaneous Tissue and Fascia, Face **4** Subcutaneous Tissue and Fascia, Right Neck **5** Subcutaneous Tissue and Fascia, Left Neck **6** Subcutaneous Tissue and Fascia, Chest **7** Subcutaneous Tissue and Fascia, Back **8** Subcutaneous Tissue and Fascia, Abdomen **9** Subcutaneous Tissue and Fascia, Buttock **B** Subcutaneous Tissue and Fascia, Perineum **C** Subcutaneous Tissue and Fascia, Pelvic Region **D** Subcutaneous Tissue and Fascia, Right Upper Arm **F** Subcutaneous Tissue and Fascia, Left Upper Arm **G** Subcutaneous Tissue and Fascia, Right Lower Arm **H** Subcutaneous Tissue and Fascia, Left Lower Arm **J** Subcutaneous Tissue and Fascia, Right Hand **K** Subcutaneous Tissue and Fascia, Left Hand **L** Subcutaneous Tissue and Fascia, Right Upper Leg **M** Subcutaneous Tissue and Fascia, Left Upper Leg **N** Subcutaneous Tissue and Fascia, Right Lower Leg **P** Subcutaneous Tissue and Fascia, Left Lower Leg **Q** Subcutaneous Tissue and Fascia, Right Foot **R** Subcutaneous Tissue and Fascia, Left Foot	**0** Open **3** Percutaneous	**Z** No Device	**B** Skin and Subcutaneous Tissue **C** Skin, Subcutaneous Tissue and Fascia **Z** No Qualifier

NOTES

Muscles 0K2-0KX

0 Medical and Surgical
K Muscles
2 **Change:** Taking out or off a device from a body part and putting back an identical or similar device in or on the same body part without cutting or puncturing the skin or a mucous membrane

Body Part	Approach	Device	Qualifier
Character 4	Character 5	Character 6	Character 7
X Upper Muscle **Y** Lower Muscle	**X** External	**0** Drainage Device **Y** Other Device	**Z** No Qualifier

0 Medical and Surgical
K Muscles
5 **Destruction:** Physical eradication of all or a portion of a body part by the direct use of energy, force, or a destructive agent

Body Part	Approach	Device	Qualifier
Character 4	Character 5	Character 6	Character 7
0 Head Muscle **1** Facial Muscle **2** Neck Muscle, Right **3** Neck Muscle, Left **4** Tongue, Palate, Pharynx Muscle **5** Shoulder Muscle, Right **6** Shoulder Muscle, Left **7** Upper Arm Muscle, Right **8** Upper Arm Muscle, Left **9** Lower Arm and Wrist Muscle, Right **B** Lower Arm and Wrist Muscle, Left **C** Hand Muscle, Right **D** Hand Muscle, Left **F** Trunk Muscle, Right **G** Trunk Muscle, Left **H** Thorax Muscle, Right **J** Thorax Muscle, Left **K** Abdomen Muscle, Right **L** Abdomen Muscle, Left **M** Perineum Muscle **N** Hip Muscle, Right **P** Hip Muscle, Left **Q** Upper Leg Muscle, Right **R** Upper Leg Muscle, Left **S** Lower Leg Muscle, Right **T** Lower Leg Muscle, Left **V** Foot Muscle, Right **W** Foot Muscle, Left	**0** Open **3** Percutaneous **4** Percutaneous Endoscopic	**Z** No Device	**Z** No Qualifier

LC Limited Coverage   NC Noncovered   HAC HAC-associated Procedure   CC Combination Cluster - See Appendix G for code lists
DRG Non-OR-Affecting MS-DRG Assignment   New/Revised Text in **Orange**   ♂ Male   ♀ Female

0 Medical and Surgical
K Muscles
8 Division: Cutting into a body part, without draining fluids and/or gases from the body part, in order to separate or transect a body part

Body Part	Approach	Device	Qualifier
Character 4	Character 5	Character 6	Character 7
0 Head Muscle	0 Open	Z No Device	Z No Qualifier
1 Facial Muscle	3 Percutaneous		
2 Neck Muscle, Right	4 Percutaneous Endoscopic		
3 Neck Muscle, Left			
4 Tongue, Palate, Pharynx Muscle			
5 Shoulder Muscle, Right			
6 Shoulder Muscle, Left			
7 Upper Arm Muscle, Right			
8 Upper Arm Muscle, Left			
9 Lower Arm and Wrist Muscle, Right			
B Lower Arm and Wrist Muscle, Left			
C Hand Muscle, Right			
D Hand Muscle, Left			
F Trunk Muscle, Right			
G Trunk Muscle, Left			
H Thorax Muscle, Right			
J Thorax Muscle, Left			
K Abdomen Muscle, Right			
L Abdomen Muscle, Left			
M Perineum Muscle			
N Hip Muscle, Right			
P Hip Muscle, Left			
Q Upper Leg Muscle, Right			
R Upper Leg Muscle, Left			
S Lower Leg Muscle, Right			
T Lower Leg Muscle, Left			
V Foot Muscle, Right			
W Foot Muscle, Left			

0 **Medical and Surgical**

K **Muscles**

9 **Drainage:** Taking or letting out fluids and/or gases from a body part

Body Part	Approach	Device	Qualifier
Character 4	Character 5	Character 6	Character 7
0 Head Muscle 1 Facial Muscle 2 Neck Muscle, Right 3 Neck Muscle, Left 4 Tongue, Palate, Pharynx Muscle 5 Shoulder Muscle, Right 6 Shoulder Muscle, Left 7 Upper Arm Muscle, Right 8 Upper Arm Muscle, Left 9 Lower Arm and Wrist Muscle, Right B Lower Arm and Wrist Muscle, Left C Hand Muscle, Right D Hand Muscle, Left F Trunk Muscle, Right G Trunk Muscle, Left H Thorax Muscle, Right J Thorax Muscle, Left K Abdomen Muscle, Right L Abdomen Muscle, Left M Perineum Muscle N Hip Muscle, Right P Hip Muscle, Left Q Upper Leg Muscle, Right R Upper Leg Muscle, Left S Lower Leg Muscle, Right T Lower Leg Muscle, Left V Foot Muscle, Right W Foot Muscle, Left	0 Open 3 Percutaneous 4 Percutaneous Endoscopic	0 Drainage Device	Z No Qualifier
0 Head Muscle 1 Facial Muscle 2 Neck Muscle, Right 3 Neck Muscle, Left 4 Tongue, Palate, Pharynx Muscle 5 Shoulder Muscle, Right 6 Shoulder Muscle, Left 7 Upper Arm Muscle, Right 8 Upper Arm Muscle, Left 9 Lower Arm and Wrist Muscle, Right B Lower Arm and Wrist Muscle, Left C Hand Muscle, Right D Hand Muscle, Left F Trunk Muscle, Right G Trunk Muscle, Left H Thorax Muscle, Right J Thorax Muscle, Left K Abdomen Muscle, Right L Abdomen Muscle, Left M Perineum Muscle N Hip Muscle, Right P Hip Muscle, Left Q Upper Leg Muscle, Right R Upper Leg Muscle, Left S Lower Leg Muscle, Right T Lower Leg Muscle, Left V Foot Muscle, Right W Foot Muscle, Left	0 Open 3 Percutaneous 4 Percutaneous Endoscopic	Z No Device	X Diagnostic Z No Qualifier

0 **Medical and Surgical**
K **Muscles**
B **Excision:** Cutting out or off, without replacement, a portion of a body part

Body Part	Approach	Device	Qualifier
Character 4	Character 5	Character 6	Character 7
0 Head Muscle 1 Facial Muscle 2 Neck Muscle, Right 3 Neck Muscle, Left 4 Tongue, Palate, Pharynx Muscle 5 Shoulder Muscle, Right 6 Shoulder Muscle, Left 7 Upper Arm Muscle, Right 8 Upper Arm Muscle, Left 9 Lower Arm and Wrist Muscle, Right B Lower Arm and Wrist Muscle, Left C Hand Muscle, Right D Hand Muscle, Left F Trunk Muscle, Right G Trunk Muscle, Left H Thorax Muscle, Right J Thorax Muscle, Left K Abdomen Muscle, Right L Abdomen Muscle, Left M Perineum Muscle N Hip Muscle, Right P Hip Muscle, Left Q Upper Leg Muscle, Right R Upper Leg Muscle, Left S Lower Leg Muscle, Right T Lower Leg Muscle, Left V Foot Muscle, Right W Foot Muscle, Left	0 Open 3 Percutaneous 4 Percutaneous Endoscopic	Z No Device	X Diagnostic Z No Qualifier

0 **Medical and Surgical**
K **Muscles**
C **Extirpation:** Taking or cutting out solid matter from a body part

Body Part	Approach	Device	Qualifier
Character 4	Character 5	Character 6	Character 7
0 Head Muscle 1 Facial Muscle 2 Neck Muscle, Right 3 Neck Muscle, Left 4 Tongue, Palate, Pharynx Muscle 5 Shoulder Muscle, Right 6 Shoulder Muscle, Left 7 Upper Arm Muscle, Right 8 Upper Arm Muscle, Left 9 Lower Arm and Wrist Muscle, Right B Lower Arm and Wrist Muscle, Left C Hand Muscle, Right D Hand Muscle, Left F Trunk Muscle, Right G Trunk Muscle, Left H Thorax Muscle, Right J Thorax Muscle, Left K Abdomen Muscle, Right L Abdomen Muscle, Left M Perineum Muscle N Hip Muscle, Right P Hip Muscle, Left Q Upper Leg Muscle, Right R Upper Leg Muscle, Left S Lower Leg Muscle, Right T Lower Leg Muscle, Left V Foot Muscle, Right W Foot Muscle, Left	0 Open 3 Percutaneous 4 Percutaneous Endoscopic	Z No Device	Z No Qualifier

LC Limited Coverage   NC Noncovered   HAC HAC-associated Procedure   CC Combination Cluster - See Appendix G for code lists
DRG Non-OR-Affecting MS-DRG Assignment   New/Revised Text in Orange   ♂ Male   ♀ Female

394

2018 ICD-10-PCS

0   Medical and Surgical
K   Muscles
D   Extraction: Pulling or stripping out or off all or a portion of a body part by the use of force

Body Part	Approach	Device	Qualifier
Character 4	Character 5	Character 6	Character 7
0 Head Muscle	0 Open	Z No Device	Z No Qualifier
1 Facial Muscle			
2 Neck Muscle, Right			
3 Neck Muscle, Left			
4 Tongue, Palate, Pharynx Muscle			
5 Shoulder Muscle, Right			
6 Shoulder Muscle, Left			
7 Upper Arm Muscle, Right			
8 Upper Arm Muscle, Left			
9 Lower Arm and Wrist Muscle, Right			
B Lower Arm and Wrist Muscle, Left			
C Hand Muscle, Right			
D Hand Muscle, Left			
F Trunk Muscle, Right			
G Trunk Muscle, Left			
H Thorax Muscle, Right			
J Thorax Muscle, Left			
K Abdomen Muscle, Right			
L Abdomen Muscle, Left			
M Perineum Muscle			
N Hip Muscle, Right			
P Hip Muscle, Left			
Q Upper Leg Muscle, Right			
R Upper Leg Muscle, Left			
S Lower Leg Muscle, Right			
T Lower Leg Muscle, Left			
V Foot Muscle, Right			
W Foot Muscle, Left			

0   Medical and Surgical
K   Muscles
H   Insertion: Putting in a nonbiological appliance that monitors, assists, performs, or prevents a physiological function but does not physically take the place of a body part

Body Part	Approach	Device	Qualifier
Character 4	Character 5	Character 6	Character 7
X Upper Muscle	0 Open	M Stimulator Lead	Z No Qualifier
Y Lower Muscle	3 Percutaneous	Y Other Device	
	4 Percutaneous Endoscopic		

0   Medical and Surgical
K   Muscles
J   Inspection: Visually and/or manually exploring a body part

Body Part	Approach	Device	Qualifier
Character 4	Character 5	Character 6	Character 7
X Upper Muscle	0 Open	Z No Device	Z No Qualifier
Y Lower Muscle	3 Percutaneous		
	4 Percutaneous Endoscopic		
	X External		

0 **Medical and Surgical**
K **Muscles**
M **Reattachment:** Putting back in or on all or a portion of a separated body part to its normal location or other suitable location

Body Part	Approach	Device	Qualifier
Character 4	Character 5	Character 6	Character 7
0 Head Muscle 1 Facial Muscle 2 Neck Muscle, Right 3 Neck Muscle, Left 4 Tongue, Palate, Pharynx Muscle 5 Shoulder Muscle, Right 6 Shoulder Muscle, Left 7 Upper Arm Muscle, Right 8 Upper Arm Muscle, Left 9 Lower Arm and Wrist Muscle, Right B Lower Arm and Wrist Muscle, Left C Hand Muscle, Right D Hand Muscle, Left F Trunk Muscle, Right G Trunk Muscle, Left H Thorax Muscle, Right J Thorax Muscle, Left K Abdomen Muscle, Right L Abdomen Muscle, Left M Perineum Muscle N Hip Muscle, Right P Hip Muscle, Left Q Upper Leg Muscle, Right R Upper Leg Muscle, Left S Lower Leg Muscle, Right T Lower Leg Muscle, Left V Foot Muscle, Right W Foot Muscle, Left	0 Open 4 Percutaneous Endoscopic	Z No Device	Z No Qualifier

LC Limited Coverage   NC Noncovered   HAC HAC-associated Procedure   CC Combination Cluster - See Appendix G for code lists
DRG Non-OR-Affecting MS-DRG Assignment   New/Revised Text in **Orange**   ♂ Male   ♀ Female

396

2018 ICD-10-PCS

MUSCLES 0K2-0KX

0 Medical and Surgical
K Muscles
N Release: Freeing a body part from an abnormal physical constraint by cutting or by the use of force

Body Part	Approach	Device	Qualifier
Character 4	Character 5	Character 6	Character 7
0 Head Muscle 1 Facial Muscle 2 Neck Muscle, Right 3 Neck Muscle, Left 4 Tongue, Palate, Pharynx Muscle 5 Shoulder Muscle, Right 6 Shoulder Muscle, Left 7 Upper Arm Muscle, Right 8 Upper Arm Muscle, Left 9 Lower Arm and Wrist Muscle, Right B Lower Arm and Wrist Muscle, Left C Hand Muscle, Right D Hand Muscle, Left F Trunk Muscle, Right G Trunk Muscle, Left H Thorax Muscle, Right J Thorax Muscle, Left K Abdomen Muscle, Right L Abdomen Muscle, Left M Perineum Muscle N Hip Muscle, Right P Hip Muscle, Left Q Upper Leg Muscle, Right R Upper Leg Muscle, Left S Lower Leg Muscle, Right T Lower Leg Muscle, Left V Foot Muscle, Right W Foot Muscle, Left	0 Open 3 Percutaneous 4 Percutaneous Endoscopic X External	Z No Device	Z No Qualifier

0 Medical and Surgical
K Muscles
P Removal: Taking out or off a device from a body part

Body Part	Approach	Device	Qualifier
Character 4	Character 5	Character 6	Character 7
X Upper Muscle Y Lower Muscle	0 Open 3 Percutaneous 4 Percutaneous Endoscopic	0 Drainage Device 7 Autologous Tissue Substitute J Synthetic Substitute K Nonautologous Tissue Substitute M Stimulator Lead Y Other Device	Z No Qualifier
X Upper Muscle Y Lower Muscle	X External	0 Drainage Device M Stimulator Lead	Z No Qualifier

LC Limited Coverage NC Noncovered HAC HAC-associated Procedure CC Combination Cluster - See Appendix G for code lists
DRG Non-OR-Affecting MS-DRG Assignment New/Revised Text in **Orange** ♂ Male ♀ Female

2018 ICD-10-PCS

397

MUSCLES 0K2-0KX

0   **Medical and Surgical**
K   **Muscles**
Q   **Repair:** Restoring, to the extent possible, a body part to its normal anatomic structure and function

Body Part	Approach	Device	Qualifier
Character 4	Character 5	Character 6	Character 7
0 Head Muscle 1 Facial Muscle 2 Neck Muscle, Right 3 Neck Muscle, Left 4 Tongue, Palate, Pharynx Muscle 5 Shoulder Muscle, Right 6 Shoulder Muscle, Left 7 Upper Arm Muscle, Right 8 Upper Arm Muscle, Left 9 Lower Arm and Wrist Muscle, Right B Lower Arm and Wrist Muscle, Left C Hand Muscle, Right D Hand Muscle, Left F Trunk Muscle, Right G Trunk Muscle, Left H Thorax Muscle, Right J Thorax Muscle, Left K Abdomen Muscle, Right L Abdomen Muscle, Left M Perineum Muscle N Hip Muscle, Right P Hip Muscle, Left Q Upper Leg Muscle, Right R Upper Leg Muscle, Left S Lower Leg Muscle, Right T Lower Leg Muscle, Left V Foot Muscle, Right W Foot Muscle, Left	0 Open 3 Percutaneous 4 Percutaneous Endoscopic	Z No Device	Z No Qualifier

0   **Medical and Surgical**
K   **Muscles**
R   **Replacement:** Putting in or on biological or synthetic material that physically takes the place and/or function of all or a portion of a body part

Body Part	Approach	Device	Qualifier
Character 4	Character 5	Character 6	Character 7
0 Head Muscle 1 Facial Muscle 2 Neck Muscle, Right 3 Neck Muscle, Left 4 Tongue, Palate, Pharynx Muscle 5 Shoulder Muscle, Right 6 Shoulder Muscle, Left 7 Upper Arm Muscle, Right 8 Upper Arm Muscle, Left 9 Lower Arm and Wrist Muscle, Right B Lower Arm and Wrist Muscle, Left C Hand Muscle, Right D Hand Muscle, Left F Trunk Muscle, Right G Trunk Muscle, Left H Thorax Muscle, Right J Thorax Muscle, Left K Abdomen Muscle, Right L Abdomen Muscle, Left M Perineum Muscle N Hip Muscle, Right P Hip Muscle, Left Q Upper Leg Muscle, Right R Upper Leg Muscle, Left S Lower Leg Muscle, Right T Lower Leg Muscle, Left V Foot Muscle, Right W Foot Muscle, Left	0 Open 4 Percutaneous Endoscopic	7 Autologous Tissue Substitute J Synthetic Substitute K Nonautologous Tissue Substitute	Z No Qualifier

LC Limited Coverage   NC Noncovered   HAC HAC-associated Procedure   CC Combination Cluster - See Appendix G for code lists
Non-OR-Affecting MS-DRG Assignment   New/Revised Text in **Orange**   ♂ Male   ♀ Female

398

2018 ICD-10-PCS

0 **Medical and Surgical**
K **Muscles**
S **Reposition:** Moving to its normal location, or other suitable location, all or a portion of a body part

Body Part	Approach	Device	Qualifier
Character 4	Character 5	Character 6	Character 7
0 Head Muscle 1 Facial Muscle 2 Neck Muscle, Right 3 Neck Muscle, Left 4 Tongue, Palate, Pharynx Muscle 5 Shoulder Muscle, Right 6 Shoulder Muscle, Left 7 Upper Arm Muscle, Right 8 Upper Arm Muscle, Left 9 Lower Arm and Wrist Muscle, Right B Lower Arm and Wrist Muscle, Left C Hand Muscle, Right D Hand Muscle, Left F Trunk Muscle, Right G Trunk Muscle, Left H Thorax Muscle, Right J Thorax Muscle, Left K Abdomen Muscle, Right L Abdomen Muscle, Left M Perineum Muscle N Hip Muscle, Right P Hip Muscle, Left Q Upper Leg Muscle, Right R Upper Leg Muscle, Left S Lower Leg Muscle, Right T Lower Leg Muscle, Left V Foot Muscle, Right W Foot Muscle, Left	0 Open 4 Percutaneous Endoscopic	Z No Device	Z No Qualifier

0 **Medical and Surgical**
K **Muscles**
T **Resection:** Cutting out or off, without replacement, all of a body part

Body Part	Approach	Device	Qualifier
Character 4	Character 5	Character 6	Character 7
0 Head Muscle 1 Facial Muscle 2 Neck Muscle, Right 3 Neck Muscle, Left 4 Tongue, Palate, Pharynx Muscle 5 Shoulder Muscle, Right 6 Shoulder Muscle, Left 7 Upper Arm Muscle, Right 8 Upper Arm Muscle, Left 9 Lower Arm and Wrist Muscle, Right B Lower Arm and Wrist Muscle, Left C Hand Muscle, Right D Hand Muscle, Left F Trunk Muscle, Right G Trunk Muscle, Left H Thorax Muscle, Right LC J Thorax Muscle, Left LC K Abdomen Muscle, Right L Abdomen Muscle, Left M Perineum Muscle N Hip Muscle, Right P Hip Muscle, Left Q Upper Leg Muscle, Right R Upper Leg Muscle, Left S Lower Leg Muscle, Right T Lower Leg Muscle, Left V Foot Muscle, Right W Foot Muscle, Left	0 Open 4 Percutaneous Endoscopic	Z No Device	Z No Qualifier

LC 0KTH0ZZ   0KTJ0ZZ

LC Limited Coverage   NC Noncovered   HAC HAC-associated Procedure   CC Combination Cluster - See Appendix G for code lists
DRG Non-OR-Affecting MS-DRG Assignment   New/Revised Text in **Orange**   ♂ Male   ♀ Female

0 Medical and Surgical
K Muscles
U Supplement: Putting in or on biological or synthetic material that physically reinforces and/or augments the function of a portion of a body part

Body Part	Approach	Device	Qualifier
Character 4	Character 5	Character 6	Character 7
0 Head Muscle 1 Facial Muscle 2 Neck Muscle, Right 3 Neck Muscle, Left 4 Tongue, Palate, Pharynx Muscle 5 Shoulder Muscle, Right 6 Shoulder Muscle, Left 7 Upper Arm Muscle, Right 8 Upper Arm Muscle, Left 9 Lower Arm and Wrist Muscle, Right B Lower Arm and Wrist Muscle, Left C Hand Muscle, Right D Hand Muscle, Left F Trunk Muscle, Right G Trunk Muscle, Left H Thorax Muscle, Right J Thorax Muscle, Left K Abdomen Muscle, Right L Abdomen Muscle, Left M Perineum Muscle N Hip Muscle, Right P Hip Muscle, Left Q Upper Leg Muscle, Right R Upper Leg Muscle, Left S Lower Leg Muscle, Right T Lower Leg Muscle, Left V Foot Muscle, Right W Foot Muscle, Left	0 Open 4 Percutaneous Endoscopic	7 Autologous Tissue Substitute J Synthetic Substitute K Nonautologous Tissue Substitute	Z No Qualifier

0 Medical and Surgical
K Muscles
W Revision: Correcting, to the extent possible, a portion of a malfunctioning device or the position of a displaced device

Body Part	Approach	Device	Qualifier
Character 4	Character 5	Character 6	Character 7
X Upper Muscle Y Lower Muscle	0 Open 3 Percutaneous 4 Percutaneous Endoscopic	0 Drainage Device 7 Autologous Tissue Substitute J Synthetic Substitute K Nonautologous Tissue Substitute M Stimulator Lead Y Other Device	Z No Qualifier
X Upper Muscle Y Lower Muscle	X External	0 Drainage Device 7 Autologous Tissue Substitute J Synthetic Substitute K Nonautologous Tissue Substitute M Stimulator Lead	Z No Qualifier

LC Limited Coverage   NC Noncovered   HAC HAC-associated Procedure   CC Combination Cluster - See Appendix G for code lists
DRG Non-OR-Affecting MS-DRG Assignment   New/Revised Text in Orange   ♂ Male   ♀ Female

400

2018 ICD-10-PCS

0 **Medical and Surgical**
K **Muscles**
X **Transfer:** Moving, without taking out, all or a portion of a body part to another location to take over the function of all or a portion of a body part

Body Part	Approach	Device	Qualifier
Character 4	Character 5	Character 6	Character 7
0 Head Muscle 1 Facial Muscle 2 Neck Muscle, Right 3 Neck Muscle, Left 4 Tongue, Palate, Pharynx Muscle 5 Shoulder Muscle, Right 6 Shoulder Muscle, Left 7 Upper Arm Muscle, Right 8 Upper Arm Muscle, Left 9 Lower Arm and Wrist Muscle, Right B Lower Arm and Wrist Muscle, Left C Hand Muscle, Right D Hand Muscle, Left H Thorax Muscle, Right J Thorax Muscle, Left M Perineum Muscle N Hip Muscle, Right P Hip Muscle, Left Q Upper Leg Muscle, Right R Upper Leg Muscle, Left S Lower Leg Muscle, Right T Lower Leg Muscle, Left V Foot Muscle, Right W Foot Muscle, Left	0 Open 4 Percutaneous Endoscopic	Z No Device	0 Skin 1 Subcutaneous Tissue 2 Skin and Subcutaneous Tissue Z No Qualifier
F Trunk Muscle, Right G Trunk Muscle, Left	0 Open 4 Percutaneous Endoscopic	Z No Device	0 Skin 1 Subcutaneous Tissue 2 Skin and Subcutaneous Tissue 5 Latissimus Dorsi Myocutaneous Flap 7 Deep Inferior Epigastric Artery Perforator Flap 8 Superficial Inferior Epigastric Artery Flap 9 Gluteal Artery Perforator Flap Z No Qualifier
K Abdomen Muscle, Right L Abdomen Muscle, Left	0 Open 4 Percutaneous Endoscopic	Z No Device	0 Skin 1 Subcutaneous Tissue 2 Skin and Subcutaneous Tissue 6 Transverse Rectus Abdominis Myocutaneous Flap Z No Qualifier

LC Limited Coverage   NC Noncovered   HAC HAC-associated Procedure   CC Combination Cluster - See Appendix G for code lists
DRG Non-OR-Affecting MS-DRG Assignment   New/Revised Text in **Orange**   ♂ Male   ♀ Female

2018 ICD-10-PCS

401

MUSCLES 0K2-0KX

NOTES

Tendons 0L2-0LX

0 Medical and Surgical
L Tendons
2 Change: Taking out or off a device from a body part and putting back an identical or similar device in or on the same body part without cutting or puncturing the skin or a mucous membrane

Body Part	Approach	Device	Qualifier
Character 4	Character 5	Character 6	Character 7
X Upper Tendon Y Lower Tendon	X External	0 Drainage Device Y Other Device	Z No Qualifier

0 Medical and Surgical
L Tendons
5 Destruction: Physical eradication of all or a portion of a body part by the direct use of energy, force, or a destructive agent

Body Part	Approach	Device	Qualifier
Character 4	Character 5	Character 6	Character 7
0 Head and Neck Tendon 1 Shoulder Tendon, Right 2 Shoulder Tendon, Left 3 Upper Arm Tendon, Right 4 Upper Arm Tendon, Left 5 Lower Arm and Wrist Tendon, Right 6 Lower Arm and Wrist Tendon, Left 7 Hand Tendon, Right 8 Hand Tendon, Left 9 Trunk Tendon, Right B Trunk Tendon, Left C Thorax Tendon, Right D Thorax Tendon, Left F Abdomen Tendon, Right G Abdomen Tendon, Left H Perineum Tendon J Hip Tendon, Right K Hip Tendon, Left L Upper Leg Tendon, Right M Upper Leg Tendon, Left N Lower Leg Tendon, Right P Lower Leg Tendon, Left Q Knee Tendon, Right R Knee Tendon, Left S Ankle Tendon, Right T Ankle Tendon, Left V Foot Tendon, Right W Foot Tendon, Left	0 Open 3 Percutaneous 4 Percutaneous Endoscopic	Z No Device	Z No Qualifier

0   Medical and Surgical
L   Tendons
8   Division: Cutting into a body part, without draining fluids and/or gases from the body part, in order to separate or transect a body part

Body Part	Approach	Device	Qualifier
Character 4	Character 5	Character 6	Character 7
0 Head and Neck Tendon	0 Open	Z No Device	Z No Qualifier
1 Shoulder Tendon, Right	3 Percutaneous		
2 Shoulder Tendon, Left	4 Percutaneous Endoscopic		
3 Upper Arm Tendon, Right			
4 Upper Arm Tendon, Left			
5 Lower Arm and Wrist Tendon, Right			
6 Lower Arm and Wrist Tendon, Left			
7 Hand Tendon, Right			
8 Hand Tendon, Left			
9 Trunk Tendon, Right			
B Trunk Tendon, Left			
C Thorax Tendon, Right			
D Thorax Tendon, Left			
F Abdomen Tendon, Right			
G Abdomen Tendon, Left			
H Perineum Tendon			
J Hip Tendon, Right			
K Hip Tendon, Left			
L Upper Leg Tendon, Right			
M Upper Leg Tendon, Left			
N Lower Leg Tendon, Right			
P Lower Leg Tendon, Left			
Q Knee Tendon, Right			
R Knee Tendon, Left			
S Ankle Tendon, Right			
T Ankle Tendon, Left			
V Foot Tendon, Right			
W Foot Tendon, Left			

0 **Medical and Surgical**
L **Tendons**
9 **Drainage:** Taking or letting out fluids and/or gases from a body part

Body Part	Approach	Device	Qualifier
Character 4	Character 5	Character 6	Character 7
0 Head and Neck Tendon 1 Shoulder Tendon, Right 2 Shoulder Tendon, Left 3 Upper Arm Tendon, Right 4 Upper Arm Tendon, Left 5 Lower Arm and Wrist Tendon, Right 6 Lower Arm and Wrist Tendon, Left 7 Hand Tendon, Right 8 Hand Tendon, Left 9 Trunk Tendon, Right B Trunk Tendon, Left C Thorax Tendon, Right D Thorax Tendon, Left F Abdomen Tendon, Right G Abdomen Tendon, Left H Perineum Tendon J Hip Tendon, Right K Hip Tendon, Left L Upper Leg Tendon, Right M Upper Leg Tendon, Left N Lower Leg Tendon, Right P Lower Leg Tendon, Left Q Knee Tendon, Right R Knee Tendon, Left S Ankle Tendon, Right T Ankle Tendon, Left V Foot Tendon, Right W Foot Tendon, Left	0 Open 3 Percutaneous 4 Percutaneous Endoscopic	0 Drainage Device	Z No Qualifier
0 Head and Neck Tendon 1 Shoulder Tendon, Right 2 Shoulder Tendon, Left 3 Upper Arm Tendon, Right 4 Upper Arm Tendon, Left 5 Lower Arm and Wrist Tendon, Right 6 Lower Arm and Wrist Tendon, Left 7 Hand Tendon, Right 8 Hand Tendon, Left 9 Trunk Tendon, Right B Trunk Tendon, Left C Thorax Tendon, Right D Thorax Tendon, Left F Abdomen Tendon, Right G Abdomen Tendon, Left H Perineum Tendon J Hip Tendon, Right K Hip Tendon, Left L Upper Leg Tendon, Right M Upper Leg Tendon, Left N Lower Leg Tendon, Right P Lower Leg Tendon, Left Q Knee Tendon, Right R Knee Tendon, Left S Ankle Tendon, Right T Ankle Tendon, Left V Foot Tendon, Right W Foot Tendon, Left	0 Open 3 Percutaneous 4 Percutaneous Endoscopic	Z No Device	X Diagnostic Z No Qualifier

LC Limited Coverage NC Noncovered HAC HAC-associated Procedure CC Combination Cluster - See Appendix G for code lists
Non-OR-Affecting MS-DRG Assignment New/Revised Text in Orange ♂ Male ♀ Female

2018 ICD-10-PCS

405

0 Medical and Surgical
L Tendons
B Excision: Cutting out or off, without replacement, a portion of a body part

Body Part	Approach	Device	Qualifier
Character 4	Character 5	Character 6	Character 7
0 Head and Neck Tendon **1** Shoulder Tendon, Right **2** Shoulder Tendon, Left **3** Upper Arm Tendon, Right **4** Upper Arm Tendon, Left **5** Lower Arm and Wrist Tendon, Right **6** Lower Arm and Wrist Tendon, Left **7** Hand Tendon, Right **8** Hand Tendon, Left **9** Trunk Tendon, Right **B** Trunk Tendon, Left **C** Thorax Tendon, Right **D** Thorax Tendon, Left **F** Abdomen Tendon, Right **G** Abdomen Tendon, Left **H** Perineum Tendon **J** Hip Tendon, Right **K** Hip Tendon, Left **L** Upper Leg Tendon, Right **M** Upper Leg Tendon, Left **N** Lower Leg Tendon, Right **P** Lower Leg Tendon, Left **Q** Knee Tendon, Right **R** Knee Tendon, Left **S** Ankle Tendon, Right **T** Ankle Tendon, Left **V** Foot Tendon, Right **W** Foot Tendon, Left	**0** Open **3** Percutaneous **4** Percutaneous Endoscopic	**Z** No Device	**X** Diagnostic **Z** No Qualifier

0 Medical and Surgical
L Tendons
C Extirpation: Taking or cutting out solid matter from a body part

Body Part	Approach	Device	Qualifier
Character 4	Character 5	Character 6	Character 7
0 Head and Neck Tendon **1** Shoulder Tendon, Right **2** Shoulder Tendon, Left **3** Upper Arm Tendon, Right **4** Upper Arm Tendon, Left **5** Lower Arm and Wrist Tendon, Right **6** Lower Arm and Wrist Tendon, Left **7** Hand Tendon, Right **8** Hand Tendon, Left **9** Trunk Tendon, Right **B** Trunk Tendon, Left **C** Thorax Tendon, Right **D** Thorax Tendon, Left **F** Abdomen Tendon, Right **G** Abdomen Tendon, Left **H** Perineum Tendon **J** Hip Tendon, Right **K** Hip Tendon, Left **L** Upper Leg Tendon, Right **M** Upper Leg Tendon, Left **N** Lower Leg Tendon, Right **P** Lower Leg Tendon, Left **Q** Knee Tendon, Right **R** Knee Tendon, Left **S** Ankle Tendon, Right **T** Ankle Tendon, Left **V** Foot Tendon, Right **W** Foot Tendon, Left	**0** Open **3** Percutaneous **4** Percutaneous Endoscopic	**Z** No Device	**Z** No Qualifier

LC Limited Coverage NC Noncovered HAC HAC-associated Procedure CC Combination Cluster - See Appendix G for code lists
Non-OR-Affecting MS-DRG Assignment New/Revised Text in Orange ♂ Male ♀ Female

406

2018 ICD-10-PCS

0   Medical and Surgical
L   Tendons
D   Extraction: Pulling or stripping out or off all or a portion of a body part by the use of force

Body Part	Approach	Device	Qualifier
Character 4	Character 5	Character 6	Character 7
0 Head and Neck Tendon	0 Open	Z No Device	Z No Qualifier
1 Shoulder Tendon, Right			
2 Shoulder Tendon, Left			
3 Upper Arm Tendon, Right			
4 Upper Arm Tendon, Left			
5 Lower Arm and Wrist Tendon, Right			
6 Lower Arm and Wrist Tendon, Left			
7 Hand Tendon, Right			
8 Hand Tendon, Left			
9 Trunk Tendon, Right			
B Trunk Tendon, Left			
C Thorax Tendon, Right			
D Thorax Tendon, Left			
F Abdomen Tendon, Right			
G Abdomen Tendon, Left			
H Perineum Tendon			
J Hip Tendon, Right			
K Hip Tendon, Left			
L Upper Leg Tendon, Right			
M Upper Leg Tendon, Left			
N Lower Leg Tendon, Right			
P Lower Leg Tendon, Left			
Q Knee Tendon, Right			
R Knee Tendon, Left			
S Ankle Tendon, Right			
T Ankle Tendon, Left			
V Foot Tendon, Right			
W Foot Tendon, Left			

0   Medical and Surgical
L   Tendons
H   Insertion: Putting in a nonbiological appliance that monitors, assists, performs, or prevents a physiological function but does not physically take the place of a body part

Body Part	Approach	Device	Qualifier
Character 4	Character 5	Character 6	Character 7
X Upper Tendon	0 Open	Y Other Device	Z No Qualifier
Y Lower Tendon	3 Percutaneous		
	4 Percutaneous Endoscopic		

0   Medical and Surgical
L   Tendons
J   Inspection: Visually and/or manually exploring a body part

Body Part	Approach	Device	Qualifier
Character 4	Character 5	Character 6	Character 7
X Upper Tendon	0 Open	Z No Device	Z No Qualifier
Y Lower Tendon	3 Percutaneous		
	4 Percutaneous Endoscopic		
	X External		

ᴸᶜ Limited Coverage   ᴺᶜ Noncovered   ᴴᴬᶜ HAC-associated Procedure   ᶜᶜ Combination Cluster - See Appendix G for code lists
ᴰᴿᴳ Non-OR-Affecting MS-DRG Assignment   New/Revised Text in **Orange**   ♂ Male   ♀ Female

2018 ICD-10-PCS   **407**

0 Medical and Surgical
L Tendons
M Reattachment: Putting back in or on all or a portion of a separated body part to its normal location or other suitable location

Body Part	Approach	Device	Qualifier
Character 4	Character 5	Character 6	Character 7
0 Head and Neck Tendon 1 Shoulder Tendon, Right 2 Shoulder Tendon, Left 3 Upper Arm Tendon, Right 4 Upper Arm Tendon, Left 5 Lower Arm and Wrist Tendon, Right 6 Lower Arm and Wrist Tendon, Left 7 Hand Tendon, Right 8 Hand Tendon, Left 9 Trunk Tendon, Right B Trunk Tendon, Left C Thorax Tendon, Right D Thorax Tendon, Left F Abdomen Tendon, Right G Abdomen Tendon, Left H Perineum Tendon J Hip Tendon, Right K Hip Tendon, Left L Upper Leg Tendon, Right M Upper Leg Tendon, Left N Lower Leg Tendon, Right P Lower Leg Tendon, Left Q Knee Tendon, Right R Knee Tendon, Left S Ankle Tendon, Right T Ankle Tendon, Left V Foot Tendon, Right W Foot Tendon, Left	0 Open 4 Percutaneous Endoscopic	Z No Device	Z No Qualifier

0   Medical and Surgical
L   Tendons
N   Release: Freeing a body part from an abnormal physical constraint by cutting or by the use of force

Body Part	Approach	Device	Qualifier
Character 4	Character 5	Character 6	Character 7
0 Head and Neck Tendon **1** Shoulder Tendon, Right **2** Shoulder Tendon, Left **3** Upper Arm Tendon, Right **4** Upper Arm Tendon, Left **5** Lower Arm and Wrist Tendon, Right **6** Lower Arm and Wrist Tendon, Left **7** Hand Tendon, Right **8** Hand Tendon, Left **9** Trunk Tendon, Right **B** Trunk Tendon, Left **C** Thorax Tendon, Right **D** Thorax Tendon, Left **F** Abdomen Tendon, Right **G** Abdomen Tendon, Left **H** Perineum Tendon **J** Hip Tendon, Right **K** Hip Tendon, Left **L** Upper Leg Tendon, Right **M** Upper Leg Tendon, Left **N** Lower Leg Tendon, Right **P** Lower Leg Tendon, Left **Q** Knee Tendon, Right **R** Knee Tendon, Left **S** Ankle Tendon, Right **T** Ankle Tendon, Left **V** Foot Tendon, Right **W** Foot Tendon, Left	**0** Open **3** Percutaneous **4** Percutaneous Endoscopic **X** External	**Z** No Device	**Z** No Qualifier

0   Medical and Surgical
L   Tendons
P   Removal: Taking out or off a device from a body part

Body Part	Approach	Device	Qualifier
Character 4	Character 5	Character 6	Character 7
X Upper Tendon **Y** Lower Tendon	**0** Open **3** Percutaneous **4** Percutaneous Endoscopic	**0** Drainage Device **7** Autologous Tissue Substitute **J** Synthetic Substitute **K** Nonautologous Tissue Substitute **Y** Other Device	**Z** No Qualifier
X Upper Tendon **Y** Lower Tendon	**X** External	**0** Drainage Device	**Z** No Qualifier

0 Medical and Surgical
L Tendons
Q Repair: Restoring, to the extent possible, a body part to its normal anatomic structure and function

Body Part	Approach	Device	Qualifier
Character 4	Character 5	Character 6	Character 7
0 Head and Neck Tendon 1 Shoulder Tendon, Right 2 Shoulder Tendon, Left 3 Upper Arm Tendon, Right 4 Upper Arm Tendon, Left 5 Lower Arm and Wrist Tendon, Right 6 Lower Arm and Wrist Tendon, Left 7 Hand Tendon, Right 8 Hand Tendon, Left 9 Trunk Tendon, Right B Trunk Tendon, Left C Thorax Tendon, Right D Thorax Tendon, Left F Abdomen Tendon, Right G Abdomen Tendon, Left H Perineum Tendon J Hip Tendon, Right K Hip Tendon, Left L Upper Leg Tendon, Right M Upper Leg Tendon, Left N Lower Leg Tendon, Right P Lower Leg Tendon, Left Q Knee Tendon, Right R Knee Tendon, Left S Ankle Tendon, Right T Ankle Tendon, Left V Foot Tendon, Right W Foot Tendon, Left	0 Open 3 Percutaneous 4 Percutaneous Endoscopic	Z No Device	Z No Qualifier

0 Medical and Surgical
L Tendons
R Replacement: Putting in or on biological or synthetic material that physically takes the place and/or function of all or a portion of a body part

Body Part	Approach	Device	Qualifier
Character 4	Character 5	Character 6	Character 7
0 Head and Neck Tendon 1 Shoulder Tendon, Right 2 Shoulder Tendon, Left 3 Upper Arm Tendon, Right 4 Upper Arm Tendon, Left 5 Lower Arm and Wrist Tendon, Right 6 Lower Arm and Wrist Tendon, Left 7 Hand Tendon, Right 8 Hand Tendon, Left 9 Trunk Tendon, Right B Trunk Tendon, Left C Thorax Tendon, Right D Thorax Tendon, Left F Abdomen Tendon, Right G Abdomen Tendon, Left H Perineum Tendon J Hip Tendon, Right K Hip Tendon, Left L Upper Leg Tendon, Right M Upper Leg Tendon, Left N Lower Leg Tendon, Right P Lower Leg Tendon, Left Q Knee Tendon, Right R Knee Tendon, Left S Ankle Tendon, Right T Ankle Tendon, Left V Foot Tendon, Right W Foot Tendon, Left	0 Open 4 Percutaneous Endoscopic	7 Autologous Tissue Substitute J Synthetic Substitute K Nonautologous Tissue Substitute	Z No Qualifier

0　**Medical and Surgical**
L　**Tendons**
S　**Reposition:** Moving to its normal location, or other suitable location, all or a portion of a body part

Body Part	Approach	Device	Qualifier
Character 4	Character 5	Character 6	Character 7
0 Head and Neck Tendon 1 Shoulder Tendon, Right 2 Shoulder Tendon, Left 3 Upper Arm Tendon, Right 4 Upper Arm Tendon, Left 5 Lower Arm and Wrist Tendon, Right 6 Lower Arm and Wrist Tendon, Left 7 Hand Tendon, Right 8 Hand Tendon, Left 9 Trunk Tendon, Right B Trunk Tendon, Left C Thorax Tendon, Right D Thorax Tendon, Left F Abdomen Tendon, Right G Abdomen Tendon, Left H Perineum Tendon J Hip Tendon, Right K Hip Tendon, Left L Upper Leg Tendon, Right M Upper Leg Tendon, Left N Lower Leg Tendon, Right P Lower Leg Tendon, Left Q Knee Tendon, Right R Knee Tendon, Left S Ankle Tendon, Right T Ankle Tendon, Left V Foot Tendon, Right W Foot Tendon, Left	0 Open 4 Percutaneous Endoscopic	Z No Device	Z No Qualifier

0　**Medical and Surgical**
L　**Tendons**
T　**Resection:** Cutting out or off, without replacement, all of a body part

Body Part	Approach	Device	Qualifier
Character 4	Character 5	Character 6	Character 7
0 Head and Neck Tendon 1 Shoulder Tendon, Right 2 Shoulder Tendon, Left 3 Upper Arm Tendon, Right 4 Upper Arm Tendon, Left 5 Lower Arm and Wrist Tendon, Right 6 Lower Arm and Wrist Tendon, Left 7 Hand Tendon, Right 8 Hand Tendon, Left 9 Trunk Tendon, Right B Trunk Tendon, Left C Thorax Tendon, Right D Thorax Tendon, Left F Abdomen Tendon, Right G Abdomen Tendon, Left H Perineum Tendon J Hip Tendon, Right K Hip Tendon, Left L Upper Leg Tendon, Right M Upper Leg Tendon, Left N Lower Leg Tendon, Right P Lower Leg Tendon, Left Q Knee Tendon, Right R Knee Tendon, Left S Ankle Tendon, Right T Ankle Tendon, Left V Foot Tendon, Right W Foot Tendon, Left	0 Open 4 Percutaneous Endoscopic	Z No Device	Z No Qualifier

0   **Medical and Surgical**
L   **Tendons**
U   **Supplement:** Putting in or on biological or synthetic material that physically reinforces and/or augments the function of a portion of a body part

Body Part	Approach	Device	Qualifier
Character 4	Character 5	Character 6	Character 7
0 Head and Neck Tendon 1 Shoulder Tendon, Right 2 Shoulder Tendon, Left 3 Upper Arm Tendon, Right 4 Upper Arm Tendon, Left 5 Lower Arm and Wrist Tendon, Right 6 Lower Arm and Wrist Tendon, Left 7 Hand Tendon, Right 8 Hand Tendon, Left 9 Trunk Tendon, Right B Trunk Tendon, Left C Thorax Tendon, Right D Thorax Tendon, Left F Abdomen Tendon, Right G Abdomen Tendon, Left H Perineum Tendon J Hip Tendon, Right K Hip Tendon, Left L Upper Leg Tendon, Right M Upper Leg Tendon, Left N Lower Leg Tendon, Right P Lower Leg Tendon, Left Q Knee Tendon, Right R Knee Tendon, Left S Ankle Tendon, Right T Ankle Tendon, Left V Foot Tendon, Right W Foot Tendon, Left	0 Open 4 Percutaneous Endoscopic	7 Autologous Tissue Substitute J Synthetic Substitute K Nonautologous Tissue Substitute	Z No Qualifier

0   **Medical and Surgical**
L   **Tendons**
W   **Revision:** Correcting, to the extent possible, a portion of a malfunctioning device or the position of a displaced device

Body Part	Approach	Device	Qualifier
Character 4	Character 5	Character 6	Character 7
X Upper Tendon Y Lower Tendon	0 Open 3 Percutaneous 4 Percutaneous Endoscopic	0 Drainage Device 7 Autologous Tissue Substitute J Synthetic Substitute K Nonautologous Tissue Substitute Y Other Device	Z No Qualifier
X Upper Tendon Y Lower Tendon	X External	0 Drainage Device 7 Autologous Tissue Substitute J Synthetic Substitute K Nonautologous Tissue Substitute	Z No Qualifier

LC Limited Coverage   NC Noncovered   HAC HAC-associated Procedure   CC Combination Cluster - See Appendix G for code lists
DRG Non-OR-Affecting MS-DRG Assignment   New/Revised Text in **Orange**   ♂ Male   ♀ Female

412

2018 ICD-10-PCS

0   Medical and Surgical
L   Tendons
X   Transfer: Moving, without taking out, all or a portion of a body part to another location to take over the function of all or a portion of a body part

Body Part	Approach	Device	Qualifier
Character 4	Character 5	Character 6	Character 7
0 Head and Neck Tendon **1** Shoulder Tendon, Right **2** Shoulder Tendon, Left **3** Upper Arm Tendon, Right **4** Upper Arm Tendon, Left **5** Lower Arm and Wrist Tendon, Right **6** Lower Arm and Wrist Tendon, Left **7** Hand Tendon, Right **8** Hand Tendon, Left **9** Trunk Tendon, Right **B** Trunk Tendon, Left **C** Thorax Tendon, Right **D** Thorax Tendon, Left **F** Abdomen Tendon, Right **G** Abdomen Tendon, Left **H** Perineum Tendon **J** Hip Tendon, Right **K** Hip Tendon, Left **L** Upper Leg Tendon, Right **M** Upper Leg Tendon, Left **N** Lower Leg Tendon, Right **P** Lower Leg Tendon, Left **Q** Knee Tendon, Right **R** Knee Tendon, Left **S** Ankle Tendon, Right **T** Ankle Tendon, Left **V** Foot Tendon, Right **W** Foot Tendon, Left	**0** Open **4** Percutaneous Endoscopic	**Z** No Device	**Z** No Qualifier

---

LC Limited Coverage   NC Noncovered   HAC HAC-associated Procedure   CC Combination Cluster - See Appendix G for code lists
DRG Non-OR-Affecting MS-DRG Assignment   New/Revised Text in Orange   ♂ Male   ♀ Female

2018 ICD-10-PCS

413

TENDONS 0L2-0LX

NOTES

Bursae and Ligaments 0M2-0MX

0   Medical and Surgical
M   Bursae and Ligaments
2   Change: Taking out or off a device from a body part and putting back an identical or similar device in or on the same body part without cutting or puncturing the skin or a mucous membrane

Body Part	Approach	Device	Qualifier
Character 4	Character 5	Character 6	Character 7
X Upper Bursa and Ligament **Y** Lower Bursa and Ligament	**X** External	**0** Drainage Device **Y** Other Device	**Z** No Qualifier

0   Medical and Surgical
M   Bursae and Ligaments
5   Destruction: Physical eradication of all or a portion of a body part by the direct use of energy, force, or a destructive agent

Body Part	Approach	Device	Qualifier
Character 4	Character 5	Character 6	Character 7
0 Head and Neck Bursa and Ligament **1** Shoulder Bursa and Ligament, Right **2** Shoulder Bursa and Ligament, Left **3** Elbow Bursa and Ligament, Right **4** Elbow Bursa and Ligament, Left **5** Wrist Bursa and Ligament, Right **6** Wrist Bursa and Ligament, Left **7** Hand Bursa and Ligament, Right **8** Hand Bursa and Ligament, Left **9** Upper Extremity Bursa and Ligament, Right **B** Upper Extremity Bursa and Ligament, Left **C** Upper Spine Bursa and Ligament **D** Lower Spine Bursa and Ligament **F** Sternum Bursa and Ligament **G** Rib(s) Bursa and Ligament **H** Abdomen Bursa and Ligament, Right **J** Abdomen Bursa and Ligament, Left **K** Perineum Bursa and Ligament **L** Hip Bursa and Ligament, Right **M** Hip Bursa and Ligament, Left **N** Knee Bursa and Ligament, Right **P** Knee Bursa and Ligament, Left **Q** Ankle Bursa and Ligament, Right **R** Ankle Bursa and Ligament, Left **S** Foot Bursa and Ligament, Right **T** Foot Bursa and Ligament, Left **V** Lower Extremity Bursa and Ligament, Right **W** Lower Extremity Bursa and Ligament, Left	**0** Open **3** Percutaneous **4** Percutaneous Endoscopic	**Z** No Device	**Z** No Qualifier

LC Limited Coverage   **NC** Noncovered   **HAC** HAC-associated Procedure   **CC** Combination Cluster - See Appendix G for code lists

DRG Non-OR-Affecting MS-DRG Assignment   New/Revised Text in **Orange**   ♂ Male   ♀ Female

2018 ICD-10-PCS

415

BURSAE AND LIGAMENTS 0M2-0MX

0 **Medical and Surgical**
M **Bursae and Ligaments**
8 **Division:** Cutting into a body part, without draining fluids and/or gases from the body part, in order to separate or transect a body part

Body Part	Approach	Device	Qualifier
Character 4	**Character 5**	**Character 6**	**Character 7**
0 Head and Neck Bursa and Ligament 1 Shoulder Bursa and Ligament, Right 2 Shoulder Bursa and Ligament, Left 3 Elbow Bursa and Ligament, Right 4 Elbow Bursa and Ligament, Left 5 Wrist Bursa and Ligament, Right 6 Wrist Bursa and Ligament, Left 7 Hand Bursa and Ligament, Right 8 Hand Bursa and Ligament, Left 9 Upper Extremity Bursa and Ligament, Right B Upper Extremity Bursa and Ligament, Left C Upper Spine Bursa and Ligament D Lower Spine Bursa and Ligament F Sternum Bursa and Ligament G Rib(s) Bursa and Ligament H Abdomen Bursa and Ligament, Right J Abdomen Bursa and Ligament, Left K Perineum Bursa and Ligament L Hip Bursa and Ligament, Right M Hip Bursa and Ligament, Left N Knee Bursa and Ligament, Right P Knee Bursa and Ligament, Left Q Ankle Bursa and Ligament, Right R Ankle Bursa and Ligament, Left S Foot Bursa and Ligament, Right T Foot Bursa and Ligament, Left V Lower Extremity Bursa and Ligament, Right W Lower Extremity Bursa and Ligament, Left	0 Open 3 Percutaneous 4 Percutaneous Endoscopic	Z No Device	Z No Qualifier

LC Limited Coverage   NC Noncovered   HAC HAC-associated Procedure   CC Combination Cluster - See Appendix G for code lists
DRG Non-OR-Affecting MS-DRG Assignment   New/Revised Text in Orange   ♂ Male   ♀ Female

416

2018 ICD-10-PCS

BURSAE AND LIGAMENTS 0M2-0MX

0 **Medical and Surgical**
M **Bursae and Ligaments**
9 **Drainage:** Taking or letting out fluids and/or gases from a body part

Body Part	Approach	Device	Qualifier
Character 4	Character 5	Character 6	Character 7
0 Head and Neck Bursa and Ligament	0 Open	0 Drainage Device	Z No Qualifier
1 Shoulder Bursa and Ligament, Right	3 Percutaneous		
2 Shoulder Bursa and Ligament, Left	4 Percutaneous Endoscopic		
3 Elbow Bursa and Ligament, Right			
4 Elbow Bursa and Ligament, Left			
5 Wrist Bursa and Ligament, Right			
6 Wrist Bursa and Ligament, Left			
7 Hand Bursa and Ligament, Right			
8 Hand Bursa and Ligament, Left			
9 Upper Extremity Bursa and Ligament, Right			
B Upper Extremity Bursa and Ligament, Left			
C Upper Spine Bursa and Ligament			
D Lower Spine Bursa and Ligament			
F Sternum Bursa and Ligament			
G Rib(s) Bursa and Ligament			
H Abdomen Bursa and Ligament, Right			
J Abdomen Bursa and Ligament, Left			
K Perineum Bursa and Ligament			
L Hip Bursa and Ligament, Right			
M Hip Bursa and Ligament, Left			
N Knee Bursa and Ligament, Right			
P Knee Bursa and Ligament, Left			
Q Ankle Bursa and Ligament, Right			
R Ankle Bursa and Ligament, Left			
S Foot Bursa and Ligament, Right			
T Foot Bursa and Ligament, Left			
V Lower Extremity Bursa and Ligament, Right			
W Lower Extremity Bursa and Ligament, Left			

0M9 continued on next page

0 **Medical and Surgical**
M **Bursae and Ligaments**
9 **Drainage:** Taking or letting out fluids and/or gases from a body part

0M9 continued from previous page

Body Part	Approach	Device	Qualifier
Character 4	Character 5	Character 6	Character 7
0 Head and Neck Bursa and Ligament	0 Open	Z No Device	X Diagnostic
1 Shoulder Bursa and Ligament, Right	3 Percutaneous		Z No Qualifier
2 Shoulder Bursa and Ligament, Left	4 Percutaneous Endoscopic		
3 Elbow Bursa and Ligament, Right			
4 Elbow Bursa and Ligament, Left			
5 Wrist Bursa and Ligament, Right			
6 Wrist Bursa and Ligament, Left			
7 Hand Bursa and Ligament, Right			
8 Hand Bursa and Ligament, Left			
9 Upper Extremity Bursa and Ligament, Right			
B Upper Extremity Bursa and Ligament, Left			
C Upper Spine Bursa and Ligament			
D Lower Spine Bursa and Ligament			
F Sternum Bursa and Ligament			
G Rib(s) Bursa and Ligament			
H Abdomen Bursa and Ligament, Right			
J Abdomen Bursa and Ligament, Left			
K Perineum Bursa and Ligament			
L Hip Bursa and Ligament, Right			
M Hip Bursa and Ligament, Left			
N Knee Bursa and Ligament, Right			
P Knee Bursa and Ligament, Left			
Q Ankle Bursa and Ligament, Right			
R Ankle Bursa and Ligament, Left			
S Foot Bursa and Ligament, Right			
T Foot Bursa and Ligament, Left			
V Lower Extremity Bursa and Ligament, Right			
W Lower Extremity Bursa and Ligament, Left			

0 Medical and Surgical
M Bursae and Ligaments
B Excision: Cutting out or off, without replacement, a portion of a body part

Body Part	Approach	Device	Qualifier
Character 4	Character 5	Character 6	Character 7
0 Head and Neck Bursa and Ligament **1** Shoulder Bursa and Ligament, Right **2** Shoulder Bursa and Ligament, Left **3** Elbow Bursa and Ligament, Right **4** Elbow Bursa and Ligament, Left **5** Wrist Bursa and Ligament, Right **6** Wrist Bursa and Ligament, Left **7** Hand Bursa and Ligament, Right **8** Hand Bursa and Ligament, Left **9** Upper Extremity Bursa and Ligament, Right **B** Upper Extremity Bursa and Ligament, Left **C** Upper Spine Bursa and Ligament **D** Lower Spine Bursa and Ligament **F** Sternum Bursa and Ligament **G** Rib(s) Bursa and Ligament **H** Abdomen Bursa and Ligament, Right **J** Abdomen Bursa and Ligament, Left **K** Perineum Bursa and Ligament **L** Hip Bursa and Ligament, Right **M** Hip Bursa and Ligament, Left **N** Knee Bursa and Ligament, Right **P** Knee Bursa and Ligament, Left **Q** Ankle Bursa and Ligament, Right **R** Ankle Bursa and Ligament, Left **S** Foot Bursa and Ligament, Right **T** Foot Bursa and Ligament, Left **V** Lower Extremity Bursa and Ligament, Right **W** Lower Extremity Bursa and Ligament, Left	**0** Open **3** Percutaneous **4** Percutaneous Endoscopic	**Z** No Device	**X** Diagnostic **Z** No Qualifier

LC Limited Coverage   **NC** Noncovered   **HAC** HAC-associated Procedure   **CC** Combination Cluster - See Appendix G for code lists
DRG Non-OR-Affecting MS-DRG Assignment   New/Revised Text in **Orange**   ♂ Male   ♀ Female

2018 ICD-10-PCS

419

0 **Medical and Surgical**
M **Bursae and Ligaments**
C **Extirpation:** Taking or cutting out solid matter from a body part

Body Part	Approach	Device	Qualifier
Character 4	Character 5	Character 6	Character 7
0 Head and Neck Bursa and Ligament 1 Shoulder Bursa and Ligament, Right 2 Shoulder Bursa and Ligament, Left 3 Elbow Bursa and Ligament, Right 4 Elbow Bursa and Ligament, Left 5 Wrist Bursa and Ligament, Right 6 Wrist Bursa and Ligament, Left 7 Hand Bursa and Ligament, Right 8 Hand Bursa and Ligament, Left 9 Upper Extremity Bursa and Ligament, Right B Upper Extremity Bursa and Ligament, Left C Upper Spine Bursa and Ligament D Lower Spine Bursa and Ligament F Sternum Bursa and Ligament G Rib(s) Bursa and Ligament H Abdomen Bursa and Ligament, Right J Abdomen Bursa and Ligament, Left K Perineum Bursa and Ligament L Hip Bursa and Ligament, Right M Hip Bursa and Ligament, Left N Knee Bursa and Ligament, Right P Knee Bursa and Ligament, Left Q Ankle Bursa and Ligament, Right R Ankle Bursa and Ligament, Left S Foot Bursa and Ligament, Right T Foot Bursa and Ligament, Left V Lower Extremity Bursa and Ligament, Right W Lower Extremity Bursa and Ligament, Left	0 Open 3 Percutaneous 4 Percutaneous Endoscopic	Z No Device	Z No Qualifier

LC Limited Coverage   NC Noncovered   HAC HAC-associated Procedure   CC Combination Cluster - See Appendix G for code lists
DRG Non-OR-Affecting MS-DRG Assignment   New/Revised Text in **Orange**   ♂ Male   ♀ Female

420

2018 ICD-10-PCS

BURSAE AND LIGAMENTS 0M2-0MX

0 **Medical and Surgical**
M **Bursae and Ligaments**
D **Extraction:** Pulling or stripping out or off all or a portion of a body part by the use of force

Body Part	Approach	Device	Qualifier
Character 4	Character 5	Character 6	Character 7
0 Head and Neck Bursa and Ligament 1 Shoulder Bursa and Ligament, Right 2 Shoulder Bursa and Ligament, Left 3 Elbow Bursa and Ligament, Right 4 Elbow Bursa and Ligament, Left 5 Wrist Bursa and Ligament, Right 6 Wrist Bursa and Ligament, Left 7 Hand Bursa and Ligament, Right 8 Hand Bursa and Ligament, Left 9 Upper Extremity Bursa and Ligament, Right B Upper Extremity Bursa and Ligament, Left C Upper Spine Bursa and Ligament D Lower Spine Bursa and Ligament F Sternum Bursa and Ligament G Rib(s) Bursa and Ligament H Abdomen Bursa and Ligament, Right J Abdomen Bursa and Ligament, Left K Perineum Bursa and Ligament L Hip Bursa and Ligament, Right M Hip Bursa and Ligament, Left N Knee Bursa and Ligament, Right P Knee Bursa and Ligament, Left Q Ankle Bursa and Ligament, Right R Ankle Bursa and Ligament, Left S Foot Bursa and Ligament, Right T Foot Bursa and Ligament, Left V Lower Extremity Bursa and Ligament, Right W Lower Extremity Bursa and Ligament, Left	0 Open 3 Percutaneous 4 Percutaneous Endoscopic	Z No Device	Z No Qualifier

0 **Medical and Surgical**
M **Bursae and Ligaments**
H **Insertion:** Putting in a nonbiological appliance that monitors, assists, performs, or prevents a physiological function but does not physically take the place of a body part

Body Part	Approach	Device	Qualifier
Character 4	Character 5	Character 6	Character 7
X Upper Bursa and Ligament Y Lower Bursa and Ligament	0 Open 3 Percutaneous 4 Percutaneous Endoscopic	Y Other Device	Z No Qualifier

0 Medical and Surgical
M Bursae and Ligaments
J Inspection: Visually and/or manually exploring a body part

Body Part	Approach	Device	Qualifier
Character 4	Character 5	Character 6	Character 7
X Upper Bursa and Ligament Y Lower Bursa and Ligament	0 Open 3 Percutaneous 4 Percutaneous Endoscopic X External	Z No Device	Z No Qualifier

0 Medical and Surgical
M Bursae and Ligaments
M Reattachment: Putting back in or on all or a portion of a separated body part to its normal location or other suitable location

Body Part	Approach	Device	Qualifier
Character 4	Character 5	Character 6	Character 7
0 Head and Neck Bursa and Ligament 1 Shoulder Bursa and Ligament, Right 2 Shoulder Bursa and Ligament, Left 3 Elbow Bursa and Ligament, Right 4 Elbow Bursa and Ligament, Left 5 Wrist Bursa and Ligament, Right 6 Wrist Bursa and Ligament, Left 7 Hand Bursa and Ligament, Right 8 Hand Bursa and Ligament, Left 9 Upper Extremity Bursa and Ligament, Right B Upper Extremity Bursa and Ligament, Left C Upper Spine Bursa and Ligament D Lower Spine Bursa and Ligament F Sternum Bursa and Ligament G Rib(s) Bursa and Ligament H Abdomen Bursa and Ligament, Right J Abdomen Bursa and Ligament, Left K Perineum Bursa and Ligament L Hip Bursa and Ligament, Right M Hip Bursa and Ligament, Left N Knee Bursa and Ligament, Right P Knee Bursa and Ligament, Left Q Ankle Bursa and Ligament, Right R Ankle Bursa and Ligament, Left S Foot Bursa and Ligament, Right T Foot Bursa and Ligament, Left V Lower Extremity Bursa and Ligament, Right W Lower Extremity Bursa and Ligament, Left	0 Open 4 Percutaneous Endoscopic	Z No Device	Z No Qualifier

LC Limited Coverage   NC Noncovered   HAC HAC-associated Procedure   CC Combination Cluster - See Appendix G for code lists
DRG Non-OR-Affecting MS-DRG Assignment   New/Revised Text in Orange   ♂ Male   ♀ Female

422

2018 ICD-10-PCS

0 Medical and Surgical
M Bursae and Ligaments
N Release: Freeing a body part from an abnormal physical constraint by cutting or by the use of force

Body Part	Approach	Device	Qualifier
Character 4	Character 5	Character 6	Character 7
0 Head and Neck Bursa and Ligament **1** Shoulder Bursa and Ligament, Right **2** Shoulder Bursa and Ligament, Left **3** Elbow Bursa and Ligament, Right **4** Elbow Bursa and Ligament, Left **5** Wrist Bursa and Ligament, Right **6** Wrist Bursa and Ligament, Left **7** Hand Bursa and Ligament, Right **8** Hand Bursa and Ligament, Left **9** Upper Extremity Bursa and Ligament, Right **B** Upper Extremity Bursa and Ligament, Left **C** Upper Spine Bursa and Ligament **D** Lower Spine Bursa and Ligament **F** Sternum Bursa and Ligament **G** Rib(s) Bursa and Ligament **H** Abdomen Bursa and Ligament, Right **J** Abdomen Bursa and Ligament, Left **K** Perineum Bursa and Ligament **L** Hip Bursa and Ligament, Right **M** Hip Bursa and Ligament, Left **N** Knee Bursa and Ligament, Right **P** Knee Bursa and Ligament, Left **Q** Ankle Bursa and Ligament, Right **R** Ankle Bursa and Ligament, Left **S** Foot Bursa and Ligament, Right **T** Foot Bursa and Ligament, Left **V** Lower Extremity Bursa and Ligament, Right **W** Lower Extremity Bursa and Ligament, Left	**0** Open **3** Percutaneous **4** Percutaneous Endoscopic **X** External	**Z** No Device	**Z** No Qualifier

0 Medical and Surgical
M Bursae and Ligaments
P Removal: Taking out or off a device from a body part

Body Part	Approach	Device	Qualifier
Character 4	Character 5	Character 6	Character 7
X Upper Bursa and Ligament **Y** Lower Bursa and Ligament	**0** Open **3** Percutaneous **4** Percutaneous Endoscopic	**0** Drainage Device **7** Autologous Tissue Substitute **J** Synthetic Substitute **K** Nonautologous Tissue Substitute **Y** Other Device	**Z** No Qualifier
X Upper Bursa and Ligament **Y** Lower Bursa and Ligament	**X** External	**0** Drainage Device	**Z** No Qualifier

0 Medical and Surgical
M Bursae and Ligaments
Q Repair: Restoring, to the extent possible, a body part to its normal anatomic structure and function

Body Part	Approach	Device	Qualifier
Character 4	Character 5	Character 6	Character 7
0 Head and Neck Bursa and Ligament	0 Open	Z No Device	Z No Qualifier
1 Shoulder Bursa and Ligament, Right	3 Percutaneous		
2 Shoulder Bursa and Ligament, Left	4 Percutaneous Endoscopic		
3 Elbow Bursa and Ligament, Right			
4 Elbow Bursa and Ligament, Left			
5 Wrist Bursa and Ligament, Right			
6 Wrist Bursa and Ligament, Left			
7 Hand Bursa and Ligament, Right			
8 Hand Bursa and Ligament, Left			
9 Upper Extremity Bursa and Ligament, Right			
B Upper Extremity Bursa and Ligament, Left			
C Upper Spine Bursa and Ligament			
D Lower Spine Bursa and Ligament			
F Sternum Bursa and Ligament			
G Rib(s) Bursa and Ligament			
H Abdomen Bursa and Ligament, Right			
J Abdomen Bursa and Ligament, Left			
K Perineum Bursa and Ligament			
L Hip Bursa and Ligament, Right			
M Hip Bursa and Ligament, Left			
N Knee Bursa and Ligament, Right			
P Knee Bursa and Ligament, Left			
Q Ankle Bursa and Ligament, Right			
R Ankle Bursa and Ligament, Left			
S Foot Bursa and Ligament, Right			
T Foot Bursa and Ligament, Left			
V Lower Extremity Bursa and Ligament, Right			
W Lower Extremity Bursa and Ligament, Left			

0 **Medical and Surgical**
M **Bursae and Ligaments**
R **Replacement:** Putting in or on biological or synthetic material that physically takes the place and/or function of all or a portion of a body part

Body Part	Approach	Device	Qualifier
Character 4	Character 5	Character 6	Character 7
0 Head and Neck Bursa and Ligament 1 Shoulder Bursa and Ligament, Right 2 Shoulder Bursa and Ligament, Left 3 Elbow Bursa and Ligament, Right 4 Elbow Bursa and Ligament, Left 5 Wrist Bursa and Ligament, Right 6 Wrist Bursa and Ligament, Left 7 Hand Bursa and Ligament, Right 8 Hand Bursa and Ligament, Left 9 Upper Extremity Bursa and Ligament, Right B Upper Extremity Bursa and Ligament, Left C Upper Spine Bursa and Ligament D Lower Spine Bursa and Ligament F Sternum Bursa and Ligament G Rib(s) Bursa and Ligament H Abdomen Bursa and Ligament, Right J Abdomen Bursa and Ligament, Left K Perineum Bursa and Ligament L Hip Bursa and Ligament, Right M Hip Bursa and Ligament, Left N Knee Bursa and Ligament, Right P Knee Bursa and Ligament, Left Q Ankle Bursa and Ligament, Right R Ankle Bursa and Ligament, Left S Foot Bursa and Ligament, Right T Foot Bursa and Ligament, Left V Lower Extremity Bursa and Ligament, Right W Lower Extremity Bursa and Ligament, Left	0 Open 4 Percutaneous Endoscopic	7 Autologous Tissue Substitute J Synthetic Substitute K Nonautologous Tissue Substitute	Z No Qualifier

---

LC Limited Coverage   NC Noncovered   HAC HAC-associated Procedure   CC Combination Cluster - See Appendix G for code lists
DRG Non-OR-Affecting MS-DRG Assignment   New/Revised Text in **Orange**   ♂ Male   ♀ Female

0 **Medical and Surgical**
M **Bursae and Ligaments**
S **Reposition:** Moving to its normal location, or other suitable location, all or a portion of a body part

Body Part	Approach	Device	Qualifier
Character 4	Character 5	Character 6	Character 7
0 Head and Neck Bursa and Ligament 1 Shoulder Bursa and Ligament, Right 2 Shoulder Bursa and Ligament, Left 3 Elbow Bursa and Ligament, Right 4 Elbow Bursa and Ligament, Left 5 Wrist Bursa and Ligament, Right 6 Wrist Bursa and Ligament, Left 7 Hand Bursa and Ligament, Right 8 Hand Bursa and Ligament, Left 9 Upper Extremity Bursa and Ligament, Right B Upper Extremity Bursa and Ligament, Left C Upper Spine Bursa and Ligament D Lower Spine Bursa and Ligament F Sternum Bursa and Ligament G Rib(s) Bursa and Ligament H Abdomen Bursa and Ligament, Right J Abdomen Bursa and Ligament, Left K Perineum Bursa and Ligament L Hip Bursa and Ligament, Right M Hip Bursa and Ligament, Left N Knee Bursa and Ligament, Right P Knee Bursa and Ligament, Left Q Ankle Bursa and Ligament, Right R Ankle Bursa and Ligament, Left S Foot Bursa and Ligament, Right T Foot Bursa and Ligament, Left V Lower Extremity Bursa and Ligament, Right W Lower Extremity Bursa and Ligament, Left	0 Open 4 Percutaneous Endoscopic	Z No Device	Z No Qualifier

0 Medical and Surgical
M Bursae and Ligaments
T Resection: Cutting out or off, without replacement, all of a body part

Body Part	Approach	Device	Qualifier
Character 4	Character 5	Character 6	Character 7
0 Head and Neck Bursa and Ligament **1** Shoulder Bursa and Ligament, Right **2** Shoulder Bursa and Ligament, Left **3** Elbow Bursa and Ligament, Right **4** Elbow Bursa and Ligament, Left **5** Wrist Bursa and Ligament, Right **6** Wrist Bursa and Ligament, Left **7** Hand Bursa and Ligament, Right **8** Hand Bursa and Ligament, Left **9** Upper Extremity Bursa and Ligament, Right **B** Upper Extremity Bursa and Ligament, Left **C** Upper Spine Bursa and Ligament **D** Lower Spine Bursa and Ligament **F** Sternum Bursa and Ligament **G** Rib(s) Bursa and Ligament **H** Abdomen Bursa and Ligament, Right **J** Abdomen Bursa and Ligament, Left **K** Perineum Bursa and Ligament **L** Hip Bursa and Ligament, Right **M** Hip Bursa and Ligament, Left **N** Knee Bursa and Ligament, Right **P** Knee Bursa and Ligament, Left **Q** Ankle Bursa and Ligament, Right **R** Ankle Bursa and Ligament, Left **S** Foot Bursa and Ligament, Right **T** Foot Bursa and Ligament, Left **V** Lower Extremity Bursa and Ligament, Right **W** Lower Extremity Bursa and Ligament, Left	**0** Open **4** Percutaneous Endoscopic	**Z** No Device	**Z** No Qualifier

0 Medical and Surgical
M Bursae and Ligaments
U Supplement: Putting in or on biological or synthetic material that physically reinforces and/or augments the function of a portion of a body part

Body Part	Approach	Device	Qualifier
Character 4	Character 5	Character 6	Character 7
0 Head and Neck Bursa and Ligament 1 Shoulder Bursa and Ligament, Right 2 Shoulder Bursa and Ligament, Left 3 Elbow Bursa and Ligament, Right 4 Elbow Bursa and Ligament, Left 5 Wrist Bursa and Ligament, Right 6 Wrist Bursa and Ligament, Left 7 Hand Bursa and Ligament, Right 8 Hand Bursa and Ligament, Left 9 Upper Extremity Bursa and Ligament, Right B Upper Extremity Bursa and Ligament, Left C Upper Spine Bursa and Ligament D Lower Spine Bursa and Ligament F Sternum Bursa and Ligament G Rib(s) Bursa and Ligament H Abdomen Bursa and Ligament, Right J Abdomen Bursa and Ligament, Left K Perineum Bursa and Ligament L Hip Bursa and Ligament, Right M Hip Bursa and Ligament, Left N Knee Bursa and Ligament, Right P Knee Bursa and Ligament, Left Q Ankle Bursa and Ligament, Right R Ankle Bursa and Ligament, Left S Foot Bursa and Ligament, Right T Foot Bursa and Ligament, Left V Lower Extremity Bursa and Ligament, Right W Lower Extremity Bursa and Ligament, Left	0 Open 4 Percutaneous Endoscopic	7 Autologous Tissue Substitute J Synthetic Substitute K Nonautologous Tissue Substitute	Z No Qualifier

0 Medical and Surgical
M Bursae and Ligaments
W Revision: Correcting, to the extent possible, a portion of a malfunctioning device or the position of a displaced device

Body Part	Approach	Device	Qualifier
Character 4	Character 5	Character 6	Character 7
X Upper Bursa and Ligament Y Lower Bursa and Ligament	0 Open 3 Percutaneous 4 Percutaneous Endoscopic	0 Drainage Device 7 Autologous Tissue Substitute J Synthetic Substitute K Nonautologous Tissue Substitute Y Other Device	Z No Qualifier
X Upper Bursa and Ligament Y Lower Bursa and Ligament	X External	0 Drainage Device 7 Autologous Tissue Substitute J Synthetic Substitute K Nonautologous Tissue Substitute	Z No Qualifier

0   Medical and Surgical
M   Bursae and Ligaments
X   Transfer: Moving, without taking out, all or a portion of a body part to another location to take over the function of all or a portion of a body part

Body Part	Approach	Device	Qualifier
Character 4	**Character 5**	**Character 6**	**Character 7**
0 Head and Neck Bursa and Ligament	**0** Open	**Z** No Device	**Z** No Qualifier
1 Shoulder Bursa and Ligament, Right	**4** Percutaneous Endoscopic		
2 Shoulder Bursa and Ligament, Left			
3 Elbow Bursa and Ligament, Right			
4 Elbow Bursa and Ligament, Left			
5 Wrist Bursa and Ligament, Right			
6 Wrist Bursa and Ligament, Left			
7 Hand Bursa and Ligament, Right			
8 Hand Bursa and Ligament, Left			
9 Upper Extremity Bursa and Ligament, Right			
B Upper Extremity Bursa and Ligament, Left			
C Upper Spine Bursa and Ligament			
D Lower Spine Bursa and Ligament			
F Sternum Bursa and Ligament			
G Rib(s) Bursa and Ligament			
H Abdomen Bursa and Ligament, Right			
J Abdomen Bursa and Ligament, Left			
K Perineum Bursa and Ligament			
L Hip Bursa and Ligament, Right			
M Hip Bursa and Ligament, Left			
N Knee Bursa and Ligament, Right			
P Knee Bursa and Ligament, Left			
Q Ankle Bursa and Ligament, Right			
R Ankle Bursa and Ligament, Left			
S Foot Bursa and Ligament, Right			
T Foot Bursa and Ligament, Left			
V Lower Extremity Bursa and Ligament, Right			
W Lower Extremity Bursa and Ligament, Left			

LC Limited Coverage   NC Noncovered   HAC HAC-associated Procedure   CC Combination Cluster - See Appendix G for code lists
DRG Non-OR-Affecting MS-DRG Assignment   New/Revised Text in **Orange**   ♂ Male   ♀ Female

2018 ICD-10-PCS

429

BURSAE AND LIGAMENTS 0M2-0MX

NOTES

Head and Facial Bones 0N2-0NW

0 **Medical and Surgical**
N **Head and Facial Bones**
2 **Change:** Taking out or off a device from a body part and putting back an identical or similar device in or on the same body part without cutting or puncturing the skin or a mucous membrane

Body Part	Approach	Device	Qualifier
Character 4	Character 5	Character 6	Character 7
0 Skull **B** Nasal Bone **W** Facial Bone	**X** External	**0** Drainage Device **Y** Other Device	**Z** No Qualifier

0 **Medical and Surgical**
N **Head and Facial Bones**
5 **Destruction:** Physical eradication of all or a portion of a body part by the direct use of energy, force, or a destructive agent

Body Part	Approach	Device	Qualifier
Character 4	Character 5	Character 6	Character 7
0 Skull **1** Frontal Bone **3** Parietal Bone, Right **4** Parietal Bone, Left **5** Temporal Bone, Right **6** Temporal Bone, Left **7** Occipital Bone **B** Nasal Bone **C** Sphenoid Bone **F** Ethmoid Bone, Right **G** Ethmoid Bone, Left **H** Lacrimal Bone, Right **J** Lacrimal Bone, Left **K** Palatine Bone, Right **L** Palatine Bone, Left **M** Zygomatic Bone, Right **N** Zygomatic Bone, Left **P** Orbit, Right **Q** Orbit, Left **R** Maxilla **T** Mandible, Right **V** Mandible, Left **X** Hyoid Bone	**0** Open **3** Percutaneous **4** Percutaneous Endoscopic	**Z** No Device	**Z** No Qualifier

0 **Medical and Surgical**
N **Head and Facial Bones**
8 **Division:** Cutting into a body part, without draining fluids and/or gases from the body part, in order to separate or transect a body part

Body Part	Approach	Device	Qualifier
Character 4	**Character 5**	**Character 6**	**Character 7**
0 Skull 1 Frontal Bone **3** Parietal Bone, Right **4** Parietal Bone, Left **5** Temporal Bone, Right **6** Temporal Bone, Left 7 Occipital Bone **B** Nasal Bone C Sphenoid Bone **F** Ethmoid Bone, Right **G** Ethmoid Bone, Left **H** Lacrimal Bone, Right **J** Lacrimal Bone, Left **K** Palatine Bone, Right **L** Palatine Bone, Left **M** Zygomatic Bone, Right **N** Zygomatic Bone, Left **P** Orbit, Right **Q** Orbit, Left R Maxilla **T** Mandible, Right **V** Mandible, Left **X** Hyoid Bone	**0** Open **3** Percutaneous **4** Percutaneous Endoscopic	**Z** No Device	**Z** No Qualifier

0 **Medical and Surgical**
N **Head and Facial Bones**
9 **Drainage:** Taking or letting out fluids and/or gases from a body part

Body Part	Approach	Device	Qualifier
Character 4	Character 5	Character 6	Character 7
0 Skull 1 Frontal Bone 3 Parietal Bone, Right 4 Parietal Bone, Left 5 Temporal Bone, Right 6 Temporal Bone, Left 7 Occipital Bone B Nasal Bone C Sphenoid Bone F Ethmoid Bone, Right G Ethmoid Bone, Left H Lacrimal Bone, Right J Lacrimal Bone, Left K Palatine Bone, Right L Palatine Bone, Left M Zygomatic Bone, Right N Zygomatic Bone, Left P Orbit, Right Q Orbit, Left R Maxilla T Mandible, Right V Mandible, Left X Hyoid Bone	0 Open 3 Percutaneous 4 Percutaneous Endoscopic	0 Drainage Device	Z No Qualifier
0 Skull 1 Frontal Bone 3 Parietal Bone, Right 4 Parietal Bone, Left 5 Temporal Bone, Right 6 Temporal Bone, Left 7 Occipital Bone B Nasal Bone C Sphenoid Bone F Ethmoid Bone, Right G Ethmoid Bone, Left H Lacrimal Bone, Right J Lacrimal Bone, Left K Palatine Bone, Right L Palatine Bone, Left M Zygomatic Bone, Right N Zygomatic Bone, Left P Orbit, Right Q Orbit, Left R Maxilla T Mandible, Right V Mandible, Left X Hyoid Bone	0 Open 3 Percutaneous 4 Percutaneous Endoscopic	Z No Device	X Diagnostic Z No Qualifier

0   Medical and Surgical
N   Head and Facial Bones
B   Excision: Cutting out or off, without replacement, a portion of a body part

Body Part	Approach	Device	Qualifier
Character 4	Character 5	Character 6	Character 7
0 Skull	0 Open	Z No Device	X Diagnostic
1 Frontal Bone	3 Percutaneous		Z No Qualifier
3 Parietal Bone, Right	4 Percutaneous Endoscopic		
4 Parietal Bone, Left			
5 Temporal Bone, Right			
6 Temporal Bone, Left			
7 Occipital Bone			
B Nasal Bone			
C Sphenoid Bone			
F Ethmoid Bone, Right			
G Ethmoid Bone, Left			
H Lacrimal Bone, Right			
J Lacrimal Bone, Left			
K Palatine Bone, Right			
L Palatine Bone, Left			
M Zygomatic Bone, Right			
N Zygomatic Bone, Left			
P Orbit, Right			
Q Orbit, Left			
R Maxilla			
T Mandible, Right			
V Mandible, Left			
X Hyoid Bone			

0   Medical and Surgical
N   Head and Facial Bones
C   Extirpation: Taking or cutting out solid matter from a body part

Body Part	Approach	Device	Qualifier
Character 4	Character 5	Character 6	Character 7
1 Frontal Bone	0 Open	Z No Device	Z No Qualifier
3 Parietal Bone, Right	3 Percutaneous		
4 Parietal Bone, Left	4 Percutaneous Endoscopic		
5 Temporal Bone, Right			
6 Temporal Bone, Left			
7 Occipital Bone			
B Nasal Bone			
C Sphenoid Bone			
F Ethmoid Bone, Right			
G Ethmoid Bone, Left			
H Lacrimal Bone, Right			
J Lacrimal Bone, Left			
K Palatine Bone, Right			
L Palatine Bone, Left			
M Zygomatic Bone, Right			
N Zygomatic Bone, Left			
P Orbit, Right			
Q Orbit, Left			
R Maxilla			
T Mandible, Right			
V Mandible, Left			
X Hyoid Bone			

LC Limited Coverage NC Noncovered HAC HAC-associated Procedure CC Combination Cluster - See Appendix G for code lists
DRG Non-OR-Affecting MS-DRG Assignment   New/Revised Text in Orange   ♂ Male   ♀ Female

434   **2018 ICD-10-PCS**

0 **Medical and Surgical**
N **Head and Facial Bones**
D **Extraction:** Pulling or stripping out or off all or a portion of a body part by the use of force

Body Part	Approach	Device	Qualifier
Character 4	Character 5	Character 6	Character 7
0 Skull	0 Open	Z No Device	Z No Qualifier
1 Frontal Bone			
3 Parietal Bone, Right			
4 Parietal Bone, Left			
5 Temporal Bone, Right			
6 Temporal Bone, Left			
7 Occipital Bone			
B Nasal Bone			
C Sphenoid Bone			
F Ethmoid Bone, Right			
G Ethmoid Bone, Left			
H Lacrimal Bone, Right			
J Lacrimal Bone, Left			
K Palatine Bone, Right			
L Palatine Bone, Left			
M Zygomatic Bone, Right			
N Zygomatic Bone, Left			
P Orbit, Right			
Q Orbit, Left			
R Maxilla			
T Mandible, Right			
V Mandible, Left			
X Hyoid Bone			

LC Limited Coverage   NC Noncovered   HAC HAC-associated Procedure   CC Combination Cluster - See Appendix G for code lists
DRG Non-OR-Affecting MS-DRG Assignment   New/Revised Text in **Orange**   ♂ Male   ♀ Female

2018 ICD-10-PCS

435

0ND

HEAD AND FACIAL BONES 0N2-0NW

0 Medical and Surgical
N Head and Facial Bones
H Insertion: Putting in a nonbiological appliance that monitors, assists, performs, or prevents a physiological function but does not physically take the place of a body part

Body Part	Approach	Device	Qualifier
Character 4	**Character 5**	**Character 6**	**Character 7**
0 Skull 🄲🄲	**0** Open	**4** Internal Fixation Device **5** External Fixation Device **M** Bone Growth Stimulator **N** Neurostimulator Generator	**Z** No Qualifier
0 Skull	**3** Percutaneous **4** Percutaneous Endoscopic	**4** Internal Fixation Device **5** External Fixation Device **M** Bone Growth Stimulator	**Z** No Qualifier
1 Frontal Bone **3** Parietal Bone, Right **4** Parietal Bone, Left **7** Occipital Bone **C** Sphenoid Bone **F** Ethmoid Bone, Right **G** Ethmoid Bone, Left **H** Lacrimal Bone, Right **J** Lacrimal Bone, Left **K** Palatine Bone, Right **L** Palatine Bone, Left **M** Zygomatic Bone, Right **N** Zygomatic Bone, Left **P** Orbit, Right **Q** Orbit, Left **X** Hyoid Bone	**0** Open **3** Percutaneous **4** Percutaneous Endoscopic	**4** Internal Fixation Device	**Z** No Qualifier
5 Temporal Bone, Right **6** Temporal Bone, Left	**0** Open **3** Percutaneous **4** Percutaneous Endoscopic	**4** Internal Fixation Device **S** Hearing Device	**Z** No Qualifier
B Nasal Bone	**0** Open **3** Percutaneous **4** Percutaneous Endoscopic	**4** Internal Fixation Device **M** Bone Growth Stimulator	**Z** No Qualifier
R Maxilla **T** Mandible, Right **V** Mandible, Left	**0** Open **3** Percutaneous **4** Percutaneous Endoscopic	**4** Internal Fixation Device **5** External Fixation Device	**Z** No Qualifier
W Facial Bone	**0** Open **3** Percutaneous **4** Percutaneous Endoscopic	**M** Bone Growth Stimulator	**Z** No Qualifier

🄲🄲 0NH00NZ

0 Medical and Surgical
N Head and Facial Bones
J Inspection: Visually and/or manually exploring a body part

Body Part	Approach	Device	Qualifier
Character 4	**Character 5**	**Character 6**	**Character 7**
0 Skull **B** Nasal Bone **W** Facial Bone	**0** Open **3** Percutaneous **4** Percutaneous Endoscopic **X** External	**Z** No Device	**Z** No Qualifier

0 Medical and Surgical
N Head and Facial Bones
N Release: Freeing a body part from an abnormal physical constraint by cutting or by the use of force

Body Part	Approach	Device	Qualifier
Character 4	Character 5	Character 6	Character 7
1 Frontal Bone 3 Parietal Bone, Right 4 Parietal Bone, Left 5 Temporal Bone, Right 6 Temporal Bone, Left 7 Occipital Bone B Nasal Bone C Sphenoid Bone F Ethmoid Bone, Right G Ethmoid Bone, Left H Lacrimal Bone, Right J Lacrimal Bone, Left K Palatine Bone, Right L Palatine Bone, Left M Zygomatic Bone, Right N Zygomatic Bone, Left P Orbit, Right Q Orbit, Left R Maxilla T Mandible, Right V Mandible, Left X Hyoid Bone	0 Open 3 Percutaneous 4 Percutaneous Endoscopic	Z No Device	Z No Qualifier

0 Medical and Surgical
N Head and Facial Bones
P Removal: Taking out or off a device from a body part

Body Part	Approach	Device	Qualifier
Character 4	Character 5	Character 6	Character 7
0 Skull	0 Open	0 Drainage Device 4 Internal Fixation Device 5 External Fixation Device 7 Autologous Tissue Substitute J Synthetic Substitute K Nonautologous Tissue Substitute M Bone Growth Stimulator N Neurostimulator Generator S Hearing Device	Z No Qualifier
0 Skull	3 Percutaneous 4 Percutaneous Endoscopic	0 Drainage Device 4 Internal Fixation Device 5 External Fixation Device 7 Autologous Tissue Substitute J Synthetic Substitute K Nonautologous Tissue Substitute M Bone Growth Stimulator S Hearing Device	Z No Qualifier
0 Skull	X External	0 Drainage Device 4 Internal Fixation Device 5 External Fixation Device M Bone Growth Stimulator S Hearing Device	Z No Qualifier
B Nasal Bone W Facial Bone	0 Open 3 Percutaneous 4 Percutaneous Endoscopic	0 Drainage Device 4 Internal Fixation Device 7 Autologous Tissue Substitute J Synthetic Substitute K Nonautologous Tissue Substitute M Bone Growth Stimulator	Z No Qualifier
B Nasal Bone W Facial Bone	X External	0 Drainage Device 4 Internal Fixation Device M Bone Growth Stimulator	Z No Qualifier

0 Medical and Surgical
N Head and Facial Bones
Q Repair: Restoring, to the extent possible, a body part to its normal anatomic structure and function

Body Part	Approach	Device	Qualifier
Character 4	Character 5	Character 6	Character 7
0 Skull 1 Frontal Bone 3 Parietal Bone, Right 4 Parietal Bone, Left 5 Temporal Bone, Right 6 Temporal Bone, Left 7 Occipital Bone B Nasal Bone C Sphenoid Bone F Ethmoid Bone, Right G Ethmoid Bone, Left H Lacrimal Bone, Right J Lacrimal Bone, Left K Palatine Bone, Right L Palatine Bone, Left M Zygomatic Bone, Right N Zygomatic Bone, Left P Orbit, Right Q Orbit, Left R Maxilla T Mandible, Right V Mandible, Left X Hyoid Bone	0 Open 3 Percutaneous 4 Percutaneous Endoscopic X External	Z No Device	Z No Qualifier

0 Medical and Surgical
N Head and Facial Bones
R Replacement: Putting in or on biological or synthetic material that physically takes the place and/or function of all or a portion of a body part

Body Part	Approach	Device	Qualifier
Character 4	Character 5	Character 6	Character 7
0 Skull 1 Frontal Bone 3 Parietal Bone, Right 4 Parietal Bone, Left 5 Temporal Bone, Right 6 Temporal Bone, Left 7 Occipital Bone B Nasal Bone C Sphenoid Bone F Ethmoid Bone, Right G Ethmoid Bone, Left H Lacrimal Bone, Right J Lacrimal Bone, Left K Palatine Bone, Right L Palatine Bone, Left M Zygomatic Bone, Right N Zygomatic Bone, Left P Orbit, Right Q Orbit, Left R Maxilla T Mandible, Right V Mandible, Left X Hyoid Bone	0 Open 3 Percutaneous 4 Percutaneous Endoscopic	7 Autologous Tissue Substitute J Synthetic Substitute K Nonautologous Tissue Substitute	Z No Qualifier

0   Medical and Surgical
N   Head and Facial Bones
S   Reposition: Moving to its normal location, or other suitable location, all or a portion of a body part

Body Part	Approach	Device	Qualifier
Character 4	Character 5	Character 6	Character 7
0 Skull **R** Maxilla **T** Mandible, Right **V** Mandible, Left	**0** Open **3** Percutaneous **4** Percutaneous Endoscopic	**4** Internal Fixation Device **5** External Fixation Device **Z** No Device	**Z** No Qualifier
0 Skull **R** Maxilla **T** Mandible, Right **V** Mandible, Left	**X** External	**Z** No Device	**Z** No Qualifier
1 Frontal Bone **3** Parietal Bone, Right **4** Parietal Bone, Left **5** Temporal Bone, Right **6** Temporal Bone, Left **7** Occipital Bone **B** Nasal Bone **C** Sphenoid Bone **F** Ethmoid Bone, Right **G** Ethmoid Bone, Left **H** Lacrimal Bone, Right **J** Lacrimal Bone, Left **K** Palatine Bone, Right **L** Palatine Bone, Left **M** Zygomatic Bone, Right **N** Zygomatic Bone, Left **P** Orbit, Right **Q** Orbit, Left **X** Hyoid Bone	**0** Open **3** Percutaneous **4** Percutaneous Endoscopic	**4** Internal Fixation Device **Z** No Device	**Z** No Qualifier
1 Frontal Bone **3** Parietal Bone, Right **4** Parietal Bone, Left **5** Temporal Bone, Right **6** Temporal Bone, Left **7** Occipital Bone **B** Nasal Bone **C** Sphenoid Bone **F** Ethmoid Bone, Right **G** Ethmoid Bone, Left **H** Lacrimal Bone, Right **J** Lacrimal Bone, Left **K** Palatine Bone, Right **L** Palatine Bone, Left **M** Zygomatic Bone, Right **N** Zygomatic Bone, Left **P** Orbit, Right **Q** Orbit, Left **X** Hyoid Bone	**X** External	**Z** No Device	**Z** No Qualifier

LC Limited Coverage   **NC** Noncovered   **HAC** HAC-associated Procedure   **CC** Combination Cluster - See Appendix G for code lists
DRG Non-OR-Affecting MS-DRG Assignment   New/Revised Text in **Orange**   ♂ Male   ♀ Female

2018 ICD-10-PCS   **439**

0 Medical and Surgical
N Head and Facial Bones
T Resection: Cutting out or off, without replacement, all of a body part

Body Part	Approach	Device	Qualifier
Character 4	Character 5	Character 6	Character 7
1 Frontal Bone 3 Parietal Bone, Right 4 Parietal Bone, Left 5 Temporal Bone, Right 6 Temporal Bone, Left 7 Occipital Bone B Nasal Bone C Sphenoid Bone F Ethmoid Bone, Right G Ethmoid Bone, Left H Lacrimal Bone, Right J Lacrimal Bone, Left K Palatine Bone, Right L Palatine Bone, Left M Zygomatic Bone, Right N Zygomatic Bone, Left P Orbit, Right Q Orbit, Left R Maxilla T Mandible, Right V Mandible, Left X Hyoid Bone	0 Open	Z No Device	Z No Qualifier

0 Medical and Surgical
N Head and Facial Bones
U Supplement: Putting in or on biological or synthetic material that physically reinforces and/or augments the function of a portion of a body part

Body Part	Approach	Device	Qualifier
Character 4	Character 5	Character 6	Character 7
0 Skull 1 Frontal Bone 3 Parietal Bone, Right 4 Parietal Bone, Left 5 Temporal Bone, Right 6 Temporal Bone, Left 7 Occipital Bone B Nasal Bone C Sphenoid Bone F Ethmoid Bone, Right G Ethmoid Bone, Left H Lacrimal Bone, Right J Lacrimal Bone, Left K Palatine Bone, Right L Palatine Bone, Left M Zygomatic Bone, Right N Zygomatic Bone, Left P Orbit, Right Q Orbit, Left R Maxilla T Mandible, Right V Mandible, Left X Hyoid Bone	0 Open 3 Percutaneous 4 Percutaneous Endoscopic	7 Autologous Tissue Substitute J Synthetic Substitute K Nonautologous Tissue Substitute	Z No Qualifier

0 **Medical and Surgical**
N **Head and Facial Bones**
W **Revision:** Correcting, to the extent possible, a portion of a malfunctioning device or the position of a displaced device

Body Part	Approach	Device	Qualifier
Character 4	Character 5	Character 6	Character 7
0 Skull	**0** Open	**0** Drainage Device **4** Internal Fixation Device **5** External Fixation Device **7** Autologous Tissue Substitute **J** Synthetic Substitute **K** Nonautologous Tissue Substitute **M** Bone Growth Stimulator **N** Neurostimulator Generator **S** Hearing Device	**Z** No Qualifier
0 Skull	**3** Percutaneous **4** Percutaneous Endoscopic **X** External	**0** Drainage Device **4** Internal Fixation Device **5** External Fixation Device **7** Autologous Tissue Substitute **J** Synthetic Substitute **K** Nonautologous Tissue Substitute **M** Bone Growth Stimulator **S** Hearing Device	**Z** No Qualifier
B Nasal Bone **W** Facial Bone	**0** Open **3** Percutaneous **4** Percutaneous Endoscopic **X** External	**0** Drainage Device **4** Internal Fixation Device **7** Autologous Tissue Substitute **J** Synthetic Substitute **K** Nonautologous Tissue Substitute **M** Bone Growth Stimulator	**Z** No Qualifier

LC Limited Coverage   **NC** Noncovered   **HAC** HAC-associated Procedure   **CC** Combination Cluster - See Appendix G for code lists
DRG Non-OR-Affecting MS-DRG Assignment   New/Revised Text in **Orange**   ♂ Male   ♀ Female

2018 ICD-10-PCS

441

NOTES

Upper Bones 0P2-0PW

0 Medical and Surgical
P Upper Bones
2 **Change:** Taking out or off a device from a body part and putting back an identical or similar device in or on the same body part without cutting or puncturing the skin or a mucous membrane

Body Part	Approach	Device	Qualifier
Character 4	Character 5	Character 6	Character 7
Y Upper Bone	**X** External	**0** Drainage Device **Y** Other Device	**Z** No Qualifier

0 Medical and Surgical
P Upper Bones
5 **Destruction:** Physical eradication of all or a portion of a body part by the direct use of energy, force, or a destructive agent

Body Part	Approach	Device	Qualifier
Character 4	Character 5	Character 6	Character 7
0 Sternum **1** Ribs, 1 to 2 **2** Ribs, 3 or More **3** Cervical Vertebra **4** Thoracic Vertebra **5** Scapula, Right **6** Scapula, Left **7** Glenoid Cavity, Right **8** Glenoid Cavity, Left **9** Clavicle, Right **B** Clavicle, Left **C** Humeral Head, Right **D** Humeral Head, Left **F** Humeral Shaft, Right **G** Humeral Shaft, Left **H** Radius, Right **J** Radius, Left **K** Ulna, Right **L** Ulna, Left **M** Carpal, Right **N** Carpal, Left **P** Metacarpal, Right **Q** Metacarpal, Left **R** Thumb Phalanx, Right **S** Thumb Phalanx, Left **T** Finger Phalanx, Right **V** Finger Phalanx, Left	**0** Open **3** Percutaneous **4** Percutaneous Endoscopic	**Z** No Device	**Z** No Qualifier

---

0 **Medical and Surgical**
P **Upper Bones**
8 **Division:** Cutting into a body part, without draining fluids and/or gases from the body part, in order to separate or transect a body part

Body Part	Approach	Device	Qualifier
Character 4	Character 5	Character 6	Character 7
0 Sternum	**0** Open	**Z** No Device	**Z** No Qualifier
1 Ribs, 1 to 2	**3** Percutaneous		
2 Ribs, 3 or More	**4** Percutaneous Endoscopic		
3 Cervical Vertebra			
4 Thoracic Vertebra			
5 Scapula, Right			
6 Scapula, Left			
7 Glenoid Cavity, Right			
8 Glenoid Cavity, Left			
9 Clavicle, Right			
B Clavicle, Left			
C Humeral Head, Right			
D Humeral Head, Left			
F Humeral Shaft, Right			
G Humeral Shaft, Left			
H Radius, Right			
J Radius, Left			
K Ulna, Right			
L Ulna, Left			
M Carpal, Right			
N Carpal, Left			
P Metacarpal, Right			
Q Metacarpal, Left			
R Thumb Phalanx, Right			
S Thumb Phalanx, Left			
T Finger Phalanx, Right			
V Finger Phalanx, Left			

LC Limited Coverage   NC Noncovered   HAC HAC-associated Procedure   CC Combination Cluster - See Appendix G for code lists
DRG Non-OR-Affecting MS-DRG Assignment   New/Revised Text in **Orange**   ♂ Male   ♀ Female

444

2018 ICD-10-PCS

UPPER BONES 0P2-0PW

0 **Medical and Surgical**
P **Upper Bones**
9 **Drainage:** Taking or letting out fluids and/or gases from a body part

Body Part	Approach	Device	Qualifier
Character 4	**Character 5**	**Character 6**	**Character 7**
0 Sternum 1 Ribs, 1 to 2 2 Ribs, 3 or More 3 Cervical Vertebra 4 Thoracic Vertebra 5 Scapula, Right 6 Scapula, Left 7 Glenoid Cavity, Right 8 Glenoid Cavity, Left 9 Clavicle, Right B Clavicle, Left C Humeral Head, Right D Humeral Head, Left F Humeral Shaft, Right G Humeral Shaft, Left H Radius, Right J Radius, Left K Ulna, Right L Ulna, Left M Carpal, Right N Carpal, Left P Metacarpal, Right Q Metacarpal, Left R Thumb Phalanx, Right S Thumb Phalanx, Left T Finger Phalanx, Right V Finger Phalanx, Left	0 Open 3 Percutaneous 4 Percutaneous Endoscopic	0 Drainage Device	Z No Qualifier
0 Sternum 1 Ribs, 1 to 2 2 Ribs, 3 or More 3 Cervical Vertebra 4 Thoracic Vertebra 5 Scapula, Right 6 Scapula, Left 7 Glenoid Cavity, Right 8 Glenoid Cavity, Left 9 Clavicle, Right B Clavicle, Left C Humeral Head, Right D Humeral Head, Left F Humeral Shaft, Right G Humeral Shaft, Left H Radius, Right J Radius, Left K Ulna, Right L Ulna, Left M Carpal, Right N Carpal, Left P Metacarpal, Right Q Metacarpal, Left R Thumb Phalanx, Right S Thumb Phalanx, Left T Finger Phalanx, Right V Finger Phalanx, Left	0 Open 3 Percutaneous 4 Percutaneous Endoscopic	Z No Device	X Diagnostic Z No Qualifier

LC Limited Coverage NC Noncovered HAC HAC-associated Procedure CC Combination Cluster - See Appendix G for code lists
DRG Non-OR-Affecting MS-DRG Assignment New/Revised Text in **Orange** ♂ Male ♀ Female

2018 ICD-10-PCS

445

UPPER BONES 0P2-0PW

0   **Medical and Surgical**
P   **Upper Bones**
B   **Excision:** Cutting out or off, without replacement, a portion of a body part

Body Part	Approach	Device	Qualifier
Character 4	Character 5	Character 6	Character 7
0 Sternum 1 Ribs, 1 to 2 2 Ribs, 3 or More 3 Cervical Vertebra 4 Thoracic Vertebra 5 Scapula, Right 6 Scapula, Left 7 Glenoid Cavity, Right 8 Glenoid Cavity, Left 9 Clavicle, Right B Clavicle, Left C Humeral Head, Right D Humeral Head, Left F Humeral Shaft, Right G Humeral Shaft, Left H Radius, Right J Radius, Left K Ulna, Right L Ulna, Left M Carpal, Right N Carpal, Left P Metacarpal, Right Q Metacarpal, Left R Thumb Phalanx, Right S Thumb Phalanx, Left T Finger Phalanx, Right V Finger Phalanx, Left	0 Open 3 Percutaneous 4 Percutaneous Endoscopic	Z No Device	X Diagnostic Z No Qualifier

0   **Medical and Surgical**
P   **Upper Bones**
C   **Extirpation:** Taking or cutting out solid matter from a body part

Body Part	Approach	Device	Qualifier
Character 4	Character 5	Character 6	Character 7
0 Sternum 1 Ribs, 1 to 2 2 Ribs, 3 or More 3 Cervical Vertebra 4 Thoracic Vertebra 5 Scapula, Right 6 Scapula, Left 7 Glenoid Cavity, Right 8 Glenoid Cavity, Left 9 Clavicle, Right B Clavicle, Left C Humeral Head, Right D Humeral Head, Left F Humeral Shaft, Right G Humeral Shaft, Left H Radius, Right J Radius, Left K Ulna, Right L Ulna, Left M Carpal, Right N Carpal, Left P Metacarpal, Right Q Metacarpal, Left R Thumb Phalanx, Right S Thumb Phalanx, Left T Finger Phalanx, Right V Finger Phalanx, Left	0 Open 3 Percutaneous 4 Percutaneous Endoscopic	Z No Device	Z No Qualifier

LC Limited Coverage **NC** Noncovered **HAC** HAC-associated Procedure **CC** Combination Cluster - See Appendix G for code lists
non-OR Non-OR-Affecting MS-DRG Assignment New/Revised Text in **Orange** ♂ Male ♀ Female

UPPER BONES 0P2-0PW

446

2018 ICD-10-PCS

0 Medical and Surgical
P Upper Bones
D Extraction: Pulling or stripping out or off all or a portion of a body part by the use of force

Body Part	Approach	Device	Qualifier
Character 4	Character 5	Character 6	Character 7
0 Sternum	0 Open	Z No Device	Z No Qualifier
1 Ribs, 1 to 2			
2 Ribs, 3 or More			
3 Cervical Vertebra			
4 Thoracic Vertebra			
5 Scapula, Right			
6 Scapula, Left			
7 Glenoid Cavity, Right			
8 Glenoid Cavity, Left			
9 Clavicle, Right			
B Clavicle, Left			
C Humeral Head, Right			
D Humeral Head, Left			
F Humeral Shaft, Right			
G Humeral Shaft, Left			
H Radius, Right			
J Radius, Left			
K Ulna, Right			
L Ulna, Left			
M Carpal, Right			
N Carpal, Left			
P Metacarpal, Right			
Q Metacarpal, Left			
R Thumb Phalanx, Right			
S Thumb Phalanx, Left			
T Finger Phalanx, Right			
V Finger Phalanx, Left			

Limited Coverage Noncovered HAC HAC-associated Procedure Combination Cluster - See Appendix G for code lists
Non-OR-Affecting MS-DRG Assignment New/Revised Text in **Orange** ♂ Male ♀ Female

2018 ICD-10-PCS 447

UPPER BONES 0P2-0PW

0 **Medical and Surgical**
P **Upper Bones**
H **Insertion:** Putting in a nonbiological appliance that monitors, assists, performs, or prevents a physiological function but does not physically take the place of a body part

Body Part	Approach	Device	Qualifier
Character 4	Character 5	Character 6	Character 7
0 Sternum	**0** Open **3** Percutaneous **4** Percutaneous Endoscopic	**0** Internal Fixation Device, Rigid Plate **4** Internal Fixation Device	**Z** No Qualifier
1 Ribs, 1 to 2 **2** Ribs, 3 or More **3** Cervical Vertebra **4** Thoracic Vertebra **5** Scapula, Right **6** Scapula, Left **7** Glenoid Cavity, Right **8** Glenoid Cavity, Left **9** Clavicle, Right **B** Clavicle, Left	**0** Open **3** Percutaneous **4** Percutaneous Endoscopic	**4** Internal Fixation Device	**Z** No Qualifier
C Humeral Head, Right **D** Humeral Head, Left **F** Humeral Shaft, Right **G** Humeral Shaft, Left **H** Radius, Right **J** Radius, Left **K** Ulna, Right **L** Ulna, Left	**0** Open **3** Percutaneous **4** Percutaneous Endoscopic	**4** Internal Fixation Device **5** External Fixation Device **6** Internal Fixation Device, Intramedullary **8** External Fixation Device, Limb Lengthening **B** External Fixation Device, Monoplanar **C** External Fixation Device, Ring **D** External Fixation Device, Hybrid	**Z** No Qualifier
M Carpal, Right **N** Carpal, Left **P** Metacarpal, Right **Q** Metacarpal, Left **R** Thumb Phalanx, Right **S** Thumb Phalanx, Left **T** Finger Phalanx, Right **V** Finger Phalanx, Left	**0** Open **3** Percutaneous **4** Percutaneous Endoscopic	**4** Internal Fixation Device **5** External Fixation Device	**Z** No Qualifier
Y Upper Bone	**0** Open **3** Percutaneous **4** Percutaneous Endoscopic	**M** Bone Growth Stimulator	**Z** No Qualifier

0 **Medical and Surgical**
P **Upper Bones**
J **Inspection:** Visually and/or manually exploring a body part

Body Part	Approach	Device	Qualifier
Character 4	Character 5	Character 6	Character 7
Y Upper Bone	**0** Open **3** Percutaneous **4** Percutaneous Endoscopic **X** External	**Z** No Device	**Z** No Qualifier

0 **Medical and Surgical**
P **Upper Bones**
N **Release:** Freeing a body part from an abnormal physical constraint by cutting or by the use of force

Body Part	Approach	Device	Qualifier
Character 4	Character 5	Character 6	Character 7
0 Sternum 1 Ribs, 1 to 2 2 Ribs, 3 or More 3 Cervical Vertebra 4 Thoracic Vertebra 5 Scapula, Right 6 Scapula, Left 7 Glenoid Cavity, Right 8 Glenoid Cavity, Left 9 Clavicle, Right B Clavicle, Left C Humeral Head, Right D Humeral Head, Left F Humeral Shaft, Right G Humeral Shaft, Left H Radius, Right J Radius, Left K Ulna, Right L Ulna, Left M Carpal, Right N Carpal, Left P Metacarpal, Right Q Metacarpal, Left R Thumb Phalanx, Right S Thumb Phalanx, Left T Finger Phalanx, Right V Finger Phalanx, Left	0 Open 3 Percutaneous 4 Percutaneous Endoscopic	Z No Device	Z No Qualifier

0 **Medical and Surgical**
P **Upper Bones**
P **Removal:** Taking out or off a device from a body part

Body Part	Approach	Device	Qualifier
Character 4	Character 5	Character 6	Character 7
0 Sternum 1 Ribs, 1 to 2 2 Ribs, 3 or More 3 Cervical Vertebra 4 Thoracic Vertebra 5 Scapula, Right 6 Scapula, Left 7 Glenoid Cavity, Right 8 Glenoid Cavity, Left 9 Clavicle, Right B Clavicle, Left	0 Open 3 Percutaneous 4 Percutaneous Endoscopic	4 Internal Fixation Device 7 Autologous Tissue Substitute J Synthetic Substitute K Nonautologous Tissue Substitute	Z No Qualifier
0 Sternum 1 Ribs, 1 to 2 2 Ribs, 3 or More 3 Cervical Vertebra 4 Thoracic Vertebra 5 Scapula, Right 6 Scapula, Left 7 Glenoid Cavity, Right 8 Glenoid Cavity, Left 9 Clavicle, Right B Clavicle, Left	X External	4 Internal Fixation Device	Z No Qualifier

0PP continued on next page

0 **Medical and Surgical**
P **Upper Bones**

0PP continued from previous page

P **Removal:** Taking out or off a device from a body part

Body Part	Approach	Device	Qualifier
Character 4	Character 5	Character 6	Character 7
C Humeral Head, Right D Humeral Head, Left F Humeral Shaft, Right G Humeral Shaft, Left H Radius, Right J Radius, Left K Ulna, Right L Ulna, Left M Carpal, Right N Carpal, Left P Metacarpal, Right Q Metacarpal, Left R Thumb Phalanx, Right S Thumb Phalanx, Left T Finger Phalanx, Right V Finger Phalanx, Left	0 Open 3 Percutaneous 4 Percutaneous Endoscopic	4 Internal Fixation Device 5 External Fixation Device 7 Autologous Tissue Substitute J Synthetic Substitute K Nonautologous Tissue Substitute	Z No Qualifier
C Humeral Head, Right D Humeral Head, Left F Humeral Shaft, Right G Humeral Shaft, Left H Radius, Right J Radius, Left K Ulna, Right L Ulna, Left M Carpal, Right N Carpal, Left P Metacarpal, Right Q Metacarpal, Left R Thumb Phalanx, Right S Thumb Phalanx, Left T Finger Phalanx, Right V Finger Phalanx, Left	X External	4 Internal Fixation Device 5 External Fixation Device	Z No Qualifier
Y Upper Bone	0 Open 3 Percutaneous 4 Percutaneous Endoscopic X External	0 Drainage Device M Bone Growth Stimulator	Z No Qualifier

LC Limited Coverage   NC Noncovered   HAC HAC-associated Procedure   CC Combination Cluster - See Appendix G for code lists
Non-OR-Affecting MS-DRG Assignment   New/Revised Text in Orange   ♂ Male   ♀ Female

450

2018 ICD-10-PCS

0 **Medical and Surgical**
P **Upper Bones**
Q **Repair:** Restoring, to the extent possible, a body part to its normal anatomic structure and function

Body Part	Approach	Device	Qualifier
Character 4	**Character 5**	**Character 6**	**Character 7**
0 Sternum	0 Open	Z No Device	Z No Qualifier
1 Ribs, 1 to 2	3 Percutaneous		
2 Ribs, 3 or More	4 Percutaneous Endoscopic		
3 Cervical Vertebra	X External		
4 Thoracic Vertebra			
5 Scapula, Right			
6 Scapula, Left			
7 Glenoid Cavity, Right			
8 Glenoid Cavity, Left			
9 Clavicle, Right			
B Clavicle, Left			
C Humeral Head, Right			
D Humeral Head, Left			
F Humeral Shaft, Right			
G Humeral Shaft, Left			
H Radius, Right			
J Radius, Left			
K Ulna, Right			
L Ulna, Left			
M Carpal, Right			
N Carpal, Left			
P Metacarpal, Right			
Q Metacarpal, Left			
R Thumb Phalanx, Right			
S Thumb Phalanx, Left			
T Finger Phalanx, Right			
V Finger Phalanx, Left			

0 **Medical and Surgical**
P **Upper Bones**
R **Replacement:** Putting in or on biological or synthetic material that physically takes the place and/or function of all or a portion of a body part

Body Part	Approach	Device	Qualifier
Character 4	**Character 5**	**Character 6**	**Character 7**
0 Sternum	0 Open	7 Autologous Tissue Substitute	Z No Qualifier
1 Ribs, 1 to 2	3 Percutaneous	J Synthetic Substitute	
2 Ribs, 3 or More	4 Percutaneous Endoscopic	K Nonautologous Tissue Substitute	
3 Cervical Vertebra			
4 Thoracic Vertebra			
5 Scapula, Right			
6 Scapula, Left			
7 Glenoid Cavity, Right			
8 Glenoid Cavity, Left			
9 Clavicle, Right			
B Clavicle, Left			
C Humeral Head, Right			
D Humeral Head, Left			
F Humeral Shaft, Right			
G Humeral Shaft, Left			
H Radius, Right			
J Radius, Left			
K Ulna, Right			
L Ulna, Left			
M Carpal, Right			
N Carpal, Left			
P Metacarpal, Right			
Q Metacarpal, Left			
R Thumb Phalanx, Right			
S Thumb Phalanx, Left			
T Finger Phalanx, Right			
V Finger Phalanx, Left			

0 **Medical and Surgical**
P **Upper Bones**
S **Reposition:** Moving to its normal location, or other suitable location, all or a portion of a body part

Body Part	Approach	Device	Qualifier
Character 4	Character 5	Character 6	Character 7
0 Sternum	0 Open 3 Percutaneous 4 Percutaneous Endoscopic	0 Internal Fixation Device, Rigid Plate 4 Internal Fixation Device Z No Device	Z No Qualifier
0 Sternum	X External	Z No Device	Z No Qualifier
1 Ribs, 1 to 2 2 Ribs, 3 or More 3 Cervical Vertebra ᴄᴄ 4 Thoracic Vertebra ᴄᴄ 5 Scapula, Right 6 Scapula, Left 7 Glenoid Cavity, Right 8 Glenoid Cavity, Left 9 Clavicle, Right B Clavicle, Left	0 Open 3 Percutaneous 4 Percutaneous Endoscopic	4 Internal Fixation Device Z No Device	Z No Qualifier
1 Ribs, 1 to 2 2 Ribs, 3 or More 3 Cervical Vertebra 4 Thoracic Vertebra 5 Scapula, Right 6 Scapula, Left 7 Glenoid Cavity, Right 8 Glenoid Cavity, Left 9 Clavicle, Right B Clavicle, Left	X External	Z No Device	Z No Qualifier
C Humeral Head, Right D Humeral Head, Left F Humeral Shaft, Right G Humeral Shaft, Left H Radius, Right J Radius, Left K Ulna, Right L Ulna, Left	0 Open 3 Percutaneous 4 Percutaneous Endoscopic	4 Internal Fixation Device 5 External Fixation Device 6 Internal Fixation Device, Intramedullary B External Fixation Device, Monoplanar C External Fixation Device, Ring D External Fixation Device, Hybrid Z No Device	Z No Qualifier
C Humeral Head, Right D Humeral Head, Left F Humeral Shaft, Right G Humeral Shaft, Left H Radius, Right J Radius, Left K Ulna, Right L Ulna, Left	X External	Z No Device	Z No Qualifier
M Carpal, Right N Carpal, Left P Metacarpal, Right Q Metacarpal, Left R Thumb Phalanx, Right S Thumb Phalanx, Left T Finger Phalanx, Right V Finger Phalanx, Left	0 Open 3 Percutaneous 4 Percutaneous Endoscopic	4 Internal Fixation Device 5 External Fixation Device Z No Device	Z No Qualifier
M Carpal, Right N Carpal, Left P Metacarpal, Right Q Metacarpal, Left R Thumb Phalanx, Right S Thumb Phalanx, Left T Finger Phalanx, Right V Finger Phalanx, Left	X External	Z No Device	Z No Qualifier

ᴄᴄ 0PS33ZZ   0PS43ZZ

ᴸᶜ Limited Coverage   ᴺᶜ Noncovered   ᴴᴬᶜ HAC-associated Procedure   ᴄᴄ Combination Cluster - See Appendix G for code lists
ᴰᴿᴳ Non-OR-Affecting MS-DRG Assignment   New/Revised Text in Orange   ♂ Male   ♀ Female

452

UPPER BONES 0P2-0PW

2018 ICD-10-PCS

0 **Medical and Surgical**

P **Upper Bones**

T **Resection:** Cutting out or off, without replacement, all of a body part

Body Part	Approach	Device	Qualifier
Character 4	Character 5	Character 6	Character 7
0 Sternum	0 Open	Z No Device	Z No Qualifier
1 Ribs, 1 to 2			
2 Ribs, 3 or More			
5 Scapula, Right			
6 Scapula, Left			
7 Glenoid Cavity, Right			
8 Glenoid Cavity, Left			
9 Clavicle, Right			
B Clavicle, Left			
C Humeral Head, Right			
D Humeral Head, Left			
F Humeral Shaft, Right			
G Humeral Shaft, Left			
H Radius, Right			
J Radius, Left			
K Ulna, Right			
L Ulna, Left			
M Carpal, Right			
N Carpal, Left			
P Metacarpal, Right			
Q Metacarpal, Left			
R Thumb Phalanx, Right			
S Thumb Phalanx, Left			
T Finger Phalanx, Right			
V Finger Phalanx, Left			

0 **Medical and Surgical**

P **Upper Bones**

U **Supplement:** Putting in or on biological or synthetic material that physically reinforces and/or augments the function of a portion of a body part

Body Part	Approach	Device	Qualifier
Character 4	Character 5	Character 6	Character 7
0 Sternum	0 Open	7 Autologous Tissue Substitute	Z No Qualifier
1 Ribs, 1 to 2	3 Percutaneous	J Synthetic Substitute	
2 Ribs, 3 or More	4 Percutaneous Endoscopic	K Nonautologous Tissue Substitute	
3 Cervical Vertebra CC			
4 Thoracic Vertebra CC			
5 Scapula, Right			
6 Scapula, Left			
7 Glenoid Cavity, Right			
8 Glenoid Cavity, Left			
9 Clavicle, Right			
B Clavicle, Left			
C Humeral Head, Right			
D Humeral Head, Left			
F Humeral Shaft, Right			
G Humeral Shaft, Left			
H Radius, Right			
J Radius, Left			
K Ulna, Right			
L Ulna, Left			
M Carpal, Right			
N Carpal, Left			
P Metacarpal, Right			
Q Metacarpal, Left			
R Thumb Phalanx, Right			
S Thumb Phalanx, Left			
T Finger Phalanx, Right			
V Finger Phalanx, Left			

CC 0PU33JZ   0PU43JZ

0 **Medical and Surgical**
P **Upper Bones**
W **Revision:** Correcting, to the extent possible, a portion of a malfunctioning device or the position of a displaced device

Body Part	Approach	Device	Qualifier
Character 4	Character 5	Character 6	Character 7
0 Sternum 1 Ribs, 1 to 2 2 Ribs, 3 or More 3 Cervical Vertebra 4 Thoracic Vertebra 5 Scapula, Right 6 Scapula, Left 7 Glenoid Cavity, Right 8 Glenoid Cavity, Left 9 Clavicle, Right B Clavicle, Left	0 Open 3 Percutaneous 4 Percutaneous Endoscopic X External	4 Internal Fixation Device 7 Autologous Tissue Substitute J Synthetic Substitute K Nonautologous Tissue Substitute	Z No Qualifier
C Humeral Head, Right D Humeral Head, Left F Humeral Shaft, Right G Humeral Shaft, Left H Radius, Right J Radius, Left K Ulna, Right L Ulna, Left M Carpal, Right N Carpal, Left P Metacarpal, Right Q Metacarpal, Left R Thumb Phalanx, Right S Thumb Phalanx, Left T Finger Phalanx, Right V Finger Phalanx, Left	0 Open 3 Percutaneous 4 Percutaneous Endoscopic X External	4 Internal Fixation Device 5 External Fixation Device 7 Autologous Tissue Substitute J Synthetic Substitute K Nonautologous Tissue Substitute	Z No Qualifier
Y Upper Bone	0 Open 3 Percutaneous 4 Percutaneous Endoscopic X External	0 Drainage Device M Bone Growth Stimulator	Z No Qualifier

LC Limited Coverage   NC Noncovered   HAC HAC-associated Procedure   CC Combination Cluster - See Appendix G for code lists
DRG Non-OR-Affecting MS-DRG Assignment   New/Revised Text in Orange   ♂ Male   ♀ Female

454

2018 ICD-10-PCS

UPPER BONES 0P2-0PW

NOTES

NOTES

Lower Bones 0Q2-0QW

0 Medical and Surgical
Q Lower Bones
2 Change: Taking out or off a device from a body part and putting back an identical or similar device in or on the same body part without cutting or puncturing the skin or a mucous membrane

Body Part	Approach	Device	Qualifier
Character 4	Character 5	Character 6	Character 7
Y Lower Bone	**X** External	**0** Drainage Device **Y** Other Device	**Z** No Qualifier

0 Medical and Surgical
Q Lower Bones
5 Destruction: Physical eradication of all or a portion of a body part by the direct use of energy, force, or a destructive agent

Body Part	Approach	Device	Qualifier
Character 4	Character 5	Character 6	Character 7
0 Lumbar Vertebra **1** Sacrum **2** Pelvic Bone, Right **3** Pelvic Bone, Left **4** Acetabulum, Right **5** Acetabulum, Left **6** Upper Femur, Right **7** Upper Femur, Left **8** Femoral Shaft, Right **9** Femoral Shaft, Left **B** Lower Femur, Right **C** Lower Femur, Left **D** Patella, Right **F** Patella, Left **G** Tibia, Right **H** Tibia, Left **J** Fibula, Right **K** Fibula, Left **L** Tarsal, Right **M** Tarsal, Left **N** Metatarsal, Right **P** Metatarsal, Left **Q** Toe Phalanx, Right **R** Toe Phalanx, Left **S** Coccyx	**0** Open **3** Percutaneous **4** Percutaneous Endoscopic	**Z** No Device	**Z** No Qualifier

0 Medical and Surgical
Q Lower Bones
8 Division: Cutting into a body part, without draining fluids and/or gases from the body part, in order to separate or transect a body part

Body Part	Approach	Device	Qualifier
Character 4	Character 5	Character 6	Character 7
0 Lumbar Vertebra 1 Sacrum 2 Pelvic Bone, Right 3 Pelvic Bone, Left 4 Acetabulum, Right 5 Acetabulum, Left 6 Upper Femur, Right 7 Upper Femur, Left 8 Femoral Shaft, Right 9 Femoral Shaft, Left B Lower Femur, Right C Lower Femur, Left D Patella, Right F Patella, Left G Tibia, Right H Tibia, Left J Fibula, Right K Fibula, Left L Tarsal, Right M Tarsal, Left N Metatarsal, Right P Metatarsal, Left Q Toe Phalanx, Right R Toe Phalanx, Left S Coccyx	0 Open 3 Percutaneous 4 Percutaneous Endoscopic	Z No Device	Z No Qualifier

LC Limited Coverage   NC Noncovered   HAC HAC-associated Procedure   CC Combination Cluster - See Appendix G for code lists
DRG Non-OR-Affecting MS-DRG Assignment   New/Revised Text in Orange   ♂ Male   ♀ Female

458

2018 ICD-10-PCS

0 Medical and Surgical
Q Lower Bones
9 Drainage: Taking or letting out fluids and/or gases from a body part

Body Part	Approach	Device	Qualifier
Character 4	Character 5	Character 6	Character 7
0 Lumbar Vertebra **1** Sacrum **2** Pelvic Bone, Right **3** Pelvic Bone, Left **4** Acetabulum, Right **5** Acetabulum, Left **6** Upper Femur, Right **7** Upper Femur, Left **8** Femoral Shaft, Right **9** Femoral Shaft, Left **B** Lower Femur, Right **C** Lower Femur, Left **D** Patella, Right **F** Patella, Left **G** Tibia, Right **H** Tibia, Left **J** Fibula, Right **K** Fibula, Left **L** Tarsal, Right **M** Tarsal, Left **N** Metatarsal, Right **P** Metatarsal, Left **Q** Toe Phalanx, Right **R** Toe Phalanx, Left **S** Coccyx	**0** Open **3** Percutaneous **4** Percutaneous Endoscopic	**0** Drainage Device	**Z** No Qualifier
0 Lumbar Vertebra **1** Sacrum **2** Pelvic Bone, Right **3** Pelvic Bone, Left **4** Acetabulum, Right **5** Acetabulum, Left **6** Upper Femur, Right **7** Upper Femur, Left **8** Femoral Shaft, Right **9** Femoral Shaft, Left **B** Lower Femur, Right **C** Lower Femur, Left **D** Patella, Right **F** Patella, Left **G** Tibia, Right **H** Tibia, Left **J** Fibula, Right **K** Fibula, Left **L** Tarsal, Right **M** Tarsal, Left **N** Metatarsal, Right **P** Metatarsal, Left **Q** Toe Phalanx, Right **R** Toe Phalanx, Left **S** Coccyx	**0** Open **3** Percutaneous **4** Percutaneous Endoscopic	**Z** No Device	**X** Diagnostic **Z** No Qualifier

0 Medical and Surgical
Q Lower Bones
B Excision: Cutting out or off, without replacement, a portion of a body part

Body Part	Approach	Device	Qualifier
Character 4	Character 5	Character 6	Character 7
0 Lumbar Vertebra 1 Sacrum 2 Pelvic Bone, Right 3 Pelvic Bone, Left 4 Acetabulum, Right 5 Acetabulum, Left 6 Upper Femur, Right 7 Upper Femur, Left 8 Femoral Shaft, Right 9 Femoral Shaft, Left B Lower Femur, Right C Lower Femur, Left D Patella, Right F Patella, Left G Tibia, Right H Tibia, Left J Fibula, Right K Fibula, Left L Tarsal, Right M Tarsal, Left N Metatarsal, Right P Metatarsal, Left Q Toe Phalanx, Right R Toe Phalanx, Left S Coccyx	0 Open 3 Percutaneous 4 Percutaneous Endoscopic	Z No Device	X Diagnostic Z No Qualifier

0 Medical and Surgical
Q Lower Bones
C Extirpation: Taking or cutting out solid matter from a body part

Body Part	Approach	Device	Qualifier
Character 4	Character 5	Character 6	Character 7
0 Lumbar Vertebra 1 Sacrum 2 Pelvic Bone, Right 3 Pelvic Bone, Left 4 Acetabulum, Right 5 Acetabulum, Left 6 Upper Femur, Right 7 Upper Femur, Left 8 Femoral Shaft, Right 9 Femoral Shaft, Left B Lower Femur, Right C Lower Femur, Left D Patella, Right F Patella, Left G Tibia, Right H Tibia, Left J Fibula, Right K Fibula, Left L Tarsal, Right M Tarsal, Left N Metatarsal, Right P Metatarsal, Left Q Toe Phalanx, Right R Toe Phalanx, Left S Coccyx	0 Open 3 Percutaneous 4 Percutaneous Endoscopic	Z No Device	Z No Qualifier

0 **Medical and Surgical**
Q **Lower Bones**
D **Extraction:** Pulling or stripping out or off all or a portion of a body part by the use of force

Body Part	Approach	Device	Qualifier
Character 4	Character 5	Character 6	Character 7
0 Lumbar Vertebra 1 Sacrum 2 Pelvic Bone, Right 3 Pelvic Bone, Left 4 Acetabulum, Right 5 Acetabulum, Left 6 Upper Femur, Right 7 Upper Femur, Left 8 Femoral Shaft, Right 9 Femoral Shaft, Left B Lower Femur, Right C Lower Femur, Left D Patella, Right F Patella, Left G Tibia, Right H Tibia, Left J Fibula, Right K Fibula, Left L Tarsal, Right M Tarsal, Left N Metatarsal, Right P Metatarsal, Left Q Toe Phalanx, Right R Toe Phalanx, Left S Coccyx	0 Open	Z No Device	Z No Qualifier

0 **Medical and Surgical**
Q **Lower Bones**
H **Insertion:** Putting in a nonbiological appliance that monitors, assists, performs, or prevents a physiological function but does not physically take the place of a body part

Body Part	Approach	Device	Qualifier
Character 4	Character 5	Character 6	Character 7
0 Lumbar Vertebra 1 Sacrum 2 Pelvic Bone, Right 3 Pelvic Bone, Left 4 Acetabulum, Right 5 Acetabulum, Left D Patella, Right F Patella, Left L Tarsal, Right M Tarsal, Left N Metatarsal, Right P Metatarsal, Left Q Toe Phalanx, Right R Toe Phalanx, Left S Coccyx	0 Open 3 Percutaneous 4 Percutaneous Endoscopic	4 Internal Fixation Device 5 External Fixation Device	Z No Qualifier
6 Upper Femur, Right 7 Upper Femur, Left 8 Femoral Shaft, Right 9 Femoral Shaft, Left B Lower Femur, Right C Lower Femur, Left G Tibia, Right H Tibia, Left J Fibula, Right K Fibula, Left	0 Open 3 Percutaneous 4 Percutaneous Endoscopic	4 Internal Fixation Device 5 External Fixation Device 6 Internal Fixation Device, Intramedullary 8 External Fixation Device, Limb Lengthening B External Fixation Device, Monoplanar C External Fixation Device, Ring D External Fixation Device, Hybrid	Z No Qualifier

0QH continued on next page

0 Medical and Surgical
Q Lower Bones
H Insertion: Putting in a nonbiological appliance that monitors, assists, performs, or prevents a physiological function but does not physically take the place of a body part

0QH continued from previous page

Body Part	Approach	Device	Qualifier
Character 4	Character 5	Character 6	Character 7
Y Lower Bone	0 Open 3 Percutaneous 4 Percutaneous Endoscopic	M Bone Growth Stimulator	Z No Qualifier

0 Medical and Surgical
Q Lower Bones
J Inspection: Visually and/or manually exploring a body part

Body Part	Approach	Device	Qualifier
Character 4	Character 5	Character 6	Character 7
Y Lower Bone	0 Open 3 Percutaneous 4 Percutaneous Endoscopic X External	Z No Device	Z No Qualifier

0 Medical and Surgical
Q Lower Bones
N Release: Freeing a body part from an abnormal physical constraint by cutting or by the use of force

Body Part	Approach	Device	Qualifier
Character 4	Character 5	Character 6	Character 7
0 Lumbar Vertebra 1 Sacrum 2 Pelvic Bone, Right 3 Pelvic Bone, Left 4 Acetabulum, Right 5 Acetabulum, Left 6 Upper Femur, Right 7 Upper Femur, Left 8 Femoral Shaft, Right 9 Femoral Shaft, Left B Lower Femur, Right C Lower Femur, Left D Patella, Right F Patella, Left G Tibia, Right H Tibia, Left J Fibula, Right K Fibula, Left L Tarsal, Right M Tarsal, Left N Metatarsal, Right P Metatarsal, Left Q Toe Phalanx, Right R Toe Phalanx, Left S Coccyx	0 Open 3 Percutaneous 4 Percutaneous Endoscopic	Z No Device	Z No Qualifier

LC Limited Coverage   **NC** Noncovered   **HAC** HAC-associated Procedure   **CC** Combination Cluster - See Appendix G for code lists

DNR Non-OR-Affecting MS-DRG Assignment   New/Revised Text in Orange   ♂ Male   ♀ Female

462

2018 ICD-10-PCS

0   **Medical and Surgical**
Q   **Lower Bones**
P   **Removal:** Taking out or off a device from a body part

Body Part	Approach	Device	Qualifier
Character 4	**Character 5**	**Character 6**	**Character 7**
0 Lumbar Vertebra 1 Sacrum 4 Acetabulum, Right 5 Acetabulum, Left S Coccyx	0 Open 3 Percutaneous 4 Percutaneous Endoscopic	4 Internal Fixation Device 7 Autologous Tissue Substitute J Synthetic Substitute K Nonautologous Tissue Substitute	Z No Qualifier
0 Lumbar Vertebra 1 Sacrum 4 Acetabulum, Right 5 Acetabulum, Left S Coccyx	X External	4 Internal Fixation Device	Z No Qualifier
2 Pelvic Bone, Right 3 Pelvic Bone, Left 6 Upper Femur, Right 7 Upper Femur, Left 8 Femoral Shaft, Right 9 Femoral Shaft, Left B Lower Femur, Right C Lower Femur, Left D Patella, Right F Patella, Left G Tibia, Right H Tibia, Left J Fibula, Right K Fibula, Left L Tarsal, Right M Tarsal, Left N Metatarsal, Right P Metatarsal, Left Q Toe Phalanx, Right R Toe Phalanx, Left	0 Open 3 Percutaneous 4 Percutaneous Endoscopic	4 Internal Fixation Device 5 External Fixation Device 7 Autologous Tissue Substitute J Synthetic Substitute K Nonautologous Tissue Substitute	Z No Qualifier
2 Pelvic Bone, Right 3 Pelvic Bone, Left 6 Upper Femur, Right 7 Upper Femur, Left 8 Femoral Shaft, Right 9 Femoral Shaft, Left B Lower Femur, Right C Lower Femur, Left D Patella, Right F Patella, Left G Tibia, Right H Tibia, Left J Fibula, Right K Fibula, Left L Tarsal, Right M Tarsal, Left N Metatarsal, Right P Metatarsal, Left Q Toe Phalanx, Right R Toe Phalanx, Left	X External	4 Internal Fixation Device 5 External Fixation Device	Z No Qualifier
Y Lower Bone	0 Open 3 Percutaneous 4 Percutaneous Endoscopic X External	0 Drainage Device M Bone Growth Stimulator	Z No Qualifier

LC Limited Coverage   NC Noncovered   HAC HAC-associated Procedure   CC Combination Cluster - See Appendix G for code lists
DRG Non-OR-Affecting MS-DRG Assignment   New/Revised Text in Orange   ♂ Male   ♀ Female

2018 ICD-10-PCS

463

LOWER BONES 0Q2-0QW

0 **Medical and Surgical**

Q **Lower Bones**

Q **Repair:** Restoring, to the extent possible, a body part to its normal anatomic structure and function

Body Part	Approach	Device	Qualifier
Character 4	Character 5	Character 6	Character 7
0 Lumbar Vertebra 1 Sacrum 2 Pelvic Bone, Right 3 Pelvic Bone, Left 4 Acetabulum, Right 5 Acetabulum, Left 6 Upper Femur, Right 7 Upper Femur, Left 8 Femoral Shaft, Right 9 Femoral Shaft, Left B Lower Femur, Right C Lower Femur, Left D Patella, Right F Patella, Left G Tibia, Right H Tibia, Left J Fibula, Right K Fibula, Left L Tarsal, Right M Tarsal, Left N Metatarsal, Right P Metatarsal, Left Q Toe Phalanx, Right R Toe Phalanx, Left S Coccyx	0 Open 3 Percutaneous 4 Percutaneous Endoscopic X External	Z No Device	Z No Qualifier

0 **Medical and Surgical**

Q **Lower Bones**

R **Replacement:** Putting in or on biological or synthetic material that physically takes the place and/or function of all or a portion of a body part

Body Part	Approach	Device	Qualifier
Character 4	Character 5	Character 6	Character 7
0 Lumbar Vertebra 1 Sacrum 2 Pelvic Bone, Right 3 Pelvic Bone, Left 4 Acetabulum, Right 5 Acetabulum, Left 6 Upper Femur, Right 7 Upper Femur, Left 8 Femoral Shaft, Right 9 Femoral Shaft, Left B Lower Femur, Right C Lower Femur, Left D Patella, Right F Patella, Left G Tibia, Right H Tibia, Left J Fibula, Right K Fibula, Left L Tarsal, Right M Tarsal, Left N Metatarsal, Right P Metatarsal, Left Q Toe Phalanx, Right R Toe Phalanx, Left S Coccyx	0 Open 3 Percutaneous 4 Percutaneous Endoscopic	7 Autologous Tissue Substitute J Synthetic Substitute K Nonautologous Tissue Substitute	Z No Qualifier

LC Limited Coverage   NC Noncovered   HAC HAC-associated Procedure   CC Combination Cluster - See Appendix G for code lists
DRG Non-OR-Affecting MS-DRG Assignment   New/Revised Text in Orange   ♂ Male   ♀ Female

464

2018 ICD-10-PCS

0 Medical and Surgical
Q Lower Bones
S Reposition: Moving to its normal location, or other suitable location, all or a portion of a body part

Body Part	Approach	Device	Qualifier
Character 4	Character 5	Character 6	Character 7
0 Lumbar Vertebra ᴸᶜ **1** Sacrum ᴸᶜ **4** Acetabulum, Right **5** Acetabulum, Left **S** Coccyx ᴸᶜ	**0** Open **3** Percutaneous **4** Percutaneous Endoscopic	**4** Internal Fixation Device **Z** No Device	**Z** No Qualifier
0 Lumbar Vertebra **1** Sacrum **4** Acetabulum, Right **5** Acetabulum, Left **S** Coccyx	**X** External	**Z** No Device	**Z** No Qualifier
2 Pelvic Bone, Right **3** Pelvic Bone, Left **D** Patella, Right **F** Patella, Left **L** Tarsal, Right **M** Tarsal, Left **Q** Toe Phalanx, Right **R** Toe Phalanx, Left	**0** Open **3** Percutaneous **4** Percutaneous Endoscopic	**4** Internal Fixation Device **5** External Fixation Device **Z** No Device	**Z** No Qualifier
2 Pelvic Bone, Right **3** Pelvic Bone, Left **D** Patella, Right **F** Patella, Left **L** Tarsal, Right **M** Tarsal, Left **Q** Toe Phalanx, Right **R** Toe Phalanx, Left	**X** External	**Z** No Device	**Z** No Qualifier
6 Upper Femur, Right **7** Upper Femur, Left **8** Femoral Shaft, Right **9** Femoral Shaft, Left **B** Lower Femur, Right **C** Lower Femur, Left **G** Tibia, Right **H** Tibia, Left **J** Fibula, Right **K** Fibula, Left	**0** Open **3** Percutaneous **4** Percutaneous Endoscopic	**4** Internal Fixation Device **5** External Fixation Device **6** Internal Fixation Device, Intramedullary **B** External Fixation Device, Monoplanar **C** External Fixation Device, Ring **D** External Fixation Device, Hybrid **Z** No Device	**Z** No Qualifier
6 Upper Femur, Right **7** Upper Femur, Left **8** Femoral Shaft, Right **9** Femoral Shaft, Left **B** Lower Femur, Right **C** Lower Femur, Left **G** Tibia, Right **H** Tibia, Left **J** Fibula, Right **K** Fibula, Left	**X** External	**Z** No Device	**Z** No Qualifier
N Metatarsal, Right **P** Metatarsal, Left	**0** Open **3** Percutaneous **4** Percutaneous Endoscopic	**4** Internal Fixation Device **5** External Fixation Device **Z** No Device	**2** Sesamoid Bone(s) 1st Toe **Z** No Qualifier
N Metatarsal, Right **P** Metatarsal, Left	**X** External	**Z** No Device	**2** Sesamoid Bone(s) 1st Toe **Z** No Qualifier

ᴸᶜ 0QS03ZZ   0QS13ZZ   0QSS3ZZ

ᴸᶜ Limited Coverage   ᴺᶜ Noncovered   ᴴᴬᶜ HAC-associated Procedure   ᶜᶜ Combination Cluster - See Appendix G for code lists
ᴰᴿᴳ Non-OR-Affecting MS-DRG Assignment   New/Revised Text in **Orange**   ♂ Male   ♀ Female

2018 ICD-10-PCS   465

LOWER BONES 0Q2-0QW

0   Medical and Surgical
Q   Lower Bones
T   Resection: Cutting out or off, without replacement, all of a body part

Body Part	Approach	Device	Qualifier
Character 4	Character 5	Character 6	Character 7
2 Pelvic Bone, Right	**0** Open	**Z** No Device	**Z** No Qualifier
3 Pelvic Bone, Left			
4 Acetabulum, Right			
5 Acetabulum, Left			
6 Upper Femur, Right			
7 Upper Femur, Left			
8 Femoral Shaft, Right			
9 Femoral Shaft, Left			
B Lower Femur, Right			
C Lower Femur, Left			
D Patella, Right			
F Patella, Left			
G Tibia, Right			
H Tibia, Left			
J Fibula, Right			
K Fibula, Left			
L Tarsal, Right			
M Tarsal, Left			
N Metatarsal, Right			
P Metatarsal, Left			
Q Toe Phalanx, Right			
R Toe Phalanx, Left			
S Coccyx			

0   Medical and Surgical
Q   Lower Bones
U   Supplement: Putting in or on biological or synthetic material that physically reinforces and/or augments the function of a portion of a body part

Body Part	Approach	Device	Qualifier
Character 4	Character 5	Character 6	Character 7
0 Lumbar Vertebra ᴸᶜ	**0** Open	**7** Autologous Tissue Substitute	**Z** No Qualifier
1 Sacrum ᴸᶜ	**3** Percutaneous	**J** Synthetic Substitute	
2 Pelvic Bone, Right	**4** Percutaneous Endoscopic	**K** Nonautologous Tissue Substitute	
3 Pelvic Bone, Left			
4 Acetabulum, Right			
5 Acetabulum, Left			
6 Upper Femur, Right			
7 Upper Femur, Left			
8 Femoral Shaft, Right			
9 Femoral Shaft, Left			
B Lower Femur, Right			
C Lower Femur, Left			
D Patella, Right			
F Patella, Left			
G Tibia, Right			
H Tibia, Left			
J Fibula, Right			
K Fibula, Left			
L Tarsal, Right			
M Tarsal, Left			
N Metatarsal, Right			
P Metatarsal, Left			
Q Toe Phalanx, Right			
R Toe Phalanx, Left			
S Coccyx ᴸᶜ			

ᴸᶜ 0QU03JZ   0QU13JZ   0QUS3JZ

ᴸᶜ Limited Coverage   ᴺᶜ Noncovered   ᴴᴬᶜ HAC-associated Procedure   ᴄᴄ Combination Cluster - See Appendix G for code lists
ᴰᴿᴳ Non-OR-Affecting MS-DRG Assignment   New/Revised Text in **Orange**   ♂ Male   ♀ Female

466   **2018 ICD-10-PCS**

0   Medical and Surgical
Q   Lower Bones
W   Revision: Correcting, to the extent possible, a portion of a malfunctioning device or the position of a displaced device

Body Part	Approach	Device	Qualifier
Character 4	**Character 5**	**Character 6**	**Character 7**
0 Lumbar Vertebra 1 Sacrum 4 Acetabulum, Right 5 Acetabulum, Left S Coccyx	0 Open 3 Percutaneous 4 Percutaneous Endoscopic X External	4 Internal Fixation Device 7 Autologous Tissue Substitute J Synthetic Substitute K Nonautologous Tissue Substitute	Z No Qualifier
2 Pelvic Bone, Right 3 Pelvic Bone, Left 6 Upper Femur, Right 7 Upper Femur, Left 8 Femoral Shaft, Right 9 Femoral Shaft, Left B Lower Femur, Right C Lower Femur, Left D Patella, Right F Patella, Left G Tibia, Right H Tibia, Left J Fibula, Right K Fibula, Left L Tarsal, Right M Tarsal, Left N Metatarsal, Right P Metatarsal, Left Q Toe Phalanx, Right R Toe Phalanx, Left	0 Open 3 Percutaneous 4 Percutaneous Endoscopic X External	4 Internal Fixation Device 5 External Fixation Device 7 Autologous Tissue Substitute J Synthetic Substitute K Nonautologous Tissue Substitute	Z No Qualifier
Y Lower Bone	0 Open 3 Percutaneous 4 Percutaneous Endoscopic X External	0 Drainage Device M Bone Growth Stimulator	Z No Qualifier

LC Limited Coverage   NC Noncovered   HAC HAC-associated Procedure   CC Combination Cluster - See Appendix G for code lists
DRG Non-OR-Affecting MS-DRG Assignment   New/Revised Text in Orange   ♂ Male   ♀ Female

2018 ICD-10-PCS

467

NOTES

Upper Joints 0R2-0RW

0 Medical and Surgical
R Upper Joints
2 Change: Taking out or off a device from a body part and putting back an identical or similar device in or on the same body part without cutting or puncturing the skin or a mucous membrane

Body Part	Approach	Device	Qualifier
Character 4	Character 5	Character 6	Character 7
Y Upper Joint	X External	0 Drainage Device Y Other Device	Z No Qualifier

0 Medical and Surgical
R Upper Joints
5 Destruction: Physical eradication of all or a portion of a body part by the direct use of energy, force, or a destructive agent

Body Part	Approach	Device	Qualifier
Character 4	Character 5	Character 6	Character 7
0 Occipital-cervical Joint 1 Cervical Vertebral Joint 3 Cervical Vertebral Disc 4 Cervicothoracic Vertebral Joint 5 Cervicothoracic Vertebral Disc 6 Thoracic Vertebral Joint 9 Thoracic Vertebral Disc A Thoracolumbar Vertebral Joint B Thoracolumbar Vertebral Disc C Temporomandibular Joint, Right D Temporomandibular Joint, Left E Sternoclavicular Joint, Right F Sternoclavicular Joint, Left G Acromioclavicular Joint, Right H Acromioclavicular Joint, Left J Shoulder Joint, Right K Shoulder Joint, Left L Elbow Joint, Right M Elbow Joint, Left N Wrist Joint, Right P Wrist Joint, Left Q Carpal Joint, Right R Carpal Joint, Left S Carpometacarpal Joint, Right T Carpometacarpal Joint, Left U Metacarpophalangeal Joint, Right V Metacarpophalangeal Joint, Left W Finger Phalangeal Joint, Right X Finger Phalangeal Joint, Left	0 Open 3 Percutaneous 4 Percutaneous Endoscopic	Z No Device	Z No Qualifier

0 **Medical and Surgical**
R **Upper Joints**
9 **Drainage:** Taking or letting out fluids and/or gases from a body part

Body Part	Approach	Device	Qualifier
Character 4	Character 5	Character 6	Character 7
0 Occipital-cervical Joint 1 Cervical Vertebral Joint 3 Cervical Vertebral Disc 4 Cervicothoracic Vertebral Joint 5 Cervicothoracic Vertebral Disc 6 Thoracic Vertebral Joint 9 Thoracic Vertebral Disc A Thoracolumbar Vertebral Joint B Thoracolumbar Vertebral Disc C Temporomandibular Joint, Right D Temporomandibular Joint, Left E Sternoclavicular Joint, Right F Sternoclavicular Joint, Left G Acromioclavicular Joint, Right H Acromioclavicular Joint, Left J Shoulder Joint, Right K Shoulder Joint, Left L Elbow Joint, Right M Elbow Joint, Left N Wrist Joint, Right P Wrist Joint, Left Q Carpal Joint, Right R Carpal Joint, Left S Carpometacarpal Joint, Right T Carpometacarpal Joint, Left U Metacarpophalangeal Joint, Right V Metacarpophalangeal Joint, Left W Finger Phalangeal Joint, Right X Finger Phalangeal Joint, Left	0 Open 3 Percutaneous 4 Percutaneous Endoscopic	0 Drainage Device	Z No Qualifier
0 Occipital-cervical Joint 1 Cervical Vertebral Joint 3 Cervical Vertebral Disc 4 Cervicothoracic Vertebral Joint 5 Cervicothoracic Vertebral Disc 6 Thoracic Vertebral Joint 9 Thoracic Vertebral Disc A Thoracolumbar Vertebral Joint B Thoracolumbar Vertebral Disc C Temporomandibular Joint, Right D Temporomandibular Joint, Left E Sternoclavicular Joint, Right F Sternoclavicular Joint, Left G Acromioclavicular Joint, Right H Acromioclavicular Joint, Left J Shoulder Joint, Right K Shoulder Joint, Left L Elbow Joint, Right M Elbow Joint, Left N Wrist Joint, Right P Wrist Joint, Left Q Carpal Joint, Right R Carpal Joint, Left S Carpometacarpal Joint, Right T Carpometacarpal Joint, Left U Metacarpophalangeal Joint, Right V Metacarpophalangeal Joint, Left W Finger Phalangeal Joint, Right X Finger Phalangeal Joint, Left	0 Open 3 Percutaneous 4 Percutaneous Endoscopic	Z No Device	X Diagnostic Z No Qualifier

LC Limited Coverage   **NC** Noncovered   **HAC** HAC-associated Procedure   **CC** Combination Cluster - See Appendix G for code lists
⊛ Non-OR-Affecting MS-DRG Assignment   New/Revised Text in **Orange**   ♂ Male   ♀ Female

470

2018 ICD-10-PCS

0 **Medical and Surgical**
R **Upper Joints**
B **Excision:** Cutting out or off, without replacement, a portion of a body part

Body Part	Approach	Device	Qualifier
Character 4	Character 5	Character 6	Character 7
0 Occipital-cervical Joint	0 Open	Z No Device	X Diagnostic
1 Cervical Vertebral Joint	3 Percutaneous		Z No Qualifier
3 Cervical Vertebral Disc	4 Percutaneous Endoscopic		
4 Cervicothoracic Vertebral Joint			
5 Cervicothoracic Vertebral Disc			
6 Thoracic Vertebral Joint			
9 Thoracic Vertebral Disc			
A Thoracolumbar Vertebral Joint			
B Thoracolumbar Vertebral Disc			
C Temporomandibular Joint, Right			
D Temporomandibular Joint, Left			
E Sternoclavicular Joint, Right			
F Sternoclavicular Joint, Left			
G Acromioclavicular Joint, Right			
H Acromioclavicular Joint, Left			
J Shoulder Joint, Right			
K Shoulder Joint, Left			
L Elbow Joint, Right			
M Elbow Joint, Left			
N Wrist Joint, Right			
P Wrist Joint, Left			
Q Carpal Joint, Right			
R Carpal Joint, Left			
S Carpometacarpal Joint, Right			
T Carpometacarpal Joint, Left			
U Metacarpophalangeal Joint, Right			
V Metacarpophalangeal Joint, Left			
W Finger Phalangeal Joint, Right			
X Finger Phalangeal Joint, Left			

LC Limited Coverage   NC Noncovered   HAC HAC-associated Procedure   CC Combination Cluster - See Appendix G for code lists
DRG Non-OR-Affecting MS-DRG Assignment   New/Revised Text in **Orange**   ♂ Male   ♀ Female

2018 ICD-10-PCS

471

0 Medical and Surgical
R Upper Joints
C Extirpation: Taking or cutting out solid matter from a body part

Body Part	Approach	Device	Qualifier
Character 4	Character 5	Character 6	Character 7
0 Occipital-cervical Joint	0 Open	Z No Device	Z No Qualifier
1 Cervical Vertebral Joint	3 Percutaneous		
3 Cervical Vertebral Disc	4 Percutaneous Endoscopic		
4 Cervicothoracic Vertebral Joint			
5 Cervicothoracic Vertebral Disc			
6 Thoracic Vertebral Joint			
9 Thoracic Vertebral Disc			
A Thoracolumbar Vertebral Joint			
B Thoracolumbar Vertebral Disc			
C Temporomandibular Joint, Right			
D Temporomandibular Joint, Left			
E Sternoclavicular Joint, Right			
F Sternoclavicular Joint, Left			
G Acromioclavicular Joint, Right			
H Acromioclavicular Joint, Left			
J Shoulder Joint, Right			
K Shoulder Joint, Left			
L Elbow Joint, Right			
M Elbow Joint, Left			
N Wrist Joint, Right			
P Wrist Joint, Left			
Q Carpal Joint, Right			
R Carpal Joint, Left			
S Carpometacarpal Joint, Right			
T Carpometacarpal Joint, Left			
U Metacarpophalangeal Joint, Right			
V Metacarpophalangeal Joint, Left			
W Finger Phalangeal Joint, Right			
X Finger Phalangeal Joint, Left			

0 Medical and Surgical
R Upper Joints
G Fusion: Joining together portions of an articular body part rendering the articular body part immobile

Body Part	Approach	Device	Qualifier
Character 4	Character 5	Character 6	Character 7
0 Occipital-cervical Joint HAC	0 Open	7 Autologous Tissue Substitute	0 Anterior Approach, Anterior Column
1 Cervical Vertebral Joint HAC	3 Percutaneous	J Synthetic Substitute	1 Posterior Approach, Posterior Column
2 Cervical Vertebral Joints, 2 or more HAC	4 Percutaneous Endoscopic	K Nonautologous Tissue Substitute	J Posterior Approach, Anterior Column
4 Cervicothoracic Vertebral Joint HAC		Z No Device	
6 Thoracic Vertebral Joint HAC			
7 Thoracic Vertebral Joints, 2 to 7 CC HAC			
8 Thoracic Vertebral Joints, 8 or more HAC			
A Thoracolumbar Vertebral Joint HAC			
0 Occipital-cervical Joint HAC	0 Open	A Interbody Fusion Device	0 Anterior Approach, Anterior Column
1 Cervical Vertebral Joint HAC	3 Percutaneous		J Posterior Approach, Anterior Column
2 Cervical Vertebral Joints, 2 or more HAC	4 Percutaneous Endoscopic		
4 Cervicothoracic Vertebral Joint HAC			
6 Thoracic Vertebral Joint HAC			
7 Thoracic Vertebral Joints, 2 to 7 CC HAC			
8 Thoracic Vertebral Joints, 8 or more HAC			
A Thoracolumbar Vertebral Joint HAC			

0RG continued on next page

0 **Medical and Surgical**
R **Upper Joints**
G **Fusion:** Joining together portions of an articular body part rendering the articular body part immobile

0RG continued from previous page

Body Part	Approach	Device	Qualifier
Character 4	Character 5	Character 6	Character 7
C Temporomandibular Joint, Right D Temporomandibular Joint, Left E Sternoclavicular Joint, Right ᴴᴬᶜ F Sternoclavicular Joint, Left ᴴᴬᶜ G Acromioclavicular Joint, Right ᴴᴬᶜ H Acromioclavicular Joint, Left ᴴᴬᶜ J Shoulder Joint, Right ᴴᴬᶜ K Shoulder Joint, Left ᴴᴬᶜ	0 Open 3 Percutaneous 4 Percutaneous Endoscopic	4 Internal Fixation Device 7 Autologous Tissue Substitute J Synthetic Substitute K Nonautologous Tissue Substitute Z No Device	Z No Qualifier
L Elbow Joint, Right ᴴᴬᶜ M Elbow Joint, Left ᴴᴬᶜ N Wrist Joint, Right P Wrist Joint, Left Q Carpal Joint, Right R Carpal Joint, Left S Carpometacarpal Joint, Right T Carpometacarpal Joint, Left U Metacarpophalangeal Joint, Right V Metacarpophalangeal Joint, Left W Finger Phalangeal Joint, Right X Finger Phalangeal Joint, Left	0 Open 3 Percutaneous 4 Percutaneous Endoscopic	4 Internal Fixation Device 5 External Fixation Device 7 Autologous Tissue Substitute J Synthetic Substitute K Nonautologous Tissue Substitute Z No Device	Z No Qualifier

ᶜᶜ 0RG7070 0RG7071 0RG707J 0RG70A0 0RG70AJ 0RG70J0 0RG70J1 0RG70JJ 0RG70K0 0RG70K1 0RG70KJ 0RG70Z0 0RG70Z1
0RG70ZJ 0RG7370 0RG7371 0RG737J 0RG73A0 0RG73AJ 0RG73J0 0RG73J1 0RG73JJ 0RG73K0 0RG73K1 0RG73KJ 0RG73Z0
0RG73Z1 0RG73ZJ 0RG7470 0RG7471 0RG747J 0RG74A0 0RG74AJ 0RG74J0 0RG74J1 0RG74JJ 0RG74K0 0RG74K1 0RG74KJ
0RG74Z0 0RG74Z1 0RG74ZJ
ᴴᴬᶜ 0RG0070 0RG0071 0RG007J 0RG00A0 0RG00AJ 0RG00J0 0RG00J1 0RG00JJ 0RG00K0 0RG00K1 0RG00KJ 0RG00Z0 0RG00Z1
0RG00ZJ 0RG0370 0RG0371 0RG037J 0RG03A0 0RG03AJ 0RG03J0 0RG03J1 0RG03JJ 0RG03K0 0RG03K1 0RG03KJ 0RG03Z0
0RG03Z1 0RG03ZJ 0RG0470 0RG0471 0RG047J 0RG04A0 0RG04AJ 0RG04J0 0RG04J1 0RG04JJ 0RG04K0 0RG04K1 0RG04KJ
0RG04Z0 0RG04Z1 0RG04ZJ 0RG1070 0RG1071 0RG107J 0RG10A0 0RG10AJ 0RG10J0 0RG10J1 0RG10JJ 0RG10K0 0RG10K1
0RG10KJ 0RG10Z0 0RG10Z1 0RG10ZJ 0RG1370 0RG1371 0RG137J 0RG13A0 0RG13AJ 0RG13J0 0RG13J1 0RG13JJ 0RG13K0
0RG13K1 0RG13KJ 0RG13Z0 0RG13Z1 0RG13ZJ 0RG1470 0RG1471 0RG147J 0RG14A0 0RG14AJ 0RG14J0 0RG14J1 0RG14JJ
0RG14K0 0RG14K1 0RG14KJ 0RG14Z0 0RG14Z1 0RG14ZJ 0RG2070 0RG2071 0RG207J 0RG20A0 0RG20AJ 0RG20J0 0RG20J1
0RG20JJ 0RG20K0 0RG20K1 0RG20KJ 0RG20Z0 0RG20Z1 0RG20ZJ 0RG2370 0RG2371 0RG237J 0RG23A0 0RG23AJ 0RG23J0
0RG23J1 0RG23JJ 0RG23K0 0RG23K1 0RG23KJ 0RG23Z0 0RG23Z1 0RG23ZJ 0RG2470 0RG2471 0RG247J 0RG24A0 0RG24AJ
0RG24J0 0RG24J1 0RG24JJ 0RG24K0 0RG24K1 0RG24KJ 0RG24Z0 0RG24Z1 0RG24ZJ 0RG4070 0RG4071 0RG407J 0RG40A0
0RG40AJ 0RG40J0 0RG40J1 0RG40JJ 0RG40K0 0RG40K1 0RG40KJ 0RG40Z0 0RG40Z1 0RG40ZJ 0RG4370 0RG4371 0RG437J
0RG43A0 0RG43AJ 0RG43J0 0RG43J1 0RG43JJ 0RG43K0 0RG43K1 0RG43KJ 0RG43Z0 0RG43Z1 0RG43ZJ 0RG4470 0RG4471
0RG447J 0RG44A0 0RG44AJ 0RG44J0 0RG44J1 0RG44JJ 0RG44K0 0RG44K1 0RG44KJ 0RG44Z0 0RG44Z1 0RG44ZJ 0RG6070
0RG6071 0RG607J 0RG60A0 0RG60AJ 0RG60J0 0RG60J1 0RG60JJ 0RG60K0 0RG60K1 0RG60KJ 0RG60Z0 0RG60Z1 0RG60ZJ
0RG6370 0RG6371 0RG637J 0RG63A0 0RG63AJ 0RG63J0 0RG63J1 0RG63JJ 0RG63K0 0RG63K1 0RG63KJ 0RG63Z0 0RG63Z1
0RG63ZJ 0RG6470 0RG6471 0RG647J 0RG64A0 0RG64AJ 0RG64J0 0RG64J1 0RG64JJ 0RG64K0 0RG64K1 0RG64KJ 0RG64Z0
0RG64Z1 0RG64ZJ 0RG7070 0RG7071 0RG707J 0RG70A0 0RG70AJ 0RG70J0 0RG70J1 0RG70JJ 0RG70K0 0RG70K1 0RG70KJ
0RG70Z0 0RG70Z1 0RG70ZJ 0RG7370 0RG7371 0RG737J 0RG73A0 0RG73AJ 0RG73J0 0RG73J1 0RG73JJ 0RG73K0 0RG73K1
0RG73KJ 0RG73Z0 0RG73Z1 0RG73ZJ 0RG7470 0RG7471 0RG747J 0RG74A0 0RG74AJ 0RG74J0 0RG74J1 0RG74JJ 0RG74K0
0RG74K1 0RG74KJ 0RG74Z0 0RG74Z1 0RG74ZJ 0RG8070 0RG8071 0RG807J 0RG80A0 0RG80AJ 0RG80J0 0RG80J1 0RG80JJ
0RG80K0 0RG80K1 0RG80KJ 0RG80Z0 0RG80Z1 0RG80ZJ 0RG8370 0RG8371 0RG837J 0RG83A0 0RG83AJ 0RG83J0 0RG83J1
0RG83JJ 0RG83K0 0RG83K1 0RG83KJ 0RG83Z0 0RG83Z1 0RG83ZJ 0RG8470 0RG8471 0RG847J 0RG84A0 0RG84AJ 0RG84J0
0RG84J1 0RG84JJ 0RG84K0 0RG84K1 0RG84KJ 0RG84Z0 0RG84Z1 0RG84ZJ 0RGA070 0RGA071 0RGA07J 0RGA0A0 0RGA0AJ
0RGA0J0 0RGA0J1 0RGA0JJ 0RGA0K0 0RGA0K1 0RGA0KJ 0RGA0Z0 0RGA0Z1 0RGA0ZJ 0RGA370 0RGA371 0RGA37J 0RGA3A0
0RGA3AJ 0RGA3J0 0RGA3J1 0RGA3JJ 0RGA3K0 0RGA3K1 0RGA3KJ 0RGA3Z0 0RGA3Z1 0RGA3ZJ 0RGA470 0RGA471 0RGA47J
0RGA4A0 0RGA4AJ 0RGA4J0 0RGA4J1 0RGA4JJ 0RGA4K0 0RGA4K1 0RGA4KJ 0RGA4Z0 0RGA4Z1 0RGA4ZJ 0RGE04Z 0RGE07Z
0RGE0JZ 0RGE0KZ 0RGE0ZZ 0RGE34Z 0RGE37Z 0RGE3JZ 0RGE3KZ 0RGE3ZZ 0RGE44Z 0RGE47Z 0RGE4JZ 0RGE4KZ 0RGE4ZZ
0RGF04Z 0RGF07Z 0RGF0JZ 0RGF0KZ 0RGF0ZZ 0RGF34Z 0RGF37Z 0RGF3JZ 0RGF3KZ 0RGF3ZZ 0RGF44Z 0RGF47Z 0RGF4JZ
0RGF4KZ 0RGF4ZZ 0RGG04Z 0RGG07Z 0RGG0JZ 0RGG0KZ 0RGG0ZZ 0RGG34Z 0RGG37Z 0RGG3JZ 0RGG3KZ 0RGG3ZZ 0RGG44Z
0RGG47Z 0RGG4JZ 0RGG4KZ 0RGG4ZZ 0RGH04Z 0RGH07Z 0RGH0JZ 0RGH0KZ 0RGH0ZZ 0RGH34Z 0RGH37Z 0RGH3JZ 0RGH3KZ
0RGH3ZZ 0RGH44Z 0RGH47Z 0RGH4JZ 0RGH4KZ 0RGH4ZZ 0RGJ04Z 0RGJ07Z 0RGJ0JZ 0RGJ0KZ 0RGJ0ZZ 0RGJ34Z 0RGJ37Z
0RGJ3JZ 0RGJ3KZ 0RGJ3ZZ 0RGJ44Z 0RGJ47Z 0RGJ4JZ 0RGJ4KZ 0RGJ4ZZ 0RGK04Z 0RGK07Z 0RGK0JZ 0RGK0KZ 0RGK0ZZ
0RGK34Z 0RGK37Z 0RGK3JZ 0RGK3KZ 0RGK3ZZ 0RGK44Z 0RGK47Z 0RGK4JZ 0RGK4KZ 0RGK4ZZ 0RGL04Z 0RGL05Z 0RGL07Z
0RGL0JZ 0RGL0KZ 0RGL0ZZ 0RGL34Z 0RGL35Z 0RGL37Z 0RGL3JZ 0RGL3KZ 0RGL3ZZ 0RGL44Z 0RGL45Z 0RGL47Z 0RGL4JZ
0RGL4KZ 0RGL4ZZ 0RGM04Z 0RGM05Z 0RGM07Z 0RGM0JZ 0RGM0KZ 0RGM0ZZ 0RGM34Z 0RGM35Z 0RGM37Z 0RGM3JZ 0RGM3KZ
0RGM3ZZ 0RGM44Z 0RGM45Z 0RGM47Z 0RGM4JZ 0RGM4KZ 0RGM4ZZ

Surgical site infection following certain orthopedic procedures of spine, shoulder or elbow procedures and secondary diagnosis K68.11, T84.60XA, T84.610A, T84.611A, T84.612A, T84.613, T84.614A, T84.615A, T84.619A, T84.63XA, T84.69XA, T84.7XXA, T81.4XXA.

0 Medical and Surgical
R Upper Joints
H Insertion: Putting in a nonbiological appliance that monitors, assists, performs, or prevents a physiological function but does not physically take the place of a body part

Body Part	Approach	Device	Qualifier
Character 4	Character 5	Character 6	Character 7
0 Occipital-cervical Joint 1 Cervical Vertebral Joint 4 Cervicothoracic Vertebral Joint 6 Thoracic Vertebral Joint A Thoracolumbar Vertebral Joint	0 Open 3 Percutaneous 4 Percutaneous Endoscopic	3 Infusion Device 4 Internal Fixation Device 8 Spacer B Spinal Stabilization Device, Interspinous Process C Spinal Stabilization Device, Pedicle-Based D Spinal Stabilization Device, Facet Replacement	Z No Qualifier
3 Cervical Vertebral Disc 5 Cervicothoracic Vertebral Disc 9 Thoracic Vertebral Disc B Thoracolumbar Vertebral Disc	0 Open 3 Percutaneous 4 Percutaneous Endoscopic	3 Infusion Device	Z No Qualifier
C Temporomandibular Joint, Right D Temporomandibular Joint, Left E Sternoclavicular Joint, Right F Sternoclavicular Joint, Left G Acromioclavicular Joint, Right H Acromioclavicular Joint, Left J Shoulder Joint, Right K Shoulder Joint, Left	0 Open 3 Percutaneous 4 Percutaneous Endoscopic	3 Infusion Device 4 Internal Fixation Device 8 Spacer	Z No Qualifier
L Elbow Joint, Right M Elbow Joint, Left N Wrist Joint, Right P Wrist Joint, Left Q Carpal Joint, Right R Carpal Joint, Left S Carpometacarpal Joint, Right T Carpometacarpal Joint, Left U Metacarpophalangeal Joint, Right V Metacarpophalangeal Joint, Left W Finger Phalangeal Joint, Right X Finger Phalangeal Joint, Left	0 Open 3 Percutaneous 4 Percutaneous Endoscopic	3 Infusion Device 4 Internal Fixation Device 5 External Fixation Device 8 Spacer	Z No Qualifier

0RG continued on next page

LC Limited Coverage   NC Noncovered   HAC HAC-associated Procedure   CC Combination Cluster - See Appendix G for code lists
DRG Non-OR-Affecting MS-DRG Assignment   New/Revised Text in **Orange**   ♂ Male   ♀ Female

UPPER JOINTS 0R2-0RW

474

2018 ICD-10-PCS

0   **Medical and Surgical**
R   **Upper Joints**
J   **Inspection:** Visually and/or manually exploring a body part

Body Part	Approach	Device	Qualifier
Character 4	Character 5	Character 6	Character 7
0 Occipital-cervical Joint **1** Cervical Vertebral Joint **3** Cervical Vertebral Disc **4** Cervicothoracic Vertebral Joint **5** Cervicothoracic Vertebral Disc **6** Thoracic Vertebral Joint **9** Thoracic Vertebral Disc **A** Thoracolumbar Vertebral Joint **B** Thoracolumbar Vertebral Disc **C** Temporomandibular Joint, Right **D** Temporomandibular Joint, Left **E** Sternoclavicular Joint, Right **F** Sternoclavicular Joint, Left **G** Acromioclavicular Joint, Right **H** Acromioclavicular Joint, Left **J** Shoulder Joint, Right **K** Shoulder Joint, Left **L** Elbow Joint, Right **M** Elbow Joint, Left **N** Wrist Joint, Right **P** Wrist Joint, Left **Q** Carpal Joint, Right **R** Carpal Joint, Left **S** Carpometacarpal Joint, Right **T** Carpometacarpal Joint, Left **U** Metacarpophalangeal Joint, Right **V** Metacarpophalangeal Joint, Left **W** Finger Phalangeal Joint, Right **X** Finger Phalangeal Joint, Left	**0** Open **3** Percutaneous **4** Percutaneous Endoscopic **X** External	**Z** No Device	**Z** No Qualifier

0 Medical and Surgical
R Upper Joints
N Release: Freeing a body part from an abnormal physical constraint by cutting or by the use of force

Body Part	Approach	Device	Qualifier
Character 4	Character 5	Character 6	Character 7
0 Occipital-cervical Joint 1 Cervical Vertebral Joint 3 Cervical Vertebral Disc 4 Cervicothoracic Vertebral Joint 5 Cervicothoracic Vertebral Disc 6 Thoracic Vertebral Joint 9 Thoracic Vertebral Disc A Thoracolumbar Vertebral Joint B Thoracolumbar Vertebral Disc C Temporomandibular Joint, Right D Temporomandibular Joint, Left E Sternoclavicular Joint, Right F Sternoclavicular Joint, Left G Acromioclavicular Joint, Right H Acromioclavicular Joint, Left J Shoulder Joint, Right K Shoulder Joint, Left L Elbow Joint, Right M Elbow Joint, Left N Wrist Joint, Right P Wrist Joint, Left Q Carpal Joint, Right R Carpal Joint, Left S Carpometacarpal Joint, Right T Carpometacarpal Joint, Left U Metacarpophalangeal Joint, Right V Metacarpophalangeal Joint, Left W Finger Phalangeal Joint, Right X Finger Phalangeal Joint, Left	0 Open 3 Percutaneous 4 Percutaneous Endoscopic X External	Z No Device	Z No Qualifier

0 Medical and Surgical
R Upper Joints
P Removal: Taking out or off a device from a body part

Body Part	Approach	Device	Qualifier
Character 4	Character 5	Character 6	Character 7
0 Occipital-cervical Joint 1 Cervical Vertebral Joint 4 Cervicothoracic Vertebral Joint 6 Thoracic Vertebral Joint A Thoracolumbar Vertebral Joint	0 Open 3 Percutaneous 4 Percutaneous Endoscopic	0 Drainage Device 3 Infusion Device 4 Internal Fixation Device 7 Autologous Tissue Substitute 8 Spacer A Interbody Fusion Device J Synthetic Substitute K Nonautologous Tissue Substitute	Z No Qualifier
0 Occipital-cervical Joint 1 Cervical Vertebral Joint 4 Cervicothoracic Vertebral Joint 6 Thoracic Vertebral Joint A Thoracolumbar Vertebral Joint	X External	0 Drainage Device 3 Infusion Device 4 Internal Fixation Device	Z No Qualifier
3 Cervical Vertebral Disc 5 Cervicothoracic Vertebral Disc 9 Thoracic Vertebral Disc B Thoracolumbar Vertebral Disc	0 Open 3 Percutaneous 4 Percutaneous Endoscopic	0 Drainage Device 3 Infusion Device 7 Autologous Tissue Substitute J Synthetic Substitute K Nonautologous Tissue Substitute	Z No Qualifier

0RP continued on next page

LC Limited Coverage   NC Noncovered   HAC HAC-associated Procedure   CC Combination Cluster - See Appendix G for code lists
DRG Non-OR-Affecting MS-DRG Assignment   New/Revised Text in Orange   ♂ Male   ♀ Female

0 **Medical and Surgical**
R **Upper Joints**
P **Removal:** Taking out or off a device from a body part

0RP continued from previous page

Body Part	Approach	Device	Qualifier
Character 4	Character 5	Character 6	Character 7
3 Cervical Vertebral Disc **5** Cervicothoracic Vertebral Disc **9** Thoracic Vertebral Disc **B** Thoracolumbar Vertebral Disc	**X** External	**0** Drainage Device **3** Infusion Device	**Z** No Qualifier
C Temporomandibular Joint, Right **D** Temporomandibular Joint, Left **E** Sternoclavicular Joint, Right **F** Sternoclavicular Joint, Left **G** Acromioclavicular Joint, Right **H** Acromioclavicular Joint, Left **J** Shoulder Joint, Right **K** Shoulder Joint, Left	**0** Open **3** Percutaneous **4** Percutaneous Endoscopic	**0** Drainage Device **3** Infusion Device **4** Internal Fixation Device **7** Autologous Tissue Substitute **8** Spacer **J** Synthetic Substitute **K** Nonautologous Tissue Substitute	**Z** No Qualifier
C Temporomandibular Joint, Right **D** Temporomandibular Joint, Left **E** Sternoclavicular Joint, Right **F** Sternoclavicular Joint, Left **G** Acromioclavicular Joint, Right **H** Acromioclavicular Joint, Left **J** Shoulder Joint, Right **K** Shoulder Joint, Left	**X** External	**0** Drainage Device **3** Infusion Device **4** Internal Fixation Device	**Z** No Qualifier
L Elbow Joint, Right **M** Elbow Joint, Left **N** Wrist Joint, Right **P** Wrist Joint, Left **Q** Carpal Joint, Right **R** Carpal Joint, Left **S** Carpometacarpal Joint, Right **T** Carpometacarpal Joint, Left **U** Metacarpophalangeal Joint, Right **V** Metacarpophalangeal Joint, Left **W** Finger Phalangeal Joint, Right **X** Finger Phalangeal Joint, Left	**0** Open **3** Percutaneous **4** Percutaneous Endoscopic	**0** Drainage Device **3** Infusion Device **4** Internal Fixation Device **5** External Fixation Device **7** Autologous Tissue Substitute **8** Spacer **J** Synthetic Substitute **K** Nonautologous Tissue Substitute	**Z** No Qualifier
L Elbow Joint, Right **M** Elbow Joint, Left **N** Wrist Joint, Right **P** Wrist Joint, Left **Q** Carpal Joint, Right **R** Carpal Joint, Left **S** Carpometacarpal Joint, Right **T** Carpometacarpal Joint, Left **U** Metacarpophalangeal Joint, Right **V** Metacarpophalangeal Joint, Left **W** Finger Phalangeal Joint, Right **X** Finger Phalangeal Joint, Left	**X** External	**0** Drainage Device **3** Infusion Device **4** Internal Fixation Device **5** External Fixation Device	**Z** No Qualifier

ORQ

0 Medical and Surgical
R Upper Joints
Q Repair: Restoring, to the extent possible, a body part to its normal anatomic structure and function

Body Part	Approach	Device	Qualifier
Character 4	Character 5	Character 6	Character 7
0 Occipital-cervical Joint 1 Cervical Vertebral Joint 3 Cervical Vertebral Disc 4 Cervicothoracic Vertebral Joint 5 Cervicothoracic Vertebral Disc 6 Thoracic Vertebral Joint 9 Thoracic Vertebral Disc A Thoracolumbar Vertebral Joint B Thoracolumbar Vertebral Disc C Temporomandibular Joint, Right D Temporomandibular Joint, Left E Sternoclavicular Joint, Right ᴴᴬᶜ F Sternoclavicular Joint, Left ᴴᴬᶜ G Acromioclavicular Joint, Right ᴴᴬᶜ H Acromioclavicular Joint, Left ᴴᴬᶜ J Shoulder Joint, Right ᴴᴬᶜ K Shoulder Joint, Left ᴴᴬᶜ L Elbow Joint, Right ᴴᴬᶜ M Elbow Joint, Left ᴴᴬᶜ N Wrist Joint, Right P Wrist Joint, Left Q Carpal Joint, Right R Carpal Joint, Left S Carpometacarpal Joint, Right T Carpometacarpal Joint, Left U Metacarpophalangeal Joint, Right V Metacarpophalangeal Joint, Left W Finger Phalangeal Joint, Right X Finger Phalangeal Joint, Left	0 Open 3 Percutaneous 4 Percutaneous Endoscopic X External	Z No Device	Z No Qualifier

ᴴᴬᶜ 0RQE0ZZ   0RQE3ZZ   0RQE4ZZ   0RQEXZZ   0RQF0ZZ   0RQF3ZZ   0RQF4ZZ   0RQFXZZ   0RQG0ZZ   0RQG3ZZ   0RQG4ZZ   0RQGXZZ   0RQH0ZZ
0RQH3ZZ   0RQH4ZZ   0RQHXZZ   0RQJ0ZZ   0RQJ3ZZ   0RQJ4ZZ   0RQJXZZ   0RQK0ZZ   0RQK3ZZ   0RQK4ZZ   0RQKXZZ   0RQL0ZZ   0RQL3ZZ
0RQL4ZZ   0RQLXZZ   0RQM0ZZ   0RQM3ZZ   0RQM4ZZ   0RQMXZZ
Surgical site infection following certain orthopedic procedures of spine, shoulder or elbow procedures and secondary diagnosis K68.11, T84.60XA, T84.610A, T84.611A, T84.612A, T84.613, T84.614A, T84.615A, T84.619A, T84.63XA, T84.69XA, T84.7XXA, T81.4XXA.

ᴸᶜ Limited Coverage   ᴺᶜ Noncovered   ᴴᴬᶜ HAC-associated Procedure   ᶜᶜ Combination Cluster - See Appendix G for code lists
ᴰᴿᴳ Non-OR-Affecting MS-DRG Assignment   New/Revised Text in Orange   ♂ Male   ♀ Female

478

2018 ICD-10-PCS

0 **Medical and Surgical**
R **Upper Joints**
R **Replacement:** Putting in or on biological or synthetic material that physically takes the place and/or function of all or a portion of a body part

Body Part	Approach	Device	Qualifier
Character 4	Character 5	Character 6	Character 7
0 Occipital-cervical Joint **1** Cervical Vertebral Joint **3** Cervical Vertebral Disc **4** Cervicothoracic Vertebral Joint **5** Cervicothoracic Vertebral Disc **6** Thoracic Vertebral Joint **9** Thoracic Vertebral Disc **A** Thoracolumbar Vertebral Joint **B** Thoracolumbar Vertebral Disc **C** Temporomandibular Joint, Right **D** Temporomandibular Joint, Left **E** Sternoclavicular Joint, Right **F** Sternoclavicular Joint, Left **G** Acromioclavicular Joint, Right **H** Acromioclavicular Joint, Left **L** Elbow Joint, Right **M** Elbow Joint, Left **N** Wrist Joint, Right **P** Wrist Joint, Left **Q** Carpal Joint, Right **R** Carpal Joint, Left **S** Carpometacarpal Joint, Right **T** Carpometacarpal Joint, Left **U** Metacarpophalangeal Joint, Right **V** Metacarpophalangeal Joint, Left **W** Finger Phalangeal Joint, Right **X** Finger Phalangeal Joint, Left	**0** Open	**7** Autologous Tissue Substitute **J** Synthetic Substitute **K** Nonautologous Tissue Substitute	**Z** No Qualifier
J Shoulder Joint, Right **K** Shoulder Joint, Left	**0** Open	**0** Synthetic Substitute, Reverse Ball and Socket **7** Autologous Tissue Substitute **K** Nonautologous Tissue Substitute	**Z** No Qualifier
J Shoulder Joint, Right **K** Shoulder Joint, Left	**0** Open	**J** Synthetic Substitute	**6** Humeral Surface **7** Glenoid Surface **Z** No Qualifier

0　**Medical and Surgical**
R　**Upper Joints**
S　**Reposition:** Moving to its normal location, or other suitable location, all or a portion of a body part

Body Part	Approach	Device	Qualifier
Character 4	Character 5	Character 6	Character 7
0 Occipital-cervical Joint **1** Cervical Vertebral Joint **4** Cervicothoracic Vertebral Joint **6** Thoracic Vertebral Joint **A** Thoracolumbar Vertebral Joint **C** Temporomandibular Joint, Right **D** Temporomandibular Joint, Left **E** Sternoclavicular Joint, Right **F** Sternoclavicular Joint, Left **G** Acromioclavicular Joint, Right **H** Acromioclavicular Joint, Left **J** Shoulder Joint, Right **K** Shoulder Joint, Left	**0** Open **3** Percutaneous **4** Percutaneous Endoscopic **X** External	**4** Internal Fixation Device **Z** No Device	**Z** No Qualifier
L Elbow Joint, Right **M** Elbow Joint, Left **N** Wrist Joint, Right **P** Wrist Joint, Left **Q** Carpal Joint, Right **R** Carpal Joint, Left **S** Carpometacarpal Joint, Right **T** Carpometacarpal Joint, Left **U** Metacarpophalangeal Joint, Right **V** Metacarpophalangeal Joint, Left **W** Finger Phalangeal Joint, Right **X** Finger Phalangeal Joint, Left	**0** Open **3** Percutaneous **4** Percutaneous Endoscopic **X** External	**4** Internal Fixation Device **5** External Fixation Device **Z** No Device	**Z** No Qualifier

LC Limited Coverage　**NC** Noncovered　**HAC** HAC-associated Procedure　**CC** Combination Cluster - See Appendix G for code lists
DRG Non-OR-Affecting MS-DRG Assignment　New/Revised Text in **Orange**　♂ Male　♀ Female

480　　　　　　　　　　　　　　　　　　　　　　　　　　　　　　　　　　　**2018 ICD-10-PCS**

0 Medical and Surgical
R Upper Joints
T Resection: Cutting out or off, without replacement, all of a body part

Body Part	Approach	Device	Qualifier
Character 4	Character 5	Character 6	Character 7
3 Cervical Vertebral Disc	0 Open	Z No Device	Z No Qualifier
4 Cervicothoracic Vertebral Joint			
5 Cervicothoracic Vertebral Disc			
9 Thoracic Vertebral Disc			
B Thoracolumbar Vertebral Disc			
C Temporomandibular Joint, Right			
D Temporomandibular Joint, Left			
E Sternoclavicular Joint, Right			
F Sternoclavicular Joint, Left			
G Acromioclavicular Joint, Right			
H Acromioclavicular Joint, Left			
J Shoulder Joint, Right			
K Shoulder Joint, Left			
L Elbow Joint, Right			
M Elbow Joint, Left			
N Wrist Joint, Right			
P Wrist Joint, Left			
Q Carpal Joint, Right			
R Carpal Joint, Left			
S Carpometacarpal Joint, Right			
T Carpometacarpal Joint, Left			
U Metacarpophalangeal Joint, Right			
V Metacarpophalangeal Joint, Left			
W Finger Phalangeal Joint, Right			
X Finger Phalangeal Joint, Left			

0 Medical and Surgical

R Upper Joints

U Supplement: Putting in or on biological or synthetic material that physically reinforces and/or augments the function of a portion of a body part

Body Part	Approach	Device	Qualifier
Character 4	Character 5	Character 6	Character 7
0 Occipital-cervical Joint 1 Cervical Vertebral Joint 3 Cervical Vertebral Disc 4 Cervicothoracic Vertebral Joint 5 Cervicothoracic Vertebral Disc 6 Thoracic Vertebral Joint 9 Thoracic Vertebral Disc A Thoracolumbar Vertebral Joint B Thoracolumbar Vertebral Disc C Temporomandibular Joint, Right D Temporomandibular Joint, Left E Sternoclavicular Joint, Right ᴴᴬᶜ F Sternoclavicular Joint, Left ᴴᴬᶜ G Acromioclavicular Joint, Right ᴴᴬᶜ H Acromioclavicular Joint, Left ᴴᴬᶜ J Shoulder Joint, Right ᴴᴬᶜ K Shoulder Joint, Left ᴴᴬᶜ L Elbow Joint, Right ᴴᴬᶜ M Elbow Joint, Left ᴴᴬᶜ N Wrist Joint, Right P Wrist Joint, Left Q Carpal Joint, Right R Carpal Joint, Left S Carpometacarpal Joint, Right T Carpometacarpal Joint, Left U Metacarpophalangeal Joint, Right V Metacarpophalangeal Joint, Left W Finger Phalangeal Joint, Right X Finger Phalangeal Joint, Left	0 Open 3 Percutaneous 4 Percutaneous Endoscopic	7 Autologous Tissue Substitute J Synthetic Substitute K Nonautologous Tissue Substitute	Z No Qualifier

ᴴᴬᶜ 0RUE07Z   0RUE0JZ   0RUE0KZ   0RUE37Z   0RUE3JZ   0RUE3KZ   0RUE47Z   0RUE4JZ   0RUE4KZ   0RUF07Z   0RUF0JZ   0RUF0KZ   0RUF37Z
0RUF3JZ   0RUF3KZ   0RUF47Z   0RUF4JZ   0RUF4KZ   0RUG07Z   0RUG0JZ   0RUG0KZ   0RUG37Z   0RUG3JZ   0RUG3KZ   0RUG47Z   0RUG4JZ
0RUG4KZ   0RUH07Z   0RUH0JZ   0RUH0KZ   0RUH37Z   0RUH3JZ   0RUH3KZ   0RUH47Z   0RUH4JZ   0RUH4KZ   0RUJ07Z   0RUJ0JZ   0RUJ0KZ
0RUJ37Z   0RUJ3JZ   0RUJ3KZ   0RUJ47Z   0RUJ4JZ   0RUJ4KZ   0RUK07Z   0RUK0JZ   0RUK0KZ   0RUK37Z   0RUK3JZ   0RUK3KZ   0RUK47Z
0RUK4JZ   0RUK4KZ   0RUL07Z   0RUL0JZ   0RUL0KZ   0RUL37Z   0RUL3JZ   0RUL47Z   0RUL4JZ   0RUL4KZ   0RUM07Z   0RUM0JZ
0RUM0KZ   0RUM37Z   0RUM3JZ   0RUM3KZ   0RUM47Z   0RUM4JZ   0RUM4KZ

Surgical site infection following certain orthopedic procedures of spine, shoulder or elbow procedures and secondary diagnosis K68.11, T84.60XA, T84.610A, T84.611A, T84.612A, T84.613, T84.614A, T84.615A, T84.619A, T84.63XA, T84.69XA, T84.7XXA, T81.4XXA.

0 **Medical and Surgical**
R **Upper Joints**
W **Revision:** Correcting, to the extent possible, a portion of a malfunctioning device or the position of a displaced device

Body Part	Approach	Device	Qualifier
Character 4	**Character 5**	**Character 6**	**Character 7**
0 Occipital-cervical Joint **1** Cervical Vertebral Joint **4** Cervicothoracic Vertebral Joint **6** Thoracic Vertebral Joint **A** Thoracolumbar Vertebral Joint	**0** Open **3** Percutaneous **4** Percutaneous Endoscopic **X** External	**0** Drainage Device **3** Infusion Device **4** Internal Fixation Device **7** Autologous Tissue Substitute **8** Spacer **A** Interbody Fusion Device **J** Synthetic Substitute **K** Nonautologous Tissue Substitute	**Z** No Qualifier
3 Cervical Vertebral Disc **5** Cervicothoracic Vertebral Disc **9** Thoracic Vertebral Disc **B** Thoracolumbar Vertebral Disc	**0** Open **3** Percutaneous **4** Percutaneous Endoscopic **X** External	**0** Drainage Device **3** Infusion Device **7** Autologous Tissue Substitute **J** Synthetic Substitute **K** Nonautologous Tissue Substitute	**Z** No Qualifier
C Temporomandibular Joint, Right **D** Temporomandibular Joint, Left **E** Sternoclavicular Joint, Right **F** Sternoclavicular Joint, Left **G** Acromioclavicular Joint, Right **H** Acromioclavicular Joint, Left **J** Shoulder Joint, Right **K** Shoulder Joint, Left	**0** Open **3** Percutaneous **4** Percutaneous Endoscopic **X** External	**0** Drainage Device **3** Infusion Device **4** Internal Fixation Device **7** Autologous Tissue Substitute **8** Spacer **J** Synthetic Substitute **K** Nonautologous Tissue Substitute	**Z** No Qualifier
L Elbow Joint, Right **M** Elbow Joint, Left **N** Wrist Joint, Right **P** Wrist Joint, Left **Q** Carpal Joint, Right **R** Carpal Joint, Left **S** Carpometacarpal Joint, Right **T** Carpometacarpal Joint, Left **U** Metacarpophalangeal Joint, Right **V** Metacarpophalangeal Joint, Left **W** Finger Phalangeal Joint, Right **X** Finger Phalangeal Joint, Left	**0** Open **3** Percutaneous **4** Percutaneous Endoscopic **X** External	**0** Drainage Device **3** Infusion Device **4** Internal Fixation Device **5** External Fixation Device **7** Autologous Tissue Substitute **8** Spacer **J** Synthetic Substitute **K** Nonautologous Tissue Substitute	**Z** No Qualifier

NOTES

Lower Joints 0S2-0SW

0 Medical and Surgical
S Lower Joints
2 Change: Taking out or off a device from a body part and putting back an identical or similar device in or on the same body part without cutting or puncturing the skin or a mucous membrane

Body Part	Approach	Device	Qualifier
Character 4	Character 5	Character 6	Character 7
Y Lower Joint	X External	0 Drainage Device Y Other Device	Z No Qualifier

0 Medical and Surgical
S Lower Joints
5 Destruction: Physical eradication of all or a portion of a body part by the direct use of energy, force, or a destructive agent

Body Part	Approach	Device	Qualifier
Character 4	Character 5	Character 6	Character 7
0 Lumbar Vertebral Joint 2 Lumbar Vertebral Disc 3 Lumbosacral Joint 4 Lumbosacral Disc 5 Sacrococcygeal Joint 6 Coccygeal Joint 7 Sacroiliac Joint, Right 8 Sacroiliac Joint, Left 9 Hip Joint, Right B Hip Joint, Left C Knee Joint, Right D Knee Joint, Left F Ankle Joint, Right G Ankle Joint, Left H Tarsal Joint, Right J Tarsal Joint, Left K Tarsometatarsal Joint, Right L Tarsometatarsal Joint, Left M Metatarsal-Phalangeal Joint, Right N Metatarsal-Phalangeal Joint, Left P Toe Phalangeal Joint, Right Q Toe Phalangeal Joint, Left	0 Open 3 Percutaneous 4 Percutaneous Endoscopic	Z No Device	Z No Qualifier

0 **Medical and Surgical**
S **Lower Joints**
9 **Drainage:** Taking or letting out fluids and/or gases from a body part

Body Part	Approach	Device	Qualifier
Character 4	Character 5	Character 6	Character 7
0 Lumbar Vertebral Joint	**0** Open	**0** Drainage Device	**Z** No Qualifier
2 Lumbar Vertebral Disc	**3** Percutaneous		
3 Lumbosacral Joint	**4** Percutaneous Endoscopic		
4 Lumbosacral Disc			
5 Sacrococcygeal Joint			
6 Coccygeal Joint			
7 Sacroiliac Joint, Right			
8 Sacroiliac Joint, Left			
9 Hip Joint, Right			
B Hip Joint, Left			
C Knee Joint, Right			
D Knee Joint, Left			
F Ankle Joint, Right			
G Ankle Joint, Left			
H Tarsal Joint, Right			
J Tarsal Joint, Left			
K Tarsometatarsal Joint, Right			
L Tarsometatarsal Joint, Left			
M Metatarsal-Phalangeal Joint, Right			
N Metatarsal-Phalangeal Joint, Left			
P Toe Phalangeal Joint, Right			
Q Toe Phalangeal Joint, Left			
0 Lumbar Vertebral Joint	**0** Open	**Z** No Device	**X** Diagnostic
2 Lumbar Vertebral Disc	**3** Percutaneous		**Z** No Qualifier
3 Lumbosacral Joint	**4** Percutaneous Endoscopic		
4 Lumbosacral Disc			
5 Sacrococcygeal Joint			
6 Coccygeal Joint			
7 Sacroiliac Joint, Right			
8 Sacroiliac Joint, Left			
9 Hip Joint, Right			
B Hip Joint, Left			
C Knee Joint, Right			
D Knee Joint, Left			
F Ankle Joint, Right			
G Ankle Joint, Left			
H Tarsal Joint, Right			
J Tarsal Joint, Left			
K Tarsometatarsal Joint, Right			
L Tarsometatarsal Joint, Left			
M Metatarsal-Phalangeal Joint, Right			
N Metatarsal-Phalangeal Joint, Left			
P Toe Phalangeal Joint, Right			
Q Toe Phalangeal Joint, Left			

LC Limited Coverage   **NC** Noncovered   **HAC** HAC-associated Procedure   **CC** Combination Cluster - See Appendix G for code lists
DRG Non-OR-Affecting MS-DRG Assignment   New/Revised Text in **Orange**   ♂ Male   ♀ Female

486

2018 ICD-10-PCS

0 Medical and Surgical
S Lower Joints
B Excision: Cutting out or off, without replacement, a portion of a body part

Body Part	Approach	Device	Qualifier
Character 4	Character 5	Character 6	Character 7
0 Lumbar Vertebral Joint **2** Lumbar Vertebral Disc **3** Lumbosacral Joint **4** Lumbosacral Disc **5** Sacrococcygeal Joint **6** Coccygeal Joint **7** Sacroiliac Joint, Right **8** Sacroiliac Joint, Left **9** Hip Joint, Right **B** Hip Joint, Left **C** Knee Joint, Right **D** Knee Joint, Left **F** Ankle Joint, Right **G** Ankle Joint, Left **H** Tarsal Joint, Right **J** Tarsal Joint, Left **K** Tarsometatarsal Joint, Right **L** Tarsometatarsal Joint, Left **M** Metatarsal-Phalangeal Joint, Right **N** Metatarsal-Phalangeal Joint, Left **P** Toe Phalangeal Joint, Right **Q** Toe Phalangeal Joint, Left	**0** Open **3** Percutaneous **4** Percutaneous Endoscopic	**Z** No Device	**X** Diagnostic **Z** No Qualifier

[LC] Limited Coverage [NC] Noncovered [HAC] HAC-associated Procedure [CC] Combination Cluster - See Appendix G for code lists
[DRG] Non-OR-Affecting MS-DRG Assignment New/Revised Text in **Orange** ♂ Male ♀ Female

2018 ICD-10-PCS

487

LOWER JOINTS 0S2-0SW

0 **Medical and Surgical**
S **Lower Joints**
C **Extirpation:** Taking or cutting out solid matter from a body part

Body Part	Approach	Device	Qualifier
Character 4	Character 5	Character 6	Character 7
0 Lumbar Vertebral Joint 2 Lumbar Vertebral Disc 3 Lumbosacral Joint 4 Lumbosacral Disc 5 Sacrococcygeal Joint 6 Coccygeal Joint 7 Sacroiliac Joint, Right 8 Sacroiliac Joint, Left 9 Hip Joint, Right B Hip Joint, Left C Knee Joint, Right D Knee Joint, Left F Ankle Joint, Right G Ankle Joint, Left H Tarsal Joint, Right J Tarsal Joint, Left K Tarsometatarsal Joint, Right L Tarsometatarsal Joint, Left M Metatarsal-Phalangeal Joint, Right N Metatarsal-Phalangeal Joint, Left P Toe Phalangeal Joint, Right Q Toe Phalangeal Joint, Left	0 Open 3 Percutaneous 4 Percutaneous Endoscopic	Z No Device	Z No Qualifier

0 **Medical and Surgical**
S **Lower Joints**
G **Fusion:** Joining together portions of an articular body part rendering the articular body part immobile

Body Part	Approach	Device	Qualifier
Character 4	Character 5	Character 6	Character 7
0 Lumbar Vertebral Joint HAC 1 Lumbar Vertebral Joints, 2 or more CC HAC 3 Lumbosacral Joint HAC	0 Open 3 Percutaneous 4 Percutaneous Endoscopic	7 Autologous Tissue Substitute J Synthetic Substitute K Nonautologous Tissue Substitute Z No Device	0 Anterior Approach, Anterior Column 1 Posterior Approach, Posterior Column J Posterior Approach, Anterior Column
0 Lumbar Vertebral Joint HAC 1 Lumbar Vertebral Joints, 2 or more CC HAC 3 Lumbosacral Joint HAC	0 Open 3 Percutaneous 4 Percutaneous Endoscopic	A Interbody Fusion Device	0 Anterior Approach, Anterior Column J Posterior Approach, Anterior Column
5 Sacrococcygeal Joint 6 Coccygeal Joint 7 Sacroiliac Joint, Right HAC 8 Sacroiliac Joint, Left HAC	0 Open 3 Percutaneous 4 Percutaneous Endoscopic	4 Internal Fixation Device 7 Autologous Tissue Substitute J Synthetic Substitute K Nonautologous Tissue Substitute Z No Device	Z No Qualifier
9 Hip Joint, Right B Hip Joint, Left C Knee Joint, Right D Knee Joint, Left F Ankle Joint, Right G Ankle Joint, Left H Tarsal Joint, Right J Tarsal Joint, Left K Tarsometatarsal Joint, Right L Tarsometatarsal Joint, Left M Metatarsal-Phalangeal Joint, Right N Metatarsal-Phalangeal Joint, Left P Toe Phalangeal Joint, Right Q Toe Phalangeal Joint, Left	0 Open 3 Percutaneous 4 Percutaneous Endoscopic	4 Internal Fixation Device 5 External Fixation Device 7 Autologous Tissue Substitute J Synthetic Substitute K Nonautologous Tissue Substitute Z No Device	Z No Qualifier

0SG continued on next page

0SG continued from previous page

0SG1070	0SG1071	0SG107J	0SG10A0	0SG10AJ	0SG10J0	0SG10J1	0SG10JJ	0SG10K0	0SG10K1	0SG10KJ	0SG10Z0	0SG10Z1
0SG10ZJ	0SG1370	0SG1371	0SG137J	0SG13A0	0SG13AJ	0SG13J0	0SG13J1	0SG13JJ	0SG13K0	0SG13K1	0SG13KJ	0SG13Z0
0SG13Z1	0SG13ZJ	0SG1470	0SG1471	0SG147J	0SG14A0	0SG14AJ	0SG14J0	0SG14J1	0SG14JJ	0SG14K0	0SG14K1	0SG14KJ
0SG14Z0	0SG14Z1	0SG14ZJ										

HAC

0SG0070	0SG0071	0SG007J	0SG00A0	0SG00AJ	0SG00J0	0SG00J1	0SG00JJ	0SG00K0	0SG00K1	0SG00KJ	0SG00Z0	0SG00Z1
0SG00ZJ	0SG0370	0SG0371	0SG037J	0SG03A0	0SG03AJ	0SG03J0	0SG03J1	0SG03JJ	0SG03K0	0SG03K1	0SG03KJ	0SG03Z0
0SG03Z1	0SG03ZJ	0SG0470	0SG0471	0SG047J	0SG04A0	0SG04AJ	0SG04J0	0SG04J1	0SG04JJ	0SG04K0	0SG04K1	0SG04KJ
0SG04Z0	0SG04Z1	0SG04ZJ	0SG1070	0SG1071	0SG107J	0SG10A0	0SG10AJ	0SG10J0	0SG10J1	0SG10JJ	0SG10K0	0SG10K1
0SG10KJ	0SG10Z0	0SG10Z1	0SG10ZJ	0SG1370	0SG1371	0SG137J	0SG13A0	0SG13AJ	0SG13J0	0SG13J1	0SG13JJ	0SG13K0
0SG13K1	0SG13KJ	0SG13Z0	0SG13Z1	0SG13ZJ	0SG1470	0SG1471	0SG147J	0SG14A0	0SG14AJ	0SG14J0	0SG14J1	0SG14JJ
0SG14K0	0SG14K1	0SG14KJ	0SG14Z0	0SG14Z1	0SG14ZJ	0SG3070	0SG3071	0SG307J	0SG30A0	0SG30AJ	0SG30J0	0SG30J1
0SG30JJ	0SG30K0	0SG30K1	0SG30KJ	0SG30Z0	0SG30Z1	0SG30ZJ	0SG3370	0SG3371	0SG337J	0SG33A0	0SG33AJ	0SG33J0
0SG33J1	0SG33JJ	0SG33K0	0SG33K1	0SG33KJ	0SG33Z0	0SG33Z1	0SG33ZJ	0SG3470	0SG3471	0SG347J	0SG34A0	0SG34AJ
0SG34J0	0SG34J1	0SG34JJ	0SG34K0	0SG34K1	0SG34KJ	0SG34Z0	0SG34Z1	0SG34ZJ	0SG704Z	0SG707Z	0SG70JZ	0SG70KZ
0SG70ZZ	0SG734Z	0SG737Z	0SG73JZ	0SG73KZ	0SG73ZZ	0SG744Z	0SG747Z	0SG74JZ	0SG74KZ	0SG74ZZ	0SG804Z	0SG807Z
0SG80JZ	0SG80KZ	0SG80ZZ	0SG834Z	0SG837Z	0SG83JZ	0SG83KZ	0SG83ZZ	0SG844Z	0SG847Z	0SG84JZ	0SG84KZ	0SG84ZZ

Surgical site infection following certain orthopedic procedures of spine, shoulder or elbow procedures and secondary diagnosis K68.11, T84.60XA, T84.610A, T84.611A, T84.612A, T84.613, T84.614A, T84.615A, T84.619A, T84.63XA, T84.69XA, T84.7XXA, T81.4XXA.

0 **Medical and Surgical**
S **Lower Joints**
H **Insertion:** Putting in a nonbiological appliance that monitors, assists, performs, or prevents a physiological function but does not physically take the place of a body part

Body Part	Approach	Device	Qualifier
Character 4	**Character 5**	**Character 6**	**Character 7**
0 Lumbar Vertebral Joint **3** Lumbosacral Joint	**0** Open **3** Percutaneous **4** Percutaneous Endoscopic	**3** Infusion Device **4** Internal Fixation Device **8** Spacer **B** Spinal Stabilization Device, Interspinous Process **C** Spinal Stabilization Device, Pedicle-Based **D** Spinal Stabilization Device, Facet Replacement	**Z** No Qualifier
2 Lumbar Vertebral Disc **4** Lumbosacral Disc	**0** Open **3** Percutaneous **4** Percutaneous Endoscopic	**3** Infusion Device **8** Spacer	**Z** No Qualifier
5 Sacrococcygeal Joint **6** Coccygeal Joint **7** Sacroiliac Joint, Right **8** Sacroiliac Joint, Left	**0** Open **3** Percutaneous **4** Percutaneous Endoscopic	**3** Infusion Device **4** Internal Fixation Device **8** Spacer	**Z** No Qualifier
9 Hip Joint, Right **B** Hip Joint, Left **C** Knee Joint, Right **D** Knee Joint, Left **F** Ankle Joint, Right **G** Ankle Joint, Left **H** Tarsal Joint, Right **J** Tarsal Joint, Left **K** Tarsometatarsal Joint, Right **L** Tarsometatarsal Joint, Left **M** Metatarsal-Phalangeal Joint, Right **N** Metatarsal-Phalangeal Joint, Left **P** Toe Phalangeal Joint, Right **Q** Toe Phalangeal Joint, Left	**0** Open **3** Percutaneous **4** Percutaneous Endoscopic	**3** Infusion Device **4** Internal Fixation Device **5** External Fixation Device **8** Spacer	**Z** No Qualifier

0 **Medical and Surgical**
S **Lower Joints**
J **Inspection:** Visually and/or manually exploring a body part

Body Part	Approach	Device	Qualifier
Character 4	Character 5	Character 6	Character 7
0 Lumbar Vertebral Joint 2 Lumbar Vertebral Disc 3 Lumbosacral Joint 4 Lumbosacral Disc 5 Sacrococcygeal Joint 6 Coccygeal Joint 7 Sacroiliac Joint, Right 8 Sacroiliac Joint, Left 9 Hip Joint, Right B Hip Joint, Left C Knee Joint, Right D Knee Joint, Left F Ankle Joint, Right G Ankle Joint, Left H Tarsal Joint, Right J Tarsal Joint, Left K Tarsometatarsal Joint, Right L Tarsometatarsal Joint, Left M Metatarsal-Phalangeal Joint, Right N Metatarsal-Phalangeal Joint, Left P Toe Phalangeal Joint, Right Q Toe Phalangeal Joint, Left	0 Open 3 Percutaneous 4 Percutaneous Endoscopic X External	Z No Device	Z No Qualifier

0 **Medical and Surgical**
S **Lower Joints**
N **Release:** Freeing a body part from an abnormal physical constraint by cutting or by the use of force

Body Part	Approach	Device	Qualifier
Character 4	Character 5	Character 6	Character 7
0 Lumbar Vertebral Joint 2 Lumbar Vertebral Disc 3 Lumbosacral Joint 4 Lumbosacral Disc 5 Sacrococcygeal Joint 6 Coccygeal Joint 7 Sacroiliac Joint, Right 8 Sacroiliac Joint, Left 9 Hip Joint, Right B Hip Joint, Left C Knee Joint, Right D Knee Joint, Left F Ankle Joint, Right G Ankle Joint, Left H Tarsal Joint, Right J Tarsal Joint, Left K Tarsometatarsal Joint, Right L Tarsometatarsal Joint, Left M Metatarsal-Phalangeal Joint, Right N Metatarsal-Phalangeal Joint, Left P Toe Phalangeal Joint, Right Q Toe Phalangeal Joint, Left	0 Open 3 Percutaneous 4 Percutaneous Endoscopic X External	Z No Device	Z No Qualifier

0 **Medical and Surgical**
S **Lower Joints**
P **Removal:** Taking out or off a device from a body part

Body Part	Approach	Device	Qualifier
Character 4	**Character 5**	**Character 6**	**Character 7**
0 Lumbar Vertebral Joint 3 Lumbosacral Joint	0 Open 3 Percutaneous 4 Percutaneous Endoscopic	0 Drainage Device 3 Infusion Device 4 Internal Fixation Device 7 Autologous Tissue Substitute 8 Spacer A Interbody Fusion Device J Synthetic Substitute K Nonautologous Tissue Substitute	Z No Qualifier
0 Lumbar Vertebral Joint 3 Lumbosacral Joint	X External	0 Drainage Device 3 Infusion Device 4 Internal Fixation Device	Z No Qualifier
2 Lumbar Vertebral Disc 4 Lumbosacral Disc	0 Open 3 Percutaneous 4 Percutaneous Endoscopic	0 Drainage Device 3 Infusion Device 7 Autologous Tissue Substitute J Synthetic Substitute K Nonautologous Tissue Substitute	Z No Qualifier
2 Lumbar Vertebral Disc 4 Lumbosacral Disc	X External	0 Drainage Device 3 Infusion Device	Z No Qualifier
5 Sacrococcygeal Joint 6 Coccygeal Joint 7 Sacroiliac Joint, Right 8 Sacroiliac Joint, Left	0 Open 3 Percutaneous 4 Percutaneous Endoscopic	0 Drainage Device 3 Infusion Device 4 Internal Fixation Device 7 Autologous Tissue Substitute 8 Spacer J Synthetic Substitute K Nonautologous Tissue Substitute	Z No Qualifier
5 Sacrococcygeal Joint 6 Coccygeal Joint 7 Sacroiliac Joint, Right 8 Sacroiliac Joint, Left	X External	0 Drainage Device 3 Infusion Device 4 Internal Fixation Device	Z No Qualifier
9 Hip Joint, Right CC B Hip Joint, Left CC	0 Open	0 Drainage Device 3 Infusion Device 4 Internal Fixation Device 5 External Fixation Device 7 Autologous Tissue Substitute 8 Spacer 9 Liner B Resurfacing Device J Synthetic Substitute K Nonautologous Tissue Substitute	Z No Qualifier
9 Hip Joint, Right CC B Hip Joint, Left CC	3 Percutaneous 4 Percutaneous Endoscopic	0 Drainage Device 3 Infusion Device 4 Internal Fixation Device 5 External Fixation Device 7 Autologous Tissue Substitute 8 Spacer J Synthetic Substitute K Nonautologous Tissue Substitute	Z No Qualifier
9 Hip Joint, Right B Hip Joint, Left	X External	0 Drainage Device 3 Infusion Device 4 Internal Fixation Device 5 External Fixation Device	Z No Qualifier

0SP continued on next page

0 **Medical and Surgical**
S **Lower Joints**
P **Removal:** Taking out or off a device from a body part

0SP continued from previous page

Body Part		Approach		Device		Qualifier	
Character 4		**Character 5**		**Character 6**		**Character 7**	
A	Hip Joint, Acetabular Surface, Right [CC]	0	Open	J	Synthetic Substitute	Z	No Qualifier
E	Hip Joint, Acetabular Surface, Left [CC]	3	Percutaneous				
R	Hip Joint, Femoral Surface, Right [CC]	4	Percutaneous Endoscopic				
S	Hip Joint, Femoral Surface, Left [CC]						
T	Knee Joint, Femoral Surface, Right [CC]						
U	Knee Joint, Femoral Surface, Left [CC]						
V	Knee Joint, Tibial Surface, Right [CC]						
W	Knee Joint, Tibial Surface, Left [CC]						
C	Knee Joint, Right [CC]	0	Open	0	Drainage Device	Z	No Qualifier
D	Knee Joint, Left [CC]			3	Infusion Device		
				4	Internal Fixation Device		
				5	External Fixation Device		
				7	Autologous Tissue Substitute		
				8	Spacer		
				9	Liner		
				K	Nonautologous Tissue Substitute		
C	Knee Joint, Right [CC]	0	Open	J	Synthetic Substitute	C	Patellar Surface
D	Knee Joint, Left [CC]					Z	No Qualifier
C	Knee Joint, Right [CC]	3	Percutaneous	0	Drainage Device	Z	No Qualifier
D	Knee Joint, Left [CC]	4	Percutaneous Endoscopic	3	Infusion Device		
				4	Internal Fixation Device		
				5	External Fixation Device		
				7	Autologous Tissue Substitute		
				8	Spacer		
				K	Nonautologous Tissue Substitute		
C	Knee Joint, Right [CC]	3	Percutaneous	J	Synthetic Substitute	C	Patellar Surface
D	Knee Joint, Left [CC]	4	Percutaneous Endoscopic			Z	No Qualifier
C	Knee Joint, Right	X	External	0	Drainage Device	Z	No Qualifier
D	Knee Joint, Left			3	Infusion Device		
				4	Internal Fixation Device		
				5	External Fixation Device		
F	Ankle Joint, Right	0	Open	0	Drainage Device	Z	No Qualifier
G	Ankle Joint, Left	3	Percutaneous	3	Infusion Device		
H	Tarsal Joint, Right	4	Percutaneous Endoscopic	4	Internal Fixation Device		
J	Tarsal Joint, Left			5	External Fixation Device		
K	Tarsometatarsal Joint, Right			7	Autologous Tissue Substitute		
L	Tarsometatarsal Joint, Left			8	Spacer		
M	Metatarsal-Phalangeal Joint, Right			J	Synthetic Substitute		
N	Metatarsal-Phalangeal Joint, Left			K	Nonautologous Tissue Substitute		
P	Toe Phalangeal Joint, Right						
Q	Toe Phalangeal Joint, Left						

0SP continued on next page

0 Medical and Surgical
S Lower Joints
P **Removal:** Taking out or off a device from a body part

0SP continued from previous page

Body Part	Approach	Device	Qualifier
Character 4	**Character 5**	**Character 6**	**Character 7**
F Ankle Joint, Right **G** Ankle Joint, Left **H** Tarsal Joint, Right **J** Tarsal Joint, Left **K** Tarsometatarsal Joint, Right **L** Tarsometatarsal Joint, Left **M** Metatarsal-Phalangeal Joint, Right **N** Metatarsal-Phalangeal Joint, Left **P** Toe Phalangeal Joint, Right **Q** Toe Phalangeal Joint, Left	**X** External	**0** Drainage Device **3** Infusion Device **4** Internal Fixation Device **5** External Fixation Device	**Z** No Qualifier

CC 0SP908Z   0SP909Z   0SP90BZ   0SP90JZ   0SP948Z   0SP94JZ   0SPA0JZ   0SPA4JZ   0SPB08Z   0SPB09Z   0SPB0BZ   0SPB0JZ   0SPB48Z
0SPB4JZ   0SPC08Z   0SPC09Z   0SPC0JC   0SPC0JZ   0SPC38Z   0SPC48Z   0SPC4JC   0SPC4JZ   0SPD08Z   0SPD09Z   0SPD0JC   0SPD0JZ
0SPD38Z   0SPD48Z   0SPD4JC   0SPD4JZ   0SPE0JZ   0SPE4JZ   0SPR0JZ   0SPR4JZ   0SPS0JZ   0SPS4JZ   0SPT0JZ   0SPT4JZ   0SPU0JZ
0SPU4JZ   0SPV0JZ   0SPV4JZ   0SPW0JZ   0SPW4JZ

0 Medical and Surgical
S Lower Joints
Q **Repair:** Restoring, to the extent possible, a body part to its normal anatomic structure and function

Body Part	Approach	Device	Qualifier
Character 4	**Character 5**	**Character 6**	**Character 7**
0 Lumbar Vertebral Joint **2** Lumbar Vertebral Disc **3** Lumbosacral Joint **4** Lumbosacral Disc **5** Sacrococcygeal Joint **6** Coccygeal Joint **7** Sacroiliac Joint, Right **8** Sacroiliac Joint, Left **9** Hip Joint, Right **B** Hip Joint, Left **C** Knee Joint, Right **D** Knee Joint, Left **F** Ankle Joint, Right **G** Ankle Joint, Left **H** Tarsal Joint, Right **J** Tarsal Joint, Left **K** Tarsometatarsal Joint, Right **L** Tarsometatarsal Joint, Left **M** Metatarsal-Phalangeal Joint, Right **N** Metatarsal-Phalangeal Joint, Left **P** Toe Phalangeal Joint, Right **Q** Toe Phalangeal Joint, Left	**0** Open **3** Percutaneous **4** Percutaneous Endoscopic **X** External	**Z** No Device	**Z** No Qualifier

0 Medical and Surgical
S Lower Joints
R Replacement: Putting in or on biological or synthetic material that physically takes the place and/or function of all or a portion of a body part

Body Part	Approach	Device	Qualifier
Character 4	Character 5	Character 6	Character 7
0 Lumbar Vertebral Joint **2** Lumbar Vertebral Disc NC **3** Lumbosacral Joint **4** Lumbosacral Disc NC **5** Sacrococcygeal Joint **6** Coccygeal Joint **7** Sacroiliac Joint, Right **8** Sacroiliac Joint, Left **H** Tarsal Joint, Right **J** Tarsal Joint, Left **K** Tarsometatarsal Joint, Right **L** Tarsometatarsal Joint, Left **M** Metatarsal-Phalangeal Joint, Right **N** Metatarsal-Phalangeal Joint, Left **P** Toe Phalangeal Joint, Right **Q** Toe Phalangeal Joint, Left	**0** Open	**7** Autologous Tissue Substitute **J** Synthetic Substitute **K** Nonautologous Tissue Substitute	**Z** No Qualifier
9 Hip Joint, Right CC HAC **B** Hip Joint, Left CC HAC	**0** Open	**1** Synthetic Substitute, Metal **2** Synthetic Substitute, Metal on Polyethylene **3** Synthetic Substitute, Ceramic **4** Synthetic Substitute, Ceramic on Polyethylene **6** Synthetic Substitute, Oxidized Zirconium on Polyethylene **J** Synthetic Substitute	**9** Cemented **A** Uncemented **Z** No Qualifier
9 Hip Joint, Right HAC **B** Hip Joint, Left HAC	**0** Open	**7** Autologous Tissue Substitute **K** Nonautologous Tissue Substitute	**Z** No Qualifier
A Hip Joint, Acetabular Surface, Right CC HAC **E** Hip Joint, Acetabular Surface, Left CC HAC	**0** Open	**0** Synthetic Substitute, Polyethylene **1** Synthetic Substitute, Metal **3** Synthetic Substitute, Ceramic **J** Synthetic Substitute	**9** Cemented **A** Uncemented **Z** No Qualifier
A Hip Joint, Acetabular Surface, Right HAC **E** Hip Joint, Acetabular Surface, Left HAC	**0** Open	**7** Autologous Tissue Substitute **K** Nonautologous Tissue Substitute	**Z** No Qualifier
C Knee Joint, Right CC HAC **D** Knee Joint, Left CC HAC	**0** Open	**6** Synthetic Substitute, Oxidized Zirconium on Polyethylene **J** Synthetic Substitute **L** Synthetic Substitute, Unicondylar	**9** Cemented **A** Uncemented **Z** No Qualifier
C Knee Joint, Right HAC **D** Knee Joint, Left HAC	**0** Open	**7** Autologous Tissue Substitute **K** Nonautologous Tissue Substitute	**Z** No Qualifier
F Ankle Joint, Right **G** Ankle Joint, Left **T** Knee Joint, Femoral Surface, Right HAC **U** Knee Joint, Femoral Surface, Left HAC **V** Knee Joint, Tibial Surface, Right HAC **W** Knee Joint, Tibial Surface, Left HAC	**0** Open	**7** Autologous Tissue Substitute **K** Nonautologous Tissue Substitute	**Z** No Qualifier

0SR continued on next page

LC Limited Coverage   NC Noncovered   HAC HAC-associated Procedure   CC Combination Cluster – See Appendix G for code lists
DRG Non-OR-Affecting MS-DRG Assignment   New/Revised Text in Orange   ♂ Male   ♀ Female

0 **Medical and Surgical**
S **Lower Joints**
R **Replacement:** Putting in or on biological or synthetic material that physically takes the place and/or function of all or a portion of a body part

0SR continued from previous page

Body Part	Approach	Device	Qualifier
Character 4	**Character 5**	**Character 6**	**Character 7**
F Ankle Joint, Right G Ankle Joint, Left T Knee Joint, Femoral Surface, Right **CC HAC** U Knee Joint, Femoral Surface, Left **CC HAC** V Knee Joint, Tibial Surface, Right **CC HAC** W Knee Joint, Tibial Surface, Left **CC HAC**	0 Open	J Synthetic Substitute	9 Cemented A Uncemented Z No Qualifier
R Hip Joint, Femoral Surface, Right **CC HAC** S Hip Joint, Femoral Surface, Left **CC HAC**	0 Open	1 Synthetic Substitute, Metal 3 Synthetic Substitute, Ceramic J Synthetic Substitute	9 Cemented A Uncemented Z No Qualifier
R Hip Joint, Femoral Surface, Right **HAC** S Hip Joint, Femoral Surface, Left **HAC**	0 Open	7 Autologous Tissue Substitute K Nonautologous Tissue Substitute	Z No Qualifier

CC 0SR9019 0SR901A 0SR901Z 0SR9029 0SR902A 0SR902Z 0SR9039 0SR903A 0SR903Z 0SR9049 0SR904A 0SR904Z 0SR90J9
0SR90JA 0SR90JZ 0SRA009 0SRA00A 0SRA00Z 0SRA019 0SRA01A 0SRA01Z 0SRA039 0SRA03A 0SRA03Z 0SRA0J9 0SRA0JA
0SRA0JZ 0SRB019 0SRB01A 0SRB01Z 0SRB029 0SRB02A 0SRB02Z 0SRB039 0SRB03A 0SRB03Z 0SRB049 0SRB04A 0SRB04Z
0SRB0J9 0SRB0JA 0SRB0JZ 0SRC0J9 0SRC0JA 0SRC0JZ 0SRC0L9 0SRC0LA 0SRC0LZ 0SRD0J9 0SRD0JA 0SRD0JZ 0SRD0L9
0SRD0LA 0SRD0LZ 0SRE009 0SRE00A 0SRE00Z 0SRE019 0SRE01A 0SRE01Z 0SRE039 0SRE03A 0SRE03Z 0SRE0J9 0SRE0JA
0SRE0JZ 0SRR019 0SRR01A 0SRR01Z 0SRR039 0SRR03A 0SRR03Z 0SRR0J9 0SRR0JA 0SRR0JZ 0SRS019 0SRS01A 0SRS01Z
0SRS039 0SRS03A 0SRS03Z 0SRS0J9 0SRS0JA 0SRS0JZ 0SRT0J9 0SRT0JA 0SRT0JZ 0SRU0J9 0SRU0JA 0SRU0JZ 0SRV0J9
0SRV0JA 0SRV0JZ 0SRW0J9 0SRW0JA 0SRW0JZ

NC 0SR20JZ 0SR40JZ

When the beneficiary is over age 60.

HAC 0SR9019 0SR901A 0SR901Z 0SR9029 0SR902A 0SR902Z 0SR9039 0SR903A 0SR903Z 0SR9049 0SR904A 0SR904Z 0SR907Z
0SR90J9 0SR90JA 0SR90JZ 0SR90KZ 0SRA009 0SRA00A 0SRA00Z 0SRA019 0SRA01A 0SRA01Z 0SRA039 0SRA03A 0SRA03Z
0SRA07Z 0SRA0J9 0SRA0JA 0SRA0JZ 0SRA0KZ 0SRB019 0SRB01A 0SRB01Z 0SRB029 0SRB02A 0SRB02Z 0SRB039 0SRB03A
0SRB03Z 0SRB049 0SRB04A 0SRB04Z 0SRB07Z 0SRB0J9 0SRB0JA 0SRB0JZ 0SRB0KZ 0SRC07Z 0SRC0J9 0SRC0JA 0SRC0JZ
0SRC0KZ 0SRC0L9 0SRC0LA 0SRC0LZ 0SRD07Z 0SRD0J9 0SRD0JA 0SRD0JZ 0SRD0KZ 0SRD0L9 0SRD0LA 0SRD0LZ 0SRE009
0SRE00A 0SRE00Z 0SRE019 0SRE01A 0SRE01Z 0SRE039 0SRE03A 0SRE03Z 0SRE07Z 0SRE0J9 0SRE0JA 0SRE0JZ 0SRE0KZ
0SRR019 0SRR01A 0SRR01Z 0SRR039 0SRR03A 0SRR03Z 0SRR07Z 0SRR0J9 0SRR0JA 0SRR0JZ 0SRR0KZ 0SRS019 0SRS01A
0SRS01Z 0SRS039 0SRS03A 0SRS03Z 0SRS07Z 0SRS0J9 0SRS0JZ 0SRS0KZ 0SRT07Z 0SRT0J9 0SRT0JA 0SRT0JZ
0SRT0KZ 0SRU07Z 0SRU0J9 0SRU0JA 0SRU0JZ 0SRU0KZ 0SRV07Z 0SRV0J9 0SRV0JA 0SRV0JZ 0SRV0KZ 0SRW07Z 0SRW0J9
0SRW0JA 0SRW0JZ 0SRW0KZ

Srgical site infection, mediastinitis, following coronary artery bypass graft (CABG) and secondary diagnosis I26.02, I26.09, I26.92, I26.99, I82.401, I82.402, I82.403, I82.409, I82.411, I82.412, I82.413, I82.419, I82.421, I82.422, I82.423, I82.429, I82.431, I82.432, I82.433, I82.439, I82.441, I82.442, I82.443, I82.449, I82.491, I82.492, I82.493, I82.499, I82.4Y1, I82.4Y2, I82.4Y3, I82.4Y9, I82.4Z1, I82.4Z2, I82.4Z3, I82.4Z9.

0 Medical and Surgical
S Lower Joints
S Reposition: Moving to its normal location, or other suitable location, all or a portion of a body part

Body Part	Approach	Device	Qualifier
Character 4	Character 5	Character 6	Character 7
0 Lumbar Vertebral Joint 3 Lumbosacral Joint 5 Sacrococcygeal Joint 6 Coccygeal Joint 7 Sacroiliac Joint, Right 8 Sacroiliac Joint, Left	0 Open 3 Percutaneous 4 Percutaneous Endoscopic X External	4 Internal Fixation Device Z No Device	Z No Qualifier
9 Hip Joint, Right B Hip Joint, Left C Knee Joint, Right D Knee Joint, Left F Ankle Joint, Right G Ankle Joint, Left H Tarsal Joint, Right J Tarsal Joint, Left K Tarsometatarsal Joint, Right L Tarsometatarsal Joint, Left M Metatarsal-Phalangeal Joint, Right N Metatarsal-Phalangeal Joint, Left P Toe Phalangeal Joint, Right Q Toe Phalangeal Joint, Left	0 Open 3 Percutaneous 4 Percutaneous Endoscopic X External	4 Internal Fixation Device 5 External Fixation Device Z No Device	Z No Qualifier

0 Medical and Surgical
S Lower Joints
T Resection: Cutting out or off, without replacement, all of a body part

Body Part	Approach	Device	Qualifier
Character 4	Character 5	Character 6	Character 7
2 Lumbar Vertebral Disc 4 Lumbosacral Disc 5 Sacrococcygeal Joint 6 Coccygeal Joint 7 Sacroiliac Joint, Right 8 Sacroiliac Joint, Left 9 Hip Joint, Right B Hip Joint, Left C Knee Joint, Right D Knee Joint, Left F Ankle Joint, Right G Ankle Joint, Left H Tarsal Joint, Right J Tarsal Joint, Left K Tarsometatarsal Joint, Right L Tarsometatarsal Joint, Left M Metatarsal-Phalangeal Joint, Right N Metatarsal-Phalangeal Joint, Left P Toe Phalangeal Joint, Right Q Toe Phalangeal Joint, Left	0 Open	Z No Device	Z No Qualifier

0 Medical and Surgical
S Lower Joints
U Supplement: Putting in or on biological or synthetic material that physically reinforces and/or augments the function of a portion of a body part

Body Part	Approach	Device	Qualifier
Character 4	Character 5	Character 6	Character 7
0 Lumbar Vertebral Joint **2** Lumbar Vertebral Disc **3** Lumbosacral Joint **4** Lumbosacral Disc **5** Sacrococcygeal Joint **6** Coccygeal Joint **7** Sacroiliac Joint, Right **8** Sacroiliac Joint, Left **F** Ankle Joint, Right **G** Ankle Joint, Left **H** Tarsal Joint, Right **J** Tarsal Joint, Left **K** Tarsometatarsal Joint, Right **L** Tarsometatarsal Joint, Left **M** Metatarsal-Phalangeal Joint, Right **N** Metatarsal-Phalangeal Joint, Left **P** Toe Phalangeal Joint, Right **Q** Toe Phalangeal Joint, Left	**0** Open **3** Percutaneous **4** Percutaneous Endoscopic	**7** Autologous Tissue Substitute **J** Synthetic Substitute **K** Nonautologous Tissue Substitute	**Z** No Qualifier
9 Hip Joint, Right ☒ HAC **B** Hip Joint, Left ☒ HAC	**0** Open	**7** Autologous Tissue Substitute **9** Liner **B** Resurfacing Device **J** Synthetic Substitute **K** Nonautologous Tissue Substitute	**Z** No Qualifier
9 Hip Joint, Right **B** Hip Joint, Left	**3** Percutaneous **4** Percutaneous Endoscopic	**7** Autologous Tissue Substitute **J** Synthetic Substitute **K** Nonautologous Tissue Substitute	**Z** No Qualifier
A Hip Joint, Acetabular Surface, Right ☒ HAC **E** Hip Joint, Acetabular Surface, Left ☒ HAC **R** Hip Joint, Femoral Surface, Right ☒ HAC **S** Hip Joint, Femoral Surface, Left ☒ HAC	**0** Open	**9** Liner **B** Resurfacing Device	**Z** No Qualifier
C Knee Joint, Right **D** Knee Joint, Left	**0** Open	**7** Autologous Tissue Substitute **J** Synthetic Substitute **K** Nonautologous Tissue Substitute	**Z** No Qualifier
C Knee Joint, Right **D** Knee Joint, Left	**0** Open	**9** Liner	**C** Patellar Surface **Z** No Qualifier
C Knee Joint, Right **D** Knee Joint, Left	**3** Percutaneous **4** Percutaneous Endoscopic	**7** Autologous Tissue Substitute **J** Synthetic Substitute **K** Nonautologous Tissue Substitute	**Z** No Qualifier
T Knee Joint, Femoral Surface, Right **U** Knee Joint, Femoral Surface, Left **V** Knee Joint, Tibial Surface, Right ☒ **W** Knee Joint, Tibial Surface, Left ☒	**0** Open	**9** Liner	**Z** No Qualifier

☒ 0SU909Z 0SUA09Z 0SUB09Z 0SUE09Z 0SUR09Z 0SUS09Z 0SUV09Z 0SUW09Z
HAC 0SU90BZ 0SUA0BZ 0SUB0BZ 0SUE0BZ 0SUR0BZ 0SUS0BZ
Srgical site infection, mediastinitis, following coronary artery bypass graft (CABG) and secondary diagnosis I26.02, I26.09, I26.92, I26.99, I82.401, I82.402, I82.403, I82.409, I82.411, I82.412, I82.413, I82.419, I82.421, I82.422, I82.423, I82.429, I82.431, I82.432, I82.433, I82.439, I82.441, I82.442, I82.443, I82.449, I82.491, I82.492, I82.493, I82.499, I82.4Y1, I82.4Y2, I82.4Y3, I82.4Y9, I82.4Z1, I82.4Z2, I82.4Z3, I82.4Z9.

0 Medical and Surgical
S Lower Joints
W Revision: Correcting, to the extent possible, a portion of a malfunctioning device or the position of a displaced device

Body Part	Approach	Device	Qualifier
Character 4	Character 5	Character 6	Character 7
0 Lumbar Vertebral Joint 3 Lumbosacral Joint	0 Open 3 Percutaneous 4 Percutaneous Endoscopic X External	0 Drainage Device 3 Infusion Device 4 Internal Fixation Device 7 Autologous Tissue Substitute 8 Spacer A Interbody Fusion Device J Synthetic Substitute K Nonautologous Tissue Substitute	Z No Qualifier
2 Lumbar Vertebral Disc 4 Lumbosacral Disc	0 Open 3 Percutaneous 4 Percutaneous Endoscopic X External	0 Drainage Device 3 Infusion Device 7 Autologous Tissue Substitute J Synthetic Substitute K Nonautologous Tissue Substitute	Z No Qualifier
5 Sacrococcygeal Joint 6 Coccygeal Joint 7 Sacroiliac Joint, Right 8 Sacroiliac Joint, Left	0 Open 3 Percutaneous 4 Percutaneous Endoscopic X External	0 Drainage Device 3 Infusion Device 4 Internal Fixation Device 7 Autologous Tissue Substitute 8 Spacer J Synthetic Substitute K Nonautologous Tissue Substitute	Z No Qualifier
9 Hip Joint, Right B Hip Joint, Left	0 Open	0 Drainage Device 3 Infusion Device 4 Internal Fixation Device 5 External Fixation Device 7 Autologous Tissue Substitute 8 Spacer 9 Liner B Resurfacing Device J Synthetic Substitute K Nonautologous Tissue Substitute	Z No Qualifier
9 Hip Joint, Right B Hip Joint, Left	3 Percutaneous 4 Percutaneous Endoscopic X External	0 Drainage Device 3 Infusion Device 4 Internal Fixation Device 5 External Fixation Device 7 Autologous Tissue Substitute 8 Spacer J Synthetic Substitute K Nonautologous Tissue Substitute	Z No Qualifier
A Hip Joint, Acetabular Surface, Right E Hip Joint, Acetabular Surface, Left R Hip Joint, Femoral Surface, Right S Hip Joint, Femoral Surface, Left T Knee Joint, Femoral Surface, Right U Knee Joint, Femoral Surface, Left V Knee Joint, Tibial Surface, Right W Knee Joint, Tibial Surface, Left	0 Open 3 Percutaneous 4 Percutaneous Endoscopic X External	J Synthetic Substitute	Z No Qualifier

0SW continued on next page

0 **Medical and Surgical**
S **Lower Joints**
W **Revision:** Correcting, to the extent possible, a portion of a malfunctioning device or the position of a displaced device

0SW continued from previous page

Body Part	Approach	Device	Qualifier
Character 4	Character 5	Character 6	Character 7
C Knee Joint, Right D Knee Joint, Left	0 Open	0 Drainage Device 3 Infusion Device 4 Internal Fixation Device 5 External Fixation Device 7 Autologous Tissue Substitute 8 Spacer 9 Liner K Nonautologous Tissue Substitute	Z No Qualifier
C Knee Joint, Right D Knee Joint, Left	0 Open	J Synthetic Substitute	C Patellar Surface Z No Qualifier
C Knee Joint, Right D Knee Joint, Left	3 Percutaneous 4 Percutaneous Endoscopic X External	0 Drainage Device 3 Infusion Device 4 Internal Fixation Device 5 External Fixation Device 7 Autologous Tissue Substitute 8 Spacer K Nonautologous Tissue Substitute	Z No Qualifier
C Knee Joint, Right D Knee Joint, Left	3 Percutaneous 4 Percutaneous Endoscopic X External	J Synthetic Substitute	C Patellar Surface Z No Qualifier
F Ankle Joint, Right G Ankle Joint, Left H Tarsal Joint, Right J Tarsal Joint, Left K Tarsometatarsal Joint, Right L Tarsometatarsal Joint, Left M Metatarsal-Phalangeal Joint, Right N Metatarsal-Phalangeal Joint, Left P Toe Phalangeal Joint, Right Q Toe Phalangeal Joint, Left	0 Open 3 Percutaneous 4 Percutaneous Endoscopic X External	0 Drainage Device 3 Infusion Device 4 Internal Fixation Device 5 External Fixation Device 7 Autologous Tissue Substitute 8 Spacer J Synthetic Substitute K Nonautologous Tissue Substitute	Z No Qualifier

NOTES

Urinary System 0T1-0TY

0 Medical and Surgical
T Urinary System
1 **Bypass:** Altering the route of passage of the contents of a tubular body part

Body Part	Approach	Device	Qualifier
Character 4	Character 5	Character 6	Character 7
3 Kidney Pelvis, Right 4 Kidney Pelvis, Left	0 Open 4 Percutaneous Endoscopic	7 Autologous Tissue Substitute J Synthetic Substitute K Nonautologous Tissue Substitute Z No Device	3 Kidney Pelvis, Right 4 Kidney Pelvis, Left 6 Ureter, Right 7 Ureter, Left 8 Colon 9 Colocutaneous A Ileum B Bladder C Ileocutaneous D Cutaneous
3 Kidney Pelvis, Right 4 Kidney Pelvis, Left	3 Percutaneous	J Synthetic Substitute	D Cutaneous
6 Ureter, Right 7 Ureter, Left 8 Ureters, Bilateral	0 Open 4 Percutaneous Endoscopic	7 Autologous Tissue Substitute J Synthetic Substitute K Nonautologous Tissue Substitute Z No Device	6 Ureter, Right 7 Ureter, Left 8 Colon 9 Colocutaneous A Ileum B Bladder C Ileocutaneous D Cutaneous
6 Ureter, Right 7 Ureter, Left 8 Ureters, Bilateral	3 Percutaneous	J Synthetic Substitute	D Cutaneous
B Bladder	0 Open 4 Percutaneous Endoscopic	7 Autologous Tissue Substitute J Synthetic Substitute K Nonautologous Tissue Substitute Z No Device	9 Colocutaneous C Ileocutaneous D Cutaneous
B Bladder	3 Percutaneous	J Synthetic Substitute	D Cutaneous

0 Medical and Surgical
T Urinary System
2 **Change:** Taking out or off a device from a body part and putting back an identical or similar device in or on the same body part without cutting or puncturing the skin or a mucous membrane

Body Part	Approach	Device	Qualifier
Character 4	Character 5	Character 6	Character 7
5 Kidney 9 Ureter B Bladder D Urethra	X External	0 Drainage Device Y Other Device	Z No Qualifier

0 Medical and Surgical
T Urinary System
5 Destruction: Physical eradication of all or a portion of a body part by the direct use of energy, force, or a destructive agent

Body Part	Approach	Device	Qualifier
Character 4	Character 5	Character 6	Character 7
0 Kidney, Right 1 Kidney, Left 3 Kidney Pelvis, Right 4 Kidney Pelvis, Left 6 Ureter, Right 7 Ureter, Left B Bladder C Bladder Neck	0 Open 3 Percutaneous 4 Percutaneous Endoscopic 7 Via Natural or Artificial Opening 8 Via Natural or Artificial Opening Endoscopic	Z No Device	Z No Qualifier
D Urethra	0 Open 3 Percutaneous 4 Percutaneous Endoscopic 7 Via Natural or Artificial Opening 8 Via Natural or Artificial Opening Endoscopic X External	Z No Device	Z No Qualifier

0 Medical and Surgical
T Urinary System
7 Dilation: Expanding an orifice or the lumen of a tubular body part

Body Part	Approach	Device	Qualifier
Character 4	Character 5	Character 6	Character 7
3 Kidney Pelvis, Right 4 Kidney Pelvis, Left 6 Ureter, Right 7 Ureter, Left 8 Ureters, Bilateral B Bladder C Bladder Neck D Urethra	0 Open 3 Percutaneous 4 Percutaneous Endoscopic 7 Via Natural or Artificial Opening 8 Via Natural or Artificial Opening Endoscopic	D Intraluminal Device Z No Device	Z No Qualifier

0 Medical and Surgical
T Urinary System
8 Division: Cutting into a body part, without draining fluids and/or gases from the body part, in order to separate or transect a body part

Body Part	Approach	Device	Qualifier
Character 4	Character 5	Character 6	Character 7
2 Kidneys, Bilateral C Bladder Neck	0 Open 3 Percutaneous 4 Percutaneous Endoscopic	Z No Device	Z No Qualifier

LC Limited Coverage   NC Noncovered   HAC HAC-associated Procedure   CC Combination Cluster - See Appendix G for code lists
DRG Non-OR-Affecting MS-DRG Assignment   New/Revised Text in **Orange**   ♂ Male   ♀ Female

502

2018 ICD-10-PCS

0 **Medical and Surgical**
T **Urinary System**
9 **Drainage:** Taking or letting out fluids and/or gases from a body part

Body Part	Approach	Device	Qualifier
Character 4	Character 5	Character 6	Character 7
0 Kidney, Right **1** Kidney, Left **3** Kidney Pelvis, Right ᴰᴿᴳ **4** Kidney Pelvis, Left ᴰᴿᴳ **6** Ureter, Right **7** Ureter, Left **8** Ureters, Bilateral **B** Bladder **C** Bladder Neck	**0** Open **3** Percutaneous **4** Percutaneous Endoscopic **7** Via Natural or Artificial Opening **8** Via Natural or Artificial Opening Endoscopic	**0** Drainage Device	**Z** No Qualifier
0 Kidney, Right **1** Kidney, Left **3** Kidney Pelvis, Right **4** Kidney Pelvis, Left **6** Ureter, Right **7** Ureter, Left **8** Ureters, Bilateral **B** Bladder **C** Bladder Neck	**0** Open **3** Percutaneous **4** Percutaneous Endoscopic **7** Via Natural or Artificial Opening **8** Via Natural or Artificial Opening Endoscopic	**Z** No Device	**X** Diagnostic **Z** No Qualifier
D Urethra	**0** Open **3** Percutaneous **4** Percutaneous Endoscopic **7** Via Natural or Artificial Opening **8** Via Natural or Artificial Opening Endoscopic **X** External	**0** Drainage Device	**Z** No Qualifier
D Urethra	**0** Open **3** Percutaneous **4** Percutaneous Endoscopic **7** Via Natural or Artificial Opening **8** Via Natural or Artificial Opening Endoscopic **X** External	**Z** No Device	**X** Diagnostic **Z** No Qualifier

ᴰᴿᴳ 0T9330Z   0T9430Z

0 **Medical and Surgical**
T **Urinary System**
B **Excision:** Cutting out or off, without replacement, a portion of a body part

Body Part	Approach	Device	Qualifier
Character 4	Character 5	Character 6	Character 7
0 Kidney, Right **1** Kidney, Left **3** Kidney Pelvis, Right **4** Kidney Pelvis, Left **6** Ureter, Right **7** Ureter, Left **B** Bladder **C** Bladder Neck	**0** Open **3** Percutaneous **4** Percutaneous Endoscopic **7** Via Natural or Artificial Opening **8** Via Natural or Artificial Opening Endoscopic	**Z** No Device	**X** Diagnostic **Z** No Qualifier
D Urethra	**0** Open **3** Percutaneous **4** Percutaneous Endoscopic **7** Via Natural or Artificial Opening **8** Via Natural or Artificial Opening Endoscopic **X** External	**Z** No Device	**X** Diagnostic **Z** No Qualifier

ᴸᶜ Limited Coverage   ᴺᶜ Noncovered   ᴴᴬᶜ HAC-associated Procedure   ᶜᶜ Combination Cluster - See Appendix G for code lists
ᴰᴿᴳ Non-OR-Affecting MS-DRG Assignment   New/Revised Text in **Orange**   ♂ Male   ♀ Female

0 Medical and Surgical
T Urinary System
C Extirpation: Taking or cutting out solid matter from a body part

Body Part	Approach	Device	Qualifier
Character 4	Character 5	Character 6	Character 7
0 Kidney, Right 1 Kidney, Left 3 Kidney Pelvis, Right 4 Kidney Pelvis, Left 6 Ureter, Right 7 Ureter, Left B Bladder C Bladder Neck	0 Open 3 Percutaneous 4 Percutaneous Endoscopic 7 Via Natural or Artificial Opening 8 Via Natural or Artificial Opening Endoscopic	Z No Device	Z No Qualifier
D Urethra	0 Open 3 Percutaneous 4 Percutaneous Endoscopic 7 Via Natural or Artificial Opening 8 Via Natural or Artificial Opening Endoscopic X External	Z No Device	Z No Qualifier

0 Medical and Surgical
T Urinary System
D Extraction: Pulling or stripping out or off all or a portion of a body part by the use of force

Body Part	Approach	Device	Qualifier
Character 4	Character 5	Character 6	Character 7
0 Kidney, Right 1 Kidney, Left	0 Open 3 Percutaneous 4 Percutaneous Endoscopic	Z No Device	Z No Qualifier

0 Medical and Surgical
T Urinary System
F Fragmentation: Breaking solid matter in a body part into pieces

Body Part	Approach	Device	Qualifier
Character 4	Character 5	Character 6	Character 7
3 Kidney Pelvis, Right 4 Kidney Pelvis, Left 6 Ureter, Right 7 Ureter, Left B Bladder C Bladder Neck D Urethra ▨	0 Open 3 Percutaneous 4 Percutaneous Endoscopic 7 Via Natural or Artificial Opening 8 Via Natural or Artificial Opening Endoscopic X External	Z No Device	Z No Qualifier

▨ 0TFDXZZ

▨ Limited Coverage   ▨ Noncovered   ▨ HAC-associated Procedure   ▨ Combination Cluster - See Appendix G for code lists
▨ Non-OR-Affecting MS-DRG Assignment   New/Revised Text in **Orange**   ♂ Male   ♀ Female

504

2018 ICD-10-PCS

0 Medical and Surgical
T Urinary System
H Insertion: Putting in a nonbiological appliance that monitors, assists, performs, or prevents a physiological function but does not physically take the place of a body part

Body Part	Approach	Device	Qualifier
Character 4	**Character 5**	**Character 6**	**Character 7**
5 Kidney	0 Open 3 Percutaneous 4 Percutaneous Endoscopic 7 Via Natural or Artificial Opening 8 Via Natural or Artificial Opening Endoscopic	2 Monitoring Device 3 Infusion Device Y Other Device	Z No Qualifier
9 Ureter	0 Open 3 Percutaneous 4 Percutaneous Endoscopic 7 Via Natural or Artificial Opening 8 Via Natural or Artificial Opening Endoscopic	2 Monitoring Device 3 Infusion Device M Stimulator Lead Y Other Device	Z No Qualifier
B Bladder ᴺᶜ	0 Open 3 Percutaneous 4 Percutaneous Endoscopic 7 Via Natural or Artificial Opening 8 Via Natural or Artificial Opening Endoscopic	2 Monitoring Device 3 Infusion Device L Artificial Sphincter M Stimulator Lead Y Other Device	Z No Qualifier
C Bladder Neck	0 Open 3 Percutaneous 4 Percutaneous Endoscopic 7 Via Natural or Artificial Opening 8 Via Natural or Artificial Opening Endoscopic	L Artificial Sphincter	Z No Qualifier
D Urethra	0 Open 3 Percutaneous 4 Percutaneous Endoscopic 7 Via Natural or Artificial Opening 8 Via Natural or Artificial Opening Endoscopic	2 Monitoring Device 3 Infusion Device L Artificial Sphincter Y Other Device	Z No Qualifier
D Urethra	X External	2 Monitoring Device 3 Infusion Device L Artificial Sphincter	Z No Qualifier

ᴺᶜ 0THB0MZ 0THB3MZ 0THB4MZ 0THB7MZ 0THB8MZ

0 Medical and Surgical
T Urinary System
J Inspection: Visually and/or manually exploring a body part

Body Part	Approach	Device	Qualifier
Character 4	**Character 5**	**Character 6**	**Character 7**
5 Kidney 9 Ureter B Bladder D Urethra	0 Open 3 Percutaneous 4 Percutaneous Endoscopic 7 Via Natural or Artificial Opening 8 Via Natural or Artificial Opening Endoscopic X External	Z No Device	Z No Qualifier

0 Medical and Surgical
T Urinary System
L Occlusion: Completely closing an orifice or the lumen of a tubular body part

Body Part	Approach	Device	Qualifier
Character 4	Character 5	Character 6	Character 7
3 Kidney Pelvis, Right 4 Kidney Pelvis, Left 6 Ureter, Right 7 Ureter, Left B Bladder C Bladder Neck	0 Open 3 Percutaneous 4 Percutaneous Endoscopic	C Extraluminal Device D Intraluminal Device Z No Device	Z No Qualifier
3 Kidney Pelvis, Right 4 Kidney Pelvis, Left 6 Ureter, Right 7 Ureter, Left B Bladder C Bladder Neck	7 Via Natural or Artificial Opening 8 Via Natural or Artificial Opening Endoscopic	D Intraluminal Device Z No Device	Z No Qualifier
D Urethra	0 Open 3 Percutaneous 4 Percutaneous Endoscopic X External	C Extraluminal Device D Intraluminal Device Z No Device	Z No Qualifier
D Urethra	7 Via Natural or Artificial Opening 8 Via Natural or Artificial Opening Endoscopic	D Intraluminal Device Z No Device	Z No Qualifier

0 Medical and Surgical
T Urinary System
M Reattachment: Putting back in or on all or a portion of a separated body part to its normal location or other suitable location

Body Part	Approach	Device	Qualifier
Character 4	Character 5	Character 6	Character 7
0 Kidney, Right 1 Kidney, Left 2 Kidneys, Bilateral 3 Kidney Pelvis, Right 4 Kidney Pelvis, Left 6 Ureter, Right 7 Ureter, Left 8 Ureters, Bilateral B Bladder C Bladder Neck D Urethra	0 Open 4 Percutaneous Endoscopic	Z No Device	Z No Qualifier

0 Medical and Surgical
T Urinary System
N Release: Freeing a body part from an abnormal physical constraint by cutting or by the use of force

Body Part	Approach	Device	Qualifier
Character 4	Character 5	Character 6	Character 7
0 Kidney, Right 1 Kidney, Left 3 Kidney Pelvis, Right 4 Kidney Pelvis, Left 6 Ureter, Right 7 Ureter, Left B Bladder C Bladder Neck	0 Open 3 Percutaneous 4 Percutaneous Endoscopic 7 Via Natural or Artificial Opening 8 Via Natural or Artificial Opening Endoscopic	Z No Device	Z No Qualifier
D Urethra	0 Open 3 Percutaneous 4 Percutaneous Endoscopic 7 Via Natural or Artificial Opening 8 Via Natural or Artificial Opening Endoscopic X External	Z No Device	Z No Qualifier

LC Limited Coverage   NC Noncovered   HAC HAC-associated Procedure   CC Combination Cluster - See Appendix G for code lists
DRG Non-OR-Affecting MS-DRG Assignment   New/Revised Text in **Orange**   ♂ Male   ♀ Female

506

2018 ICD-10-PCS

0   Medical and Surgical
T   Urinary System
P   Removal: Taking out or off a device from a body part

Body Part	Approach	Device	Qualifier
Character 4	**Character 5**	**Character 6**	**Character 7**
5 Kidney	0 Open 3 Percutaneous 4 Percutaneous Endoscopic 7 Via Natural or Artificial Opening 8 Via Natural or Artificial Opening Endoscopic	0 Drainage Device 2 Monitoring Device 3 Infusion Device 7 Autologous Tissue Substitute C Extraluminal Device D Intraluminal Device J Synthetic Substitute K Nonautologous Tissue Substitute Y Other Device	Z No Qualifier
5 Kidney	X External	0 Drainage Device 2 Monitoring Device 3 Infusion Device D Intraluminal Device	Z No Qualifier
9 Ureter	0 Open 3 Percutaneous 4 Percutaneous Endoscopic 7 Via Natural or Artificial Opening 8 Via Natural or Artificial Opening Endoscopic	0 Drainage Device 2 Monitoring Device 3 Infusion Device 7 Autologous Tissue Substitute C Extraluminal Device D Intraluminal Device J Synthetic Substitute K Nonautologous Tissue Substitute M Stimulator Lead Y Other Device	Z No Qualifier
9 Ureter	X External	0 Drainage Device 2 Monitoring Device 3 Infusion Device D Intraluminal Device M Stimulator Lead	Z No Qualifier
B Bladder NC	0 Open 3 Percutaneous 4 Percutaneous Endoscopic 7 Via Natural or Artificial Opening 8 Via Natural or Artificial Opening Endoscopic	0 Drainage Device 2 Monitoring Device 3 Infusion Device 7 Autologous Tissue Substitute C Extraluminal Device D Intraluminal Device J Synthetic Substitute K Nonautologous Tissue Substitute L Artificial Sphincter M Stimulator Lead Y Other Device	Z No Qualifier
B Bladder	X External	0 Drainage Device 2 Monitoring Device 3 Infusion Device D Intraluminal Device L Artificial Sphincter M Stimulator Lead	Z No Qualifier
D Urethra	0 Open 3 Percutaneous 4 Percutaneous Endoscopic 7 Via Natural or Artificial Opening 8 Via Natural or Artificial Opening Endoscopic	0 Drainage Device 2 Monitoring Device 3 Infusion Device 7 Autologous Tissue Substitute C Extraluminal Device D Intraluminal Device J Synthetic Substitute K Nonautologous Tissue Substitute L Artificial Sphincter Y Other Device	Z No Qualifier

0TP continued on next page

LC Limited Coverage   NC Noncovered   HAC HAC-associated Procedure   CC Combination Cluster - See Appendix G for code lists
Non-OR-Affecting MS-DRG Assignment   New/Revised Text in **Orange**   ♂ Male   ♀ Female

0 Medical and Surgical
T Urinary System
P Removal: Taking out or off a device from a body part

0TP continued from previous page

Body Part	Approach	Device	Qualifier
Character 4	**Character 5**	**Character 6**	**Character 7**
D Urethra	**X** External	**0** Drainage Device **2** Monitoring Device **3** Infusion Device **D** Intraluminal Device **L** Artificial Sphincter	**Z** No Qualifier

NC 0TPB0MZ 0TPB3MZ 0TPB4MZ 0TPB7MZ 0TPB8MZ

0 Medical and Surgical
T Urinary System
Q Repair: Restoring, to the extent possible, a body part to its normal anatomic structure and function

Body Part	Approach	Device	Qualifier
Character 4	**Character 5**	**Character 6**	**Character 7**
0 Kidney, Right **1** Kidney, Left **3** Kidney Pelvis, Right **4** Kidney Pelvis, Left **6** Ureter, Right **7** Ureter, Left **B** Bladder CC **C** Bladder Neck	**0** Open **3** Percutaneous **4** Percutaneous Endoscopic **7** Via Natural or Artificial Opening **8** Via Natural or Artificial Opening Endoscopic	**Z** No Device	**Z** No Qualifier
D Urethra	**0** Open **3** Percutaneous **4** Percutaneous Endoscopic **7** Via Natural or Artificial Opening **8** Via Natural or Artificial Opening Endoscopic **X** External	**Z** No Device	**Z** No Qualifier

CC 0TQB0ZZ 0TQB3ZZ 0TQB4ZZ

0 Medical and Surgical
T Urinary System
R Replacement: Putting in or on biological or synthetic material that physically takes the place and/or function of all or a portion of a body part

Body Part	Approach	Device	Qualifier
Character 4	**Character 5**	**Character 6**	**Character 7**
3 Kidney Pelvis, Right **4** Kidney Pelvis, Left **6** Ureter, Right **7** Ureter, Left **B** Bladder **C** Bladder Neck	**0** Open **4** Percutaneous Endoscopic **7** Via Natural or Artificial Opening **8** Via Natural or Artificial Opening Endoscopic	**7** Autologous Tissue Substitute **J** Synthetic Substitute **K** Nonautologous Tissue Substitute	**Z** No Qualifier
D Urethra	**0** Open **4** Percutaneous Endoscopic **7** Via Natural or Artificial Opening **8** Via Natural or Artificial Opening Endoscopic **X** External	**7** Autologous Tissue Substitute **J** Synthetic Substitute **K** Nonautologous Tissue Substitute	**Z** No Qualifier

0 **Medical and Surgical**
T **Urinary System**
S **Reposition:** Moving to its normal location, or other suitable location, all or a portion of a body part

Body Part	Approach	Device	Qualifier
Character 4	Character 5	Character 6	Character 7
0 Kidney, Right **1** Kidney, Left **2** Kidneys, Bilateral **3** Kidney Pelvis, Right **4** Kidney Pelvis, Left **6** Ureter, Right **7** Ureter, Left **8** Ureters, Bilateral **B** Bladder **C** Bladder Neck **D** Urethra	**0** Open **4** Percutaneous Endoscopic	**Z** No Device	**Z** No Qualifier

0 **Medical and Surgical**
T **Urinary System**
T **Resection:** Cutting out or off, without replacement, all of a body part

Body Part	Approach	Device	Qualifier
Character 4	Character 5	Character 6	Character 7
0 Kidney, Right **1** Kidney, Left **2** Kidneys, Bilateral	**0** Open **4** Percutaneous Endoscopic	**Z** No Device	**Z** No Qualifier
3 Kidney Pelvis, Right **4** Kidney Pelvis, Left **6** Ureter, Right **7** Ureter, Left **B** Bladder ⟦CC⟧ **C** Bladder Neck **D** Urethra ⟦CC⟧	**0** Open **4** Percutaneous Endoscopic **7** Via Natural or Artificial Opening **8** Via Natural or Artificial Opening Endoscopic	**Z** No Device	**Z** No Qualifier

⟦CC⟧ 0TTB0ZZ   0TTD0ZZ

0 **Medical and Surgical**
T **Urinary System**
U **Supplement:** Putting in or on biological or synthetic material that physically reinforces and/or augments the function of a portion of a body part

Body Part	Approach	Device	Qualifier
Character 4	Character 5	Character 6	Character 7
3 Kidney Pelvis, Right **4** Kidney Pelvis, Left **6** Ureter, Right **7** Ureter, Left **B** Bladder **C** Bladder Neck	**0** Open **4** Percutaneous Endoscopic **7** Via Natural or Artificial Opening **8** Via Natural or Artificial Opening Endoscopic	**7** Autologous Tissue Substitute **J** Synthetic Substitute **K** Nonautologous Tissue Substitute	**Z** No Qualifier
D Urethra	**0** Open **4** Percutaneous Endoscopic **7** Via Natural or Artificial Opening **8** Via Natural or Artificial Opening Endoscopic **X** External	**7** Autologous Tissue Substitute **J** Synthetic Substitute **K** Nonautologous Tissue Substitute	**Z** No Qualifier

⟦LC⟧ Limited Coverage   ⟦NC⟧ Noncovered   ⟦HAC⟧ HAC-associated Procedure   ⟦CC⟧ Combination Cluster - See Appendix G for code lists
⟦DRG⟧ Non-OR-Affecting MS-DRG Assignment   New/Revised Text in Orange   ♂ Male   ♀ Female

2018 ICD-10-PCS

509

0 Medical and Surgical
T Urinary System
V Restriction: Partially closing an orifice or the lumen of a tubular body part

Body Part	Approach	Device	Qualifier
Character 4	Character 5	Character 6	Character 7
3 Kidney Pelvis, Right 4 Kidney Pelvis, Left 6 Ureter, Right 7 Ureter, Left B Bladder C Bladder Neck	0 Open 3 Percutaneous 4 Percutaneous Endoscopic	C Extraluminal Device D Intraluminal Device Z No Device	Z No Qualifier
3 Kidney Pelvis, Right 4 Kidney Pelvis, Left 6 Ureter, Right 7 Ureter, Left B Bladder C Bladder Neck	7 Via Natural or Artificial Opening 8 Via Natural or Artificial Opening Endoscopic	D Intraluminal Device Z No Device	Z No Qualifier
D Urethra	0 Open 3 Percutaneous 4 Percutaneous Endoscopic	C Extraluminal Device D Intraluminal Device Z No Device	Z No Qualifier
D Urethra	7 Via Natural or Artificial Opening 8 Via Natural or Artificial Opening Endoscopic	D Intraluminal Device Z No Device	Z No Qualifier
D Urethra	X External	Z No Device	Z No Qualifier

0 Medical and Surgical
T Urinary System
W Revision: Correcting, to the extent possible, a portion of a malfunctioning device or the position of a displaced device

Body Part	Approach	Device	Qualifier
Character 4	Character 5	Character 6	Character 7
5 Kidney	0 Open 3 Percutaneous 4 Percutaneous Endoscopic 7 Via Natural or Artificial Opening 8 Via Natural or Artificial Opening Endoscopic	0 Drainage Device 2 Monitoring Device 3 Infusion Device 7 Autologous Tissue Substitute C Extraluminal Device D Intraluminal Device J Synthetic Substitute K Nonautologous Tissue Substitute Y Other Device	Z No Qualifier
5 Kidney	X External	0 Drainage Device 2 Monitoring Device 3 Infusion Device 7 Autologous Tissue Substitute C Extraluminal Device D Intraluminal Device J Synthetic Substitute K Nonautologous Tissue Substitute	Z No Qualifier
9 Ureter	0 Open 3 Percutaneous 4 Percutaneous Endoscopic 7 Via Natural or Artificial Opening 8 Via Natural or Artificial Opening Endoscopic	0 Drainage Device 2 Monitoring Device 3 Infusion Device 7 Autologous Tissue Substitute C Extraluminal Device D Intraluminal Device J Synthetic Substitute K Nonautologous Tissue Substitute M Stimulator Lead Y Other Device	Z No Qualifier
9 Ureter	X External	0 Drainage Device 2 Monitoring Device 3 Infusion Device 7 Autologous Tissue Substitute C Extraluminal Device D Intraluminal Device J Synthetic Substitute K Nonautologous Tissue Substitute M Stimulator Lead	Z No Qualifier

0TW continued on next page

LC Limited Coverage   NC Noncovered   HAC HAC-associated Procedure   CC Combination Cluster - See Appendix G for code lists
DRG Non-OR-Affecting MS-DRG Assignment   New/Revised Text in **Orange**   ♂ Male   ♀ Female

0 Medical and Surgical
T Urinary System
W Revision: Correcting, to the extent possible, a portion of a malfunctioning device or the position of a displaced device

0TW continued from previous page

Body Part	Approach	Device	Qualifier
Character 4	**Character 5**	**Character 6**	**Character 7**
B Bladder	**0** Open **3** Percutaneous **4** Percutaneous Endoscopic **7** Via Natural or Artificial Opening **8** Via Natural or Artificial Opening Endoscopic	**0** Drainage Device **2** Monitoring Device **3** Infusion Device **7** Autologous Tissue Substitute **C** Extraluminal Device **D** Intraluminal Device **J** Synthetic Substitute **K** Nonautologous Tissue Substitute **L** Artificial Sphincter **M** Stimulator Lead Y Other Device	**Z** No Qualifier
B Bladder	**X** External	**0** Drainage Device **2** Monitoring Device **3** Infusion Device **7** Autologous Tissue Substitute **C** Extraluminal Device **D** Intraluminal Device **J** Synthetic Substitute **K** Nonautologous Tissue Substitute **L** Artificial Sphincter **M** Stimulator Lead	**Z** No Qualifier
D Urethra	**0** Open **3** Percutaneous **4** Percutaneous Endoscopic **7** Via Natural or Artificial Opening **8** Via Natural or Artificial Opening Endoscopic	**0** Drainage Device **2** Monitoring Device **3** Infusion Device **7** Autologous Tissue Substitute **C** Extraluminal Device **D** Intraluminal Device **J** Synthetic Substitute **K** Nonautologous Tissue Substitute **L** Artificial Sphincter Y Other Device	**Z** No Qualifier
D Urethra	**X** External	**0** Drainage Device **2** Monitoring Device **3** Infusion Device **7** Autologous Tissue Substitute **C** Extraluminal Device **D** Intraluminal Device **J** Synthetic Substitute **K** Nonautologous Tissue Substitute **L** Artificial Sphincter	**Z** No Qualifier

0 Medical and Surgical
T Urinary System
Y Transplantation: Putting in or on all or a portion of a living body part taken from another individual or animal to physically take the place and/or function of all or a portion of a similar body part

Body Part	Approach	Device	Qualifier
Character 4	**Character 5**	**Character 6**	**Character 7**
0 Kidney, Right 🅻🅲 🅲🅲 **1** Kidney, Left 🅻🅲 🅲🅲	**0** Open	**Z** No Device	**0** Allogeneic **1** Syngeneic **2** Zooplastic

🅻🅲 0TY00Z0   0TY00Z1   0TY00Z2   0TY10Z0   0TY10Z1   0TY10Z2
🅲🅲 0TY00Z0   0TY00Z1   0TY00Z2   0TY10Z0   0TY10Z1   0TY10Z2

🅻🅲 Limited Coverage   🅽🅲 Noncovered   HAC HAC-associated Procedure   🅲🅲 Combination Cluster - See Appendix G for code lists
DRG Non-OR-Affecting MS-DRG Assignment   New/Revised Text in **Orange**   ♂ Male   ♀ Female

2018 ICD-10-PCS   511

NOTES

Female Reproductive System 0U1-0UY

0   Medical and Surgical
U   Female Reproductive System
1   Bypass: Altering the route of passage of the contents of a tubular body part

Body Part	Approach	Device	Qualifier
Character 4	Character 5	Character 6	Character 7
5 Fallopian Tube, Right ♀ 6 Fallopian Tube, Left ♀	0 Open 4 Percutaneous Endoscopic	7 Autologous Tissue Substitute J Synthetic Substitute K Nonautologous Tissue Substitute Z No Device	5 Fallopian Tube, Right 6 Fallopian Tube, Left 9 Uterus

♀ 0U15075   0U15076   0U15079   0U150J5   0U150J6   0U150J9   0U150K5   0U150K6   0U150K9   0U150Z5   0U150Z6   0U150Z9   0U15475
0U15476   0U15479   0U154J5   0U154J6   0U154J9   0U154K5   0U154K6   0U154K9   0U154Z5   0U154Z6   0U154Z9   0U16075   0U16076
0U16079   0U160J5   0U160J6   0U160J9   0U160K5   0U160K6   0U160K9   0U160Z5   0U160Z6   0U160Z9   0U16475   0U16476   0U16479
0U164J5   0U164J6   0U164J9   0U164K5   0U164K6   0U164K9   0U164Z5   0U164Z6   0U164Z9

0   Medical and Surgical
U   Female Reproductive System
2   Change: Taking out or off a device from a body part and putting back an identical or similar device in or on the same body part without cutting or puncturing the skin or a mucous membrane

Body Part	Approach	Device	Qualifier
Character 4	Character 5	Character 6	Character 7
3 Ovary ♀ 8 Fallopian Tube ♀ M Vulva ♀	X External	0 Drainage Device Y Other Device	Z No Qualifier
D Uterus and Cervix ♀	X External	0 Drainage Device H Contraceptive Device Y Other Device	Z No Qualifier
H Vagina and Cul-de-sac ♀	X External	0 Drainage Device G Intraluminal Device, Pessary Y Other Device	Z No Qualifier

♀ 0U23X0Z   0U23XYZ   0U28X0Z   0U28XYZ   0U2DX0Z   0U2DXHZ   0U2DXYZ   0U2HX0Z   0U2HXGZ   0U2HXYZ   0U2MX0Z   0U2MXYZ

0   Medical and Surgical
U   Female Reproductive System
5   Destruction: Physical eradication of all or a portion of a body part by the direct use of energy, force, or a destructive agent

Body Part	Approach	Device	Qualifier
Character 4	Character 5	Character 6	Character 7
0 Ovary, Right ♀ 1 Ovary, Left ♀ 2 Ovaries, Bilateral ♀ 4 Uterine Supporting Structure ♀	0 Open 3 Percutaneous 4 Percutaneous Endoscopic 8 Via Natural or Artificial Opening Endoscopic	Z No Device	Z No Qualifier
5 Fallopian Tube, Right ♀ 6 Fallopian Tube, Left ♀ 7 Fallopian Tubes, Bilateral ♀ 9 Uterus ♀ B Endometrium ♀ C Cervix ♀ F Cul-de-sac ♀	0 Open 3 Percutaneous 4 Percutaneous Endoscopic 7 Via Natural or Artificial Opening 8 Via Natural or Artificial Opening Endoscopic	Z No Device	Z No Qualifier
G Vagina ♀ K Hymen ♀	0 Open 3 Percutaneous 4 Percutaneous Endoscopic 7 Via Natural or Artificial Opening 8 Via Natural or Artificial Opening Endoscopic X External	Z No Device	Z No Qualifier

0U5 continued on next page

0U5-0U8

0 **Medical and Surgical**
U **Female Reproductive System**

0U5 continued from previous page

5 **Destruction:** Physical eradication of all or a portion of a body part by the direct use of energy, force, or a destructive agent

Body Part	Approach	Device	Qualifier
Character 4	Character 5	Character 6	Character 7
J Clitoris ♀ **L** Vestibular Gland ♀ **M** Vulva ♀	**0** Open **X** External	**Z** No Device	**Z** No Qualifier

♀ 0U500ZZ 0U503ZZ 0U504ZZ 0U508ZZ 0U510ZZ 0U513ZZ 0U514ZZ 0U518ZZ 0U520ZZ 0U523ZZ 0U524ZZ 0U528ZZ 0U540ZZ
0U543ZZ 0U544ZZ 0U548ZZ 0U550ZZ 0U553ZZ 0U554ZZ 0U557ZZ 0U558ZZ 0U560ZZ 0U563ZZ 0U564ZZ 0U567ZZ 0U568ZZ
0U570ZZ 0U573ZZ 0U574ZZ 0U577ZZ 0U578ZZ 0U590ZZ 0U593ZZ 0U594ZZ 0U597ZZ 0U598ZZ 0U5B0ZZ 0U5B3ZZ 0U5B4ZZ
0U5B7ZZ 0U5B8ZZ 0U5C0ZZ 0U5C3ZZ 0U5C4ZZ 0U5C7ZZ 0U5C8ZZ 0U5F0ZZ 0U5F3ZZ 0U5F4ZZ 0U5F7ZZ 0U5F8ZZ 0U5G0ZZ
0U5G3ZZ 0U5G4ZZ 0U5G7ZZ 0U5G8ZZ 0U5GXZZ 0U5J0ZZ 0U5JXZZ 0U5K0ZZ 0U5K3ZZ 0U5K4ZZ 0U5K7ZZ 0U5K8ZZ 0U5KXZZ
0U5L0ZZ 0U5LXZZ 0U5M0ZZ 0U5MXZZ

0 **Medical and Surgical**
U **Female Reproductive System**
7 **Dilation:** Expanding an orifice or the lumen of a tubular body part

Body Part	Approach	Device	Qualifier
Character 4	Character 5	Character 6	Character 7
5 Fallopian Tube, Right ♀ **6** Fallopian Tube, Left ♀ **7** Fallopian Tubes, Bilateral ♀ **9** Uterus ♀ **C** Cervix ♀ **G** Vagina ♀	**0** Open **3** Percutaneous **4** Percutaneous Endoscopic **7** Via Natural or Artificial Opening **8** Via Natural or Artificial Opening Endoscopic	**D** Intraluminal Device **Z** No Device	**Z** No Qualifier
K Hymen ♀	**0** Open **3** Percutaneous **4** Percutaneous Endoscopic **7** Via Natural or Artificial Opening **8** Via Natural or Artificial Opening Endoscopic **X** External	**D** Intraluminal Device **Z** No Device	**Z** No Qualifier

♀ 0U750DZ 0U750ZZ 0U753DZ 0U753ZZ 0U754DZ 0U754ZZ 0U757DZ 0U757ZZ 0U758DZ 0U758ZZ 0U760DZ 0U760ZZ 0U763DZ
0U763ZZ 0U764DZ 0U764ZZ 0U767DZ 0U767ZZ 0U768DZ 0U768ZZ 0U770DZ 0U770ZZ 0U773DZ 0U773ZZ 0U774DZ 0U774ZZ
0U777DZ 0U777ZZ 0U778DZ 0U778ZZ 0U790DZ 0U790ZZ 0U793DZ 0U793ZZ 0U794DZ 0U794ZZ 0U797DZ 0U797ZZ 0U798DZ
0U798ZZ 0U7C0DZ 0U7C0ZZ 0U7C3DZ 0U7C3ZZ 0U7C4DZ 0U7C4ZZ 0U7C7DZ 0U7C7ZZ 0U7C8DZ 0U7C8ZZ 0U7G0DZ 0U7G0ZZ
0U7G3DZ 0U7G3ZZ 0U7G4DZ 0U7G4ZZ 0U7G7DZ 0U7G7ZZ 0U7G8DZ 0U7G8ZZ 0U7K0DZ 0U7K0ZZ 0U7K3DZ 0U7K3ZZ 0U7K4DZ
0U7K4ZZ 0U7K7DZ 0U7K7ZZ 0U7K8DZ 0U7K8ZZ 0U7KXDZ 0U7KXZZ

0 **Medical and Surgical**
U **Female Reproductive System**
8 **Division:** Cutting into a body part, without draining fluids and/or gases from the body part, in order to separate or transect a body part

Body Part	Approach	Device	Qualifier
Character 4	Character 5	Character 6	Character 7
0 Ovary, Right ♀ **1** Ovary, Left ♀ **2** Ovaries, Bilateral ♀ **4** Uterine Supporting Structure ♀	**0** Open **3** Percutaneous **4** Percutaneous Endoscopic	**Z** No Device	**Z** No Qualifier
K Hymen ♀	**7** Via Natural or Artificial Opening **8** Via Natural or Artificial Opening Endoscopic **X** External	**Z** No Device	**Z** No Qualifier

♀ 0U800ZZ 0U803ZZ 0U804ZZ 0U810ZZ 0U813ZZ 0U814ZZ 0U820ZZ 0U823ZZ 0U824ZZ 0U840ZZ 0U843ZZ 0U844ZZ 0U8K7ZZ
0U8K8ZZ 0U8KXZZ

LC Limited Coverage **NC** Noncovered **HAC** HAC-associated Procedure **CC** Combination Cluster - See Appendix G for code lists
DNA Non-OR-Affecting MS-DRG Assignment New/Revised Text in **Orange** ♂ Male ♀ Female

514

2018 ICD-10-PCS

0 Medical and Surgical
U Female Reproductive System
9 Drainage: Taking or letting out fluids and/or gases from a body part

Body Part	Approach	Device	Qualifier
Character 4	Character 5	Character 6	Character 7
0 Ovary, Right ♀ **1** Ovary, Left ♀ **2** Ovaries, Bilateral ♀	**0** Open **3** Percutaneous **4** Percutaneous Endoscopic **8** Via Natural or Artificial Opening Endoscopic	**0** Drainage Device	**Z** No Qualifier
0 Ovary, Right ♀ **1** Ovary, Left ♀ **2** Ovaries, Bilateral ♀	**0** Open **3** Percutaneous **4** Percutaneous Endoscopic **8** Via Natural or Artificial Opening Endoscopic	**Z** No Device	**X** Diagnostic **Z** No Qualifier
0 Ovary, Right ♀ **1** Ovary, Left ♀ **2** Ovaries, Bilateral ♀	**X** External	**Z** No Device	**Z** No Qualifier
4 Uterine Supporting Structure ♀	**0** Open **3** Percutaneous **4** Percutaneous Endoscopic **8** Via Natural or Artificial Opening Endoscopic	**0** Drainage Device	**Z** No Qualifier
4 Uterine Supporting Structure ♀	**0** Open **3** Percutaneous **4** Percutaneous Endoscopic **8** Via Natural or Artificial Opening Endoscopic	**Z** No Device	**X** Diagnostic **Z** No Qualifier
5 Fallopian Tube, Right ♀ **6** Fallopian Tube, Left ♀ **7** Fallopian Tubes, Bilateral ♀ **9** Uterus ♀ **C** Cervix ♀ **F** Cul-de-sac ♀	**0** Open **3** Percutaneous **4** Percutaneous Endoscopic **7** Via Natural or Artificial Opening **8** Via Natural or Artificial Opening Endoscopic	**0** Drainage Device	**Z** No Qualifier
5 Fallopian Tube, Right ♀ **6** Fallopian Tube, Left ♀ **7** Fallopian Tubes, Bilateral ♀ **9** Uterus ♀ **C** Cervix ♀ **F** Cul-de-sac ♀	**0** Open **3** Percutaneous **4** Percutaneous Endoscopic **7** Via Natural or Artificial Opening **8** Via Natural or Artificial Opening Endoscopic	**Z** No Device	**X** Diagnostic **Z** No Qualifier
G Vagina ♀ **K** Hymen ♀	**0** Open **3** Percutaneous **4** Percutaneous Endoscopic **7** Via Natural or Artificial Opening **8** Via Natural or Artificial Opening Endoscopic **X** External	**0** Drainage Device	**Z** No Qualifier
G Vagina ♀ **K** Hymen ♀	**0** Open **3** Percutaneous **4** Percutaneous Endoscopic **7** Via Natural or Artificial Opening **8** Via Natural or Artificial Opening Endoscopic **X** External	**Z** No Device	**X** Diagnostic **Z** No Qualifier
J Clitoris ♀ **L** Vestibular Gland ♀ **M** Vulva ♀	**0** Open **X** External	**0** Drainage Device	**Z** No Qualifier
J Clitoris ♀ **L** Vestibular Gland ♀ **M** Vulva ♀	**0** Open **X** External	**Z** No Device	**X** Diagnostic **Z** No Qualifier

0U9 continued on next page

0U9 continued from previous page

♀ 0U9000Z 0U900ZX 0U900ZZ 0U9030Z 0U903ZX 0U903ZZ 0U9040Z 0U904ZX 0U904ZZ 0U9080Z 0U908ZX 0U908ZZ 0U90XZZ
0U9100Z 0U910ZX 0U910ZZ 0U9130Z 0U913ZX 0U913ZZ 0U9140Z 0U914ZX 0U914ZZ 0U9180Z 0U918ZX 0U918ZZ 0U91XZZ
0U9200Z 0U920ZX 0U920ZZ 0U9230Z 0U923ZX 0U923ZZ 0U9240Z 0U924ZX 0U924ZZ 0U9280Z 0U928ZX 0U928ZZ 0U92XZZ
0U9400Z 0U940ZX 0U940ZZ 0U9430Z 0U943ZX 0U943ZZ 0U9440Z 0U944ZX 0U944ZZ 0U9480Z 0U948ZX 0U948ZZ 0U9500Z
0U950ZX 0U950ZZ 0U9530Z 0U953ZX 0U953ZZ 0U9540Z 0U954ZX 0U954ZZ 0U9570Z 0U957ZX 0U957ZZ 0U9580Z 0U958ZX
0U958ZZ 0U9600Z 0U960ZX 0U960ZZ 0U9630Z 0U963ZX 0U963ZZ 0U9640Z 0U964ZX 0U964ZZ 0U9670Z 0U967ZX 0U967ZZ
0U9680Z 0U968ZX 0U968ZZ 0U9700Z 0U970ZX 0U970ZZ 0U9730Z 0U973ZX 0U973ZZ 0U9740Z 0U974ZX 0U974ZZ 0U9770Z
0U977ZX 0U977ZZ 0U9780Z 0U978ZX 0U978ZZ 0U9900Z 0U990ZX 0U990ZZ 0U9930Z 0U993ZX 0U993ZZ 0U9940Z 0U994ZX
0U994ZZ 0U9970Z 0U997ZX 0U997ZZ 0U9980Z 0U998ZX 0U998ZZ 0U9C00Z 0U9C0ZX 0U9C0ZZ 0U9C30Z 0U9C3ZX 0U9C3ZZ
0U9C40Z 0U9C4ZX 0U9C4ZZ 0U9C70Z 0U9C7ZX 0U9C7ZZ 0U9C80Z 0U9C8ZX 0U9C8ZZ 0U9F00Z 0U9F0ZX 0U9F0ZZ 0U9F30Z
0U9F3ZX 0U9F3ZZ 0U9F40Z 0U9F4ZX 0U9F4ZZ 0U9F70Z 0U9F7ZX 0U9F7ZZ 0U9F80Z 0U9F8ZX 0U9F8ZZ 0U9G00Z 0U9G0ZX
0U9G0ZZ 0U9G30Z 0U9G3ZX 0U9G3ZZ 0U9G40Z 0U9G4ZX 0U9G70Z 0U9G7ZX 0U9G7ZZ 0U9G80Z 0U9G8ZX 0U9G8ZZ
0U9GX0Z 0U9GXZX 0U9GXZZ 0U9J00Z 0U9J0ZX 0U9J0ZZ 0U9JX0Z 0U9JXZX 0U9JXZZ 0U9K00Z 0U9K0ZX 0U9K0ZZ 0U9K30Z
0U9K3ZX 0U9K3ZZ 0U9K40Z 0U9K4ZX 0U9K4ZZ 0U9K70Z 0U9K7ZX 0U9K7ZZ 0U9K80Z 0U9K8ZX 0U9K8ZZ 0U9KX0Z 0U9KXZX
0U9KXZZ 0U9L00Z 0U9L0ZX 0U9L0ZZ 0U9LX0Z 0U9LXZX 0U9LXZZ 0U9M00Z 0U9M0ZX 0U9M0ZZ 0U9MX0Z 0U9MXZX 0U9MXZZ

0 **Medical and Surgical**
U **Female Reproductive System**
B **Excision:** Cutting out or off, without replacement, a portion of a body part

Body Part	Approach	Device	Qualifier
Character 4	Character 5	Character 6	Character 7
0 Ovary, Right ♀ **1** Ovary, Left ♀ **2** Ovaries, Bilateral ♀ **4** Uterine Supporting Structure ♀ **5** Fallopian Tube, Right ♀ **6** Fallopian Tube, Left ♀ **7** Fallopian Tubes, Bilateral ♀ **9** Uterus ♀ **C** Cervix ♀ **F** Cul-de-sac ♀	**0** Open **3** Percutaneous **4** Percutaneous Endoscopic **7** Via Natural or Artificial Opening **8** Via Natural or Artificial Opening Endoscopic	**Z** No Device	**X** Diagnostic **Z** No Qualifier
G Vagina ♀ **K** Hymen ♀	**0** Open **3** Percutaneous **4** Percutaneous Endoscopic **7** Via Natural or Artificial Opening **8** Via Natural or Artificial Opening Endoscopic **X** External	**Z** No Device	**X** Diagnostic **Z** No Qualifier
J Clitoris ♀ **L** Vestibular Gland ♀ **M** Vulva ♀	**0** Open **X** External	**Z** No Device	**X** Diagnostic **Z** No Qualifier

♀ 0UB00ZX 0UB00ZZ 0UB03ZX 0UB03ZZ 0UB04ZX 0UB04ZZ 0UB07ZX 0UB07ZZ 0UB08ZX 0UB08ZZ 0UB10ZX 0UB10ZZ 0UB13ZX
0UB13ZZ 0UB14ZX 0UB14ZZ 0UB17ZX 0UB17ZZ 0UB18ZX 0UB18ZZ 0UB20ZX 0UB20ZZ 0UB23ZX 0UB23ZZ 0UB24ZX 0UB24ZZ
0UB27ZX 0UB27ZZ 0UB28ZX 0UB28ZZ 0UB40ZX 0UB40ZZ 0UB43ZX 0UB43ZZ 0UB44ZX 0UB44ZZ 0UB47ZX 0UB47ZZ 0UB48ZX
0UB48ZZ 0UB50ZX 0UB50ZZ 0UB53ZX 0UB53ZZ 0UB54ZX 0UB54ZZ 0UB57ZX 0UB57ZZ 0UB58ZX 0UB58ZZ 0UB60ZX 0UB60ZZ
0UB63ZX 0UB63ZZ 0UB64ZX 0UB64ZZ 0UB67ZX 0UB67ZZ 0UB68ZX 0UB68ZZ 0UB70ZX 0UB70ZZ 0UB73ZX 0UB73ZZ 0UB74ZX
0UB74ZZ 0UB77ZX 0UB77ZZ 0UB78ZX 0UB78ZZ 0UB90ZX 0UB90ZZ 0UB93ZX 0UB93ZZ 0UB94ZX 0UB94ZZ 0UB97ZX 0UB97ZZ
0UB98ZX 0UB98ZZ 0UBC0ZX 0UBC0ZZ 0UBC3ZX 0UBC3ZZ 0UBC4ZX 0UBC4ZZ 0UBC7ZX 0UBC7ZZ 0UBC8ZX 0UBC8ZZ 0UBF0ZX
0UBF0ZZ 0UBF3ZX 0UBF3ZZ 0UBF4ZX 0UBF4ZZ 0UBF7ZX 0UBF7ZZ 0UBF8ZX 0UBF8ZZ 0UBG0ZX 0UBG0ZZ 0UBG3ZX 0UBG3ZZ
0UBG4ZX 0UBG4ZZ 0UBG7ZX 0UBG7ZZ 0UBG8ZZ 0UBGXZX 0UBGXZZ 0UBJ0ZX 0UBJ0ZZ 0UBJXZX 0UBJXZZ 0UBK0ZX
0UBK0ZZ 0UBK3ZX 0UBK3ZZ 0UBK4ZX 0UBK4ZZ 0UBK7ZX 0UBK7ZZ 0UBK8ZX 0UBK8ZZ 0UBKXZX 0UBKXZZ 0UBL0ZX 0UBL0ZZ
0UBLXZX 0UBLXZZ 0UBM0ZX 0UBM0ZZ 0UBMXZX 0UBMXZZ

0 Medical and Surgical
U Female Reproductive System
C Extirpation: Taking or cutting out solid matter from a body part

Body Part	Approach	Device	Qualifier
Character 4	Character 5	Character 6	Character 7
0 Ovary, Right ♀ **1** Ovary, Left ♀ **2** Ovaries, Bilateral ♀ **4** Uterine Supporting Structure ♀	**0** Open **3** Percutaneous **4** Percutaneous Endoscopic **8** Via Natural or Artificial Opening Endoscopic	**Z** No Device	**Z** No Qualifier
5 Fallopian Tube, Right ♀ **6** Fallopian Tube, Left ♀ **7** Fallopian Tubes, Bilateral ♀ **9** Uterus ♀ **B** Endometrium ♀ **C** Cervix ♀ **F** Cul-de-sac ♀	**0** Open **3** Percutaneous **4** Percutaneous Endoscopic **7** Via Natural or Artificial Opening **8** Via Natural or Artificial Opening Endoscopic	**Z** No Device	**Z** No Qualifier
G Vagina ♀ **K** Hymen ♀	**0** Open **3** Percutaneous **4** Percutaneous Endoscopic **7** Via Natural or Artificial Opening **8** Via Natural or Artificial Opening Endoscopic **X** External	**Z** No Device	**Z** No Qualifier
J Clitoris ♀ **L** Vestibular Gland ♀ **M** Vulva ♀	**0** Open **X** External	**Z** No Device	**Z** No Qualifier

♀ 0UC00ZZ 0UC03ZZ 0UC04ZZ 0UC08ZZ 0UC10ZZ 0UC13ZZ 0UC14ZZ 0UC18ZZ 0UC20ZZ 0UC23ZZ 0UC24ZZ 0UC28ZZ 0UC40ZZ
0UC43ZZ 0UC44ZZ 0UC48ZZ 0UC50ZZ 0UC53ZZ 0UC54ZZ 0UC57ZZ 0UC58ZZ 0UC60ZZ 0UC63ZZ 0UC64ZZ 0UC67ZZ 0UC68ZZ
0UC70ZZ 0UC73ZZ 0UC74ZZ 0UC77ZZ 0UC78ZZ 0UC90ZZ 0UC93ZZ 0UC94ZZ 0UC97ZZ 0UC98ZZ 0UCB0ZZ 0UCB3ZZ 0UCB4ZZ
0UCB7ZZ 0UCB8ZZ 0UCC0ZZ 0UCC3ZZ 0UCC4ZZ 0UCC7ZZ 0UCC8ZZ 0UCF0ZZ 0UCF3ZZ 0UCF4ZZ 0UCF7ZZ 0UCF8ZZ 0UCG0ZZ
0UCG3ZZ 0UCG4ZZ 0UCG7ZZ 0UCG8ZZ 0UCGXZZ 0UCJ0ZZ 0UCJXZZ 0UCK0ZZ 0UCK3ZZ 0UCK4ZZ 0UCK7ZZ 0UCK8ZZ 0UCKXZZ
0UCL0ZZ 0UCLXZZ 0UCM0ZZ 0UCMXZZ

0 Medical and Surgical
U Female Reproductive System
D Extraction: Pulling or stripping out or off all or a portion of a body part by the use of force

Body Part	Approach	Device	Qualifier
Character 4	Character 5	Character 6	Character 7
B Endometrium ♀	**7** Via Natural or Artificial Opening **8** Via Natural or Artificial Opening Endoscopic	**Z** No Device	**X** Diagnostic **Z** No Qualifier
N Ova ♀	**0** Open **3** Percutaneous **4** Percutaneous Endoscopic	**Z** No Device	**Z** No Qualifier

♀ 0UDB7ZX 0UDB7ZZ 0UDB8ZX 0UDB8ZZ 0UDN0ZZ 0UDN3ZZ 0UDN4ZZ

0 Medical and Surgical
U Female Reproductive System
F Fragmentation: Breaking solid matter in a body part into pieces

Body Part	Approach	Device	Qualifier
Character 4	Character 5	Character 6	Character 7
5 Fallopian Tube, Right NC ♀ **6** Fallopian Tube, Left NC ♀ **7** Fallopian Tubes, Bilateral NC ♀ **9** Uterus NC ♀	**0** Open **3** Percutaneous **4** Percutaneous Endoscopic **7** Via Natural or Artificial Opening **8** Via Natural or Artificial Opening Endoscopic **X** External	**Z** No Device	**Z** No Qualifier

♀ 0UF50ZZ 0UF53ZZ 0UF54ZZ 0UF57ZZ 0UF58ZZ 0UF5XZZ 0UF60ZZ 0UF63ZZ 0UF64ZZ 0UF67ZZ 0UF68ZZ 0UF6XZZ 0UF70ZZ
0UF73ZZ 0UF74ZZ 0UF77ZZ 0UF78ZZ 0UF7XZZ 0UF90ZZ 0UF93ZZ 0UF94ZZ 0UF97ZZ 0UF98ZZ 0UF9XZZ
NC 0UF5XZZ 0UF6XZZ 0UF7XZZ 0UF9XZZ

0 **Medical and Surgical**
U **Female Reproductive System**
H **Insertion:** Putting in a nonbiological appliance that monitors, assists, performs, or prevents a physiological function but does not physically take the place of a body part

Body Part	Approach	Device	Qualifier
Character 4	Character 5	Character 6	Character 7
3 Ovary ♀	0 Open 3 Percutaneous 4 Percutaneous Endoscopic	3 Infusion Device Y Other Device	Z No Qualifier
3 Ovary ♀	7 Via Natural or Artificial Opening 8 Via Natural or Artificial Opening Endoscopic	Y Other Device	Z No Qualifier
8 Fallopian Tube ♀ D Uterus and Cervix ♀ H Vagina and Cul-de-sac ♀	0 Open 3 Percutaneous 4 Percutaneous Endoscopic 7 Via Natural or Artificial Opening 8 Via Natural or Artificial Opening Endoscopic	3 Infusion Device Y Other Device	Z No Qualifier
9 Uterus ♀	0 Open 7 Via Natural or Artificial Opening 8 Via Natural or Artificial Opening Endoscopic	H Contraceptive Device	Z No Qualifier
C Cervix ♀	0 Open 3 Percutaneous 4 Percutaneous Endoscopic	1 Radioactive Element	Z No Qualifier
C Cervix ♀	7 Via Natural or Artificial Opening 8 Via Natural or Artificial Opening Endoscopic	1 Radioactive Element H Contraceptive Device	Z No Qualifier
F Cul-de-sac ♀	7 Via Natural or Artificial Opening 8 Via Natural or Artificial Opening Endoscopic	G Intraluminal Device, Pessary	Z No Qualifier
G Vagina ♀	0 Open 3 Percutaneous 4 Percutaneous Endoscopic X External	1 Radioactive Element	Z No Qualifier
G Vagina ♀	7 Via Natural or Artificial Opening 8 Via Natural or Artificial Opening Endoscopic	1 Radioactive Element G Intraluminal Device, Pessary	Z No Qualifier

♀ 0UH303Z   0UH30YZ   0UH333Z   0UH33YZ   0UH343Z   0UH34YZ   0UH37YZ   0UH38YZ   0UH803Z   0UH80YZ   0UH833Z   0UH83YZ   0UH843Z
0UH84YZ   0UH873Z   0UH87YZ   0UH883Z   0UH88YZ   0UH90HZ   0UH97HZ   0UH98HZ   0UHC01Z   0UHC31Z   0UHC41Z   0UHC71Z   0UHC7HZ
0UHC81Z   0UHC8HZ   0UHD03Z   0UHD0YZ   0UHD33Z   0UHD3YZ   0UHD43Z   0UHD4YZ   0UHD73Z   0UHD7YZ   0UHD83Z   0UHD8YZ   0UHF7GZ
0UHF8GZ   0UHG01Z   0UHG31Z   0UHG41Z   0UHG71Z   0UHG7GZ   0UHG81Z   0UHG8GZ   0UHGX1Z   0UHH03Z   0UHH0YZ   0UHH33Z   0UHH3YZ
0UHH43Z   0UHH4YZ   0UHH73Z   0UHH7YZ   0UHH83Z   0UHH8YZ

0 **Medical and Surgical**
U **Female Reproductive System**
J **Inspection:** Visually and/or manually exploring a body part

Body Part	Approach	Device	Qualifier
Character 4	Character 5	Character 6	Character 7
3 Ovary ♀	0 Open 3 Percutaneous 4 Percutaneous Endoscopic 8 Via Natural or Artificial Opening Endoscopic X External	Z No Device	Z No Qualifier

0UJ continued on next page

0 **Medical and Surgical**
U **Female Reproductive System**
J **Inspection:** Visually and/or manually exploring a body part

0UJ continued from previous page

Body Part	Approach	Device	Qualifier
Character 4	Character 5	Character 6	Character 7
8 Fallopian Tube ♀ **D** Uterus and Cervix ♀ **H** Vagina and Cul-de-sac ♀	**0** Open **3** Percutaneous **4** Percutaneous Endoscopic **7** Via Natural or Artificial Opening **8** Via Natural or Artificial Opening Endoscopic **X** External	**Z** No Device	**Z** No Qualifier
M Vulva ♀	**0** Open **X** External	**Z** No Device	**Z** No Qualifier

♀ 0UJ30ZZ   0UJ33ZZ   0UJ34ZZ   0UJ38ZZ   0UJ3XZZ   0UJ80ZZ   0UJ83ZZ   0UJ84ZZ   0UJ87ZZ   0UJ88ZZ   0UJ8XZZ   0UJD0ZZ   0UJD3ZZ
0UJD4ZZ   0UJD7ZZ   0UJD8ZZ   0UJDXZZ   0UJH0ZZ   0UJH3ZZ   0UJH4ZZ   0UJH7ZZ   0UJH8ZZ   0UJHXZZ   0UJM0ZZ   0UJMXZZ

0 **Medical and Surgical**
U **Female Reproductive System**
L **Occlusion:** Completely closing an orifice or the lumen of a tubular body part

Body Part	Approach	Device	Qualifier
Character 4	Character 5	Character 6	Character 7
5 Fallopian Tube, Right ♀ **6** Fallopian Tube, Left ♀ **7** Fallopian Tubes, Bilateral ♀	**0** Open **3** Percutaneous **4** Percutaneous Endoscopic	**C** Extraluminal Device **D** Intraluminal Device **Z** No Device	**Z** No Qualifier
5 Fallopian Tube, Right ♀ **6** Fallopian Tube, Left ♀ **7** Fallopian Tubes, Bilateral ♀	**7** Via Natural or Artificial Opening **8** Via Natural or Artificial Opening Endoscopic	**D** Intraluminal Device **Z** No Device	**Z** No Qualifier
F Cul-de-sac ♀ **G** Vagina ♀	**7** Via Natural or Artificial Opening **8** Via Natural or Artificial Opening Endoscopic	**D** Intraluminal Device **Z** No Device	**Z** No Qualifier

♀ 0UL50CZ   0UL50DZ   0UL50ZZ   0UL53CZ   0UL53DZ   0UL53ZZ   0UL54CZ   0UL54DZ   0UL54ZZ   0UL57DZ   0UL57ZZ   0UL58DZ   0UL58ZZ
0UL60CZ   0UL60DZ   0UL60ZZ   0UL63CZ   0UL63DZ   0UL63ZZ   0UL64CZ   0UL64DZ   0UL64ZZ   0UL67DZ   0UL67ZZ   0UL68DZ   0UL68ZZ
0UL70CZ   0UL70DZ   0UL70ZZ   0UL73CZ   0UL73DZ   0UL73ZZ   0UL74CZ   0UL74DZ   0UL74ZZ   0UL77DZ   0UL77ZZ   0UL78DZ   0UL78ZZ
0ULF7DZ   0ULF7ZZ   0ULF8DZ   0ULF8ZZ   0ULG7DZ   0ULG7ZZ   0ULG8DZ   0ULG8ZZ

0 **Medical and Surgical**
U **Female Reproductive System**
M **Reattachment:** Putting back in or on all or a portion of a separated body part to its normal location or other suitable location

Body Part	Approach	Device	Qualifier
Character 4	Character 5	Character 6	Character 7
0 Ovary, Right ♀ **1** Ovary, Left ♀ **2** Ovaries, Bilateral ♀ **4** Uterine Supporting Structure ♀ **5** Fallopian Tube, Right ♀ **6** Fallopian Tube, Left ♀ **7** Fallopian Tubes, Bilateral ♀ **9** Uterus ♀ **C** Cervix ♀ **F** Cul-de-sac ♀ **G** Vagina ♀	**0** Open **4** Percutaneous Endoscopic	**Z** No Device	**Z** No Qualifier
J Clitoris ♀ **M** Vulva ♀	**X** External	**Z** No Device	**Z** No Qualifier
K Hymen ♀	**0** Open **4** Percutaneous Endoscopic **X** External	**Z** No Device	**Z** No Qualifier

♀ 0UM00ZZ   0UM04ZZ   0UM10ZZ   0UM14ZZ   0UM20ZZ   0UM24ZZ   0UM40ZZ   0UM44ZZ   0UM50ZZ   0UM54ZZ   0UM60ZZ   0UM64ZZ   0UM70ZZ
0UM74ZZ   0UM90ZZ   0UM94ZZ   0UMC0ZZ   0UMC4ZZ   0UMF0ZZ   0UMF4ZZ   0UMG0ZZ   0UMG4ZZ   0UMJXZZ   0UMK0ZZ   0UMK4ZZ   0UMKXZZ
0UMMXZZ

[LC] Limited Coverage   [NC] Noncovered   [HAC] HAC-associated Procedure   [CC] Combination Cluster - See Appendix G for code lists
[DRG] Non-OR-Affecting MS-DRG Assignment   New/Revised Text in **Orange**   ♂ Male   ♀ Female

2018 ICD-10-PCS

519

0 Medical and Surgical
U Female Reproductive System
N Release: Freeing a body part from an abnormal physical constraint by cutting or by the use of force

Body Part	Approach	Device	Qualifier
Character 4	Character 5	Character 6	Character 7
0 Ovary, Right ♀ 1 Ovary, Left ♀ 2 Ovaries, Bilateral ♀ 4 Uterine Supporting Structure ♀	0 Open 3 Percutaneous 4 Percutaneous Endoscopic 8 Via Natural or Artificial Opening Endoscopic	Z No Device	Z No Qualifier
5 Fallopian Tube, Right ♀ 6 Fallopian Tube, Left ♀ 7 Fallopian Tubes, Bilateral ♀ 9 Uterus ♀ C Cervix ♀ F Cul-de-sac ♀	0 Open 3 Percutaneous 4 Percutaneous Endoscopic 7 Via Natural or Artificial Opening 8 Via Natural or Artificial Opening Endoscopic	Z No Device	Z No Qualifier
G Vagina ♀ K Hymen ♀	0 Open 3 Percutaneous 4 Percutaneous Endoscopic 7 Via Natural or Artificial Opening 8 Via Natural or Artificial Opening Endoscopic X External	Z No Device	Z No Qualifier
J Clitoris ♀ L Vestibular Gland ♀ M Vulva ♀	0 Open X External	Z No Device	Z No Qualifier

♀ 0UN00ZZ 0UN03ZZ 0UN04ZZ 0UN08ZZ 0UN10ZZ 0UN13ZZ 0UN14ZZ 0UN18ZZ 0UN20ZZ 0UN23ZZ 0UN24ZZ 0UN28ZZ 0UN40ZZ
0UN43ZZ 0UN44ZZ 0UN48ZZ 0UN50ZZ 0UN53ZZ 0UN54ZZ 0UN57ZZ 0UN58ZZ 0UN60ZZ 0UN63ZZ 0UN64ZZ 0UN67ZZ 0UN68ZZ
0UN70ZZ 0UN73ZZ 0UN74ZZ 0UN77ZZ 0UN78ZZ 0UN90ZZ 0UN93ZZ 0UN94ZZ 0UN97ZZ 0UN98ZZ 0UNC0ZZ 0UNC3ZZ 0UNC4ZZ
0UNC7ZZ 0UNC8ZZ 0UNF0ZZ 0UNF3ZZ 0UNF4ZZ 0UNF7ZZ 0UNF8ZZ 0UNG0ZZ 0UNG3ZZ 0UNG4ZZ 0UNG7ZZ 0UNG8ZZ 0UNGXZZ
0UNJ0ZZ 0UNJXZZ 0UNK0ZZ 0UNK3ZZ 0UNK4ZZ 0UNK7ZZ 0UNK8ZZ 0UNKXZZ 0UNL0ZZ 0UNLXZZ 0UNM0ZZ 0UNMXZZ

0 Medical and Surgical
U Female Reproductive System
P Removal: Taking out or off a device from a body part

Body Part	Approach	Device	Qualifier
Character 4	Character 5	Character 6	Character 7
3 Ovary ♀	0 Open 3 Percutaneous 4 Percutaneous Endoscopic	0 Drainage Device 3 Infusion Device Y Other Device	Z No Qualifier
3 Ovary ♀	7 Via Natural or Artificial Opening 8 Via Natural or Artificial Opening Endoscopic	Y Other Device	Z No Qualifier
3 Ovary ♀	X External	0 Drainage Device 3 Infusion Device	Z No Qualifier
8 Fallopian Tube ♀	0 Open 3 Percutaneous 4 Percutaneous Endoscopic 7 Via Natural or Artificial Opening 8 Via Natural or Artificial Opening Endoscopic	0 Drainage Device 3 Infusion Device 7 Autologous Tissue Substitute C Extraluminal Device D Intraluminal Device J Synthetic Substitute K Nonautologous Tissue Substitute Y Other Device	Z No Qualifier
8 Fallopian Tube ♀	X External	0 Drainage Device 3 Infusion Device D Intraluminal Device	Z No Qualifier

0UP continued on next page

LC Limited Coverage   NC Noncovered   HAC HAC-associated Procedure   CC Combination Cluster - See Appendix G for code lists
DRG Non-OR-Affecting MS-DRG Assignment   New/Revised Text in **Orange**   ♂ Male   ♀ Female

0 **Medical and Surgical**
U **Female Reproductive System**
P **Removal:** Taking out or off a device from a body part

0UP continued from previous page

Body Part	Approach	Device	Qualifier
Character 4	Character 5	Character 6	Character 7
D Uterus and Cervix ♀	**0** Open **3** Percutaneous **4** Percutaneous Endoscopic **7** Via Natural or Artificial Opening **8** Via Natural or Artificial Opening Endoscopic	**0** Drainage Device **1** Radioactive Element **3** Infusion Device **7** Autologous Tissue Substitute **C** Extraluminal Device **D** Intraluminal Device **H** Contraceptive Device **J** Synthetic Substitute **K** Nonautologous Tissue Substitute **Y** Other Device	**Z** No Qualifier
D Uterus and Cervix ♀	**X** External	**0** Drainage Device **3** Infusion Device **D** Intraluminal Device **H** Contraceptive Device	**Z** No Qualifier
H Vagina and Cul-de-sac ♀	**0** Open **3** Percutaneous **4** Percutaneous Endoscopic **7** Via Natural or Artificial Opening **8** Via Natural or Artificial Opening Endoscopic	**0** Drainage Device **1** Radioactive Element **3** Infusion Device **7** Autologous Tissue Substitute **D** Intraluminal Device **J** Synthetic Substitute **K** Nonautologous Tissue Substitute **Y** Other Device	**Z** No Qualifier
H Vagina and Cul-de-sac ♀	**X** External	**0** Drainage Device **1** Radioactive Element **3** Infusion Device **D** Intraluminal Device	**Z** No Qualifier
M Vulva ♀	**0** Open	**0** Drainage Device **7** Autologous Tissue Substitute **J** Synthetic Substitute **K** Nonautologous Tissue Substitute	**Z** No Qualifier
M Vulva ♀	**X** External	**0** Drainage Device	**Z** No Qualifier

♀ 0UP300Z 0UP303Z 0UP30YZ 0UP330Z 0UP333Z 0UP33YZ 0UP340Z 0UP343Z 0UP34YZ 0UP37YZ 0UP38YZ 0UP3X0Z 0UP3X3Z
0UP800Z 0UP803Z 0UP807Z 0UP80CZ 0UP80DZ 0UP80JZ 0UP80KZ 0UP80YZ 0UP830Z 0UP833Z 0UP837Z 0UP83CZ 0UP83DZ
0UP83JZ 0UP83KZ 0UP83YZ 0UP840Z 0UP843Z 0UP847Z 0UP84CZ 0UP84DZ 0UP84JZ 0UP84KZ 0UP84YZ 0UP870Z 0UP873Z
0UP877Z 0UP87CZ 0UP87DZ 0UP87JZ 0UP87KZ 0UP87YZ 0UP880Z 0UP883Z 0UP887Z 0UP88CZ 0UP88DZ 0UP88JZ 0UP88KZ
0UP88YZ 0UP8X0Z 0UP8X3Z 0UP8XDZ 0UPD00Z 0UPD01Z 0UPD03Z 0UPD07Z 0UPD0CZ 0UPD0DZ 0UPD0HZ 0UPD0JZ 0UPD0KZ
0UPD0YZ 0UPD30Z 0UPD31Z 0UPD33Z 0UPD37Z 0UPD3CZ 0UPD3DZ 0UPD3HZ 0UPD3JZ 0UPD3KZ 0UPD3YZ 0UPD40Z 0UPD41Z
0UPD43Z 0UPD47Z 0UPD4CZ 0UPD4DZ 0UPD4HZ 0UPD4JZ 0UPD4KZ 0UPD4YZ 0UPD70Z 0UPD71Z 0UPD73Z 0UPD77Z 0UPD7CZ
0UPD7DZ 0UPD7HZ 0UPD7JZ 0UPD7KZ 0UPD7YZ 0UPD80Z 0UPD81Z 0UPD83Z 0UPD87Z 0UPD8CZ 0UPD8DZ 0UPD8HZ 0UPD8JZ
0UPD8KZ 0UPD8YZ 0UPDX0Z 0UPDX3Z 0UPDXDZ 0UPDXHZ 0UPH00Z 0UPH01Z 0UPH03Z 0UPH07Z 0UPH0DZ 0UPH0JZ 0UPH0KZ
0UPH0YZ 0UPH30Z 0UPH31Z 0UPH33Z 0UPH37Z 0UPH3DZ 0UPH3JZ 0UPH3KZ 0UPH3YZ 0UPH40Z 0UPH41Z 0UPH43Z 0UPH47Z
0UPH4DZ 0UPH4JZ 0UPH4KZ 0UPH4YZ 0UPH70Z 0UPH71Z 0UPH73Z 0UPH77Z 0UPH7DZ 0UPH7JZ 0UPH7KZ 0UPH7YZ 0UPH80Z
0UPH81Z 0UPH83Z 0UPH87Z 0UPH8DZ 0UPH8JZ 0UPH8KZ 0UPH8YZ 0UPHX0Z 0UPHX1Z 0UPHX3Z 0UPHXDZ 0UPM00Z 0UPM07Z
0UPM0JZ 0UPM0KZ 0UPMX0Z

0 **Medical and Surgical**
U **Female Reproductive System**
Q **Repair:** Restoring, to the extent possible, a body part to its normal anatomic structure and function

Body Part	Approach	Device	Qualifier
Character 4	Character 5	Character 6	Character 7
0 Ovary, Right ♀ 1 Ovary, Left ♀ 2 Ovaries, Bilateral ♀ 4 Uterine Supporting Structure ♀	0 Open 3 Percutaneous 4 Percutaneous Endoscopic 8 Via Natural or Artificial Opening Endoscopic	Z No Device	Z No Qualifier
5 Fallopian Tube, Right ♀ 6 Fallopian Tube, Left ♀ 7 Fallopian Tubes, Bilateral ♀ 9 Uterus ♀ C Cervix ♀ F Cul-de-sac ♀	0 Open 3 Percutaneous 4 Percutaneous Endoscopic 7 Via Natural or Artificial Opening 8 Via Natural or Artificial Opening Endoscopic	Z No Device	Z No Qualifier
G Vagina ♀ K Hymen ♀	0 Open 3 Percutaneous 4 Percutaneous Endoscopic 7 Via Natural or Artificial Opening 8 Via Natural or Artificial Opening Endoscopic X External	Z No Device	Z No Qualifier
J Clitoris ♀ L Vestibular Gland ♀ M Vulva ♀	0 Open X External	Z No Device	Z No Qualifier

♀ 0UQ00ZZ 0UQ03ZZ 0UQ04ZZ 0UQ08ZZ 0UQ10ZZ 0UQ13ZZ 0UQ14ZZ 0UQ18ZZ 0UQ20ZZ 0UQ23ZZ 0UQ24ZZ 0UQ28ZZ 0UQ40ZZ
0UQ43ZZ 0UQ44ZZ 0UQ48ZZ 0UQ50ZZ 0UQ53ZZ 0UQ54ZZ 0UQ57ZZ 0UQ58ZZ 0UQ60ZZ 0UQ63ZZ 0UQ64ZZ 0UQ67ZZ 0UQ68ZZ
0UQ70ZZ 0UQ73ZZ 0UQ74ZZ 0UQ77ZZ 0UQ78ZZ 0UQ90ZZ 0UQ93ZZ 0UQ94ZZ 0UQ97ZZ 0UQ98ZZ 0UQC0ZZ 0UQC3ZZ 0UQC4ZZ
0UQC7ZZ 0UQC8ZZ 0UQF0ZZ 0UQF3ZZ 0UQF4ZZ 0UQF7ZZ 0UQF8ZZ 0UQG0ZZ 0UQG3ZZ 0UQG4ZZ 0UQG7ZZ 0UQG8ZZ 0UQGXZZ
0UQJ0ZZ 0UQJXZZ 0UQK0ZZ 0UQK3ZZ 0UQK4ZZ 0UQK7ZZ 0UQK8ZZ 0UQKXZZ 0UQL0ZZ 0UQLXZZ 0UQM0ZZ 0UQMXZZ

0 **Medical and Surgical**
U **Female Reproductive System**
S **Reposition:** Moving to its normal location, or other suitable location, all or a portion of a body part

Body Part	Approach	Device	Qualifier
Character 4	Character 5	Character 6	Character 7
0 Ovary, Right ♀ 1 Ovary, Left ♀ 2 Ovaries, Bilateral ♀ 4 Uterine Supporting Structure ♀ 5 Fallopian Tube, Right ♀ 6 Fallopian Tube, Left ♀ 7 Fallopian Tubes, Bilateral ♀ C Cervix ♀ F Cul-de-sac ♀	0 Open 4 Percutaneous Endoscopic 8 Via Natural or Artificial Opening Endoscopic	Z No Device	Z No Qualifier
9 Uterus ♀ G Vagina ♀	0 Open 4 Percutaneous Endoscopic 7 Via Natural or Artificial Opening 8 Via Natural or Artificial Opening Endoscopic X External	Z No Device	Z No Qualifier

♀ 0US00ZZ 0US04ZZ 0US08ZZ 0US10ZZ 0US14ZZ 0US18ZZ 0US20ZZ 0US24ZZ 0US28ZZ 0US40ZZ 0US44ZZ 0US48ZZ 0US50ZZ
0US54ZZ 0US58ZZ 0US60ZZ 0US64ZZ 0US68ZZ 0US70ZZ 0US74ZZ 0US78ZZ 0US90ZZ 0US94ZZ 0US97ZZ 0US98ZZ 0US9XZZ
0USC0ZZ 0USC4ZZ 0USC8ZZ 0USF0ZZ 0USF4ZZ 0USF8ZZ 0USG0ZZ 0USG4ZZ 0USG7ZZ 0USG8ZZ 0USGXZZ

LC Limited Coverage **NC** Noncovered **HAC** HAC-associated Procedure **CC** Combination Cluster - See Appendix G for code lists
DRG Non-OR-Affecting MS-DRG Assignment New/Revised Text in **Orange** ♂ Male ♀ Female

522

2018 ICD-10-PCS

0 Medical and Surgical
U Female Reproductive System
T Resection: Cutting out or off, without replacement, all of a body part

Body Part	Approach	Device	Qualifier
Character 4	Character 5	Character 6	Character 7
0 Ovary, Right ♀ **1** Ovary, Left ♀ **2** Ovaries, Bilateral ⦶ ♀ **5** Fallopian Tube, Right ♀ **6** Fallopian Tube, Left ♀ **7** Fallopian Tubes, Bilateral ⦶ ♀	**0** Open **4** Percutaneous Endoscopic **7** Via Natural or Artificial Opening **8** Via Natural or Artificial Opening Endoscopic **F** Via Natural or Artificial Opening With Percutaneous Endoscopic Assistance	**Z** No Device	**Z** No Qualifier
4 Uterine Supporting Structure ⦶ ♀ **C** Cervix ⦶ ♀ **F** Cul-de-sac ♀ **G** Vagina ⦶ ♀	**0** Open **4** Percutaneous Endoscopic **7** Via Natural or Artificial Opening **8** Via Natural or Artificial Opening Endoscopic	**Z** No Device	**Z** No Qualifier
9 Uterus ⦶ ♀	**0** Open **4** Percutaneous Endoscopic **7** Via Natural or Artificial Opening **8** Via Natural or Artificial Opening Endoscopic **F** Via Natural or Artificial Opening With Percutaneous Endoscopic Assistance	**Z** No Device	**L** Supracervical **Z** No Qualifier
J Clitoris ♀ **L** Vestibular Gland ♀ **M** Vulva ⦶ ♀	**0** Open **X** External	**Z** No Device	**Z** No Qualifier
K Hymen ♀	**0** Open **4** Percutaneous Endoscopic **7** Via Natural or Artificial Opening **8** Via Natural or Artificial Opening Endoscopic **X** External	**Z** No Device	**Z** No Qualifier

♀ 0UT00ZZ 0UT04ZZ 0UT07ZZ 0UT08ZZ 0UT0FZZ 0UT10ZZ 0UT14ZZ 0UT17ZZ 0UT18ZZ 0UT1FZZ 0UT20ZZ 0UT24ZZ 0UT27ZZ
0UT28ZZ 0UT2FZZ 0UT40ZZ 0UT44ZZ 0UT47ZZ 0UT48ZZ 0UT50ZZ 0UT54ZZ 0UT57ZZ 0UT58ZZ 0UT5FZZ 0UT60ZZ 0UT64ZZ
0UT67ZZ 0UT68ZZ 0UT6FZZ 0UT70ZZ 0UT74ZZ 0UT77ZZ 0UT78ZZ 0UT7FZZ 0UT90ZL 0UT90ZZ 0UT94ZL 0UT94ZZ 0UT97ZL
0UT97ZZ 0UT98ZL 0UT98ZZ 0UT9FZL 0UT9FZZ 0UTC0ZZ 0UTC4ZZ 0UTC7ZZ 0UTC8ZZ 0UTF0ZZ 0UTF4ZZ 0UTF7ZZ 0UTF8ZZ
0UTG0ZZ 0UTG4ZZ 0UTG7ZZ 0UTG8ZZ 0UTJ0ZZ 0UTJXZZ 0UTK0ZZ 0UTK4ZZ 0UTK7ZZ 0UTK8ZZ 0UTKXZZ 0UTL0ZZ 0UTLXZZ
0UTM0ZZ 0UTMXZZ

⦶ 0UT20ZZ 0UT40ZZ 0UT44ZZ 0UT47ZZ 0UT48ZZ 0UT70ZZ 0UT90ZZ 0UT94ZZ 0UT97ZZ 0UT98ZZ 0UT9FZZ 0UTC0ZZ 0UTC4ZZ
0UTC7ZZ 0UTC8ZZ 0UTG0ZZ 0UTM0ZZ 0UTMXZZ

0 Medical and Surgical
U Female Reproductive System
U Supplement: Putting in or on biological or synthetic material that physically reinforces and/or augments the function of a portion of a body part

Body Part	Approach	Device	Qualifier
Character 4	Character 5	Character 6	Character 7
4 Uterine Supporting Structure ♀	**0** Open **4** Percutaneous Endoscopic	**7** Autologous Tissue Substitute **J** Synthetic Substitute **K** Nonautologous Tissue Substitute	**Z** No Qualifier
5 Fallopian Tube, Right ♀ **6** Fallopian Tube, Left ♀ **7** Fallopian Tubes, Bilateral ♀ **F** Cul-de-sac ♀	**0** Open **4** Percutaneous Endoscopic **7** Via Natural or Artificial Opening **8** Via Natural or Artificial Opening Endoscopic	**7** Autologous Tissue Substitute **J** Synthetic Substitute **K** Nonautologous Tissue Substitute	**Z** No Qualifier
G Vagina ♀ **K** Hymen ♀	**0** Open **4** Percutaneous Endoscopic **7** Via Natural or Artificial Opening **8** Via Natural or Artificial Opening Endoscopic **X** External	**7** Autologous Tissue Substitute **J** Synthetic Substitute **K** Nonautologous Tissue Substitute	**Z** No Qualifier

0UU continued on next page

0 **Medical and Surgical**
U **Female Reproductive System**
U **Supplement:** Putting in or on biological or synthetic material that physically reinforces and/or augments the function of a portion of a body part

0UU continued from previous page

Body Part	Approach	Device	Qualifier
Character 4	Character 5	Character 6	Character 7
J Clitoris ♀ M Vulva ♀	0 Open X External	7 Autologous Tissue Substitute J Synthetic Substitute K Nonautologous Tissue Substitute	Z No Qualifier

♀ 0UU407Z 0UU40JZ 0UU40KZ 0UU447Z 0UU44JZ 0UU44KZ 0UU507Z 0UU50JZ 0UU50KZ 0UU547Z 0UU54JZ 0UU54KZ 0UU577Z
0UU57JZ 0UU57KZ 0UU587Z 0UU58JZ 0UU58KZ 0UU607Z 0UU60JZ 0UU60KZ 0UU647Z 0UU64JZ 0UU64KZ 0UU677Z 0UU67JZ
0UU67KZ 0UU687Z 0UU68JZ 0UU68KZ 0UU707Z 0UU70JZ 0UU70KZ 0UU747Z 0UU74JZ 0UU74KZ 0UU777Z 0UU77JZ 0UU77KZ
0UU787Z 0UU78JZ 0UU78KZ 0UUF07Z 0UUF0JZ 0UUF0KZ 0UUF47Z 0UUF4JZ 0UUF4KZ 0UUF77Z 0UUF7JZ 0UUF7KZ 0UUF87Z
0UUF8JZ 0UUF8KZ 0UUG07Z 0UUG0JZ 0UUG0KZ 0UUG47Z 0UUG4JZ 0UUG4KZ 0UUG77Z 0UUG7JZ 0UUG7KZ 0UUG87Z 0UUG8JZ
0UUG8KZ 0UUGX7Z 0UUGXJZ 0UUGXKZ 0UUJ07Z 0UUJ0JZ 0UUJ0KZ 0UUJX7Z 0UUJXJZ 0UUJXKZ 0UUK07Z 0UUK0JZ 0UUK0KZ
0UUK47Z 0UUK4JZ 0UUK4KZ 0UUK77Z 0UUK7JZ 0UUK7KZ 0UUK87Z 0UUK8JZ 0UUK8KZ 0UUKX7Z 0UUKXJZ 0UUKXKZ 0UUM07Z
0UUM0JZ 0UUM0KZ 0UUMX7Z 0UUMXJZ 0UUMXKZ

0 **Medical and Surgical**
U **Female Reproductive System**
V **Restriction:** Partially closing an orifice or the lumen of a tubular body part

Body Part	Approach	Device	Qualifier
Character 4	Character 5	Character 6	Character 7
C Cervix ♀	0 Open 3 Percutaneous 4 Percutaneous Endoscopic	C Extraluminal Device D Intraluminal Device Z No Device	Z No Qualifier
C Cervix ♀	7 Via Natural or Artificial Opening 8 Via Natural or Artificial Opening Endoscopic	D Intraluminal Device Z No Device	Z No Qualifier

♀ 0UVC0CZ 0UVC0DZ 0UVC0ZZ 0UVC3CZ 0UVC3DZ 0UVC3ZZ 0UVC4CZ 0UVC4DZ 0UVC4ZZ 0UVC7DZ 0UVC7ZZ 0UVC8DZ 0UVC8ZZ

0 **Medical and Surgical**
U **Female Reproductive System**
W **Revision:** Correcting, to the extent possible, a portion of a malfunctioning device or the position of a displaced device

Body Part	Approach	Device	Qualifier
Character 4	Character 5	Character 6	Character 7
3 Ovary ♀	0 Open 3 Percutaneous 4 Percutaneous Endoscopic	0 Drainage Device 3 Infusion Device Y Other Device	Z No Qualifier
3 Ovary ♀	7 Via Natural or Artificial Opening 8 Via Natural or Artificial Opening Endoscopic	Y Other Device	Z No Qualifier
3 Ovary ♀	X External	0 Drainage Device 3 Infusion Device	Z No Qualifier
8 Fallopian Tube ♀	0 Open 3 Percutaneous 4 Percutaneous Endoscopic 7 Via Natural or Artificial Opening 8 Via Natural or Artificial Opening Endoscopic	0 Drainage Device 3 Infusion Device 7 Autologous Tissue Substitute C Extraluminal Device D Intraluminal Device J Synthetic Substitute K Nonautologous Tissue Substitute Y Other Device	Z No Qualifier
8 Fallopian Tube ♀	X External	0 Drainage Device 3 Infusion Device 7 Autologous Tissue Substitute C Extraluminal Device D Intraluminal Device J Synthetic Substitute K Nonautologous Tissue Substitute	Z No Qualifier

0UW continued on next page

LC Limited Coverage   NC Noncovered   HAC HAC-associated Procedure   CC Combination Cluster - See Appendix G for code lists
DRG Non-OR-Affecting MS-DRG Assignment   New/Revised Text in **Orange**   ♂ Male   ♀ Female

524

2018 ICD-10-PCS

0 **Medical and Surgical**
U **Female Reproductive System**
W **Revision:** Correcting, to the extent possible, a portion of a malfunctioning device or the position of a displaced device

0UW continued from previous page

Body Part	Approach	Device	Qualifier
Character 4	Character 5	Character 6	Character 7
D Uterus and Cervix ♀	**0** Open **3** Percutaneous **4** Percutaneous Endoscopic **7** Via Natural or Artificial Opening **8** Via Natural or Artificial Opening Endoscopic	**0** Drainage Device **1** Radioactive Element **3** Infusion Device **7** Autologous Tissue Substitute **C** Extraluminal Device **D** Intraluminal Device **H** Contraceptive Device **J** Synthetic Substitute **K** Nonautologous Tissue Substitute **Y** Other Device	**Z** No Qualifier
D Uterus and Cervix ♀	**X** External	**0** Drainage Device **3** Infusion Device **7** Autologous Tissue Substitute **C** Extraluminal Device **D** Intraluminal Device **H** Contraceptive Device **J** Synthetic Substitute **K** Nonautologous Tissue Substitute	**Z** No Qualifier
H Vagina and Cul-de-sac ♀	**0** Open **3** Percutaneous **4** Percutaneous Endoscopic **7** Via Natural or Artificial Opening **8** Via Natural or Artificial Opening Endoscopic	**0** Drainage Device **1** Radioactive Element **3** Infusion Device **7** Autologous Tissue Substitute **D** Intraluminal Device **J** Synthetic Substitute **K** Nonautologous Tissue Substitute **Y** Other Device	**Z** No Qualifier
H Vagina and Cul-de-sac ♀	**X** External	**0** Drainage Device **3** Infusion Device **7** Autologous Tissue Substitute **D** Intraluminal Device **J** Synthetic Substitute **K** Nonautologous Tissue Substitute	**Z** No Qualifier
M Vulva ♀	**0** Open **X** External	**0** Drainage Device **7** Autologous Tissue Substitute **J** Synthetic Substitute **K** Nonautologous Tissue Substitute	**Z** No Qualifier

♀ 0UW300Z 0UW303Z 0UW30YZ 0UW330Z 0UW333Z 0UW33YZ 0UW340Z 0UW343Z 0UW34YZ 0UW37YZ 0UW38YZ 0UW3X0Z 0UW3X3Z
0UW800Z 0UW803Z 0UW807Z 0UW80CZ 0UW80DZ 0UW80JZ 0UW80KZ 0UW80YZ 0UW830Z 0UW833Z 0UW837Z 0UW83CZ 0UW83DZ
0UW83JZ 0UW83KZ 0UW83YZ 0UW840Z 0UW843Z 0UW847Z 0UW84CZ 0UW84DZ 0UW84JZ 0UW84KZ 0UW84YZ 0UW870Z 0UW873Z
0UW877Z 0UW87CZ 0UW87DZ 0UW87JZ 0UW87KZ 0UW87YZ 0UW880Z 0UW883Z 0UW887Z 0UW88CZ 0UW88DZ 0UW88JZ 0UW88KZ
0UW88YZ 0UW8X0Z 0UW8X3Z 0UW8X7Z 0UW8XCZ 0UW8XDZ 0UW8XJZ 0UW8XKZ 0UWD00Z 0UWD01Z 0UWD03Z 0UWD07Z 0UWD0CZ
0UWD0DZ 0UWD0HZ 0UWD0JZ 0UWD0KZ 0UWD0YZ 0UWD30Z 0UWD31Z 0UWD33Z 0UWD37Z 0UWD3CZ 0UWD3DZ 0UWD3HZ 0UWD3JZ
0UWD3KZ 0UWD3YZ 0UWD40Z 0UWD41Z 0UWD43Z 0UWD47Z 0UWD4CZ 0UWD4DZ 0UWD4HZ 0UWD4JZ 0UWD4KZ 0UWD4YZ 0UWD70Z
0UWD71Z 0UWD73Z 0UWD77Z 0UWD7CZ 0UWD7DZ 0UWD7HZ 0UWD7JZ 0UWD7KZ 0UWD7YZ 0UWD80Z 0UWD81Z 0UWD83Z 0UWD87Z
0UWD8CZ 0UWD8DZ 0UWD8HZ 0UWD8JZ 0UWD8KZ 0UWD8YZ 0UWDX0Z 0UWDX3Z 0UWDX7Z 0UWDXCZ 0UWDXDZ 0UWDXHZ 0UWDXJZ
0UWDXKZ 0UWH00Z 0UWH01Z 0UWH03Z 0UWH07Z 0UWH0DZ 0UWH0JZ 0UWH0KZ 0UWH0YZ 0UWH30Z 0UWH31Z 0UWH33Z 0UWH37Z
0UWH3DZ 0UWH3JZ 0UWH3KZ 0UWH3YZ 0UWH40Z 0UWH41Z 0UWH43Z 0UWH47Z 0UWH4DZ 0UWH4JZ 0UWH4KZ 0UWH4YZ 0UWH70Z
0UWH71Z 0UWH73Z 0UWH77Z 0UWH7DZ 0UWH7JZ 0UWH7KZ 0UWH7YZ 0UWH80Z 0UWH81Z 0UWH83Z 0UWH87Z 0UWH8DZ 0UWH8JZ
0UWH8KZ 0UWH8YZ 0UWHX0Z 0UWHX3Z 0UWHX7Z 0UWHXDZ 0UWHXJZ 0UWHXKZ 0UWM00Z 0UWM07Z 0UWM0JZ 0UWM0KZ 0UWMX0Z
0UWMX7Z 0UWMXJZ 0UWMXKZ

0 **Medical and Surgical**
U **Female Reproductive System**
Y **Transplantation:** Putting in or on all or a portion of a living body part taken from another individual or animal to physically take the place and/or function of all or a portion of a similar body part

Body Part	Approach	Device	Qualifier
Character 4	**Character 5**	**Character 6**	**Character 7**
0 Ovary, Right ♀ **1** Ovary, Left ♀	**0** Open	**Z** No Device	**0** Allogeneic **1** Syngeneic **2** Zooplastic

♀ 0UY00Z0   0UY00Z1   0UY00Z2   0UY10Z0   0UY10Z1   0UY10Z2

Ⓛ Limited Coverage   Ⓝ Noncovered   Ⓗ HAC-associated Procedure   Ⓒ Combination Cluster - See Appendix G for code lists
Ⓝ Non-OR-Affecting MS-DRG Assignment   New/Revised Text in **Orange**   ♂ Male   ♀ Female

526

2018 ICD-10-PCS

NOTES

NOTES

Male Reproductive System 0V1-0VW

0 Medical and Surgical
V Male Reproductive System
1 Bypass: Altering the route of passage of the contents of a tubular body part

Body Part	Approach	Device	Qualifier
Character 4	Character 5	Character 6	Character 7
N Vas Deferens, Right ♂ **P** Vas Deferens, Left ♂ **Q** Vas Deferens, Bilateral ♂	**0** Open **4** Percutaneous Endoscopic	**7** Autologous Tissue Substitute **J** Synthetic Substitute **K** Nonautologous Tissue Substitute **Z** No Device	**J** Epididymis, Right **K** Epididymis, Left **N** Vas Deferens, Right **P** Vas Deferens, Left

♂ 0V1N07J 0V1N07K 0V1N07N 0V1N07P 0V1N0JJ 0V1N0JK 0V1N0JN 0V1N0JP 0V1N0KJ 0V1N0KK 0V1N0KN 0V1N0KP 0V1N0ZJ
0V1N0ZK 0V1N0ZN 0V1N0ZP 0V1N47J 0V1N47K 0V1N47N 0V1N47P 0V1N4JJ 0V1N4JK 0V1N4JN 0V1N4JP 0V1N4KJ 0V1N4KK
0V1N4KN 0V1N4KP 0V1N4ZJ 0V1N4ZK 0V1N4ZN 0V1N4ZP 0V1P07J 0V1P07K 0V1P07N 0V1P07P 0V1P0JJ 0V1P0JK 0V1P0JN
0V1P0JP 0V1P0KJ 0V1P0KK 0V1P0KN 0V1P0KP 0V1P0ZJ 0V1P0ZK 0V1P0ZN 0V1P0ZP 0V1P47J 0V1P47K 0V1P47N 0V1P47P
0V1P4JJ 0V1P4JK 0V1P4JN 0V1P4JP 0V1P4KJ 0V1P4KK 0V1P4KN 0V1P4KP 0V1P4ZJ 0V1P4ZK 0V1P4ZN 0V1P4ZP 0V1Q07J
0V1Q07K 0V1Q07N 0V1Q07P 0V1Q0JJ 0V1Q0JK 0V1Q0JN 0V1Q0JP 0V1Q0KJ 0V1Q0KK 0V1Q0KN 0V1Q0KP 0V1Q0ZJ 0V1Q0ZK
0V1Q0ZN 0V1Q0ZP 0V1Q47J 0V1Q47K 0V1Q47N 0V1Q47P 0V1Q4JJ 0V1Q4JK 0V1Q4JN 0V1Q4JP 0V1Q4KJ 0V1Q4KK 0V1Q4KN
0V1Q4KP 0V1Q4ZJ 0V1Q4ZK 0V1Q4ZN 0V1Q4ZP

0 Medical and Surgical
V Male Reproductive System
2 Change: Taking out or off a device from a body part and putting back an identical or similar device in or on the same body part without cutting or puncturing the skin or a mucous membrane

Body Part	Approach	Device	Qualifier
Character 4	Character 5	Character 6	Character 7
4 Prostate and Seminal Vesicles ♂ **8** Scrotum and Tunica Vaginalis ♂ **D** Testis ♂ **M** Epididymis and Spermatic Cord ♂ **R** Vas Deferens ♂ **S** Penis ♂	**X** External	**0** Drainage Device **Y** Other Device	**Z** No Qualifier

♂ 0V24X0Z 0V24XYZ 0V28X0Z 0V28XYZ 0V2DX0Z 0V2DXYZ 0V2MX0Z 0V2MXYZ 0V2RX0Z 0V2RXYZ 0V2SX0Z 0V2SXYZ

0V5-0V7

0   Medical and Surgical
V   Male Reproductive System
5   Destruction: Physical eradication of all or a portion of a body part by the direct use of energy, force, or a destructive agent

Body Part	Approach	Device	Qualifier
Character 4	Character 5	Character 6	Character 7
0 Prostate ♂	**0** Open **3** Percutaneous **4** Percutaneous Endoscopic **7** Via Natural or Artificial Opening **8** Via Natural or Artificial Opening Endoscopic	**Z** No Device	**Z** No Qualifier
1 Seminal Vesicle, Right ♂ **2** Seminal Vesicle, Left ♂ **3** Seminal Vesicles, Bilateral ♂ **6** Tunica Vaginalis, Right ♂ **7** Tunica Vaginalis, Left ♂ **9** Testis, Right ♂ **B** Testis, Left ♂ **C** Testes, Bilateral ♂	**0** Open **3** Percutaneous **4** Percutaneous Endoscopic	**Z** No Device	**Z** No Qualifier
5 Scrotum ♂ **S** Penis ♂ **T** Prepuce ♂	**0** Open **3** Percutaneous **4** Percutaneous Endoscopic **X** External	**Z** No Device	**Z** No Qualifier
F Spermatic Cord, Right ♂ **G** Spermatic Cord, Left ♂ **H** Spermatic Cords, Bilateral ♂ **J** Epididymis, Right ♂ **K** Epididymis, Left ♂ **L** Epididymis, Bilateral ♂ **N** Vas Deferens, Right ♂ **P** Vas Deferens, Left ♂ **Q** Vas Deferens, Bilateral ♂	**0** Open **3** Percutaneous **4** Percutaneous Endoscopic **8** Via Natural or Artificial Opening Endoscopic	**Z** No Device	**Z** No Qualifier

♂ 0V500ZZ   0V503ZZ   0V504ZZ   0V507ZZ   0V508ZZ   0V510ZZ   0V513ZZ   0V514ZZ   0V520ZZ   0V523ZZ   0V524ZZ   0V530ZZ   0V533ZZ
    0V534ZZ   0V550ZZ   0V553ZZ   0V554ZZ   0V55XZZ   0V560ZZ   0V563ZZ   0V564ZZ   0V570ZZ   0V573ZZ   0V574ZZ   0V590ZZ   0V593ZZ
    0V594ZZ   0V5B0ZZ   0V5B3ZZ   0V5B4ZZ   0V5C0ZZ   0V5C3ZZ   0V5C4ZZ   0V5F0ZZ   0V5F3ZZ   0V5F4ZZ   0V5F8ZZ   0V5G0ZZ   0V5G3ZZ
    0V5G4ZZ   0V5G8ZZ   0V5H0ZZ   0V5H3ZZ   0V5H4ZZ   0V5H8ZZ   0V5J0ZZ   0V5J3ZZ   0V5J4ZZ   0V5J8ZZ   0V5K0ZZ   0V5K3ZZ   0V5K4ZZ
    0V5K8ZZ   0V5L0ZZ   0V5L3ZZ   0V5L4ZZ   0V5L8ZZ   0V5N0ZZ   0V5N3ZZ   0V5N4ZZ   0V5N8ZZ   0V5P0ZZ   0V5P3ZZ   0V5P4ZZ   0V5P8ZZ
    0V5Q0ZZ   0V5Q3ZZ   0V5Q4ZZ   0V5Q8ZZ   0V5S0ZZ   0V5S3ZZ   0V5S4ZZ   0V5SXZZ   0V5T0ZZ   0V5T3ZZ   0V5T4ZZ   0V5TXZZ

0   Medical and Surgical
V   Male Reproductive System
7   Dilation: Expanding an orifice or the lumen of a tubular body part

Body Part	Approach	Device	Qualifier
Character 4	Character 5	Character 6	Character 7
N Vas Deferens, Right ♂ **P** Vas Deferens, Left ♂ **Q** Vas Deferens, Bilateral ♂	**0** Open **3** Percutaneous **4** Percutaneous Endoscopic	**D** Intraluminal Device **Z** No Device	**Z** No Qualifier

♂ 0V7N0DZ   0V7N0ZZ   0V7N3DZ   0V7N3ZZ   0V7N4DZ   0V7N4ZZ   0V7P0DZ   0V7P0ZZ   0V7P3DZ   0V7P3ZZ   0V7P4DZ   0V7P4ZZ   0V7Q0DZ
    0V7Q0ZZ   0V7Q3DZ   0V7Q3ZZ   0V7Q4DZ   0V7Q4ZZ

LC Limited Coverage   **NC** Noncovered   **HAC** HAC-associated Procedure   **CC** Combination Cluster - See Appendix G for code lists
DNR Non-OR-Affecting MS-DRG Assignment   New/Revised Text in **Orange**   ♂ Male   ♀ Female

530   **2018 ICD-10-PCS**

0 Medical and Surgical
V Male Reproductive System
9 **Drainage:** Taking or letting out fluids and/or gases from a body part

Body Part	Approach	Device	Qualifier
Character 4	Character 5	Character 6	Character 7
0 Prostate ♂	**0** Open **3** Percutaneous **4** Percutaneous Endoscopic **7** Via Natural or Artificial Opening **8** Via Natural or Artificial Opening Endoscopic	**0** Drainage Device	**Z** No Qualifier
0 Prostate ♂	**0** Open **3** Percutaneous **4** Percutaneous Endoscopic **7** Via Natural or Artificial Opening **8** Via Natural or Artificial Opening Endoscopic	**Z** No Device	**X** Diagnostic **Z** No Qualifier
1 Seminal Vesicle, Right ♂ **2** Seminal Vesicle, Left ♂ **3** Seminal Vesicles, Bilateral ♂ **6** Tunica Vaginalis, Right ♂ **7** Tunica Vaginalis, Left ♂ **9** Testis, Right ♂ **B** Testis, Left ♂ **C** Testes, Bilateral ♂ **F** Spermatic Cord, Right ♂ **G** Spermatic Cord, Left ♂ **H** Spermatic Cords, Bilateral ♂ **J** Epididymis, Right ♂ **K** Epididymis, Left ♂ **L** Epididymis, Bilateral ♂ **N** Vas Deferens, Right ♂ **P** Vas Deferens, Left ♂ **Q** Vas Deferens, Bilateral ♂	**0** Open **3** Percutaneous **4** Percutaneous Endoscopic	**0** Drainage Device	**Z** No Qualifier
1 Seminal Vesicle, Right ♂ **2** Seminal Vesicle, Left ♂ **3** Seminal Vesicles, Bilateral ♂ **6** Tunica Vaginalis, Right ♂ **7** Tunica Vaginalis, Left ♂ **9** Testis, Right ♂ **B** Testis, Left ♂ **C** Testes, Bilateral ♂ **F** Spermatic Cord, Right ♂ **G** Spermatic Cord, Left ♂ **H** Spermatic Cords, Bilateral ♂ **J** Epididymis, Right ♂ **K** Epididymis, Left ♂ **L** Epididymis, Bilateral ♂ **N** Vas Deferens, Right ♂ **P** Vas Deferens, Left ♂ **Q** Vas Deferens, Bilateral ♂	**0** Open **3** Percutaneous **4** Percutaneous Endoscopic	**Z** No Device	**X** Diagnostic **Z** No Qualifier
5 Scrotum ♂ **S** Penis ♂ **T** Prepuce ♂	**0** Open **3** Percutaneous **4** Percutaneous Endoscopic **X** External	**0** Drainage Device	**Z** No Qualifier
5 Scrotum ♂ **S** Penis ♂ **T** Prepuce ♂	**0** Open **3** Percutaneous **4** Percutaneous Endoscopic **X** External	**Z** No Device	**X** Diagnostic **Z** No Qualifier

♂ 0V9000Z 0V900ZX 0V900ZZ 0V9030Z 0V903ZX 0V903ZZ 0V9040Z 0V904ZX 0V904ZZ 0V9070Z 0V907ZX 0V907ZZ 0V9080Z
0V908ZX 0V908ZZ 0V9100Z 0V910ZX 0V910ZZ 0V9130Z 0V913ZX 0V913ZZ 0V9140Z 0V914ZX 0V914ZZ 0V9200Z 0V920ZX
0V920ZZ 0V9230Z 0V923ZX 0V923ZZ 0V9240Z 0V924ZX 0V924ZZ 0V9300Z 0V930ZX 0V930ZZ 0V9330Z 0V933ZX 0V933ZZ
0V9340Z 0V934ZX 0V934ZZ 0V9500Z 0V950ZX 0V950ZZ 0V9530Z 0V953ZX 0V953ZZ 0V9540Z 0V954ZX 0V954ZZ 0V95X0Z

0V9 continued on next page

LC Limited Coverage   NC Noncovered   HAC HAC-associated Procedure   CC Combination Cluster - See Appendix G for code lists
DRG Non-OR-Affecting MS-DRG Assignment   New/Revised Text in Orange   ♂ Male   ♀ Female

0V9 continued from previous page

0V95XZX	0V95XZZ	0V9600Z	0V960ZX	0V960ZZ	0V9630Z	0V963ZX	0V963ZZ	0V9640Z	0V964ZX	0V964ZZ	0V9700Z	0V970ZX
0V970ZZ	0V9730Z	0V973ZX	0V973ZZ	0V9740Z	0V974ZX	0V974ZZ	0V9900Z	0V990ZX	0V990ZZ	0V9930Z	0V993ZX	0V993ZZ
0V9940Z	0V994ZX	0V994ZZ	0V9B00Z	0V9B0ZX	0V9B0ZZ	0V9B30Z	0V9B3ZX	0V9B3ZZ	0V9B40Z	0V9B4ZX	0V9B4ZZ	0V9C00Z
0V9C0ZX	0V9C0ZZ	0V9C30Z	0V9C3ZX	0V9C3ZZ	0V9C40Z	0V9C4ZX	0V9C4ZZ	0V9F00Z	0V9F0ZX	0V9F0ZZ	0V9F30Z	0V9F3ZX
0V9F3ZZ	0V9F40Z	0V9F4ZX	0V9F4ZZ	0V9G00Z	0V9G0ZX	0V9G0ZZ	0V9G30Z	0V9G3ZX	0V9G3ZZ	0V9G40Z	0V9G4ZX	0V9G4ZZ
0V9H00Z	0V9H0ZX	0V9H0ZZ	0V9H30Z	0V9H3ZX	0V9H3ZZ	0V9H40Z	0V9H4ZX	0V9H4ZZ	0V9J00Z	0V9J0ZX	0V9J0ZZ	0V9J30Z
0V9J3ZX	0V9J3ZZ	0V9J40Z	0V9J4ZX	0V9J4ZZ	0V9K00Z	0V9K0ZX	0V9K0ZZ	0V9K30Z	0V9K3ZX	0V9K3ZZ	0V9K40Z	0V9K4ZX
0V9K4ZZ	0V9L00Z	0V9L0ZX	0V9L0ZZ	0V9L30Z	0V9L3ZX	0V9L3ZZ	0V9L40Z	0V9L4ZX	0V9L4ZZ	0V9N00Z	0V9N0ZX	0V9N0ZZ
0V9N30Z	0V9N3ZX	0V9N3ZZ	0V9N40Z	0V9N4ZX	0V9N4ZZ	0V9P00Z	0V9P0ZX	0V9P0ZZ	0V9P30Z	0V9P3ZX	0V9P3ZZ	0V9P40Z
0V9P4ZX	0V9P4ZZ	0V9Q00Z	0V9Q0ZX	0V9Q0ZZ	0V9Q30Z	0V9Q3ZX	0V9Q3ZZ	0V9Q40Z	0V9Q4ZX	0V9Q4ZZ	0V9S00Z	0V9S0ZX
0V9S0ZZ	0V9S30Z	0V9S3ZX	0V9S3ZZ	0V9S40Z	0V9S4ZX	0V9S4ZZ	0V9SX0Z	0V9SXZX	0V9SXZZ	0V9T00Z	0V9T0ZX	0V9T0ZZ
0V9T30Z	0V9T3ZX	0V9T3ZZ	0V9T40Z	0V9T4ZX	0V9T4ZZ	0V9TX0Z	0V9TXZX	0V9TXZZ				

0   **Medical and Surgical**
V   **Male Reproductive System**
B   **Excision:** Cutting out or off, without replacement, a portion of a body part

Body Part		Approach		Device		Qualifier	
Character 4		**Character 5**		**Character 6**		**Character 7**	
0	Prostate ♂	**0** **3** **4** **7** **8**	Open Percutaneous Percutaneous Endoscopic Via Natural or Artificial Opening Via Natural or Artificial Opening Endoscopic	**Z**	No Device	**X** **Z**	Diagnostic No Qualifier
1 **2** **3** **6** **7** **9** **B** **C**	Seminal Vesicle, Right ♂ Seminal Vesicle, Left ♂ Seminal Vesicles, Bilateral ♂ Tunica Vaginalis, Right ♂ Tunica Vaginalis, Left ♂ Testis, Right ♂ Testis, Left ♂ Testes, Bilateral ♂	**0** **3** **4**	Open Percutaneous Percutaneous Endoscopic	**Z**	No Device	**X** **Z**	Diagnostic No Qualifier
5 **S** **T**	Scrotum ♂ Penis ♂ Prepuce ♂	**0** **3** **4** **X**	Open Percutaneous Percutaneous Endoscopic External	**Z**	No Device	**X** **Z**	Diagnostic No Qualifier
F **G** **H** **J** **K** **L** **N** **P** **Q**	Spermatic Cord, Right ♂ Spermatic Cord, Left ♂ Spermatic Cords, Bilateral ♂ Epididymis, Right ♂ Epididymis, Left ♂ Epididymis, Bilateral ♂ Vas Deferens, Right ♂ Vas Deferens, Left ♂ Vas Deferens, Bilateral ♂	**0** **3** **4** **8**	Open Percutaneous Percutaneous Endoscopic Via Natural or Artificial Opening Endoscopic	**Z**	No Device	**X** **Z**	Diagnostic No Qualifier

♂												
0VB00ZX	0VB00ZZ	0VB03ZX	0VB03ZZ	0VB04ZX	0VB04ZZ	0VB07ZX	0VB07ZZ	0VB08ZX	0VB08ZZ	0VB10ZX	0VB10ZZ	0VB13ZX
0VB13ZZ	0VB14ZX	0VB14ZZ	0VB20ZX	0VB20ZZ	0VB23ZX	0VB23ZZ	0VB24ZX	0VB24ZZ	0VB30ZX	0VB30ZZ	0VB33ZX	0VB33ZZ
0VB34ZX	0VB34ZZ	0VB50ZX	0VB50ZZ	0VB53ZX	0VB53ZZ	0VB54ZX	0VB54ZZ	0VB5XZX	0VB5XZZ	0VB60ZX	0VB60ZZ	0VB63ZX
0VB63ZZ	0VB64ZX	0VB64ZZ	0VB70ZX	0VB70ZZ	0VB73ZX	0VB73ZZ	0VB74ZX	0VB74ZZ	0VB90ZX	0VB90ZZ	0VB93ZX	0VB93ZZ
0VB94ZX	0VB94ZZ	0VBB0ZX	0VBB0ZZ	0VBB3ZX	0VBB3ZZ	0VBB4ZX	0VBB4ZZ	0VBC0ZX	0VBC0ZZ	0VBC3ZX	0VBC3ZZ	0VBC4ZX
0VBC4ZZ	0VBF0ZX	0VBF0ZZ	0VBF3ZX	0VBF3ZZ	0VBF4ZX	0VBF4ZZ	0VBF8ZX	0VBF8ZZ	0VBG0ZX	0VBG0ZZ	0VBG3ZX	0VBG3ZZ
0VBG4ZX	0VBG4ZZ	0VBG8ZX	0VBG8ZZ	0VBH0ZX	0VBH0ZZ	0VBH3ZX	0VBH3ZZ	0VBH4ZX	0VBH4ZZ	0VBH8ZX	0VBH8ZZ	0VBJ0ZX
0VBJ0ZZ	0VBJ3ZX	0VBJ3ZZ	0VBJ4ZX	0VBJ4ZZ	0VBJ8ZX	0VBJ8ZZ	0VBK0ZX	0VBK0ZZ	0VBK3ZX	0VBK3ZZ	0VBK4ZX	0VBK4ZZ
0VBK8ZX	0VBK8ZZ	0VBL0ZX	0VBL0ZZ	0VBL3ZX	0VBL3ZZ	0VBL4ZX	0VBL4ZZ	0VBL8ZX	0VBL8ZZ	0VBN0ZX	0VBN0ZZ	0VBN3ZX
0VBN3ZZ	0VBN4ZX	0VBN4ZZ	0VBN8ZX	0VBN8ZZ	0VBP0ZX	0VBP0ZZ	0VBP3ZX	0VBP3ZZ	0VBP4ZX	0VBP4ZZ	0VBP8ZX	0VBP8ZZ
0VBQ0ZX	0VBQ0ZZ	0VBQ3ZX	0VBQ3ZZ	0VBQ4ZX	0VBQ4ZZ	0VBQ8ZX	0VBQ8ZZ	0VBS0ZX	0VBS0ZZ	0VBS3ZX	0VBS3ZZ	0VBS4ZX
0VBS4ZZ	0VBSXZX	0VBSXZZ	0VBT0ZX	0VBT0ZZ	0VBT3ZX	0VBT3ZZ	0VBT4ZX	0VBT4ZZ	0VBTXZX	0VBTXZZ		

0 Medical and Surgical
V Male Reproductive System
C Extirpation: Taking or cutting out solid matter from a body part

Body Part	Approach	Device	Qualifier
Character 4	Character 5	Character 6	Character 7
0 Prostate ♂	**0** Open **3** Percutaneous **4** Percutaneous Endoscopic **7** Via Natural or Artificial Opening **8** Via Natural or Artificial Opening Endoscopic	**Z** No Device	**Z** No Qualifier
1 Seminal Vesicle, Right ♂ **2** Seminal Vesicle, Left ♂ **3** Seminal Vesicles, Bilateral ♂ **6** Tunica Vaginalis, Right ♂ **7** Tunica Vaginalis, Left ♂ **9** Testis, Right ♂ **B** Testis, Left ♂ **C** Testes, Bilateral ♂ **F** Spermatic Cord, Right ♂ **G** Spermatic Cord, Left ♂ **H** Spermatic Cords, Bilateral ♂ **J** Epididymis, Right ♂ **K** Epididymis, Left ♂ **L** Epididymis, Bilateral ♂ **N** Vas Deferens, Right ♂ **P** Vas Deferens, Left ♂ **Q** Vas Deferens, Bilateral ♂	**0** Open **3** Percutaneous **4** Percutaneous Endoscopic	**Z** No Device	**Z** No Qualifier
5 Scrotum ♂ **S** Penis ♂ **T** Prepuce ♂	**0** Open **3** Percutaneous **4** Percutaneous Endoscopic **X** External	**Z** No Device	**Z** No Qualifier

♂ 0VC00ZZ 0VC03ZZ 0VC04ZZ 0VC07ZZ 0VC08ZZ 0VC10ZZ 0VC13ZZ 0VC14ZZ 0VC20ZZ 0VC23ZZ 0VC24ZZ 0VC30ZZ 0VC33ZZ
0VC34ZZ 0VC50ZZ 0VC53ZZ 0VC54ZZ 0VC5XZZ 0VC60ZZ 0VC63ZZ 0VC64ZZ 0VC70ZZ 0VC73ZZ 0VC74ZZ 0VC90ZZ 0VC93ZZ
0VC94ZZ 0VCB0ZZ 0VCB3ZZ 0VCB4ZZ 0VCC0ZZ 0VCC3ZZ 0VCC4ZZ 0VCF0ZZ 0VCF3ZZ 0VCF4ZZ 0VCG0ZZ 0VCG3ZZ 0VCG4ZZ
0VCH0ZZ 0VCH3ZZ 0VCH4ZZ 0VCJ0ZZ 0VCJ3ZZ 0VCJ4ZZ 0VCK0ZZ 0VCK3ZZ 0VCK4ZZ 0VCL0ZZ 0VCL3ZZ 0VCL4ZZ 0VCN0ZZ
0VCN3ZZ 0VCN4ZZ 0VCP0ZZ 0VCP3ZZ 0VCP4ZZ 0VCQ0ZZ 0VCQ3ZZ 0VCQ4ZZ 0VCS0ZZ 0VCS3ZZ 0VCS4ZZ 0VCSXZZ 0VCT0ZZ
0VCT3ZZ 0VCT4ZZ 0VCTXZZ

0 **Medical and Surgical**
V **Male Reproductive System**
H **Insertion:** Putting in a nonbiological appliance that monitors, assists, performs, or prevents a physiological function but does not physically take the place of a body part

Body Part	Approach	Device	Qualifier
Character 4	Character 5	Character 6	Character 7
0 Prostate ♂	**0** Open **3** Percutaneous **4** Percutaneous Endoscopic **7** Via Natural or Artificial Opening **8** Via Natural or Artificial Opening Endoscopic	**1** Radioactive Element	**Z** No Qualifier
4 Prostate and Seminal Vesicles ♂ **8** Scrotum and Tunica Vaginalis ♂ **D** Testis ♂ **M** Epididymis and Spermatic Cord ♂ **R** Vas Deferens ♂	**0** Open **3** Percutaneous **4** Percutaneous Endoscopic **7** Via Natural or Artificial Opening **8** Via Natural or Artificial Opening Endoscopic	**3** Infusion Device **Y** Other Device	**Z** No Qualifier
S Penis ♂	**0** Open **3** Percutaneous **4** Percutaneous Endoscopic	**3** Infusion Device **Y** Other Device	**Z** No Qualifier
S Penis ♂	**7** Via Natural or Artificial Opening **8** Via Natural or Artificial Opening Endoscopic	**Y** Other Device	**Z** No Qualifier
S Penis ♂	**X** External	**3** Infusion Device	**Z** No Qualifier

♂ 0VH001Z 0VH031Z 0VH041Z 0VH071Z 0VH081Z 0VH403Z 0VH40YZ 0VH433Z 0VH43YZ 0VH443Z 0VH44YZ 0VH473Z 0VH47YZ
0VH483Z 0VH48YZ 0VH803Z 0VH80YZ 0VH833Z 0VH83YZ 0VH843Z 0VH84YZ 0VH873Z 0VH87YZ 0VH883Z 0VH88YZ 0VHD03Z
0VHD0YZ 0VHD33Z 0VHD3YZ 0VHD43Z 0VHD4YZ 0VHD73Z 0VHD7YZ 0VHD83Z 0VHD8YZ 0VHM03Z 0VHM0YZ 0VHM33Z 0VHM3YZ
0VHM43Z 0VHM4YZ 0VHM73Z 0VHM7YZ 0VHM83Z 0VHM8YZ 0VHR03Z 0VHR0YZ 0VHR33Z 0VHR3YZ 0VHR43Z 0VHR4YZ 0VHR73Z
0VHR7YZ 0VHR83Z 0VHR8YZ 0VHS03Z 0VHS0YZ 0VHS33Z 0VHS3YZ 0VHS43Z 0VHS4YZ 0VHS7YZ 0VHS8YZ 0VHSX3Z

0 **Medical and Surgical**
V **Male Reproductive System**
J **Inspection:** Visually and/or manually exploring a body part

Body Part	Approach	Device	Qualifier
Character 4	Character 5	Character 6	Character 7
4 Prostate and Seminal Vesicles ♂ **8** Scrotum and Tunica Vaginalis ♂ **D** Testis ♂ **M** Epididymis and Spermatic Cord ♂ **R** Vas Deferens ♂ **S** Penis ♂	**0** Open **3** Percutaneous **4** Percutaneous Endoscopic **X** External	**Z** No Device	**Z** No Qualifier

♂ 0VJ40ZZ 0VJ43ZZ 0VJ44ZZ 0VJ4XZZ 0VJ80ZZ 0VJ83ZZ 0VJ84ZZ 0VJ8XZZ 0VJD0ZZ 0VJD3ZZ 0VJD4ZZ 0VJDXZZ 0VJM0ZZ
0VJM3ZZ 0VJM4ZZ 0VJMXZZ 0VJR0ZZ 0VJR3ZZ 0VJR4ZZ 0VJRXZZ 0VJS0ZZ 0VJS3ZZ 0VJS4ZZ 0VJSXZZ

LC Limited Coverage   NC Noncovered   HAC HAC-associated Procedure   CC Combination Cluster - See Appendix G for code lists
DRG Non-OR-Affecting MS-DRG Assignment   New/Revised Text in Orange   ♂ Male   ♀ Female

534   2018 ICD-10-PCS

0 **Medical and Surgical**
V **Male Reproductive System**
L **Occlusion:** Completely closing an orifice or the lumen of a tubular body part

Body Part	Approach	Device	Qualifier
Character 4	Character 5	Character 6	Character 7
F Spermatic Cord, Right♂ **G** Spermatic Cord, Left ♂ **H** Spermatic Cords, Bilateral ♂ **N** Vas Deferens, Right ♂ **P** Vas Deferens, Left ♂ **Q** Vas Deferens, Bilateral ♂	**0** Open **3** Percutaneous **4** Percutaneous Endoscopic **8** Via Natural or Artificial Opening Endoscopic	**C** Extraluminal Device **D** Intraluminal Device **Z** No Device	**Z** No Qualifier

♂ 0VLF0CZ 0VLF0DZ 0VLF0ZZ 0VLF3CZ 0VLF3DZ 0VLF3ZZ 0VLF4CZ 0VLF4DZ 0VLF4ZZ 0VLF8CZ 0VLF8DZ 0VLF8ZZ 0VLG0CZ
0VLG0DZ 0VLG0ZZ 0VLG3CZ 0VLG3DZ 0VLG3ZZ 0VLG4CZ 0VLG4DZ 0VLG4ZZ 0VLG8CZ 0VLG8DZ 0VLG8ZZ 0VLH0CZ 0VLH0DZ
0VLH0ZZ 0VLH3CZ 0VLH3DZ 0VLH3ZZ 0VLH4CZ 0VLH4DZ 0VLH4ZZ 0VLH8CZ 0VLH8DZ 0VLH8ZZ 0VLN0CZ 0VLN0DZ 0VLN0ZZ
0VLN3CZ 0VLN3DZ 0VLN3ZZ 0VLN4CZ 0VLN4DZ 0VLN4ZZ 0VLN8CZ 0VLN8DZ 0VLN8ZZ 0VLP0CZ 0VLP0DZ 0VLP0ZZ 0VLP3CZ
0VLP3DZ 0VLP3ZZ 0VLP4CZ 0VLP4DZ 0VLP4ZZ 0VLP8CZ 0VLP8DZ 0VLP8ZZ 0VLQ0CZ 0VLQ0DZ 0VLQ0ZZ 0VLQ3CZ 0VLQ3DZ
0VLQ3ZZ 0VLQ4CZ 0VLQ4DZ 0VLQ4ZZ 0VLQ8CZ 0VLQ8DZ 0VLQ8ZZ

0 **Medical and Surgical**
V **Male Reproductive System**
M **Reattachment:** Putting back in or on all or a portion of a separated body part to its normal location or other suitable location

Body Part	Approach	Device	Qualifier
Character 4	Character 5	Character 6	Character 7
5 Scrotum ♂ **S** Penis ♂	**X** External	**Z** No Device	**Z** No Qualifier
6 Tunica Vaginalis, Right ♂ **7** Tunica Vaginalis, Left ♂ **9** Testis, Right ♂ **B** Testis, Left ♂ **C** Testes, Bilateral ♂ **F** Spermatic Cord, Right ♂ **G** Spermatic Cord, Left ♂ **H** Spermatic Cords, Bilateral ♂	**0** Open **4** Percutaneous Endoscopic	**Z** No Device	**Z** No Qualifier

♂ 0VM5XZZ 0VM60ZZ 0VM64ZZ 0VM70ZZ 0VM74ZZ 0VM90ZZ 0VM94ZZ 0VMB0ZZ 0VMB4ZZ 0VMC0ZZ 0VMC4ZZ 0VMF0ZZ 0VMF4ZZ
0VMG0ZZ 0VMG4ZZ 0VMH0ZZ 0VMH4ZZ 0VMSXZZ

LC Limited Coverage **NC** Noncovered **HAC** HAC-associated Procedure **CC** Combination Cluster - See Appendix G for code lists
drg Non-OR-Affecting MS-DRG Assignment New/Revised Text in **Orange** ♂ Male ♀ Female

2018 ICD-10-PCS

535

0 **Medical and Surgical**
V **Male Reproductive System**
N **Release:** Freeing a body part from an abnormal physical constraint by cutting or by the use of force

Body Part		Approach		Device		Qualifier	
Character 4		**Character 5**		**Character 6**		**Character 7**	
0 Prostate ♂		**0** Open **3** Percutaneous **4** Percutaneous Endoscopic **7** Via Natural or Artificial Opening **8** Via Natural or Artificial Opening Endoscopic		**Z** No Device		**Z** No Qualifier	
1 Seminal Vesicle, Right ♂ **2** Seminal Vesicle, Left ♂ **3** Seminal Vesicles, Bilateral ♂ **6** Tunica Vaginalis, Right ♂ **7** Tunica Vaginalis, Left ♂ **9** Testis, Right ♂ **B** Testis, Left ♂ **C** Testes, Bilateral ♂		**0** Open **3** Percutaneous **4** Percutaneous Endoscopic		**Z** No Device		**Z** No Qualifier	
5 Scrotum ♂ **S** Penis ♂ **T** Prepuce ♂		**0** Open **3** Percutaneous **4** Percutaneous Endoscopic **X** External		**Z** No Device		**Z** No Qualifier	
F Spermatic Cord, Right ♂ **G** Spermatic Cord, Left ♂ **H** Spermatic Cords, Bilateral ♂ **J** Epididymis, Right ♂ **K** Epididymis, Left ♂ **L** Epididymis, Bilateral ♂ **N** Vas Deferens, Right ♂ **P** Vas Deferens, Left ♂ **Q** Vas Deferens, Bilateral ♂		**0** Open **3** Percutaneous **4** Percutaneous Endoscopic **8** Via Natural or Artificial Opening Endoscopic		**Z** No Device		**Z** No Qualifier	

♂ 0VN00ZZ 0VN03ZZ 0VN04ZZ 0VN07ZZ 0VN08ZZ 0VN10ZZ 0VN13ZZ 0VN14ZZ 0VN20ZZ 0VN23ZZ 0VN24ZZ 0VN30ZZ 0VN33ZZ
0VN34ZZ 0VN50ZZ 0VN53ZZ 0VN54ZZ 0VN5XZZ 0VN60ZZ 0VN63ZZ 0VN64ZZ 0VN70ZZ 0VN73ZZ 0VN74ZZ 0VN90ZZ 0VN93ZZ
0VN94ZZ 0VNB0ZZ 0VNB3ZZ 0VNB4ZZ 0VNC0ZZ 0VNC3ZZ 0VNC4ZZ 0VNF0ZZ 0VNF3ZZ 0VNF4ZZ 0VNF8ZZ 0VNG0ZZ 0VNG3ZZ
0VNG4ZZ 0VNG8ZZ 0VNH0ZZ 0VNH3ZZ 0VNH4ZZ 0VNH8ZZ 0VNJ0ZZ 0VNJ3ZZ 0VNJ4ZZ 0VNJ8ZZ 0VNK0ZZ 0VNK3ZZ 0VNK4ZZ
0VNK8ZZ 0VNL0ZZ 0VNL3ZZ 0VNL4ZZ 0VNL8ZZ 0VNN0ZZ 0VNN3ZZ 0VNN4ZZ 0VNN8ZZ 0VNP0ZZ 0VNP3ZZ 0VNP4ZZ 0VNP8ZZ
0VNQ0ZZ 0VNQ3ZZ 0VNQ4ZZ 0VNQ8ZZ 0VNS0ZZ 0VNS3ZZ 0VNS4ZZ 0VNSXZZ 0VNT0ZZ 0VNT3ZZ 0VNT4ZZ 0VNTXZZ

LC Limited Coverage **NC** Noncovered **HAC** HAC-associated Procedure **CC** Combination Cluster - See Appendix G for code lists
DRG Non-OR-Affecting MS-DRG Assignment New/Revised Text in **Orange** ♂ Male ♀ Female

536

2018 ICD-10-PCS

0 **Medical and Surgical**
V **Male Reproductive System**
P **Removal:** Taking out or off a device from a body part

Body Part	Approach	Device	Qualifier
Character 4	Character 5	Character 6	Character 7
4 Prostate and Seminal Vesicles ♂	**0** Open **3** Percutaneous **4** Percutaneous Endoscopic **7** Via Natural or Artificial Opening **8** Via Natural or Artificial Opening Endoscopic	**0** Drainage Device **1** Radioactive Element **3** Infusion Device **7** Autologous Tissue Substitute **J** Synthetic Substitute **K** Nonautologous Tissue Substitute **Y** Other Device	**Z** No Qualifier
4 Prostate and Seminal Vesicles ♂	**X** External	**0** Drainage Device **1** Radioactive Element **3** Infusion Device	**Z** No Qualifier
8 Scrotum and Tunica Vaginalis ♂ **D** Testis ♂ **S** Penis ♂	**0** Open **3** Percutaneous **4** Percutaneous Endoscopic **7** Via Natural or Artificial Opening **8** Via Natural or Artificial Opening Endoscopic	**0** Drainage Device **3** Infusion Device **7** Autologous Tissue Substitute **J** Synthetic Substitute **K** Nonautologous Tissue Substitute **Y** Other Device	**Z** No Qualifier
8 Scrotum and Tunica Vaginalis ♂ **D** Testis ♂ **S** Penis ♂	**X** External	**0** Drainage Device **3** Infusion Device	**Z** No Qualifier
M Epididymis and Spermatic Cord ♂	**0** Open **3** Percutaneous **4** Percutaneous Endoscopic **7** Via Natural or Artificial Opening **8** Via Natural or Artificial Opening Endoscopic	**0** Drainage Device **3** Infusion Device **7** Autologous Tissue Substitute **C** Extraluminal Device **J** Synthetic Substitute **K** Nonautologous Tissue Substitute **Y** Other Device	**Z** No Qualifier
M Epididymis and Spermatic Cord ♂	**X** External	**0** Drainage Device **3** Infusion Device	**Z** No Qualifier
R Vas Deferens ♂	**0** Open **3** Percutaneous **4** Percutaneous Endoscopic **7** Via Natural or Artificial Opening **8** Via Natural or Artificial Opening Endoscopic	**0** Drainage Device **3** Infusion Device **7** Autologous Tissue Substitute **C** Extraluminal Device **D** Intraluminal Device **J** Synthetic Substitute **K** Nonautologous Tissue Substitute **Y** Other Device	**Z** No Qualifier
R Vas Deferens ♂	**X** External	**0** Drainage Device **3** Infusion Device **D** Intraluminal Device	**Z** No Qualifier

♂ 0VP400Z 0VP401Z 0VP403Z 0VP407Z 0VP40JZ 0VP40KZ 0VP40YZ 0VP430Z 0VP431Z 0VP433Z 0VP437Z 0VP43JZ 0VP43KZ
0VP43YZ 0VP440Z 0VP441Z 0VP443Z 0VP447Z 0VP44JZ 0VP44KZ 0VP44YZ 0VP470Z 0VP471Z 0VP473Z 0VP477Z 0VP47JZ
0VP47KZ 0VP47YZ 0VP480Z 0VP481Z 0VP483Z 0VP487Z 0VP48JZ 0VP48KZ 0VP48YZ 0VP4X0Z 0VP4X1Z 0VP4X3Z 0VP800Z
0VP803Z 0VP807Z 0VP80JZ 0VP80KZ 0VP80YZ 0VP830Z 0VP833Z 0VP837Z 0VP83JZ 0VP83KZ 0VP83YZ 0VP840Z 0VP843Z
0VP847Z 0VP84JZ 0VP84KZ 0VP84YZ 0VP870Z 0VP873Z 0VP877Z 0VP87JZ 0VP87KZ 0VP87YZ 0VP880Z 0VP883Z 0VP887Z
0VP88JZ 0VP88KZ 0VP88YZ 0VP8X0Z 0VP8X3Z 0VPD00Z 0VPD03Z 0VPD07Z 0VPD0JZ 0VPD0KZ 0VPD0YZ 0VPD30Z 0VPD33Z
0VPD37Z 0VPD3JZ 0VPD3KZ 0VPD3YZ 0VPD40Z 0VPD43Z 0VPD47Z 0VPD4JZ 0VPD4KZ 0VPD4YZ 0VPD70Z 0VPD73Z 0VPD77Z
0VPD7JZ 0VPD7KZ 0VPD7YZ 0VPD80Z 0VPD83Z 0VPD87Z 0VPD8JZ 0VPD8KZ 0VPD8YZ 0VPDX0Z 0VPDX3Z 0VPM00Z 0VPM03Z
0VPM07Z 0VPM0CZ 0VPM0JZ 0VPM0KZ 0VPM0YZ 0VPM30Z 0VPM33Z 0VPM37Z 0VPM3CZ 0VPM3JZ 0VPM3KZ 0VPM3YZ 0VPM40Z
0VPM43Z 0VPM47Z 0VPM4CZ 0VPM4JZ 0VPM4KZ 0VPM4YZ 0VPM70Z 0VPM73Z 0VPM77Z 0VPM7CZ 0VPM7JZ 0VPM7KZ 0VPM7YZ
0VPM80Z 0VPM83Z 0VPM87Z 0VPM8CZ 0VPM8JZ 0VPM8KZ 0VPM8YZ 0VPMX0Z 0VPMX3Z 0VPR00Z 0VPR03Z 0VPR07Z 0VPR0CZ
0VPR0DZ 0VPR0JZ 0VPR0KZ 0VPR0YZ 0VPR30Z 0VPR33Z 0VPR37Z 0VPR3CZ 0VPR3DZ 0VPR3JZ 0VPR3KZ 0VPR3YZ 0VPR40Z
0VPR43Z 0VPR47Z 0VPR4CZ 0VPR4DZ 0VPR4JZ 0VPR4KZ 0VPR4YZ 0VPR70Z 0VPR73Z 0VPR77Z 0VPR7CZ 0VPR7DZ 0VPR7JZ
0VPR7KZ 0VPR7YZ 0VPR80Z 0VPR83Z 0VPR87Z 0VPR8CZ 0VPR8DZ 0VPR8JZ 0VPR8KZ 0VPR8YZ 0VPRX0Z 0VPRX3Z 0VPRXDZ
0VPS00Z 0VPS03Z 0VPS07Z 0VPS0JZ 0VPS0KZ 0VPS0YZ 0VPS30Z 0VPS33Z 0VPS37Z 0VPS3JZ 0VPS3KZ 0VPS3YZ 0VPS40Z
0VPS43Z 0VPS47Z 0VPS4JZ 0VPS4KZ 0VPS4YZ 0VPS70Z 0VPS73Z 0VPS77Z 0VPS7JZ 0VPS7KZ 0VPS7YZ 0VPS80Z 0VPS83Z
0VPS87Z 0VPS8JZ 0VPS8KZ 0VPS8YZ 0VPSX0Z 0VPSX3Z

0 **Medical and Surgical**
V **Male Reproductive System**
Q **Repair:** Restoring, to the extent possible, a body part to its normal anatomic structure and function

Body Part	Approach	Device	Qualifier
Character 4	Character 5	Character 6	Character 7
0 Prostate ♂	0 Open 3 Percutaneous 4 Percutaneous Endoscopic 7 Via Natural or Artificial Opening 8 Via Natural or Artificial Opening Endoscopic	Z No Device	Z No Qualifier
1 Seminal Vesicle, Right ♂ 2 Seminal Vesicle, Left ♂ 3 Seminal Vesicles, Bilateral ♂ 6 Tunica Vaginalis, Right ♂ 7 Tunica Vaginalis, Left ♂ 9 Testis, Right ♂ B Testis, Left ♂ C Testes, Bilateral ♂	0 Open 3 Percutaneous 4 Percutaneous Endoscopic	Z No Device	Z No Qualifier
5 Scrotum ♂ S Penis ♂ T Prepuce ♂	0 Open 3 Percutaneous 4 Percutaneous Endoscopic X External	Z No Device	Z No Qualifier
F Spermatic Cord, Right ♂ G Spermatic Cord, Left ♂ H Spermatic Cords, Bilateral ♂ J Epididymis, Right ♂ K Epididymis, Left ♂ L Epididymis, Bilateral ♂ N Vas Deferens, Right ♂ P Vas Deferens, Left ♂ Q Vas Deferens, Bilateral ♂	0 Open 3 Percutaneous 4 Percutaneous Endoscopic 8 Via Natural or Artificial Opening Endoscopic	Z No Device	Z No Qualifier

♂ 0VQ00ZZ 0VQ03ZZ 0VQ04ZZ 0VQ07ZZ 0VQ08ZZ 0VQ10ZZ 0VQ13ZZ 0VQ14ZZ 0VQ20ZZ 0VQ23ZZ 0VQ24ZZ 0VQ30ZZ 0VQ33ZZ
0VQ34ZZ 0VQ50ZZ 0VQ53ZZ 0VQ54ZZ 0VQ5XZZ 0VQ60ZZ 0VQ63ZZ 0VQ64ZZ 0VQ70ZZ 0VQ73ZZ 0VQ74ZZ 0VQ90ZZ 0VQ93ZZ
0VQ94ZZ 0VQB0ZZ 0VQB3ZZ 0VQB4ZZ 0VQC0ZZ 0VQC3ZZ 0VQC4ZZ 0VQF0ZZ 0VQF3ZZ 0VQF4ZZ 0VQF8ZZ 0VQG0ZZ 0VQG3ZZ
0VQG4ZZ 0VQG8ZZ 0VQH0ZZ 0VQH3ZZ 0VQH4ZZ 0VQH8ZZ 0VQJ0ZZ 0VQJ3ZZ 0VQJ4ZZ 0VQJ8ZZ 0VQK0ZZ 0VQK3ZZ 0VQK4ZZ
0VQK8ZZ 0VQL0ZZ 0VQL3ZZ 0VQL4ZZ 0VQL8ZZ 0VQN0ZZ 0VQN3ZZ 0VQN4ZZ 0VQN8ZZ 0VQP0ZZ 0VQP3ZZ 0VQP4ZZ 0VQP8ZZ
0VQQ0ZZ 0VQQ3ZZ 0VQQ4ZZ 0VQQ8ZZ 0VQS0ZZ 0VQS3ZZ 0VQS4ZZ 0VQSXZZ 0VQT0ZZ 0VQT3ZZ 0VQT4ZZ 0VQTXZZ

0 **Medical and Surgical**
V **Male Reproductive System**
R **Replacement:** Putting in or on biological or synthetic material that physically takes the place and/or function of all or a portion of a body part

Body Part	Approach	Device	Qualifier
Character 4	Character 5	Character 6	Character 7
9 Testis, Right ♂ B Testis, Left ♂ C Testes, Bilateral ♂	0 Open	J Synthetic Substitute	Z No Qualifier

♂ 0VR90JZ 0VRB0JZ 0VRC0JZ

🅛🅒 Limited Coverage 🅝🅒 Noncovered 🅗🅐🅒 HAC-associated Procedure 🅒🅒 Combination Cluster - See Appendix G for code lists
🅝🅡🅖 Non-OR-Affecting MS-DRG Assignment New/Revised Text in **Orange** ♂ Male ♀ Female

538   2018 ICD-10-PCS

0 **Medical and Surgical**
V **Male Reproductive System**
S **Reposition:** Moving to its normal location, or other suitable location, all or a portion of a body part

Body Part	Approach	Device	Qualifier
Character 4	Character 5	Character 6	Character 7
9 Testis, Right ♂ B Testis, Left ♂ C Testes, Bilateral ♂ F Spermatic Cord, Right ♂ G Spermatic Cord, Left ♂ H Spermatic Cords, Bilateral ♂	0 Open 3 Percutaneous 4 Percutaneous Endoscopic 8 Via Natural or Artificial Opening Endoscopic	Z No Device	Z No Qualifier

♂ 0VS90ZZ 0VS93ZZ 0VS94ZZ 0VS98ZZ 0VSB0ZZ 0VSB3ZZ 0VSB4ZZ 0VSB8ZZ 0VSC0ZZ 0VSC3ZZ 0VSC4ZZ 0VSC8ZZ 0VSF0ZZ
0VSF3ZZ 0VSF4ZZ 0VSF8ZZ 0VSG0ZZ 0VSG3ZZ 0VSG4ZZ 0VSG8ZZ 0VSH0ZZ 0VSH3ZZ 0VSH4ZZ 0VSH8ZZ

0 **Medical and Surgical**
V **Male Reproductive System**
T **Resection:** Cutting out or off, without replacement, all of a body part

Body Part	Approach	Device	Qualifier
Character 4	Character 5	Character 6	Character 7
0 Prostate ⬛ ♂	0 Open 4 Percutaneous Endoscopic 7 Via Natural or Artificial Opening 8 Via Natural or Artificial Opening Endoscopic	Z No Device	Z No Qualifier
1 Seminal Vesicle, Right ♂ 2 Seminal Vesicle, Left ♂ 3 Seminal Vesicles, Bilateral ⬛ ♂ 6 Tunica Vaginalis, Right ♂ 7 Tunica Vaginalis, Left ♂ 9 Testis, Right ♂ B Testis, Left ♂ C Testes, Bilateral ♂ F Spermatic Cord, Right ♂ G Spermatic Cord, Left ♂ H Spermatic Cords, Bilateral ♂ J Epididymis, Right ♂ K Epididymis, Left ♂ L Epididymis, Bilateral ♂ N Vas Deferens, Right ♂ P Vas Deferens, Left ♂ Q Vas Deferens, Bilateral ♂	0 Open 4 Percutaneous Endoscopic	Z No Device	Z No Qualifier
5 Scrotum ♂ S Penis ♂ T Prepuce ♂	0 Open 4 Percutaneous Endoscopic X External	Z No Device	Z No Qualifier

♂ 0VT00ZZ 0VT04ZZ 0VT07ZZ 0VT08ZZ 0VT10ZZ 0VT14ZZ 0VT20ZZ 0VT24ZZ 0VT30ZZ 0VT34ZZ 0VT50ZZ 0VT54ZZ 0VT5XZZ
0VT60ZZ 0VT64ZZ 0VT70ZZ 0VT74ZZ 0VT90ZZ 0VT94ZZ 0VTB0ZZ 0VTB4ZZ 0VTC0ZZ 0VTC4ZZ 0VTF0ZZ 0VTF4ZZ 0VTG0ZZ
0VTG4ZZ 0VTH0ZZ 0VTH4ZZ 0VTJ0ZZ 0VTJ4ZZ 0VTK0ZZ 0VTK4ZZ 0VTL0ZZ 0VTL4ZZ 0VTN0ZZ 0VTN4ZZ 0VTP0ZZ 0VTP4ZZ
0VTQ0ZZ 0VTQ4ZZ 0VTS0ZZ 0VTS4ZZ 0VTSXZZ 0VTT0ZZ 0VTT4ZZ 0VTTXZZ
⬛ 0VT00ZZ 0VT04ZZ 0VT07ZZ 0VT08ZZ 0VT30ZZ 0VT34ZZ

⬛ Limited Coverage ⬛ Noncovered ⬛ HAC-associated Procedure ⬛ Combination Cluster - See Appendix G for code lists
⬛ Non-OR-Affecting MS-DRG Assignment New/Revised Text in Orange ♂ Male ♀ Female

2018 ICD-10-PCS

539

0 Medical and Surgical
V Male Reproductive System
U Supplement: Putting in or on biological or synthetic material that physically reinforces and/or augments the function of a portion of a body part

Body Part	Approach	Device	Qualifier
Character 4	Character 5	Character 6	Character 7
1 Seminal Vesicle, Right ♂ 2 Seminal Vesicle, Left ♂ 3 Seminal Vesicles, Bilateral ♂ 6 Tunica Vaginalis, Right ♂ 7 Tunica Vaginalis, Left ♂ F Spermatic Cord, Right ♂ G Spermatic Cord, Left ♂ H Spermatic Cords, Bilateral ♂ J Epididymis, Right ♂ K Epididymis, Left ♂ L Epididymis, Bilateral ♂ N Vas Deferens, Right ♂ P Vas Deferens, Left ♂ Q Vas Deferens, Bilateral ♂	0 Open 4 Percutaneous Endoscopic 8 Via Natural or Artificial Opening Endoscopic	7 Autologous Tissue Substitute J Synthetic Substitute K Nonautologous Tissue Substitute	Z No Qualifier
5 Scrotum ♂ S Penis ♂ T Prepuce ♂	0 Open 4 Percutaneous Endoscopic X External	7 Autologous Tissue Substitute J Synthetic Substitute K Nonautologous Tissue Substitute	Z No Qualifier
9 Testis, Right ♂ B Testis, Left ♂ C Testes, Bilateral ♂	0 Open	7 Autologous Tissue Substitute J Synthetic Substitute K Nonautologous Tissue Substitute	Z No Qualifier

♂ 0VU107Z 0VU10JZ 0VU10KZ 0VU147Z 0VU14JZ 0VU14KZ 0VU187Z 0VU18JZ 0VU18KZ 0VU207Z 0VU20JZ 0VU20KZ 0VU247Z
0VU24JZ 0VU24KZ 0VU287Z 0VU28JZ 0VU28KZ 0VU307Z 0VU30JZ 0VU30KZ 0VU347Z 0VU34JZ 0VU34KZ 0VU387Z 0VU38JZ
0VU38KZ 0VU507Z 0VU50JZ 0VU50KZ 0VU547Z 0VU54JZ 0VU54KZ 0VU5X7Z 0VU5XJZ 0VU5XKZ 0VU607Z 0VU60JZ 0VU60KZ
0VU647Z 0VU64JZ 0VU64KZ 0VU687Z 0VU68JZ 0VU68KZ 0VU707Z 0VU70JZ 0VU70KZ 0VU747Z 0VU74JZ 0VU74KZ 0VU787Z
0VU78JZ 0VU78KZ 0VU907Z 0VU90JZ 0VU90KZ 0VUB07Z 0VUB0JZ 0VUB0KZ 0VUC07Z 0VUC0JZ 0VUC0KZ 0VUF07Z 0VUF0JZ
0VUF0KZ 0VUF47Z 0VUF4JZ 0VUF4KZ 0VUF87Z 0VUF8JZ 0VUF8KZ 0VUG07Z 0VUG0JZ 0VUG0KZ 0VUG47Z 0VUG4JZ 0VUG4KZ
0VUG87Z 0VUG8JZ 0VUG8KZ 0VUH07Z 0VUH0JZ 0VUH0KZ 0VUH47Z 0VUH4JZ 0VUH4KZ 0VUH87Z 0VUH8JZ 0VUH8KZ 0VUJ07Z
0VUJ0JZ 0VUJ0KZ 0VUJ47Z 0VUJ4JZ 0VUJ4KZ 0VUJ87Z 0VUJ8JZ 0VUJ8KZ 0VUK07Z 0VUK0JZ 0VUK0KZ 0VUK47Z 0VUK4JZ
0VUK4KZ 0VUK87Z 0VUK8JZ 0VUK8KZ 0VUL07Z 0VUL0JZ 0VUL0KZ 0VUL47Z 0VUL4JZ 0VUL4KZ 0VUL87Z 0VUL8JZ 0VUL8KZ
0VUN07Z 0VUN0JZ 0VUN0KZ 0VUN47Z 0VUN4JZ 0VUN4KZ 0VUN87Z 0VUN8JZ 0VUN8KZ 0VUP07Z 0VUP0JZ 0VUP0KZ 0VUP47Z
0VUP4JZ 0VUP4KZ 0VUP87Z 0VUP8JZ 0VUP8KZ 0VUQ07Z 0VUQ0JZ 0VUQ0KZ 0VUQ47Z 0VUQ4JZ 0VUQ4KZ 0VUQ87Z 0VUQ8JZ
0VUQ8KZ 0VUS07Z 0VUS0JZ 0VUS0KZ 0VUS47Z 0VUS4JZ 0VUS4KZ 0VUSX7Z 0VUSXJZ 0VUSXKZ 0VUT07Z 0VUT0JZ 0VUT0KZ
0VUT47Z 0VUT4JZ 0VUT4KZ 0VUTX7Z 0VUTXJZ 0VUTXKZ

LC Limited Coverage   NC Noncovered   HAC HAC-associated Procedure   CC Combination Cluster - See Appendix G for code lists
DRG Non-OR-Affecting MS-DRG Assignment   New/Revised Text in **Orange**   ♂ Male   ♀ Female

540   **2018 ICD-10-PCS**

0 Medical and Surgical
V Male Reproductive System
W Revision: Correcting, to the extent possible, a portion of a malfunctioning device or the position of a displaced device

Body Part	Approach	Device	Qualifier
Character 4	Character 5	Character 6	Character 7
4 Prostate and Seminal Vesicles ♂ 8 Scrotum and Tunica Vaginalis ♂ D Testis ♂ S Penis ♂	0 Open 3 Percutaneous 4 Percutaneous Endoscopic 7 Via Natural or Artificial Opening 8 Via Natural or Artificial Opening Endoscopic	0 Drainage Device 3 Infusion Device 7 Autologous Tissue Substitute J Synthetic Substitute K Nonautologous Tissue Substitute Y Other Device	Z No Qualifier
4 Prostate and Seminal Vesicles ♂ 8 Scrotum and Tunica Vaginalis ♂ D Testis ♂ S Penis ♂	X External	0 Drainage Device 3 Infusion Device 7 Autologous Tissue Substitute J Synthetic Substitute K Nonautologous Tissue Substitute	Z No Qualifier
M Epididymis and Spermatic Cord ♂	0 Open 3 Percutaneous 4 Percutaneous Endoscopic 7 Via Natural or Artificial Opening 8 Via Natural or Artificial Opening Endoscopic	0 Drainage Device 3 Infusion Device 7 Autologous Tissue Substitute C Extraluminal Device J Synthetic Substitute K Nonautologous Tissue Substitute Y Other Device	Z No Qualifier
M Epididymis and Spermatic Cord ♂	X External	0 Drainage Device 3 Infusion Device 7 Autologous Tissue Substitute C Extraluminal Device J Synthetic Substitute K Nonautologous Tissue Substitute	Z No Qualifier
R Vas Deferens ♂	0 Open 3 Percutaneous 4 Percutaneous Endoscopic 7 Via Natural or Artificial Opening 8 Via Natural or Artificial Opening Endoscopic	0 Drainage Device 3 Infusion Device 7 Autologous Tissue Substitute C Extraluminal Device D Intraluminal Device J Synthetic Substitute K Nonautologous Tissue Substitute Y Other Device	Z No Qualifier
R Vas Deferens ♂	X External	0 Drainage Device 3 Infusion Device 7 Autologous Tissue Substitute C Extraluminal Device D Intraluminal Device J Synthetic Substitute K Nonautologous Tissue Substitute	Z No Qualifier

♂ 0VW400Z 0VW403Z 0VW407Z 0VW40JZ 0VW40KZ 0VW40YZ 0VW430Z 0VW433Z 0VW437Z 0VW43JZ 0VW43KZ 0VW43YZ 0VW440Z
0VW443Z 0VW447Z 0VW44JZ 0VW44KZ 0VW44YZ 0VW470Z 0VW473Z 0VW477Z 0VW47JZ 0VW47KZ 0VW47YZ 0VW480Z 0VW483Z
0VW487Z 0VW48JZ 0VW48KZ 0VW48YZ 0VW4X0Z 0VW4X3Z 0VW4X7Z 0VW4XJZ 0VW4XKZ 0VW800Z 0VW803Z 0VW807Z 0VW80JZ
0VW80KZ 0VW80YZ 0VW830Z 0VW833Z 0VW837Z 0VW83JZ 0VW83KZ 0VW83YZ 0VW840Z 0VW843Z 0VW847Z 0VW84JZ 0VW84KZ
0VW84YZ 0VW870Z 0VW873Z 0VW877Z 0VW87JZ 0VW87KZ 0VW87YZ 0VW880Z 0VW883Z 0VW887Z 0VW88JZ 0VW88KZ 0VW88YZ
0VW8X0Z 0VW8X3Z 0VW8X7Z 0VW8XJZ 0VW8XKZ 0VWD00Z 0VWD03Z 0VWD07Z 0VWD0JZ 0VWD0KZ 0VWD0YZ 0VWD30Z 0VWD33Z
0VWD37Z 0VWD3JZ 0VWD3KZ 0VWD3YZ 0VWD40Z 0VWD43Z 0VWD47Z 0VWD4JZ 0VWD4KZ 0VWD4YZ 0VWD70Z 0VWD73Z 0VWD77Z
0VWD7JZ 0VWD7KZ 0VWD7YZ 0VWD80Z 0VWD83Z 0VWD87Z 0VWD8JZ 0VWD8KZ 0VWD8YZ 0VWDX0Z 0VWDX3Z 0VWDX7Z 0VWDXJZ
0VWDXKZ 0VWM00Z 0VWM03Z 0VWM07Z 0VWM0CZ 0VWM0JZ 0VWM0KZ 0VWM0YZ 0VWM30Z 0VWM33Z 0VWM37Z 0VWM3CZ 0VWM3JZ
0VWM3KZ 0VWM3YZ 0VWM40Z 0VWM43Z 0VWM47Z 0VWM4CZ 0VWM4JZ 0VWM4KZ 0VWM4YZ 0VWM70Z 0VWM73Z 0VWM77Z 0VWM7CZ
0VWM7JZ 0VWM7KZ 0VWM7YZ 0VWM80Z 0VWM83Z 0VWM87Z 0VWM8CZ 0VWM8JZ 0VWM8KZ 0VWM8YZ 0VWMX0Z 0VWMX3Z 0VWMX7Z
0VWMXCZ 0VWMXJZ 0VWMXKZ 0VWR00Z 0VWR03Z 0VWR07Z 0VWR0CZ 0VWR0DZ 0VWR0JZ 0VWR0KZ 0VWR0YZ 0VWR30Z 0VWR33Z
0VWR37Z 0VWR3CZ 0VWR3DZ 0VWR3JZ 0VWR3KZ 0VWR3YZ 0VWR40Z 0VWR43Z 0VWR47Z 0VWR4CZ 0VWR4DZ 0VWR4JZ 0VWR4KZ
0VWR4YZ 0VWR70Z 0VWR73Z 0VWR77Z 0VWR7CZ 0VWR7DZ 0VWR7JZ 0VWR7KZ 0VWR7YZ 0VWR80Z 0VWR83Z 0VWR87Z 0VWR8CZ
0VWR8DZ 0VWR8JZ 0VWR8KZ 0VWR8YZ 0VWRX0Z 0VWRX3Z 0VWRX7Z 0VWRXCZ 0VWRXDZ 0VWRXJZ 0VWRXKZ 0VWS00Z 0VWS03Z
0VWS07Z 0VWS0JZ 0VWS0KZ 0VWS0YZ 0VWS30Z 0VWS33Z 0VWS37Z 0VWS3JZ 0VWS3KZ 0VWS3YZ 0VWS40Z 0VWS43Z 0VWS47Z
0VWS4JZ 0VWS4KZ 0VWS4YZ 0VWS70Z 0VWS73Z 0VWS77Z 0VWS7JZ 0VWS7KZ 0VWS7YZ 0VWS80Z 0VWS83Z 0VWS87Z 0VWS8JZ
0VWS8KZ 0VWS8YZ 0VWSX0Z 0VWSX3Z 0VWSX7Z 0VWSXJZ 0VWSXKZ

LC Limited Coverage   NC Noncovered   HAC HAC-associated Procedure   CC Combination Cluster - See Appendix G for code lists
DRG Non-OR-Affecting MS-DRG Assignment   New/Revised Text in Orange   ♂ Male   ♀ Female

2018 ICD-10-PCS

541

MALE REPRODUCTIVE SYSTEM 0V1-0VW

NOTES

Anatomical Regions, General 0W0-0WY

0 Medical and Surgical
W Anatomical Regions, General
0 Alteration: Modifying the anatomic structure of a body part without affecting the function of the body part

Body Part	Approach	Device	Qualifier
Character 4	Character 5	Character 6	Character 7
0 Head **2** Face **4** Upper Jaw **5** Lower Jaw **6** Neck **8** Chest Wall **F** Abdominal Wall **K** Upper Back **L** Lower Back **M** Perineum, Male ♂ **N** Perineum, Female ♀	**0** Open **3** Percutaneous **4** Percutaneous Endoscopic	**7** Autologous Tissue Substitute **J** Synthetic Substitute **K** Nonautologous Tissue Substitute **Z** No Device	**Z** No Qualifier

♂ 0W0M07Z 0W0M0JZ 0W0M0KZ 0W0M0ZZ 0W0M37Z 0W0M3JZ 0W0M3KZ 0W0M3ZZ 0W0M47Z 0W0M4JZ 0W0M4KZ 0W0M4ZZ
♀ 0W0N07Z 0W0N0JZ 0W0N0KZ 0W0N0ZZ 0W0N37Z 0W0N3JZ 0W0N3KZ 0W0N3ZZ 0W0N47Z 0W0N4JZ 0W0N4KZ 0W0N4ZZ

0 Medical and Surgical
W Anatomical Regions, General
1 Bypass: Altering the route of passage of the contents of a tubular body part

Body Part	Approach	Device	Qualifier
Character 4	Character 5	Character 6	Character 7
1 Cranial Cavity	**0** Open	**J** Synthetic Substitute	**9** Pleural Cavity, Right **B** Pleural Cavity, Left **G** Peritoneal Cavity **J** Pelvic Cavity
9 Pleural Cavity, Right **B** Pleural Cavity, Left **G** Peritoneal Cavity **J** Pelvic Cavity	**0** Open **4** Percutaneous Endoscopic	**J** Synthetic Substitute	**4** Cutaneous **9** Pleural Cavity, Right **B** Pleural Cavity, Left **G** Peritoneal Cavity **J** Pelvic Cavity **Y** Lower Vein
9 Pleural Cavity, Right **B** Pleural Cavity, Left **G** Peritoneal Cavity **J** Pelvic Cavity	**3** Percutaneous	**J** Synthetic Substitute	**4** Cutaneous

LC Limited Coverage   **NC** Noncovered   **HAC** HAC-associated Procedure   **CC** Combination Cluster - See Appendix G for code lists
DRG Non-OR-Affecting MS-DRG Assignment   New/Revised Text in **Orange**   ♂ Male   ♀ Female

2018 ICD-10-PCS

543

ANATOMICAL REGIONS, GENERAL 0W0-0WY

0 Medical and Surgical

W Anatomical Regions, General

2 Change: Taking out or off a device from a body part and putting back an identical or similar device in or on the same body part without cutting or puncturing the skin or a mucous membrane

Body Part	Approach	Device	Qualifier
Character 4	Character 5	Character 6	Character 7
0 Head 1 Cranial Cavity 2 Face 4 Upper Jaw 5 Lower Jaw 6 Neck 8 Chest Wall 9 Pleural Cavity, Right B Pleural Cavity, Left C Mediastinum D Pericardial Cavity F Abdominal Wall G Peritoneal Cavity H Retroperitoneum J Pelvic Cavity K Upper Back L Lower Back M Perineum, Male ♂ N Perineum, Female ♀	X External	0 Drainage Device Y Other Device	Z No Qualifier

♂ 0W2MX0Z 0W2MXYZ

♀ 0W2NX0Z 0W2NXYZ

0 Medical and Surgical

W Anatomical Regions, General

3 Control: Stopping, or attempting to stop, postprocedural or other acute bleeding

Body Part	Approach	Device	Qualifier
Character 4	Character 5	Character 6	Character 7
0 Head 1 Cranial Cavity 2 Face 4 Upper Jaw 5 Lower Jaw 6 Neck 8 Chest Wall 9 Pleural Cavity, Right B Pleural Cavity, Left C Mediastinum D Pericardial Cavity F Abdominal Wall G Peritoneal Cavity H Retroperitoneum J Pelvic Cavity K Upper Back L Lower Back M Perineum, Male ♂ N Perineum, Female ♀	0 Open 3 Percutaneous 4 Percutaneous Endoscopic	Z No Device	Z No Qualifier
3 Oral Cavity and Throat	0 Open 3 Percutaneous 4 Percutaneous Endoscopic 7 Via Natural or Artificial Opening 8 Via Natural or Artificial Opening Endoscopic X External	Z No Device	Z No Qualifier
P Gastrointestinal Tract Q Respiratory Tract R Genitourinary Tract	0 Open 3 Percutaneous 4 Percutaneous Endoscopic 7 Via Natural or Artificial Opening 8 Via Natural or Artificial Opening Endoscopic	Z No Device	Z No Qualifier

♂ 0W3M0ZZ 0W3M3ZZ 0W3M4ZZ

♀ 0W3N0ZZ 0W3N3ZZ 0W3N4ZZ

0 Medical and Surgical
W Anatomical Regions, General
4 Creation: Putting in or on biological or synthetic material to form a new body part that to the extent possible replicates the anatomic structure or function of an absent body part

Body Part	Approach	Device	Qualifier
Character 4	Character 5	Character 6	Character 7
M Perineum, Male ♂ NC	0 Open	7 Autologous Tissue Substitute J Synthetic Substitute K Nonautologous Tissue Substitute Z No Device	0 Vagina
N Perineum, Female ♀ NC	0 Open	7 Autologous Tissue Substitute J Synthetic Substitute K Nonautologous Tissue Substitute Z No Device	1 Penis

♂ 0W4M070 0W4M0J0 0W4M0K0 0W4M0Z0
♀ 0W4N071 0W4N0J1 0W4N0K1 0W4N0Z1
NC 0W4M070 0W4M0J0 0W4M0K0 0W4M0Z0 0W4N071 0W4N0J1 0W4N0K1 0W4N0Z1

0 Medical and Surgical
W Anatomical Regions, General
8 Division: Cutting into a body part, without draining fluids and/or gases from the body part, in order to separate or transect a body part

Body Part	Approach	Device	Qualifier
Character 4	Character 5	Character 6	Character 7
N Perineum, Female ♀	X External	Z No Device	Z No Qualifier

♀ 0W8NXZZ

0 Medical and Surgical
W Anatomical Regions, General
9 Drainage: Taking or letting out fluids and/or gases from a body part

Body Part	Approach	Device	Qualifier
Character 4	Character 5	Character 6	Character 7
0 Head 1 Cranial Cavity 2 Face 3 Oral Cavity and Throat 4 Upper Jaw 5 Lower Jaw 6 Neck 8 Chest Wall 9 Pleural Cavity, Right B Pleural Cavity, Left C Mediastinum D Pericardial Cavity F Abdominal Wall G Peritoneal Cavity H Retroperitoneum J Pelvic Cavity K Upper Back L Lower Back M Perineum, Male ♂ N Perineum, Female ♀	0 Open 3 Percutaneous 4 Percutaneous Endoscopic	0 Drainage Device	Z No Qualifier

0W9 continued on next page

0 Medical and Surgical
W Anatomical Regions, General
9 Drainage: Taking or letting out fluids and/or gases from a body part

0W9 continued from previous page

Body Part	Approach	Device	Qualifier
Character 4	Character 5	Character 6	Character 7
0 Head	0 Open	Z No Device	X Diagnostic
1 Cranial Cavity	3 Percutaneous		Z No Qualifier
2 Face	4 Percutaneous Endoscopic		
3 Oral Cavity and Throat			
4 Upper Jaw			
5 Lower Jaw			
6 Neck			
8 Chest Wall			
9 Pleural Cavity, Right			
B Pleural Cavity, Left			
C Mediastinum			
D Pericardial Cavity			
F Abdominal Wall			
G Peritoneal Cavity			
H Retroperitoneum			
J Pelvic Cavity			
K Upper Back			
L Lower Back			
M Perineum, Male ♂			
N Perineum, Female ♀			

♂ 0W9M00Z 0W9M0ZX 0W9M0ZZ 0W9M30Z 0W9M3ZX 0W9M3ZZ 0W9M40Z 0W9M4ZX 0W9M4ZZ
♀ 0W9N00Z 0W9N0ZX 0W9N0ZZ 0W9N30Z 0W9N3ZX 0W9N3ZZ 0W9N40Z 0W9N4ZZ

0 Medical and Surgical
W Anatomical Regions, General
B Excision: Cutting out or off, without replacement, a portion of a body part

Body Part	Approach	Device	Qualifier
Character 4	Character 5	Character 6	Character 7
0 Head	0 Open	Z No Device	X Diagnostic
2 Face	3 Percutaneous		Z No Qualifier
3 Oral Cavity and Throat	4 Percutaneous Endoscopic		
4 Upper Jaw	X External		
5 Lower Jaw			
8 Chest Wall			
K Upper Back			
L Lower Back			
M Perineum, Male ♂			
N Perineum, Female ♀			
6 Neck	0 Open	Z No Device	X Diagnostic
F Abdominal Wall	3 Percutaneous		Z No Qualifier
	4 Percutaneous Endoscopic		
6 Neck	X External	Z No Device	2 Stoma
F Abdominal Wall			X Diagnostic
			Z No Qualifier
C Mediastinum	0 Open	Z No Device	X Diagnostic
H Retroperitoneum	3 Percutaneous		Z No Qualifier
	4 Percutaneous Endoscopic		

♂ 0WBM0ZX 0WBM0ZZ 0WBM3ZX 0WBM3ZZ 0WBM4ZX 0WBM4ZZ 0WBMXZX 0WBMXZZ
♀ 0WBN0ZX 0WBN0ZZ 0WBN3ZX 0WBN3ZZ 0WBN4ZX 0WBN4ZZ 0WBNXZX 0WBNXZZ

0 Medical and Surgical
W Anatomical Regions, General
C Extirpation: Taking or cutting out solid matter from a body part

Body Part	Approach	Device	Qualifier
Character 4	Character 5	Character 6	Character 7
1 Cranial Cavity 3 Oral Cavity and Throat 9 Pleural Cavity, Right B Pleural Cavity, Left C Mediastinum D Pericardial Cavity G Peritoneal Cavity H Retroperitoneum J Pelvic Cavity	0 Open 3 Percutaneous 4 Percutaneous Endoscopic X External	Z No Device	Z No Qualifier
P Gastrointestinal Tract Q Respiratory Tract R Genitourinary Tract	0 Open 3 Percutaneous 4 Percutaneous Endoscopic 7 Via Natural or Artificial Opening 8 Via Natural or Artificial Opening Endoscopic X External	Z No Device	Z No Qualifier

0 Medical and Surgical
W Anatomical Regions, General
F Fragmentation: Breaking solid matter in a body part into pieces

Body Part	Approach	Device	Qualifier
Character 4	Character 5	Character 6	Character 7
1 Cranial Cavity � NC 3 Oral Cavity and Throat NC 9 Pleural Cavity, Right NC B Pleural Cavity, Left NC C Mediastinum NC D Pericardial Cavity G Peritoneal Cavity NC J Pelvic Cavity NC	0 Open 3 Percutaneous 4 Percutaneous Endoscopic X External	Z No Device	Z No Qualifier
P Gastrointestinal Tract NC Q Respiratory Tract NC R Genitourinary Tract	0 Open 3 Percutaneous 4 Percutaneous Endoscopic 7 Via Natural or Artificial Opening 8 Via Natural or Artificial Opening Endoscopic X External	Z No Device	Z No Qualifier

NC 0WF1XZZ   0WF3XZZ   0WF9XZZ   0WFBXZZ   0WFCXZZ   0WFGXZZ   0WFJXZZ   0WFPXZZ   0WFQXZZ

0   Medical and Surgical
W   Anatomical Regions, General
H   Insertion: Putting in a nonbiological appliance that monitors, assists, performs, or prevents a physiological function but does not physically take the place of a body part

Body Part	Approach	Device	Qualifier
Character 4	Character 5	Character 6	Character 7
0 Head ᴼᴿᴳ 1 Cranial Cavity 2 Face ᴼᴿᴳ 3 Oral Cavity and Throat 4 Upper Jaw ᴼᴿᴳ 5 Lower Jaw ᴼᴿᴳ 6 Neck ᴼᴿᴳ 8 Chest Wall 9 Pleural Cavity, Right B Pleural Cavity, Left C Mediastinum D Pericardial Cavity F Abdominal Wall G Peritoneal Cavity H Retroperitoneum J Pelvic Cavity K Upper Back ᴼᴿᴳ L Lower Back ᴼᴿᴳ M Perineum, Male ♂ ᴼᴿᴳ N Perineum, Female ♀	0 Open 3 Percutaneous 4 Percutaneous Endoscopic	1 Radioactive Element 3 Infusion Device Y Other Device	Z No Qualifier
P Gastrointestinal Tract Q Respiratory Tract R Genitourinary Tract	0 Open 3 Percutaneous 4 Percutaneous Endoscopic 7 Via Natural or Artificial Opening 8 Via Natural or Artificial Opening Endoscopic	1 Radioactive Element 3 Infusion Device Y Other Device	Z No Qualifier

♀ 0WHN03Z 0WHN0YZ 0WHN33Z 0WHN3YZ 0WHN43Z 0WHN4YZ
ᴼᴿᴳ 0WH043Z 0WH04YZ 0WH203Z 0WH20YZ 0WH233Z 0WH23YZ 0WH243Z 0WH24YZ 0WH403Z 0WH40YZ 0WH433Z 0WH43YZ 0WH443Z
      0WH44YZ 0WH503Z 0WH50YZ 0WH533Z 0WH53YZ 0WH543Z 0WH54YZ 0WH603Z 0WH60YZ 0WH633Z 0WH63YZ 0WH643Z 0WH64YZ
      0WHK03Z 0WHK0YZ 0WHK33Z 0WHK3YZ 0WHK43Z 0WHK4YZ 0WHL03Z 0WHL0YZ 0WHL33Z 0WHL3YZ 0WHL43Z 0WHL4YZ 0WHM03Z
      0WHM0YZ 0WHM33Z 0WHM3YZ 0WHM43Z 0WHM4YZ

ᴵᶜ Limited Coverage   ᴺᶜ Noncovered   ᴴᴬᶜ HAC-associated Procedure   ᶜᶜ Combination Cluster - See Appendix G for code lists
ᴼᴿᴳ Non-OR-Affecting MS-DRG Assignment   New/Revised Text in **Orange**   ♂ Male   ♀ Female

548

2018 ICD-10-PCS

0 **Medical and Surgical**
W **Anatomical Regions, General**
J **Inspection:** Visually and/or manually exploring a body part

Body Part	Approach	Device	Qualifier
Character 4	Character 5	Character 6	Character 7
0 Head ᴰᴿᴳ 2 Face ᴰᴿᴳ 3 Oral Cavity and Throat 4 Upper Jaw ᴰᴿᴳ 5 Lower Jaw ᴰᴿᴳ 6 Neck 8 Chest Wall F Abdominal Wall K Upper Back L Lower Back M Perineum, Male ♂ N Perineum, Female ♀	0 Open 3 Percutaneous 4 Percutaneous Endoscopic X External	Z No Device	Z No Qualifier
1 Cranial Cavity ᴰᴿᴳ 9 Pleural Cavity, Right B Pleural Cavity, Left C Mediastinum D Pericardial Cavity G Peritoneal Cavity H Retroperitoneum J Pelvic Cavity	0 Open 3 Percutaneous 4 Percutaneous Endoscopic	Z No Device	Z No Qualifier
P Gastrointestinal Tract Q Respiratory Tract R Genitourinary Tract	0 Open 3 Percutaneous 4 Percutaneous Endoscopic 7 Via Natural or Artificial Opening 8 Via Natural or Artificial Opening Endoscopic	Z No Device	Z No Qualifier

♂ 0WJM0ZZ 0WJM3ZZ 0WJM4ZZ 0WJMXZZ
♀ 0WJN0ZZ 0WJN3ZZ 0WJN4ZZ 0WJNXZZ
ᴰᴿᴳ 0WJ00ZZ 0WJ13ZZ 0WJ20ZZ 0WJ40ZZ 0WJ50ZZ

0 **Medical and Surgical**
W **Anatomical Regions, General**
M **Reattachment:** Putting back in or on all or a portion of a separated body part to its normal location or other suitable location

Body Part	Approach	Device	Qualifier
Character 4	Character 5	Character 6	Character 7
2 Face 4 Upper Jaw 5 Lower Jaw 6 Neck 8 Chest Wall F Abdominal Wall K Upper Back L Lower Back M Perineum, Male ♂ N Perineum, Female ♀	0 Open	Z No Device	Z No Qualifier

♂ 0WMM0ZZ
♀ 0WMN0ZZ

0 **Medical and Surgical**
W **Anatomical Regions, General**
P **Removal:** Taking out or off a device from a body part

Body Part	Approach	Device	Qualifier
Character 4	Character 5	Character 6	Character 7
0 Head 2 Face 4 Upper Jaw 5 Lower Jaw 6 Neck 8 Chest Wall C Mediastinum F Abdominal Wall K Upper Back L Lower Back M Perineum, Male ♂ N Perineum, Female ♀	0 Open 3 Percutaneous 4 Percutaneous Endoscopic X External	0 Drainage Device 1 Radioactive Element 3 Infusion Device 7 Autologous Tissue Substitute J Synthetic Substitute K Nonautologous Tissue Substitute Y Other Device	Z No Qualifier
1 Cranial Cavity 9 Pleural Cavity, Right B Pleural Cavity, Left G Peritoneal Cavity J Pelvic Cavity	0 Open 3 Percutaneous 4 Percutaneous Endoscopic	0 Drainage Device 1 Radioactive Element 3 Infusion Device J Synthetic Substitute Y Other Device	Z No Qualifier
1 Cranial Cavity 9 Pleural Cavity, Right B Pleural Cavity, Left G Peritoneal Cavity J Pelvic Cavity	X External	0 Drainage Device 1 Radioactive Element 3 Infusion Device	Z No Qualifier
D Pericardial Cavity H Retroperitoneum	0 Open 3 Percutaneous 4 Percutaneous Endoscopic	0 Drainage Device 1 Radioactive Element 3 Infusion Device Y Other Device	Z No Qualifier
D Pericardial Cavity H Retroperitoneum	X External	0 Drainage Device 1 Radioactive Element 3 Infusion Device	Z No Qualifier
P Gastrointestinal Tract Q Respiratory Tract R Genitourinary Tract	0 Open 3 Percutaneous 4 Percutaneous Endoscopic 7 Via Natural or Artificial Opening 8 Via Natural or Artificial Opening Endoscopic X External	1 Radioactive Element 3 Infusion Device Y Other Device	Z No Qualifier

♂ 0WPM00Z 0WPM01Z 0WPM03Z 0WPM07Z 0WPM0JZ 0WPM0KZ 0WPM0YZ 0WPM30Z 0WPM31Z 0WPM33Z 0WPM37Z 0WPM3JZ 0WPM3KZ 0WPM3YZ 0WPM40Z 0WPM41Z 0WPM43Z 0WPM47Z 0WPM4JZ 0WPM4KZ 0WPM4YZ 0WPMX0Z 0WPMX1Z 0WPMX3Z 0WPMX7Z 0WPMXJZ 0WPMXKZ 0WPMXYZ

♀ 0WPN00Z 0WPN01Z 0WPN03Z 0WPN07Z 0WPN0JZ 0WPN0KZ 0WPN0YZ 0WPN30Z 0WPN31Z 0WPN33Z 0WPN37Z 0WPN3JZ 0WPN3KZ 0WPN3YZ 0WPN40Z 0WPN41Z 0WPN43Z 0WPN47Z 0WPN4JZ 0WPN4KZ 0WPN4YZ 0WPNX0Z 0WPNX1Z 0WPNX3Z 0WPNX7Z 0WPNXJZ 0WPNXKZ 0WPNXYZ

LC Limited Coverage   **NC** Noncovered   **HAC** HAC-associated Procedure   **CC** Combination Cluster - See Appendix G for code lists

ORG Non-OR-Affecting MS-DRG Assignment   New/Revised Text in **Orange**   ♂ Male   ♀ Female

550

2018 ICD-10-PCS

ANATOMICAL REGIONS, GENERAL 0W0-0WY

0   **Medical and Surgical**
W   **Anatomical Regions, General**
Q   **Repair:** Restoring, to the extent possible, a body part to its normal anatomic structure and function

Body Part	Approach	Device	Qualifier
Character 4	Character 5	Character 6	Character 7
0 Head 2 Face 3 Oral Cavity and Throat 4 Upper Jaw 5 Lower Jaw 8 Chest Wall K Upper Back L Lower Back M Perineum, Male ♂ N Perineum, Female ♀	0 Open 3 Percutaneous 4 Percutaneous Endoscopic X External	Z No Device	Z No Qualifier
6 Neck F Abdominal Wall	0 Open 3 Percutaneous 4 Percutaneous Endoscopic	Z No Device	Z No Qualifier
6 Neck F Abdominal Wall 🅲🅲	X External	Z No Device	2 Stoma Z No Qualifier
C Mediastinum	0 Open 3 Percutaneous 4 Percutaneous Endoscopic	Z No Device	Z No Qualifier

♂   0WQM0ZZ   0WQM3ZZ   0WQM4ZZ   0WQMXZZ
♀   0WQN0ZZ   0WQN3ZZ   0WQN4ZZ   0WQNXZZ
🅲🅲   0WQFXZ2   0WQFXZZ

0   **Medical and Surgical**
W   **Anatomical Regions, General**
U   **Supplement:** Putting in or on biological or synthetic material that physically reinforces and/or augments the function of a portion of a body part

Body Part	Approach	Device	Qualifier
Character 4	Character 5	Character 6	Character 7
0 Head 2 Face 4 Upper Jaw 5 Lower Jaw 6 Neck 8 Chest Wall C Mediastinum F Abdominal Wall K Upper Back L Lower Back M Perineum, Male ♂ N Perineum, Female ♀	0 Open 4 Percutaneous Endoscopic	7 Autologous Tissue Substitute J Synthetic Substitute K Nonautologous Tissue Substitute	Z No Qualifier

♂   0WUM07Z   0WUM0JZ   0WUM0KZ   0WUM47Z   0WUM4JZ   0WUM4KZ
♀   0WUN07Z   0WUN0JZ   0WUN0KZ   0WUN47Z   0WUN4JZ   0WUN4KZ

0 Medical and Surgical
W Anatomical Regions, General
W Revision: Correcting, to the extent possible, a portion of a malfunctioning device or the position of a displaced device

Body Part	Approach	Device	Qualifier
Character 4	Character 5	Character 6	Character 7
0 Head ᴼᴿᴳ 2 Face ᴼᴿᴳ 4 Upper Jaw ᴼᴿᴳ 5 Lower Jaw ᴼᴿᴳ 6 Neck ᴼᴿᴳ 8 Chest Wall C Mediastinum F Abdominal Wall K Upper Back L Lower Back M Perineum, Male ♂ N Perineum, Female ♀	0 Open 3 Percutaneous 4 Percutaneous Endoscopic X External	0 Drainage Device 1 Radioactive Element 3 Infusion Device 7 Autologous Tissue Substitute J Synthetic Substitute K Nonautologous Tissue Substitute Y Other Device	Z No Qualifier
1 Cranial Cavity 9 Pleural Cavity, Right B Pleural Cavity, Left G Peritoneal Cavity J Pelvic Cavity	0 Open 3 Percutaneous 4 Percutaneous Endoscopic X External	0 Drainage Device 1 Radioactive Element 3 Infusion Device J Synthetic Substitute Y Other Device	Z No Qualifier
D Pericardial Cavity H Retroperitoneum	0 Open 3 Percutaneous 4 Percutaneous Endoscopic X External	0 Drainage Device 1 Radioactive Element 3 Infusion Device Y Other Device	Z No Qualifier
P Gastrointestinal Tract Q Respiratory Tract R Genitourinary Tract	0 Open 3 Percutaneous 4 Percutaneous Endoscopic 7 Via Natural or Artificial Opening 8 Via Natural or Artificial Opening Endoscopic X External	1 Radioactive Element 3 Infusion Device Y Other Device	Z No Qualifier

♂ 0WWM00Z 0WWM01Z 0WWM03Z 0WWM07Z 0WWM0JZ 0WWM0KZ 0WWM0YZ 0WWM30Z 0WWM31Z 0WWM33Z 0WWM37Z 0WWM3JZ 0WWM3KZ 0WWM3YZ 0WWM40Z 0WWM41Z 0WWM43Z 0WWM47Z 0WWM4JZ 0WWM4KZ 0WWM4YZ 0WWMX0Z 0WWMX1Z 0WWMX3Z 0WWMX7Z 0WWMXJZ 0WWMXKZ 0WWMXYZ

♀ 0WWN00Z 0WWN01Z 0WWN03Z 0WWN07Z 0WWN0JZ 0WWN0KZ 0WWN0YZ 0WWN30Z 0WWN31Z 0WWN33Z 0WWN37Z 0WWN3JZ 0WWN3KZ 0WWN3YZ 0WWN40Z 0WWN41Z 0WWN43Z 0WWN47Z 0WWN4JZ 0WWN4KZ 0WWN4YZ 0WWNX0Z 0WWNX1Z 0WWNX3Z 0WWNX7Z 0WWNXJZ 0WWNXKZ 0WWNXYZ

ᴼᴿᴳ 0WW000Z 0WW001Z 0WW003Z 0WW007Z 0WW00JZ 0WW00KZ 0WW00YZ 0WW030Z 0WW031Z 0WW033Z 0WW037Z 0WW03JZ 0WW03KZ 0WW03YZ 0WW040Z 0WW041Z 0WW043Z 0WW047Z 0WW04JZ 0WW04KZ 0WW04YZ 0WW200Z 0WW201Z 0WW203Z 0WW207Z 0WW20JZ 0WW20KZ 0WW20YZ 0WW230Z 0WW231Z 0WW233Z 0WW237Z 0WW23JZ 0WW23KZ 0WW23YZ 0WW240Z 0WW241Z 0WW243Z 0WW247Z 0WW24JZ 0WW24KZ 0WW24YZ 0WW400Z 0WW401Z 0WW403Z 0WW407Z 0WW40JZ 0WW40KZ 0WW40YZ 0WW430Z 0WW431Z 0WW433Z 0WW437Z 0WW43JZ 0WW43KZ 0WW43YZ 0WW440Z 0WW441Z 0WW443Z 0WW447Z 0WW44JZ 0WW44KZ 0WW44YZ 0WW500Z 0WW501Z 0WW503Z 0WW507Z 0WW50JZ 0WW50KZ 0WW50YZ 0WW530Z 0WW531Z 0WW533Z 0WW537Z 0WW53JZ 0WW53KZ 0WW53YZ 0WW540Z 0WW541Z 0WW543Z 0WW547Z 0WW54JZ 0WW54KZ 0WW54YZ 0WW600Z 0WW601Z 0WW603Z 0WW607Z 0WW60JZ 0WW60KZ 0WW60YZ 0WW630Z 0WW631Z 0WW633Z 0WW637Z 0WW63JZ 0WW63KZ 0WW63YZ 0WW640Z 0WW641Z 0WW643Z 0WW647Z 0WW64JZ 0WW64KZ 0WW64YZ

0 Medical and Surgical
W Anatomical Regions, General
Y Transplantation: Putting in or on all or a portion of a living body part taken from another individual or animal to physically take the place and/or function of all or a portion of a similar body part

Body Part	Approach	Device	Qualifier
Character 4	Character 5	Character 6	Character 7
2 Face	0 Open	Z No Device	0 Allogeneic 1 Syngeneic

NOTES

NOTES

Anatomical Regions, Upper Extremities 0X0-0XY

0 **Medical and Surgical**
X **Anatomical Regions, Upper Extremities**
0 **Alteration:** Modifying the anatomic structure of a body part without affecting the function of the body part

Body Part	Approach	Device	Qualifier
Character 4	**Character 5**	**Character 6**	**Character 7**
2 Shoulder Region, Right **3** Shoulder Region, Left **4** Axilla, Right **5** Axilla, Left **6** Upper Extremity, Right **7** Upper Extremity, Left **8** Upper Arm, Right **9** Upper Arm, Left **B** Elbow Region, Right **C** Elbow Region, Left **D** Lower Arm, Right **F** Lower Arm, Left **G** Wrist Region, Right **H** Wrist Region, Left	**0** Open **3** Percutaneous **4** Percutaneous Endoscopic	**7** Autologous Tissue Substitute **J** Synthetic Substitute **K** Nonautologous Tissue Substitute **Z** No Device	**Z** No Qualifier

0 **Medical and Surgical**
X **Anatomical Regions, Upper Extremities**
2 **Change:** Taking out or off a device from a body part and putting back an identical or similar device in or on the same body part without cutting or puncturing the skin or a mucous membrane

Body Part	Approach	Device	Qualifier
Character 4	**Character 5**	**Character 6**	**Character 7**
6 Upper Extremity, Right **7** Upper Extremity, Left	**X** External	**0** Drainage Device **Y** Other Device	**Z** No Qualifier

0 **Medical and Surgical**
X **Anatomical Regions, Upper Extremities**
3 **Control:** Stopping, or attempting to stop, postprocedural or other acute bleeding

Body Part	Approach	Device	Qualifier
Character 4	**Character 5**	**Character 6**	**Character 7**
2 Shoulder Region, Right **3** Shoulder Region, Left **4** Axilla, Right **5** Axilla, Left **6** Upper Extremity, Right **7** Upper Extremity, Left **8** Upper Arm, Right **9** Upper Arm, Left **B** Elbow Region, Right **C** Elbow Region, Left **D** Lower Arm, Right **F** Lower Arm, Left **G** Wrist Region, Right **H** Wrist Region, Left **J** Hand, Right **K** Hand, Left	**0** Open **3** Percutaneous **4** Percutaneous Endoscopic	**Z** No Device	**Z** No Qualifier

0 Medical and Surgical
X Anatomical Regions, Upper Extremities
6 Detachment: Cutting off all or a portion of the upper or lower extremities

Body Part	Approach	Device	Qualifier
Character 4	Character 5	Character 6	Character 7
0 Forequarter, Right **1** Forequarter, Left **2** Shoulder Region, Right **3** Shoulder Region, Left **B** Elbow Region, Right **C** Elbow Region, Left	**0** Open	**Z** No Device	**Z** No Qualifier
8 Upper Arm, Right **9** Upper Arm, Left **D** Lower Arm, Right **F** Lower Arm, Left	**0** Open	**Z** No Device	**1** High **2** Mid **3** Low
J Hand, Right **K** Hand, Left	**0** Open	**Z** No Device	**0** Complete **4** Complete 1st Ray **5** Complete 2nd Ray **6** Complete 3rd Ray **7** Complete 4th Ray **8** Complete 5th Ray **9** Partial 1st Ray **B** Partial 2nd Ray **C** Partial 3rd Ray **D** Partial 4th Ray **F** Partial 5th Ray
L Thumb, Right **M** Thumb, Left **N** Index Finger, Right **P** Index Finger, Left **Q** Middle Finger, Right **R** Middle Finger, Left **S** Ring Finger, Right **T** Ring Finger, Left **V** Little Finger, Right **W** Little Finger, Left	**0** Open	**Z** No Device	**0** Complete **1** High **2** Mid **3** Low

0 **Medical and Surgical**
X **Anatomical Regions, Upper Extremities**
9 **Drainage:** Taking or letting out fluids and/or gases from a body part

Body Part	Approach	Device	Qualifier
Character 4	Character 5	Character 6	Character 7
2 Shoulder Region, Right 3 Shoulder Region, Left 4 Axilla, Right 5 Axilla, Left 6 Upper Extremity, Right 7 Upper Extremity, Left 8 Upper Arm, Right 9 Upper Arm, Left B Elbow Region, Right C Elbow Region, Left D Lower Arm, Right F Lower Arm, Left G Wrist Region, Right H Wrist Region, Left J Hand, Right K Hand, Left	0 Open 3 Percutaneous 4 Percutaneous Endoscopic	0 Drainage Device	Z No Qualifier
2 Shoulder Region, Right 3 Shoulder Region, Left 4 Axilla, Right 5 Axilla, Left 6 Upper Extremity, Right 7 Upper Extremity, Left 8 Upper Arm, Right 9 Upper Arm, Left B Elbow Region, Right C Elbow Region, Left D Lower Arm, Right F Lower Arm, Left G Wrist Region, Right H Wrist Region, Left J Hand, Right K Hand, Left	0 Open 3 Percutaneous 4 Percutaneous Endoscopic	Z No Device	X Diagnostic Z No Qualifier

LC Limited Coverage   NC Noncovered   HAC HAC-associated Procedure   CC Combination Cluster - See Appendix G for code lists
Non-OR-Affecting MS-DRG Assignment   New/Revised Text in Orange   ♂ Male   ♀ Female

2018 ICD-10-PCS

557

0 Medical and Surgical
X Anatomical Regions, Upper Extremities
B Excision: Cutting out or off, without replacement, a portion of a body part

Body Part	Approach	Device	Qualifier
Character 4	Character 5	Character 6	Character 7
2 Shoulder Region, Right **3** Shoulder Region, Left **4** Axilla, Right **5** Axilla, Left **6** Upper Extremity, Right **7** Upper Extremity, Left **8** Upper Arm, Right **9** Upper Arm, Left **B** Elbow Region, Right **C** Elbow Region, Left **D** Lower Arm, Right **F** Lower Arm, Left **G** Wrist Region, Right **H** Wrist Region, Left **J** Hand, Right **K** Hand, Left	**0** Open **3** Percutaneous **4** Percutaneous Endoscopic	**Z** No Device	**X** Diagnostic **Z** No Qualifier

0 Medical and Surgical
X Anatomical Regions, Upper Extremities
H Insertion: Putting in a nonbiological appliance that monitors, assists, performs, or prevents a physiological function but does not physically take the place of a body part

Body Part	Approach	Device	Qualifier
Character 4	Character 5	Character 6	Character 7
2 Shoulder Region, Right **3** Shoulder Region, Left **4** Axilla, Right **5** Axilla, Left **6** Upper Extremity, Right **7** Upper Extremity, Left **8** Upper Arm, Right **9** Upper Arm, Left **B** Elbow Region, Right **C** Elbow Region, Left **D** Lower Arm, Right **F** Lower Arm, Left **G** Wrist Region, Right **H** Wrist Region, Left **J** Hand, Right **K** Hand, Left	**0** Open **3** Percutaneous **4** Percutaneous Endoscopic	**1** Radioactive Element **3** Infusion Device **Y** Other Device	**Z** No Qualifier

0 Medical and Surgical
X Anatomical Regions, Upper Extremities
J Inspection: Visually and/or manually exploring a body part

Body Part	Approach	Device	Qualifier
Character 4	Character 5	Character 6	Character 7
2 Shoulder Region, Right **3** Shoulder Region, Left **4** Axilla, Right **5** Axilla, Left **6** Upper Extremity, Right **7** Upper Extremity, Left **8** Upper Arm, Right **9** Upper Arm, Left **B** Elbow Region, Right **C** Elbow Region, Left **D** Lower Arm, Right **F** Lower Arm, Left **G** Wrist Region, Right **H** Wrist Region, Left **J** Hand, Right **K** Hand, Left	**0** Open **3** Percutaneous **4** Percutaneous Endoscopic **X** External	**Z** No Device	**Z** No Qualifier

0 Medical and Surgical
X Anatomical Regions, Upper Extremities
M Reattachment: Putting back in or on all or a portion of a separated body part to its normal location or other suitable location

Body Part	Approach	Device	Qualifier
Character 4	Character 5	Character 6	Character 7
0 Forequarter, Right **1** Forequarter, Left **2** Shoulder Region, Right **3** Shoulder Region, Left **4** Axilla, Right **5** Axilla, Left **6** Upper Extremity, Right **7** Upper Extremity, Left **8** Upper Arm, Right **9** Upper Arm, Left **B** Elbow Region, Right **C** Elbow Region, Left **D** Lower Arm, Right **F** Lower Arm, Left **G** Wrist Region, Right **H** Wrist Region, Left **J** Hand, Right **K** Hand, Left **L** Thumb, Right **M** Thumb, Left **N** Index Finger, Right **P** Index Finger, Left **Q** Middle Finger, Right **R** Middle Finger, Left **S** Ring Finger, Right **T** Ring Finger, Left **V** Little Finger, Right **W** Little Finger, Left	**0** Open	**Z** No Device	**Z** No Qualifier

LC Limited Coverage   NC Noncovered   HAC HAC-associated Procedure   CC Combination Cluster - See Appendix G for code lists
DRG Non-OR-Affecting MS-DRG Assignment   New/Revised Text in Orange   ♂ Male   ♀ Female

2018 ICD-10-PCS

559

0 Medical and Surgical
X Anatomical Regions, Upper Extremities
P Removal: Taking out or off a device from a body part

Body Part	Approach	Device	Qualifier
Character 4	Character 5	Character 6	Character 7
6 Upper Extremity, Right 7 Upper Extremity, Left	0 Open 3 Percutaneous 4 Percutaneous Endoscopic X External	0 Drainage Device 1 Radioactive Element 3 Infusion Device 7 Autologous Tissue Substitute J Synthetic Substitute K Nonautologous Tissue Substitute Y Other Device	Z No Qualifier

0 Medical and Surgical
X Anatomical Regions, Upper Extremities
Q Repair: Restoring, to the extent possible, a body part to its normal anatomic structure and function

Body Part	Approach	Device	Qualifier
Character 4	Character 5	Character 6	Character 7
2 Shoulder Region, Right 3 Shoulder Region, Left 4 Axilla, Right 5 Axilla, Left 6 Upper Extremity, Right 7 Upper Extremity, Left 8 Upper Arm, Right 9 Upper Arm, Left B Elbow Region, Right C Elbow Region, Left D Lower Arm, Right F Lower Arm, Left G Wrist Region, Right H Wrist Region, Left J Hand, Right K Hand, Left L Thumb, Right M Thumb, Left N Index Finger, Right P Index Finger, Left Q Middle Finger, Right R Middle Finger, Left S Ring Finger, Right T Ring Finger, Left V Little Finger, Right W Little Finger, Left	0 Open 3 Percutaneous 4 Percutaneous Endoscopic X External	Z No Device	Z No Qualifier

0 Medical and Surgical
X Anatomical Regions, Upper Extremities
R Replacement: Putting in or on biological or synthetic material that physically takes the place and/or function of all or a portion of a body part

Body Part	Approach	Device	Qualifier
Character 4	Character 5	Character 6	Character 7
L Thumb, Right M Thumb, Left	0 Open 4 Percutaneous Endoscopic	7 Autologous Tissue Substitute	N Toe, Right P Toe, Left

0 Medical and Surgical
X Anatomical Regions, Upper Extremities
U Supplement: Putting in or on biological or synthetic material that physically reinforces and/or augments the function of a portion of a body part

Body Part	Approach	Device	Qualifier
Character 4	Character 5	Character 6	Character 7
2 Shoulder Region, Right **3** Shoulder Region, Left **4** Axilla, Right **5** Axilla, Left **6** Upper Extremity, Right **7** Upper Extremity, Left **8** Upper Arm, Right **9** Upper Arm, Left **B** Elbow Region, Right **C** Elbow Region, Left **D** Lower Arm, Right **F** Lower Arm, Left **G** Wrist Region, Right **H** Wrist Region, Left **J** Hand, Right **K** Hand, Left **L** Thumb, Right **M** Thumb, Left **N** Index Finger, Right **P** Index Finger, Left **Q** Middle Finger, Right **R** Middle Finger, Left **S** Ring Finger, Right **T** Ring Finger, Left **V** Little Finger, Right **W** Little Finger, Left	**0** Open **4** Percutaneous Endoscopic	**7** Autologous Tissue Substitute **J** Synthetic Substitute **K** Nonautologous Tissue Substitute	**Z** No Qualifier

0 Medical and Surgical
X Anatomical Regions, Upper Extremities
W Revision: Correcting, to the extent possible, a portion of a malfunctioning device or the position of a displaced device

Body Part	Approach	Device	Qualifier
Character 4	Character 5	Character 6	Character 7
6 Upper Extremity, Right **7** Upper Extremity, Left	**0** Open **3** Percutaneous **4** Percutaneous Endoscopic **X** External	**0** Drainage Device **3** Infusion Device **7** Autologous Tissue Substitute **J** Synthetic Substitute **K** Nonautologous Tissue Substitute **Y** Other Device	**Z** No Qualifier

0 Medical and Surgical
X Anatomical Regions, Upper Extremities
X Transfer: Moving, without taking out, all or a portion of a body part to another location to take over the function of all or a portion of a body part

Body Part	Approach	Device	Qualifier
Character 4	Character 5	Character 6	Character 7
N Index Finger, Right	**0** Open	**Z** No Device	**L** Thumb, Right
P Index Finger, Left	**0** Open	**Z** No Device	**M** Thumb, Left

0 Medical and Surgical
X Anatomical Regions, Upper Extremities
Y Transplantation: Putting in or on all or a portion of a living body part taken from another individual or animal to physically take the place and/or function of all or a portion of a similar body part

Body Part	Approach	Device	Qualifier
Character 4	Character 5	Character 6	Character 7
J Hand, Right **K** Hand, Left	**0** Open	**Z** No Device	**0** Allogeneic **1** Syngeneic

NOTES

0 Medical and Surgical
Y Anatomical Regions, Lower Extremities
0 Alteration: Modifying the anatomic structure of a body part without affecting the function of the body part

Body Part — Character 4	Approach — Character 5	Device — Character 6	Qualifier — Character 7
0 Buttock, Right 1 Buttock, Left 9 Lower Extremity, Right B Lower Extremity, Left C Upper Leg, Right D Upper Leg, Left F Knee Region, Right G Knee Region, Left H Lower Leg, Right J Lower Leg, Left K Ankle Region, Right L Ankle Region, Left	0 Open 3 Percutaneous 4 Percutaneous Endoscopic	7 Autologous Tissue Substitute J Synthetic Substitute K Nonautologous Tissue Substitute Z No Device	Z No Qualifier

0 Medical and Surgical
Y Anatomical Regions, Lower Extremities
2 Change: Taking out or off a device from a body part and putting back an identical or similar device in or on the same body part without cutting or puncturing the skin or a mucous membrane

Body Part — Character 4	Approach — Character 5	Device — Character 6	Qualifier — Character 7
9 Lower Extremity, Right B Lower Extremity, Left	X External	0 Drainage Device Y Other Device	Z No Qualifier

0 Medical and Surgical
Y Anatomical Regions, Lower Extremities
3 Control: Stopping, or attempting to stop, postprocedural or other acute bleeding

Body Part — Character 4	Approach — Character 5	Device — Character 6	Qualifier — Character 7
0 Buttock, Right 1 Buttock, Left 5 Inguinal Region, Right 6 Inguinal Region, Left 7 Femoral Region, Right 8 Femoral Region, Left 9 Lower Extremity, Right B Lower Extremity, Left C Upper Leg, Right D Upper Leg, Left F Knee Region, Right G Knee Region, Left H Lower Leg, Right J Lower Leg, Left K Ankle Region, Right L Ankle Region, Left M Foot, Right N Foot, Left	0 Open 3 Percutaneous 4 Percutaneous Endoscopic	Z No Device	Z No Qualifier

LC Limited Coverage   NC Noncovered   HAC HAC-associated Procedure   CC Combination Cluster - See Appendix G for code lists
Non-OR-Affecting MS-DRG Assignment   New/Revised Text in Orange   ♂ Male   ♀ Female

2018 ICD-10-PCS

563

ANATOMICAL REGIONS, LOWER EXTREMITIES 0Y0-0YW

0 Medical and Surgical
Y Anatomical Regions, Lower Extremities
6 **Detachment:** Cutting off all or a portion of the upper or lower extremities

Body Part	Approach	Device	Qualifier
Character 4	**Character 5**	**Character 6**	**Character 7**
2 Hindquarter, Right **3** Hindquarter, Left **4** Hindquarter, Bilateral **7** Femoral Region, Right **8** Femoral Region, Left **F** Knee Region, Right **G** Knee Region, Left	**0** Open	**Z** No Device	**Z** No Qualifier
C Upper Leg, Right **D** Upper Leg, Left **H** Lower Leg, Right **J** Lower Leg, Left	**0** Open	**Z** No Device	**1** High **2** Mid **3** Low
M Foot, Right **N** Foot, Left	**0** Open	**Z** No Device	**0** Complete **4** Complete 1st Ray **5** Complete 2nd Ray **6** Complete 3rd Ray **7** Complete 4th Ray **8** Complete 5th Ray **9** Partial 1st Ray **B** Partial 2nd Ray **C** Partial 3rd Ray **D** Partial 4th Ray **F** Partial 5th Ray
P 1st Toe, Right **Q** 1st Toe, Left **R** 2nd Toe, Right **S** 2nd Toe, Left **T** 3rd Toe, Right **U** 3rd Toe, Left **V** 4th Toe, Right **W** 4th Toe, Left **X** 5th Toe, Right **Y** 5th Toe, Left	**0** Open	**Z** No Device	**0** Complete **1** High **2** Mid **3** Low

0 **Medical and Surgical**
Y **Anatomical Regions, Lower Extremities**
9 **Drainage:** Taking or letting out fluids and/or gases from a body part

Body Part	Approach	Device	Qualifier
Character 4	Character 5	Character 6	Character 7
0 Buttock, Right **1** Buttock, Left **5** Inguinal Region, Right **6** Inguinal Region, Left **7** Femoral Region, Right **8** Femoral Region, Left **9** Lower Extremity, Right **B** Lower Extremity, Left **C** Upper Leg, Right **D** Upper Leg, Left **F** Knee Region, Right **G** Knee Region, Left **H** Lower Leg, Right **J** Lower Leg, Left **K** Ankle Region, Right **L** Ankle Region, Left **M** Foot, Right **N** Foot, Left	**0** Open **3** Percutaneous **4** Percutaneous Endoscopic	**0** Drainage Device	**Z** No Qualifier
0 Buttock, Right **1** Buttock, Left **5** Inguinal Region, Right **6** Inguinal Region, Left **7** Femoral Region, Right **8** Femoral Region, Left **9** Lower Extremity, Right **B** Lower Extremity, Left **C** Upper Leg, Right **D** Upper Leg, Left **F** Knee Region, Right **G** Knee Region, Left **H** Lower Leg, Right **J** Lower Leg, Left **K** Ankle Region, Right **L** Ankle Region, Left **M** Foot, Right **N** Foot, Left	**0** Open **3** Percutaneous **4** Percutaneous Endoscopic	**Z** No Device	**X** Diagnostic **Z** No Qualifier

0 **Medical and Surgical**
Y **Anatomical Regions, Lower Extremities**
B **Excision:** Cutting out or off, without replacement, a portion of a body part

Body Part	Approach	Device	Qualifier
Character 4	Character 5	Character 6	Character 7
0 Buttock, Right **1** Buttock, Left **5** Inguinal Region, Right **6** Inguinal Region, Left **7** Femoral Region, Right **8** Femoral Region, Left **9** Lower Extremity, Right **B** Lower Extremity, Left **C** Upper Leg, Right **D** Upper Leg, Left **F** Knee Region, Right **G** Knee Region, Left **H** Lower Leg, Right **J** Lower Leg, Left **K** Ankle Region, Right **L** Ankle Region, Left **M** Foot, Right **N** Foot, Left	**0** Open **3** Percutaneous **4** Percutaneous Endoscopic	**Z** No Device	**X** Diagnostic **Z** No Qualifier

0 Medical and Surgical
Y Anatomical Regions, Lower Extremities
H Insertion: Putting in a nonbiological appliance that monitors, assists, performs, or prevents a physiological function but does not physically take the place of a body part

Body Part	Approach	Device	Qualifier
Character 4	Character 5	Character 6	Character 7
0 Buttock, Right ᴰᴿᴳ 1 Buttock, Left ᴰᴿᴳ 5 Inguinal Region, Right ᴰᴿᴳ 6 Inguinal Region, Left ᴰᴿᴳ 7 Femoral Region, Right ᴰᴿᴳ 8 Femoral Region, Left ᴰᴿᴳ 9 Lower Extremity, Right ᴰᴿᴳ B Lower Extremity, Left ᴰᴿᴳ C Upper Leg, Right ᴰᴿᴳ D Upper Leg, Left ᴰᴿᴳ F Knee Region, Right ᴰᴿᴳ G Knee Region, Left ᴰᴿᴳ H Lower Leg, Right ᴰᴿᴳ J Lower Leg, Left ᴰᴿᴳ K Ankle Region, Right ᴰᴿᴳ L Ankle Region, Left ᴰᴿᴳ M Foot, Right ᴰᴿᴳ N Foot, Left ᴰᴿᴳ	0 Open 3 Percutaneous 4 Percutaneous Endoscopic	1 Radioactive Element 3 Infusion Device Y Other Device	Z No Qualifier

ᴰᴿᴳ

0YH003Z	0YH00YZ	0YH033Z	0YH03YZ	0YH043Z	0YH04YZ	0YH103Z	0YH10YZ	0YH133Z	0YH13YZ	0YH143Z	0YH14YZ	0YH503Z
0YH50YZ	0YH533Z	0YH53YZ	0YH543Z	0YH54YZ	0YH603Z	0YH60YZ	0YH633Z	0YH63YZ	0YH643Z	0YH64YZ	0YH703Z	0YH70YZ
0YH733Z	0YH73YZ	0YH743Z	0YH74YZ	0YH803Z	0YH80YZ	0YH833Z	0YH83YZ	0YH843Z	0YH84YZ	0YH903Z	0YH90YZ	0YH933Z
0YH93YZ	0YH943Z	0YH94YZ	0YHB03Z	0YHB0YZ	0YHB33Z	0YHB3YZ	0YHB43Z	0YHB4YZ	0YHC03Z	0YHC0YZ	0YHC33Z	0YHC3YZ
0YHC43Z	0YHC4YZ	0YHD03Z	0YHD0YZ	0YHD33Z	0YHD3YZ	0YHD43Z	0YHD4YZ	0YHF03Z	0YHF0YZ	0YHF33Z	0YHF3YZ	0YHF43Z
0YHF4YZ	0YHG03Z	0YHG0YZ	0YHG33Z	0YHG3YZ	0YHG43Z	0YHG4YZ	0YHH03Z	0YHH0YZ	0YHH33Z	0YHH3YZ	0YHH43Z	0YHH4YZ
0YHJ03Z	0YHJ0YZ	0YHJ33Z	0YHJ3YZ	0YHJ43Z	0YHJ4YZ	0YHK03Z	0YHK0YZ	0YHK33Z	0YHK3YZ	0YHK43Z	0YHK4YZ	0YHL03Z
0YHL0YZ	0YHL33Z	0YHL3YZ	0YHL43Z	0YHL4YZ	0YHM03Z	0YHM0YZ	0YHM33Z	0YHM3YZ	0YHM43Z	0YHM4YZ	0YHN03Z	0YHN0YZ
0YHN33Z	0YHN3YZ	0YHN43Z	0YHN4YZ									

0 Medical and Surgical
Y Anatomical Regions, Lower Extremities
J Inspection: Visually and/or manually exploring a body part

Body Part	Approach	Device	Qualifier
Character 4	Character 5	Character 6	Character 7
0 Buttock, Right ᴰᴿᴳ 1 Buttock, Left ᴰᴿᴳ 5 Inguinal Region, Right ᴰᴿᴳ 6 Inguinal Region, Left ᴰᴿᴳ 7 Femoral Region, Right ᴰᴿᴳ 8 Femoral Region, Left ᴰᴿᴳ 9 Lower Extremity, Right ᴰᴿᴳ A Inguinal Region, Bilateral ᴰᴿᴳ B Lower Extremity, Left ᴰᴿᴳ C Upper Leg, Right ᴰᴿᴳ D Upper Leg, Left ᴰᴿᴳ E Femoral Region, Bilateral ᴰᴿᴳ F Knee Region, Right ᴰᴿᴳ G Knee Region, Left ᴰᴿᴳ H Lower Leg, Right ᴰᴿᴳ J Lower Leg, Left ᴰᴿᴳ K Ankle Region, Right ᴰᴿᴳ L Ankle Region, Left ᴰᴿᴳ M Foot, Right ᴰᴿᴳ N Foot, Left ᴰᴿᴳ	0 Open 3 Percutaneous 4 Percutaneous Endoscopic X External	Z No Device	Z No Qualifier

ᴰᴿᴳ

0YJ00ZZ	0YJ10ZZ	0YJ53ZZ	0YJ63ZZ	0YJ73ZZ	0YJ80ZZ	0YJ83ZZ	0YJ90ZZ	0YJA3ZZ	0YJB0ZZ	0YJC0ZZ	0YJD0ZZ	0YJE0ZZ
0YJE3ZZ	0YJF0ZZ	0YJG0ZZ	0YJH0ZZ	0YJJ0ZZ	0YJK0ZZ	0YJL0ZZ	0YJM0ZZ	0YJN0ZZ				

ᴸᶜ Limited Coverage   ᴺᶜ Noncovered   ᴴᴬᶜ HAC-associated Procedure   ᶜᶜ Combination Cluster - See Appendix G for code lists
ᴰᴿᴳ Non-OR-Affecting MS-DRG Assignment   New/Revised Text in **Orange**   ♂ Male   ♀ Female

566

2018 ICD-10-PCS

0 Medical and Surgical
Y Anatomical Regions, Lower Extremities
M Reattachment: Putting back in or on all or a portion of a separated body part to its normal location or other suitable location

Body Part	Approach	Device	Qualifier
Character 4	Character 5	Character 6	Character 7
0 Buttock, Right	0 Open	Z No Device	Z No Qualifier
1 Buttock, Left			
2 Hindquarter, Right			
3 Hindquarter, Left			
4 Hindquarter, Bilateral			
5 Inguinal Region, Right			
6 Inguinal Region, Left			
7 Femoral Region, Right			
8 Femoral Region, Left			
9 Lower Extremity, Right			
B Lower Extremity, Left			
C Upper Leg, Right			
D Upper Leg, Left			
F Knee Region, Right			
G Knee Region, Left			
H Lower Leg, Right			
J Lower Leg, Left			
K Ankle Region, Right			
L Ankle Region, Left			
M Foot, Right			
N Foot, Left			
P 1st Toe, Right			
Q 1st Toe, Left			
R 2nd Toe, Right			
S 2nd Toe, Left			
T 3rd Toe, Right			
U 3rd Toe, Left			
V 4th Toe, Right			
W 4th Toe, Left			
X 5th Toe, Right			
Y 5th Toe, Left			

0 Medical and Surgical
Y Anatomical Regions, Lower Extremities
P Removal: Taking out or off a device from a body part

Body Part	Approach	Device	Qualifier
Character 4	Character 5	Character 6	Character 7
9 Lower Extremity, Right	0 Open	0 Drainage Device	Z No Qualifier
B Lower Extremity, Left	3 Percutaneous	1 Radioactive Element	
	4 Percutaneous Endoscopic	3 Infusion Device	
	X External	7 Autologous Tissue Substitute	
		J Synthetic Substitute	
		K Nonautologous Tissue Substitute	
		Y Other Device	

0 Medical and Surgical
Y Anatomical Regions, Lower Extremities
Q Repair: Restoring, to the extent possible, a body part to its normal anatomic structure and function

Body Part		Approach	Device	Qualifier
Character 4		**Character 5**	**Character 6**	**Character 7**
0 Buttock, Right		0 Open	Z No Device	Z No Qualifier
1 Buttock, Left		3 Percutaneous		
5 Inguinal Region, Right		4 Percutaneous Endoscopic		
6 Inguinal Region, Left		X External		
7 Femoral Region, Right				
8 Femoral Region, Left				
9 Lower Extremity, Right				
A Inguinal Region, Bilateral				
B Lower Extremity, Left				
C Upper Leg, Right				
D Upper Leg, Left				
E Femoral Region, Bilateral				
F Knee Region, Right				
G Knee Region, Left				
H Lower Leg, Right				
J Lower Leg, Left				
K Ankle Region, Right				
L Ankle Region, Left				
M Foot, Right				
N Foot, Left				
P 1st Toe, Right				
Q 1st Toe, Left				
R 2nd Toe, Right				
S 2nd Toe, Left				
T 3rd Toe, Right				
U 3rd Toe, Left				
V 4th Toe, Right				
W 4th Toe, Left				
X 5th Toe, Right				
Y 5th Toe, Left				

LC Limited Coverage   NC Noncovered   HAC HAC-associated Procedure   CC Combination Cluster - See Appendix G for code lists
DRG Non-OR-Affecting MS-DRG Assignment   New/Revised Text in **Orange**   ♂ Male   ♀ Female

0 **Medical and Surgical**
Y **Anatomical Regions, Lower Extremities**
U **Supplement:** Putting in or on biological or synthetic material that physically reinforces and/or augments the function of a portion of a body part

Body Part	Approach	Device	Qualifier
Character 4	Character 5	Character 6	Character 7
0 Buttock, Right 1 Buttock, Left 5 Inguinal Region, Right 6 Inguinal Region, Left 7 Femoral Region, Right 8 Femoral Region, Left 9 Lower Extremity, Right A Inguinal Region, Bilateral B Lower Extremity, Left C Upper Leg, Right D Upper Leg, Left E Femoral Region, Bilateral F Knee Region, Right G Knee Region, Left H Lower Leg, Right J Lower Leg, Left K Ankle Region, Right L Ankle Region, Left M Foot, Right N Foot, Left P 1st Toe, Right Q 1st Toe, Left R 2nd Toe, Right S 2nd Toe, Left T 3rd Toe, Right U 3rd Toe, Left V 4th Toe, Right W 4th Toe, Left X 5th Toe, Right Y 5th Toe, Left	0 Open 4 Percutaneous Endoscopic	7 Autologous Tissue Substitute J Synthetic Substitute K Nonautologous Tissue Substitute	Z No Qualifier

0 **Medical and Surgical**
Y **Anatomical Regions, Lower Extremities**
W **Revision:** Correcting, to the extent possible, a portion of a malfunctioning device or the position of a displaced device

Body Part	Approach	Device	Qualifier
Character 4	Character 5	Character 6	Character 7
9 Lower Extremity, Right B Lower Extremity, Left	0 Open 3 Percutaneous 4 Percutaneous Endoscopic X External	0 Drainage Device 3 Infusion Device 7 Autologous Tissue Substitute J Synthetic Substitute K Nonautologous Tissue Substitute Y Other Device	Z No Qualifier

LC Limited Coverage   NC Noncovered   HAC HAC-associated Procedure   CC Combination Cluster - See Appendix G for code lists
DRG Non-OR-Affecting MS-DRG Assignment   New/Revised Text in Orange   ♂ Male   ♀ Female

2018 ICD-10-PCS

569

ANATOMICAL REGIONS, LOWER EXTREMITIES 0Y0-0YW

NOTES

1 Obstetrics
0 Pregnancy
2 Change: Taking out or off a device from a body part and putting back an identical or similar device in or on the same body part without cutting or puncturing the skin or a mucous membrane

Body Part	Approach	Device	Qualifier
Character 4	Character 5	Character 6	Character 7
0 Products of Conception ♀	**7** Via Natural or Artificial Opening	**3** Monitoring Electrode **Y** Other Device	**Z** No Qualifier

♀ 102073Z   10207YZ

1 Obstetrics
0 Pregnancy
9 Drainage: Taking or letting out fluids and/or gases from a body part

Body Part	Approach	Device	Qualifier
Character 4	Character 5	Character 6	Character 7
0 Products of Conception ♀	**0** Open **3** Percutaneous **4** Percutaneous Endoscopic **7** Via Natural or Artificial Opening **8** Via Natural or Artificial Opening Endoscopic	**Z** No Device	**9** Fetal Blood **A** Fetal Cerebrospinal Fluid **B** Fetal Fluid, Other **C** Amniotic Fluid, Therapeutic **D** Fluid, Other **U** Amniotic Fluid, Diagnostic

♀ 10900Z9   10900ZA   10900ZB   10900ZC   10900ZD   10900ZU   10903Z9   10903ZA   10903ZB   10903ZC   10903ZD   10903ZU   10904Z9
    10904ZA   10904ZB   10904ZC   10904ZD   10904ZU   10907Z9   10907ZA   10907ZB   10907ZC   10907ZD   10907ZU   10908Z9   10908ZA
    10908ZB   10908ZC   10908ZD   10908ZU

1 Obstetrics
0 Pregnancy
A Abortion: Artificially terminating a pregnancy

Body Part	Approach	Device	Qualifier
Character 4	Character 5	Character 6	Character 7
0 Products of Conception ♀	**0** Open **3** Percutaneous **4** Percutaneous Endoscopic **8** Via Natural or Artificial Opening Endoscopic	**Z** No Device	**Z** No Qualifier
0 Products of Conception ♀	**7** Via Natural or Artificial Opening	**Z** No Device	**6** Vacuum **W** Laminaria **X** Abortifacient **Z** No Qualifier

♀ 10A00ZZ   10A03ZZ   10A04ZZ   10A07Z6   10A07ZW   10A07ZX   10A07ZZ   10A08ZZ

1 Obstetrics

0 Pregnancy

D Extraction: Pulling or stripping out or off all or a portion of a body part by the use of force

Body Part	Approach	Device	Qualifier
Character 4	Character 5	Character 6	Character 7
0 Products of Conception ♀	**0** Open	**Z** No Device	**0** Classical **1** Low Cervical **2** Extraperitoneal
0 Products of Conception ♀	**7** Via Natural or Artificial Opening	**Z** No Device	**3** Low Forceps **4** Mid Forceps **5** High Forceps **6** Vacuum **7** Internal Version **8** Other
1 Products of Conception, Retained ♀	**7** Via Natural or Artificial Opening **8** Via Natural or Artificial Opening Endoscopic	**Z** No Device	**9** Manual **Z** No Qualifier
2 Products of Conception, Ectopic ♀	**7** Via Natural or Artificial Opening **8** Via Natural or Artificial Opening Endoscopic	**Z** No Device	**Z** No Qualifier

♀ 10D00Z0   10D00Z1   10D00Z2   10D07Z3   10D07Z4   10D07Z5   10D07Z6   10D07Z7   10D07Z8   10D17ZZ   10D18ZZ   10D27ZZ   10D28ZZ

1 Obstetrics

0 Pregnancy

E Delivery: Assisting the passage of the products of conception from the genital canal

Body Part	Approach	Device	Qualifier
Character 4	Character 5	Character 6	Character 7
0 Products of Conception ♀	**X** External	**Z** No Device	**Z** No Qualifier

♀ 10E0XZZ

1 Obstetrics

0 Pregnancy

H Insertion: Putting in a nonbiological appliance that monitors, assists, performs, or prevents a physiological function but does not physically take the place of a body part

Body Part	Approach	Device	Qualifier
Character 4	Character 5	Character 6	Character 7
0 Products of Conception ♀	**0** Open **7** Via Natural or Artificial Opening	**3** Monitoring Electrode **Y** Other Device	**Z** No Qualifier

♀ 10H003Z   10H00YZ   10H073Z   10H07YZ

1 Obstetrics

0 Pregnancy

J Inspection: Visually and/or manually exploring a body part

Body Part	Approach	Device	Qualifier
Character 4	Character 5	Character 6	Character 7
0 Products of Conception ♀ **1** Products of Conception, Retained ♀ **2** Products of Conception, Ectopic ♀	**0** Open **3** Percutaneous **4** Percutaneous Endoscopic **7** Via Natural or Artificial Opening **8** Via Natural or Artificial Opening Endoscopic **X** External	**Z** No Device	**Z** No Qualifier

♀ 10J00ZZ   10J03ZZ   10J04ZZ   10J07ZZ   10J08ZZ   10J0XZZ   10J10ZZ   10J13ZZ   10J14ZZ   10J17ZZ   10J18ZZ   10J1XZZ   10J20ZZ
10J23ZZ   10J24ZZ   10J27ZZ   10J28ZZ   10J2XZZ

LC Limited Coverage   **NC** Noncovered   **HAC** HAC-associated Procedure   **CC** Combination Cluster - See Appendix G for code lists
DRG Non-OR-Affecting MS-DRG Assignment   New/Revised Text in **Orange**   ♂ Male   ♀ Female

572

2018 ICD-10-PCS

1 Obstetrics
0 Pregnancy
P Removal: Taking out or off a device from a body part, region, or orifice

Body Part	Approach	Device	Qualifier
Character 4	Character 5	Character 6	Character 7
0 Products of Conception ♀	**0** Open **7** Via Natural or Artificial Opening	**3** Monitoring Electrode **Y** Other Device	**Z** No Qualifier

♀ 10P003Z 10P00YZ 10P073Z 10P07YZ

1 Obstetrics
0 Pregnancy
Q Repair: Restoring, to the extent possible, a body part to its normal anatomic structure and function

Body Part	Approach	Device	Qualifier
Character 4	Character 5	Character 6	Character 7
0 Products of Conception ♀	**0** Open **3** Percutaneous **4** Percutaneous Endoscopic **7** Via Natural or Artificial Opening **8** Via Natural or Artificial Opening Endoscopic	**Y** Other Device **Z** No Device	**E** Nervous System **F** Cardiovascular System **G** Lymphatics and Hemic **H** Eye **J** Ear, Nose and Sinus **K** Respiratory System **L** Mouth and Throat **M** Gastrointestinal System **N** Hepatobiliary and Pancreas **P** Endocrine System **Q** Skin **R** Musculoskeletal System **S** Urinary System **T** Female Reproductive System **V** Male Reproductive System **Y** Other Body System

♀ 10Q00YE 10Q00YF 10Q00YG 10Q00YH 10Q00YJ 10Q00YK 10Q00YL 10Q00YM 10Q00YN 10Q00YP 10Q00YQ 10Q00YR 10Q00YS
10Q00YT 10Q00YV 10Q00YY 10Q00ZE 10Q00ZF 10Q00ZG 10Q00ZH 10Q00ZJ 10Q00ZK 10Q00ZL 10Q00ZM 10Q00ZN 10Q00ZP
10Q00ZQ 10Q00ZR 10Q00ZS 10Q00ZT 10Q00ZV 10Q00ZY 10Q03YE 10Q03YF 10Q03YG 10Q03YH 10Q03YJ 10Q03YK 10Q03YL
10Q03YM 10Q03YN 10Q03YP 10Q03YQ 10Q03YR 10Q03YS 10Q03YT 10Q03YV 10Q03YY 10Q03ZE 10Q03ZF 10Q03ZG 10Q03ZH
10Q03ZJ 10Q03ZK 10Q03ZL 10Q03ZM 10Q03ZN 10Q03ZP 10Q03ZQ 10Q03ZR 10Q03ZS 10Q03ZT 10Q03ZV 10Q03ZY 10Q04YE
10Q04YF 10Q04YG 10Q04YH 10Q04YJ 10Q04YK 10Q04YL 10Q04YM 10Q04YN 10Q04YP 10Q04YQ 10Q04YR 10Q04YS 10Q04YT
10Q04YV 10Q04YY 10Q04ZE 10Q04ZF 10Q04ZG 10Q04ZH 10Q04ZJ 10Q04ZK 10Q04ZL 10Q04ZM 10Q04ZN 10Q04ZP 10Q04ZQ
10Q04ZR 10Q04ZS 10Q04ZT 10Q04ZV 10Q04ZY 10Q07YE 10Q07YF 10Q07YG 10Q07YH 10Q07YJ 10Q07YK 10Q07YL 10Q07YM
10Q07YN 10Q07YP 10Q07YQ 10Q07YR 10Q07YS 10Q07YT 10Q07YV 10Q07YY 10Q07ZE 10Q07ZF 10Q07ZG 10Q07ZH 10Q07ZJ
10Q07ZK 10Q07ZL 10Q07ZM 10Q07ZN 10Q07ZP 10Q07ZQ 10Q07ZR 10Q07ZS 10Q07ZT 10Q07ZV 10Q07ZY 10Q08YE 10Q08YF
10Q08YG 10Q08YH 10Q08YJ 10Q08YK 10Q08YL 10Q08YM 10Q08YN 10Q08YP 10Q08YQ 10Q08YR 10Q08YS 10Q08YT 10Q08YV
10Q08YY 10Q08ZE 10Q08ZF 10Q08ZG 10Q08ZH 10Q08ZJ 10Q08ZK 10Q08ZL 10Q08ZM 10Q08ZN 10Q08ZP 10Q08ZQ 10Q08ZR
10Q08ZS 10Q08ZT 10Q08ZV 10Q08ZY

Limited Coverage Noncovered HAC-associated Procedure Combination Cluster - See Appendix G for code lists
Non-OR-Affecting MS-DRG Assignment New/Revised Text in **Orange** ♂ Male ♀ Female

2018 ICD-10-PCS 573

OBSTETRICS 102-10Y

1 Obstetrics
0 Pregnancy
S Reposition: Moving to its normal location, or other suitable location, all or a portion of a body part

Body Part	Approach	Device	Qualifier
Character 4	Character 5	Character 6	Character 7
0 Products of Conception 🔹♀	**7** Via Natural or Artificial Opening **X** External	**Z** No Device	**Z** No Qualifier
2 Products of Conception, Ectopic ♀	**0** Open **3** Percutaneous **4** Percutaneous Endoscopic **7** Via Natural or Artificial Opening **8** Via Natural or Artificial Opening Endoscopic	**Z** No Device	**Z** No Qualifier

♀ 10S07ZZ   10S0XZZ   10S20ZZ   10S23ZZ   10S24ZZ   10S27ZZ   10S28ZZ
🔹 10S07ZZ

1 Obstetrics
0 Pregnancy
T Resection: Cutting out or off, without replacement, all of a body part

Body Part	Approach	Device	Qualifier
Character 4	Character 5	Character 6	Character 7
2 Products of Conception, Ectopic ♀	**0** Open **3** Percutaneous **4** Percutaneous Endoscopic **7** Via Natural or Artificial Opening **8** Via Natural or Artificial Opening Endoscopic	**Z** No Device	**Z** No Qualifier

♀ 10T20ZZ   10T23ZZ   10T24ZZ   10T27ZZ   10T28ZZ

1 Obstetrics
0 Pregnancy
Y Transplantation: Putting in or on all or a portion of a living body part taken from another individual or animal to physically take the place and/or function of all or a portion of a similar body part

Body Part	Approach	Device	Qualifier
Character 4	Character 5	Character 6	Character 7
0 Products of Conception ♀	**3** Percutaneous **4** Percutaneous Endoscopic **7** Via Natural or Artificial Opening	**Z** No Device	**E** Nervous System **F** Cardiovascular System **G** Lymphatics and Hemic **H** Eye **J** Ear, Nose and Sinus **K** Respiratory System **L** Mouth and Throat **M** Gastrointestinal System **N** Hepatobiliary and Pancreas **P** Endocrine System **Q** Skin **R** Musculoskeletal System **S** Urinary System **T** Female Reproductive System **V** Male Reproductive System **Y** Other Body System

♀ 10Y03ZE   10Y03ZF   10Y03ZG   10Y03ZH   10Y03ZJ   10Y03ZK   10Y03ZL   10Y03ZM   10Y03ZN   10Y03ZP   10Y03ZQ   10Y03ZR   10Y03ZS
10Y03ZT   10Y03ZV   10Y03ZY   10Y04ZE   10Y04ZF   10Y04ZG   10Y04ZH   10Y04ZJ   10Y04ZK   10Y04ZL   10Y04ZM   10Y04ZN   10Y04ZP
10Y04ZQ   10Y04ZR   10Y04ZS   10Y04ZT   10Y04ZV   10Y04ZY   10Y07ZE   10Y07ZF   10Y07ZG   10Y07ZH   10Y07ZJ   10Y07ZK   10Y07ZL
10Y07ZM   10Y07ZN   10Y07ZP   10Y07ZQ   10Y07ZR   10Y07ZS   10Y07ZT   10Y07ZV   10Y07ZY

NOTES

NOTES

Placement-Anatomical Regions 2W0-2W6

2 Placement
W Anatomical Regions
0 Change: Taking out or off a device from a body part and putting back an identical or similar device in or on the same body part without cutting or puncturing the skin or a mucous membrane

Body Region	Approach	Device	Qualifier
Character 4	Character 5	Character 6	Character 7
0 Head	X External	0 Traction Apparatus	Z No Qualifier
2 Neck		1 Splint	
3 Abdominal Wall		2 Cast	
4 Chest Wall		3 Brace	
5 Back		4 Bandage	
6 Inguinal Region, Right		5 Packing Material	
7 Inguinal Region, Left		6 Pressure Dressing	
8 Upper Extremity, Right		7 Intermittent Pressure Device	
9 Upper Extremity, Left		Y Other Device	
A Upper Arm, Right			
B Upper Arm, Left			
C Lower Arm, Right			
D Lower Arm, Left			
E Hand, Right			
F Hand, Left			
G Thumb, Right			
H Thumb, Left			
J Finger, Right			
K Finger, Left			
L Lower Extremity, Right			
M Lower Extremity, Left			
N Upper Leg, Right			
P Upper Leg, Left			
Q Lower Leg, Right			
R Lower Leg, Left			
S Foot, Right			
T Foot, Left			
U Toe, Right			
V Toe, Left			
1 Face	X External	0 Traction Apparatus	Z No Qualifier
		1 Splint	
		2 Cast	
		3 Brace	
		4 Bandage	
		5 Packing Material	
		6 Pressure Dressing	
		7 Intermittent Pressure Device	
		9 Wire	
		Y Other Device	

2 Placement
W Anatomical Regions
1 Compression: Putting pressure on a body region

Body Region	Approach	Device	Qualifier
Character 4	Character 5	Character 6	Character 7
0 Head	X External	6 Pressure Dressing	Z No Qualifier
1 Face		7 Intermittent Pressure Device	
2 Neck			
3 Abdominal Wall			
4 Chest Wall			
5 Back			
6 Inguinal Region, Right			
7 Inguinal Region, Left			
8 Upper Extremity, Right			
9 Upper Extremity, Left			
A Upper Arm, Right			
B Upper Arm, Left			
C Lower Arm, Right			
D Lower Arm, Left			
E Hand, Right			
F Hand, Left			
G Thumb, Right			
H Thumb, Left			
J Finger, Right			
K Finger, Left			
L Lower Extremity, Right			
M Lower Extremity, Left			
N Upper Leg, Right			
P Upper Leg, Left			
Q Lower Leg, Right			
R Lower Leg, Left			
S Foot, Right			
T Foot, Left			
U Toe, Right			
V Toe, Left			

LC Limited Coverage   **NC** Noncovered   **HAC** HAC-associated Procedure   **CC** Combination Cluster - See Appendix G for code lists
DRG Non-OR-Affecting MS-DRG Assignment   New/Revised Text in **Orange**   ♂ Male   ♀ Female

578

2018 ICD-10-PCS

2 Placement
W Anatomical Regions
2 Dressing: Putting material on a body region for protection

Body Region	Approach	Device	Qualifier
Character 4	Character 5	Character 6	Character 7
0 Head	X External	4 Bandage	Z No Qualifier
1 Face			
2 Neck			
3 Abdominal Wall			
4 Chest Wall			
5 Back			
6 Inguinal Region, Right			
7 Inguinal Region, Left			
8 Upper Extremity, Right			
9 Upper Extremity, Left			
A Upper Arm, Right			
B Upper Arm, Left			
C Lower Arm, Right			
D Lower Arm, Left			
E Hand, Right			
F Hand, Left			
G Thumb, Right			
H Thumb, Left			
J Finger, Right			
K Finger, Left			
L Lower Extremity, Right			
M Lower Extremity, Left			
N Upper Leg, Right			
P Upper Leg, Left			
Q Lower Leg, Right			
R Lower Leg, Left			
S Foot, Right			
T Foot, Left			
U Toe, Right			
V Toe, Left			

2 Placement
W Anatomical Regions
3 Immobilization: Limiting or preventing motion of a body region

Body Region	Approach	Device	Qualifier
Character 4	Character 5	Character 6	Character 7
0 Head 2 Neck 3 Abdominal Wall 4 Chest Wall 5 Back 6 Inguinal Region, Right 7 Inguinal Region, Left 8 Upper Extremity, Right 9 Upper Extremity, Left A Upper Arm, Right B Upper Arm, Left C Lower Arm, Right D Lower Arm, Left E Hand, Right F Hand, Left G Thumb, Right H Thumb, Left J Finger, Right K Finger, Left L Lower Extremity, Right M Lower Extremity, Left N Upper Leg, Right P Upper Leg, Left Q Lower Leg, Right R Lower Leg, Left S Foot, Right T Foot, Left U Toe, Right V Toe, Left	X External	1 Splint 2 Cast 3 Brace Y Other Device	Z No Qualifier
1 Face	X External	1 Splint 2 Cast 3 Brace 9 Wire Y Other Device	Z No Qualifier

LC Limited Coverage   **NC** Noncovered   **HAC** HAC-associated Procedure   **CC** Combination Cluster - See Appendix G for code lists
DRG Non-OR-Affecting MS-DRG Assignment   New/Revised Text in **Orange**   ♂ Male   ♀ Female

2 Placement
W Anatomical Regions
4 Packing: Putting material in a body region or orifice

Body Region	Approach	Device	Qualifier
Character 4	Character 5	Character 6	Character 7
0 Head	X External	5 Packing Material	Z No Qualifier
1 Face			
2 Neck			
3 Abdominal Wall			
4 Chest Wall			
5 Back			
6 Inguinal Region, Right			
7 Inguinal Region, Left			
8 Upper Extremity, Right			
9 Upper Extremity, Left			
A Upper Arm, Right			
B Upper Arm, Left			
C Lower Arm, Right			
D Lower Arm, Left			
E Hand, Right			
F Hand, Left			
G Thumb, Right			
H Thumb, Left			
J Finger, Right			
K Finger, Left			
L Lower Extremity, Right			
M Lower Extremity, Left			
N Upper Leg, Right			
P Upper Leg, Left			
Q Lower Leg, Right			
R Lower Leg, Left			
S Foot, Right			
T Foot, Left			
U Toe, Right			
V Toe, Left			

LC Limited Coverage NC Noncovered HAC HAC-associated Procedure CC Combination Cluster - See Appendix G for code lists
DRG Non-OR-Affecting MS-DRG Assignment New/Revised Text in **Orange** ♂ Male ♀ Female

2018 ICD-10-PCS

581

PLACEMENT-ANATOMICAL REGIONS 2W0-2W6

2 Placement
W Anatomical Regions
5 Removal: Taking out or off a device from a body part

Body Region	Approach	Device	Qualifier
Character 4	**Character 5**	**Character 6**	**Character 7**
0 Head	X External	0 Traction Apparatus	Z No Qualifier
2 Neck		1 Splint	
3 Abdominal Wall		2 Cast	
4 Chest Wall		3 Brace	
5 Back		4 Bandage	
6 Inguinal Region, Right		5 Packing Material	
7 Inguinal Region, Left		6 Pressure Dressing	
8 Upper Extremity, Right		7 Intermittent Pressure Device	
9 Upper Extremity, Left		Y Other Device	
A Upper Arm, Right			
B Upper Arm, Left			
C Lower Arm, Right			
D Lower Arm, Left			
E Hand, Right			
F Hand, Left			
G Thumb, Right			
H Thumb, Left			
J Finger, Right			
K Finger, Left			
L Lower Extremity, Right			
M Lower Extremity, Left			
N Upper Leg, Right			
P Upper Leg, Left			
Q Lower Leg, Right			
R Lower Leg, Left			
S Foot, Right			
T Foot, Left			
U Toe, Right			
V Toe, Left			
1 Face	X External	0 Traction Apparatus	Z No Qualifier
		1 Splint	
		2 Cast	
		3 Brace	
		4 Bandage	
		5 Packing Material	
		6 Pressure Dressing	
		7 Intermittent Pressure Device	
		9 Wire	
		Y Other Device	

LC Limited Coverage **NC** Noncovered **HAC** HAC-associated Procedure **CC** Combination Cluster - See Appendix G for code lists
DRG Non-OR-Affecting MS-DRG Assignment   New/Revised Text in **Orange**   ♂ Male   ♀ Female

582

2018 ICD-10-PCS

2 **Placement**
W **Anatomical Regions**
6 **Traction:** Exerting a pulling force on a body region in a distal direction

Body Region	Approach	Device	Qualifier
Character 4	Character 5	Character 6	Character 7
0 Head 1 Face 2 Neck 3 Abdominal Wall 4 Chest Wall 5 Back 6 Inguinal Region, Right 7 Inguinal Region, Left 8 Upper Extremity, Right 9 Upper Extremity, Left A Upper Arm, Right B Upper Arm, Left C Lower Arm, Right D Lower Arm, Left E Hand, Right F Hand, Left G Thumb, Right H Thumb, Left J Finger, Right K Finger, Left L Lower Extremity, Right M Lower Extremity, Left N Upper Leg, Right P Upper Leg, Left Q Lower Leg, Right R Lower Leg, Left S Foot, Right T Foot, Left U Toe, Right V Toe, Left	X External	0 Traction Apparatus Z No Device	Z No Qualifier

NOTES

Placement-Anatomical Orifices 2Y0-2Y5

2 Placement
Y Anatomical Orifices
0 Change: Taking out or off a device from a body part and putting back an identical or similar device in or on the same body part without cutting or puncturing the skin or a mucous membrane

Body Region	Approach	Device	Qualifier
Character 4	Character 5	Character 6	Character 7
0 Mouth and Pharynx **1** Nasal **2** Ear **3** Anorectal **4** Female Genital Tract ♀ **5** Urethra	**X** External	**5** Packing Material	**Z** No Qualifier

♀ 2Y04X5Z

2 Placement
Y Anatomical Orifices
4 Packing: Putting material in a body region or orifice

Body Region	Approach	Device	Qualifier
Character 4	Character 5	Character 6	Character 7
0 Mouth and Pharynx **1** Nasal **2** Ear **3** Anorectal **4** Female Genital Tract ♀ **5** Urethra	**X** External	**5** Packing Material	**Z** No Qualifier

♀ 2Y44X5Z

2 Placement
Y Anatomical Orifices
5 Removal: Taking out or off a device from a body part

Body Region	Approach	Device	Qualifier
Character 4	Character 5	Character 6	Character 7
0 Mouth and Pharynx **1** Nasal **2** Ear **3** Anorectal **4** Female Genital Tract ♀ **5** Urethra	**X** External	**5** Packing Material	**Z** No Qualifier

♀ 2Y54X5Z

LC Limited Coverage   NC Noncovered   HAC HAC-associated Procedure   CC Combination Cluster - See Appendix G for code lists
DRG Non-OR-Affecting MS-DRG Assignment   New/Revised Text in **Orange**   ♂ Male   ♀ Female

2018 ICD-10-PCS

585

NOTES

3 Administration
0 Circulatory
2 Transfusion: Putting in blood or blood products

Body System / Region	Approach	Substance	Qualifier
Character 4	**Character 5**	**Character 6**	**Character 7**
3 Peripheral Vein NC **4** Central Vein NC	**0** Open **3** Percutaneous	**A** Stem Cells, Embryonic	**Z** No Qualifier
3 Peripheral Vein NC **4** Central Vein NC	**0** Open **3** Percutaneous	**G** Bone Marrow **X** Stem Cells, Cord Blood **Y** Stem Cells, Hematopoietic	**0** Autologous **2** Allogeneic, Related **3** Allogeneic, Unrelated **4** Allogeneic, Unspecified
3 Peripheral Vein **4** Central Vein	**0** Open **3** Percutaneous	**H** Whole Blood **J** Serum Albumin **K** Frozen Plasma **L** Fresh Plasma **M** Plasma Cryoprecipitate **N** Red Blood Cells **P** Frozen Red Cells **Q** White Cells **R** Platelets **S** Globulin **T** Fibrinogen **V** Antihemophilic Factors **W** Factor IX	**0** Autologous **1** Nonautologous
5 Peripheral Artery NC **6** Central Artery NC	**0** Open **3** Percutaneous	**G** Bone Marrow **H** Whole Blood **J** Serum Albumin **K** Frozen Plasma **L** Fresh Plasma **M** Plasma Cryoprecipitate **N** Red Blood Cells **P** Frozen Red Cells **Q** White Cells **R** Platelets **S** Globulin **T** Fibrinogen **V** Antihemophilic Factors **W** Factor IX **X** Stem Cells, Cord Blood **Y** Stem Cells, Hematopoietic	**0** Autologous **1** Nonautologous
7 Products of Conception, Circulatory ♀	**3** Percutaneous **7** Via Natural or Artificial Opening	**H** Whole Blood **J** Serum Albumin **K** Frozen Plasma **L** Fresh Plasma **M** Plasma Cryoprecipitate **N** Red Blood Cells **P** Frozen Red Cells **Q** White Cells **R** Platelets **S** Globulin **T** Fibrinogen **V** Antihemophilic Factors **W** Factor IX	**1** Nonautologous
8 Vein	**0** Open **3** Percutaneous	**B** 4-Factor Prothrombin Complex Concentrate	**1** Nonautologous

♀ 30273H1 30273J1 30273K1 30273L1 30273M1 30273N1 30273P1 30273Q1 30273R1 30273S1 30273T1 30273V1 30273W1
 30277H1 30277J1 30277K1 30277L1 30277M1 30277N1 30277P1 30277Q1 30277R1 30277S1 30277T1 30277V1 30277W1
NC 30230G2 30230G3 30230G4 30230Y2 30230Y3 30230Y4 30233G2 30233G3 30233G4 30233Y2 30233Y3 30233Y4 30240G2
 30240G3 30240G4 30240Y2 30240Y3 30240Y4 30243G2 30243G3 30243G4 30243Y2 30243Y3 30243Y4 30250G1 30250Y1
 30253G1 30253Y1 30260G1 30260Y1 30263G1 30263Y1

Codes in this list are noncovered procedures only when reported with C90.00 or C90.01 as either a principal or secondary diagnosis.

302 continued on next page

302 continued from previous page

NC 30230AZ 30230G0 30230G2 30230G3 30230G4 30230Y0 30230Y2 30230Y3 30230Y4 30233AZ 30233G0 30233G2 30233G3
30233G4 30233Y0 30233Y2 30233Y3 30233Y4 30240AZ 30240G0 30240G2 30240G3 30240G4 30240Y0 30240Y2 30240Y3
30240Y4 30243AZ 30243G0 30243G2 30243G3 30243G4 30243Y0 30243Y2 30243Y3 30243Y4 30250G0 30250G1 30250Y0
30250Y1 30253G0 30253G1 30253Y0 30253Y1 30260G0 30260G1 30260Y0 30260Y1 30263G0 30263G1 30263Y0 30263Y1

Codes in this list are noncovered procedures only when reported with C90.00, C90.01, C91.00, C92.00, C92.10, C92.11, C92.40, C92.50, C92.60, C92.A0, C93.00, C94.00, or C95.00 as either a principal or secondary diagnosis.

3 Administration
C Indwelling Device
1 Irrigation: Putting in or on a cleansing substance

Body System / Region	Approach	Substance	Qualifier
Character 4	Character 5	Character 6	Character 7
Z None	X External	8 Irrigating Substance	Z No Qualifier

3 Administration
E Physiological Systems and Anatomical Regions
0 Introduction: Putting in or on a therapeutic, diagnostic, nutritional, physiological, or prophylactic substance except blood or blood products

Body System / Region	Approach	Substance	Qualifier
Character 4	Character 5	Character 6	Character 7
0 Skin and Mucous Membranes	X External	0 Antineoplastic	5 Other Antineoplastic M Monoclonal Antibody
0 Skin and Mucous Membranes	X External	2 Anti-infective	8 Oxazolidinones 9 Other Anti-infective
0 Skin and Mucous Membranes	X External	3 Anti-inflammatory 4 Serum, Toxoid and Vaccine B Anesthetic Agent K Other Diagnostic Substance M Pigment N Analgesics, Hypnotics, Sedatives T Destructive Agent	Z No Qualifier
0 Skin and Mucous Membranes	X External	G Other Therapeutic Substance	C Other Substance
1 Subcutaneous Tissue	0 Open	2 Anti-infective	A Anti-Infective Envelope
1 Subcutaneous Tissue	3 Percutaneous	0 Antineoplastic	5 Other Antineoplastic M Monoclonal Antibody
1 Subcutaneous Tissue	3 Percutaneous	2 Anti-infective	8 Oxazolidinones 9 Other Anti-infective A Anti-Infective Envelope
1 Subcutaneous Tissue	3 Percutaneous	3 Anti-inflammatory 6 Nutritional Substance 7 Electrolytic and Water Balance Substance B Anesthetic Agent H Radioactive Substance K Other Diagnostic Substance N Analgesics, Hypnotics, Sedatives T Destructive Agent	Z No Qualifier
1 Subcutaneous Tissue	3 Percutaneous	4 Serum, Toxoid and Vaccine	0 Influenza Vaccine Z No Qualifier
1 Subcutaneous Tissue	3 Percutaneous	G Other Therapeutic Substance	C Other Substance
1 Subcutaneous Tissue	3 Percutaneous	V Hormone	G Insulin J Other Hormone
2 Muscle	3 Percutaneous	0 Antineoplastic	5 Other Antineoplastic M Monoclonal Antibody
2 Muscle	3 Percutaneous	2 Anti-infective	8 Oxazolidinones 9 Other Anti-infective

3E0 continued on next page

3 **Administration**
E **Physiological Systems and Anatomical Regions**
0 **Introduction:** Putting in or on a therapeutic, diagnostic, nutritional, physiological, or prophylactic substance except blood or blood products

Body System / Region	Approach	Substance	Qualifier
Character 4	Character 5	Character 6	Character 7
2 Muscle	3 Percutaneous	3 Anti-inflammatory 4 Serum, Toxoid and Vaccine 6 Nutritional Substance 7 Electrolytic and Water Balance Substance B Anesthetic Agent H Radioactive Substance K Other Diagnostic Substance N Analgesics, Hypnotics, Sedatives T Destructive Agent	Z No Qualifier
2 Muscle	3 Percutaneous	G Other Therapeutic Substance	C Other Substance
3 Peripheral Vein DRG	0 Open	0 Antineoplastic	2 High-dose Interleukin-2 3 Low-dose Interleukin-2 5 Other Antineoplastic M Monoclonal Antibody P Clofarabine
3 Peripheral Vein DRG	0 Open	1 Thrombolytic	6 Recombinant Human-activated Protein C 7 Other Thrombolytic
3 Peripheral Vein	0 Open	2 Anti-infective	8 Oxazolidinones 9 Other Anti-infective
3 Peripheral Vein	0 Open	3 Anti-inflammatory 4 Serum, Toxoid and Vaccine 6 Nutritional Substance 7 Electrolytic and Water Balance Substance F Intracirculatory Anesthetic H Radioactive Substance K Other Diagnostic Substance N Analgesics, Hypnotics, Sedatives P Platelet Inhibitor R Antiarrhythmic T Destructive Agent X Vasopressor	Z No Qualifier
3 Peripheral Vein	0 Open	G Other Therapeutic Substance	C Other Substance N Blood Brain Barrier Disruption
3 Peripheral Vein DRG	0 Open	U Pancreatic Islet Cells	0 Autologous 1 Nonautologous
3 Peripheral Vein	0 Open	V Hormone	G Insulin H Human B -type Natriuretic Peptide J Other Hormone
3 Peripheral Vein	0 Open	W Immunotherapeutic	K Immunostimulator L Immunosuppressive
3 Peripheral Vein DRG	3 Percutaneous	0 Antineoplastic	2 High-dose Interleukin-2 3 Low-dose Interleukin-2 5 Other Antineoplastic M Monoclonal Antibody P Clofarabine

3E0 continued on next page

3 Administration
E Physiological Systems and Anatomical Regions
0 Introduction: Putting in or on a therapeutic, diagnostic, nutritional, physiological, or prophylactic substance except blood or blood products

3E0 continued from previous page

Body System / Region	Approach	Substance	Qualifier
Character 4	Character 5	Character 6	Character 7
3 Peripheral Vein ᴰᴿᴳ	3 Percutaneous	1 Thrombolytic	6 Recombinant Human-activated Protein C 7 Other Thrombolytic
3 Peripheral Vein	3 Percutaneous	2 Anti-infective	8 Oxazolidinones 9 Other Anti-infective
3 Peripheral Vein	3 Percutaneous	3 Anti-inflammatory 4 Serum, Toxoid and Vaccine 6 Nutritional Substance 7 Electrolytic and Water Balance Substance F Intracirculatory Anesthetic H Radioactive Substance K Other Diagnostic Substance N Analgesics, Hypnotics, Sedatives P Platelet Inhibitor R Antiarrhythmic T Destructive Agent X Vasopressor	Z No Qualifier
3 Peripheral Vein	3 Percutaneous	G Other Therapeutic Substance	C Other Substance N Blood Brain Barrier Disruption Q Glucarpidase
3 Peripheral Vein ᴰᴿᴳ	3 Percutaneous	U Pancreatic Islet Cells	0 Autologous 1 Nonautologous
3 Peripheral Vein	3 Percutaneous	V Hormone	G Insulin H Human B-type Natriuretic Peptide J Other Hormone
3 Peripheral Vein	3 Percutaneous	W Immunotherapeutic	K Immunostimulator L Immunosuppressive
4 Central Vein ᴰᴿᴳ	0 Open	0 Antineoplastic	2 High-dose Interleukin-2 3 Low-dose Interleukin-2 5 Other Antineoplastic M Monoclonal Antibody P Clofarabine
4 Central Vein ᴰᴿᴳ	0 Open	1 Thrombolytic	6 Recombinant Human-activated Protein C 7 Other Thrombolytic
4 Central Vein	0 Open	2 Anti-infective	8 Oxazolidinones 9 Other Anti-infective
4 Central Vein ᴰᴿᴳ	0 Open	3 Anti-inflammatory 4 Serum, Toxoid and Vaccine 6 Nutritional Substance 7 Electrolytic and Water Balance Substance F Intracirculatory Anesthetic H Radioactive Substance K Other Diagnostic Substance N Analgesics, Hypnotics, Sedatives P Platelet Inhibitor R Antiarrhythmic T Destructive Agent X Vasopressor	Z No Qualifier
4 Central Vein	0 Open	G Other Therapeutic Substance	C Other Substance N Blood Brain Barrier Disruption

3E0 continued on next page

ᴸᶜ Limited Coverage   ᴺᶜ Noncovered   ᴴᴬᶜ HAC-associated Procedure   ᶜᶜ Combination Cluster - See Appendix G for code lists
ᴰᴿᴳ Non-OR-Affecting MS-DRG Assignment   New/Revised Text in **Orange**   ♂ Male   ♀ Female

3 **Administration**
E **Physiological Systems and Anatomical Regions**
0 **Introduction:** Putting in or on a therapeutic, diagnostic, nutritional, physiological, or prophylactic substance except blood or blood products

Body System / Region	Approach	Substance	Qualifier
Character 4	Character 5	Character 6	Character 7
4 Central Vein	0 Open	V Hormone	G Insulin H Human B-type Natriuretic Peptide J Other Hormone
4 Central Vein	0 Open	W Immunotherapeutic	K Immunostimulator L Immunosuppressive
4 Central Vein ᴰᴿᴳ	3 Percutaneous	0 Antineoplastic	2 High-dose Interleukin-2 3 Low-dose Interleukin-2 5 Other Antineoplastic M Monoclonal Antibody P Clofarabine
4 Central Vein ᴰᴿᴳ	3 Percutaneous	1 Thrombolytic	6 Recombinant Human-activated Protein C 7 Other Thrombolytic
4 Central Vein	3 Percutaneous	2 Anti-infective	8 Oxazolidinones 9 Other Anti-infective
4 Central Vein	3 Percutaneous	3 Anti-inflammatory 4 Serum, Toxoid and Vaccine 6 Nutritional Substance 7 Electrolytic and Water Balance Substance F Intracirculatory Anesthetic H Radioactive Substance K Other Diagnostic Substance N Analgesics, Hypnotics, Sedatives P Platelet Inhibitor R Antiarrhythmic T Destructive Agent X Vasopressor	Z No Qualifier
4 Central Vein	3 Percutaneous	G Other Therapeutic Substance	C Other Substance N Blood Brain Barrier Disruption Q Glucarpidase
4 Central Vein	3 Percutaneous	V Hormone	G Insulin H Human B-type Natriuretic Peptide J Other Hormone
4 Central Vein	3 Percutaneous	W Immunotherapeutic	K Immunostimulator L Immunosuppressive
5 Peripheral Artery ᴰᴿᴳ 6 Central Artery ᴰᴿᴳ	0 Open 3 Percutaneous	0 Antineoplastic	2 High-dose Interleukin-2 3 Low-dose Interleukin-2 5 Other Antineoplastic M Monoclonal Antibody P Clofarabine
5 Peripheral Artery ᴰᴿᴳ 6 Central Artery ᴰᴿᴳ	0 Open 3 Percutaneous	1 Thrombolytic	6 Recombinant Human-activated Protein C 7 Other Thrombolytic
5 Peripheral Artery 6 Central Artery	0 Open 3 Percutaneous	2 Anti-infective	8 Oxazolidinones 9 Other Anti-infective

3E0 continued on next page

3 **Administration**
E **Physiological Systems and Anatomical Regions**
0 **Introduction:** Putting in or on a therapeutic, diagnostic, nutritional, physiological, or prophylactic substance except blood or blood products

3E0 continued from previous page

Body System / Region	Approach	Substance	Qualifier
Character 4	Character 5	Character 6	Character 7
5 Peripheral Artery 6 Central Artery	0 Open 3 Percutaneous	3 Anti-inflammatory 4 Serum, Toxoid and Vaccine 6 Nutritional Substance 7 Electrolytic and Water Balance Substance F Intracirculatory Anesthetic H Radioactive Substance K Other Diagnostic Substance N Analgesics, Hypnotics, Sedatives P Platelet Inhibitor R Antiarrhythmic T Destructive Agent X Vasopressor	Z No Qualifier
5 Peripheral Artery 6 Central Artery	0 Open 3 Percutaneous	G Other Therapeutic Substance	C Other Substance N Blood Brain Barrier Disruption
5 Peripheral Artery 6 Central Artery	0 Open 3 Percutaneous	V Hormone	G Insulin H Human B-type Natriuretic Peptide J Other Hormone
5 Peripheral Artery 6 Central Artery	0 Open 3 Percutaneous	W Immunotherapeutic	K Immunostimulator L Immunosuppressive
7 Coronary Artery 8 Heart ᴰᴿᴳ	0 Open 3 Percutaneous	1 Thrombolytic	6 Recombinant Human-activated Protein C 7 Other Thrombolytic
7 Coronary Artery 8 Heart	0 Open 3 Percutaneous	G Other Therapeutic Substance	C Other Substance
7 Coronary Artery 8 Heart	0 Open 3 Percutaneous	K Other Diagnostic Substance P Platelet Inhibitor	Z No Qualifier
7 Coronary Artery 8 Heart	4 Percutaneous Endoscopic	G Other Therapeutic Substance	C Other Substance
9 Nose	3 Percutaneous 7 Via Natural or Artificial Opening X External	0 Antineoplastic	5 Other Antineoplastic M Monoclonal Antibody
9 Nose	3 Percutaneous 7 Via Natural or Artificial Opening X External	2 Anti-infective	8 Oxazolidinones 9 Other Anti-infective
9 Nose	3 Percutaneous 7 Via Natural or Artificial Opening X External	3 Anti-inflammatory 4 Serum, Toxoid and Vaccine B Anesthetic Agent H Radioactive Substance K Other Diagnostic Substance N Analgesics, Hypnotics, Sedatives T Destructive Agent	Z No Qualifier
9 Nose	3 Percutaneous 7 Via Natural or Artificial Opening X External	G Other Therapeutic Substance	C Other Substance
A Bone Marrow	3 Percutaneous	0 Antineoplastic	5 Other Antineoplastic M Monoclonal Antibody
A Bone Marrow	3 Percutaneous	G Other Therapeutic Substance	C Other Substance
B Ear	3 Percutaneous 7 Via Natural or Artificial Opening X External	0 Antineoplastic	4 Liquid Brachytherapy Radioisotope 5 Other Antineoplastic M Monoclonal Antibody

3E0 continued on next page

3 Administration
E Physiological Systems and Anatomical Regions
0 Introduction: Putting in or on a therapeutic, diagnostic, nutritional, physiological, or prophylactic substance except blood or blood products

Body System / Region	Approach	Substance	Qualifier
Character 4	**Character 5**	**Character 6**	**Character 7**
B Ear	**3** Percutaneous **7** Via Natural or Artificial Opening **X** External	**2** Anti-infective	**8** Oxazolidinones **9** Other Anti-infective
B Ear	**3** Percutaneous **7** Via Natural or Artificial Opening **X** External	**3** Anti-inflammatory **B** Anesthetic Agent **H** Radioactive Substance **K** Other Diagnostic Substance **N** Analgesics, Hypnotics, Sedatives **T** Destructive Agent	**Z** No Qualifier
B Ear	**3** Percutaneous **7** Via Natural or Artificial Opening **X** External	**G** Other Therapeutic Substance	**C** Other Substance
C Eye	**3** Percutaneous **7** Via Natural or Artificial Opening **X** External	**0** Antineoplastic	**4** Liquid Brachytherapy Radioisotope **5** Other Antineoplastic **M** Monoclonal Antibody
C Eye	**3** Percutaneous **7** Via Natural or Artificial Opening **X** External	**2** Anti-infective	**8** Oxazolidinones **9** Other Anti-infective
C Eye	**3** Percutaneous **7** Via Natural or Artificial Opening **X** External	**3** Anti-inflammatory **B** Anesthetic Agent **H** Radioactive Substance **K** Other Diagnostic Substance **M** Pigment **N** Analgesics, Hypnotics, Sedatives **T** Destructive Agent	**Z** No Qualifier
C Eye	**3** Percutaneous **7** Via Natural or Artificial Opening **X** External	**G** Other Therapeutic Substance	**C** Other Substance
C Eye	**3** Percutaneous **7** Via Natural or Artificial Opening **X** External	**S** Gas	**F** Other Gas
D Mouth and Pharynx	**3** Percutaneous **7** Via Natural or Artificial Opening **X** External	**0** Antineoplastic	**4** Liquid Brachytherapy Radioisotope **5** Other Antineoplastic **M** Monoclonal Antibody
D Mouth and Pharynx	**3** Percutaneous **7** Via Natural or Artificial Opening **X** External	**2** Anti-infective	**8** Oxazolidinones **9** Other Anti-infective
D Mouth and Pharynx	**3** Percutaneous **7** Via Natural or Artificial Opening **X** External	**3** Anti-inflammatory **4** Serum, Toxoid and Vaccine **6** Nutritional Substance **7** Electrolytic and Water Balance Substance **B** Anesthetic Agent **H** Radioactive Substance **K** Other Diagnostic Substance **N** Analgesics, Hypnotics, Sedatives **R** Antiarrhythmic **T** Destructive Agent	**Z** No Qualifier
D Mouth and Pharynx	**3** Percutaneous **7** Via Natural or Artificial Opening **X** External	**G** Other Therapeutic Substance	**C** Other Substance

3E0 continued on next page

LC Limited Coverage **NC** Noncovered **HAC** HAC-associated Procedure **CC** Combination Cluster - See Appendix G for code lists
DRG Non-OR-Affecting MS-DRG Assignment New/Revised Text in **Orange** ♂ Male ♀ Female

3 **Administration**

3E0 continued from previous page

E **Physiological Systems and Anatomical Regions**

0 **Introduction:** Putting in or on a therapeutic, diagnostic, nutritional, physiological, or prophylactic substance except blood or blood products

Body System / Region	Approach	Substance	Qualifier
Character 4	Character 5	Character 6	Character 7
E Products of Conception ♀ G Upper GI H Lower GI K Genitourinary Tract N Male Reproductive ♂	3 Percutaneous 7 Via Natural or Artificial Opening 8 Via Natural or Artificial Opening Endoscopic	0 Antineoplastic	4 Liquid Brachytherapy Radioisotope 5 Other Antineoplastic M Monoclonal Antibody
E Products of Conception ♀ G Upper GI H Lower GI K Genitourinary Tract N Male Reproductive ♂	3 Percutaneous 7 Via Natural or Artificial Opening 8 Via Natural or Artificial Opening Endoscopic	2 Anti-infective	8 Oxazolidinones 9 Other Anti-infective
E Products of Conception ♀ G Upper GI H Lower GI K Genitourinary Tract N Male Reproductive ♂	3 Percutaneous 7 Via Natural or Artificial Opening 8 Via Natural or Artificial Opening Endoscopic	3 Anti-inflammatory 6 Nutritional Substance 7 Electrolytic and Water Balance Substance B Anesthetic Agent H Radioactive Substance K Other Diagnostic Substance N Analgesics, Hypnotics, Sedatives T Destructive Agent	Z No Qualifier
E Products of Conception ♀ G Upper GI H Lower GI K Genitourinary Tract N Male Reproductive ♂	3 Percutaneous 7 Via Natural or Artificial Opening 8 Via Natural or Artificial Opening Endoscopic	G Other Therapeutic Substance	C Other Substance
E Products of Conception ♀ G Upper GI H Lower GI K Genitourinary Tract N Male Reproductive ♂	3 Percutaneous 7 Via Natural or Artificial Opening 8 Via Natural or Artificial Opening Endoscopic	S Gas	F Other Gas
E Products of Conception ♀ G Upper GI H Lower GI K Genitourinary Tract N Male Reproductive ♂	4 Percutaneous Endoscopic	G Other Therapeutic Substance	C Other Substance
F Respiratory Tract	3 Percutaneous 7 Via Natural or Artificial Opening 8 Via Natural or Artificial Opening Endoscopic	0 Antineoplastic	4 Liquid Brachytherapy Radioisotope 5 Other Antineoplastic M Monoclonal Antibody
F Respiratory Tract	3 Percutaneous 7 Via Natural or Artificial Opening 8 Via Natural or Artificial Opening Endoscopic	2 Anti-infective	8 Oxazolidinones 9 Other Anti-infective
F Respiratory Tract	3 Percutaneous 7 Via Natural or Artificial Opening 8 Via Natural or Artificial Opening Endoscopic	3 Anti-inflammatory 6 Nutritional Substance 7 Electrolytic and Water Balance Substance B Anesthetic Agent H Radioactive Substance K Other Diagnostic Substance N Analgesics, Hypnotics, Sedatives T Destructive Agent	Z No Qualifier
F Respiratory Tract	3 Percutaneous 7 Via Natural or Artificial Opening 8 Via Natural or Artificial Opening Endoscopic	G Other Therapeutic Substance	C Other Substance

3E0 continued on next page

3 **Administration**
E **Physiological Systems and Anatomical Regions**

3E0 continued from previous page

0 **Introduction:** Putting in or on a therapeutic, diagnostic, nutritional, physiological, or prophylactic substance except blood or blood products

Body System / Region	Approach	Substance	Qualifier
Character 4	**Character 5**	**Character 6**	**Character 7**
F Respiratory Tract	**3** Percutaneous **7** Via Natural or Artificial Opening **8** Via Natural or Artificial Opening Endoscopic	**S** Gas	**D** Nitric Oxide **F** Other Gas
F Respiratory Tract	**4** Percutaneous Endoscopic	**G** Other Therapeutic Substance	**C** Other Substance
J Biliary and Pancreatic Tract	**3** Percutaneous **7** Via Natural or Artificial Opening **8** Via Natural or Artificial Opening Endoscopic	**0** Antineoplastic	**4** Liquid Brachytherapy Radioisotope **5** Other Antineoplastic **M** Monoclonal Antibody
J Biliary and Pancreatic Tract	**3** Percutaneous **7** Via Natural or Artificial Opening **8** Via Natural or Artificial Opening Endoscopic	**2** Anti-infective	**8** Oxazolidinones **9** Other Anti-infective
J Biliary and Pancreatic Tract	**3** Percutaneous **7** Via Natural or Artificial Opening **8** Via Natural or Artificial Opening Endoscopic	**3** Anti-inflammatory **6** Nutritional Substance **7** Electrolytic and Water Balance Substance **B** Anesthetic Agent **H** Radioactive Substance **K** Other Diagnostic Substance **N** Analgesics, Hypnotics, Sedatives **T** Destructive Agent	**Z** No Qualifier
J Biliary and Pancreatic Tract	**3** Percutaneous **7** Via Natural or Artificial Opening **8** Via Natural or Artificial Opening Endoscopic	**G** Other Therapeutic Substance	**C** Other Substance
J Biliary and Pancreatic Tract	**3** Percutaneous **7** Via Natural or Artificial Opening **8** Via Natural or Artificial Opening Endoscopic	**S** Gas	**F** Other Gas
J Biliary and Pancreatic Tract ᴰᴿᴳ	**3** Percutaneous **7** Via Natural or Artificial Opening **8** Via Natural or Artificial Opening Endoscopic	**U** Pancreatic Islet Cells	**0** Autologous **1** Nonautologous
J Biliary and Pancreatic Tract	**4** Percutaneous Endoscopic	**G** Other Therapeutic Substance	**C** Other Substance
L Pleural Cavity **M** Peritoneal Cavity	**0** Open	**5** Adhesion Barrier	**Z** No Qualifier
L Pleural Cavity **M** Peritoneal Cavity	**3** Percutaneous	**0** Antineoplastic	**4** Liquid Brachytherapy Radioisotope **5** Other Antineoplastic **M** Monoclonal Antibody
L Pleural Cavity **M** Peritoneal Cavity	**3** Percutaneous	**2** Anti-infective	**8** Oxazolidinones **9** Other Anti-infective
L Pleural Cavity **M** Peritoneal Cavity	**3** Percutaneous	**3** Anti-inflammatory **5** Adhesion Barrier **6** Nutritional Substance **7** Electrolytic and Water Balance Substance **B** Anesthetic Agent **H** Radioactive Substance **K** Other Diagnostic Substance **N** Analgesics, Hypnotics, Sedatives **T** Destructive Agent	**Z** No Qualifier
L Pleural Cavity **M** Peritoneal Cavity	**3** Percutaneous	**G** Other Therapeutic Substance	**C** Other Substance

3E0 continued on next page

ᴸᶜ Limited Coverage   ᴺᶜ Noncovered   ᴴᴬᶜ HAC-associated Procedure   ᶜᶜ Combination Cluster - See Appendix G for code lists

ᴰᴿᴳ Non-OR-Affecting MS-DRG Assignment   New/Revised Text in **Orange**   ♂ Male   ♀ Female

3 **Administration**
E **Physiological Systems and Anatomical Regions**

3E0 continued from previous page

0 **Introduction:** Putting in or on a therapeutic, diagnostic, nutritional, physiological, or prophylactic substance except blood or blood products

Body System / Region	Approach	Substance	Qualifier
Character 4	Character 5	Character 6	Character 7
L Pleural Cavity M Peritoneal Cavity	3 Percutaneous	S Gas	F Other Gas
L Pleural Cavity M Peritoneal Cavity	4 Percutaneous Endoscopic	5 Adhesion Barrier	Z No Qualifier
L Pleural Cavity M Peritoneal Cavity	4 Percutaneous Endoscopic	G Other Therapeutic Substance	C Other Substance
L Pleural Cavity M Peritoneal Cavity	7 Via Natural or Artificial Opening	0 Antineoplastic	4 Liquid Brachytherapy Radioisotope 5 Other Antineoplastic M Monoclonal Antibody
L Pleural Cavity M Peritoneal Cavity	7 Via Natural or Artificial Opening	S Gas	F Other Gas
P Female Reproductive ♀	0 Open	5 Adhesion Barrier	Z No Qualifier
P Female Reproductive ♀	3 Percutaneous	0 Antineoplastic	4 Liquid Brachytherapy Radioisotope 5 Other Antineoplastic M Monoclonal Antibody
P Female Reproductive ♀	3 Percutaneous	2 Anti-infective	8 Oxazolidinones 9 Other Anti-infective
P Female Reproductive ♀	3 Percutaneous	3 Anti-inflammatory 5 Adhesion Barrier 6 Nutritional Substance 7 Electrolytic and Water Balance Substance B Anesthetic Agent H Radioactive Substance K Other Diagnostic Substance L Sperm N Analgesics, Hypnotics, Sedatives T Destructive Agent V Hormone	Z No Qualifier
P Female Reproductive ♀	3 Percutaneous	G Other Therapeutic Substance	C Other Substance
P Female Reproductive ♀	3 Percutaneous	Q Fertilized Ovum	0 Autologous 1 Nonautologous
P Female Reproductive ♀	3 Percutaneous	S Gas	F Other Gas
P Female Reproductive ♀	4 Percutaneous Endoscopic	5 Adhesion Barrier	Z No Qualifier
P Female Reproductive ♀	4 Percutaneous Endoscopic	G Other Therapeutic Substance	C Other Substance
P Female Reproductive ♀	7 Via Natural or Artificial Opening	0 Antineoplastic	4 Liquid Brachytherapy Radioisotope 5 Other Antineoplastic M Monoclonal Antibody
P Female Reproductive ♀	7 Via Natural or Artificial Opening	2 Anti-infective	8 Oxazolidinones 9 Other Anti-infective
P Female Reproductive ♀	7 Via Natural or Artificial Opening	3 Anti-inflammatory 6 Nutritional Substance 7 Electrolytic and Water Balance Substance B Anesthetic Agent H Radioactive Substance K Other Diagnostic Substance L Sperm N Analgesics, Hypnotics, Sedatives T Destructive Agent V Hormone	Z No Qualifier

3E0 continued on next page

🄻 Limited Coverage   🄽🄲 Noncovered   🄷🄰🄲 HAC-associated Procedure   🄻🄲 Combination Cluster - See Appendix G for code lists
🄓🄗🄘 Non-OR-Affecting MS-DRG Assignment   New/Revised Text in **Orange**   ♂ Male   ♀ Female

3   Administration
E   Physiological Systems and Anatomical Regions
0   Introduction: Putting in or on a therapeutic, diagnostic, nutritional, physiological, or prophylactic substance except blood or blood products

3E0 continued from previous page

Body System / Region	Approach	Substance	Qualifier
Character 4	Character 5	Character 6	Character 7
P Female Reproductive ♀	7 Via Natural or Artificial Opening	G Other Therapeutic Substance	C Other Substance
P Female Reproductive ♀	7 Via Natural or Artificial Opening	Q Fertilized Ovum	0 Autologous 1 Nonautologous
P Female Reproductive ♀	7 Via Natural or Artificial Opening	S Gas	F Other Gas
P Female Reproductive ♀	8 Via Natural or Artificial Opening Endoscopic	0 Antineoplastic	4 Liquid Brachytherapy Radioisotope 5 Other Antineoplastic M Monoclonal Antibody
P Female Reproductive ♀	8 Via Natural or Artificial Opening Endoscopic	2 Anti-infective	8 Oxazolidinones 9 Other Anti-infective
P Female Reproductive ♀	8 Via Natural or Artificial Opening Endoscopic	3 Anti-inflammatory 6 Nutritional Substance 7 Electrolytic and Water Balance Substance B Anesthetic Agent H Radioactive Substance K Other Diagnostic Substance N Analgesics, Hypnotics, Sedatives T Destructive Agent	Z No Qualifier
P Female Reproductive ♀	8 Via Natural or Artificial Opening Endoscopic	G Other Therapeutic Substance	C Other Substance
P Female Reproductive ♀	8 Via Natural or Artificial Opening Endoscopic	S Gas	F Other Gas
Q Cranial Cavity and Brain 🄾🅁🄶	0 Open 3 Percutaneous	0 Antineoplastic	4 Liquid Brachytherapy Radioisotope 5 Other Antineoplastic M Monoclonal Antibody
Q Cranial Cavity and Brain	0 Open 3 Percutaneous	2 Anti-infective	8 Oxazolidinones 9 Other Anti-infective
Q Cranial Cavity and Brain	0 Open 3 Percutaneous	3 Anti-inflammatory 6 Nutritional Substance 7 Electrolytic and Water Balance Substance A Stem Cells, Embryonic B Anesthetic Agent H Radioactive Substance K Other Diagnostic Substance N Analgesics, Hypnotics, Sedatives T Destructive Agent	Z No Qualifier
Q Cranial Cavity and Brain	0 Open 3 Percutaneous	E Stem Cells, Somatic	0 Autologous 1 Nonautologous
Q Cranial Cavity and Brain	0 Open 3 Percutaneous	G Other Therapeutic Substance	C Other Substance
Q Cranial Cavity and Brain	0 Open 3 Percutaneous	S Gas	F Other Gas
Q Cranial Cavity and Brain 🄾🅁🄶	7 Via Natural or Artificial Opening	0 Antineoplastic	4 Liquid Brachytherapy Radioisotope 5 Other Antineoplastic M Monoclonal Antibody
Q Cranial Cavity and Brain	7 Via Natural or Artificial Opening	S Gas	F Other Gas
R Spinal Canal	0 Open	A Stem Cells, Embryonic	Z No Qualifier
R Spinal Canal	0 Open	E Stem Cells, Somatic	0 Autologous 1 Nonautologous

3E0 continued on next page

3 Administration
E Physiological Systems and Anatomical Regions
0 Introduction: Putting in or on a therapeutic, diagnostic, nutritional, physiological, or prophylactic substance except blood or blood products

3E0 continued from previous page

Body System / Region	Approach	Substance	Qualifier
Character 4	Character 5	Character 6	Character 7
R Spinal Canal ᴅʀɢ	3 Percutaneous	0 Antineoplastic	2 High-dose Interleukin-2 3 Low-dose Interleukin-2 4 Liquid Brachytherapy Radioisotope 5 Other Antineoplastic M Monoclonal Antibody
R Spinal Canal	3 Percutaneous	2 Anti-infective	8 Oxazolidinones 9 Other Anti-infective
R Spinal Canal	3 Percutaneous	3 Anti-inflammatory 6 Nutritional Substance 7 Electrolytic and Water Balance Substance A Stem Cells, Embryonic B Anesthetic Agent H Radioactive Substance K Other Diagnostic Substance N Analgesics, Hypnotics, Sedatives T Destructive Agent	Z No Qualifier
R Spinal Canal	3 Percutaneous	E Stem Cells, Somatic	0 Autologous 1 Nonautologous
R Spinal Canal	3 Percutaneous	G Other Therapeutic Substance	C Other Substance
R Spinal Canal	3 Percutaneous	S Gas	F Other Gas
R Spinal Canal	7 Via Natural or Artificial Opening	S Gas	F Other Gas
S Epidural Space ᴅʀɢ	3 Percutaneous	0 Antineoplastic	2 High-dose Interleukin-2 3 Low-dose Interleukin-2 4 Liquid Brachytherapy Radioisotope 5 Other Antineoplastic M Monoclonal Antibody
S Epidural Space	3 Percutaneous	2 Anti-infective	8 Oxazolidinones 9 Other Anti-infective
S Epidural Space	3 Percutaneous	3 Anti-inflammatory 6 Nutritional Substance 7 Electrolytic and Water Balance Substance B Anesthetic Agent H Radioactive Substance K Other Diagnostic Substance N Analgesics, Hypnotics, Sedatives T Destructive Agent	Z No Qualifier
S Epidural Space	3 Percutaneous	G Other Therapeutic Substance	C Other Substance
S Epidural Space	3 Percutaneous	S Gas	F Other Gas
S Epidural Space	7 Via Natural or Artificial Opening	S Gas	F Other Gas
T Peripheral Nerves and Plexi X Cranial Nerves	3 Percutaneous	3 Anti-inflammatory B Anesthetic Agent T Destructive Agent	Z No Qualifier
T Peripheral Nerves and Plexi X Cranial Nerves	3 Percutaneous	G Other Therapeutic Substance	C Other Substance
U Joints	0 Open	2 Anti-infective	8 Oxazolidinones 9 Other Anti-infective
U Joints	0 Open	G Other Therapeutic Substance	B Recombinant Bone Morphogenetic Protein

3E0 continued on next page

ᴸᶜ Limited Coverage   ᴺᶜ Noncovered   ᴴᴬᶜ HAC-associated Procedure   ᶜᶜ Combination Cluster - See Appendix G for code lists
ᴅʀɢ Non-OR-Affecting MS-DRG Assignment   New/Revised Text in **Orange**   ♂ Male   ♀ Female

3 Administration
E Physiological Systems and Anatomical Regions

3E0 continued from previous page

0 **Introduction:** Putting in or on a therapeutic, diagnostic, nutritional, physiological, or prophylactic substance except blood or blood products

Body System / Region	Approach	Substance	Qualifier
Character 4	Character 5	Character 6	Character 7
U Joints	3 Percutaneous	0 Antineoplastic	4 Liquid Brachytherapy Radioisotope 5 Other Antineoplastic M Monoclonal Antibody
U Joints	3 Percutaneous	2 Anti-infective	8 Oxazolidinones 9 Other Anti-infective
U Joints	3 Percutaneous	3 Anti-inflammatory 6 Nutritional Substance 7 Electrolytic and Water Balance Substance B Anesthetic Agent H Radioactive Substance K Other Diagnostic Substance N Analgesics, Hypnotics, Sedatives T Destructive Agent	Z No Qualifier
U Joints	3 Percutaneous	G Other Therapeutic Substance	B Recombinant Bone Morphogenetic Protein C Other Substance
U Joints	3 Percutaneous	S Gas	F Other Gas
U Joints	4 Percutaneous Endoscopic	G Other Therapeutic Substance	C Other Substance
V Bones	0 Open	G Other Therapeutic Substance	B Recombinant Bone Morphogenetic Protein
V Bones	3 Percutaneous	0 Antineoplastic	5 Other Antineoplastic M Monoclonal Antibody
V Bones	3 Percutaneous	2 Anti-infective	8 Oxazolidinones 9 Other Anti-infective
V Bones	3 Percutaneous	3 Anti-inflammatory 6 Nutritional Substance 7 Electrolytic and Water Balance Substance B Anesthetic Agent H Radioactive Substance K Other Diagnostic Substance N Analgesics, Hypnotics, Sedatives T Destructive Agent	Z No Qualifier
V Bones	3 Percutaneous	G Other Therapeutic Substance	B Recombinant Bone Morphogenetic Protein C Other Substance
W Lymphatics	3 Percutaneous	0 Antineoplastic	5 Other Antineoplastic M Monoclonal Antibody
W Lymphatics	3 Percutaneous	2 Anti-infective	8 Oxazolidinones 9 Other Anti-infective
W Lymphatics	3 Percutaneous	3 Anti-inflammatory 6 Nutritional Substance 7 Electrolytic and Water Balance Substance B Anesthetic Agent H Radioactive Substance K Other Diagnostic Substance N Analgesics, Hypnotics, Sedatives T Destructive Agent	Z No Qualifier
W Lymphatics	3 Percutaneous	G Other Therapeutic Substance	C Other Substance

3E0 continued on next page

3 Administration
E Physiological Systems and Anatomical Regions
0 Introduction: Putting in or on a therapeutic, diagnostic, nutritional, physiological, or prophylactic substance except blood or blood products

3E0 continued from previous page

Body System / Region	Approach	Substance	Qualifier
Character 4	Character 5	Character 6	Character 7
Y Pericardial Cavity	3 Percutaneous	0 Antineoplastic	4 Liquid Brachytherapy Radioisotope 5 Other Antineoplastic M Monoclonal Antibody
Y Pericardial Cavity	3 Percutaneous	2 Anti-infective	8 Oxazolidinones 9 Other Anti-infective
Y Pericardial Cavity	3 Percutaneous	3 Anti-inflammatory 6 Nutritional Substance 7 Electrolytic and Water Balance Substance B Anesthetic Agent H Radioactive Substance K Other Diagnostic Substance N Analgesics, Hypnotics, Sedatives T Destructive Agent	Z No Qualifier
Y Pericardial Cavity	3 Percutaneous	G Other Therapeutic Substance	C Other Substance
Y Pericardial Cavity	3 Percutaneous	S Gas	F Other Gas
Y Pericardial Cavity	4 Percutaneous Endoscopic	G Other Therapeutic Substance	C Other Substance
Y Pericardial Cavity	7 Via Natural or Artificial Opening	0 Antineoplastic	4 Liquid Brachytherapy Radioisotope 5 Other Antineoplastic M Monoclonal Antibody
Y Pericardial Cavity	7 Via Natural or Artificial Opening	S Gas	F Other Gas

♂ 3E0N304 3E0N305 3E0N30M 3E0N328 3E0N329 3E0N33Z 3E0N36Z 3E0N37Z 3E0N3BZ 3E0N3GC 3E0N3HZ 3E0N3KZ 3E0N3NZ
3E0N3SF 3E0N3TZ 3E0N704 3E0N705 3E0N70M 3E0N728 3E0N729 3E0N73Z 3E0N76Z 3E0N77Z 3E0N7BZ 3E0N7GC 3E0N7HZ
3E0N7KZ 3E0N7NZ 3E0N7SF 3E0N7TZ 3E0N804 3E0N805 3E0N80M 3E0N828 3E0N829 3E0N83Z 3E0N86Z 3E0N87Z 3E0N8BZ
3E0N8GC 3E0N8HZ 3E0N8KZ 3E0N8NZ 3E0N8SF 3E0N8TZ

♀ 3E0E304 3E0E305 3E0E30M 3E0E328 3E0E329 3E0E33Z 3E0E36Z 3E0E37Z 3E0E3BZ 3E0E3GC 3E0E3HZ 3E0E3KZ 3E0E3NZ
3E0E3SF 3E0E3TZ 3E0E704 3E0E705 3E0E70M 3E0E728 3E0E729 3E0E73Z 3E0E76Z 3E0E77Z 3E0E7BZ 3E0E7GC 3E0E7HZ
3E0E7KZ 3E0E7NZ 3E0E7SF 3E0E7TZ 3E0E804 3E0E805 3E0E80M 3E0E828 3E0E829 3E0E83Z 3E0E86Z 3E0E87Z 3E0E8BZ
3E0E8GC 3E0E8HZ 3E0E8KZ 3E0E8NZ 3E0E8SF 3E0E8TZ 3E0P05Z 3E0P304 3E0P305 3E0P30M 3E0P328 3E0P329 3E0P33Z
3E0P36Z 3E0P37Z 3E0P3BZ 3E0P3GC 3E0P3HZ 3E0P3KZ 3E0P3LZ 3E0P3NZ 3E0P3Q0 3E0P3Q1 3E0P3SF 3E0P3TZ 3E0P704
3E0P705 3E0P70M 3E0P728 3E0P729 3E0P73Z 3E0P76Z 3E0P77Z 3E0P7BZ 3E0P7GC 3E0P7HZ 3E0P7KZ 3E0P7LZ 3E0P7NZ
3E0P7Q0 3E0P7Q1 3E0P7SF 3E0P7TZ 3E0P804 3E0P805 3E0P80M 3E0P828 3E0P829 3E0P83Z 3E0P86Z 3E0P87Z 3E0P8BZ
3E0P8GC 3E0P8HZ 3E0P8KZ 3E0P8NZ 3E0P8SF 3E0P8TZ

DRG 3E03002 3E03017 3E030U0 3E030U1 3E03302 3E03317 3E033U0 3E033U1 3E04002 3E04017 3E04302 3E04317 3E05002
3E05017 3E05302 3E05317 3E06002 3E06017 3E06302 3E06317 3E08017 3E08317 3E0J3U0 3E0J3U1 3E0J7U0 3E0J7U1
3E0J8U0 3E0J8U1 3E0Q005 3E0Q305 3E0Q705 3E0R302 3E0S302

LC Limited Coverage   NC Noncovered   HAC HAC-associated Procedure   CC Combination Cluster - See Appendix G for code lists
DRG Non-OR-Affecting MS-DRG Assignment   New/Revised Text in **Orange**   ♂ Male   ♀ Female

600

2018 ICD-10-PCS

3 Administration
E Physiological Systems and Anatomical Regions
1 Irrigation: Putting in or on a cleansing substance

Body System / Region	Approach	Substance	Qualifier
Character 4	**Character 5**	**Character 6**	**Character 7**
0 Skin and Mucous Membranes **C** Eye	**3** Percutaneous **X** External	**8** Irrigating Substance	**X** Diagnostic **Z** No Qualifier
9 Nose **B** Ear **F** Respiratory Tract **G** Upper GI **H** Lower GI **J** Biliary and Pancreatic Tract **K** Genitourinary Tract **N** Male Reproductive ♂ **P** Female Reproductive ♀	**3** Percutaneous **7** Via Natural or Artificial Opening **8** Via Natural or Artificial Opening Endoscopic	**8** Irrigating Substance	**X** Diagnostic **Z** No Qualifier
L Pleural Cavity **Q** Cranial Cavity and Brain **R** Spinal Canal **S** Epidural Space **U** Joints **Y** Pericardial Cavity	**3** Percutaneous	**8** Irrigating Substance	**X** Diagnostic **Z** No Qualifier
M Peritoneal Cavity	**3** Percutaneous	**8** Irrigating Substance	**X** Diagnostic **Z** No Qualifier
M Peritoneal Cavity	**3** Percutaneous	**9** Dialysate	**Z** No Qualifier

♂ 3E1N38X 3E1N38Z 3E1N78X 3E1N78Z 3E1N88X 3E1N88Z
♀ 3E1P38X 3E1P38Z 3E1P78X 3E1P78Z 3E1P88X 3E1P88Z

LC Limited Coverage   NC Noncovered   HAC HAC-associated Procedure   CC Combination Cluster - See Appendix G for code lists
NOR Non-OR-Affecting MS-DRG Assignment   New/Revised Text in **Orange**   ♂ Male   ♀ Female

2018 ICD-10-PCS   601

NOTES

Measurement and Monitoring 4A0-4B0

4   Measurement and Monitoring
A   Physiological Systems
0   Measurement: Determining the level of a physiological or physical function at a point in time

Body System	Approach	Function/Device	Qualifier
Character 4	**Character 5**	**Character 6**	**Character 7**
0 Central Nervous	**0** Open	**2** Conductivity **4** Electrical Activity **B** Pressure	**Z** No Qualifier
0 Central Nervous	**3** Percutaneous **7** Via Natural or Artificial Opening **8** Via Natural or Artificial Opening Endoscopic	**4** Electrical Activity	**Z** No Qualifier
0 Central Nervous	**3** Percutaneous **7** Via Natural or Artificial Opening **8** Via Natural or Artificial Opening Endoscopic	**B** Pressure **K** Temperature **R** Saturation	**D** Intracranial
0 Central Nervous	**X** External	**2** Conductivity **4** Electrical Activity	**Z** No Qualifier
1 Peripheral Nervous	**0** Open **3** Percutaneous **7** Via Natural or Artificial Opening **8** Via Natural or Artificial Opening Endoscopic **X** External	**2** Conductivity	**9** Sensory **B** Motor
1 Peripheral Nervous	**0** Open **3** Percutaneous **7** Via Natural or Artificial Opening **8** Via Natural or Artificial Opening Endoscopic **X** External	**4** Electrical Activity	**Z** No Qualifier
2 Cardiac 🏷	**0** Open **3** Percutaneous **7** Via Natural or Artificial Opening **8** Via Natural or Artificial Opening Endoscopic	**4** Electrical Activity **9** Output **C** Rate **F** Rhythm **H** Sound **P** Action Currents	**Z** No Qualifier
2 Cardiac 🏷	**0** Open **3** Percutaneous **7** Via Natural or Artificial Opening **8** Via Natural or Artificial Opening Endoscopic	**N** Sampling and Pressure	**6** Right Heart **7** Left Heart **8** Bilateral
2 Cardiac	**X** External	**4** Electrical Activity	**A** Guidance **Z** No Qualifier
2 Cardiac	**X** External	**9** Output **C** Rate **F** Rhythm **H** Sound **P** Action Currents	**Z** No Qualifier
2 Cardiac	**X** External	**M** Total Activity	**4** Stress
3 Arterial	**0** Open **3** Percutaneous	**5** Flow **J** Pulse	**1** Peripheral **3** Pulmonary **C** Coronary
3 Arterial	**0** Open **3** Percutaneous	**B** Pressure	**1** Peripheral **3** Pulmonary **C** Coronary **F** Other Thoracic

4A0 continued on next page

4 Measurement and Monitoring
A Physiological Systems
0 Measurement: Determining the level of a physiological or physical function at a point in time

4A0 continued from previous page

Body System	Approach	Function/Device	Qualifier
Character 4	**Character 5**	**Character 6**	**Character 7**
3 Arterial	**0** Open **3** Percutaneous	**H** Sound **R** Saturation	**1** Peripheral
3 Arterial	**X** External	**5** Flow **B** Pressure **H** Sound **J** Pulse **R** Saturation	**1** Peripheral
4 Venous	**0** Open **3** Percutaneous	**5** Flow **B** Pressure **J** Pulse	**0** Central **1** Peripheral **2** Portal **3** Pulmonary
4 Venous	**0** Open **3** Percutaneous	**R** Saturation	**1** Peripheral
4 Venous	**X** External	**5** Flow **B** Pressure **J** Pulse **R** Saturation	**1** Peripheral
5 Circulatory	**X** External	**L** Volume	**Z** No Qualifier
6 Lymphatic	**0** Open **3** Percutaneous **7** Via Natural or Artificial Opening **8** Via Natural or Artificial Opening Endoscopic	**5** Flow **B** Pressure	**Z** No Qualifier
7 Visual	**X** External	**0** Acuity **7** Mobility **B** Pressure	**Z** No Qualifier
8 Olfactory	**X** External	**0** Acuity	**Z** No Qualifier
9 Respiratory	**7** Via Natural or Artificial Opening **8** Via Natural or Artificial Opening Endoscopic **X** External	**1** Capacity **5** Flow **C** Rate **D** Resistance **L** Volume **M** Total Activity	**Z** No Qualifier
B Gastrointestinal	**7** Via Natural or Artificial Opening **8** Via Natural or Artificial Opening Endoscopic	**8** Motility **B** Pressure **G** Secretion	**Z** No Qualifier
C Biliary	**3** Percutaneous **4** Percutaneous Endoscopic **7** Via Natural or Artificial Opening **8** Via Natural or Artificial Opening Endoscopic	**5** Flow **B** Pressure	**Z** No Qualifier
D Urinary	**7** Via Natural or Artificial Opening **8** Via Natural or Artificial Opening Endoscopic	**3** Contractility **5** Flow **B** Pressure **D** Resistance **L** Volume	**Z** No Qualifier
F Musculoskeletal	**3** Percutaneous **X** External	**3** Contractility	**Z** No Qualifier
H Products of Conception, Cardiac ♀	**7** Via Natural or Artificial Opening **8** Via Natural or Artificial Opening Endoscopic **X** External	**4** Electrical Activity **C** Rate **F** Rhythm **H** Sound	**Z** No Qualifier

4A0 continued on next page

LC Limited Coverage   **NC** Noncovered   **HAC** HAC-associated Procedure   **CC** Combination Cluster - See Appendix G for code lists
DRG Non-OR-Affecting MS-DRG Assignment   New/Revised Text in **Orange**   ♂ Male   ♀ Female

4 Measurement and Monitoring
A Physiological Systems
0 Measurement: Determining the level of a physiological or physical function at a point in time

4A0 continued from previous page

Body System	Approach	Function/Device	Qualifier
Character 4	Character 5	Character 6	Character 7
J Products of Conception, Nervous ♀	7 Via Natural or Artificial Opening 8 Via Natural or Artificial Opening Endoscopic X External	2 Conductivity 4 Electrical Activity B Pressure	Z No Qualifier
Z None	7 Via Natural or Artificial Opening	6 Metabolism K Temperature	Z No Qualifier
Z None	X External	6 Metabolism K Temperature Q Sleep	Z No Qualifier

♀ 4A0H74Z 4A0H7CZ 4A0H7FZ 4A0H7HZ 4A0H84Z 4A0H8CZ 4A0H8FZ 4A0H8HZ 4A0HX4Z 4A0HXCZ 4A0HXFZ 4A0HXHZ 4A0J72Z
4A0J74Z 4A0J7BZ 4A0J82Z 4A0J84Z 4A0J8BZ 4A0JX2Z 4A0JX4Z 4A0JXBZ
DRG 4A020N6 4A020N7 4A020N8 4A023FZ 4A023N6 4A023N7 4A023N8

4 Measurement and Monitoring
A Physiological Systems
1 Monitoring: Determining the level of a physiological or physical function repetitively over a period of time

Body System	Approach	Function/Device	Qualifier
Character 4	Character 5	Character 6	Character 7
0 Central Nervous	0 Open	2 Conductivity B Pressure	Z No Qualifier
0 Central Nervous	0 Open	4 Electrical Activity	G Intraoperative Z No Qualifier
0 Central Nervous	3 Percutaneous 7 Via Natural or Artificial Opening 8 Via Natural or Artificial Opening Endoscopic	4 Electrical Activity	G Intraoperative Z No Qualifier
0 Central Nervous	3 Percutaneous 7 Via Natural or Artificial Opening 8 Via Natural or Artificial Opening Endoscopic	B Pressure K Temperature R Saturation	D Intracranial
0 Central Nervous	X External	2 Conductivity	Z No Qualifier
0 Central Nervous	X External	4 Electrical Activity	G Intraoperative Z No Qualifier
1 Peripheral Nervous	0 Open 3 Percutaneous 7 Via Natural or Artificial Opening 8 Via Natural or Artificial Opening Endoscopic X External	2 Conductivity	9 Sensory B Motor
1 Peripheral Nervous	0 Open 3 Percutaneous 7 Via Natural or Artificial Opening 8 Via Natural or Artificial Opening Endoscopic X External	4 Electrical Activity	G Intraoperative Z No Qualifier
2 Cardiac	0 Open 3 Percutaneous 7 Via Natural or Artificial Opening 8 Via Natural or Artificial Opening Endoscopic	4 Electrical Activity 9 Output C Rate F Rhythm H Sound	Z No Qualifier
2 Cardiac	X External	4 Electrical Activity	5 Ambulatory Z No Qualifier

4A1 continued on next page

4 **Measurement and Monitoring**
A **Physiological Systems**

4A1 continued from previous page

1 **Monitoring:** Determining the level of a physiological or physical function repetitively over a period of time

Body System	Approach	Function/Device	Qualifier
Character 4	Character 5	Character 6	Character 7
2 Cardiac	X External	9 Output C Rate F Rhythm H Sound	Z No Qualifier
2 Cardiac	X External	M Total Activity	4 Stress
2 Cardiac	X External	S Vascular Perfusion	H Indocyanine Green Dye
3 Arterial	0 Open 3 Percutaneous	5 Flow B Pressure J Pulse	1 Peripheral 3 Pulmonary C Coronary
3 Arterial	0 Open 3 Percutaneous	H Sound R Saturation	1 Peripheral
3 Arterial	X External	5 Flow B Pressure H Sound J Pulse R Saturation	1 Peripheral
4 Venous	0 Open 3 Percutaneous	5 Flow B Pressure J Pulse	0 Central 1 Peripheral 2 Portal 3 Pulmonary
4 Venous	0 Open 3 Percutaneous	R Saturation	0 Central 2 Portal 3 Pulmonary
4 Venous	X External	5 Flow B Pressure J Pulse	1 Peripheral
6 Lymphatic	0 Open 3 Percutaneous 7 Via Natural or Artificial Opening 8 Via Natural or Artificial Opening Endoscopic	5 Flow B Pressure	Z No Qualifier
9 Respiratory	7 Via Natural or Artificial Opening X External	1 Capacity 5 Flow C Rate D Resistance L Volume	Z No Qualifier
B Gastrointestinal	7 Via Natural or Artificial Opening 8 Via Natural or Artificial Opening Endoscopic	8 Motility B Pressure G Secretion	Z No Qualifier
B Gastrointestinal	X External	S Vascular Perfusion	H Indocyanine Green Dye
D Urinary	7 Via Natural or Artificial Opening 8 Via Natural or Artificial Opening Endoscopic	3 Contractility 5 Flow B Pressure D Resistance L Volume	Z No Qualifier
G Skin and Breast	X External	S Vascular Perfusion	H Indocyanine Green Dye
H Products of Conception, Cardiac ♀	7 Via Natural or Artificial Opening 8 Via Natural or Artificial Opening Endoscopic X External	4 Electrical Activity C Rate F Rhythm H Sound	Z No Qualifier

4A1 continued on next page

4 Measurement and Monitoring
A Physiological Systems
1 Monitoring: Determining the level of a physiological or physical function repetitively over a period of time

4A1 continued from previous page

Body System	Approach	Function/Device	Qualifier
Character 4	Character 5	Character 6	Character 7
J Products of Conception, Nervous ♀	**7** Via Natural or Artificial Opening **8** Via Natural or Artificial Opening Endoscopic **X** External	**2** Conductivity **4** Electrical Activity **B** Pressure	**Z** No Qualifier
Z None	**7** Via Natural or Artificial Opening	**K** Temperature	**Z** No Qualifier
Z None	**X** External	**K** Temperature **Q** Sleep	**Z** No Qualifier

♀ 4A1H74Z 4A1H7CZ 4A1H7FZ 4A1H7HZ 4A1H84Z 4A1H8CZ 4A1H8FZ 4A1H8HZ 4A1HX4Z 4A1HXCZ 4A1HXFZ 4A1HXHZ 4A1J72Z
4A1J74Z 4A1J7BZ 4A1J82Z 4A1J84Z 4A1J8BZ 4A1JX2Z 4A1JX4Z 4A1JXBZ

4 Measurement and Monitoring
B Physiological Devices
0 Measurement: Determining the level of a physiological or physical function at a point in time

Body System	Approach	Function/Device	Qualifier
Character 4	Character 5	Character 6	Character 7
0 Central Nervous **1** Peripheral Nervous **F** Musculoskeletal	**X** External	**V** Stimulator	**Z** No Qualifier
2 Cardiac	**X** External	**S** Pacemaker **T** Defibrillator	**Z** No Qualifier
9 Respiratory	**X** External	**S** Pacemaker	**Z** No Qualifier

NOTES

Extracorporeal or Systemic Assistance and Performance 5A0-5A2

5 **Extracorporeal** or Systemic **Assistance and Performance**
A **Physiological Systems**
0 **Assistance:** Taking over a portion of a physiological function by extracorporeal means

Body System	Approach	Function/Device	Qualifier
Character 4	Character 5	Character 6	Character 7
2 Cardiac	1 Intermittent 2 Continuous	1 Output	0 Balloon Pump 5 Pulsatile Compression 6 Other Pump D Impeller Pump
5 Circulatory	1 Intermittent 2 Continuous	2 Oxygenation	1 Hyperbaric C Supersaturated
9 Respiratory	2 Continuous	0 Filtration	Z No Qualifier
9 Respiratory	3 Less than 24 Consecutive Hours 4 24-96 Consecutive Hours 5 Greater than 96 Consecutive Hours	5 Ventilation	7 Continuous Positive Airway Pressure 8 Intermittent Positive Airway Pressure 9 Continuous Negative Airway Pressure B Intermittent Negative Airway Pressure Z No Qualifier

5 **Extracorporeal** or Systemic **Assistance and Performance**
A **Physiological Systems**
1 **Performance:** Completely taking over a physiological function by extracorporeal means

Body System	Approach	Function/Device	Qualifier
Character 4	Character 5	Character 6	Character 7
2 Cardiac	0 Single	1 Output	2 Manual
2 Cardiac	1 Intermittent	3 Pacing	Z No Qualifier
2 Cardiac	2 Continuous	1 Output 3 Pacing	Z No Qualifier
5 Circulatory	2 Continuous	2 Oxygenation	3 Membrane
9 Respiratory	0 Single	5 Ventilation	4 Nonmechanical
9 Respiratory ᴼᴿᴳ	3 Less than 24 Consecutive Hours 4 24-96 Consecutive Hours 5 Greater than 96 Consecutive Hours	5 Ventilation	Z No Qualifier
C Biliary	0 Single 6 Multiple	0 Filtration	Z No Qualifier
D Urinary	7 Intermittent, Less than 6 Hours Per Day 8 Prolonged Intermittent, 6-18 hours Per Day 9 Continuous, Greater than 18 hours Per Day	0 Filtration	Z No Qualifier

ᴼᴿᴳ 5A1935Z   5A1945Z   5A1955Z

5 **Extracorporeal** or Systemic **Assistance and Performance**
A **Physiological Systems**
2 **Restoration:** Returning, or attempting to return, a physiological function to its original state by extracorporeal means.

Body System	Approach	Function/Device	Qualifier
Character 4	Character 5	Character 6	Character 7
2 Cardiac	0 Single	4 Rhythm	Z No Qualifier

NOTES

Extracorporeal or Systemic Therapies 6A0-6AB

6 **Extracorporeal** or Systemic **Therapies**
A **Physiological Systems**
0 **Atmospheric Control:** Extracorporeal control of atmospheric pressure and composition

Body System	Duration	Qualifier	Qualifier
Character 4	Character 5	Character 6	Character 7
Z None	**0** Single **1** Multiple	**Z** No Qualifier	**Z** No Qualifier

6 **Extracorporeal** or Systemic **Therapies**
A **Physiological Systems**
1 **Decompression:** Extracorporeal elimination of undissolved gas from body fluids

Body System	Duration	Qualifier	Qualifier
Character 4	Character 5	Character 6	Character 7
5 Circulatory	**0** Single **1** Multiple	**Z** No Qualifier	**Z** No Qualifier

6 **Extracorporeal** or Systemic **Therapies**
A **Physiological Systems**
2 **Electromagnetic Therapy:** Extracorporeal treatment by electromagnetic rays

Body System	Duration	Qualifier	Qualifier
Character 4	Character 5	Character 6	Character 7
1 Urinary **2** Central Nervous	**0** Single **1** Multiple	**Z** No Qualifier	**Z** No Qualifier

6 **Extracorporeal** or Systemic **Therapies**
A **Physiological Systems**
3 **Hyperthermia:** Extracorporeal raising of body temperature

Body System	Duration	Qualifier	Qualifier
Character 4	Character 5	Character 6	Character 7
Z None	**0** Single **1** Multiple	**Z** No Qualifier	**Z** No Qualifier

6 **Extracorporeal** or Systemic **Therapies**
A **Physiological Systems**
4 **Hypothermia:** Extracorporeal lowering of body temperature

Body System	Duration	Qualifier	Qualifier
Character 4	Character 5	Character 6	Character 7
Z None	**0** Single **1** Multiple	**Z** No Qualifier	**Z** No Qualifier

6 **Extracorporeal** or Systemic **Therapies**
A **Physiological Systems**
5 **Pheresis:** Extracorporeal separation of blood products

Body System	Duration	Qualifier	Qualifier
Character 4	Character 5	Character 6	Character 7
5 Circulatory	**0** Single **1** Multiple	**Z** No Qualifier	**0** Erythrocytes **1** Leukocytes **2** Platelets **3** Plasma **T** Stem Cells, Cord Blood **V** Stem Cells, Hematopoietic

LC Limited Coverage   **NC** Noncovered   **HAC** HAC-associated Procedure   **CC** Combination Cluster - See Appendix G for code lists
DRG Non-OR-Affecting MS-DRG Assignment   New/Revised Text in **Orange**   ♂ Male   ♀ Female

2018 ICD-10-PCS

611

6 **Extracorporeal** or Systemic **Therapies**
A **Physiological Systems**
6 **Phototherapy:** Extracorporeal treatment by light rays

Body System	Duration	Qualifier	Qualifier
Character 4	Character 5	Character 6	Character 7
0 Skin **5** Circulatory	**0** Single **1** Multiple	**Z** No Qualifier	**Z** No Qualifier

6 **Extracorporeal** or Systemic **Therapies**
A **Physiological Systems**
7 **Ultrasound Therapy:** Extracorporeal treatment by ultrasound

Body System Character 4	Duration Character 5	Qualifier Character 6	Qualifier Character 7
5 Circulatory	**0** Single **1** Multiple	**Z** No Qualifier	**4** Head and Neck Vessels **5** Heart **6** Peripheral Vessels **7** Other Vessels **Z** No Qualifier

6 **Extracorporeal** or Systemic **Therapies**
A **Physiological Systems**
8 **Ultraviolet Light Therapy:** Extracorporeal treatment by ultraviolet light

Body System	Duration	Qualifier	Qualifier
Character 4	Character 5	Character 6	Character 7
0 Skin	**0** Single **1** Multiple	**Z** No Qualifier	**Z** No Qualifier

6 **Extracorporeal** or Systemic **Therapies**
A **Physiological Systems**
9 **Shock Wave Therapy:** Extracorporeal treatment by shock waves

Body System	Duration	Qualifier	Qualifier
Character 4	Character 5	Character 6	Character 7
3 Musculoskeletal	**0** Single **1** Multiple	**Z** No Qualifier	**Z** No Qualifier

6 **Extracorporeal** or Systemic **Therapies**
A **Physiological Systems**
B **Perfusion:** Extracorporeal treatment by diffusion of therapeutic fluid

Body System	Duration	Qualifier	Qualifier
Character 4	Character 5	Character 6	Character 7
5 Circulatory **B** Respiratory System **F** Hepatobiliary System and Pancreas **T** Urinary System	**0** Single	**B** Donor Organ	**Z** No Qualifier

NOTES

NOTES

Osteopathic 7W0

7 Osteopathic
W Anatomical Regions
0 Treatment: Manual treatment to eliminate or alleviate somatic dysfunction and related disorders

Body Region	Approach	Method	Qualifier
Character 4	Character 5	Character 6	Character 7
0 Head	X External	0 Articulatory-Raising	Z None
1 Cervical		1 Fascial Release	
2 Thoracic		2 General Mobilization	
3 Lumbar		3 High Velocity-Low Amplitude	
4 Sacrum		4 Indirect	
5 Pelvis		5 Low Velocity-High Amplitude	
6 Lower Extremities		6 Lymphatic Pump	
7 Upper Extremities		7 Muscle Energy-Isometric	
8 Rib Cage		8 Muscle Energy-Isotonic	
9 Abdomen		9 Other Method	

NOTES

Other Procedures 8C0-8E0

8   Other Procedures
C   Indwelling Device
0   Other Procedures: Methodologies which attempt to remediate or cure a disorder or disease

Body Region	Approach	Method	Qualifier
Character 4	Character 5	Character 6	Character 7
1 Nervous System	X External	6 Collection	J Cerebrospinal Fluid L Other Fluid
2 Circulatory System	X External	6 Collection	K Blood L Other Fluid

8   Other Procedures
E   Physiological Systems and Anatomical Regions
0   Other Procedures: Methodologies which attempt to remediate or cure a disorder or disease

Body Region	Approach	Method	Qualifier
Character 4	Character 5	Character 6	Character 7
1 Nervous System U Female Reproductive System ♀	X External	Y Other Method	7 Examination
2 Circulatory System	3 Percutaneous	D Near Infrared Spectroscopy	Z No Qualifier
9 Head and Neck Region W Trunk Region	0 Open 3 Percutaneous 4 Percutaneous Endoscopic 7 Via Natural or Artificial Opening 8 Via Natural or Artificial Opening Endoscopic	C Robotic Assisted Procedure	Z No Qualifier
9 Head and Neck Region W Trunk Region	X External	B Computer Assisted Procedure	F With Fluoroscopy G With Computerized Tomography H With Magnetic Resonance Imaging Z No Qualifier
9 Head and Neck Region W Trunk Region	X External	C Robotic Assisted Procedure	Z No Qualifier
9 Head and Neck Region W Trunk Region	X External	Y Other Method	8 Suture Removal
H Integumentary System and Breast	3 Percutaneous	0 Acupuncture	0 Anesthesia Z No Qualifier
H Integumentary System and Breast ♀	X External	6 Collection	2 Breast Milk
H Integumentary System and Breast	X External	Y Other Method	9 Piercing
K Musculoskeletal System	X External	1 Therapeutic Massage	Z No Qualifier
K Musculoskeletal System	X External	Y Other Method	7 Examination
V Male Reproductive System ♂	X External	1 Therapeutic Massage	C Prostate D Rectum
V Male Reproductive System ♂	X External	6 Collection	3 Sperm
X Upper Extremity Y Lower Extremity	0 Open 3 Percutaneous 4 Percutaneous Endoscopic	C Robotic Assisted Procedure	Z No Qualifier
X Upper Extremity Y Lower Extremity	X External	B Computer Assisted Procedure	F With Fluoroscopy G With Computerized Tomography H With Magnetic Resonance Imaging Z No Qualifier

8E0 continued on next page

LC Limited Coverage   NC Noncovered   HAC HAC-associated Procedure   CC Combination Cluster - See Appendix G for code lists
DRG Non-OR-Affecting MS-DRG Assignment   New/Revised Text in **Orange**   ♂ Male   ♀ Female

8 **Other Procedures**
E **Physiological Systems and Anatomical Regions**
0 **Other Procedures:** Methodologies which attempt to remediate or cure a disorder or disease

8E0 continued from previous page

Body Region	Approach	Method	Qualifier
Character 4	Character 5	Character 6	Character 7
X Upper Extremity **Y** Lower Extremity	**X** External	**C** Robotic Assisted Procedure	**Z** No Qualifier
X Upper Extremity **Y** Lower Extremity	**X** External	**Y** Other Method	**8** Suture Removal
Z None	**X** External	**Y** Other Method	**1** In Vitro Fertilization **4** Yoga Therapy **5** Meditation **6** Isolation

♂ 8E0VX1C   8E0VX1D   8E0VX63
♀ 8E0HX62   8E0UXY7

NOTES

NOTES

9 Chiropractic
W Anatomical Regions
B Manipulation: Manual procedure that involves a directed thrust to move a joint past the physiological range of motion, without exceeding the anatomical limit

Body Region	Approach	Method	Qualifier
Character 4	**Character 5**	**Character 6**	**Character 7**
0 Head **1** Cervical **2** Thoracic **3** Lumbar **4** Sacrum **5** Pelvis **6** Lower Extremities **7** Upper Extremities **8** Rib Cage **9** Abdomen	**X** External	**B** Non-Manual **C** Indirect Visceral **D** Extra-Articular **F** Direct Visceral **G** Long Lever Specific Contact **H** Short Lever Specific Contact **J** Long and Short Lever Specific Contact **K** Mechanically Assisted **L** Other Method	**Z** None

LC Limited Coverage **NC** Noncovered **HAC** HAC-associated Procedure **CC** Combination Cluster - See Appendix G for code lists
DRG Non-OR-Affecting MS-DRG Assignment New/Revised Text in **Orange** ♂ Male ♀ Female

2018 ICD-10-PCS 621

NOTES

Imaging B00-BY4

B Imaging
0 Central Nervous System
0 Plain Radiography: Planar display of an image developed from the capture of external ionizing radiation on photographic or photoconductive plate

Body Part	Contrast	Qualifier	Qualifier
Character 4	Character 5	Character 6	Character 7
B Spinal Cord	**0** High Osmolar **1** Low Osmolar **Y** Other Contrast **Z** None	**Z** None	**Z** None

B Imaging
0 Central Nervous System
1 Fluoroscopy: Single plane or bi-plane real time display of an image developed from the capture of external ionizing radiation on a fluorescent screen. The image may also be stored by either digital or analog means

Body Part	Contrast	Qualifier	Qualifier
Character 4	Character 5	Character 6	Character 7
B Spinal Cord	**0** High Osmolar **1** Low Osmolar **Y** Other Contrast **Z** None	**Z** None	**Z** None

B Imaging
0 Central Nervous System
2 Computerized Tomography (CT Scan): Computer reformatted digital display of multiplanar images developed from the capture of multiple exposures of external ionizing radiation

Body Part	Contrast	Qualifier	Qualifier
Character 4	Character 5	Character 6	Character 7
0 Brain **7** Cisterna **8** Cerebral Ventricle(s) **9** Sella Turcica/Pituitary Gland **B** Spinal Cord	**0** High Osmolar **1** Low Osmolar **Y** Other Contrast	**0** Unenhanced and Enhanced **Z** None	**Z** None
0 Brain **7** Cisterna **8** Cerebral Ventricle(s) **9** Sella Turcica/Pituitary Gland **B** Spinal Cord	**Z** None	**Z** None	**Z** None

B Imaging
0 Central Nervous System
3 Magnetic Resonance Imaging (MRI): Computer reformatted digital display of multiplanar images developed from the capture of radiofrequency signals emitted by nuclei in a body site excited within a magnetic field

Body Part	Contrast	Qualifier	Qualifier
Character 4	Character 5	Character 6	Character 7
0 Brain **9** Sella Turcica/Pituitary Gland **B** Spinal Cord **C** Acoustic Nerves	**Y** Other Contrast	**0** Unenhanced and Enhanced **Z** None	**Z** None
0 Brain **9** Sella Turcica/Pituitary Gland **B** Spinal Cord **C** Acoustic Nerves	**Z** None	**Z** None	**Z** None

B Imaging
0 Central Nervous System
4 Ultrasonography: Real time display of images of anatomy or flow information developed from the capture of reflected and attenuated high frequency sound waves

Body Part	Contrast	Qualifier	Qualifier
Character 4	Character 5	Character 6	Character 7
0 Brain **B** Spinal Cord	**Z** None	**Z** None	**Z** None

B Imaging
2 Heart
0 Plain Radiography: Planar display of an image developed from the capture of external ionizing radiation on photographic or photoconductive plate

Body Part	Contrast	Qualifier	Qualifier
Character 4	Character 5	Character 6	Character 7
0 Coronary Artery, Single ᴰᴿᴳ **1** Coronary Arteries, Multiple ᴰᴿᴳ **2** Coronary Artery Bypass Graft, Single ᴰᴿᴳ **3** Coronary Artery Bypass Grafts, Multiple ᴰᴿᴳ **4** Heart, Right ᴰᴿᴳ **5** Heart, Left **6** Heart, Right and Left **7** Internal Mammary Bypass Graft, Right **8** Internal Mammary Bypass Graft, Left **F** Bypass Graft, Other	**0** High Osmolar **1** Low Osmolar **Y** Other Contrast	**Z** None	**Z** None

ᴰᴿᴳ B2000ZZ   B2001ZZ   B200YZZ   B2010ZZ   B2011ZZ   B201YZZ   B2020ZZ   B2021ZZ   B202YZZ   B2030ZZ   B2031ZZ   B203YZZ   B2040ZZ   B2041ZZ

B Imaging
2 Heart
1 Fluoroscopy: Single plane or bi-plane real time display of an image developed from the capture of external ionizing radiation on a fluorescent screen. The image may also be stored by either digital or analog means

Body Part	Contrast	Qualifier	Qualifier
Character 4	Character 5	Character 6	Character 7
0 Coronary Artery, Single **1** Coronary Arteries, Multiple **2** Coronary Artery Bypass Graft, Single **3** Coronary Artery Bypass Grafts, Multiple	**0** High Osmolar **1** Low Osmolar **Y** Other Contrast	**1** Laser	**0** Intraoperative
0 Coronary Artery, Single **1** Coronary Arteries, Multiple **2** Coronary Artery Bypass Graft, Single **3** Coronary Artery Bypass Grafts, Multiple	**0** High Osmolar **1** Low Osmolar **Y** Other Contrast	**Z** None	**Z** None
4 Heart, Right **5** Heart, Left **6** Heart, Right and Left **7** Internal Mammary Bypass Graft, Right **8** Internal Mammary Bypass Graft, Left **F** Bypass Graft, Other	**0** High Osmolar **1** Low Osmolar **Y** Other Contrast	**Z** None	**Z** None

B   Imaging
2   Heart
2   Computerized Tomography (CT Scan): Computer reformatted digital display of multiplanar images developed from the capture of multiple exposures of external ionizing radiation

Body Part	Contrast	Qualifier	Qualifier
Character 4	Character 5	Character 6	Character 7
1 Coronary Arteries, Multiple 3 Coronary Artery Bypass Grafts, Multiple 6 Heart, Right and Left	0 High Osmolar 1 Low Osmolar Y Other Contrast	0 Unenhanced and Enhanced Z None	Z None
1 Coronary Arteries, Multiple 3 Coronary Artery Bypass Grafts, Multiple 6 Heart, Right and Left	Z None	2 Intravascular Optical Coherence Z None	Z None

B   Imaging
2   Heart
3   Magnetic Resonance Imaging (MRI): Computer reformatted digital display of multiplanar images developed from the capture of radiofrequency signals emitted by nuclei in a body site excited within a magnetic field

Body Part	Contrast	Qualifier	Qualifier
Character 4	Character 5	Character 6	Character 7
1 Coronary Arteries, Multiple 3 Coronary Artery Bypass Grafts, Multiple 6 Heart, Right and Left	Y Other Contrast	0 Unenhanced and Enhanced Z None	Z None
1 Coronary Arteries, Multiple 3 Coronary Artery Bypass Grafts, Multiple 6 Heart, Right and Left	Z None	Z None	Z None

B   Imaging
2   Heart
4   Ultrasonography: Real time display of images of anatomy or flow information developed from the capture of reflected and attenuated high frequency sound waves

Body Part	Contrast	Qualifier	Qualifier
Character 4	Character 5	Character 6	Character 7
0 Coronary Artery, Single 1 Coronary Arteries, Multiple 4 Heart, Right 5 Heart, Left 6 Heart, Right and Left B Heart with Aorta C Pericardium D Pediatric Heart	Y Other Contrast	Z None	Z None
0 Coronary Artery, Single 1 Coronary Arteries, Multiple 4 Heart, Right 5 Heart, Left 6 Heart, Right and Left B Heart with Aorta C Pericardium D Pediatric Heart	Z None	Z None	3 Intravascular 4 Transesophageal Z None

B Imaging
3 Upper Arteries
0 Plain Radiography: Planar display of an image developed from the capture of external ionizing radiation on photographic or photoconductive plate

Body Part	Contrast	Qualifier	Qualifier
Character 4	Character 5	Character 6	Character 7
0 Thoracic Aorta 1 Brachiocephalic-Subclavian Artery, Right 2 Subclavian Artery, Left 3 Common Carotid Artery, Right 4 Common Carotid Artery, Left 5 Common Carotid Arteries, Bilateral 6 Internal Carotid Artery, Right 7 Internal Carotid Artery, Left 8 Internal Carotid Arteries, Bilateral 9 External Carotid Artery, Right B External Carotid Artery, Left C External Carotid Arteries, Bilateral D Vertebral Artery, Right F Vertebral Artery, Left G Vertebral Arteries, Bilateral H Upper Extremity Arteries, Right J Upper Extremity Arteries, Left K Upper Extremity Arteries, Bilateral L Intercostal and Bronchial Arteries M Spinal Arteries N Upper Arteries, Other P Thoraco-Abdominal Aorta Q Cervico-Cerebral Arch R Intracranial Arteries S Pulmonary Artery, Right T Pulmonary Artery, Left	0 High Osmolar 1 Low Osmolar Y Other Contrast Z None	Z None	Z None

B Imaging
3 Upper Arteries
1 Fluoroscopy: Single plane or bi-plane real time display of an image developed from the capture of external ionizing radiation on a fluorescent screen. The image may also be stored by either digital or analog means

Body Part	Contrast	Qualifier	Qualifier
Character 4	Character 5	Character 6	Character 7
0 Thoracic Aorta	**0** High Osmolar	**1** Laser	**0** Intraoperative
1 Brachiocephalic-Subclavian Artery, Right	**1** Low Osmolar		
2 Subclavian Artery, Left	**Y** Other Contrast		
3 Common Carotid Artery, Right			
4 Common Carotid Artery, Left			
5 Common Carotid Arteries, Bilateral			
6 Internal Carotid Artery, Right			
7 Internal Carotid Artery, Left			
8 Internal Carotid Arteries, Bilateral			
9 External Carotid Artery, Right			
B External Carotid Artery, Left			
C External Carotid Arteries, Bilateral			
D Vertebral Artery, Right			
F Vertebral Artery, Left			
G Vertebral Arteries, Bilateral			
H Upper Extremity Arteries, Right			
J Upper Extremity Arteries, Left			
K Upper Extremity Arteries, Bilateral			
L Intercostal and Bronchial Arteries			
M Spinal Arteries			
N Upper Arteries, Other			
P Thoraco-Abdominal Aorta			
Q Cervico-Cerebral Arch			
R Intracranial Arteries			
S Pulmonary Artery, Right			
T Pulmonary Artery, Left			
U Pulmonary Trunk			

B31 continued on next page

B Imaging
3 Upper Arteries

B31 continued from previous page

1 Fluoroscopy: Single plane or bi-plane real time display of an image developed from the capture of external ionizing radiation on a fluorescent screen. The image may also be stored by either digital or analog means

Body Part	Contrast	Qualifier	Qualifier
Character 4	Character 5	Character 6	Character 7
0 Thoracic Aorta 1 Brachiocephalic-Subclavian Artery, Right 2 Subclavian Artery, Left 3 Common Carotid Artery, Right 4 Common Carotid Artery, Left 5 Common Carotid Arteries, Bilateral 6 Internal Carotid Artery, Right 7 Internal Carotid Artery, Left 8 Internal Carotid Arteries, Bilateral 9 External Carotid Artery, Right B External Carotid Artery, Left C External Carotid Arteries, Bilateral D Vertebral Artery, Right F Vertebral Artery, Left G Vertebral Arteries, Bilateral H Upper Extremity Arteries, Right J Upper Extremity Arteries, Left K Upper Extremity Arteries, Bilateral L Intercostal and Bronchial Arteries M Spinal Arteries N Upper Arteries, Other P Thoraco-Abdominal Aorta Q Cervico-Cerebral Arch R Intracranial Arteries S Pulmonary Artery, Right T Pulmonary Artery, Left U Pulmonary Trunk	0 High Osmolar 1 Low Osmolar Y Other Contrast	Z None	Z None

B31 continued on next page

B Imaging
3 Upper Arteries

B31 continued from previous page

1 **Fluoroscopy:** Single plane or bi-plane real time display of an image developed from the capture of external ionizing radiation on a fluorescent screen. The image may also be stored by either digital or analog means

Body Part	Contrast	Qualifier	Qualifier
Character 4	Character 5	Character 6	Character 7
0 Thoracic Aorta 1 Brachiocephalic-Subclavian Artery, Right 2 Subclavian Artery, Left 3 Common Carotid Artery, Right 4 Common Carotid Artery, Left 5 Common Carotid Arteries, Bilateral 6 Internal Carotid Artery, Right 7 Internal Carotid Artery, Left 8 Internal Carotid Arteries, Bilateral 9 External Carotid Artery, Right B External Carotid Artery, Left C External Carotid Arteries, Bilateral D Vertebral Artery, Right F Vertebral Artery, Left G Vertebral Arteries, Bilateral H Upper Extremity Arteries, Right J Upper Extremity Arteries, Left K Upper Extremity Arteries, Bilateral L Intercostal and Bronchial Arteries M Spinal Arteries N Upper Arteries, Other P Thoraco-Abdominal Aorta Q Cervico-Cerebral Arch R Intracranial Arteries S Pulmonary Artery, Right T Pulmonary Artery, Left U Pulmonary Trunk	Z None	Z None	Z None

B Imaging
3 Upper Arteries

2 **Computerized Tomography (CT Scan):** Computer reformatted digital display of multiplanar images developed from the capture of multiple exposures of external ionizing radiation

Body Part	Contrast	Qualifier	Qualifier
Character 4	Character 5	Character 6	Character 7
0 Thoracic Aorta 5 Common Carotid Arteries, Bilateral 8 Internal Carotid Arteries, Bilateral G Vertebral Arteries, Bilateral R Intracranial Arteries S Pulmonary Artery, Right T Pulmonary Artery, Left	0 High Osmolar 1 Low Osmolar Y Other Contrast	Z None	Z None
0 Thoracic Aorta 5 Common Carotid Arteries, Bilateral 8 Internal Carotid Arteries, Bilateral G Vertebral Arteries, Bilateral R Intracranial Arteries S Pulmonary Artery, Right T Pulmonary Artery, Left	Z None	2 Intravascular Optical Coherence Z None	Z None

B Imaging
3 Upper Arteries
3 Magnetic Resonance Imaging (MRI): Computer reformatted digital display of multiplanar images developed from the capture of radiofrequency signals emitted by nuclei in a body site excited within a magnetic field

Body Part	Contrast	Qualifier	Qualifier
Character 4	Character 5	Character 6	Character 7
0 Thoracic Aorta 5 Common Carotid Arteries, Bilateral 8 Internal Carotid Arteries, Bilateral G Vertebral Arteries, Bilateral H Upper Extremity Arteries, Right J Upper Extremity Arteries, Left K Upper Extremity Arteries, Bilateral M Spinal Arteries Q Cervico-Cerebral Arch R Intracranial Arteries	Y Other Contrast	0 Unenhanced and Enhanced Z None	Z None
0 Thoracic Aorta 5 Common Carotid Arteries, Bilateral 8 Internal Carotid Arteries, Bilateral G Vertebral Arteries, Bilateral H Upper Extremity Arteries, Right J Upper Extremity Arteries, Left K Upper Extremity Arteries, Bilateral M Spinal Arteries Q Cervico-Cerebral Arch R Intracranial Arteries	Z None	Z None	Z None

B Imaging
3 Upper Arteries
4 Ultrasonography: Real time display of images of anatomy or flow information developed from the capture of reflected and attenuated high frequency sound waves

Body Part	Contrast	Qualifier	Qualifier
Character 4	Character 5	Character 6	Character 7
0 Thoracic Aorta 1 Brachiocephalic-Subclavian Artery, Right 2 Subclavian Artery, Left 3 Common Carotid Artery, Right 4 Common Carotid Artery, Left 5 Common Carotid Arteries, Bilateral 6 Internal Carotid Artery, Right 7 Internal Carotid Artery, Left 8 Internal Carotid Arteries, Bilateral H Upper Extremity Arteries, Right J Upper Extremity Arteries, Left K Upper Extremity Arteries, Bilateral R Intracranial Arteries S Pulmonary Artery, Right T Pulmonary Artery, Left V Ophthalmic Arteries	Z None	Z None	3 Intravascular Z None

B Imaging
4 Lower Arteries
0 Plain Radiography: Planar display of an image developed from the capture of external ionizing radiation on photographic or photoconductive plate

Body Part	Contrast	Qualifier	Qualifier
Character 4	Character 5	Character 6	Character 7
0 Abdominal Aorta **2** Hepatic Artery **3** Splenic Arteries **4** Superior Mesenteric Artery **5** Inferior Mesenteric Artery **6** Renal Artery, Right **7** Renal Artery, Left **8** Renal Arteries, Bilateral **9** Lumbar Arteries **B** Intra-Abdominal Arteries, Other **C** Pelvic Arteries **D** Aorta and Bilateral Lower Extremity Arteries **F** Lower Extremity Arteries, Right **G** Lower Extremity Arteries, Left **J** Lower Arteries, Other **M** Renal Artery Transplant	**0** High Osmolar **1** Low Osmolar **Y** Other Contrast	**Z** None	**Z** None

B **Imaging**
4 **Lower Arteries**
1 **Fluoroscopy:** Single plane or bi-plane real time display of an image developed from the capture of external ionizing radiation on a fluorescent screen. The image may also be stored by either digital or analog means

Body Part	Contrast	Qualifier	Qualifier
Character 4	Character 5	Character 6	Character 7
0 Abdominal Aorta **2** Hepatic Artery **3** Splenic Arteries **4** Superior Mesenteric Artery **5** Inferior Mesenteric Artery **6** Renal Artery, Right **7** Renal Artery, Left **8** Renal Arteries, Bilateral **9** Lumbar Arteries **B** Intra-Abdominal Arteries, Other **C** Pelvic Arteries **D** Aorta and Bilateral Lower Extremity Arteries **F** Lower Extremity Arteries, Right **G** Lower Extremity Arteries, Left **J** Lower Arteries, Other	**0** High Osmolar **1** Low Osmolar **Y** Other Contrast	**1** Laser	**0** Intraoperative
0 Abdominal Aorta **2** Hepatic Artery **3** Splenic Arteries **4** Superior Mesenteric Artery **5** Inferior Mesenteric Artery **6** Renal Artery, Right **7** Renal Artery, Left **8** Renal Arteries, Bilateral **9** Lumbar Arteries **B** Intra-Abdominal Arteries, Other **C** Pelvic Arteries **D** Aorta and Bilateral Lower Extremity Arteries **F** Lower Extremity Arteries, Right **G** Lower Extremity Arteries, Left **J** Lower Arteries, Other	**0** High Osmolar **1** Low Osmolar **Y** Other Contrast	**Z** None	**Z** None
0 Abdominal Aorta **2** Hepatic Artery **3** Splenic Arteries **4** Superior Mesenteric Artery **5** Inferior Mesenteric Artery **6** Renal Artery, Right **7** Renal Artery, Left **8** Renal Arteries, Bilateral **9** Lumbar Arteries **B** Intra-Abdominal Arteries, Other **C** Pelvic Arteries **D** Aorta and Bilateral Lower Extremity Arteries **F** Lower Extremity Arteries, Right **G** Lower Extremity Arteries, Left **J** Lower Arteries, Other	**Z** None	**Z** None	**Z** None

LC Limited Coverage   **NC** Noncovered   **HAC** HAC-associated Procedure   **CC** Combination Cluster - See Appendix G for code lists
DRG Non-OR-Affecting MS-DRG Assignment   New/Revised Text in **Orange**   ♂ Male   ♀ Female

632

2018 ICD-10-PCS

B Imaging
4 Lower Arteries
2 Computerized Tomography (CT Scan): Computer reformatted digital display of multiplanar images developed from the capture of multiple exposures of external ionizing radiation

Body Part	Contrast	Qualifier	Qualifier
Character 4	Character 5	Character 6	Character 7
0 Abdominal Aorta 1 Celiac Artery 4 Superior Mesenteric Artery 8 Renal Arteries, Bilateral C Pelvic Arteries F Lower Extremity Arteries, Right G Lower Extremity Arteries, Left H Lower Extremity Arteries, Bilateral M Renal Artery Transplant	0 High Osmolar 1 Low Osmolar Y Other Contrast	Z None	Z None
0 Abdominal Aorta 1 Celiac Artery 4 Superior Mesenteric Artery 8 Renal Arteries, Bilateral C Pelvic Arteries F Lower Extremity Arteries, Right G Lower Extremity Arteries, Left H Lower Extremity Arteries, Bilateral M Renal Artery Transplant	Z None	2 Intravascular Optical Coherence Z None	Z None

B Imaging
4 Lower Arteries
3 Magnetic Resonance Imaging (MRI): Computer reformatted digital display of multiplanar images developed from the capture of radiofrequency signals emitted by nuclei in a body site excited within a magnetic field

Body Part	Contrast	Qualifier	Qualifier
Character 4	Character 5	Character 6	Character 7
0 Abdominal Aorta 1 Celiac Artery 4 Superior Mesenteric Artery 8 Renal Arteries, Bilateral C Pelvic Arteries F Lower Extremity Arteries, Right G Lower Extremity Arteries, Left H Lower Extremity Arteries, Bilateral	Y Other Contrast	0 Unenhanced and Enhanced Z None	Z None
0 Abdominal Aorta 1 Celiac Artery 4 Superior Mesenteric Artery 8 Renal Arteries, Bilateral C Pelvic Arteries F Lower Extremity Arteries, Right G Lower Extremity Arteries, Left H Lower Extremity Arteries, Bilateral	Z None	Z None	Z None

LC Limited Coverage   NC Noncovered   HAC HAC-associated Procedure   CC Combination Cluster - See Appendix G for code lists
DRG Non-OR-Affecting MS-DRG Assignment   New/Revised Text in Orange   ♂ Male   ♀ Female

2018 ICD-10-PCS   **633**

IMAGING B00-BY4

B Imaging

4 Lower Arteries

4 Ultrasonography: Real time display of images of anatomy or flow information developed from the capture of reflected and attenuated high frequency sound waves

Body Part	Contrast	Qualifier	Qualifier
Character 4	Character 5	Character 6	Character 7
0 Abdominal Aorta 4 Superior Mesenteric Artery 5 Inferior Mesenteric Artery 6 Renal Artery, Right 7 Renal Artery, Left 8 Renal Arteries, Bilateral B Intra-Abdominal Arteries, Other F Lower Extremity Arteries, Right G Lower Extremity Arteries, Left H Lower Extremity Arteries, Bilateral K Celiac and Mesenteric Arteries L Femoral Artery N Penile Arteries	Z None	Z None	3 Intravascular Z None

B Imaging

5 Veins

0 Plain Radiography: Planar display of an image developed from the capture of external ionizing radiation on photographic or photoconductive plate

Body Part	Contrast	Qualifier	Qualifier
Character 4	Character 5	Character 6	Character 7
0 Epidural Veins 1 Cerebral and Cerebellar Veins 2 Intracranial Sinuses 3 Jugular Veins, Right 4 Jugular Veins, Left 5 Jugular Veins, Bilateral 6 Subclavian Vein, Right 7 Subclavian Vein, Left 8 Superior Vena Cava 9 Inferior Vena Cava B Lower Extremity Veins, Right C Lower Extremity Veins, Left D Lower Extremity Veins, Bilateral F Pelvic (Iliac) Veins, Right G Pelvic (Iliac) Veins, Left H Pelvic (Iliac) Veins, Bilateral J Renal Vein, Right K Renal Vein, Left L Renal Veins, Bilateral M Upper Extremity Veins, Right N Upper Extremity Veins, Left P Upper Extremity Veins, Bilateral Q Pulmonary Vein, Right R Pulmonary Vein, Left S Pulmonary Veins, Bilateral T Portal and Splanchnic Veins V Veins, Other W Dialysis Shunt/Fistula	0 High Osmolar 1 Low Osmolar Y Other Contrast	Z None	Z None

B Imaging
5 Veins
1 Fluoroscopy: Single plane or bi-plane real time display of an image developed from the capture of external ionizing radiation on a fluorescent screen. The image may also be stored by either digital or analog means

Body Part	Contrast	Qualifier	Qualifier
Character 4	Character 5	Character 6	Character 7
0 Epidural Veins	0 High Osmolar	Z None	A Guidance
1 Cerebral and Cerebellar Veins	1 Low Osmolar		Z None
2 Intracranial Sinuses	Y Other Contrast		
3 Jugular Veins, Right	Z None		
4 Jugular Veins, Left			
5 Jugular Veins, Bilateral			
6 Subclavian Vein, Right			
7 Subclavian Vein, Left			
8 Superior Vena Cava			
9 Inferior Vena Cava			
B Lower Extremity Veins, Right			
C Lower Extremity Veins, Left			
D Lower Extremity Veins, Bilateral			
F Pelvic (Iliac) Veins, Right			
G Pelvic (Iliac) Veins, Left			
H Pelvic (Iliac) Veins, Bilateral			
J Renal Vein, Right			
K Renal Vein, Left			
L Renal Veins, Bilateral			
M Upper Extremity Veins, Right			
N Upper Extremity Veins, Left			
P Upper Extremity Veins, Bilateral			
Q Pulmonary Vein, Right			
R Pulmonary Vein, Left			
S Pulmonary Veins, Bilateral			
T Portal and Splanchnic Veins			
V Veins, Other			
W Dialysis Shunt/Fistula			

LC Limited Coverage   NC Noncovered   HAC HAC-associated Procedure   CC Combination Cluster - See Appendix G for code lists
DRG Non-OR-Affecting MS-DRG Assignment   New/Revised Text in **Orange**   ♂ Male   ♀ Female

2018 ICD-10-PCS   635

IMAGING B00-BY4

B Imaging
5 Veins
2 Computerized Tomography (CT Scan): Computer reformatted digital display of multiplanar images developed from the capture of multiple exposures of external ionizing radiation

Body Part	Contrast	Qualifier	Qualifier
Character 4	Character 5	Character 6	Character 7
2 Intracranial Sinuses **8** Superior Vena Cava **9** Inferior Vena Cava **F** Pelvic (Iliac) Veins, Right **G** Pelvic (Iliac) Veins, Left **H** Pelvic (Iliac) Veins, Bilateral **J** Renal Vein, Right **K** Renal Vein, Left **L** Renal Veins, Bilateral **Q** Pulmonary Vein, Right **R** Pulmonary Vein, Left **S** Pulmonary Veins, Bilateral **T** Portal and Splanchnic Veins	**0** High Osmolar **1** Low Osmolar **Y** Other Contrast	**0** Unenhanced and Enhanced **Z** None	**Z** None
2 Intracranial Sinuses **8** Superior Vena Cava **9** Inferior Vena Cava **F** Pelvic (Iliac) Veins, Right **G** Pelvic (Iliac) Veins, Left **H** Pelvic (Iliac) Veins, Bilateral **J** Renal Vein, Right **K** Renal Vein, Left **L** Renal Veins, Bilateral **Q** Pulmonary Vein, Right **R** Pulmonary Vein, Left **S** Pulmonary Veins, Bilateral **T** Portal and Splanchnic Veins	**Z** None	**2** Intravascular Optical Coherence **Z** None	**Z** None

IC Limited Coverage   **NC** Noncovered   **HAC** HAC-associated Procedure   **CC** Combination Cluster - See Appendix G for code lists
DRG Non-OR-Affecting MS-DRG Assignment   New/Revised Text in **Orange**   ♂ Male   ♀ Female

636   **2018 ICD-10-PCS**

B Imaging
5 Veins
3 **Magnetic Resonance Imaging (MRI):** Computer reformatted digital display of multiplanar images developed from the capture of radiofrequency signals emitted by nuclei in a body site excited within a magnetic field

Body Part	Contrast	Qualifier	Qualifier
Character 4	Character 5	Character 6	Character 7
1 Cerebral and Cerebellar Veins **2** Intracranial Sinuses **5** Jugular Veins, Bilateral **8** Superior Vena Cava **9** Inferior Vena Cava **B** Lower Extremity Veins, Right **C** Lower Extremity Veins, Left **D** Lower Extremity Veins, Bilateral **H** Pelvic (Iliac) Veins, Bilateral **L** Renal Veins, Bilateral **M** Upper Extremity Veins, Right **N** Upper Extremity Veins, Left **P** Upper Extremity Veins, Bilateral **S** Pulmonary Veins, Bilateral **T** Portal and Splanchnic Veins **V** Veins, Other	**Y** Other Contrast	**0** Unenhanced and Enhanced **Z** None	**Z** None
1 Cerebral and Cerebellar Veins **2** Intracranial Sinuses **5** Jugular Veins, Bilateral **8** Superior Vena Cava **9** Inferior Vena Cava **B** Lower Extremity Veins, Right **C** Lower Extremity Veins, Left **D** Lower Extremity Veins, Bilateral **H** Pelvic (Iliac) Veins, Bilateral **L** Renal Veins, Bilateral **M** Upper Extremity Veins, Right **N** Upper Extremity Veins, Left **P** Upper Extremity Veins, Bilateral **S** Pulmonary Veins, Bilateral **T** Portal and Splanchnic Veins **V** Veins, Other	**Z** None	**Z** None	**Z** None

LC Limited Coverage   NC Noncovered   HAC HAC-associated Procedure   CC Combination Cluster - See Appendix G for code lists
DRG Non-OR-Affecting MS-DRG Assignment   New/Revised Text in **Orange**   ♂ Male   ♀ Female

2018 ICD-10-PCS

637

IMAGING B00-BY4

B Imaging
5 Veins
4 Ultrasonography: Real time display of images of anatomy or flow information developed from the capture of reflected and attenuated high frequency sound waves

Body Part	Contrast	Qualifier	Qualifier
Character 4	Character 5	Character 6	Character 7
3 Jugular Veins, Right	Z None	Z None	3 Intravascular
4 Jugular Veins, Left			A Guidance
6 Subclavian Vein, Right			Z None
7 Subclavian Vein, Left			
8 Superior Vena Cava			
9 Inferior Vena Cava			
B Lower Extremity Veins, Right			
C Lower Extremity Veins, Left			
D Lower Extremity Veins, Bilateral			
J Renal Vein, Right			
K Renal Vein, Left			
L Renal Veins, Bilateral			
M Upper Extremity Veins, Right			
N Upper Extremity Veins, Left			
P Upper Extremity Veins, Bilateral			
T Portal and Splanchnic Veins			

B Imaging
7 Lymphatic System
0 Plain Radiography: Planar display of an image developed from the capture of external ionizing radiation on photographic or photoconductive plate

Body Part	Contrast	Qualifier	Qualifier
Character 4	Character 5	Character 6	Character 7
0 Abdominal/Retroperitoneal Lymphatics, Unilateral	0 High Osmolar	Z None	Z None
1 Abdominal/Retroperitoneal Lymphatics, Bilateral	1 Low Osmolar		
4 Lymphatics, Head and Neck	Y Other Contrast		
5 Upper Extremity Lymphatics, Right			
6 Upper Extremity Lymphatics, Left			
7 Upper Extremity Lymphatics, Bilateral			
8 Lower Extremity Lymphatics, Right			
9 Lower Extremity Lymphatics, Left			
B Lower Extremity Lymphatics, Bilateral			
C Lymphatics, Pelvic			

LC Limited Coverage   NC Noncovered   HAC HAC-associated Procedure   CC Combination Cluster - See Appendix G for code lists
DRG Non-OR-Affecting MS-DRG Assignment   New/Revised Text in Orange   ♂ Male   ♀ Female

638   2018 ICD-10-PCS

IMAGING B00-BY4

B Imaging
8 Eye
0 Plain Radiography: Planar display of an image developed from the capture of external ionizing radiation on photographic or photoconductive plate

Body Part	Contrast	Qualifier	Qualifier
Character 4	Character 5	Character 6	Character 7
0 Lacrimal Duct, Right 1 Lacrimal Duct, Left 2 Lacrimal Ducts, Bilateral	0 High Osmolar 1 Low Osmolar Y Other Contrast	Z None	Z None
3 Optic Foramina, Right 4 Optic Foramina, Left 5 Eye, Right 6 Eye, Left 7 Eyes, Bilateral	Z None	Z None	Z None

B Imaging
8 Eye
2 Computerized Tomography (CT Scan): Computer reformatted digital display of multiplanar images developed from the capture of multiple exposures of external ionizing radiation

Body Part	Contrast	Qualifier	Qualifier
Character 4	Character 5	Character 6	Character 7
5 Eye, Right 6 Eye, Left 7 Eyes, Bilateral	0 High Osmolar 1 Low Osmolar Y Other Contrast	0 Unenhanced and Enhanced Z None	Z None
5 Eye, Right 6 Eye, Left 7 Eyes, Bilateral	Z None	Z None	Z None

B Imaging
8 Eye
3 Magnetic Resonance Imaging (MRI): Computer reformatted digital display of multiplanar images developed from the capture of radiofrequency signals emitted by nuclei in a body site excited within a magnetic field

Body Part	Contrast	Qualifier	Qualifier
Character 4	Character 5	Character 6	Character 7
5 Eye, Right 6 Eye, Left 7 Eyes, Bilateral	Y Other Contrast	0 Unenhanced and Enhanced Z None	Z None
5 Eye, Right 6 Eye, Left 7 Eyes, Bilateral	Z None	Z None	Z None

B Imaging
8 Eye
4 Ultrasonography: Real time display of images of anatomy or flow information developed from the capture of reflected and attenuated high frequency sound waves

Body Part	Contrast	Qualifier	Qualifier
Character 4	Character 5	Character 6	Character 7
5 Eye, Right 6 Eye, Left 7 Eyes, Bilateral	Z None	Z None	Z None

B Imaging
9 Ear, Nose, Mouth and Throat
0 Plain Radiography: Planar display of an image developed from the capture of external ionizing radiation on photographic or photoconductive plate

Body Part	Contrast	Qualifier	Qualifier
Character 4	Character 5	Character 6	Character 7
2 Paranasal Sinuses F Nasopharynx/Oropharynx H Mastoids	Z None	Z None	Z None
4 Parotid Gland, Right 5 Parotid Gland, Left 6 Parotid Glands, Bilateral 7 Submandibular Gland, Right 8 Submandibular Gland, Left 9 Submandibular Glands, Bilateral B Salivary Gland, Right C Salivary Gland, Left D Salivary Glands, Bilateral	0 High Osmolar 1 Low Osmolar Y Other Contrast	Z None	Z None

B Imaging
9 Ear, Nose, Mouth and Throat
1 Fluoroscopy: Single plane or bi-plane real time display of an image developed from the capture of external ionizing radiation on a fluorescent screen. The image may also be stored by either digital or analog means

Body Part	Contrast	Qualifier	Qualifier
Character 4	Character 5	Character 6	Character 7
G Pharynx and Epiglottis J Larynx	Y Other Contrast Z None	Z None	Z None

B Imaging
9 Ear, Nose, Mouth and Throat
2 Computerized Tomography (CT Scan): Computer reformatted digital display of multiplanar images developed from the capture of multiple exposures of external ionizing radiation

Body Part	Contrast	Qualifier	Qualifier
Character 4	Character 5	Character 6	Character 7
0 Ear 2 Paranasal Sinuses 6 Parotid Glands, Bilateral 9 Submandibular Glands, Bilateral D Salivary Glands, Bilateral F Nasopharynx/Oropharynx J Larynx	0 High Osmolar 1 Low Osmolar Y Other Contrast	0 Unenhanced and Enhanced Z None	Z None
0 Ear 2 Paranasal Sinuses 6 Parotid Glands, Bilateral 9 Submandibular Glands, Bilateral D Salivary Glands, Bilateral F Nasopharynx/Oropharynx J Larynx	Z None	Z None	Z None

B Imaging
9 Ear, Nose, Mouth and Throat
3 Magnetic Resonance Imaging (MRI): Computer reformatted digital display of multiplanar images developed from the capture of radiofrequency signals emitted by nuclei in a body site excited within a magnetic field

Body Part	Contrast	Qualifier	Qualifier
Character 4	Character 5	Character 6	Character 7
0 Ear **2** Paranasal Sinuses **6** Parotid Glands, Bilateral **9** Submandibular Glands, Bilateral **D** Salivary Glands, Bilateral **F** Nasopharynx/Oropharynx **J** Larynx	**Y** Other Contrast	**0** Unenhanced and Enhanced **Z** None	**Z** None
0 Ear **2** Paranasal Sinuses **6** Parotid Glands, Bilateral **9** Submandibular Glands, Bilateral **D** Salivary Glands, Bilateral **F** Nasopharynx/Oropharynx **J** Larynx	**Z** None	**Z** None	**Z** None

B Imaging
B Respiratory System
0 Plain Radiography: Planar display of an image developed from the capture of external ionizing radiation on photographic or photoconductive plate

Body Part	Contrast	Qualifier	Qualifier
Character 4	Character 5	Character 6	Character 7
7 Tracheobronchial Tree, Right **8** Tracheobronchial Tree, Left **9** Tracheobronchial Trees, Bilateral	**Y** Other Contrast	**Z** None	**Z** None
D Upper Airways	**Z** None	**Z** None	**Z** None

B Imaging
B Respiratory System
1 Fluoroscopy: Single plane or bi-plane real time display of an image developed from the capture of external ionizing radiation on a fluorescent screen. The image may also be stored by either digital or analog means

Body Part	Contrast	Qualifier	Qualifier
Character 4	Character 5	Character 6	Character 7
2 Lung, Right **3** Lung, Left **4** Lungs, Bilateral **6** Diaphragm **C** Mediastinum **D** Upper Airways	**Z** None	**Z** None	**Z** None
7 Tracheobronchial Tree, Right **8** Tracheobronchial Tree, Left **9** Tracheobronchial Trees, Bilateral	**Y** Other Contrast	**Z** None	**Z** None

BB2-BD1

B Imaging
B Respiratory System
2 Computerized Tomography (CT Scan): Computer reformatted digital display of multiplanar images developed from the capture of multiple exposures of external ionizing radiation

Body Part	Contrast	Qualifier	Qualifier
Character 4	Character 5	Character 6	Character 7
4 Lungs, Bilateral 7 Tracheobronchial Tree, Right 8 Tracheobronchial Tree, Left 9 Tracheobronchial Trees, Bilateral F Trachea/Airways	0 High Osmolar 1 Low Osmolar Y Other Contrast	0 Unenhanced and Enhanced Z None	Z None
4 Lungs, Bilateral 7 Tracheobronchial Tree, Right 8 Tracheobronchial Tree, Left 9 Tracheobronchial Trees, Bilateral F Trachea/Airways	Z None	Z None	Z None

B Imaging
B Respiratory System
3 Magnetic Resonance Imaging (MRI): Computer reformatted digital display of multiplanar images developed from the capture of radiofrequency signals emitted by nuclei in a body site excited within a magnetic field

Body Part	Contrast	Qualifier	Qualifier
Character 4	Character 5	Character 6	Character 7
G Lung Apices	Y Other Contrast	0 Unenhanced and Enhanced Z None	Z None
G Lung Apices	Z None	Z None	Z None

B Imaging
B Respiratory System
4 Ultrasonography: Real time display of images of anatomy or flow information developed from the capture of reflected and attenuated high frequency sound waves

Body Part	Contrast	Qualifier	Qualifier
Character 4	Character 5	Character 6	Character 7
B Pleura C Mediastinum	Z None	Z None	Z None

B Imaging
D Gastrointestinal System
1 Fluoroscopy: Single plane or bi-plane real time display of an image developed from the capture of external ionizing radiation on a fluorescent screen. The image may also be stored by either digital or analog means

Body Part	Contrast	Qualifier	Qualifier
Character 4	Character 5	Character 6	Character 7
1 Esophagus 2 Stomach 3 Small Bowel 4 Colon 5 Upper GI 6 Upper GI and Small Bowel 9 Duodenum B Mouth/Oropharynx	Y Other Contrast Z None	Z None	Z None

B **Imaging**
D **Gastrointestinal System**
2 **Computerized Tomography (CT Scan):** Computer reformatted digital display of multiplanar images developed from the capture of multiple exposures of external ionizing radiation

Body Part	Contrast	Qualifier	Qualifier
Character 4	Character 5	Character 6	Character 7
4 Colon	**0** High Osmolar **1** Low Osmolar **Y** Other Contrast	**0** Unenhanced and Enhanced **Z** None	**Z** None
4 Colon	**Z** None	**Z** None	**Z** None

B **Imaging**
D **Gastrointestinal System**
4 **Ultrasonography:** Real time display of images of anatomy or flow information developed from the capture of reflected and attenuated high frequency sound waves

Body Part	Contrast	Qualifier	Qualifier
Character 4	Character 5	Character 6	Character 7
1 Esophagus **2** Stomach **7** Gastrointestinal Tract **8** Appendix **9** Duodenum **C** Rectum	**Z** None	**Z** None	**Z** None

B **Imaging**
F **Hepatobiliary System and Pancreas**
0 **Plain Radiography:** Planar display of an image developed from the capture of external ionizing radiation on photographic or photoconductive plate

Body Part	Contrast	Qualifier	Qualifier
Character 4	Character 5	Character 6	Character 7
0 Bile Ducts **3** Gallbladder and Bile Ducts **C** Hepatobiliary System, All	**0** High Osmolar **1** Low Osmolar **Y** Other Contrast	**Z** None	**Z** None

B **Imaging**
F **Hepatobiliary System and Pancreas**
1 **Fluoroscopy:** Single plane or bi-plane real time display of an image developed from the capture of external ionizing radiation on a fluorescent screen. The image may also be stored by either digital or analog means

Body Part	Contrast	Qualifier	Qualifier
Character 4	Character 5	Character 6	Character 7
0 Bile Ducts **1** Biliary and Pancreatic Ducts **2** Gallbladder **3** Gallbladder and Bile Ducts **4** Gallbladder, Bile Ducts and Pancreatic Ducts **8** Pancreatic Ducts	**0** High Osmolar **1** Low Osmolar **Y** Other Contrast	**Z** None	**Z** None

LC Limited Coverage   **NC** Noncovered   **HAC** HAC-associated Procedure   **CC** Combination Cluster - See Appendix G for code lists
DRG Non-OR-Affecting MS-DRG Assignment   New/Revised Text in **Orange**   ♂ Male   ♀ Female

2018 ICD-10-PCS   **643**

IMAGING B00-BY4

B Imaging
F Hepatobiliary System and Pancreas
2 **Computerized Tomography (CT Scan):** Computer reformatted digital display of multiplanar images developed from the capture of multiple exposures of external ionizing radiation

Body Part	Contrast	Qualifier	Qualifier
Character 4	Character 5	Character 6	Character 7
5 Liver 6 Liver and Spleen 7 Pancreas C Hepatobiliary System, All	0 High Osmolar 1 Low Osmolar Y Other Contrast	0 Unenhanced and Enhanced Z None	Z None
5 Liver 6 Liver and Spleen 7 Pancreas C Hepatobiliary System, All	Z None	Z None	Z None

B Imaging
F Hepatobiliary System and Pancreas
3 **Magnetic Resonance Imaging (MRI):** Computer reformatted digital display of multiplanar images developed from the capture of radiofrequency signals emitted by nuclei in a body site excited within a magnetic field

Body Part	Contrast	Qualifier	Qualifier
Character 4	Character 5	Character 6	Character 7
5 Liver 6 Liver and Spleen 7 Pancreas	Y Other Contrast	0 Unenhanced and Enhanced Z None	Z None
5 Liver 6 Liver and Spleen 7 Pancreas	Z None	Z None	Z None

B Imaging
F Hepatobiliary System and Pancreas
4 **Ultrasonography:** Real time display of images of anatomy or flow information developed from the capture of reflected and attenuated high frequency sound waves

Body Part	Contrast	Qualifier	Qualifier
Character 4	Character 5	Character 6	Character 7
0 Bile Ducts 2 Gallbladder 3 Gallbladder and Bile Ducts 5 Liver 6 Liver and Spleen 7 Pancreas C Hepatobiliary System, All	Z None	Z None	Z None

B Imaging
G Endocrine System
2 **Computerized Tomography (CT Scan):** Computer reformatted digital display of multiplanar images developed from the capture of multiple exposures of external ionizing radiation

Body Part	Contrast	Qualifier	Qualifier
Character 4	Character 5	Character 6	Character 7
2 Adrenal Glands, Bilateral 3 Parathyroid Glands 4 Thyroid Gland	0 High Osmolar 1 Low Osmolar Y Other Contrast	0 Unenhanced and Enhanced Z None	Z None
2 Adrenal Glands, Bilateral 3 Parathyroid Glands 4 Thyroid Gland	Z None	Z None	Z None

LC Limited Coverage   NC Noncovered   HAC HAC-associated Procedure   CC Combination Cluster - See Appendix G for code lists
DRG Non-OR-Affecting MS-DRG Assignment   New/Revised Text in **Orange**   ♂ Male   ♀ Female

644

2018 ICD-10-PCS

B Imaging
G Endocrine System
3 Magnetic Resonance Imaging (MRI): Computer reformatted digital display of multiplanar images developed from the capture of radiofrequency signals emitted by nuclei in a body site excited within a magnetic field

Body Part	Contrast	Qualifier	Qualifier
Character 4	Character 5	Character 6	Character 7
2 Adrenal Glands, Bilateral **3** Parathyroid Glands **4** Thyroid Gland	**Y** Other Contrast	**0** Unenhanced and Enhanced **Z** None	**Z** None
2 Adrenal Glands, Bilateral **3** Parathyroid Glands **4** Thyroid Gland	**Z** None	**Z** None	**Z** None

B Imaging
G Endocrine System
4 Ultrasonography: Real time display of images of anatomy or flow information developed from the capture of reflected and attenuated high frequency sound waves

Body Part	Contrast	Qualifier	Qualifier
Character 4	Character 5	Character 6	Character 7
0 Adrenal Gland, Right **1** Adrenal Gland, Left **2** Adrenal Glands, Bilateral **3** Parathyroid Glands **4** Thyroid Gland	**Z** None	**Z** None	**Z** None

B Imaging
H Skin, Subcutaneous Tissue and Breast
0 Plain Radiography: Planar display of an image developed from the capture of external ionizing radiation on photographic or photoconductive plate

Body Part	Contrast	Qualifier	Qualifier
Character 4	Character 5	Character 6	Character 7
0 Breast, Right **1** Breast, Left **2** Breasts, Bilateral	**Z** None	**Z** None	**Z** None
3 Single Mammary Duct, Right **4** Single Mammary Duct, Left **5** Multiple Mammary Ducts, Right **6** Multiple Mammary Ducts, Left	**0** High Osmolar **1** Low Osmolar **Y** Other Contrast **Z** None	**Z** None	**Z** None

LC Limited Coverage   **NC** Noncovered   **HAC** HAC-associated Procedure   **CC** Combination Cluster - See Appendix G for code lists
DRG Non-OR-Affecting MS-DRG Assignment   New/Revised Text in **Orange**   ♂ Male   ♀ Female

2018 ICD-10-PCS

645

B Imaging
H Skin, Subcutaneous Tissue and Breast
3 **Magnetic Resonance Imaging (MRI):** Computer reformatted digital display of multiplanar images developed from the capture of radiofrequency signals emitted by nuclei in a body site excited within a magnetic field

Body Part	Contrast	Qualifier	Qualifier
Character 4	**Character 5**	**Character 6**	**Character 7**
0 Breast, Right **1** Breast, Left **2** Breasts, Bilateral **D** Subcutaneous Tissue, Head/ Neck **F** Subcutaneous Tissue, Upper Extremity **G** Subcutaneous Tissue, Thorax **H** Subcutaneous Tissue, Abdomen and Pelvis **J** Subcutaneous Tissue, Lower Extremity	**Y** Other Contrast	**0** Unenhanced and Enhanced **Z** None	**Z** None
0 Breast, Right **1** Breast, Left **2** Breasts, Bilateral **D** Subcutaneous Tissue, Head/ Neck **F** Subcutaneous Tissue, Upper Extremity **G** Subcutaneous Tissue, Thorax **H** Subcutaneous Tissue, Abdomen and Pelvis **J** Subcutaneous Tissue, Lower Extremity	**Z** None	**Z** None	**Z** None

B Imaging
H Skin, Subcutaneous Tissue and Breast
4 **Ultrasonography:** Real time display of images of anatomy or flow information developed from the capture of reflected and attenuated high frequency sound waves

Body Part	Contrast	Qualifier	Qualifier
Character 4	**Character 5**	**Character 6**	**Character 7**
0 Breast, Right **1** Breast, Left **2** Breasts, Bilateral **7** Extremity, Upper **8** Extremity, Lower **9** Abdominal Wall **B** Chest Wall **C** Head and Neck	**Z** None	**Z** None	**Z** None

B Imaging
L Connective Tissue
3 Magnetic Resonance Imaging (MRI): Computer reformatted digital display of multiplanar images developed from the capture of radiofrequency signals emitted by nuclei in a body site excited within a magnetic field

Body Part	Contrast	Qualifier	Qualifier
Character 4	Character 5	Character 6	Character 7
0 Connective Tissue, Upper Extremity 1 Connective Tissue, Lower Extremity 2 Tendons, Upper Extremity 3 Tendons, Lower Extremity	Y Other Contrast	0 Unenhanced and Enhanced Z None	Z None
0 Connective Tissue, Upper Extremity 1 Connective Tissue, Lower Extremity 2 Tendons, Upper Extremity 3 Tendons, Lower Extremity	Z None	Z None	Z None

B Imaging
L Connective Tissue
4 Ultrasonography: Real time display of images of anatomy or flow information developed from the capture of reflected and attenuated high frequency sound waves

Body Part	Contrast	Qualifier	Qualifier
Character 4	Character 5	Character 6	Character 7
0 Connective Tissue, Upper Extremity 1 Connective Tissue, Lower Extremity 2 Tendons, Upper Extremity 3 Tendons, Lower Extremity	Z None	Z None	Z None

B Imaging
N Skull and Facial Bones
0 Plain Radiography: Planar display of an image developed from the capture of external ionizing radiation on photographic or photoconductive plate

Body Part	Contrast	Qualifier	Qualifier
Character 4	Character 5	Character 6	Character 7
0 Skull 1 Orbit, Right 2 Orbit, Left 3 Orbits, Bilateral 4 Nasal Bones 5 Facial Bones 6 Mandible B Zygomatic Arch, Right C Zygomatic Arch, Left D Zygomatic Arches, Bilateral G Tooth, Single H Teeth, Multiple J Teeth, All	Z None	Z None	Z None
7 Temporomandibular Joint, Right 8 Temporomandibular Joint, Left 9 Temporomandibular Joints, Bilateral	0 High Osmolar 1 Low Osmolar Y Other Contrast Z None	Z None	Z None

LC Limited Coverage   NC Noncovered   HAC HAC-associated Procedure   CC Combination Cluster - See Appendix G for code lists
Non-OR-Affecting MS-DRG Assignment   New/Revised Text in Orange   ♂ Male   ♀ Female

2018 ICD-10-PCS

647

B Imaging
N Skull and Facial Bones
1 Fluoroscopy: Single plane or bi-plane real time display of an image developed from the capture of external ionizing radiation on a fluorescent screen. The image may also be stored by either digital or analog means

Body Part	Contrast	Qualifier	Qualifier
Character 4	Character 5	Character 6	Character 7
7 Temporomandibular Joint, Right 8 Temporomandibular Joint, Left 9 Temporomandibular Joints, Bilateral	0 High Osmolar 1 Low Osmolar Y Other Contrast Z None	Z None	Z None

B Imaging
N Skull and Facial Bones
2 Computerized Tomography (CT Scan): Computer reformatted digital display of multiplanar images developed from the capture of multiple exposures of external ionizing radiation

Body Part	Contrast	Qualifier	Qualifier
Character 4	Character 5	Character 6	Character 7
0 Skull 3 Orbits, Bilateral 5 Facial Bones 6 Mandible 9 Temporomandibular Joints, Bilateral F Temporal Bones	0 High Osmolar 1 Low Osmolar Y Other Contrast Z None	Z None	Z None

B Imaging
N Skull and Facial Bones
3 Magnetic Resonance Imaging (MRI): Computer reformatted digital display of multiplanar images developed from the capture of radiofrequency signals emitted by nuclei in a body site excited within a magnetic field

Body Part	Contrast	Qualifier	Qualifier
Character 4	Character 5	Character 6	Character 7
9 Temporomandibular Joints, Bilateral	Y Other Contrast Z None	Z None	Z None

B Imaging
P Non-Axial Upper Bones
0 Plain Radiography: Planar display of an image developed from the capture of external ionizing radiation on photographic or photoconductive plate

Body Part	Contrast	Qualifier	Qualifier
Character 4	Character 5	Character 6	Character 7

0 Sternoclavicular Joint, Right
1 Sternoclavicular Joint, Left
2 Sternoclavicular Joints,
    Bilateral
3 Acromioclavicular Joints,
    Bilateral
4 Clavicle, Right
5 Clavicle, Left
6 Scapula, Right
7 Scapula, Left
A Humerus, Right
B Humerus, Left
E Upper Arm, Right
F Upper Arm, Left
J Forearm, Right
K Forearm, Left
N Hand, Right
P Hand, Left
R Finger(s), Right
S Finger(s), Left
X Ribs, Right
Y Ribs, Left
	Z None	Z None	Z None

BP0 continued on next page

B   Imaging
P   Non-Axial Upper Bones
0   Plain Radiography: Planar display of an image developed from the capture of external ionizing radiation on photographic or photoconductive plate

BP0 continued from previous page

Body Part	Contrast	Qualifier	Qualifier
Character 4	Character 5	Character 6	Character 7
8 Shoulder, Right 9 Shoulder, Left C Hand/Finger Joint, Right D Hand/Finger Joint, Left G Elbow, Right H Elbow, Left L Wrist, Right M Wrist, Left	0 High Osmolar 1 Low Osmolar Y Other Contrast Z None	Z None	Z None

B   Imaging
P   Non-Axial Upper Bones
1   Fluoroscopy: Single plane or bi-plane real time display of an image developed from the capture of external ionizing radiation on a fluorescent screen. The image may also be stored by either digital or analog means

Body Part	Contrast	Qualifier	Qualifier
Character 4	Character 5	Character 6	Character 7
0 Sternoclavicular Joint, Right 1 Sternoclavicular Joint, Left 2 Sternoclavicular Joints, Bilateral 3 Acromioclavicular Joints, Bilateral 4 Clavicle, Right 5 Clavicle, Left 6 Scapula, Right 7 Scapula, Left A Humerus, Right B Humerus, Left E Upper Arm, Right F Upper Arm, Left J Forearm, Right K Forearm, Left N Hand, Right P Hand, Left R Finger(s), Right S Finger(s), Left X Ribs, Right Y Ribs, Left	Z None	Z None	Z None
8 Shoulder, Right 9 Shoulder, Left L Wrist, Right M Wrist, Left	0 High Osmolar 1 Low Osmolar Y Other Contrast Z None	Z None	Z None
C Hand/Finger Joint, Right D Hand/Finger Joint, Left G Elbow, Right H Elbow, Left	0 High Osmolar 1 Low Osmolar Y Other Contrast	Z None	Z None

B Imaging
P Non-Axial Upper Bones
2 Computerized Tomography (CT Scan): Computer reformatted digital display of multiplanar images developed from the capture of multiple exposures of external ionizing radiation

Body Part	Contrast	Qualifier	Qualifier
Character 4	Character 5	Character 6	Character 7
0 Sternoclavicular Joint, Right 1 Sternoclavicular Joint, Left W Thorax	0 High Osmolar 1 Low Osmolar Y Other Contrast	Z None	Z None
2 Sternoclavicular Joints, Bilateral 3 Acromioclavicular Joints, Bilateral 4 Clavicle, Right 5 Clavicle, Left 6 Scapula, Right 7 Scapula, Left 8 Shoulder, Right 9 Shoulder, Left A Humerus, Right B Humerus, Left E Upper Arm, Right F Upper Arm, Left G Elbow, Right H Elbow, Left J Forearm, Right K Forearm, Left L Wrist, Right M Wrist, Left N Hand, Right P Hand, Left Q Hands and Wrists, Bilateral R Finger(s), Right S Finger(s), Left T Upper Extremity, Right U Upper Extremity, Left V Upper Extremities, Bilateral X Ribs, Right Y Ribs, Left	0 High Osmolar 1 Low Osmolar Y Other Contrast Z None	Z None	Z None
C Hand/Finger Joint, Right D Hand/Finger Joint, Left	Z None	Z None	Z None

B Imaging
P Non-Axial Upper Bones
3 Magnetic Resonance Imaging (MRI): Computer reformatted digital display of multiplanar images developed from the capture of radiofrequency signals emitted by nuclei in a body site excited within a magnetic field

Body Part	Contrast	Qualifier	Qualifier
Character 4	Character 5	Character 6	Character 7
8 Shoulder, Right 9 Shoulder, Left C Hand/Finger Joint, Right D Hand/Finger Joint, Left E Upper Arm, Right F Upper Arm, Left G Elbow, Right H Elbow, Left J Forearm, Right K Forearm, Left L Wrist, Right M Wrist, Left	Y Other Contrast	0 Unenhanced and Enhanced Z None	Z None

BP3 continued on next page

B Imaging
P Non-Axial Upper Bones

BP3 continued from previous page

3 Magnetic Resonance Imaging (MRI): Computer reformatted digital display of multiplanar images developed from the capture of radiofrequency signals emitted by nuclei in a body site excited within a magnetic field

Body Part	Contrast	Qualifier	Qualifier
Character 4	Character 5	Character 6	Character 7
8 Shoulder, Right 9 Shoulder, Left C Hand/Finger Joint, Right D Hand/Finger Joint, Left E Upper Arm, Right F Upper Arm, Left G Elbow, Right H Elbow, Left J Forearm, Right K Forearm, Left L Wrist, Right M Wrist, Left	Z None	Z None	Z None

B Imaging
P Non-Axial Upper Bones
4 Ultrasonography: Real time display of images of anatomy or flow information developed from the capture of reflected and attenuated high frequency sound waves

Body Part	Contrast	Qualifier	Qualifier
Character 4	Character 5	Character 6	Character 7
8 Shoulder, Right 9 Shoulder, Left G Elbow, Right H Elbow, Left L Wrist, Right M Wrist, Left N Hand, Right P Hand, Left	Z None	Z None	1 Densitometry Z None

B Imaging
Q Non-Axial Lower Bones
0 Plain Radiography: Planar display of an image developed from the capture of external ionizing radiation on photographic or photoconductive plate

Body Part	Contrast	Qualifier	Qualifier
Character 4	Character 5	Character 6	Character 7
0 Hip, Right 1 Hip, Left	0 High Osmolar 1 Low Osmolar Y Other Contrast	Z None	Z None
0 Hip, Right 1 Hip, Left	Z None	Z None	1 Densitometry Z None
3 Femur, Right 4 Femur, Left	Z None	Z None	1 Densitometry Z None
7 Knee, Right 8 Knee, Left G Ankle, Right H Ankle, Left	0 High Osmolar 1 Low Osmolar Y Other Contrast Z None	Z None	Z None
D Lower Leg, Right F Lower Leg, Left J Calcaneus, Right K Calcaneus, Left L Foot, Right M Foot, Left P Toe(s), Right Q Toe(s), Left V Patella, Right W Patella, Left	Z None	Z None	Z None
X Foot/Toe Joint, Right Y Foot/Toe Joint, Left	0 High Osmolar 1 Low Osmolar Y Other Contrast	Z None	Z None

LC Limited Coverage   NC Noncovered   HAC HAC-associated Procedure   CC Combination Cluster - See Appendix G for code lists
DRG Non-OR-Affecting MS-DRG Assignment   New/Revised Text in Orange   ♂ Male   ♀ Female

2018 ICD-10-PCS

651

B **Imaging**
Q **Non-Axial Lower Bones**
1 **Fluoroscopy:** Single plane or bi-plane real time display of an image developed from the capture of external ionizing radiation on a fluorescent screen. The image may also be stored by either digital or analog means

Body Part	Contrast	Qualifier	Qualifier
Character 4	Character 5	Character 6	Character 7
0 Hip, Right 1 Hip, Left 7 Knee, Right 8 Knee, Left G Ankle, Right H Ankle, Left X Foot/Toe Joint, Right Y Foot/Toe Joint, Left	0 High Osmolar 1 Low Osmolar Y Other Contrast Z None	Z None	Z None
3 Femur, Right 4 Femur, Left D Lower Leg, Right F Lower Leg, Left J Calcaneus, Right K Calcaneus, Left L Foot, Right M Foot, Left P Toe(s), Right Q Toe(s), Left V Patella, Right W Patella, Left	Z None	Z None	Z None

B **Imaging**
Q **Non-Axial Lower Bones**
2 **Computerized Tomography (CT Scan):** Computer reformatted digital display of multiplanar images developed from the capture of multiple exposures of external ionizing radiation

Body Part	Contrast	Qualifier	Qualifier
Character 4	Character 5	Character 6	Character 7
0 Hip, Right 1 Hip, Left 3 Femur, Right 4 Femur, Left 7 Knee, Right 8 Knee, Left D Lower Leg, Right F Lower Leg, Left G Ankle, Right H Ankle, Left J Calcaneus, Right K Calcaneus, Left L Foot, Right M Foot, Left P Toe(s), Right Q Toe(s), Left R Lower Extremity, Right S Lower Extremity, Left V Patella, Right W Patella, Left X Foot/Toe Joint, Right Y Foot/Toe Joint, Left	0 High Osmolar 1 Low Osmolar Y Other Contrast Z None	Z None	Z None
B Tibia/Fibula, Right C Tibia/Fibula, Left	0 High Osmolar 1 Low Osmolar Y Other Contrast	Z None	Z None

LC Limited Coverage   NC Noncovered   HAC HAC-associated Procedure   CC Combination Cluster - See Appendix G for code lists
DRG Non-OR-Affecting MS-DRG Assignment   New/Revised Text in Orange   ♂ Male   ♀ Female

652   2018 ICD-10-PCS

B Imaging
Q Non-Axial Lower Bones
3 Magnetic Resonance Imaging (MRI): Computer reformatted digital display of multiplanar images developed from the capture of radiofrequency signals emitted by nuclei in a body site excited within a magnetic field

Body Part	Contrast	Qualifier	Qualifier
Character 4	Character 5	Character 6	Character 7
0 Hip, Right 1 Hip, Left 3 Femur, Right 4 Femur, Left 7 Knee, Right 8 Knee, Left D Lower Leg, Right F Lower Leg, Left G Ankle, Right H Ankle, Left J Calcaneus, Right K Calcaneus, Left L Foot, Right M Foot, Left P Toe(s), Right Q Toe(s), Left V Patella, Right W Patella, Left	Y Other Contrast	0 Unenhanced and Enhanced Z None	Z None
0 Hip, Right 1 Hip, Left 3 Femur, Right 4 Femur, Left 7 Knee, Right 8 Knee, Left D Lower Leg, Right F Lower Leg, Left G Ankle, Right H Ankle, Left J Calcaneus, Right K Calcaneus, Left L Foot, Right M Foot, Left P Toe(s), Right Q Toe(s), Left V Patella, Right W Patella, Left	Z None	Z None	Z None

B Imaging
Q Non-Axial Lower Bones
4 Ultrasonography: Real time display of images of anatomy or flow information developed from the capture of reflected and attenuated high frequency sound waves

Body Part	Contrast	Qualifier	Qualifier
Character 4	Character 5	Character 6	Character 7
0 Hip, Right 1 Hip, Left 2 Hips, Bilateral 7 Knee, Right 8 Knee, Left 9 Knees, Bilateral	Z None	Z None	Z None

B Imaging

R Axial Skeleton, Except Skull and Facial Bones

0 Plain Radiography: Planar display of an image developed from the capture of external ionizing radiation on photographic or photoconductive plate

Body Part	Contrast	Qualifier	Qualifier
Character 4	Character 5	Character 6	Character 7
0 Cervical Spine 7 Thoracic Spine 9 Lumbar Spine G Whole Spine	Z None	Z None	1 Densitometry Z None
1 Cervical Disc(s) 2 Thoracic Disc(s) 3 Lumbar Disc(s) 4 Cervical Facet Joint(s) 5 Thoracic Facet Joint(s) 6 Lumbar Facet Joint(s) D Sacroiliac Joints	0 High Osmolar 1 Low Osmolar Y Other Contrast Z None	Z None	Z None
8 Thoracolumbar Joint B Lumbosacral Joint C Pelvis F Sacrum and Coccyx H Sternum	Z None	Z None	Z None

B Imaging

R Axial Skeleton, Except Skull and Facial Bones

1 Fluoroscopy: Single plane or bi-plane real time display of an image developed from the capture of external ionizing radiation on a fluorescent screen. The image may also be stored by either digital or analog means

Body Part	Contrast	Qualifier	Qualifier
Character 4	Character 5	Character 6	Character 7
0 Cervical Spine 1 Cervical Disc(s) 2 Thoracic Disc(s) 3 Lumbar Disc(s) 4 Cervical Facet Joint(s) 5 Thoracic Facet Joint(s) 6 Lumbar Facet Joint(s) 7 Thoracic Spine 8 Thoracolumbar Joint 9 Lumbar Spine B Lumbosacral Joint C Pelvis D Sacroiliac Joints F Sacrum and Coccyx G Whole Spine H Sternum	0 High Osmolar 1 Low Osmolar Y Other Contrast Z None	Z None	Z None

B Imaging

R Axial Skeleton, Except Skull and Facial Bones

2 Computerized Tomography (CT Scan): Computer reformatted digital display of multiplanar images developed from the capture of multiple exposures of external ionizing radiation

Body Part	Contrast	Qualifier	Qualifier
Character 4	Character 5	Character 6	Character 7
0 Cervical Spine 7 Thoracic Spine 9 Lumbar Spine C Pelvis D Sacroiliac Joints F Sacrum and Coccyx	0 High Osmolar 1 Low Osmolar Y Other Contrast Z None	Z None	Z None

LC Limited Coverage   **NC** Noncovered   **HAC** HAC-associated Procedure   **CC** Combination Cluster - See Appendix G for code lists
DNH Non-OR-Affecting MS-DRG Assignment   New/Revised Text in Orange   ♂ Male   ♀ Female

654   2018 ICD-10-PCS

B Imaging
R Axial Skeleton, Except Skull and Facial Bones
3 Magnetic Resonance Imaging (MRI): Computer reformatted digital display of multiplanar images developed from the capture of radiofrequency signals emitted by nuclei in a body site excited within a magnetic field

Body Part	Contrast	Qualifier	Qualifier
Character 4	Character 5	Character 6	Character 7
0 Cervical Spine 1 Cervical Disc(s) 2 Thoracic Disc(s) 3 Lumbar Disc(s) 7 Thoracic Spine 9 Lumbar Spine C Pelvis F Sacrum and Coccyx	Y Other Contrast	0 Unenhanced and Enhanced Z None	Z None
0 Cervical Spine 1 Cervical Disc(s) 2 Thoracic Disc(s) 3 Lumbar Disc(s) 7 Thoracic Spine 9 Lumbar Spine C Pelvis F Sacrum and Coccyx	Z None	Z None	Z None

B Imaging
R Axial Skeleton, Except Skull and Facial Bones
4 Ultrasonography: Real time display of images of anatomy or flow information developed from the capture of reflected and attenuated high frequency sound waves

Body Part	Contrast	Qualifier	Qualifier
Character 4	Character 5	Character 6	Character 7
0 Cervical Spine 7 Thoracic Spine 9 Lumbar Spine F Sacrum and Coccyx	Z None	Z None	Z None

B Imaging
T Urinary System
0 Plain Radiography: Planar display of an image developed from the capture of external ionizing radiation on photographic or photoconductive plate

Body Part	Contrast	Qualifier	Qualifier
Character 4	Character 5	Character 6	Character 7
0 Bladder 1 Kidney, Right 2 Kidney, Left 3 Kidneys, Bilateral 4 Kidneys, Ureters and Bladder 5 Urethra 6 Ureter, Right 7 Ureter, Left 8 Ureters, Bilateral B Bladder and Urethra C Ileal Diversion Loop	0 High Osmolar 1 Low Osmolar Y Other Contrast Z None	Z None	Z None

LC Limited Coverage   **NC** Noncovered   **HAC** HAC-associated Procedure   **CC** Combination Cluster - See Appendix G for code lists
DRG Non-OR-Affecting MS-DRG Assignment   New/Revised Text in **Orange**   ♂ Male   ♀ Female

2018 ICD-10-PCS

655

IMAGING B00-BY4

B Imaging
T Urinary System
1 Fluoroscopy: Single plane or bi-plane real time display of an image developed from the capture of external ionizing radiation on a fluorescent screen. The image may also be stored by either digital or analog means

Body Part	Contrast	Qualifier	Qualifier
Character 4	Character 5	Character 6	Character 7
0 Bladder 1 Kidney, Right 2 Kidney, Left 3 Kidneys, Bilateral 4 Kidneys, Ureters and Bladder 5 Urethra 6 Ureter, Right 7 Ureter, Left B Bladder and Urethra C Ileal Diversion Loop D Kidney, Ureter and Bladder, Right F Kidney, Ureter and Bladder, Left G Ileal Loop, Ureters and Kidneys	0 High Osmolar 1 Low Osmolar Y Other Contrast Z None	Z None	Z None

B Imaging
T Urinary System
2 Computerized Tomography (CT Scan): Computer reformatted digital display of multiplanar images developed from the capture of multiple exposures of external ionizing radiation

Body Part	Contrast	Qualifier	Qualifier
Character 4	Character 5	Character 6	Character 7
0 Bladder 1 Kidney, Right 2 Kidney, Left 3 Kidneys, Bilateral 9 Kidney Transplant	0 High Osmolar 1 Low Osmolar Y Other Contrast	0 Unenhanced and Enhanced Z None	Z None
0 Bladder 1 Kidney, Right 2 Kidney, Left 3 Kidneys, Bilateral 9 Kidney Transplant	Z None	Z None	Z None

B Imaging
T Urinary System
3 Magnetic Resonance Imaging (MRI): Computer reformatted digital display of multiplanar images developed from the capture of radiofrequency signals emitted by nuclei in a body site excited within a magnetic field

Body Part	Contrast	Qualifier	Qualifier
Character 4	Character 5	Character 6	Character 7
0 Bladder 1 Kidney, Right 2 Kidney, Left 3 Kidneys, Bilateral 9 Kidney Transplant	Y Other Contrast	0 Unenhanced and Enhanced Z None	Z None
0 Bladder 1 Kidney, Right 2 Kidney, Left 3 Kidneys, Bilateral 9 Kidney Transplant	Z None	Z None	Z None

LC Limited Coverage   NC Noncovered   HAC HAC-associated Procedure   CC Combination Cluster - See Appendix G for code lists
DRG Non-OR-Affecting MS-DRG Assignment   New/Revised Text in Orange   ♂ Male   ♀ Female

656

2018 ICD-10-PCS

B   Imaging
T   Urinary System
4   Ultrasonography: Real time display of images of anatomy or flow information developed from the capture of reflected and attenuated high frequency sound waves

Body Part	Contrast	Qualifier	Qualifier
Character 4	Character 5	Character 6	Character 7
0 Bladder **1** Kidney, Right **2** Kidney, Left **3** Kidneys, Bilateral **5** Urethra **6** Ureter, Right **7** Ureter, Left **8** Ureters, Bilateral **9** Kidney Transplant **J** Kidneys and Bladder	**Z** None	**Z** None	**Z** None

B   Imaging
U   Female Reproductive System
0   Plain Radiography: Planar display of an image developed from the capture of external ionizing radiation on photographic or photoconductive plate

Body Part	Contrast	Qualifier	Qualifier
Character 4	Character 5	Character 6	Character 7
0 Fallopian Tube, Right ♀ **1** Fallopian Tube, Left ♀ **2** Fallopian Tubes, Bilateral ♀ **6** Uterus ♀ **8** Uterus and Fallopian Tubes ♀ **9** Vagina ♀	**0** High Osmolar **1** Low Osmolar **Y** Other Contrast	**Z** None	**Z** None

♀ BU000ZZ   BU001ZZ   BU00YZZ   BU010ZZ   BU011ZZ   BU01YZZ   BU020ZZ   BU021ZZ   BU02YZZ   BU060ZZ   BU061ZZ   BU06YZZ   BU080ZZ
   BU081ZZ   BU08YZZ   BU090ZZ   BU091ZZ   BU09YZZ

B   Imaging
U   Female Reproductive System
1   Fluoroscopy: Single plane or bi-plane real time display of an image developed from the capture of external ionizing radiation on a fluorescent screen. The image may also be stored by either digital or analog means

Body Part	Contrast	Qualifier	Qualifier
Character 4	Character 5	Character 6	Character 7
0 Fallopian Tube, Right ♀ **1** Fallopian Tube, Left ♀ **2** Fallopian Tubes, Bilateral ♀ **6** Uterus ♀ **8** Uterus and Fallopian Tubes ♀ **9** Vagina ♀	**0** High Osmolar **1** Low Osmolar **Y** Other Contrast **Z** None	**Z** None	**Z** None

♀ BU100ZZ   BU101ZZ   BU10YZZ   BU10ZZZ   BU110ZZ   BU111ZZ   BU11YZZ   BU11ZZZ   BU120ZZ   BU121ZZ   BU12YZZ   BU12ZZZ   BU160ZZ
   BU161ZZ   BU16YZZ   BU16ZZZ   BU180ZZ   BU181ZZ   BU18YZZ   BU18ZZZ   BU190ZZ   BU191ZZ   BU19YZZ   BU19ZZZ

LC Limited Coverage   **NC** Noncovered   **HAC** HAC-associated Procedure   **CC** Combination Cluster - See Appendix G for code lists
DRG Non-OR-Affecting MS-DRG Assignment   New/Revised Text in Orange   ♂ Male   ♀ Female

2018 ICD-10-PCS

657

IMAGING B00-BY4

B Imaging
U Female Reproductive System
3 Magnetic Resonance Imaging (MRI): Computer reformatted digital display of multiplanar images developed from the capture of radiofrequency signals emitted by nuclei in a body site excited within a magnetic field

Body Part	Contrast	Qualifier	Qualifier
Character 4	Character 5	Character 6	Character 7
3 Ovary, Right ♀ 4 Ovary, Left ♀ 5 Ovaries, Bilateral ♀ 6 Uterus ♀ 9 Vagina ♀ B Pregnant Uterus ♀ C Uterus and Ovaries ♀	Y Other Contrast	0 Unenhanced and Enhanced Z None	Z None
3 Ovary, Right ♀ 4 Ovary, Left ♀ 5 Ovaries, Bilateral ♀ 6 Uterus ♀ 9 Vagina ♀ B Pregnant Uterus ♀ C Uterus and Ovaries ♀	Z None	Z None	Z None

♀ BU33Y0Z BU33YZZ BU33ZZZ BU34Y0Z BU34YZZ BU34ZZZ BU35Y0Z BU35YZZ BU35ZZZ BU36Y0Z BU36YZZ BU36ZZZ BU39Y0Z
BU39YZZ BU39ZZZ BU3BY0Z BU3BYZZ BU3BZZZ BU3CY0Z BU3CYZZ BU3CZZZ

B Imaging
U Female Reproductive System
4 Ultrasonography: Real time display of images of anatomy or flow information developed from the capture of reflected and attenuated high frequency sound waves

Body Part	Contrast	Qualifier	Qualifier
Character 4	Character 5	Character 6	Character 7
0 Fallopian Tube, Right ♀ 1 Fallopian Tube, Left ♀ 2 Fallopian Tubes, Bilateral ♀ 3 Ovary, Right ♀ 4 Ovary, Left ♀ 5 Ovaries, Bilateral ♀ 6 Uterus ♀ C Uterus and Ovaries ♀	Y Other Contrast Z None	Z None	Z None

♀ BU40YZZ BU40ZZZ BU41YZZ BU41ZZZ BU42YZZ BU42ZZZ BU43YZZ BU43ZZZ BU44YZZ BU44ZZZ BU45YZZ BU45ZZZ BU46YZZ
BU46ZZZ BU4CYZZ BU4CZZZ

B Imaging
V Male Reproductive System
0 Plain Radiography: Planar display of an image developed from the capture of external ionizing radiation on photographic or photoconductive plate

Body Part	Contrast	Qualifier	Qualifier
Character 4	Character 5	Character 6	Character 7
0 Corpora Cavernosa ♂ 1 Epididymis, Right ♂ 2 Epididymis, Left ♂ 3 Prostate ♂ 5 Testicle, Right ♂ 6 Testicle, Left ♂ 8 Vasa Vasorum ♂	0 High Osmolar 1 Low Osmolar Y Other Contrast	Z None	Z None

♂ BV000ZZ BV001ZZ BV00YZZ BV010ZZ BV011ZZ BV01YZZ BV020ZZ BV021ZZ BV02YZZ BV030ZZ BV031ZZ BV03YZZ BV050ZZ
BV051ZZ BV05YZZ BV060ZZ BV061ZZ BV06YZZ BV080ZZ BV081ZZ BV08YZZ

LC Limited Coverage   NC Noncovered   HAC HAC-associated Procedure   CC Combination Cluster - See Appendix G for code lists
DRG Non-OR-Affecting MS-DRG Assignment   New/Revised Text in Orange   ♂ Male   ♀ Female

658

2018 ICD-10-PCS

IMAGING B00-BY4

B Imaging
V Male Reproductive System
1 **Fluoroscopy:** Single plane or bi-plane real time display of an image developed from the capture of external ionizing radiation on a fluorescent screen. The image may also be stored by either digital or analog means

Body Part	Contrast	Qualifier	Qualifier
Character 4	Character 5	Character 6	Character 7
0 Corpora Cavernosa ♂ **8** Vasa Vasorum ♂	**0** High Osmolar **1** Low Osmolar **Y** Other Contrast **Z** None	**Z** None	**Z** None

♂ BV100ZZ   BV101ZZ   BV10YZZ   BV10ZZZ   BV180ZZ   BV181ZZ   BV18YZZ   BV18ZZZ

B Imaging
V Male Reproductive System
2 **Computerized Tomography (CT Scan):** Computer reformatted digital display of multiplanar images developed from the capture of multiple exposures of external ionizing radiation

Body Part	Contrast	Qualifier	Qualifier
Character 4	Character 5	Character 6	Character 7
3 Prostate ♂	**0** High Osmolar **1** Low Osmolar **Y** Other Contrast	**0** Unenhanced and Enhanced **Z** None	**Z** None
3 Prostate ♂	**Z** None	**Z** None	**Z** None

♂ BV2300Z   BV230ZZ   BV2310Z   BV23Y0Z   BV23YZZ   BV23ZZZ

B Imaging
V Male Reproductive System
3 **Magnetic Resonance Imaging (MRI):** Computer reformatted digital display of multiplanar images developed from the capture of radiofrequency signals emitted by nuclei in a body site excited within a magnetic field

Body Part	Contrast	Qualifier	Qualifier
Character 4	Character 5	Character 6	Character 7
0 Corpora Cavernosa ♂ **3** Prostate ♂ **4** Scrotum ♂ **5** Testicle, Right ♂ **6** Testicle, Left ♂ **7** Testicles, Bilateral ♂	**Y** Other Contrast	**0** Unenhanced and Enhanced **Z** None	**Z** None
0 Corpora Cavernosa ♂ **3** Prostate ♂ **4** Scrotum ♂ **5** Testicle, Right ♂ **6** Testicle, Left ♂ **7** Testicles, Bilateral ♂	**Z** None	**Z** None	**Z** None

♂ BV30Y0Z   BV30YZZ   BV30ZZZ   BV33Y0Z   BV33YZZ   BV33ZZZ   BV34Y0Z   BV34YZZ   BV34ZZZ   BV35Y0Z   BV35YZZ   BV35ZZZ   BV36Y0Z
  BV36YZZ   BV36ZZZ   BV37Y0Z   BV37YZZ   BV37ZZZ

B Imaging
V Male Reproductive System
4 **Ultrasonography:** Real time display of images of anatomy or flow information developed from the capture of reflected and attenuated high frequency sound waves

Body Part	Contrast	Qualifier	Qualifier
Character 4	Character 5	Character 6	Character 7
4 Scrotum ♂ **9** Prostate and Seminal Vesicles ♂ **B** Penis ♂	**Z** None	**Z** None	**Z** None

♂ BV44ZZZ   BV49ZZZ   BV4BZZZ

B Imaging
W Anatomical Regions
0 Plain Radiography: Planar display of an image developed from the capture of external ionizing radiation on photographic or photoconductive plate

Body Part	Contrast	Qualifier	Qualifier
Character 4	Character 5	Character 6	Character 7
0 Abdomen 1 Abdomen and Pelvis 3 Chest B Long Bones, All C Lower Extremity J Upper Extremity K Whole Body L Whole Skeleton M Whole Body, Infant	Z None	Z None	Z None

B Imaging
W Anatomical Regions
1 Fluoroscopy: Single plane or bi-plane real time display of an image developed from the capture of external ionizing radiation on a fluorescent screen. The image may also be stored by either digital or analog means

Body Part	Contrast	Qualifier	Qualifier
Character 4	Character 5	Character 6	Character 7
1 Abdomen and Pelvis 9 Head and Neck C Lower Extremity J Upper Extremity	0 High Osmolar 1 Low Osmolar Y Other Contrast Z None	Z None	Z None

B Imaging
W Anatomical Regions
2 Computerized Tomography (CT Scan): Computer reformatted digital display of multiplanar images developed from the capture of multiple exposures of external ionizing radiation

Body Part	Contrast	Qualifier	Qualifier
Character 4	Character 5	Character 6	Character 7
0 Abdomen 1 Abdomen and Pelvis 4 Chest and Abdomen 5 Chest, Abdomen and Pelvis 8 Head 9 Head and Neck F Neck G Pelvic Region	0 High Osmolar 1 Low Osmolar Y Other Contrast	0 Unenhanced and Enhanced Z None	Z None
0 Abdomen 1 Abdomen and Pelvis 4 Chest and Abdomen 5 Chest, Abdomen and Pelvis 8 Head 9 Head and Neck F Neck G Pelvic Region	Z None	Z None	Z None

LC Limited Coverage   NC Noncovered   HAC HAC-associated Procedure   CC Combination Cluster - See Appendix G for code lists
DRG Non-OR-Affecting MS-DRG Assignment   New/Revised Text in **Orange**   ♂ Male   ♀ Female

660   **2018 ICD-10-PCS**

B Imaging
W Anatomical Regions
3 Magnetic Resonance Imaging (MRI): Computer reformatted digital display of multiplanar images developed from the capture of radiofrequency signals emitted by nuclei in a body site excited within a magnetic field

Body Part	Contrast	Qualifier	Qualifier
Character 4	Character 5	Character 6	Character 7
0 Abdomen **8** Head **F** Neck **G** Pelvic Region **H** Retroperitoneum **P** Brachial Plexus	**Y** Other Contrast	**0** Unenhanced and Enhanced **Z** None	**Z** None
0 Abdomen **8** Head **F** Neck **G** Pelvic Region **H** Retroperitoneum **P** Brachial Plexus	**Z** None	**Z** None	**Z** None
3 Chest	**Y** Other Contrast	**0** Unenhanced and Enhanced **Z** None	**Z** None

B Imaging
W Anatomical Regions
4 Ultrasonography: Real time display of images of anatomy or flow information developed from the capture of reflected and attenuated high frequency sound waves

Body Part	Contrast	Qualifier	Qualifier
Character 4	Character 5	Character 6	Character 7
0 Abdomen **1** Abdomen and Pelvis **F** Neck **G** Pelvic Region	**Z** None	**Z** None	**Z** None

B Imaging
Y Fetus and Obstetrical
3 Magnetic Resonance Imaging (MRI): Computer reformatted digital display of multiplanar images developed from the capture of radiofrequency signals emitted by nuclei in a body site excited within a magnetic field

Body Part	Contrast	Qualifier	Qualifier
Character 4	Character 5	Character 6	Character 7
0 Fetal Head ♀ **1** Fetal Heart ♀ **2** Fetal Thorax ♀ **3** Fetal Abdomen ♀ **4** Fetal Spine ♀ **5** Fetal Extremities ♀ **6** Whole Fetus ♀	**Y** Other Contrast	**0** Unenhanced and Enhanced **Z** None	**Z** None
0 Fetal Head ♀ **1** Fetal Heart ♀ **2** Fetal Thorax ♀ **3** Fetal Abdomen ♀ **4** Fetal Spine ♀ **5** Fetal Extremities ♀ **6** Whole Fetus ♀	**Z** None	**Z** None	**Z** None

♀ BY30Y0Z BY30YZZ BY30ZZZ BY31Y0Z BY31YZZ BY31ZZZ BY32Y0Z BY32YZZ BY32ZZZ BY33Y0Z BY33YZZ BY33ZZZ BY34YZZ
BY34ZZZ BY35Y0Z BY35YZZ BY35ZZZ BY36Y0Z BY36YZZ BY36ZZZ

B Imaging
Y Fetus and Obstetrical
4 Ultrasonography: Real time display of images of anatomy or flow information developed from the capture of reflected and attenuated high frequency sound waves

Body Part	Contrast	Qualifier	Qualifier
Character 4	Character 5	Character 6	Character 7
7 Fetal Umbilical Cord ♀ 8 Placenta ♀ 9 First Trimester, Single Fetus ♀ B First Trimester, Multiple Gestation ♀ C Second Trimester, Single Fetus ♀ D Second Trimester, Multiple Gestation ♀ F Third Trimester, Single Fetus ♀ G Third Trimester, Multiple Gestation ♀	**Z** None	**Z** None	**Z** None

♀ BY47ZZZ   BY48ZZZ   BY49ZZZ   BY4BZZZ   BY4CZZZ   BY4DZZZ   BY4FZZZ   BY4GZZZ

NOTES

NOTES

Nuclear Medicine C01-CW7

C **Nuclear Medicine**
0 **Central Nervous System**
1 **Planar Nuclear Medicine Imaging:** Introduction of radioactive materials into the body for single plane display of images developed from the capture of radioactive emissions

Body Part	Radionuclide	Qualifier	Qualifier
Character 4	Character 5	Character 6	Character 7
0 Brain	**1** Technetium 99m (Tc-99m) **Y** Other Radionuclide	**Z** None	**Z** None
5 Cerebrospinal Fluid	**D** Indium 111 (In-111) **Y** Other Radionuclide	**Z** None	**Z** None
Y Central Nervous System	**Y** Other Radionuclide	**Z** None	**Z** None

C **Nuclear Medicine**
0 **Central Nervous System**
2 **Tomographic (Tomo) Nuclear Medicine Imaging:** Introduction of radioactive materials into the body for three dimensional display of images developed from the capture of radioactive emissions

Body Part	Radionuclide	Qualifier	Qualifier
Character 4	Character 5	Character 6	Character 7
0 Brain	**1** Technetium 99m (Tc-99m) **F** Iodine 123 (I-123) **S** Thallium 201 (Tl-201) **Y** Other Radionuclide	**Z** None	**Z** None
5 Cerebrospinal Fluid	**D** Indium 111 (In-111) **Y** Other Radionuclide	**Z** None	**Z** None
Y Central Nervous System	**Y** Other Radionuclide	**Z** None	**Z** None

C **Nuclear Medicine**
0 **Central Nervous System**
3 **Positron Emission Tomographic (PET) Imaging:** Introduction of radioactive materials into the body for three dimensional display of images developed from the simultaneous capture, 180 degrees apart, of radioactive emissions

Body Part	Radionuclide	Qualifier	Qualifier
Character 4	Character 5	Character 6	Character 7
0 Brain	**B** Carbon 11 (C-11) **K** Fluorine 18 (F-18) **M** Oxygen 15 (O-15) **Y** Other Radionuclide	**Z** None	**Z** None
Y Central Nervous System	**Y** Other Radionuclide	**Z** None	**Z** None

C **Nuclear Medicine**
0 **Central Nervous System**
5 **Nonimaging Nuclear Medicine Probe:** Introduction of radioactive materials into the body for the study of distribution and fate of certain substances by the detection of radioactive emissions; or, alternatively, measurement of absorption of radioactive emissions from an external source

Body Part	Radionuclide	Qualifier	Qualifier
Character 4	Character 5	Character 6	Character 7
0 Brain	**V** Xenon 133 (Xe-133) **Y** Other Radionuclide	**Z** None	**Z** None
Y Central Nervous System	**Y** Other Radionuclide	**Z** None	**Z** None

C Nuclear Medicine
2 Heart
1 Planar Nuclear Medicine Imaging: Introduction of radioactive materials into the body for single plane display of images developed from the capture of radioactive emissions

Body Part	Radionuclide	Qualifier	Qualifier
Character 4	Character 5	Character 6	Character 7
6 Heart, Right and Left	1 Technetium 99m (Tc-99m) Y Other Radionuclide	Z None	Z None
G Myocardium	1 Technetium 99m (Tc-99m) D Indium 111 (In-111) S Thallium 201 (Tl-201) Y Other Radionuclide Z None	Z None	Z None
Y Heart	Y Other Radionuclide	Z None	Z None

C Nuclear Medicine
2 Heart
2 Tomographic (Tomo) Nuclear Medicine Imaging: Introduction of radioactive materials into the body for three dimensional display of images developed from the capture of radioactive emissions

Body Part	Radionuclide	Qualifier	Qualifier
Character 4	Character 5	Character 6	Character 7
6 Heart, Right and Left	1 Technetium 99m (Tc-99m) Y Other Radionuclide	Z None	Z None
G Myocardium	1 Technetium 99m (Tc-99m) D Indium 111 (In-111) K Fluorine 18 (F-18) S Thallium 201 (Tl-201) Y Other Radionuclide Z None	Z None	Z None
Y Heart	Y Other Radionuclide	Z None	Z None

C Nuclear Medicine
2 Heart
3 Positron Emission Tomographic (PET) Imaging: Introduction of radioactive materials into the body for three dimensional display of images developed from the simultaneous capture, 180 degrees apart, of radioactive emissions

Body Part	Radionuclide	Qualifier	Qualifier
Character 4	Character 5	Character 6	Character 7
G Myocardium	K Fluorine 18 (F-18) M Oxygen 15 (O-15) Q Rubidium 82 (Rb-82) R Nitrogen 13 (N-13) Y Other Radionuclide	Z None	Z None
Y Heart	Y Other Radionuclide	Z None	Z None

C Nuclear Medicine
2 Heart
5 Nonimaging Nuclear Medicine Probe: Introduction of radioactive materials into the body for the study of distribution and fate of certain substances by the detection of radioactive emissions; or, alternatively, measurement of absorption of radioactive emissions from an external source

Body Part	Radionuclide	Qualifier	Qualifier
Character 4	Character 5	Character 6	Character 7
6 Heart, Right and Left	1 Technetium 99m (Tc-99m) Y Other Radionuclide	Z None	Z None
Y Heart	Y Other Radionuclide	Z None	Z None

C   Nuclear Medicine
5   Veins
1   Planar Nuclear Medicine Imaging: Introduction of radioactive materials into the body for single plane display of images developed from the capture of radioactive emissions

Body Part	Radionuclide	Qualifier	Qualifier
Character 4	Character 5	Character 6	Character 7
B Lower Extremity Veins, Right **C** Lower Extremity Veins, Left **D** Lower Extremity Veins, Bilateral **N** Upper Extremity Veins, Right **P** Upper Extremity Veins, Left **Q** Upper Extremity Veins, Bilateral **R** Central Veins	**1** Technetium 99m (Tc-99m) **Y** Other Radionuclide	**Z** None	**Z** None
Y Veins	**Y** Other Radionuclide	**Z** None	**Z** None

C   Nuclear Medicine
7   Lymphatic and Hematologic System
1   Planar Nuclear Medicine Imaging: Introduction of radioactive materials into the body for single plane display of images developed from the capture of radioactive emissions

Body Part	Radionuclide	Qualifier	Qualifier
Character 4	Character 5	Character 6	Character 7
0 Bone Marrow	**1** Technetium 99m (Tc-99m) **D** Indium 111 (In-111) **Y** Other Radionuclide	**Z** None	**Z** None
2 Spleen **5** Lymphatics, Head and Neck **D** Lymphatics, Pelvic **J** Lymphatics, Head **K** Lymphatics, Neck **L** Lymphatics, Upper Chest **M** Lymphatics, Trunk **N** Lymphatics, Upper Extremity **P** Lymphatics, Lower Extremity	**1** Technetium 99m (Tc-99m) **Y** Other Radionuclide	**Z** None	**Z** None
3 Blood	**D** Indium 111 (In-111) **Y** Other Radionuclide	**Z** None	**Z** None
Y Lymphatic and Hematologic System	**Y** Other Radionuclide	**Z** None	**Z** None

C   Nuclear Medicine
7   Lymphatic and Hematologic System
2   Tomographic (Tomo) Nuclear Medicine Imaging: Introduction of radioactive materials into the body for three dimensional display of images developed from the capture of radioactive emissions

Body Part	Radionuclide	Qualifier	Qualifier
Character 4	Character 5	Character 6	Character 7
2 Spleen	**1** Technetium 99m (Tc-99m) **Y** Other Radionuclide	**Z** None	**Z** None
Y Lymphatic and Hematologic System	**Y** Other Radionuclide	**Z** None	**Z** None

LC Limited Coverage   NC Noncovered   HAC HAC-associated Procedure   CC Combination Cluster - See Appendix G for code lists
DRG Non-OR-Affecting MS-DRG Assignment   New/Revised Text in **Orange**   ♂ Male   ♀ Female

C Nuclear Medicine
7 Lymphatic and Hematologic System
5 Nonimaging Nuclear Medicine Probe: Introduction of radioactive materials into the body for the study of distribution and fate of certain substances by the detection of radioactive emissions; or, alternatively, measurement of absorption of radioactive emissions from an external source

Body Part	Radionuclide	Qualifier	Qualifier
Character 4	Character 5	Character 6	Character 7
5 Lymphatics, Head and Neck **D** Lymphatics, Pelvic **J** Lymphatics, Head **K** Lymphatics, Neck **L** Lymphatics, Upper Chest **M** Lymphatics, Trunk **N** Lymphatics, Upper Extremity **P** Lymphatics, Lower Extremity	**1** Technetium 99m (Tc-99m) **Y** Other Radionuclide	**Z** None	**Z** None
Y Lymphatic and Hematologic System	**Y** Other Radionuclide	**Z** None	**Z** None

C Nuclear Medicine
7 Lymphatic and Hematologic System
6 Nonimaging Nuclear Medicine Assay: Introduction of radioactive materials into the body for the study of body fluids and blood elements, by the detection of radioactive emissions

Body Part	Radionuclide	Qualifier	Qualifier
Character 4	Character 5	Character 6	Character 7
3 Blood	**1** Technetium 99m (Tc-99m) **7** Cobalt 58 (Co-58) **C** Cobalt 57 (Co-57) **D** Indium 111 (In-111) **H** Iodine 125 (I-125) **W** Chromium (Cr-51) **Y** Other Radionuclide	**Z** None	**Z** None
Y Lymphatic and Hematologic System	**Y** Other Radionuclide	**Z** None	**Z** None

C Nuclear Medicine
8 Eye
1 Planar Nuclear Medicine Imaging: Introduction of radioactive materials into the body for single plane display of images developed from the capture of radioactive emissions

Body Part	Radionuclide	Qualifier	Qualifier
Character 4	Character 5	Character 6	Character 7
9 Lacrimal Ducts, Bilateral	**1** Technetium 99m (Tc-99m) **Y** Other Radionuclide	**Z** None	**Z** None
Y Eye	**Y** Other Radionuclide	**Z** None	**Z** None

C Nuclear Medicine
9 Ear, Nose, Mouth and Throat
1 Planar Nuclear Medicine Imaging: Introduction of radioactive materials into the body for single plane display of images developed from the capture of radioactive emissions

Body Part	Radionuclide	Qualifier	Qualifier
Character 4	Character 5	Character 6	Character 7
B Salivary Glands, Bilateral	**1** Technetium 99m (Tc-99m) **Y** Other Radionuclide	**Z** None	**Z** None
Y Ear, Nose, Mouth and Throat	**Y** Other Radionuclide	**Z** None	**Z** None

C   Nuclear Medicine
B   Respiratory System
1   Planar Nuclear Medicine Imaging: Introduction of radioactive materials into the body for single plane display of images developed from the capture of radioactive emissions

Body Part	Radionuclide	Qualifier	Qualifier
Character 4	Character 5	Character 6	Character 7
2 Lungs and Bronchi	1 Technetium 99m (Tc-99m) 9 Krypton (Kr-81m) T Xenon 127 (Xe-127) V Xenon 133 (Xe-133) Y Other Radionuclide	Z None	Z None
Y Respiratory System	Y Other Radionuclide	Z None	Z None

C   Nuclear Medicine
B   Respiratory System
2   Tomographic (Tomo) Nuclear Medicine Imaging: Introduction of radioactive materials into the body for three dimensional display of images developed from the capture of radioactive emissions

Body Part	Radionuclide	Qualifier	Qualifier
Character 4	Character 5	Character 6	Character 7
2 Lungs and Bronchi	1 Technetium 99m (Tc-99m) 9 Krypton (Kr-81m) Y Other Radionuclide	Z None	Z None
Y Respiratory System	Y Other Radionuclide	Z None	Z None

C   Nuclear Medicine
B   Respiratory System
3   Positron Emission Tomographic (PET) Imaging: Introduction of radioactive materials into the body for three dimensional display of images developed from the simultaneous capture, 180 degrees apart, of radioactive emissions

Body Part	Radionuclide	Qualifier	Qualifier
Character 4	Character 5	Character 6	Character 7
2 Lungs and Bronchi	K Fluorine 18 (F-18) Y Other Radionuclide	Z None	Z None
Y Respiratory System	Y Other Radionuclide	Z None	Z None

C   Nuclear Medicine
D   Gastrointestinal System
1   Planar Nuclear Medicine Imaging: Introduction of radioactive materials into the body for single plane display of images developed from the capture of radioactive emissions

Body Part	Radionuclide	Qualifier	Qualifier
Character 4	Character 5	Character 6	Character 7
5 Upper Gastrointestinal Tract 7 Gastrointestinal Tract	1 Technetium 99m (Tc-99m) D Indium 111 (In-111) Y Other Radionuclide	Z None	Z None
Y Digestive System	Y Other Radionuclide	Z None	Z None

C   Nuclear Medicine
D   Gastrointestinal System
2   Tomographic (Tomo) Nuclear Medicine Imaging: Introduction of radioactive materials into the body for three dimensional display of images developed from the capture of radioactive emissions

Body Part	Radionuclide	Qualifier	Qualifier
Character 4	Character 5	Character 6	Character 7
7 Gastrointestinal Tract	1 Technetium 99m (Tc-99m) D Indium 111 (In-111) Y Other Radionuclide	Z None	Z None
Y Digestive System	Y Other Radionuclide	Z None	Z None

C Nuclear Medicine
F Hepatobiliary System and Pancreas
1 Planar Nuclear Medicine Imaging: Introduction of radioactive materials into the body for single plane display of images developed from the capture of radioactive emissions

Body Part	Radionuclide	Qualifier	Qualifier
Character 4	Character 5	Character 6	Character 7
4 Gallbladder 5 Liver 6 Liver and Spleen C Hepatobiliary System, All	1 Technetium 99m (Tc-99m) Y Other Radionuclide	Z None	Z None
Y Hepatobiliary System and Pancreas	Y Other Radionuclide	Z None	Z None

C Nuclear Medicine
F Hepatobiliary System and Pancreas
2 Tomographic (Tomo) Nuclear Medicine Imaging: Introduction of radioactive materials into the body for three dimensional display of images developed from the capture of radioactive emissions

Body Part	Radionuclide	Qualifier	Qualifier
Character 4	Character 5	Character 6	Character 7
4 Gallbladder 5 Liver 6 Liver and Spleen	1 Technetium 99m (Tc-99m) Y Other Radionuclide	Z None	Z None
Y Hepatobiliary System and Pancreas	Y Other Radionuclide	Z None	Z None

C Nuclear Medicine
G Endocrine System
1 Planar Nuclear Medicine Imaging: Introduction of radioactive materials into the body for single plane display of images developed from the capture of radioactive emissions

Body Part	Radionuclide	Qualifier	Qualifier
Character 4	Character 5	Character 6	Character 7
1 Parathyroid Glands	1 Technetium 99m (Tc-99m) S Thallium 201 (Tl-201) Y Other Radionuclide	Z None	Z None
2 Thyroid Gland	1 Technetium 99m (Tc-99m) F Iodine 123 (I-123) G Iodine 131 (I-131) Y Other Radionuclide	Z None	Z None
4 Adrenal Glands, Bilateral	G Iodine 131 (I-131) Y Other Radionuclide	Z None	Z None
Y Endocrine System	Y Other Radionuclide	Z None	Z None

C Nuclear Medicine
G Endocrine System
2 Tomographic (Tomo) Nuclear Medicine Imaging: Introduction of radioactive materials into the body for three dimensional display of images developed from the capture of radioactive emissions

Body Part	Radionuclide	Qualifier	Qualifier
Character 4	Character 5	Character 6	Character 7
1 Parathyroid Glands	1 Technetium 99m (Tc-99m) S Thallium 201 (Tl-201) Y Other Radionuclide	Z None	Z None
Y Endocrine System	Y Other Radionuclide	Z None	Z None

LC Limited Coverage   NC Noncovered   HAC HAC-associated Procedure   CC Combination Cluster - See Appendix G for code lists
DRG Non-OR-Affecting MS-DRG Assignment   New/Revised Text in Orange   ♂ Male   ♀ Female

670   2018 ICD-10-PCS

C Nuclear Medicine
G Endocrine System
4 **Nonimaging Nuclear Medicine Uptake:** Introduction of radioactive materials into the body for measurements of organ function, from the detection of radioactive emissions

Body Part	Radionuclide	Qualifier	Qualifier
Character 4	Character 5	Character 6	Character 7
2 Thyroid Gland	**1** Technetium 99m (Tc-99m) **F** Iodine 123 (I-123) **G** Iodine 131 (I-131) **Y** Other Radionuclide	**Z** None	**Z** None
Y Endocrine System	**Y** Other Radionuclide	**Z** None	**Z** None

C Nuclear Medicine
H Skin, Subcutaneous Tissue and Breast
1 **Planar Nuclear Medicine Imaging:** Introduction of radioactive materials into the body for single plane display of images developed from the capture of radioactive emissions

Body Part	Radionuclide	Qualifier	Qualifier
Character 4	Character 5	Character 6	Character 7
0 Breast, Right **1** Breast, Left **2** Breasts, Bilateral	**1** Technetium 99m (Tc-99m) **S** Thallium 201 (Tl-201) **Y** Other Radionuclide	**Z** None	**Z** None
Y Skin, Subcutaneous Tissue and Breast	**Y** Other Radionuclide	**Z** None	**Z** None

C Nuclear Medicine
H Skin, Subcutaneous Tissue and Breast
2 **Tomographic (Tomo) Nuclear Medicine Imaging:** Introduction of radioactive materials into the body for three dimensional display of images developed from the capture of radioactive emissions

Body Part	Radionuclide	Qualifier	Qualifier
Character 4	Character 5	Character 6	Character 7
0 Breast, Right **1** Breast, Left **2** Breasts, Bilateral	**1** Technetium 99m (Tc-99m) **S** Thallium 201 (Tl-201) **Y** Other Radionuclide	**Z** None	**Z** None
Y Skin, Subcutaneous Tissue and Breast	**Y** Other Radionuclide	**Z** None	**Z** None

C Nuclear Medicine
P Musculoskeletal System
1 **Planar Nuclear Medicine Imaging:** Introduction of radioactive materials into the body for single plane display of images developed from the capture of radioactive emissions

Body Part	Radionuclide	Qualifier	Qualifier
Character 4	Character 5	Character 6	Character 7
1 Skull **4** Thorax **5** Spine **6** Pelvis **7** Spine and Pelvis **8** Upper Extremity, Right **9** Upper Extremity, Left **B** Upper Extremities, Bilateral **C** Lower Extremity, Right **D** Lower Extremity, Left **F** Lower Extremities, Bilateral **Z** Musculoskeletal System, All	**1** Technetium 99m (Tc-99m) **Y** Other Radionuclide	**Z** None	**Z** None
Y Musculoskeletal System, Other	**Y** Other Radionuclide	**Z** None	**Z** None

LC Limited Coverage   NC Noncovered   HAC HAC-associated Procedure   CC Combination Cluster - See Appendix G for code lists
DRG Non-OR-Affecting MS-DRG Assignment   New/Revised Text in **Orange**   ♂ Male   ♀ Female

C Nuclear Medicine
P Musculoskeletal System
2 Tomographic (Tomo) Nuclear Medicine Imaging: Introduction of radioactive materials into the body for three dimensional display of images developed from the capture of radioactive emissions

Body Part	Radionuclide	Qualifier	Qualifier
Character 4	Character 5	Character 6	Character 7
1 Skull 2 Cervical Spine 3 Skull and Cervical Spine 4 Thorax 6 Pelvis 7 Spine and Pelvis 8 Upper Extremity, Right 9 Upper Extremity, Left B Upper Extremities, Bilateral C Lower Extremity, Right D Lower Extremity, Left F Lower Extremities, Bilateral G Thoracic Spine H Lumbar Spine J Thoracolumbar Spine	1 Technetium 99m (Tc-99m) Y Other Radionuclide	Z None	Z None
Y Musculoskeletal System, Other	Y Other Radionuclide	Z None	Z None

C Nuclear Medicine
P Musculoskeletal System
5 Nonimaging Nuclear Medicine Probe: Introduction of radioactive materials into the body for the study of distribution and fate of certain substances by the detection of radioactive emissions; or, alternatively, measurement of absorption of radioactive emissions from an external source

Body Part	Radionuclide	Qualifier	Qualifier
Character 4	Character 5	Character 6	Character 7
5 Spine N Upper Extremities P Lower Extremities	Z None	Z None	Z None
Y Musculoskeletal System, Other	Y Other Radionuclide	Z None	Z None

C Nuclear Medicine
T Urinary System
1 Planar Nuclear Medicine Imaging: Introduction of radioactive materials into the body for single plane display of images developed from the capture of radioactive emissions

Body Part	Radionuclide	Qualifier	Qualifier
Character 4	Character 5	Character 6	Character 7
3 Kidneys, Ureters and Bladder	1 Technetium 99m (Tc-99m) F Iodine 123 (I-123) G Iodine 131 (I-131) Y Other Radionuclide	Z None	Z None
H Bladder and Ureters	1 Technetium 99m (Tc-99m) Y Other Radionuclide	Z None	Z None
Y Urinary System	Y Other Radionuclide	Z None	Z None

C Nuclear Medicine
T Urinary System
2 Tomographic (Tomo) Nuclear Medicine Imaging: Introduction of radioactive materials into the body for three dimensional display of images developed from the capture of radioactive emissions

Body Part	Radionuclide	Qualifier	Qualifier
Character 4	Character 5	Character 6	Character 7
3 Kidneys, Ureters and Bladder	1 Technetium 99m (Tc-99m) Y Other Radionuclide	Z None	Z None
Y Urinary System	Y Other Radionuclide	Z None	Z None

C Nuclear Medicine
T Urinary System
6 **Nonimaging Nuclear Medicine Assay:** Introduction of radioactive materials into the body for the study of body fluids and blood elements, by the detection of radioactive emissions

Body Part	Radionuclide	Qualifier	Qualifier
Character 4	Character 5	Character 6	Character 7
3 Kidneys, Ureters and Bladder	**1** Technetium 99m (Tc-99m) **F** Iodine 123 (I-123) **G** Iodine 131 (I-131) **H** Iodine 125 (I-125) **Y** Other Radionuclide	**Z** None	**Z** None
Y Urinary System	**Y** Other Radionuclide	**Z** None	**Z** None

C Nuclear Medicine
V Male Reproductive System
1 **Planar Nuclear Medicine Imaging:** Introduction of radioactive materials into the body for single plane display of images developed from the capture of radioactive emissions

Body Part	Radionuclide	Qualifier	Qualifier
Character 4	Character 5	Character 6	Character 7
9 Testicles, Bilateral ♂	**1** Technetium 99m (Tc-99m) **Y** Other Radionuclide	**Z** None	**Z** None
Y Male Reproductive System ♂	**Y** Other Radionuclide	**Z** None	**Z** None

♂ CV191ZZ   CV19YZZ   CV1YYZZ

C Nuclear Medicine
W Anatomical Regions
1 **Planar Nuclear Medicine Imaging:** Introduction of radioactive materials into the body for single plane display of images developed from the capture of radioactive emissions

Body Part	Radionuclide	Qualifier	Qualifier
Character 4	Character 5	Character 6	Character 7
0 Abdomen **1** Abdomen and Pelvis **4** Chest and Abdomen **6** Chest and Neck **B** Head and Neck **D** Lower Extremity **J** Pelvic Region **M** Upper Extremity **N** Whole Body	**1** Technetium 99m (Tc-99m) **D** Indium 111 (In-111) **F** Iodine 123 (I-123) **G** Iodine 131 (I-131) **L** Gallium 67 (Ga-67) **S** Thallium 201 (Tl-201) **Y** Other Radionuclide	**Z** None	**Z** None
3 Chest	**1** Technetium 99m (Tc-99m) **D** Indium 111 (In-111) **F** Iodine 123 (I-123) **G** Iodine 131 (I-131) **K** Fluorine 18 (F-18) **L** Gallium 67 (Ga-67) **S** Thallium 201 (Tl-201) **Y** Other Radionuclide	**Z** None	**Z** None
Y Anatomical Regions, Multiple	**Y** Other Radionuclide	**Z** None	**Z** None
Z Anatomical Region, Other	**Z** None	**Z** None	**Z** None

LC Limited Coverage   **NC** Noncovered   **HAC** HAC-associated Procedure   **CC** Combination Cluster - See Appendix G for code lists
DRG Non-OR-Affecting MS-DRG Assignment   New/Revised Text in **Orange**   ♂ Male   ♀ Female

2018 ICD-10-PCS 673

NUCLEAR MEDICINE C01-CW7

CT6-CW1

C Nuclear Medicine
W Anatomical Regions
2 **Tomographic (Tomo) Nuclear Medicine Imaging:** Introduction of radioactive materials into the body for three dimensional display of images developed from the capture of radioactive emissions

Body Part	Radionuclide	Qualifier	Qualifier
Character 4	Character 5	Character 6	Character 7
0 Abdomen 1 Abdomen and Pelvis 3 Chest 4 Chest and Abdomen 6 Chest and Neck B Head and Neck D Lower Extremity J Pelvic Region M Upper Extremity	1 Technetium 99m (Tc-99m) D Indium 111 (In-111) F Iodine 123 (I-123) G Iodine 131 (I-131) K Fluorine 18 (F-18) L Gallium 67 (Ga-67) S Thallium 201 (Tl-201) Y Other Radionuclide	Z None	Z None
Y Anatomical Regions, Multiple	Y Other Radionuclide	Z None	Z None

C Nuclear Medicine
W Anatomical Regions
3 **Positron Emission Tomographic (PET) Imaging:** Introduction of radioactive materials into the body for three dimensional display of images developed from the simultaneous capture, 180 degrees apart, of radioactive emissions

Body Part	Radionuclide	Qualifier	Qualifier
Character 4	Character 5	Character 6	Character 7
N Whole Body	Y Other Radionuclide	Z None	Z None

C Nuclear Medicine
W Anatomical Regions
5 **Nonimaging Nuclear Medicine Probe:** Introduction of radioactive materials into the body for the study of distribution and fate of certain substances by the detection of radioactive emissions; or, alternatively, measurement of absorption of radioactive emissions from an external source

Body Part	Radionuclide	Qualifier	Qualifier
Character 4	Character 5	Character 6	Character 7
0 Abdomen 1 Abdomen and Pelvis 3 Chest 4 Chest and Abdomen 6 Chest and Neck B Head and Neck D Lower Extremity J Pelvic Region M Upper Extremity	1 Technetium 99m (Tc-99m) D Indium 111 (In-111) Y Other Radionuclide	Z None	Z None

C Nuclear Medicine
W Anatomical Regions
7 **Systemic Nuclear Medicine Therapy:** Introduction of unsealed radioactive materials into the body for treatment

Body Part	Radionuclide	Qualifier	Qualifier
Character 4	Character 5	Character 6	Character 7
0 Abdomen 3 Chest	N Phosphorus 32 (P-32) Y Other Radionuclide	Z None	Z None
G Thyroid	G Iodine 131 (I-131) Y Other Radionuclide	Z None	Z None
N Whole Body	8 Samarium 153 (Sm-153) G Iodine 131 (I-131) N Phosphorus 32 (P-32) P Strontium 89 (Sr-89) Y Other Radionuclide	Z None	Z None
Y Anatomical Regions, Multiple	Y Other Radionuclide	Z None	Z None

LC Limited Coverage   NC Noncovered   HAC HAC-associated Procedure   CC Combination Cluster - See Appendix G for code lists
DRG Non-OR-Affecting MS-DRG Assignment   New/Revised Text in **Orange**   ♂ Male   ♀ Female

674

2018 ICD-10-PCS

NOTES

NOTES

Radiation Therapy D00-DWY

D Radiation Therapy
0 Central and Peripheral Nervous System
0 Beam Radiation

Treatment Site	Modality Qualifier	Isotope	Qualifier
Character 4	**Character 5**	**Character 6**	**Character 7**
0 Brain **1** Brain Stem **6** Spinal Cord **7** Peripheral Nerve	**0** Photons <1 MeV **1** Photons 1 - 10 MeV **2** Photons >10 MeV **4** Heavy Particles (Protons, Ions) **5** Neutrons **6** Neutron Capture	**Z** None	**Z** None
0 Brain **1** Brain Stem **6** Spinal Cord **7** Peripheral Nerve	**3** Electrons	**Z** None	**0** Intraoperative **Z** None

D Radiation Therapy
0 Central and Peripheral Nervous System
1 Brachytherapy

Treatment Site	Modality Qualifier	Isotope	Qualifier
Character 4	**Character 5**	**Character 6**	**Character 7**
0 Brain **1** Brain Stem **6** Spinal Cord **7** Peripheral Nerve	**9** High Dose Rate (HDR) **B** Low Dose Rate (LDR)	**7** Cesium 137 (Cs-137) **8** Iridium 192 (Ir-192) **9** Iodine 125 (I-125) **B** Palladium 103 (Pd-103) **C** Californium 252 (Cf-252) **Y** Other Isotope	**Z** None

D Radiation Therapy
0 Central and Peripheral Nervous System
2 Stereotactic Radiosurgery

Treatment Site	Modality Qualifier	Isotope	Qualifier
Character 4	**Character 5**	**Character 6**	**Character 7**
0 Brain **1** Brain Stem **6** Spinal Cord **7** Peripheral Nerve	**D** Stereotactic Other Photon Radiosurgery **H** Stereotactic Particulate Radiosurgery **J** Stereotactic Gamma Beam Radiosurgery	**Z** None	**Z** None

D Radiation Therapy
0 Central and Peripheral Nervous System
Y Other Radiation

Treatment Site	Modality Qualifier	Isotope	Qualifier
Character 4	**Character 5**	**Character 6**	**Character 7**
0 Brain **1** Brain Stem **6** Spinal Cord **7** Peripheral Nerve	**7** Contact Radiation **8** Hyperthermia **F** Plaque Radiation **K** Laser Interstitial Thermal Therapy	**Z** None	**Z** None

LC Limited Coverage   NC Noncovered   HAC HAC-associated Procedure   CC Combination Cluster - See Appendix G for code lists
DRG Non-OR-Affecting MS-DRG Assignment   New/Revised Text in **Orange**   ♂ Male   ♀ Female

D Radiation Therapy
7 Lymphatic and Hematologic System
0 Beam Radiation

Treatment Site	Modality Qualifier	Isotope	Qualifier
Character 4	Character 5	Character 6	Character 7
0 Bone Marrow 1 Thymus 2 Spleen 3 Lymphatics, Neck 4 Lymphatics, Axillary 5 Lymphatics, Thorax 6 Lymphatics, Abdomen 7 Lymphatics, Pelvis 8 Lymphatics, Inguinal	0 Photons <1 MeV 1 Photons 1 - 10 MeV 2 Photons >10 MeV 4 Heavy Particles (Protons, Ions) 5 Neutrons 6 Neutron Capture	Z None	Z None
0 Bone Marrow 1 Thymus 2 Spleen 3 Lymphatics, Neck 4 Lymphatics, Axillary 5 Lymphatics, Thorax 6 Lymphatics, Abdomen 7 Lymphatics, Pelvis 8 Lymphatics, Inguinal	3 Electrons	Z None	0 Intraoperative Z None

D Radiation Therapy
7 Lymphatic and Hematologic System
1 Brachytherapy

Treatment Site	Modality Qualifier	Isotope	Qualifier
Character 4	Character 5	Character 6	Character 7
0 Bone Marrow 1 Thymus 2 Spleen 3 Lymphatics, Neck 4 Lymphatics, Axillary 5 Lymphatics, Thorax 6 Lymphatics, Abdomen 7 Lymphatics, Pelvis 8 Lymphatics, Inguinal	9 High Dose Rate (HDR) B Low Dose Rate (LDR)	7 Cesium 137 (Cs-137) 8 Iridium 192 (Ir-192) 9 Iodine 125 (I-125) B Palladium 103 (Pd-103) C Californium 252 (Cf-252) Y Other Isotope	Z None

D Radiation Therapy
7 Lymphatic and Hematologic System
2 Stereotactic Radiosurgery

Treatment Site	Modality Qualifier	Isotope	Qualifier
Character 4	Character 5	Character 6	Character 7
0 Bone Marrow 1 Thymus 2 Spleen 3 Lymphatics, Neck 4 Lymphatics, Axillary 5 Lymphatics, Thorax 6 Lymphatics, Abdomen 7 Lymphatics, Pelvis 8 Lymphatics, Inguinal	D Stereotactic Other Photon Radiosurgery H Stereotactic Particulate Radiosurgery J Stereotactic Gamma Beam Radiosurgery	Z None	Z None

Ⓛ Limited Coverage Ⓝ Noncovered Ⓗ HAC-associated Procedure Ⓒ Combination Cluster - See Appendix G for code lists
Ⓓ Non-OR-Affecting MS-DRG Assignment New/Revised Text in **Orange** ♂ Male ♀ Female

678

2018 ICD-10-PCS

D Radiation Therapy
7 Lymphatic and Hematologic System
Y Other Radiation

Treatment Site	Modality Qualifier	Isotope	Qualifier
Character 4	Character 5	Character 6	Character 7
0 Bone Marrow 1 Thymus 2 Spleen 3 Lymphatics, Neck 4 Lymphatics, Axillary 5 Lymphatics, Thorax 6 Lymphatics, Abdomen 7 Lymphatics, Pelvis 8 Lymphatics, Inguinal	8 Hyperthermia F Plaque Radiation	Z None	Z None

D Radiation Therapy
8 Eye
0 Beam Radiation

Treatment Site	Modality Qualifier	Isotope	Qualifier
Character 4	Character 5	Character 6	Character 7
0 Eye	0 Photons <1 MeV 1 Photons 1 - 10 MeV 2 Photons >10 MeV 4 Heavy Particles (Protons, Ions) 5 Neutrons 6 Neutron Capture	Z None	Z None
0 Eye	3 Electrons	Z None	0 Intraoperative Z None

D Radiation Therapy
8 Eye
1 Brachytherapy

Treatment Site	Modality Qualifier	Isotope	Qualifier
Character 4	Character 5	Character 6	Character 7
0 Eye	9 High Dose Rate (HDR) B Low Dose Rate (LDR)	7 Cesium 137 (Cs-137) 8 Iridium 192 (Ir-192) 9 Iodine 125 (I-125) B Palladium 103 (Pd-103) C Californium 252 (Cf-252) Y Other Isotope	Z None

D Radiation Therapy
8 Eye
2 Stereotactic Radiosurgery

Treatment Site	Modality Qualifier	Isotope	Qualifier
Character 4	Character 5	Character 6	Character 7

0 Eye	D Stereotactic Other Photon
	   Radiosurgery
	H Stereotactic Particulate
	   Radiosurgery
	J Stereotactic Gamma Beam
	   Radiosurgery
		Z None	Z None

LC Limited Coverage   NC Noncovered   HAC HAC-associated Procedure   CC Combination Cluster - See Appendix G for code lists
DRG Non-OR-Affecting MS-DRG Assignment   New/Revised Text in **Orange**   ♂ Male   ♀ Female

2018 ICD-10-PCS   679

RADIATION THERAPY D00-DWY

D Radiation Therapy
8 Eye
Y Other Radiation

Treatment Site	Modality Qualifier	Isotope	Qualifier
Character 4	Character 5	Character 6	Character 7
0 Eye	**7** Contact Radiation **8** Hyperthermia **F** Plaque Radiation	**Z** None	**Z** None

D Radiation Therapy
9 Ear, Nose, Mouth and Throat
0 Beam Radiation

Treatment Site	Modality Qualifier	Isotope	Qualifier
Character 4	Character 5	Character 6	Character 7
0 Ear **1** Nose **3** Hypopharynx **4** Mouth **5** Tongue **6** Salivary Glands **7** Sinuses **8** Hard Palate **9** Soft Palate **B** Larynx **D** Nasopharynx **F** Oropharynx	**0** Photons <1 MeV **1** Photons 1 - 10 MeV **2** Photons >10 MeV **4** Heavy Particles (Protons, Ions) **5** Neutrons **6** Neutron Capture	**Z** None	**Z** None
0 Ear **1** Nose **3** Hypopharynx **4** Mouth **5** Tongue **6** Salivary Glands **7** Sinuses **8** Hard Palate **9** Soft Palate **B** Larynx **D** Nasopharynx **F** Oropharynx	**3** Electrons	**Z** None	**0** Intraoperative **Z** None

D Radiation Therapy
9 Ear, Nose, Mouth and Throat
1 Brachytherapy

Treatment Site	Modality Qualifier	Isotope	Qualifier
Character 4	Character 5	Character 6	Character 7
0 Ear **1** Nose **3** Hypopharynx **4** Mouth **5** Tongue **6** Salivary Glands **7** Sinuses **8** Hard Palate **9** Soft Palate **B** Larynx **D** Nasopharynx **F** Oropharynx	**9** High Dose Rate (HDR) **B** Low Dose Rate (LDR)	**7** Cesium 137 (Cs-137) **8** Iridium 192 (Ir-192) **9** Iodine 125 (I-125) **B** Palladium 103 (Pd-103) **C** Californium 252 (Cf-252) **Y** Other Isotope	**Z** None

LC Limited Coverage   NC Noncovered   HAC HAC-associated Procedure   CC Combination Cluster - See Appendix G for code lists
DRG Non-OR-Affecting MS-DRG Assignment   New/Revised Text in **Orange**   ♂ Male   ♀ Female

680

2018 ICD-10-PCS

D Radiation Therapy
9 Ear, Nose, Mouth and Throat
2 Stereotactic Radiosurgery

Treatment Site	Modality Qualifier	Isotope	Qualifier
Character 4	Character 5	Character 6	Character 7
0 Ear 1 Nose 4 Mouth 5 Tongue 6 Salivary Glands 7 Sinuses 8 Hard Palate 9 Soft Palate B Larynx C Pharynx D Nasopharynx	D Stereotactic Other Photon Radiosurgery H Stereotactic Particulate Radiosurgery J Stereotactic Gamma Beam Radiosurgery	Z None	Z None

D Radiation Therapy
9 Ear, Nose, Mouth and Throat
Y Other Radiation

Treatment Site	Modality Qualifier	Isotope	Qualifier
Character 4	Character 5	Character 6	Character 7
0 Ear 1 Nose 5 Tongue 6 Salivary Glands 7 Sinuses 8 Hard Palate 9 Soft Palate	7 Contact Radiation 8 Hyperthermia F Plaque Radiation	Z None	Z None
3 Hypopharynx F Oropharynx	7 Contact Radiation 8 Hyperthermia	Z None	Z None
4 Mouth B Larynx D Nasopharynx	7 Contact Radiation 8 Hyperthermia C Intraoperative Radiation Therapy (IORT) F Plaque Radiation	Z None	Z None
C Pharynx	C Intraoperative Radiation Therapy (IORT) F Plaque Radiation	Z None	Z None

D Radiation Therapy
B Respiratory System
0 Beam Radiation

Treatment Site	Modality Qualifier	Isotope	Qualifier
Character 4	Character 5	Character 6	Character 7
0 Trachea 1 Bronchus 2 Lung 5 Pleura 6 Mediastinum 7 Chest Wall 8 Diaphragm	0 Photons <1 MeV 1 Photons 1 - 10 MeV 2 Photons >10 MeV 4 Heavy Particles (Protons, Ions) 5 Neutrons 6 Neutron Capture	Z None	Z None
0 Trachea 1 Bronchus 2 Lung 5 Pleura 6 Mediastinum 7 Chest Wall 8 Diaphragm	3 Electrons	Z None	0 Intraoperative Z None

D Radiation Therapy
B Respiratory System
1 Brachytherapy

Treatment Site	Modality Qualifier	Isotope	Qualifier
Character 4	Character 5	Character 6	Character 7
0 Trachea 1 Bronchus 2 Lung 5 Pleura 6 Mediastinum 7 Chest Wall 8 Diaphragm	9 High Dose Rate (HDR) B Low Dose Rate (LDR)	7 Cesium 137 (Cs-137) 8 Iridium 192 (Ir-192) 9 Iodine 125 (I-125) B Palladium 103 (Pd-103) C Californium 252 (Cf-252) Y Other Isotope	Z None

D Radiation Therapy
B Respiratory System
2 Stereotactic Radiosurgery

Treatment Site	Modality Qualifier	Isotope	Qualifier
Character 4	Character 5	Character 6	Character 7

0 Trachea
1 Bronchus
2 Lung
5 Pleura
6 Mediastinum
7 Chest Wall
8 Diaphragm
	D Stereotactic Other Photon
	    Radiosurgery
	H Stereotactic Particulate
	    Radiosurgery
	J Stereotactic Gamma Beam
	    Radiosurgery
		Z None	Z None

D Radiation Therapy
B Respiratory System
Y Other Radiation

Treatment Site	Modality Qualifier	Isotope	Qualifier
Character 4	Character 5	Character 6	Character 7
0 Trachea 1 Bronchus 2 Lung 5 Pleura 6 Mediastinum 7 Chest Wall 8 Diaphragm	7 Contact Radiation 8 Hyperthermia F Plaque Radiation K Laser Interstitial Thermal Therapy	Z None	Z None

D Radiation Therapy
D Gastrointestinal System
0 Beam Radiation

Treatment Site	Modality Qualifier	Isotope	Qualifier
Character 4	Character 5	Character 6	Character 7
0 Esophagus 1 Stomach 2 Duodenum 3 Jejunum 4 Ileum 5 Colon 7 Rectum	0 Photons <1 MeV 1 Photons 1 - 10 MeV 2 Photons >10 MeV 4 Heavy Particles (Protons, Ions) 5 Neutrons 6 Neutron Capture	Z None	Z None
0 Esophagus 1 Stomach 2 Duodenum 3 Jejunum 4 Ileum 5 Colon 7 Rectum	3 Electrons	Z None	0 Intraoperative Z None

D Radiation Therapy
D Gastrointestinal System
1 Brachytherapy

Treatment Site	Modality Qualifier	Isotope	Qualifier
Character 4	Character 5	Character 6	Character 7
0 Esophagus 1 Stomach 2 Duodenum 3 Jejunum 4 Ileum 5 Colon 7 Rectum	9 High Dose Rate (HDR) B Low Dose Rate (LDR)	7 Cesium 137 (Cs-137) 8 Iridium 192 (Ir-192) 9 Iodine 125 (I-125) B Palladium 103 (Pd-103) C Californium 252 (Cf-252) Y Other Isotope	Z None

D Radiation Therapy
D Gastrointestinal System
2 Stereotactic Radiosurgery

Treatment Site	Modality Qualifier	Isotope	Qualifier
Character 4	Character 5	Character 6	Character 7
0 Esophagus 1 Stomach 2 Duodenum 3 Jejunum 4 Ileum 5 Colon 7 Rectum	D Stereotactic Other Photon Radiosurgery H Stereotactic Particulate Radiosurgery J Stereotactic Gamma Beam Radiosurgery	Z None	Z None

D Radiation Therapy
D Gastrointestinal System
Y Other Radiation

Treatment Site	Modality Qualifier	Isotope	Qualifier
Character 4	Character 5	Character 6	Character 7
0 Esophagus	7 Contact Radiation 8 Hyperthermia F Plaque Radiation K Laser Interstitial Thermal Therapy	Z None	Z None
1 Stomach 2 Duodenum 3 Jejunum 4 Ileum 5 Colon 7 Rectum	7 Contact Radiation 8 Hyperthermia C Intraoperative Radiation Therapy (IORT) F Plaque Radiation K Laser Interstitial Thermal Therapy	Z None	Z None
8 Anus	C Intraoperative Radiation Therapy (IORT) F Plaque Radiation K Laser Interstitial Thermal Therapy	Z None	Z None

LC Limited Coverage   NC Noncovered   HAC HAC-associated Procedure   CC Combination Cluster - See Appendix G for code lists
DRG Non-OR-Affecting MS-DRG Assignment   New/Revised Text in **Orange**   ♂ Male   ♀ Female

2018 ICD-10-PCS

683

D Radiation Therapy
F Hepatobiliary System and Pancreas
0 Beam Radiation

Treatment Site	Modality Qualifier	Isotope	Qualifier
Character 4	Character 5	Character 6	Character 7
0 Liver 1 Gallbladder 2 Bile Ducts 3 Pancreas	0 Photons <1 MeV 1 Photons 1 - 10 MeV 2 Photons >10 MeV 4 Heavy Particles (Protons, Ions) 5 Neutrons 6 Neutron Capture	Z None	Z None
0 Liver 1 Gallbladder 2 Bile Ducts 3 Pancreas	3 Electrons	Z None	0 Intraoperative Z None

D Radiation Therapy
F Hepatobiliary System and Pancreas
1 Brachytherapy

Treatment Site	Modality Qualifier	Isotope	Qualifier
Character 4	Character 5	Character 6	Character 7
0 Liver 1 Gallbladder 2 Bile Ducts 3 Pancreas	9 High Dose Rate (HDR) B Low Dose Rate (LDR)	7 Cesium 137 (Cs-137) 8 Iridium 192 (Ir-192) 9 Iodine 125 (I-125) B Palladium 103 (Pd-103) C Californium 252 (Cf-252) Y Other Isotope	Z None

D Radiation Therapy
F Hepatobiliary System and Pancreas
2 Stereotactic Radiosurgery

Treatment Site	Modality Qualifier	Isotope	Qualifier
Character 4	Character 5	Character 6	Character 7
0 Liver 1 Gallbladder 2 Bile Ducts 3 Pancreas	D Stereotactic Other Photon Radiosurgery H Stereotactic Particulate Radiosurgery J Stereotactic Gamma Beam Radiosurgery	Z None	Z None

D Radiation Therapy
F Hepatobiliary System and Pancreas
Y Other Radiation

Treatment Site	Modality Qualifier	Isotope	Qualifier
Character 4	Character 5	Character 6	Character 7
0 Liver 1 Gallbladder 2 Bile Ducts 3 Pancreas	7 Contact Radiation 8 Hyperthermia C Intraoperative Radiation Therapy (IORT) F Plaque Radiation K Laser Interstitial Thermal Therapy	Z None	Z None

LC Limited Coverage   NC Noncovered   HAC HAC-associated Procedure   CC Combination Cluster - See Appendix G for code lists
DRG Non-OR-Affecting MS-DRG Assignment   New/Revised Text in **Orange**   ♂ Male   ♀ Female

684   2018 ICD-10-PCS

D Radiation Therapy
G Endocrine System
0 Beam Radiation

Treatment Site	Modality Qualifier	Isotope	Qualifier
Character 4	Character 5	Character 6	Character 7
0 Pituitary Gland 1 Pineal Body 2 Adrenal Glands 4 Parathyroid Glands 5 Thyroid	0 Photons <1 MeV 1 Photons 1 - 10 MeV 2 Photons >10 MeV 5 Neutrons 6 Neutron Capture	Z None	Z None
0 Pituitary Gland 1 Pineal Body 2 Adrenal Glands 4 Parathyroid Glands 5 Thyroid	3 Electrons	Z None	0 Intraoperative Z None

D Radiation Therapy
G Endocrine System
1 Brachytherapy

Treatment Site	Modality Qualifier	Isotope	Qualifier
Character 4	Character 5	Character 6	Character 7
0 Pituitary Gland 1 Pineal Body 2 Adrenal Glands 4 Parathyroid Glands 5 Thyroid	9 High Dose Rate (HDR) B Low Dose Rate (LDR)	7 Cesium 137 (Cs-137) 8 Iridium 192 (Ir-192) 9 Iodine 125 (I-125) B Palladium 103 (Pd-103) C Californium 252 (Cf-252) Y Other Isotope	Z None

D Radiation Therapy
G Endocrine System
2 Stereotactic Radiosurgery

Treatment Site	Modality Qualifier	Isotope	Qualifier
Character 4	Character 5	Character 6	Character 7

0 Pituitary Gland ᴰᴿᴳ
1 Pineal Body ᴰᴿᴳ
2 Adrenal Glands ᴰᴿᴳ
4 Parathyroid Glands ᴰᴿᴳ
5 Thyroid ᴰᴿᴳ
	D Stereotactic Other Photon
	     Radiosurgery
	H Stereotactic Particulate
	     Radiosurgery
	J Stereotactic Gamma Beam
	     Radiosurgery
		Z None	Z None

ᴰᴿᴳ DG20HZZ   DG20JZZ   DG21DZZ   DG21HZZ   DG21JZZ   DG22DZZ   DG22HZZ   DG22JZZ   DG24DZZ   DG24HZZ   DG24JZZ   DG25DZZ   DG25HZZ
DG25JZZ

D Radiation Therapy
G Endocrine System
Y Other Radiation

Treatment Site	Modality Qualifier	Isotope	Qualifier
Character 4	Character 5	Character 6	Character 7
0 Pituitary Gland 1 Pineal Body 2 Adrenal Glands 4 Parathyroid Glands 5 Thyroid	7 Contact Radiation 8 Hyperthermia F Plaque Radiation K Laser Interstitial Thermal Therapy	Z None	Z None

D Radiation Therapy
H Skin
0 Beam Radiation

Treatment Site	Modality Qualifier	Isotope	Qualifier
Character 4	**Character 5**	**Character 6**	**Character 7**
2 Skin, Face 3 Skin, Neck 4 Skin, Arm 6 Skin, Chest 7 Skin, Back 8 Skin, Abdomen 9 Skin, Buttock B Skin, Leg	0 Photons <1 MeV 1 Photons 1 - 10 MeV 2 Photons >10 MeV 4 Heavy Particles (Protons, Ions) 5 Neutrons 6 Neutron Capture	Z None	Z None
2 Skin, Face 3 Skin, Neck 4 Skin, Arm 6 Skin, Chest 7 Skin, Back 8 Skin, Abdomen 9 Skin, Buttock B Skin, Leg	3 Electrons	Z None	0 Intraoperative Z None

D Radiation Therapy
H Skin
Y Other Radiation

Treatment Site	Modality Qualifier	Isotope	Qualifier
Character 4	**Character 5**	**Character 6**	**Character 7**
2 Skin, Face 3 Skin, Neck 4 Skin, Arm 6 Skin, Chest 7 Skin, Back 8 Skin, Abdomen 9 Skin, Buttock B Skin, Leg	7 Contact Radiation 8 Hyperthermia F Plaque Radiation	Z None	Z None
5 Skin, Hand C Skin, Foot	F Plaque Radiation	Z None	Z None

D Radiation Therapy
M Breast
0 Beam Radiation

Treatment Site	Modality Qualifier	Isotope	Qualifier
Character 4	**Character 5**	**Character 6**	**Character 7**
0 Breast, Left 1 Breast, Right	0 Photons <1 MeV 1 Photons 1 - 10 MeV 2 Photons >10 MeV 4 Heavy Particles (Protons, Ions) 5 Neutrons 6 Neutron Capture	Z None	Z None
0 Breast, Left 1 Breast, Right	3 Electrons	Z None	0 Intraoperative Z None

D Radiation Therapy
M Breast
1 Brachytherapy

Treatment Site	Modality Qualifier	Isotope	Qualifier
Character 4	Character 5	Character 6	Character 7
0 Breast, Left **1** Breast, Right	**9** High Dose Rate (HDR) **B** Low Dose Rate (LDR)	**7** Cesium 137 (Cs-137) **8** Iridium 192 (Ir-192) **9** Iodine 125 (I-125) **B** Palladium 103 (Pd-103) **C** Californium 252 (Cf-252) **Y** Other Isotope	**Z** None

D Radiation Therapy
M Breast
2 Stereotactic Radiosurgery

Treatment Site	Modality Qualifier	Isotope	Qualifier
Character 4	Character 5	Character 6	Character 7
0 Breast, Left ⓓⓡⓖ **1** Breast, Right ⓓⓡⓖ	**D** Stereotactic Other Photon Radiosurgery **H** Stereotactic Particulate Radiosurgery **J** Stereotactic Gamma Beam Radiosurgery	**Z** None	**Z** None

ⓓⓡⓖ DM20DZZ DM20HZZ DM20JZZ   DM21DZZ DM21HZZ DM21JZZ

D Radiation Therapy
M Breast
Y Other Radiation

Treatment Site	Modality Qualifier	Isotope	Qualifier
Character 4	Character 5	Character 6	Character 7
0 Breast, Left **1** Breast, Right	**7** Contact Radiation **8** Hyperthermia **F** Plaque Radiation **K** Laser Interstitial Thermal Therapy	**Z** None	**Z** None

🄻🄲 Limited Coverage   🄽🄲 Noncovered   🄷🄰🄲 HAC-associated Procedure   🄲🄲 Combination Cluster - See Appendix G for code lists
ⓓⓡⓖ Non-OR-Affecting MS-DRG Assignment   New/Revised Text in **Orange**   ♂ Male   ♀ Female

2018 ICD-10-PCS

687

D Radiation Therapy
P Musculoskeletal System
0 Beam Radiation

Treatment Site	Modality Qualifier	Isotope	Qualifier
Character 4	Character 5	Character 6	Character 7
0 Skull 2 Maxilla 3 Mandible 4 Sternum 5 Rib(s) 6 Humerus 7 Radius/Ulna 8 Pelvic Bones 9 Femur B Tibia/Fibula C Other Bone	0 Photons <1 MeV 1 Photons 1 - 10 MeV 2 Photons >10 MeV 4 Heavy Particles (Protons, Ions) 5 Neutrons 6 Neutron Capture	Z None	Z None
0 Skull 2 Maxilla 3 Mandible 4 Sternum 5 Rib(s) 6 Humerus 7 Radius/Ulna 8 Pelvic Bones 9 Femur B Tibia/Fibula C Other Bone	3 Electrons	Z None	0 Intraoperative Z None

D Radiation Therapy
P Musculoskeletal System
Y Other Radiation

Treatment Site	Modality Qualifier	Isotope	Qualifier
Character 4	Character 5	Character 6	Character 7
0 Skull 2 Maxilla 3 Mandible 4 Sternum 5 Rib(s) 6 Humerus 7 Radius/Ulna 8 Pelvic Bones 9 Femur B Tibia/Fibula C Other Bone	7 Contact Radiation 8 Hyperthermia F Plaque Radiation	Z None	Z None

D Radiation Therapy
T Urinary System
0 Beam Radiation

Treatment Site	Modality Qualifier	Isotope	Qualifier
Character 4	Character 5	Character 6	Character 7
0 Kidney 1 Ureter 2 Bladder 3 Urethra	0 Photons <1 MeV 1 Photons 1 - 10 MeV 2 Photons >10 MeV 4 Heavy Particles (Protons, Ions) 5 Neutrons 6 Neutron Capture	Z None	Z None
0 Kidney 1 Ureter 2 Bladder 3 Urethra	3 Electrons	Z None	0 Intraoperative Z None

D Radiation Therapy
T Urinary System
1 Brachytherapy

Treatment Site	Modality Qualifier	Isotope	Qualifier
Character 4	Character 5	Character 6	Character 7
0 Kidney 1 Ureter 2 Bladder 3 Urethra	9 High Dose Rate (HDR) B Low Dose Rate (LDR)	7 Cesium 137 (Cs-137) 8 Iridium 192 (Ir-192) 9 Iodine 125 (I-125) B Palladium 103 (Pd-103) C Californium 252 (Cf-252) Y Other Isotope	Z None

D Radiation Therapy
T Urinary System
2 Stereotactic Radiosurgery

Treatment Site	Modality Qualifier	Isotope	Qualifier
Character 4	Character 5	Character 6	Character 7

0 Kidney Ⓓⓡⓖ
1 Ureter Ⓓⓡⓖ
2 Bladder Ⓓⓡⓖ
3 Urethra Ⓓⓡⓖ
	D Stereotactic Other Photon
	   Radiosurgery
	H Stereotactic Particulate
	   Radiosurgery
	J Stereotactic Gamma Beam
	   Radiosurgery
		Z None	Z None

ⓓⓡⓖ DT20DZZ   DT20HZZ   DT20JZZ   DT21DZZ   DT21HZZ   DT21JZZ   DT22DZZ   DT22HZZ   DT22JZZ   DT23DZZ   DT23HZZ   DT23JZZ

D Radiation Therapy
T Urinary System
Y Other Radiation

Treatment Site	Modality Qualifier	Isotope	Qualifier
Character 4	Character 5	Character 6	Character 7
0 Kidney 1 Ureter 2 Bladder 3 Urethra	7 Contact Radiation 8 Hyperthermia C Intraoperative Radiation Therapy (IORT) F Plaque Radiation	Z None	Z None

D Radiation Therapy
U Female Reproductive System
0 Beam Radiation

Treatment Site	Modality Qualifier	Isotope	Qualifier
Character 4	Character 5	Character 6	Character 7
0 Ovary ♀ 1 Cervix ♀ 2 Uterus ♀	0 Photons <1 MeV 1 Photons 1 - 10 MeV 2 Photons >10 MeV 4 Heavy Particles (Protons, Ions) 5 Neutrons 6 Neutron Capture	Z None	Z None
0 Ovary ♀ 1 Cervix ♀ 2 Uterus ♀	3 Electrons	Z None	0 Intraoperative Z None

♀ DU000ZZ   DU001ZZ   DU002ZZ   DU003Z0   DU003ZZ   DU004ZZ   DU005ZZ   DU006ZZ   DU010ZZ   DU011ZZ   DU012ZZ   DU013Z0   DU013ZZ
    DU014ZZ   DU015ZZ   DU016ZZ   DU020ZZ   DU021ZZ   DU022ZZ   DU023Z0   DU023ZZ   DU024ZZ   DU025ZZ   DU026ZZ

D Radiation Therapy
U Female Reproductive System
1 Brachytherapy

Treatment Site	Modality Qualifier	Isotope	Qualifier
Character 4	Character 5	Character 6	Character 7
0 Ovary ♀ 1 Cervix ♀ 2 Uterus ♀	9 High Dose Rate (HDR) B Low Dose Rate (LDR)	7 Cesium 137 (Cs-137) 8 Iridium 192 (Ir-192) 9 Iodine 125 (I-125) B Palladium 103 (Pd-103) C Californium 252 (Cf-252) Y Other Isotope	Z None

♀ DU1097Z   DU1098Z   DU1099Z   DU109BZ   DU109CZ   DU109YZ   DU10B7Z   DU10B8Z   DU10B9Z   DU10BBZ   DU10BCZ   DU10BYZ   DU1197Z
    DU1198Z   DU1199Z   DU119BZ   DU119CZ   DU119YZ   DU11B7Z   DU11B8Z   DU11B9Z   DU11BBZ   DU11BCZ   DU11BYZ   DU1297Z   DU1298Z
    DU1299Z   DU129BZ   DU129CZ   DU129YZ   DU12B7Z   DU12B8Z   DU12B9Z   DU12BBZ   DU12BCZ   DU12BYZ

D Radiation Therapy
U Female Reproductive System
2 Stereotactic Radiosurgery

Treatment Site	Modality Qualifier	Isotope	Qualifier
Character 4	Character 5	Character 6	Character 7

0 Ovary ♀ ᴅᴿɢ
1 Cervix ♀ ᴅᴿɢ
2 Uterus ♀ ᴅᴿɢ
	D Stereotactic Other Photon
	   Radiosurgery
	H Stereotactic Particulate
	   Radiosurgery
	J Stereotactic Gamma Beam
	   Radiosurgery
		Z None	Z None

♀   DU20DZZ   DU20HZZ   DU20JZZ   DU21DZZ   DU21HZZ   DU21JZZ   DU22DZZ   DU22HZZ   DU22JZZ
ᴅᴿɢ DU20DZZ   DU20HZZ   DU20JZZ   DU21DZZ   DU21HZZ   DU21JZZ   DU22DZZ   DU22HZZ   DU22JZZ

D Radiation Therapy
U Female Reproductive System
Y Other Radiation

Treatment Site	Modality Qualifier	Isotope	Qualifier
Character 4	Character 5	Character 6	Character 7
0 Ovary ♀ 1 Cervix ♀ 2 Uterus ♀	7 Contact Radiation 8 Hyperthermia C Intraoperative Radiation Therapy (IORT) F Plaque Radiation	Z None	Z None

♀ DUY07ZZ   DUY08ZZ   DUY0CZZ   DUY0FZZ   DUY17ZZ   DUY18ZZ   DUY1CZZ   DUY1FZZ   DUY27ZZ   DUY28ZZ   DUY2CZZ   DUY2FZZ

🄻🄲 Limited Coverage   🄽🄲 Noncovered   🄷🄰🄲 HAC-associated Procedure   🄲🄲 Combination Cluster - See Appendix G for code lists
ᴅᴿɢ Non-OR-Affecting MS-DRG Assignment   New/Revised Text in **Orange**   ♂ Male   ♀ Female

690   2018 ICD-10-PCS

D Radiation Therapy
V Male Reproductive System
0 Beam Radiation

Treatment Site	Modality Qualifier	Isotope	Qualifier
Character 4	Character 5	Character 6	Character 7
0 Prostate ♂ 1 Testis ♂	0 Photons <1 MeV 1 Photons 1 - 10 MeV 2 Photons >10 MeV 4 Heavy Particles (Protons, Ions) 5 Neutrons 6 Neutron Capture	Z None	Z None
0 Prostate ♂ 1 Testis ♂	3 Electrons	Z None	0 Intraoperative Z None

♂ DV000ZZ DV001ZZ DV002ZZ DV003Z0 DV003ZZ DV004ZZ DV005ZZ DV006ZZ DV010ZZ DV011ZZ DV012ZZ DV013Z0 DV013ZZ
  DV014ZZ DV015ZZ DV016ZZ

D Radiation Therapy
V Male Reproductive System
1 Brachytherapy

Treatment Site	Modality Qualifier	Isotope	Qualifier
Character 4	Character 5	Character 6	Character 7
0 Prostate ♂ 1 Testis ♂	9 High Dose Rate (HDR) B Low Dose Rate (LDR)	7 Cesium 137 (Cs-137) 8 Iridium 192 (Ir-192) 9 Iodine 125 (I-125) B Palladium 103 (Pd-103) C Californium 252 (Cf-252) Y Other Isotope	Z None

♂ DV1097Z DV1098Z DV1099Z DV109BZ DV109CZ DV109YZ DV10B7Z DV10B8Z DV10B9Z DV10BBZ DV10BCZ DV10BYZ DV1197Z
  DV1198Z DV1199Z DV119BZ DV119CZ DV119YZ DV11B7Z DV11B8Z DV11B9Z DV11BBZ DV11BCZ DV11BYZ

D Radiation Therapy
V Male Reproductive System
2 Stereotactic Radiosurgery

Treatment Site	Modality Qualifier	Isotope	Qualifier
Character 4	Character 5	Character 6	Character 7

0 Prostate ♂ DRG
1 Testis ♂ DRG
	D Stereotactic Other Photon
	   Radiosurgery
	H Stereotactic Particulate
	   Radiosurgery
	J Stereotactic Gamma Beam
	   Radiosurgery
		Z None	Z None

♂ DV20DZZ DV20HZZ DV20JZZ DV21DZZ DV21HZZ DV21JZZ
DRG DV20DZZ DV20HZZ DV20JZZ DV21DZZ DV21HZZ DV21JZZ

D Radiation Therapy
V Male Reproductive System
Y Other Radiation

Treatment Site	Modality Qualifier	Isotope	Qualifier
Character 4	Character 5	Character 6	Character 7

0 Prostate ♂	7 Contact Radiation
	8 Hyperthermia
	C Intraoperative Radiation
	   Therapy (IORT)
	F Plaque Radiation
	K Laser Interstitial Thermal
	   Therapy
		Z None	Z None

1 Testis ♂	7 Contact Radiation 8 Hyperthermia F Plaque Radiation	Z None	Z None

♂ DVY07ZZ DVY08ZZ DVY0CZZ DVY0FZZ DVY0KZZ DVY17ZZ DVY18ZZ DVY1FZZ

LC Limited Coverage   NC Noncovered   HAC HAC-associated Procedure   CC Combination Cluster - See Appendix G for code lists
DRG Non-OR-Affecting MS-DRG Assignment   New/Revised Text in Orange   ♂ Male   ♀ Female

D Radiation Therapy
W Anatomical Regions
0 Beam Radiation

Treatment Site	Modality Qualifier	Isotope	Qualifier
Character 4	**Character 5**	**Character 6**	**Character 7**
1 Head and Neck 2 Chest 3 Abdomen 4 Hemibody 5 Whole Body 6 Pelvic Region	0 Photons <1 MeV 1 Photons 1 - 10 MeV 2 Photons >10 MeV 4 Heavy Particles (Protons, Ions) 5 Neutrons 6 Neutron Capture	Z None	Z None
1 Head and Neck 2 Chest 3 Abdomen 4 Hemibody 5 Whole Body 6 Pelvic Region	3 Electrons	Z None	0 Intraoperative Z None

D Radiation Therapy
W Anatomical Regions
1 Brachytherapy

Treatment Site	Modality Qualifier	Isotope	Qualifier
Character 4	**Character 5**	**Character 6**	**Character 7**
1 Head and Neck 2 Chest 3 Abdomen 6 Pelvic Region	9 High Dose Rate (HDR) B Low Dose Rate (LDR)	7 Cesium 137 (Cs-137) 8 Iridium 192 (Ir-192) 9 Iodine 125 (I-125) B Palladium 103 (Pd-103) C Californium 252 (Cf-252) Y Other Isotope	Z None

D Radiation Therapy
W Anatomical Regions
2 Stereotactic Radiosurgery

Treatment Site	Modality Qualifier	Isotope	Qualifier
Character 4	**Character 5**	**Character 6**	**Character 7**
1 Head and Neck ᴰᴿᴳ 2 Chest ᴰᴿᴳ 3 Abdomen ᴰᴿᴳ 6 Pelvic Region ᴰᴿᴳ	D Stereotactic Other Photon 　Radiosurgery H Stereotactic Particulate 　Radiosurgery J Stereotactic Gamma Beam 　Radiosurgery	Z None	Z None

ᴰᴿᴳ　DW21DZZ　DW21HZZ　DW21JZZ　DW22DZZ　DW22HZZ　DW22JZZ　DW23DZZ　DW23HZZ　DW23JZZ　DW26DZZ　DW26HZZ　DW26JZZ

D Radiation Therapy
W Anatomical Regions
Y Other Radiation

Treatment Site	Modality Qualifier	Isotope	Qualifier
Character 4	**Character 5**	**Character 6**	**Character 7**
1 Head and Neck 2 Chest 3 Abdomen 4 Hemibody 6 Pelvic Region	7 Contact Radiation 8 Hyperthermia F Plaque Radiation	Z None	Z None
5 Whole Body	7 Contact Radiation 8 Hyperthermia F Plaque Radiation	Z None	Z None
5 Whole Body	G Isotope Administration	D Iodine 131 (I-131) F Phosphorus 32 (P-32) G Strontium 89 (Sr-89) H Strontium 90 (Sr-90) Y Other Isotope	Z None

ᴸᶜ Limited Coverage　ᴺᶜ Noncovered　ᴴᴬᶜ HAC-associated Procedure　ᶜᶜ Combination Cluster - See Appendix G for code lists
ᴰᴿᴳ Non-OR-Affecting MS-DRG Assignment　New/Revised Text in **Orange**　♂ Male　♀ Female

692　　　　　　　　　　　　　　　　　　　　　　　　　　　　**2018 ICD-10-PCS**

NOTES

NOTES

F   Physical Rehabilitation and Diagnostic Audiology
0   Rehabilitation
0   Speech Assessment: Measurement of speech and related functions

Body system/ Region	Type Qualifier	Equipment	Qualifier
Character 4	**Character 5**	**Character 6**	**Character 7**
3 Neurological System - Whole Body ᴰᴿᴳ	**G** Communicative/Cognitive Integration Skills	**K** Audiovisual **M** Augmentative / Alternative Communication **P** Computer **Y** Other Equipment **Z** None	**Z** None
Z None ᴰᴿᴳ	**0** Filtered Speech **3** Staggered Spondaic Word **Q** Performance Intensity Phonetically Balanced Speech Discrimination **R** Brief Tone Stimuli **S** Distorted Speech **T** Dichotic Stimuli **V** Temporal Ordering of Stimuli **W** Masking Patterns	**1** Audiometer **2** Sound Field / Booth **K** Audiovisual **Z** None	**Z** None
Z None ᴰᴿᴳ	**1** Speech Threshold **2** Speech/Word Recognition	**1** Audiometer **2** Sound Field / Booth **9** Cochlear Implant **K** Audiovisual **Z** None	**Z** None
Z None ᴰᴿᴳ	**4** Sensorineural Acuity Level	**1** Audiometer **2** Sound Field / Booth **Z** None	**Z** None
Z None ᴰᴿᴳ	**5** Synthetic Sentence Identification	**1** Audiometer **2** Sound Field / Booth **9** Cochlear Implant **K** Audiovisual	**Z** None
Z None ᴰᴿᴳ	**6** Speech and/or Language Screening **7** Nonspoken Language **8** Receptive/Expressive Language **C** Aphasia **G** Communicative/Cognitive Integration Skills **L** Augmentative/Alternative Communication System	**K** Audiovisual **M** Augmentative / Alternative Communication **P** Computer **Y** Other Equipment **Z** None	**Z** None
Z None ᴰᴿᴳ	**9** Articulation/Phonology	**K** Audiovisual **P** Computer **Q** Speech Analysis **Y** Other Equipment **Z** None	**Z** None
Z None ᴰᴿᴳ	**B** Motor Speech	**K** Audiovisual **N** Biosensory Feedback **P** Computer **Q** Speech Analysis **T** Aerodynamic Function **Y** Other Equipment **Z** None	**Z** None

F00 continued on next page

F Physical Rehabilitation and Diagnostic Audiology

F00 continued from previous page

0 Rehabilitation

0 Speech Assessment: Measurement of speech and related functions

Body system/ Region	Type Qualifier	Equipment	Qualifier
Character 4	Character 5	Character 6	Character 7
Z None ᴰᴿᴳ	D Fluency	K Audiovisual N Biosensory Feedback P Computer Q Speech Analysis S Voice Analysis T Aerodynamic Function Y Other Equipment Z None	Z None
Z None ᴰᴿᴳ	F Voice	K Audiovisual N Biosensory Feedback P Computer S Voice Analysis T Aerodynamic Function Y Other Equipment Z None	Z None
Z None ᴰᴿᴳ	H Bedside Swallowing and Oral Function P Oral Peripheral Mechanism	Y Other Equipment Z None	Z None
Z None ᴰᴿᴳ	J Instrumental Swallowing and Oral Function	T Aerodynamic Function W Swallowing Y Other Equipment	Z None
Z None ᴰᴿᴳ	K Orofacial Myofunctional	K Audiovisual P Computer Y Other Equipment Z None	Z None
Z None ᴰᴿᴳ	M Voice Prosthetic	K Audiovisual P Computer S Voice Analysis V Speech Prosthesis Y Other Equipment Z None	Z None
Z None ᴰᴿᴳ	N Non-invasive Instrumental Status	N Biosensory Feedback P Computer Q Speech Analysis S Voice Analysis T Aerodynamic Function Y Other Equipment	Z None
Z None ᴰᴿᴳ	X Other Specified Central Auditory Processing	Z None	Z None

ᴰᴿᴳ F003GKZ F003GMZ F003GPZ F003GYZ F003GZZ F00Z01Z F00Z02Z F00Z0KZ F00Z0ZZ F00Z11Z F00Z12Z F00Z19Z F00Z1KZ
F00Z1ZZ F00Z21Z F00Z22Z F00Z29Z F00Z2KZ F00Z2ZZ F00Z31Z F00Z32Z F00Z3KZ F00Z3ZZ F00Z41Z F00Z42Z F00Z4ZZ
F00Z51Z F00Z52Z F00Z59Z F00Z5KZ F00Z6KZ F00Z6MZ F00Z6PZ F00Z6YZ F00Z6ZZ F00Z7KZ F00Z7MZ F00Z7PZ F00Z7YZ
F00Z7ZZ F00Z8KZ F00Z8MZ F00Z8PZ F00Z8YZ F00Z8ZZ F00Z9KZ F00Z9PZ F00Z9QZ F00Z9YZ F00Z9ZZ F00ZBKZ F00ZBNZ
F00ZBPZ F00ZBQZ F00ZBTZ F00ZBYZ F00ZBZZ F00ZCKZ F00ZCMZ F00ZCPZ F00ZCYZ F00ZCZZ F00ZDKZ F00ZDNZ F00ZDPZ
F00ZDQZ F00ZDSZ F00ZDTZ F00ZDYZ F00ZDZZ F00ZFKZ F00ZFNZ F00ZFPZ F00ZFSZ F00ZFTZ F00ZFYZ F00ZFZZ F00ZGKZ
F00ZGMZ F00ZGPZ F00ZGYZ F00ZGZZ F00ZHYZ F00ZHZZ F00ZJTZ F00ZJWZ F00ZJYZ F00ZKKZ F00ZKPZ F00ZKYZ F00ZKZZ
F00ZLKZ F00ZLMZ F00ZLPZ F00ZLYZ F00ZLZZ F00ZMKZ F00ZMPZ F00ZMSZ F00ZMVZ F00ZMYZ F00ZMZZ F00ZNNZ F00ZNPZ
F00ZNQZ F00ZNSZ F00ZNTZ F00ZNYZ F00ZPYZ F00ZPZZ F00ZQ1Z F00ZQ2Z F00ZQKZ F00ZQZZ F00ZR1Z F00ZR2Z F00ZRKZ
F00ZRZZ F00ZS1Z F00ZS2Z F00ZSKZ F00ZSZZ F00ZT1Z F00ZT2Z F00ZTKZ F00ZTZZ F00ZV1Z F00ZV2Z F00ZVKZ F00ZVZZ
F00ZW1Z F00ZW2Z F00ZWKZ

F   **Physical Rehabilitation and Diagnostic Audiology**
0   **Rehabilitation**
1   **Motor and/or Nerve Function Assessment:** Measurement of motor, nerve, and related functions

Body system/ Region	Type Qualifier	Equipment	Qualifier
Character 4	Character 5	Character 6	Character 7
0 Neurological System - Head and Neck **1** Neurological System - Upper Back / Upper Extremity **2** Neurological System - Lower Back / Lower Extremity **3** Neurological System - Whole Body	**0** Muscle Performance	**E** Orthosis **F** Assistive, Adaptive, Supportive or Protective **U** Prosthesis **Y** Other Equipment **Z** None	**Z** None
0 Neurological System - Head and Neck **1** Neurological System - Upper Back / Upper Extremity **2** Neurological System - Lower Back / Lower Extremity **3** Neurological System - Whole Body	**1** Integumentary Integrity **3** Coordination/Dexterity **4** Motor Function **G** Reflex Integrity	**Z** None	**Z** None
0 Neurological System - Head and Neck **1** Neurological System - Upper Back / Upper Extremity **2** Neurological System - Lower Back / Lower Extremity **3** Neurological System - Whole Body	**5** Range of Motion and Joint Integrity **6** Sensory Awareness/Processing/ Integrity	**Y** Other Equipment **Z** None	**Z** None
D Integumentary System - Head and Neck **F** Integumentary System - Upper Back / Upper Extremity **G** Integumentary System - Lower Back / Lower Extremity **H** Integumentary System - Whole Body **J** Musculoskeletal System - Head and Neck **K** Musculoskeletal System - Upper Back / Upper Extremity **L** Musculoskeletal System - Lower Back / Lower Extremity **M** Musculoskeletal System - Whole Body	**0** Muscle Performance	**E** Orthosis **F** Assistive, Adaptive, Supportive or Protective **U** Prosthesis **Y** Other Equipment **Z** None	**Z** None
D Integumentary System - Head and Neck **F** Integumentary System - Upper Back / Upper Extremity **G** Integumentary System - Lower Back / Lower Extremity **H** Integumentary System - Whole Body **J** Musculoskeletal System - Head and Neck **K** Musculoskeletal System - Upper Back / Upper Extremity **L** Musculoskeletal System - Lower Back / Lower Extremity **M** Musculoskeletal System - Whole Body	**1** Integumentary Integrity	**Z** None	**Z** None

F01 continued on next page

LC Limited Coverage   NC Noncovered   HAC HAC-associated Procedure   CC Combination Cluster - See Appendix G for code lists
DRG Non-OR-Affecting MS-DRG Assignment   New/Revised Text in Orange   ♂ Male   ♀ Female

F   Physical Rehabilitation and Diagnostic Audiology   F01 continued from previous page
0   Rehabilitation
1   Motor and/or Nerve Function Assessment: Measurement of motor, nerve, and related functions

Body system/ Region	Type Qualifier	Equipment	Qualifier
Character 4	Character 5	Character 6	Character 7
D Integumentary System - Head and Neck **F** Integumentary System - Upper Back / Upper Extremity **G** Integumentary System - Lower Back / Lower Extremity **H** Integumentary System - Whole Body **J** Musculoskeletal System - Head and Neck **K** Musculoskeletal System - Upper Back / Upper Extremity **L** Musculoskeletal System - Lower Back / Lower Extremity **M** Musculoskeletal System - Whole Body	**5** Range of Motion and Joint Integrity **6** Sensory Awareness/Processing/ Integrity	**Y** Other Equipment **Z** None	**Z** None
N Genitourinary System	**0** Muscle Performance	**E** Orthosis **F** Assistive, Adaptive, Supportive or Protective **U** Prosthesis **Y** Other Equipment **Z** None	**Z** None
Z None	**2** Visual Motor Integration	**K** Audiovisual **M** Augmentative / Alternative Communication **N** Biosensory Feedback **P** Computer **Q** Speech Analysis **S** Voice Analysis **Y** Other Equipment **Z** None	**Z** None
Z None	**7** Facial Nerve Function	**7** Electrophysiologic	**Z** None
Z None	**9** Somatosensory Evoked Potentials	**J** Somatosensory	**Z** None
Z None	**B** Bed Mobility **C** Transfer **F** Wheelchair Mobility	**E** Orthosis **F** Assistive, Adaptive, Supportive or Protective **U** Prosthesis **Z** None	**Z** None
Z None	**D** Gait and/or Balance	**E** Orthosis **F** Assistive, Adaptive, Supportive or Protective **U** Prosthesis **Y** Other Equipment **Z** None	**Z** None

---

LC Limited Coverage   **NC** Noncovered   **HAC** HAC-associated Procedure   **CC** Combination Cluster - See Appendix G for code lists
DRG Non-OR-Affecting MS-DRG Assignment   New/Revised Text in **Orange**   ♂ Male   ♀ Female

698   **2018 ICD-10-PCS**

F Physical Rehabilitation and Diagnostic Audiology
0 Rehabilitation
2 Activities of Daily Living Assessment: Measurement of functional level for activities of daily living

Body system/ Region	Type Qualifier	Equipment	Qualifier
Character 4	Character 5	Character 6	Character 7
0 Neurological System - Head and Neck	**9** Cranial Nerve Integrity **D** Neuromotor Development	**Y** Other Equipment **Z** None	**Z** None
1 Neurological System - Upper Back / Upper Extremity **2** Neurological System - Lower Back / Lower Extremity **3** Neurological System - Whole Body	**D** Neuromotor Development	**Y** Other Equipment **Z** None	**Z** None
4 Circulatory System - Head and Neck **5** Circulatory System - Upper Back / Upper Extremity **6** Circulatory System - Lower Back / Lower Extremity **8** Respiratory System - Head and Neck **9** Respiratory System - Upper Back / Upper Extremity **B** Respiratory System - Lower Back / Lower Extremity	**G** Ventilation, Respiration and Circulation	**C** Mechanical **G** Aerobic Endurance and Conditioning **Y** Other Equipment **Z** None	**Z** None
7 Circulatory System - Whole Body **C** Respiratory System - Whole Body	**7** Aerobic Capacity and Endurance	**E** Orthosis **G** Aerobic Endurance and Conditioning **U** Prosthesis **Y** Other Equipment **Z** None	**Z** None
7 Circulatory System - Whole Body **C** Respiratory System - Whole Body	**G** Ventilation, Respiration and Circulation	**C** Mechanical **G** Aerobic Endurance and Conditioning **Y** Other Equipment **Z** None	**Z** None
Z None	**0** Bathing/Showering **1** Dressing **3** Grooming/Personal Hygiene **4** Home Management	**E** Orthosis **F** Assistive, Adaptive, Supportive or Protective **U** Prosthesis **Z** None	**Z** None
Z None	**2** Feeding/Eating **8** Anthropometric Characteristics **F** Pain	**Y** Other Equipment **Z** None	**Z** None
Z None	**5** Perceptual Processing	**K** Audiovisual **M** Augmentative / Alternative Communication **N** Biosensory Feedback **P** Computer **Q** Speech Analysis **S** Voice Analysis **Y** Other Equipment **Z** None	**Z** None
Z None	**6** Psychosocial Skills	**Z** None	**Z** None
Z None	**B** Environmental, Home and Work Barriers **C** Ergonomics and Body Mechanics	**E** Orthosis **F** Assistive, Adaptive, Supportive or Protective **U** Prosthesis **Y** Other Equipment **Z** None	**Z** None

F02 continued on next page

F Physical Rehabilitation and Diagnostic Audiology
0 Rehabilitation
2 Activities of Daily Living Assessment: Measurement of functional level for activities of daily living

F02 continued from previous page

Body system/ Region	Type Qualifier	Equipment	Qualifier
Character 4	**Character 5**	**Character 6**	**Character 7**
Z None	**H** Vocational Activities and Functional Community or Work Reintegration Skills	**E** Orthosis **F** Assistive, Adaptive, Supportive or Protective **G** Aerobic Endurance and Conditioning **U** Prosthesis **Y** Other Equipment **Z** None	**Z** None

F Physical Rehabilitation and Diagnostic Audiology
0 Rehabilitation
6 Speech Treatment: Application of techniques to improve, augment, or compensate for speech and related functional impairment

Body system/ Region	Type Qualifier	Equipment	Qualifier
Character 4	**Character 5**	**Character 6**	**Character 7**
3 Neurological System - Whole Body	**6** Communicative/Cognitive Integration Skills	**K** Audiovisual **M** Augmentative / Alternative Communication **P** Computer **Y** Other Equipment **Z** None	**Z** None
Z None	**0** Nonspoken Language **3** Aphasia **6** Communicative/Cognitive Integration Skills	**K** Audiovisual **M** Augmentative / Alternative Communication **P** Computer **Y** Other Equipment **Z** None	**Z** None
Z None	**1** Speech-Language Pathology and Related Disorders Counseling **2** Speech-Language Pathology and Related Disorders Prevention	**K** Audiovisual **Z** None	**Z** None
Z None	**4** Articulation/Phonology	**K** Audiovisual **P** Computer **Q** Speech Analysis **T** Aerodynamic Function **Y** Other Equipment **Z** None	**Z** None
Z None	**5** Aural Rehabilitation	**K** Audiovisual **L** Assistive Listening **M** Augmentative / Alternative Communication **N** Biosensory Feedback **P** Computer **Q** Speech Analysis **S** Voice Analysis **Y** Other Equipment **Z** None	**Z** None
Z None	**7** Fluency	**4** Electroacoustic Immittance / Acoustic Reflex **K** Audiovisual **N** Biosensory Feedback **Q** Speech Analysis **S** Voice Analysis **T** Aerodynamic Function **Y** Other Equipment **Z** None	**Z** None

F06 continued on next page

LC Limited Coverage   NC Noncovered   HAC HAC-associated Procedure   CC Combination Cluster - See Appendix G for code lists
DRG Non-OR-Affecting MS-DRG Assignment   New/Revised Text in **Orange**   ♂ Male   ♀ Female

F   **Physical Rehabilitation and Diagnostic Audiology**
0   **Rehabilitation**
6   **Speech Treatment:** Application of techniques to improve, augment, or compensate for speech and related functional impairment

F06 continued from previous page

Body system/ Region		Type Qualifier		Equipment		Qualifier	
Character 4		**Character 5**		**Character 6**		**Character 7**	
Z	None	**8**	Motor Speech	**K** **N** **P** **Q** **S** **T** **Y** **Z**	Audiovisual Biosensory Feedback Computer Speech Analysis Voice Analysis Aerodynamic Function Other Equipment None	**Z**	None
Z	None	**9**	Orofacial Myofunctional	**K** **P** **Y** **Z**	Audiovisual Computer Other Equipment None	**Z**	None
Z	None	**B**	Receptive/Expressive Language	**K** **L** **M** **P** **Y** **Z**	Audiovisual Assistive Listening Augmentative / Alternative Communication Computer Other Equipment None	**Z**	None
Z	None	**C**	Voice	**K** **N** **P** **S** **T** **V** **Y** **Z**	Audiovisual Biosensory Feedback Computer Voice Analysis Aerodynamic Function Speech Prosthesis Other Equipment None	**Z**	None
Z	None	**D**	Swallowing Dysfunction	**M** **T** **V** **Y** **Z**	Augmentative / Alternative Communication Aerodynamic Function Speech Prosthesis Other Equipment None	**Z**	None

F Physical Rehabilitation and Diagnostic Audiology
0 Rehabilitation
7 Motor Treatment: Exercise or activities to increase or facilitate motor function

Body system/ Region	Type Qualifier	Equipment	Qualifier
Character 4	**Character 5**	**Character 6**	**Character 7**
0 Neurological System - Head and Neck **1** Neurological System - Upper Back / Upper Extremity **2** Neurological System - Lower Back / Lower Extremity **3** Neurological System - Whole Body **D** Integumentary System - Head and Neck **F** Integumentary System - Upper Back / Upper Extremity **G** Integumentary System - Lower Back / Lower Extremity **H** Integumentary System - Whole Body **J** Musculoskeletal System - Head and Neck **K** Musculoskeletal System - Upper Back / Upper Extremity **L** Musculoskeletal System - Lower Back / Lower Extremity **M** Musculoskeletal System - Whole Body	**0** Range of Motion and Joint Mobility **1** Muscle Performance **2** Coordination/Dexterity **3** Motor Function	**E** Orthosis **F** Assistive, Adaptive, Supportive or Protective **U** Prosthesis **Y** Other Equipment **Z** None	**Z** None
0 Neurological System - Head and Neck **1** Neurological System - Upper Back / Upper Extremity **2** Neurological System - Lower Back / Lower Extremity **3** Neurological System - Whole Body **D** Integumentary System - Head and Neck **F** Integumentary System - Upper Back / Upper Extremity **G** Integumentary System - Lower Back / Lower Extremity **H** Integumentary System - Whole Body **J** Musculoskeletal System - Head and Neck **K** Musculoskeletal System - Upper Back / Upper Extremity **L** Musculoskeletal System - Lower Back / Lower Extremity **M** Musculoskeletal System - Whole Body	**6** Therapeutic Exercise	**B** Physical Agents **C** Mechanical **D** Electrotherapeutic **E** Orthosis **F** Assistive, Adaptive, Supportive or Protective **G** Aerobic Endurance and Conditioning **H** Mechanical or Electromechanical **U** Prosthesis **Y** Other Equipment **Z** None	**Z** None

F07 continued on next page

F **Physical Rehabilitation and Diagnostic Audiology**
0 **Rehabilitation**
7 **Motor Treatment:** Exercise or activities to increase or facilitate motor function

F07 continued from previous page

Body system/ Region	Type Qualifier	Equipment	Qualifier
Character 4	**Character 5**	**Character 6**	**Character 7**
0 Neurological System - Head and Neck 1 Neurological System - Upper Back / Upper Extremity 2 Neurological System - Lower Back / Lower Extremity 3 Neurological System - Whole Body D Integumentary System - Head and Neck F Integumentary System - Upper Back / Upper Extremity G Integumentary System - Lower Back / Lower Extremity H Integumentary System - Whole Body J Musculoskeletal System - Head and Neck K Musculoskeletal System - Upper Back / Upper Extremity L Musculoskeletal System - Lower Back / Lower Extremity M Musculoskeletal System - Whole Body	7 Manual Therapy Techniques	Z None	Z None
4 Circulatory System - Head and Neck 5 Circulatory System - Upper Back / Upper Extremity 6 Circulatory System - Lower Back / Lower Extremity 7 Circulatory System - Whole Body 8 Respiratory System - Head and Neck 9 Respiratory System - Upper Back / Upper Extremity B Respiratory System - Lower Back / Lower Extremity C Respiratory System - Whole Body	6 Therapeutic Exercise	B Physical Agents C Mechanical D Electrotherapeutic E Orthosis F Assistive, Adaptive, Supportive or Protective G Aerobic Endurance and Conditioning H Mechanical or Electromechanical U Prosthesis Y Other Equipment Z None	Z None
N Genitourinary System	1 Muscle Performance	E Orthosis F Assistive, Adaptive, Supportive or Protective U Prosthesis Y Other Equipment Z None	Z None
N Genitourinary System ᴰᴿᴳ	6 Therapeutic Exercise	B Physical Agents C Mechanical D Electrotherapeutic E Orthosis F Assistive, Adaptive, Supportive or Protective G Aerobic Endurance and Conditioning H Mechanical or Electromechanical U Prosthesis Y Other Equipment Z None	Z None

F07 continued on next page

F Physical Rehabilitation and Diagnostic Audiology   F07 continued from previous page
0 Rehabilitation
7 Motor Treatment: Exercise or activities to increase or facilitate motor function

Body system/ Region	Type Qualifier	Equipment	Qualifier
Character 4	Character 5	Character 6	Character 7
Z None ᴰᴿᴳ	4 Wheelchair Mobility	D Electrotherapeutic E Orthosis F Assistive, Adaptive, Supportive or Protective U Prosthesis Y Other Equipment Z None	Z None
Z None ᴰᴿᴳ	5 Bed Mobility	C Mechanical E Orthosis F Assistive, Adaptive, Supportive or Protective U Prosthesis Y Other Equipment Z None	Z None
Z None ᴰᴿᴳ	8 Transfer Training	C Mechanical D Electrotherapeutic E Orthosis F Assistive, Adaptive, Supportive or Protective U Prosthesis Y Other Equipment Z None	Z None

Z None ᴰᴿᴳ	9 Gait Training/Functional
	   Ambulation
		C Mechanical
		D Electrotherapeutic
		E Orthosis
		F Assistive, Adaptive, Supportive
		   or Protective
		G Aerobic Endurance and
		   Conditioning
		U Prosthesis
		Y Other Equipment
		Z None
			Z None

ᴰᴿᴳ F07N6BZ   F07N6CZ   F07N6DZ   F07N6EZ   F07N6FZ   F07N6GZ   F07N6HZ   F07N6UZ   F07N6YZ   F07N6ZZ   F07Z4DZ   F07Z4EZ   F07Z4FZ
   F07Z4UZ   F07Z4YZ   F07Z4ZZ   F07Z5CZ   F07Z5EZ   F07Z5FZ   F07Z5UZ   F07Z5YZ   F07Z5ZZ   F07Z8CZ   F07Z8DZ   F07Z8EZ   F07Z8FZ
   F07Z8UZ   F07Z8YZ   F07Z8ZZ   F07Z9CZ   F07Z9DZ   F07Z9EZ   F07Z9FZ   F07Z9GZ   F07Z9UZ   F07Z9YZ   F07Z9ZZ

F Physical Rehabilitation and Diagnostic Audiology
0 Rehabilitation
8 Activities of Daily Living Treatment: Exercise or activities to facilitate functional competence for activities of daily living

Body system/ Region	Type Qualifier	Equipment	Qualifier
Character 4	Character 5	Character 6	Character 7

D Integumentary System - Head
   and Neck ᴰᴿᴳ
F Integumentary System - Upper
   Back / Upper Extremity ᴰᴿᴳ
G Integumentary System - Lower
   Back / Lower Extremity ᴰᴿᴳ
H Integumentary System - Whole
   Body ᴰᴿᴳ
J Musculoskeletal System - Head
   and Neck ᴰᴿᴳ
K Musculoskeletal System - Upper
   Back / Upper Extremity ᴰᴿᴳ
L Musculoskeletal System - Lower
   Back / Lower Extremity ᴰᴿᴳ
M Musculoskeletal System - Whole
   Body ᴰᴿᴳ
	5 Wound Management	B Physical Agents
		C Mechanical
		D Electrotherapeutic
		E Orthosis
		F Assistive, Adaptive, Supportive
		   or Protective
		U Prosthesis
		Y Other Equipment
		Z None
			Z None

F08 continued on next page

F Physical Rehabilitation and Diagnostic Audiology
0 Rehabilitation
8 Activities of Daily Living Treatment: Exercise or activities to facilitate functional competence for activities of daily living

F08 continued from previous page

Body system/ Region	Type Qualifier	Equipment	Qualifier
Character 4	Character 5	Character 6	Character 7
Z None ᴼᴿᴳ	**0** Bathing/Showering Techniques **1** Dressing Techniques **2** Grooming/Personal Hygiene	**E** Orthosis **F** Assistive, Adaptive, Supportive or Protective **U** Prosthesis **Y** Other Equipment **Z** None	**Z** None
Z None ᴼᴿᴳ	**3** Feeding/Eating	**C** Mechanical **D** Electrotherapeutic **E** Orthosis **F** Assistive, Adaptive, Supportive or Protective **U** Prosthesis **Y** Other Equipment **Z** None	**Z** None
Z None ᴼᴿᴳ	**4** Home Management	**D** Electrotherapeutic **E** Orthosis **F** Assistive, Adaptive, Supportive or Protective **U** Prosthesis **Y** Other Equipment **Z** None	**Z** None
Z None ᴼᴿᴳ	**6** Psychosocial Skills	**Z** None	**Z** None
Z None ᴼᴿᴳ	**7** Vocational Activities and Functional Community or Work Reintegration Skills	**B** Physical Agents **C** Mechanical **D** Electrotherapeutic **E** Orthosis **F** Assistive, Adaptive, Supportive or Protective **G** Aerobic Endurance and Conditioning **U** Prosthesis **Y** Other Equipment **Z** None	**Z** None

ᴼᴿᴳ F08D5BZ F08D5CZ F08D5DZ F08D5EZ F08D5FZ F08D5UZ F08D5YZ F08D5ZZ F08F5BZ F08F5CZ F08F5DZ F08F5EZ F08F5FZ
F08F5UZ F08F5YZ F08F5ZZ F08G5BZ F08G5CZ F08G5DZ F08G5EZ F08G5FZ F08G5UZ F08G5YZ F08G5ZZ F08H5BZ F08H5CZ
F08H5DZ F08H5EZ F08H5FZ F08H5UZ F08H5YZ F08H5ZZ F08J5BZ F08J5CZ F08J5DZ F08J5EZ F08J5FZ F08J5UZ F08J5YZ
F08J5ZZ F08K5BZ F08K5CZ F08K5DZ F08K5EZ F08K5FZ F08K5UZ F08K5YZ F08K5ZZ F08L5BZ F08L5CZ F08L5DZ F08L5EZ
F08L5FZ F08L5UZ F08L5YZ F08L5ZZ F08M5BZ F08M5CZ F08M5DZ F08M5EZ F08M5FZ F08M5UZ F08M5YZ F08M5ZZ F08Z0EZ
F08Z0FZ F08Z0UZ F08Z0YZ F08Z0ZZ F08Z1EZ F08Z1FZ F08Z1UZ F08Z1YZ F08Z1ZZ F08Z2EZ F08Z2FZ F08Z2UZ F08Z2YZ
F08Z2ZZ F08Z3CZ F08Z3DZ F08Z3EZ F08Z3FZ F08Z3UZ F08Z3YZ F08Z3ZZ F08Z4DZ F08Z4EZ F08Z4FZ F08Z4UZ F08Z4YZ
F08Z4ZZ F08Z6ZZ F08Z7BZ F08Z7CZ F08Z7DZ F08Z7EZ F08Z7FZ F08Z7GZ F08Z7UZ F08Z7YZ F08Z7ZZ

F Physical Rehabilitation and Diagnostic Audiology
0 Rehabilitation
9 Hearing Treatment: Application of techniques to improve, augment, or compensate for hearing and related functional impairment

Body system/ Region	Type Qualifier	Equipment	Qualifier
Character 4	Character 5	Character 6	Character 7
Z None ᴼᴿᴳ	**0** Hearing and Related Disorders Counseling **1** Hearing and Related Disorders Prevention	**K** Audiovisual **Z** None	**Z** None
Z None ᴼᴿᴳ	**2** Auditory Processing	**K** Audiovisual **L** Assistive Listening **P** Computer **Y** Other Equipment **Z** None	**Z** None
Z None ᴼᴿᴳ	**3** Cerumen Management	**X** Cerumen Management **Z** None	**Z** None

ᴼᴿᴳ F09Z0KZ F09Z0ZZ F09Z1KZ F09Z1ZZ F09Z2KZ F09Z2LZ F09Z2PZ F09Z2YZ F09Z2ZZ F09Z3XZ F09Z3ZZ

F Physical Rehabilitation and Diagnostic Audiology
0 Rehabilitation
B Cochlear Implant Treatment: Application of techniques to improve the communication abilities of individuals with cochlear implant

Body system/ Region	Type Qualifier	Equipment	Qualifier
Character 4	Character 5	Character 6	Character 7
Z None ᴅᴿɢ	0 Cochlear Implant Rehabilitation	1 Audiometer 2 Sound Field / Booth 9 Cochlear Implant K Audiovisual P Computer Y Other Equipment	Z None

ᴅᴿɢ F0BZ01Z   F0BZ02Z   F0BZ09Z   F0BZ0KZ   F0BZ0PZ   F0BZ0YZ

F Physical Rehabilitation and Diagnostic Audiology
0 Rehabilitation
C Vestibular Treatment: Application of techniques to improve, augment, or compensate for vestibular and related functional impairment

Body system/ Region	Type Qualifier	Equipment	Qualifier
Character 4	Character 5	Character 6	Character 7
3 Neurological System - Whole Body ᴅᴿɢ H Integumentary System - Whole Body ᴅᴿɢ M Musculoskeletal System - Whole Body ᴅᴿɢ	3 Postural Control	E Orthosis F Assistive, Adaptive, Supportive or Protective U Prosthesis Y Other Equipment Z None	Z None
Z None ᴅᴿɢ	0 Vestibular	8 Vestibular / Balance Z None	Z None
Z None ᴅᴿɢ	1 Perceptual Processing 2 Visual Motor Integration	K Audiovisual L Assistive Listening N Biosensory Feedback P Computer Q Speech Analysis S Voice Analysis T Aerodynamic Function Y Other Equipment Z None	Z None

ᴅᴿɢ F0C33EZ   F0C33FZ   F0C33UZ   F0C33YZ   F0C33ZZ   F0CH3EZ   F0CH3FZ   F0CH3UZ   F0CH3YZ   F0CH3ZZ   F0CM3EZ   F0CM3FZ   F0CM3UZ
F0CM3YZ   F0CM3ZZ   F0CZ08Z   F0CZ0ZZ   F0CZ1KZ   F0CZ1LZ   F0CZ1NZ   F0CZ1PZ   F0CZ1QZ   F0CZ1SZ   F0CZ1TZ   F0CZ1YZ   F0CZ1ZZ
F0CZ2KZ   F0CZ2LZ   F0CZ2NZ   F0CZ2PZ   F0CZ2QZ   F0CZ2SZ   F0CZ2TZ   F0CZ2YZ   F0CZ2ZZ

F Physical Rehabilitation and Diagnostic Audiology
0 Rehabilitation
D Device Fitting: Fitting of a device designed to facilitate or support achievement of a higher level of function

Body system/ Region	Type Qualifier	Equipment	Qualifier
Character 4	Character 5	Character 6	Character 7
Z None ᴅᴿɢ	0 Tinnitus Masker	5 Hearing Aid Selection / Fitting / Test Z None	Z None
Z None ᴅᴿɢ	1 Monaural Hearing Aid 2 Binaural Hearing Aid 5 Assistive Listening Device	1 Audiometer 2 Sound Field / Booth 5 Hearing Aid Selection / Fitting / Test K Audiovisual L Assistive Listening Z None	Z None
Z None ᴅᴿɢ	3 Augmentative/Alternative Communication System	M Augmentative / Alternative Communication	Z None
Z None ᴅᴿɢ	4 Voice Prosthetic	S Voice Analysis V Speech Prosthesis	Z None
Z None ᴅᴿɢ	6 Dynamic Orthosis 7 Static Orthosis 8 Prosthesis 9 Assistive, Adaptive, Supportive or Protective Devices	E Orthosis F Assistive, Adaptive, Supportive or Protective U Prosthesis Z None	Z None

F0D continued on next page

ᴸᶜ Limited Coverage   ᴺᶜ Noncovered   ᴴᴬᶜ HAC-associated Procedure   ᶜᶜ Combination Cluster - See Appendix G for code lists
ᴅᴿɢ Non-OR-Affecting MS-DRG Assignment   New/Revised Text in **Orange**   ♂ Male   ♀ Female

706 **2018 ICD-10-PCS**

ᴰᴿᴳ FODZ05Z   FODZ0ZZ   FODZ11Z   FODZ12Z   FODZ15Z   FODZ1KZ   FODZ1LZ   FODZ1ZZ   FODZ21Z   FODZ22Z   FODZ25Z   FODZ2KZ   FODZ2LZ
    FODZ2ZZ   FODZ3MZ   FODZ4SZ   FODZ4VZ   FODZ51Z   FODZ52Z   FODZ55Z   FODZ5KZ   FODZ5LZ   FODZ5ZZ   FODZ6EZ   FODZ6FZ   FODZ6UZ
    FODZ6ZZ   FODZ7EZ   FODZ7FZ   FODZ7UZ   FODZ7ZZ   FODZ8EZ   FODZ8FZ   FODZ8UZ

F   Physical Rehabilitation and Diagnostic Audiology
0   Rehabilitation
F   Caregiver Training: Training in activities to support patient's optimal level of function

Body system/ Region	Type Qualifier	Equipment	Qualifier
Character 4	Character 5	Character 6	Character 7
Z None ᴰᴿᴳ	**0** Bathing/Showering Technique **1** Dressing **2** Feeding and Eating **3** Grooming/Personal Hygiene **4** Bed Mobility **5** Transfer **6** Wheelchair Mobility **7** Therapeutic Exercise **8** Airway Clearance Techniques **9** Wound Management **B** Vocational Activities and Functional Community or Work Reintegration Skills **C** Gait Training/Functional Ambulation **D** Application, Proper Use and Care of Devices **F** Application, Proper Use and Care of Orthoses **G** Application, Proper Use and Care of Prosthesis **H** Home Management	**E** Orthosis **F** Assistive, Adaptive, Supportive or Protective **U** Prosthesis **Z** None	**Z** None
Z None ᴰᴿᴳ	**J** Communication Skills	**K** Audiovisual **L** Assistive Listening **M** Augmentative / Alternative Communication **P** Computer **Z** None	**Z** None

ᴰᴿᴳ FOFZ0EZ   FOFZ0FZ   FOFZ0UZ   FOFZ0ZZ   FOFZ1EZ   FOFZ1FZ   FOFZ1UZ   FOFZ1ZZ   FOFZ2EZ   FOFZ2FZ   FOFZ2UZ   FOFZ2ZZ   FOFZ3EZ
    FOFZ3FZ   FOFZ3UZ   FOFZ3ZZ   FOFZ4EZ   FOFZ4FZ   FOFZ4UZ   FOFZ4ZZ   FOFZ5EZ   FOFZ5FZ   FOFZ5UZ   FOFZ5ZZ   FOFZ6EZ   FOFZ6FZ
    FOFZ6UZ   FOFZ6ZZ   FOFZ7EZ   FOFZ7FZ   FOFZ7UZ   FOFZ7ZZ   FOFZ8EZ   FOFZ8FZ   FOFZ8UZ   FOFZ8ZZ   FOFZ9EZ   FOFZ9FZ   FOFZ9UZ
    FOFZ9ZZ   FOFZBEZ   FOFZBFZ   FOFZBUZ   FOFZBZZ   FOFZCEZ   FOFZCFZ   FOFZCUZ   FOFZCZZ   FOFZDEZ   FOFZDFZ   FOFZDUZ   FOFZDZZ
    FOFZFEZ   FOFZFFZ   FOFZFUZ   FOFZFZZ   FOFZGEZ   FOFZGFZ   FOFZGUZ   FOFZGZZ   FOFZHEZ   FOFZHFZ   FOFZHUZ   FOFZHZZ   FOFZJKZ
    FOFZJLZ   FOFZJMZ   FOFZJPZ   FOFZJZZ

F   Physical Rehabilitation and Diagnostic Audiology
1   Diagnostic Audiology
3   Hearing Assessment: Measurement of hearing and related functions

Body system/ Region	Type Qualifier	Equipment	Qualifier
Character 4	Character 5	Character 6	Character 7
Z None	**0** Hearing Screening	**0** Occupational Hearing **1** Audiometer **2** Sound Field / Booth **3** Tympanometer **8** Vestibular / Balance **9** Cochlear Implant **Z** None	**Z** None
Z None	**1** Pure Tone Audiometry, Air **2** Pure Tone Audiometry, Air and Bone	**0** Occupational Hearing **1** Audiometer **2** Sound Field / Booth **Z** None	**Z** None

F13 continued on next page

F Physical Rehabilitation and Diagnostic Audiology
1 Diagnostic Audiology
3 Hearing Assessment: Measurement of hearing and related functions

F13 continued from previous page

Body system/ Region	Type Qualifier	Equipment	Qualifier
Character 4	**Character 5**	**Character 6**	**Character 7**
Z None	**3** Bekesy Audiometry **6** Visual Reinforcement Audiometry **9** Short Increment Sensitivity Index **B** Stenger **C** Pure Tone Stenger	**1** Audiometer **2** Sound Field / Booth **Z** None	**Z** None
Z None	**4** Conditioned Play Audiometry **5** Select Picture Audiometry	**1** Audiometer **2** Sound Field / Booth **K** Audiovisual **Z** None	**Z** None
Z None	**7** Alternate Binaural or Monaural Loudness Balance	**1** Audiometer **K** Audiovisual **Z** None	**Z** None
Z None	**8** Tone Decay **D** Tympanometry **F** Eustachian Tube Function **G** Acoustic Reflex Patterns **H** Acoustic Reflex Threshold **J** Acoustic Reflex Decay	**3** Tympanometer **4** Electroacoustic Immittance / Acoustic Reflex **Z** None	**Z** None
Z None	**K** Electrocochleography **L** Auditory Evoked Potentials	**7** Electrophysiologic **Z** None	**Z** None
Z None	**M** Evoked Otoacoustic Emissions, Screening **N** Evoked Otoacoustic Emissions, Diagnostic	**6** Otoacoustic Emission (OAE) **Z** None	**Z** None
Z None	**P** Aural Rehabilitation Status	**1** Audiometer **2** Sound Field / Booth **4** Electroacoustic Immittance / Acoustic Reflex **9** Cochlear Implant **K** Audiovisual **L** Assistive Listening **P** Computer **Z** None	**Z** None
Z None	**Q** Auditory Processing	**K** Audiovisual **P** Computer **Y** Other Equipment **Z** None	**Z** None

LC Limited Coverage   NC Noncovered   HAC HAC-associated Procedure   CC Combination Cluster - See Appendix G for code lists
DRG Non-OR-Affecting MS-DRG Assignment   New/Revised Text in **Orange**   ♂ Male   ♀ Female

708

2018 ICD-10-PCS

F **Physical Rehabilitation and Diagnostic Audiology**
1 **Diagnostic Audiology**
4 **Hearing Aid Assessment:** Measurement of the appropriateness and/or effectiveness of a hearing device

Body system/ Region	Type Qualifier	Equipment	Qualifier
Character 4	Character 5	Character 6	Character 7
Z None	0 Cochlear Implant	1 Audiometer 2 Sound Field / Booth 3 Tympanometer 4 Electroacoustic Immittance / Acoustic Reflex 5 Hearing Aid Selection / Fitting / Test 7 Electrophysiologic 9 Cochlear Implant K Audiovisual L Assistive Listening P Computer Y Other Equipment Z None	Z None
Z None	1 Ear Canal Probe Microphone 6 Binaural Electroacoustic Hearing Aid Check 8 Monaural Electroacoustic Hearing Aid Check	5 Hearing Aid Selection / Fitting / Test Z None	Z None
Z None	2 Monaural Hearing Aid 3 Binaural Hearing Aid	1 Audiometer 2 Sound Field / Booth 3 Tympanometer 4 Electroacoustic Immittance / Acoustic Reflex 5 Hearing Aid Selection / Fitting / Test K Audiovisual L Assistive Listening P Computer Z None	Z None
Z None	4 Assistive Listening System/ Device Selection	1 Audiometer 2 Sound Field / Booth 3 Tympanometer 4 Electroacoustic Immittance / Acoustic Reflex K Audiovisual L Assistive Listening Z None	Z None
Z None	5 Sensory Aids	1 Audiometer 2 Sound Field / Booth 3 Tympanometer 4 Electroacoustic Immittance / Acoustic Reflex 5 Hearing Aid Selection / Fitting / Test K Audiovisual L Assistive Listening Z None	Z None
Z None	7 Ear Protector Attenuation	0 Occupational Hearing Z None	Z None

F   Physical Rehabilitation and Diagnostic Audiology
1   Diagnostic Audiology
5   Vestibular Assessment: Measurement of the vestibular system and related functions

Body system/ Region	Type Qualifier	Equipment	Qualifier
Character 4	Character 5	Character 6	Character 7
Z None	**0** Bithermal, Binaural Caloric Irrigation **1** Bithermal, Monaural Caloric Irrigation **2** Unithermal Binaural Screen **3** Oscillating Tracking **4** Sinusoidal Vertical Axis Rotational **5** Dix-Hallpike Dynamic **6** Computerized Dynamic Posturography	**8** Vestibular / Balance **Z** None	**Z** None
Z None	**7** Tinnitus Masker	**5** Hearing Aid Selection / Fitting / Test **Z** None	**Z** None

LC Limited Coverage   NC Noncovered   HAC HAC-associated Procedure   CC Combination Cluster - See Appendix G for code lists
DRG Non-OR-Affecting MS-DRG Assignment   New/Revised Text in **Orange**   ♂ Male   ♀ Female

710

2018 ICD-10-PCS

NOTES

NOTES

Mental Health GZ1-GZJ

G Mental Health
Z None
1 **Psychological Tests:** The administration and interpretation of standardized psychological tests and measurement instruments for the assessment of psychological function

Qualifier	Qualifier	Qualifier	Qualifier
Character 4	Character 5	Character 6	Character 7
0 Developmental **1** Personality and Behavioral **2** Intellectual and Psychoeducational **3** Neuropsychological **4** Neurobehavioral and Cognitive Status	**Z** None	**Z** None	**Z** None

G Mental Health
Z None
2 **Crisis Intervention:** Treatment of a traumatized, acutely disturbed or distressed individual for the purpose of short-term stabilization

Qualifier	Qualifier	Qualifier	Qualifier
Character 4	Character 5	Character 6	Character 7
Z None	**Z** None	**Z** None	**Z** None

G Mental Health
Z None
3 **Medication Management:** Monitoring and adjusting the use of medications for the treatment of a mental health disorder

Qualifier	Qualifier	Qualifier	Qualifier
Character 4	Character 5	Character 6	Character 7
Z None	**Z** None	**Z** None	**Z** None

G Mental Health
Z None
5 **Individual Psychotherapy:** Treatment of an individual with a mental health disorder by behavioral, cognitive, psychoanalytic, psychodynamic or psychophysiological means to improve functioning or well-being

Qualifier	Qualifier	Qualifier	Qualifier
Character 4	Character 5	Character 6	Character 7
0 Interactive **1** Behavioral **2** Cognitive **3** Interpersonal **4** Psychoanalysis **5** Psychodynamic **6** Supportive **8** Cognitive-Behavioral **9** Psychophysiological	**Z** None	**Z** None	**Z** None

G Mental Health
Z None
6 **Counseling:** The application of psychological methods to treat an individual with normal developmental issues and psychological problems in order to increase function, improve well-being, alleviate distress, maladjustment or resolve crises

Qualifier	Qualifier	Qualifier	Qualifier
Character 4	Character 5	Character 6	Character 7
0 Educational **1** Vocational **3** Other Counseling	**Z** None	**Z** None	**Z** None

LC Limited Coverage   NC Noncovered   HAC HAC-associated Procedure   CC Combination Cluster - See Appendix G for code lists
DRG Non-OR-Affecting MS-DRG Assignment   New/Revised Text in **Orange**   ♂ Male   ♀ Female

G Mental Health
Z None
7 Family Psychotherapy: Treatment that includes one or more family members of an individual with a mental health disorder by behavioral, cognitive, psychoanalytic, psychodynamic or psychophysiological means to improve functioning or well-being

Qualifier	Qualifier	Qualifier	Qualifier
Character 4	Character 5	Character 6	Character 7
2 Other Family Psychotherapy	Z None	Z None	Z None

G Mental Health
Z None
B Electroconvulsive Therapy: The application of controlled electrical voltages to treat a mental health disorder

Qualifier	Qualifier	Qualifier	Qualifier
Character 4	Character 5	Character 6	Character 7
0 Unilateral-Single Seizure 1 Unilateral-Multiple Seizure 2 Bilateral-Single Seizure 3 Bilateral-Multiple Seizure 4 Other Electroconvulsive Therapy	Z None	Z None	Z None

G Mental Health
Z None
C Biofeedback: Provision of information from the monitoring and regulating of physiological processes in conjunction with cognitive-behavioral techniques to improve patient functioning or well-being

Qualifier	Qualifier	Qualifier	Qualifier
Character 4	Character 5	Character 6	Character 7
9 Other Biofeedback	Z None	Z None	Z None

G Mental Health
Z None
F Hypnosis: Induction of a state of heightened suggestibility by auditory, visual and tactile techniques to elicit an emotional or behavioral response

Qualifier	Qualifier	Qualifier	Qualifier
Character 4	Character 5	Character 6	Character 7
Z None	Z None	Z None	Z None

G Mental Health
Z None
G Narcosynthesis: Administration of intravenous barbiturates in order to release suppressed or repressed thoughts

Qualifier	Qualifier	Qualifier	Qualifier
Character 4	Character 5	Character 6	Character 7
Z None	Z None	Z None	Z None

G Mental Health
Z None
H Group Psychotherapy: Treatment of two or more individuals with a mental health disorder by behavioral, cognitive, psychoanalytic, psychodynamic or psychophysiological means to improve functioning or well-being

Qualifier	Qualifier	Qualifier	Qualifier
Character 4	Character 5	Character 6	Character 7
Z None	Z None	Z None	Z None

G Mental Health
Z None
J Light Therapy: Application of specialized light treatments to improve functioning or well-being

Qualifier	Qualifier	Qualifier	Qualifier
Character 4	Character 5	Character 6	Character 7
Z None	Z None	Z None	Z None

LC Limited Coverage   NC Noncovered   HAC HAC-associated Procedure   CC Combination Cluster - See Appendix G for code lists
DRG Non-OR-Affecting MS-DRG Assignment   New/Revised Text in Orange   ♂ Male   ♀ Female

714

2018 ICD-10-PCS

NOTES

NOTES

Substance Abuse Treatment HZ2-HZ9

H Substance Abuse Treatment
Z None
2 Detoxification Services: Detoxification from alcohol and/or drugs

Qualifier	Qualifier	Qualifier	Qualifier
Character 4	Character 5	Character 6	Character 7
Z None	**Z** None	**Z** None	**Z** None

H Substance Abuse Treatment
Z None
3 Individual Counseling: The application of psychological methods to treat an individual with addictive behavior

Qualifier	Qualifier	Qualifier	Qualifier
Character 4	Character 5	Character 6	Character 7
0 Cognitive ᴰᴿᴳ **1** Behavioral ᴰᴿᴳ **2** Cognitive-Behavioral ᴰᴿᴳ **3** 12-Step ᴰᴿᴳ **4** Interpersonal ᴰᴿᴳ **5** Vocational ᴰᴿᴳ **6** Psychoeducation ᴰᴿᴳ **7** Motivational Enhancement ᴰᴿᴳ **8** Confrontational ᴰᴿᴳ **9** Continuing Care ᴰᴿᴳ **B** Spiritual ᴰᴿᴳ **C** Pre/Post-Test Infectious Disease	**Z** None	**Z** None	**Z** None

ᴰᴿᴳ   HZ30ZZZ   HZ31ZZZ   HZ32ZZZ   HZ33ZZZ   HZ34ZZZ   HZ35ZZZ   HZ36ZZZ   HZ37ZZZ   HZ38ZZZ   HZ39ZZZ   HZ3BZZZ

H Substance Abuse Treatment
Z None
4 Group Counseling: The application of psychological methods to treat two or more individuals with addictive behavior

Qualifier	Qualifier	Qualifier	Qualifier
Character 4	Character 5	Character 6	Character 7
0 Cognitive ᴰᴿᴳ **1** Behavioral ᴰᴿᴳ **2** Cognitive-Behavioral ᴰᴿᴳ **3** 12-Step ᴰᴿᴳ **4** Interpersonal ᴰᴿᴳ **5** Vocational ᴰᴿᴳ **6** Psychoeducation ᴰᴿᴳ **7** Motivational Enhancement ᴰᴿᴳ **8** Confrontational ᴰᴿᴳ **9** Continuing Care ᴰᴿᴳ **B** Spiritual ᴰᴿᴳ **C** Pre/Post-Test Infectious Disease	**Z** None	**Z** None	**Z** None

ᴰᴿᴳ   HZ40ZZZ   HZ41ZZZ   HZ42ZZZ   HZ43ZZZ   HZ44ZZZ   HZ45ZZZ   HZ46ZZZ   HZ47ZZZ   HZ48ZZZ   HZ49ZZZ   HZ4BZZZ

ᴸᶜ Limited Coverage   ᴺᶜ Noncovered   ᴴᴬᶜ HAC-associated Procedure   ᶜᶜ Combination Cluster - See Appendix G for code lists
ᴰᴿᴳ Non-OR-Affecting MS-DRG Assignment   New/Revised Text in **Orange**   ♂ Male   ♀ Female

H Substance Abuse Treatment

Z None

5 Individual Psychotherapy: Treatment of an individual with addictive behavior by behavioral, cognitive, psychoanalytic, psychodynamic or psychophysiological means

Qualifier	Qualifier	Qualifier	Qualifier
Character 4	Character 5	Character 6	Character 7
0 Cognitive ᴼᴿᴳ **1** Behavioral ᴼᴿᴳ **2** Cognitive-Behavioral ᴼᴿᴳ **3** 12-Step ᴼᴿᴳ **4** Interpersonal ᴼᴿᴳ **5** Interactive ᴼᴿᴳ **6** Psychoeducation ᴼᴿᴳ **7** Motivational Enhancement ᴼᴿᴳ **8** Confrontational ᴼᴿᴳ **9** Supportive ᴼᴿᴳ **B** Psychoanalysis ᴼᴿᴳ **C** Psychodynamic ᴼᴿᴳ **D** Psychophysiological ᴼᴿᴳ	**Z** None	**Z** None	**Z** None

ᴼᴿᴳ HZ50ZZZ   HZ51ZZZ   HZ52ZZZ   HZ53ZZZ   HZ54ZZZ   HZ55ZZZ   HZ56ZZZ   HZ57ZZZ   HZ58ZZZ   HZ59ZZZ   HZ5BZZZ   HZ5CZZZ   HZ5DZZZ

H Substance Abuse Treatment

Z None

6 Family Counseling: The application of psychological methods that includes one or more family members to treat an individual with addictive behavior

Qualifier	Qualifier	Qualifier	Qualifier
Character 4	Character 5	Character 6	Character 7
3 Other Family Counseling	**Z** None	**Z** None	**Z** None

H Substance Abuse Treatment

Z None

8 Medication Management: Monitoring and adjusting the use of replacement medications for the treatment of addiction

Qualifier	Qualifier	Qualifier	Qualifier
Character 4	Character 5	Character 6	Character 7
0 Nicotine Replacement **1** Methadone Maintenance **2** Levo-alpha-acetyl-methadol (LAAM) **3** Antabuse **4** Naltrexone **5** Naloxone **6** Clonidine **7** Bupropion **8** Psychiatric Medication **9** Other Replacement Medication	**Z** None	**Z** None	**Z** None

H Substance Abuse Treatment
Z None
9 Pharmacotherapy: The use of replacement medications for the treatment of addiction

Qualifier	Qualifier	Qualifier	Qualifier
Character 4	**Character 5**	**Character 6**	**Character 7**
0 Nicotine Replacement **1** Methadone Maintenance **2** Levo-alpha-acetyl-methadol (LAAM) **3** Antabuse **4** Naltrexone **5** Naloxone **6** Clonidine **7** Bupropion **8** Psychiatric Medication **9** Other Replacement Medication	**Z** None	**Z** None	**Z** None

LC Limited Coverage   NC Noncovered   HAC HAC-associated Procedure   CC Combination Cluster - See Appendix G for code lists
DRG Non-OR-Affecting MS-DRG Assignment   New/Revised Text in **Orange**   ♂ Male   ♀ Female

NOTES

New Technology X2A-XY0

Cardiovascular System X2A-X2R

X New Technology
2 Cardiovascular System
A Assistance: Taking over a portion of a physiological function by extracorporeal means

Body Part	Approach	Device/Substance/Technology	Qualifier
Character 4	Character 5	Character 6	Character 7
5 Innominate Artery and Left Common Carotid Artery	**3** Percutaneous	**1** Cerebral Embolic Filtration, Dual Filter	**2** New Technology Group 2

X New Technology
2 Cardiovascular System
C Extirpation: Taking or cutting out solid matter from a body part

Body Part	Approach	Device/Substance/Technology	Qualifier
Character 4	Character 5	Character 6	Character 7
0 Coronary Artery, One Artery **1** Coronary Artery, Two Arteries **2** Coronary Artery, Three Arteries **3** Coronary Artery, Four or More Arteries	**3** Percutaneous	**6** Orbital Atherectomy Technology	**1** New Technology Group 1

X New Technology
2 Cardiovascular System
R Replacement: Putting in or on biological or synthetic material that physically takes the place and/or function of all or a portion of a body part

Body Part	Approach	Device/Substance/Technology	Qualifier
Character 4	Character 5	Character 6	Character 7
F Aortic Valve	**0** Open **3** Percutaneous **4** Percutaneous Endoscopic	**3** Zooplastic Tissue, Rapid Deployment Technique	**2** New Technology Group 2

LC Limited Coverage **NC** Noncovered **HAC** HAC-associated Procedure **CC** Combination Cluster - See Appendix G for code lists
DRG Non-OR-Affecting MS-DRG Assignment New/Revised Text in **Orange** ♂ Male ♀ Female

2018 ICD-10-PCS 721

CARDIOVASCULAR SYSTEM X2A-X2R

NOTES

Skin, Subcutaneous Tissue, Fascia, and Breast XHR

X New Technology
H Skin, Subcutaneous Tissue, Fascia and Breast
R Replacement: Putting in or on biological or synthetic material that physically takes the place and/or function of all or a portion of a body part

Body Part	Approach	Device/Substance/Technology	Qualifier
Character 4	**Character 5**	**Character 6**	**Character 7**
P Skin	**X** External	**L** Skin Substitute, Porcine Liver Derived	**2** New Technology Group 2

NOTES

Muscles, Tendons, Bursae, and Ligaments XK0

X **New Technology**
K **Muscles, Tendons, Bursae and Ligaments**
0 **Introduction:** Putting in or on a therapeutic, diagnostic, nutritional, physiological, or prophylactic substance except blood or blood products

Body Part	Approach	Device/Substance/Technology	Qualifier
Character 4	Character 5	Character 6	Character 7
2 Muscle	3 Percutaneous	0 Concentrated Bone Marrow Aspirate	3 New Technology Group 3

NOTES

Bones XNS

X New Technology
N Bones
S **Reposition:** Moving to its normal location, or other suitable location, all or a portion of a body part

Body Part	Approach	Device/Substance/Technology	Qualifier
Character 4	**Character 5**	**Character 6**	**Character 7**
0 Lumbar Vertebra **3** Cervical Vertebra **4** Thoracic Vertebra	**0** Open **3** Percutaneous	**3** Magnetically Controlled Growth Rod(s)	**2** New Technology Group 2

LC Limited Coverage   NC Noncovered   HAC HAC-associated Procedure   CC Combination Cluster - See Appendix G for code lists
DRG Non-OR-Affecting MS-DRG Assignment   New/Revised Text in **Orange**   ♂ Male   ♀ Female

2018 ICD-10-PCS

727

BONES XNS

NOTES

Joints XR2-XRG

X New Technology
R Joints
2 Monitoring: Determining the level of a physiological or physical function repetitively over a period of time

Body Part	Approach	Device/Substance/Technology	Qualifier
Character 4	**Character 5**	**Character 6**	**Character 7**
G Knee Joint, Right **H** Knee Joint, Left	**0** Open	**2** Intraoperative Knee Replacement Sensor	**1** New Technology Group 1

X New Technology
R Joints
G Fusion: Joining together portions of an articular body part rendering the articular body part immobile

Body Part	Approach	Device/Substance/Technology	Qualifier
Character 4	**Character 5**	**Character 6**	**Character 7**
0 Occipital-cervical Joint ⬛	**0** Open	**9** Interbody Fusion Device, Nanotextured Surface	**2** New Technology Group 2
0 Occipital-cervical Joint	**0** Open	**F** Interbody Fusion Device, Radiolucent Porous	**3** New Technology Group 3
1 Cervical Vertebral Joint ⬛	**0** Open	**9** Interbody Fusion Device, Nanotextured Surface	**2** New Technology Group 2
1 Cervical Vertebral Joint	**0** Open	**F** Interbody Fusion Device, Radiolucent Porous	**3** New Technology Group 3
2 Cervical Vertebral Joints, 2 or more ⬛	**0** Open	**9** Interbody Fusion Device, Nanotextured Surface	**2** New Technology Group 2
2 Cervical Vertebral Joints, 2 or more	**0** Open	**F** Interbody Fusion Device, Radiolucent Porous	**3** New Technology Group 3
4 Cervicothoracic Vertebral Joint ⬛	**0** Open	**9** Interbody Fusion Device, Nanotextured Surface	**2** New Technology Group 2
4 Cervicothoracic Vertebral Joint	**0** Open	**F** Interbody Fusion Device, Radiolucent Porous	**3** New Technology Group 3
6 Thoracic Vertebral Joint ⬛	**0** Open	**9** Interbody Fusion Device, Nanotextured Surface	**2** New Technology Group 2
6 Thoracic Vertebral Joint	**0** Open	**F** Interbody Fusion Device, Radiolucent Porous	**3** New Technology Group 3
7 Thoracic Vertebral Joints, 2 to 7 ⬛ ⬛	**0** Open	**9** Interbody Fusion Device, Nanotextured Surface	**2** New Technology Group 2
7 Thoracic Vertebral Joints, 2 to 7	**0** Open	**F** Interbody Fusion Device, Radiolucent Porous	**3** New Technology Group 3
8 Thoracic Vertebral Joints, 8 or more ⬛	**0** Open	**9** Interbody Fusion Device, Nanotextured Surface	**2** New Technology Group 2
8 Thoracic Vertebral Joints, 8 or more	**0** Open	**F** Interbody Fusion Device, Radiolucent Porous	**3** New Technology Group 3
A Thoracolumbar Vertebral Joint ⬛	**0** Open	**9** Interbody Fusion Device, Nanotextured Surface	**2** New Technology Group 2
A Thoracolumbar Vertebral Joint	**0** Open	**F** Interbody Fusion Device, Radiolucent Porous	**3** New Technology Group 3
B Lumbar Vertebral Joint ⬛	**0** Open	**9** Interbody Fusion Device, Nanotextured Surface	**2** New Technology Group 2
B Lumbar Vertebral Joint	**0** Open	**F** Interbody Fusion Device, Radiolucent Porous	**3** New Technology Group 3
C Lumbar Vertebral Joints, 2 or more ⬛ ⬛	**0** Open	**9** Interbody Fusion Device, Nanotextured Surface	**2** New Technology Group 2
C Lumbar Vertebral Joints, 2 or more	**0** Open	**F** Interbody Fusion Device, Radiolucent Porous	**3** New Technology Group 3

XRG continued on next page

X New Technology

XRG continued from previous page

R Joints

G Fusion: Joining together portions of an articular body part rendering the articular body part immobile

Body Part		Approach		Device/Substance/Technology		Qualifier	
Character 4		**Character 5**		**Character 6**		**Character 7**	
D	Lumbosacral Joint ᴴᴬᶜ	**0**	Open	**9**	Interbody Fusion Device, Nanotextured Surface	**2**	New Technology Group 2
D	Lumbosacral Joint	**0**	Open	**F**	Interbody Fusion Device, Radiolucent Porous	**3**	New Technology Group 3

ᴄᴄ XRG7092   XRGC092

ᴴᴬᶜ XRG0092   XRG1092   XRG2092   XRG4092   XRG6092   XRG7092   XRG8092   XRGA092   XRGB092   XRGC092   XRGD092
Surgical site infection following certain orthopedic procedures of spine, shoulder or elbow procedures and secondary diagnosis K68.11, T84.60XA, T84.610A, T84.611A, T84.612A, T84.613, T84.614A, T84.615A, T84.619A, T84.63XA, T84.69XA, T84.7XXA, T81.4XXA.

ᴸᶜ Limited Coverage   ᴺᶜ Noncovered   ᴴᴬᶜ HAC-associated Procedure   ᶜᶜ Combination Cluster - See Appendix G for code lists
ᴰᴿᴳ Non-OR-Affecting MS-DRG Assignment   New/Revised Text in **Orange**   ♂ Male   ♀ Female

730

2018 ICD-10-PCS

NOTES

NOTES

Anatomical Regions XW0

X New Technology
W Anatomical Regions
0 Introduction: Putting in or on a therapeutic, diagnostic, nutritional, physiological, or prophylactic substance except blood or blood products

Body Part	Approach	Device/Substance/Technology	Qualifier
Character 4	Character 5	Character 6	Character 7
3 Peripheral Vein	3 Percutaneous	2 Ceftazidime-Avibactam Anti-infective 3 Idarucizumab, Dabigatran Reversal Agent 4 Isavuconazole Anti-infective 5 Blinatumomab Antineoplastic Immunotherapy	1 New Technology Group 1
3 Peripheral Vein	3 Percutaneous	7 Andexanet Alfa, Factor Xa Inhibitor Reversal Agent 9 Defibrotide Sodium Anticoagulant	2 New Technology Group 2
3 Peripheral Vein	3 Percutaneous	A Bezlotoxumab Monoclonal Antibody B Cytarabine and Daunorubicin Liposome Antineoplastic C Engineered Autologous Chimeric Antigen Receptor T-cell Immunotherapy F Other New Technology Therapeutic Substance	3 New Technology Group 3
4 Central Vein	3 Percutaneous	2 Ceftazidime-Avibactam Anti-infective 3 Idarucizumab, Dabigatran Reversal Agent 4 Isavuconazole Antiinfective 5 Blinatumomab Antineoplastic Immunotherapy	1 New Technology Group 1
4 Central Vein	3 Percutaneous	7 Andexanet Alfa, Factor Xa Inhibitor Reversal Agent 9 Defibrotide Sodium Anticoagulant	2 New Technology Group 2
4 Central Vein	3 Percutaneous	A Bezlotoxumab Monoclonal Antibody B Cytarabine and Daunorubicin Liposome Antineoplastic C Engineered Autologous Chimeric Antigen Receptor T-cell Immunotherapy F Other New Technology Therapeutic Substance	3 New Technology Group 3
D Mouth and Pharynx	X External	8 Uridine Triacetate	2 New Technology Group 2

LC Limited Coverage   NC Noncovered   HAC HAC-associated Procedure   CC Combination Cluster - See Appendix G for code lists
Non-OR-Affecting MS-DRG Assignment   New/Revised Text in **Orange**   ♂ Male   ♀ Female

NOTES

Extracorporeal XY0

X **New Technology**
Y **Extracorporeal**
0 **Introduction:** Putting in or on a therapeutic, diagnostic, nutritional, physiological, or prophylactic substance except blood or blood products

Body Part	Approach	Device/Substance/Technology	Qualifier
Character 4	Character 5	Character 6	Character 7
V Vein Graft	**X** External	**8** Endothelial Damage Inhibitor	**3** New Technology Group 3

NOTES

Appendix A: Root Operations Definitions

0 - Medical and Surgical

Value	Root Operation	Definition/Explanation
0	Alteration	**Definition:** Modifying the anatomic structure of a body part without affecting the function of the body part **Explanation:** Principal purpose is to improve appearance **Includes/Examples:** Face lift, breast augmentation
1	Bypass	**Definition:** Altering the route of passage of the contents of a tubular body part **Explanation:** Rerouting contents of a body part to a downstream area of the normal route, to a similar route and body part, or to an abnormal route and dissimilar body part. Includes one or more anastomoses, with or without the use of a device **Includes/Examples:** Coronary artery bypass, colostomy formation
2	Change	**Definition:** Taking out or off a device from a body part and putting back an identical or similar device in or on the same body part without cutting or puncturing the skin or a mucous membrane **Explanation:** All CHANGE procedures are coded using the approach EXTERNAL **Includes/Examples:** Urinary catheter change, gastrostomy tube change
3	Control	**Definition:** Stopping, or attempting to stop, postprocedural or other acute bleeding **Explanation:** The site of the bleeding is coded as an anatomical region and not to a specific body part **Includes/Examples:** Control of post-prostatectomy hemorrhage, control of intracranial subdural hemorrhage, control of bleeding duodenal ulcer, control of retroperitoneal hemorrhage
4	Creation	**Definition:** Putting in or on biological or synthetic material to form a new body part that to the extent possible replicates the anatomic structure or function of an absent body part **Explanation:** Used for gender reassignment surgery and corrective procedures in individuals with congenital anomalies **Includes/Examples:** Creation of vagina in a male, creation of right and left atrioventricular valve from common atrioventricular valve
5	Destruction	**Definition:** Physical eradication of all or a portion of a body part by the direct use of energy, force, or a destructive agent **Explanation:** None of the body part is physically taken out **Includes/Examples:** Fulguration of rectal polyp, cautery of skin lesion
6	Detachment	**Definition:** Cutting off all or a portion of the upper or lower extremities **Explanation:** The body part value is the site of the detachment, with a qualifier if applicable to further specify the level where the extremity was detached **Includes/Examples:** Below knee amputation, disarticulation of shoulder
7	Dilation	**Definition:** Expanding an orifice or the lumen of a tubular body part **Explanation:** The orifice can be a natural orifice or an artificially created orifice. Accomplished by stretching a tubular body part using intraluminal pressure or by cutting part of the orifice or wall of the tubular body part **Includes/Examples:** Percutaneous transluminal angioplasty, internal urethrotomy
8	Division	**Definition:** Cutting into a body part, without draining fluids and/or gases from the body part, in order to separate or transect a body part **Explanation:** All or a portion of the body part is separated into two or more portions **Includes/Examples:** Spinal cordotomy, osteotomy
9	Drainage	**Definition:** Taking or letting out fluids and/or gases from a body part **Explanation:** The qualifier DIAGNOSTIC is used to identify drainage procedures that are biopsies **Includes/Examples:** Thoracentesis, incision and drainage
B	Excision	**Definition:** Cutting out or off, without replacement, a portion of a body part **Explanation:** The qualifier DIAGNOSTIC is used to identify excision procedures that are biopsies **Includes/Examples:** Partial nephrectomy, liver biopsy

Value	Root Operation	Definition/Explanation
		0 - Medical and Surgical
C	Extirpation	**Definition:** Taking or cutting out solid matter from a body part **Explanation:** The solid matter may be an abnormal byproduct of a biological function or a foreign body; it may be imbedded in a body part or in the lumen of a tubular body part. The solid matter may or may not have been previously broken into pieces **Includes/Examples:** Thrombectomy, choledocholithotomy
D	Extraction	**Definition:** Pulling or stripping out or off all or a portion of a body part by the use of force **Explanation:** The qualifier DIAGNOSTIC is used to identify extraction procedures that are biopsies **Includes/Examples:** Dilation and curettage, vein stripping
F	Fragmentation	**Definition:** Breaking solid matter in a body part into pieces **Explanation:** Physical force (e.g., manual, ultrasonic) applied directly or indirectly is used to break the solid matter into pieces. The solid matter may be an abnormal byproduct of a biological function or a foreign body. The pieces of solid matter are not taken out **Includes/Examples:** Extracorporeal shockwave lithotripsy, transurethral lithotripsy
G	Fusion	**Definition:** Joining together portions of an articular body part rendering the articular body part immobile **Explanation:** The body part is joined together by fixation device, bone graft, or other means **Includes/Examples:** Spinal fusion, ankle arthrodesis
H	Insertion	**Definition:** Putting in a nonbiological appliance that monitors, assists, performs, or prevents a physiological function but does not physically take the place of a body part **Includes/Examples:** Insertion of radioactive implant, insertion of central venous catheter
J	Inspection	**Definition:** Visually and/or manually exploring a body part **Explanation:** Visual exploration may be performed with or without optical instrumentation. Manual exploration may be performed directly or through intervening body layers **Includes/Examples:** Diagnostic arthroscopy, exploratory laparotomy
K	Map	**Definition:** Locating the route of passage of electrical impulses and/or locating functional areas in a body part **Explanation:** Applicable only to the cardiac conduction mechanism and the central nervous system **Includes/Examples:** Cardiac mapping, cortical mapping
L	Occlusion	**Definition:** Completely closing an orifice or the lumen of a tubular body part **Explanation:** The orifice can be a natural orifice or an artificially created orifice **Includes/Examples:** Fallopian tube ligation, ligation of inferior vena cava
M	Reattachment	**Definition:** Putting back in or on all or a portion of a separated body part to its normal location or other suitable location **Explanation:** Vascular circulation and nervous pathways may or may not be reestablished **Includes/Examples:** Reattachment of hand, reattachment of avulsed kidney
N	Release	**Definition:** Freeing a body part from an abnormal physical constraint by cutting or by the use of force **Explanation:** Some of the restraining tissue may be taken out but none of the body part is taken out **Includes/Examples:** Adhesiolysis, carpal tunnel release
P	Removal	**Definition:** Taking out or off a device from a body part **Explanation:** If a device is taken out and a similar device put in without cutting or puncturing the skin or mucous membrane, the procedure is coded to the root operation CHANGE. Otherwise, the procedure for taking out a device is coded to the root operation REMOVAL **Includes/Examples:** Drainage tube removal, cardiac pacemaker removal
Q	Repair	**Definition:** Restoring, to the extent possible, a body part to its normal anatomic structure and function **Explanation:** Used only when the method to accomplish the repair is not one of the other root operations **Includes/Examples:** Colostomy takedown, suture of laceration

0 - Medical and Surgical

Value	Root Operation	Definition/Explanation
R	Replacement	**Definition:** Putting in or on biological or synthetic material that physically takes the place and/or function of all or a portion of a body part **Explanation:** The body part may have been taken out or replaced, or may be taken out, physically eradicated, or rendered nonfunctional during the Replacement procedure. A Removal procedure is coded for taking out the device used in a previous replacement procedure **Includes/Examples:** Total hip replacement, bone graft, free skin graft
S	Reposition	**Definition:** Moving to its normal location, or other suitable location, all or a portion of a body part **Explanation:** The body part is moved to a new location from an abnormal location, or from a normal location where it is not functioning correctly. The body part may or may not be cut out or off to be moved to the new location **Includes/Examples:** Reposition of undescended testicle, fracture reduction
T	Resection	**Definition:** Cutting out or off, without replacement, all of a body part **Includes/Examples:** Total nephrectomy, total lobectomy of lung
V	Restriction	**Definition:** Partially closing an orifice or the lumen of a tubular body part **Explanation:** The orifice can be a natural orifice or an artificially created orifice **Includes/Examples:** Esophagogastric fundoplication, cervical cerclage
W	Revision	**Definition:** Correcting, to the extent possible, a portion of a malfunctioning device or the position of a displaced device **Explanation:** Revision can include correcting a malfunctioning or displaced device by taking out or putting in components of the device such as a screw or pin **Includes/Examples:** Adjustment of position of pacemaker lead, recementing of hip prosthesis
U	Supplement	**Definition:** Putting in or on biological or synthetic material that physically reinforces and/or augments the function of a portion of a body part **Explanation:** The biological material is non-living, or is living and from the same individual. The body part may have been previously replaced, and the Supplement procedure is performed to physically reinforce and/or augment the function of the replaced body part **Includes/Examples:** Herniorrhaphy using mesh, free nerve graft, mitral valve ring annuloplasty, put a new acetabular liner in a previous hip replacement
X	Transfer	**Definition:** Moving, without taking out, all or a portion of a body part to another location to take over the function of all or a portion of a body part **Explanation:** The body part transferred remains connected to its vascular and nervous supply **Includes/Examples:** Tendon transfer, skin pedicle flap transfer
Y	Transplantation	**Definition:** Putting in or on all or a portion of a living body part taken from another individual or animal to physically take the place and/or function of all or a portion of a similar body part **Explanation:** The native body part may or may not be taken out, and the transplanted body part may take over all or a portion of its function **Includes/Examples:** Kidney transplant, heart transplant

1 - Obstetrics

Value	Root Operation	Definition/Explanation
A	Abortion	**Definition:** Artificially terminating a pregnancy
2	Change	**Definition:** Taking out or off a device from a body part and putting back an identical or similar device in or on the same body part without cutting or puncturing the skin or a mucous membrane
E	Delivery	**Definition:** Assisting the passage of the products of conception from the genital canal
9	Drainage	**Definition:** Taking or letting out fluids and/or gases from a body part
D	Extraction	**Definition:** Pulling or stripping out or off all or a portion of a body part by the use of force

1-Obstetrics continued on next page

1-Obstetrics continued from previous page

1 - Obstetrics

Value	Root Operation	Definition/Explanation
H	Insertion	**Definition:** Putting in a nonbiological appliance that monitors, assists, performs, or prevents a physiological function but does not physically take the place of a body part
J	Inspection	**Definition:** Visually and/or manually exploring a body part **Explanation:** Visual exploration may be performed with or without optical instrumentation. Manual exploration may be performed directly or through intervening body layers
P	Removal	**Definition:** Taking out or off a device from a body part, region or orifice **Explanation:** If a device is taken out and a similar device put in without cutting or puncturing the skin or mucous membrane, the procedure is coded to the root operation CHANGE. Otherwise, the procedure for taking out a device is coded to the root operation REMOVAL
Q	Repair	**Definition:** Restoring, to the extent possible, a body part to its normal anatomic structure and function **Explanation:** Used only when the method to accomplish the repair is not one of the other root operations
S	Reposition	**Definition:** Moving to its normal location, or other suitable location, all or a portion of a body part **Explanation:** The body part is moved to a new location from an abnormal location, or from a normal location where it is not functioning correctly. The body part may or may not be cut out or off to be moved to the new location
T	Resection	**Definition:** Cutting out or off, without replacement, all of a body part
Y	Transplantation	**Definition:** Putting in or on all or a portion of a living body part taken from another individual or animal to physically take the place and/or function of all or a portion of a similar body part **Explanation:** The native body part may or may not be taken out, and the transplanted body part may take over all or a portion of its function

2 - Placement

Value	Root Operation	Definition/Explanation
0	Change	**Definition:** Taking out or off a device from a body part and putting back an identical or similar device in or on the same body part without cutting or puncturing the skin or a mucous membrane
1	Compression	**Definition:** Putting pressure on a body region
2	Dressing	**Definition:** Putting material on a body region for protection
3	Immobilization	**Definition:** Limiting or preventing motion of a body region
4	Packing	**Definition:** Putting material in a body region or orifice
5	Removal	**Definition:** Taking out or off a device from a body part
6	Traction	**Definition:** Exerting a pulling force on a body region in a distal direction

3 - Administration

Value	Root Operation	Definition/Explanation
0	Introduction	**Definition:** Putting in or on a therapeutic, diagnostic, nutritional, physiological, or prophylactic substance except blood or blood products
1	Irrigation	**Definition:** Putting in or on a cleansing substance
2	Transfusion	**Definition:** Putting in blood or blood products

4 - Measurement and Monitoring

Value	Root Operation	Definition/Explanation
0	Measurement	**Definition:** Determining the level of a physiological or physical function at a point in time
1	Monitoring	**Definition:** Determining the level of a physiological or physical function repetitively over a period of time

5 - Extracorporeal or Systemic Assistance and Performance

Value	Root Operation	Definition/Explanation
0	Assistance	**Definition:** Taking over a portion of a physiological function by extracorporeal means
1	Performance	**Definition:** Completely taking over a physiological function by extracorporeal means
2	Restoration	**Definition:** Returning, or attempting to return, a physiological function to its original state by extracorporeal means.

6 - Extracorporeal or Systemic Therapies

Value	Root Operation	Definition/Explanation
0	Atmospheric Control	**Definition:** Extracorporeal control of atmospheric pressure and composition
1	Decompression	**Definition:** Extracorporeal elimination of undissolved gas from body fluids
2	Electromagnetic Therapy	**Definition:** Extracorporeal treatment by electromagnetic rays
3	Hyperthermia	**Definition:** Extracorporeal raising of body temperature
4	Hypothermia	**Definition:** Extracorporeal lowering of body temperature
B	Perfusion	**Definition:** Extracorporeal treatment by diffusion of therapeutic fluid
5	Pheresis	**Definition:** Extracorporeal separation of blood products
6	Phototherapy	**Definition:** Extracorporeal treatment by light rays
9	Shock Wave Therapy	**Definition:** Extracorporeal treatment by shock waves
7	Ultrasound Therapy	**Definition:** Extracorporeal treatment by ultrasound
8	Ultraviolet Light Therapy	**Definition:** Extracorporeal treatment by ultraviolet light

7 - Osteopathic

Value	Root Operation	Definition/Explanation
0	Treatment	**Definition:** Manual treatment to eliminate or alleviate somatic dysfunction and related disorders

8 - Other Procedures

Value	Root Operation	Definition/Explanation
0	Other Procedures	**Definition:** Methodologies which attempt to remediate or cure a disorder or disease

9 - Chiropractic

Value	Root Operation	Definition/Explanation
B	Manipulation	**Definition:** Manual procedure that involves a directed thrust to move a joint past the physiological range of motion, without exceeding the anatomical limit

X - New Technology

Value	Root Operation	Definition/Explanation
A	Assistance	**Definition:** Taking over a portion of a physiological function by extracorporeal means
C	Extirpation	**Definition:** Taking or cutting out solid matter from a body part **Explanation:** The solid matter may be an abnormal byproduct of a biological function or a foreign body; it may be imbedded in a body part or in the lumen of a tubular body part. The solid matter may or may not have been previously broken into pieces **Includes/Examples:** Thrombectomy, choledocholithotomy
G	Fusion	**Definition:** Joining together portions of an articular body part rendering the articular body part immobile **Explanation:** The body part is joined together by fixation device, bone graft, or other means **Includes/Examples:** Spinal fusion, ankle arthrodesis
0	Introduction	**Definition:** Putting in or on a therapeutic, diagnostic, nutritional, physiological, or prophylactic substance except blood or blood products
2	Monitoring	**Definition:** Determining the level of a physiological or physical function repetitively over a period of time
R	Replacement	**Definition:** Putting in or on biological or synthetic material that physically takes the place and/or function of all or a portion of a body part **Explanation:** The body part may have been taken out or replaced, or may be taken out, physically eradicated, or rendered nonfunctional during the Replacement procedure. A Removal procedure is coded for taking out the device used in a previous replacement procedure **Includes/Examples:** Total hip replacement, bone graft, free skin graft
S	Reposition	**Definition:** Moving to its normal location, or other suitable location, all or a portion of a body part **Explanation:** The body part is moved to a new location from an abnormal location, or from a normal location where it is not functioning correctly. The body part may or may not be cut out or off to be moved to the new location **Includes/Examples:** Reposition of undescended testicle, fracture reduction

Appendix B: Body Part Key

Anatomical Term	ICD-10-PCS Value
Abdominal aortic plexus	Abdominal Sympathetic Nerve
Abdominal esophagus	Esophagus, Lower
Abductor hallucis muscle	Foot Muscle, Right
	Foot Muscle, Left
Accessory cephalic vein	Cephalic Vein, Right
	Cephalic Vein, Left
Accessory obturator nerve	Lumbar Plexus
Accessory phrenic nerve	Phrenic Nerve
Accessory spleen	Spleen
Acetabulofemoral joint	Hip Joint, Right
	Hip Joint, Left
Achilles tendon	Lower Leg Tendon, Right
	Lower Leg Tendon, Left
Acromioclavicular ligament	Shoulder Bursa and Ligament, Right
	Shoulder Bursa and Ligament, Left
Acromion (process)	Scapula, Right
	Scapula, Left
Adductor brevis muscle	Upper Leg Muscle, Right
	Upper Leg Muscle, Left
Adductor hallucis muscle	Foot Muscle, Right
	Foot Muscle, Left
Adductor longus muscle	Upper Leg Muscle, Right
	Upper Leg Muscle, Left
Adductor magnus muscle	Upper Leg Muscle, Right
	Upper Leg Muscle, Left
Adenohypophysis	Pituitary Gland
Alar ligament of axis	Head and Neck Bursa and Ligament
Alveolar process of mandible	Mandible, Right
	Mandible, Left
Alveolar process of maxilla	Maxilla
Anal orifice	Anus
Anatomical snuffbox	Lower Arm and Wrist Muscle, Right
	Lower Arm and Wrist Muscle, Left
Angular artery	Face Artery
Angular vein	Face Vein, Right
	Face Vein, Left
Annular ligament	Elbow Bursa and Ligament, Right
	Elbow Bursa and Ligament, Left
Anorectal junction	Rectum
Ansa cervicalis	Cervical Plexus
Antebrachial fascia	Subcutaneous Tissue and Fascia, Right Lower Arm
	Subcutaneous Tissue and Fascia, Left Lower Arm

Anatomical Term	ICD-10-PCS Value
Anterior (pectoral) lymph node	Lymphatic, Right Axillary
	Lymphatic, Left Axillary
Anterior cerebral artery	Intracranial Artery
Anterior cerebral vein	Intracranial Vein
Anterior choroidal artery	Intracranial Artery
Anterior circumflex humeral artery	Axillary Artery, Right
	Axillary Artery, Left
Anterior communicating artery	Intracranial Artery
Anterior cruciate ligament (ACL)	Knee Bursa and Ligament, Right
	Knee Bursa and Ligament, Left
Anterior crural nerve	Femoral Nerve
Anterior facial vein	Face Vein, Right
	Face Vein, Left
Anterior intercostal artery	Internal Mammary Artery, Right
	Internal Mammary Artery, Left
Anterior interosseous nerve	Median Nerve
Anterior lateral malleolar artery	Anterior Tibial Artery, Right
	Anterior Tibial Artery, Left
Anterior lingual gland	Minor Salivary Gland
Anterior medial malleolar artery	Anterior Tibial Artery, Right
	Anterior Tibial Artery, Left
Anterior spinal artery	Vertebral Artery, Right
	Vertebral Artery, Left
Anterior tibial recurrent artery	Anterior Tibial Artery, Right
	Anterior Tibial Artery, Left
Anterior ulnar recurrent artery	Ulnar Artery, Right
	Ulnar Artery, Left
Anterior vagal trunk	Vagus Nerve
Anterior vertebral muscle	Neck Muscle, Right
	Neck Muscle, Left
Antihelix	External Ear, Right
	External Ear, Left
	External Ear, Bilateral
Antitragus	External Ear, Right
	External Ear, Left
	External Ear, Bilateral
Antrum of Highmore	Maxillary Sinus, Right
	Maxillary Sinus, Left
Aortic annulus	Aortic Valve
Aortic arch	Thoracic Aorta, Ascending/Arch
Aortic intercostal artery	Upper Artery
Apical (subclavicular) lymph node	Lymphatic, Right Axillary
	Lymphatic, Left Axillary
Apneustic center	Pons
Aqueduct of Sylvius	Cerebral Ventricle

Anatomical Term	ICD-10-PCS Value
Aqueous humour	Anterior Chamber, Right
	Anterior Chamber, Left
Arachnoid mater, intracranial	Cerebral Meninges
Arachnoid mater, spinal	Spinal Meninges
Arcuate artery	Foot Artery, Right
	Foot Artery, Left
Areola	Nipple, Right
	Nipple, Left
Arterial canal (duct)	Pulmonary Artery, Left
Aryepiglottic fold	Larynx
Arytenoid cartilage	Larynx
Arytenoid muscle	Neck Muscle, Right
	Neck Muscle, Left
Ascending aorta	Thoracic Aorta, Ascending/Arch
Ascending palatine artery	Face Artery
Ascending pharyngeal artery	External Carotid Artery, Right
	External Carotid Artery, Left
Atlantoaxial joint	Cervical Vertebral Joint
Atrioventricular node	Conduction Mechanism
Atrium dextrum cordis	Atrium, Right
Atrium pulmonale	Atrium, Left
Auditory tube	Eustachian Tube, Right
	Eustachian Tube, Left
Auerbach's (myenteric) plexus	Abdominal Sympathetic Nerve
Auricle	External Ear, Right
	External Ear, Left
	External Ear, Bilateral
Auricularis muscle	Head Muscle
Axillary fascia	Subcutaneous Tissue and Fascia, Right Upper Arm
	Subcutaneous Tissue and Fascia, Left Upper Arm
Axillary nerve	Brachial Plexus
Bartholin's (greater vestibular) gland	Vestibular Gland
Basal (internal) cerebral vein	Intracranial Vein
Basal nuclei	Basal Ganglia
Base of Tongue	Pharynx
Basilar artery	Intracranial Artery
Basis pontis	Pons
Biceps brachii muscle	Upper Arm Muscle, Right
	Upper Arm Muscle, Left
Biceps femoris muscle	Upper Leg Muscle, Right
	Upper Leg Muscle, Left
Bicipital aponeurosis	Subcutaneous Tissue and Fascia, Right Lower Arm
	Subcutaneous Tissue and Fascia, Left Lower Arm

Anatomical Term	ICD-10-PCS Value
Bicuspid valve	Mitral Valve
Body of femur	Femoral Shaft, Right
	Femoral Shaft, Left
Body of fibula	Fibula, Right
	Fibula, Left
Bony labyrinth	Inner Ear, Right
	Inner Ear, Left
Bony orbit	Orbit, Right
	Orbit, Left
Bony vestibule	Inner Ear, Right
	Inner Ear, Left
Botallo's duct	Pulmonary Artery, Left
Brachial (lateral) lymph node	Lymphatic, Right Axillary
	Lymphatic, Left Axillary
Brachialis muscle	Upper Arm Muscle, Right
	Upper Arm Muscle, Left
Brachiocephalic artery	Innominate Artery
Brachiocephalic trunk	Innominate Artery
Brachiocephalic vein	Innominate Vein, Right
	Innominate Vein, Left
Brachioradialis muscle	Lower Arm and Wrist Muscle, Right
	Lower Arm and Wrist Muscle, Left
Broad ligament	Uterine Supporting Structure
Bronchial artery	Upper Artery
Bronchus intermedius	Main Bronchus, Right
Buccal gland	Buccal Mucosa
Buccinator lymph node	Lymphatic, Head
Buccinator muscle	Facial Muscle
Bulbospongiosus muscle	Perineum Muscle
Bulbourethral (Cowper's) gland	Urethra
Bundle of His	Conduction Mechanism
Bundle of Kent	Conduction Mechanism
Calcaneocuboid joint	Tarsal Joint, Right
	Tarsal Joint, Left
Calcaneocuboid ligament	Foot Bursa and Ligament, Right
	Foot Bursa and Ligament, Left
Calcaneofibular ligament	Ankle Bursa and Ligament, Right
	Ankle Bursa and Ligament, Left
Calcaneus	Tarsal, Right
	Tarsal, Left
Capitate bone	Carpal, Right
	Carpal, Left
Cardia	Esophagogastric Junction
Cardiac plexus	Thoracic Sympathetic Nerve
Cardioesophageal junction	Esophagogastric Junction
Caroticotympanic artery	Internal Carotid Artery, Right
	Internal Carotid Artery, Left

Anatomical Term	ICD-10-PCS Value
Carotid glomus	Carotid Body, Left
	Carotid Body, Right
	Carotid Bodies, Bilateral
Carotid sinus	Internal Carotid Artery, Right
	Internal Carotid Artery, Left
Carotid sinus nerve	Glossopharyngeal Nerve
Carpometacarpal ligament	Hand Bursa and Ligament, Right
	Hand Bursa and Ligament, Left
Cauda equina	Lumbar Spinal Cord
Cavernous plexus	Head and Neck Sympathetic Nerve
Celiac (solar) plexus	Abdominal Sympathetic Nerve
Celiac ganglion	Abdominal Sympathetic Nerve
Celiac lymph node	Lymphatic, Aortic
Celiac trunk	Celiac Artery
Central axillary lymph node	Lymphatic, Right Axillary
	Lymphatic, Left Axillary
Cerebral aqueduct (Sylvius)	Cerebral Ventricle
Cerebrum	Brain
Cervical esophagus	Esophagus, Upper
Cervical facet joint	Cervical Vertebral Joint
	Cervical Vertebral Joints, 2 or more
Cervical ganglion	Head and Neck Sympathetic Nerve
Cervical interspinous ligament	Head and Neck Bursa and Ligament
Cervical intertransverse ligament	Head and Neck Bursa and Ligament
Cervical ligamentum flavum	Head and Neck Bursa and Ligament
Cervical lymph node	Lymphatic, Right Neck
	Lymphatic, Left Neck
Cervicothoracic facet joint	Cervicothoracic Vertebral Joint
Choana	Nasopharynx
Chondroglossus muscle	Tongue, Palate, Pharynx Muscle
Chorda tympani	Facial Nerve
Choroid plexus	Cerebral Ventricle
Ciliary body	Eye, Right
	Eye, Left
Ciliary ganglion	Head and Neck Sympathetic Nerve
Circle of Willis	Intracranial Artery
Circumflex iliac artery	Femoral Artery, Right
	Femoral Artery, Left
Claustrum	Basal Ganglia
Coccygeal body	Coccygeal Glomus
Coccygeus muscle	Trunk Muscle, Right
	Trunk Muscle, Left
Cochlea	Inner Ear, Right
	Inner Ear, Left
Cochlear nerve	Acoustic Nerve

Anatomical Term	ICD-10-PCS Value
Columella	Nasal Mucosa and Soft Tissue
Common digital vein	Foot Vein, Right
	Foot Vein, Left
Common facial vein	Face Vein, Right
	Face Vein, Left
Common fibular nerve	Peroneal Nerve
Common hepatic artery	Hepatic Artery
Common iliac (subaortic) lymph node	Lymphatic, Pelvis
Common interosseous artery	Ulnar Artery, Right
	Ulnar Artery, Left
Common peroneal nerve	Peroneal Nerve
Condyloid process	Mandible, Right
	Mandible, Left
Conus arteriosus	Ventricle, Right
Conus medullaris	Lumbar Spinal Cord
Coracoacromial ligament	Shoulder Bursa and Ligament, Right
	Shoulder Bursa and Ligament, Left
Coracobrachialis muscle	Upper Arm Muscle, Right
	Upper Arm Muscle, Left
Coracoclavicular ligament	Shoulder Bursa and Ligament, Right
	Shoulder Bursa and Ligament, Left
Coracohumeral ligament	Shoulder Bursa and Ligament, Right
	Shoulder Bursa and Ligament, Left
Coracoid process	Scapula, Right
	Scapula, Left
Corniculate cartilage	Larynx
Corpus callosum	Brain
Corpus cavernosum	Penis
Corpus spongiosum	Penis
Corpus striatum	Basal Ganglia
Corrugator supercilii muscle	Facial Muscle
Costocervical trunk	Subclavian Artery, Right
	Subclavian Artery, Left
Costoclavicular ligament	Shoulder Bursa and Ligament, Right
	Shoulder Bursa and Ligament, Left
Costotransverse joint	Thoracic Vertebral Joint
Costotransverse ligament	Sternum Bursa and Ligament
	Rib(s) Bursa and Ligament
Costovertebral joint	Thoracic Vertebral Joint
Costoxiphoid ligament	Sternum Bursa and Ligament
	Rib(s) Bursa and Ligament
Cowper's (bulbourethral) gland	Urethra
Cremaster muscle	Perineum Muscle

Anatomical Term	ICD-10-PCS Value
Cribriform plate	Ethmoid Bone, Right
	Ethmoid Bone, Left
Cricoid cartilage	Trachea
Cricothyroid artery	Thyroid Artery, Right
	Thyroid Artery, Left
Cricothyroid muscle	Neck Muscle, Right
	Neck Muscle, Left
Crural fascia	Subcutaneous Tissue and Fascia, Right Upper Leg
	Subcutaneous Tissue and Fascia, Left Upper Leg
Cubital lymph node	Lymphatic, Right Upper Extremity
	Lymphatic, Left Upper Extremity
Cubital nerve	Ulnar Nerve
Cuboid bone	Tarsal, Right
	Tarsal, Left
Cuboideonavicular joint	Tarsal Joint, Right
	Tarsal Joint, Left
Culmen	Cerebellum
Cuneiform cartilage	Larynx
Cuneonavicular joint	Tarsal Joint, Right
	Tarsal Joint, Left
Cuneonavicular ligament	Foot Bursa and Ligament, Right
	Foot Bursa and Ligament, Left
Cutaneous (transverse) cervical nerve	Cervical Plexus
Deep cervical fascia	Subcutaneous Tissue and Fascia, Right Neck
	Subcutaneous Tissue and Fascia, Left Neck
Deep cervical vein	Vertebral Vein, Right
	Vertebral Vein, Left
Deep circumflex iliac artery	External Iliac Artery, Right
	External Iliac Artery, Left
Deep facial vein	Face Vein, Right
	Face Vein, Left
Deep femoral (profunda femoris) vein	Femoral Vein, Right
	Femoral Vein, Left
Deep femoral artery	Femoral Artery, Right
	Femoral Artery, Left
Deep palmar arch	Hand Artery, Right
	Hand Artery, Left
Deep transverse perineal muscle	Perineum Muscle
Deferential artery	Internal Iliac Artery, Right
	Internal Iliac Artery, Left
Deltoid fascia	Subcutaneous Tissue and Fascia, Right Upper Arm
	Subcutaneous Tissue and Fascia, Left Upper Arm

Anatomical Term	ICD-10-PCS Value
Deltoid ligament	Ankle Bursa and Ligament, Right
	Ankle Bursa and Ligament, Left
Deltoid muscle	Shoulder Muscle, Right
	Shoulder Muscle, Left
Deltopectoral (infraclavicular) lymph node	Lymphatic, Right Upper Extremity
	Lymphatic, Left Upper Extremity
Dens	Cervical Vertebra
Denticulate (dentate) ligament	Spinal Meninges
Depressor anguli oris muscle	Facial Muscle
Depressor labii inferioris muscle	Facial Muscle
Depressor septi nasi muscle	Facial Muscle
Depressor supercilii muscle	Facial Muscle
Dermis	Skin
Descending genicular artery	Femoral Artery, Right
	Femoral Artery, Left
Diaphragma sellae	Dura Mater
Distal humerus	Humeral Shaft, Right
	Humeral Shaft, Left
Distal humerus, involving joint	Elbow Joint, Right
	Elbow Joint, Left
Distal radioulnar joint	Wrist Joint, Right
	Wrist Joint, Left
Dorsal digital nerve	Radial Nerve
Dorsal metacarpal vein	Hand Vein, Right
	Hand Vein, Left
Dorsal metatarsal artery	Foot Artery, Right
	Foot Artery, Left
Dorsal metatarsal vein	Foot Vein, Right
	Foot Vein, Left
Dorsal scapular artery	Subclavian Artery, Right
	Subclavian Artery, Left
Dorsal scapular nerve	Brachial Plexus
Dorsal venous arch	Foot Vein, Right
	Foot Vein, Left
Dorsalis pedis artery	Anterior Tibial Artery, Right
	Anterior Tibial Artery, Left
Duct of Santorini	Pancreatic Duct, Accessory
Duct of Wirsung	Pancreatic Duct
Ductus deferens	Vas Deferens, Right
	Vas Deferens, Left
	Vas Deferens, Bilateral
	Vas Deferens
Duodenal ampulla	Ampulla of Vater
Duodenojejunal flexure	Jejunum
Dura mater, intracranial	Dura Mater
Dura mater, spinal	Spinal Meninges

Anatomical Term	ICD-10-PCS Value
Dural venous sinus	Intracranial Vein
Earlobe	External Ear, Right
	External Ear, Left
	External Ear, Bilateral
Eighth cranial nerve	Acoustic Nerve
Ejaculatory duct	Vas Deferens, Right
	Vas Deferens, Left
	Vas Deferens, Bilateral
	Vas Deferens
Eleventh cranial nerve	Accessory Nerve
Encephalon	Brain
Ependyma	Cerebral Ventricle
Epidermis	Skin
Epidural space, spinal	Spinal Canal
Epiploic foramen	Peritoneum
Epithalamus	Thalamus
Epitrochlear lymph node	Lymphatic, Right Upper Extremity
	Lymphatic, Left Upper Extremity
Erector spinae muscle	Trunk Muscle, Right
	Trunk Muscle, Left
Esophageal artery	Upper Artery
Esophageal plexus	Thoracic Sympathetic Nerve
Ethmoidal air cell	Ethmoid Sinus, Right
	Ethmoid Sinus, Left
Extensor carpi radialis muscle	Lower Arm and Wrist Muscle, Right
	Lower Arm and Wrist Muscle, Left
Extensor carpi ulnaris muscle	Lower Arm and Wrist Muscle, Right
	Lower Arm and Wrist Muscle, Left
Extensor digitorum brevis muscle	Foot Muscle, Right
	Foot Muscle, Left
Extensor digitorum longus muscle	Lower Leg Muscle, Right
	Lower Leg Muscle, Left
Extensor hallucis brevis muscle	Foot Muscle, Right
	Foot Muscle, Left
Extensor hallucis longus muscle	Lower Leg Muscle, Right
	Lower Leg Muscle, Left
External anal sphincter	Anal Sphincter
External auditory meatus	External Auditory Canal, Right
	External Auditory Canal, Left
External maxillary artery	Face Artery
External naris	Nasal Mucosa and Soft Tissue
External oblique aponeurosis	Subcutaneous Tissue and Fascia, Trunk
External oblique muscle	Abdomen Muscle, Right
	Abdomen Muscle, Left
External popliteal nerve	Peroneal Nerve
External pudendal artery	Femoral Artery, Right
	Femoral Artery, Left

Anatomical Term	ICD-10-PCS Value
External pudendal vein	Saphenous Vein, Right
	Saphenous Vein, Left
External urethral sphincter	Urethra
Extradural space, intracranial	Epidural Space, Intracranial
Extradural space, spinal	Spinal Canal
Facial artery	Face Artery
False vocal cord	Larynx
Falx cerebri	Dura Mater
Fascia lata	Subcutaneous Tissue and Fascia, Right Upper Leg
	Subcutaneous Tissue and Fascia, Left Upper Leg
Femoral head	Upper Femur, Right
	Upper Femur, Left
Femoral lymph node	Lymphatic, Right Lower Extremity
	Lymphatic, Left Lower Extremity
Femoropatellar joint	Knee Joint, Right
	Knee Joint, Left
	Knee Joint, Femoral Surface, Right
	Knee Joint, Femoral Surface, Left
Femorotibial joint	Knee Joint, Right
	Knee Joint, Left
	Knee Joint, Tibial Surface, Right
	Knee Joint, Tibial Surface, Left
Fibular artery	Peroneal Artery, Right
	Peroneal Artery, Left
Fibularis brevis muscle	Lower Leg Muscle, Right
	Lower Leg Muscle, Left
Fibularis longus muscle	Lower Leg Muscle, Right
	Lower Leg Muscle, Left
Fifth cranial nerve	Trigeminal Nerve
Filum terminale	Spinal Meninges
First cranial nerve	Olfactory Nerve
First intercostal nerve	Brachial Plexus
Flexor carpi radialis muscle	Lower Arm and Wrist Muscle, Right
	Lower Arm and Wrist Muscle, Left
Flexor carpi ulnaris muscle	Lower Arm and Wrist Muscle, Right
	Lower Arm and Wrist Muscle, Left
Flexor digitorum brevis muscle	Foot Muscle, Right
	Foot Muscle, Left
Flexor digitorum longus muscle	Lower Leg Muscle, Right
	Lower Leg Muscle, Left
Flexor hallucis brevis muscle	Foot Muscle, Right
	Foot Muscle, Left
Flexor hallucis longus muscle	Lower Leg Muscle, Right
	Lower Leg Muscle, Left
Flexor pollicis longus muscle	Lower Arm and Wrist Muscle, Right
	Lower Arm and Wrist Muscle, Left

Anatomical Term	ICD-10-PCS Value
Foramen magnum	Occipital Bone
Foramen of Monro (intraventricular)	Cerebral Ventricle
Foreskin	Prepuce
Fossa of Rosenmuller	Nasopharynx
Fourth cranial nerve	Trochlear Nerve
Fourth ventricle	Cerebral Ventricle
Fovea	Retina, Right
	Retina, Left
Frenulum labii inferioris	Lower Lip
Frenulum labii superioris	Upper Lip
Frenulum linguae	Tongue
Frontal lobe	Cerebral Hemisphere
Frontal vein	Face Vein, Right
	Face Vein, Left
Fundus uteri	Uterus
Galea aponeurotica	Subcutaneous Tissue and Fascia, Scalp
Ganglion impar (ganglion of Walther)	Sacral Sympathetic Nerve
Gasserian ganglion	Trigeminal Nerve
Gastric lymph node	Lymphatic, Aortic
Gastric plexus	Abdominal Sympathetic Nerve
Gastrocnemius muscle	Lower Leg Muscle, Right
	Lower Leg Muscle, Left
Gastrocolic ligament	Omentum
Gastrocolic omentum	Omentum
Gastroduodenal artery	Hepatic Artery
Gastroesophageal (GE) junction	Esophagogastric Junction
Gastrohepatic omentum	Omentum
Gastrophrenic ligament	Omentum
Gastrosplenic ligament	Omentum
Gemellus muscle	Hip Muscle, Right
	Hip Muscle, Left
Geniculate ganglion	Facial Nerve
Geniculate nucleus	Thalamus
Genioglossus muscle	Tongue, Palate, Pharynx Muscle
Genitofemoral nerve	Lumbar Plexus
Glans penis	Prepuce
Glenohumeral joint	Shoulder Joint, Right
	Shoulder Joint, Left
Glenohumeral ligament	Shoulder Bursa and Ligament, Right
	Shoulder Bursa and Ligament, Left
Glenoid fossa (of scapula)	Glenoid Cavity, Right
	Glenoid Cavity, Left
Glenoid ligament (labrum)	Shoulder Joint, Right
	Shoulder Joint, Left

Anatomical Term	ICD-10-PCS Value
Globus pallidus	Basal Ganglia
Glossoepiglottic fold	Epiglottis
Glottis	Larynx
Gluteal lymph node	Lymphatic, Pelvis
Gluteal vein	Hypogastric Vein, Right
	Hypogastric Vein, Left
Gluteus maximus muscle	Hip Muscle, Right
	Hip Muscle, Left
Gluteus medius muscle	Hip Muscle, Right
	Hip Muscle, Left
Gluteus minimus muscle	Hip Muscle, Right
	Hip Muscle, Left
Gracilis muscle	Upper Leg Muscle, Right
	Upper Leg Muscle, Left
Great auricular nerve	Cervical Plexus
Great cerebral vein	Intracranial Vein
Great(er) saphenous vein	Saphenous Vein, Right
	Saphenous Vein, Left
Greater alar cartilage	Nasal Mucosa and Soft Tissue
Greater occipital nerve	Cervical Nerve
Greater Omentum	Omentum
Greater splanchnic nerve	Thoracic Sympathetic Nerve
Greater superficial petrosal nerve	Facial Nerve
Greater trochanter	Upper Femur, Right
	Upper Femur, Left
Greater tuberosity	Humeral Head, Right
	Humeral Head, Left
Greater vestibular (Bartholin's) gland	Vestibular Gland
Greater wing	Sphenoid Bone
Hallux	1st Toe, Right
	1st Toe, Left
Hamate bone	Carpal, Right
	Carpal, Left
Head of fibula	Fibula, Right
	Fibula, Left
Helix	External Ear, Right
	External Ear, Left
	External Ear, Bilateral
Hepatic artery proper	Hepatic Artery
Hepatic flexure	Transverse Colon
Hepatic lymph node	Lymphatic, Aortic
Hepatic plexus	Abdominal Sympathetic Nerve
Hepatic portal vein	Portal Vein
Hepatogastric ligament	Omentum
Hepatopancreatic ampulla	Ampulla of Vater

APPENDIX B: BODY PART KEY

Anatomical Term	ICD-10-PCS Value
Humeroradial joint	Elbow Joint, Right
	Elbow Joint, Left
Humeroulnar joint	Elbow Joint, Right
	Elbow Joint, Left
Humerus, distal	Humeral Shaft, Right
	Humeral Shaft, Left
Hyoglossus muscle	Tongue, Palate, Pharynx Muscle
Hyoid artery	Thyroid Artery, Right
	Thyroid Artery, Left
Hypogastric artery	Internal Iliac Artery, Right
	Internal Iliac Artery, Left
Hypopharynx	Pharynx
Hypophysis	Pituitary Gland
Hypothenar muscle	Hand Muscle, Right
	Hand Muscle, Left
Ileal artery	Superior Mesenteric Artery
Ileocolic artery	Superior Mesenteric Artery
Ileocolic vein	Colic Vein
Iliac crest	Pelvic Bone, Right
	Pelvic Bone, Left
Iliac fascia	Subcutaneous Tissue and Fascia, Right Upper Leg
	Subcutaneous Tissue and Fascia, Left Upper Leg
Iliac lymph node	Lymphatic, Pelvis
Iliacus muscle	Hip Muscle, Right
	Hip Muscle, Left
Iliofemoral ligament	Hip Bursa and Ligament, Right
	Hip Bursa and Ligament, Left
Iliohypogastric nerve	Lumbar Plexus
Ilioinguinal nerve	Lumbar Plexus
Iliolumbar artery	Internal Iliac Artery, Right
	Internal Iliac Artery, Left
Iliolumbar ligament	Lower Spine Bursa and Ligament
Iliotibial tract (band)	Subcutaneous Tissue and Fascia, Right Upper Leg
	Subcutaneous Tissue and Fascia, Left Upper Leg
Ilium	Pelvic Bone, Right
	Pelvic Bone, Left
Incus	Auditory Ossicle, Right
	Auditory Ossicle, Left
Inferior cardiac nerve	Thoracic Sympathetic Nerve
Inferior cerebellar vein	Intracranial Vein
Inferior cerebral vein	Intracranial Vein
Inferior epigastric artery	External Iliac Artery, Right
	External Iliac Artery, Left
Inferior epigastric lymph node	Lymphatic, Pelvis

Anatomical Term	ICD-10-PCS Value
Inferior genicular artery	Popliteal Artery, Right
	Popliteal Artery, Left
Inferior gluteal artery	Internal Iliac Artery, Right
	Internal Iliac Artery, Left
Inferior gluteal nerve	Sacral Plexus
Inferior hypogastric plexus	Abdominal Sympathetic Nerve
Inferior labial artery	Face Artery
Inferior longitudinal muscle	Tongue, Palate, Pharynx Muscle
Inferior mesenteric ganglion	Abdominal Sympathetic Nerve
Inferior mesenteric lymph node	Lymphatic, Mesenteric
Inferior mesenteric plexus	Abdominal Sympathetic Nerve
Inferior oblique muscle	Extraocular Muscle, Right
	Extraocular Muscle, Left
Inferior pancreaticoduodenal artery	Superior Mesenteric Artery
Inferior phrenic artery	Abdominal Aorta
Inferior rectus muscle	Extraocular Muscle, Right
	Extraocular Muscle, Left
Inferior suprarenal artery	Renal Artery, Right
	Renal Artery, Left
Inferior tarsal plate	Lower Eyelid, Right
	Lower Eyelid, Left
Inferior thyroid vein	Innominate Vein, Right
	Innominate Vein, Left
Inferior tibiofibular joint	Ankle Joint, Right
	Ankle Joint, Left
Inferior turbinate	Nasal Turbinate
Inferior ulnar collateral artery	Brachial Artery, Right
	Brachial Artery, Left
Inferior vesical artery	Internal Iliac Artery, Right
	Internal Iliac Artery, Left
Infraauricular lymph node	Lymphatic, Head
Infraclavicular (deltopectoral) lymphnode	Lymphatic, Right Upper Extremity
	Lymphatic, Left Upper Extremity
Infrahyoid muscle	Neck Muscle, Right
	Neck Muscle, Left
Infraparotid lymph node	Lymphatic, Head
Infraspinatus fascia	Subcutaneous Tissue and Fascia, Right Upper Arm
	Subcutaneous Tissue and Fascia, Left Upper Arm
Infraspinatus muscle	Shoulder Muscle, Right
	Shoulder Muscle, Left
Infundibulopelvic ligament	Uterine Supporting Structure
Inguinal canal	Inguinal Region, Right
	Inguinal Region, Left
	Inguinal Region, Bilateral

Anatomical Term	ICD-10-PCS Value
Inguinal triangle	Inguinal Region, Right
	Inguinal Region, Left
	Inguinal Region, Bilateral
Interatrial septum	Atrial Septum
Intercarpal joint	Carpal Joint, Right
	Carpal Joint, Left
Intercarpal ligament	Hand Bursa and Ligament, Right
	Hand Bursa and Ligament, Left
Interclavicular ligament	Shoulder Bursa and Ligament, Right
	Shoulder Bursa and Ligament, Left
Intercostal lymph node	Lymphatic, Thorax
Intercostal muscle	Thorax Muscle, Right
	Thorax Muscle, Left
Intercostal nerve	Thoracic Nerve
Intercostobrachial nerve	Thoracic Nerve
Intercuneiform joint	Tarsal Joint, Right
	Tarsal Joint, Left
Intercuneiform ligament	Foot Bursa and Ligament, Right
	Foot Bursa and Ligament, Left
Intermediate bronchus	Main Bronchus, Right
Intermediate cuneiform bone	Tarsal, Right
	Tarsal, Left
Internal (basal) cerebral vein	Intracranial Vein
Internal anal sphincter	Anal Sphincter
Internal carotid artery, intracranial portion	Intracranial Artery
Internal carotid plexus	Head and Neck Sympathetic Nerve
Internal iliac vein	Hypogastric Vein, Right
	Hypogastric Vein, Left
Internal maxillary artery	External Carotid Artery, Right
	External Carotid Artery, Left
Internal naris	Nasal Mucosa and Soft Tissue
Internal oblique muscle	Abdomen Muscle, Right
	Abdomen Muscle, Left
Internal pudendal artery	Internal Iliac Artery, Right
	Internal Iliac Artery, Left
Internal pudendal vein	Hypogastric Vein, Right
	Hypogastric Vein, Left
Internal thoracic artery	Internal Mammary Artery, Right
	Internal Mammary Artery, Left
	Subclavian Artery, Right
	Subclavian Artery, Left
Internal urethral sphincter	Urethra
Interphalangeal (IP) joint	Finger Phalangeal Joint, Right
	Finger Phalangeal Joint, Left
	Toe Phalangeal Joint, Right
	Toe Phalangeal Joint, Left

Anatomical Term	ICD-10-PCS Value
Interphalangeal ligament	Hand Bursa and Ligament, Right
	Hand Bursa and Ligament, Left
	Foot Bursa and Ligament, Right
	Foot Bursa and Ligament, Left
Interspinalis muscle	Trunk Muscle, Right
	Trunk Muscle, Left
Interspinous ligament	Head and Neck Bursa and Ligament
	Upper Spine Bursa and Ligament
	Lower Spine Bursa and Ligament
Intertransversarius muscle	Trunk Muscle, Right
	Trunk Muscle, Left
Intertransverse ligament	Upper Spine Bursa and Ligament
	Lower Spine Bursa and Ligament
Interventricular foramen (Monro)	Cerebral Ventricle
Interventricular septum	Ventricular Septum
Intestinal lymphatic trunk	Cisterna Chyli
Ischiatic nerve	Sciatic Nerve
Ischiocavernosus muscle	Perineum Muscle
Ischiofemoral ligament	Hip Bursa and Ligament, Right
	Hip Bursa and Ligament, Left
Ischium	Pelvic Bone, Right
	Pelvic Bone, Left
Jejunal artery	Superior Mesenteric Artery
Jugular body	Glomus Jugulare
Jugular lymph node	Lymphatic, Right Neck
	Lymphatic, Left Neck
Labia majora	Vulva
Labia minora	Vulva
Labial gland	Upper Lip
	Lower Lip
Lacrimal canaliculus	Lacrimal Duct, Right
	Lacrimal Duct, Left
Lacrimal punctum	Lacrimal Duct, Right
	Lacrimal Duct, Left
Lacrimal sac	Lacrimal Duct, Right
	Lacrimal Duct, Left
Laryngopharynx	Pharynx
Lateral (brachial) lymph node	Lymphatic, Right Axillary
	Lymphatic, Left Axillary
Lateral canthus	Upper Eyelid, Right
	Upper Eyelid, Left
Lateral collateral ligament (LCL)	Knee Bursa and Ligament, Right
	Knee Bursa and Ligament, Left
Lateral condyle of femur	Lower Femur, Right
	Lower Femur, Left

Anatomical Term	ICD-10-PCS Value
Lateral condyle of tibia	Tibia, Right
	Tibia, Left
Lateral cuneiform bone	Tarsal, Right
	Tarsal, Left
Lateral epicondyle of femur	Lower Femur, Right
	Lower Femur, Left
Lateral epicondyle of humerus	Humeral Shaft, Right
	Humeral Shaft, Left
Lateral femoral cutaneous nerve	Lumbar Plexus
Lateral malleolus	Fibula, Right
	Fibula, Left
Lateral meniscus	Knee Joint, Right
	Knee Joint, Left
Lateral nasal cartilage	Nasal Mucosa and Soft Tissue
Lateral plantar artery	Foot Artery, Right
	Foot Artery, Left
Lateral plantar nerve	Tibial Nerve
Lateral rectus muscle	Extraocular Muscle, Right
	Extraocular Muscle, Left
Lateral sacral artery	Internal Iliac Artery, Right
	Internal Iliac Artery, Left
Lateral sacral vein	Hypogastric Vein, Right
	Hypogastric Vein, Left
Lateral sural cutaneous nerve	Peroneal Nerve
Lateral tarsal artery	Foot Artery, Right
	Foot Artery, Left
Lateral temporomandibular ligament	Head and Neck Bursa and Ligament
Lateral thoracic artery	Axillary Artery, Right
	Axillary Artery, Left
Latissimus dorsi muscle	Trunk Muscle, Right
	Trunk Muscle, Left
Least splanchnic nerve	Thoracic Sympathetic Nerve
Left ascending lumbar vein	Hemiazygos Vein
Left atrioventricular valve	Mitral Valve
Left auricular appendix	Atrium, Left
Left colic vein	Colic Vein
Left coronary sulcus	Heart, Left
Left gastric artery	Gastric Artery
Left gastroepiploic artery	Splenic Artery
Left gastroepiploic vein	Splenic Vein
Left inferior phrenic vein	Renal Vein, Left
Left inferior pulmonary vein	Pulmonary Vein, Left
Left jugular trunk	Thoracic Duct
Left lateral ventricle	Cerebral Ventricle
Left ovarian vein	Renal Vein, Left

Anatomical Term	ICD-10-PCS Value
Left second lumbar vein	Renal Vein, Left
Left subclavian trunk	Thoracic Duct
Left subcostal vein	Hemiazygos Vein
Left superior pulmonary vein	Pulmonary Vein, Left
Left suprarenal vein	Renal Vein, Left
Left testicular vein	Renal Vein, Left
Leptomeninges, intracranial	Cerebral Meninges
Leptomeninges, spinal	Spinal Meninges
Lesser alar cartilage	Nasal Mucosa and Soft Tissue
Lesser occipital nerve	Cervical Plexus
Lesser omentum	Omentum
Lesser saphenous vein	Saphenous Vein, Right
	Saphenous Vein, Left
Lesser splanchnic nerve	Thoracic Sympathetic Nerve
Lesser trochanter	Upper Femur, Right
	Upper Femur, Left
Lesser tuberosity	Humeral Head, Right
	Humeral Head, Left
Lesser wing	Sphenoid Bone
Levator anguli oris muscle	Facial Muscle
Levator ani muscle	Perineum Muscle
Levator labii superioris alaeque nasi muscle	Facial Muscle
Levator labii superioris muscle	Facial Muscle
Levator palpebrae superioris muscle	Upper Eyelid, Right
	Upper Eyelid, Left
Levator scapulae muscle	Neck Muscle, Right
	Neck Muscle, Left
Levator veli palatini muscle	Tongue, Palate, Pharynx Muscle
Levatores costarum muscle	Thorax Muscle, Right
	Thorax Muscle, Left
Ligament of head of fibula	Knee Bursa and Ligament, Right
	Knee Bursa and Ligament, Left
Ligament of the lateral malleolus	Ankle Bursa and Ligament, Right
	Ankle Bursa and Ligament, Left
Ligamentum flavum	Upper Spine Bursa and Ligament
	Lower Spine Bursa and Ligament
Lingual artery	External Carotid Artery, Right
	External Carotid Artery, Left
Lingual tonsil	Pharynx
Locus ceruleus	Pons
Long thoracic nerve	Brachial Plexus
Lumbar artery	Abdominal Aorta
Lumbar facet joint	Lumbar Vertebral Joint
Lumbar ganglion	Lumbar Sympathetic Nerve
Lumbar lymph node	Lymphatic, Aortic
Lumbar lymphatic trunk	Cisterna Chyli
Lumbar splanchnic nerve	Lumbar Sympathetic Nerve

Anatomical Term	ICD-10-PCS Value
Lumbosacral facet joint	Lumbosacral Joint
Lumbosacral trunk	Lumbar Nerve
Lunate bone	Carpal, Right
	Carpal, Left
Lunotriquetral ligament	Hand Bursa and Ligament, Right
	Hand Bursa and Ligament, Left
Macula	Retina, Right
	Retina, Left
Malleus	Auditory Ossicle, Right
	Auditory Ossicle, Left
Mammary duct	Breast, Right
	Breast, Left
	Breast, Bilateral
Mammary gland	Breast, Right
	Breast, Left
	Breast, Bilateral
Mammillary body	Hypothalamus
Mandibular nerve	Trigeminal Nerve
Mandibular notch	Mandible, Right
	Mandible, Left
Manubrium	Sternum
Masseter muscle	Head Muscle
Masseteric fascia	Subcutaneous Tissue and Fascia, Face
Mastoid (postauricular) lymph node	Lymphatic, Right Neck
	Lymphatic, Left Neck
Mastoid air cells	Mastoid Sinus, Right
	Mastoid Sinus, Left
Mastoid process	Temporal Bone, Right
	Temporal Bone, Left
Maxillary artery	External Carotid Artery, Right
	External Carotid Artery, Left
Maxillary nerve	Trigeminal Nerve
Medial canthus	Lower Eyelid, Right
	Lower Eyelid, Left
Medial collateral ligament (MCL)	Knee Bursa and Ligament, Right
	Knee Bursa and Ligament, Left
Medial condyle of femur	Lower Femur, Right
	Lower Femur, Left
Medial condyle of tibia	Tibia, Right
	Tibia, Left
Medial cuneiform bone	Tarsal, Right
	Tarsal, Left
Medial epicondyle of femur	Lower Femur, Right
	Lower Femur, Left
Medial epicondyle of humerus	Humeral Shaft, Right
	Humeral Shaft, Left

Anatomical Term	ICD-10-PCS Value
Medial malleolus	Tibia, Right
	Tibia, Left
Medial meniscus	Knee Joint, Right
	Knee Joint, Left
Medial plantar artery	Foot Artery, Right
	Foot Artery, Left
Medial plantar nerve	Tibial Nerve
Medial popliteal nerve	Tibial Nerve
Medial rectus muscle	Extraocular Muscle, Right
	Extraocular Muscle, Left
Medial sural cutaneous nerve	Tibial Nerve
Median antebrachial vein	Basilic Vein, Right
	Basilic Vein, Left
Median cubital vein	Basilic Vein, Right
	Basilic Vein, Left
Median sacral artery	Abdominal Aorta
Mediastinal lymph node	Lymphatic, Thorax
Meissner's (submucous) plexus	Abdominal Sympathetic Nerve
Membranous urethra	Urethra
Mental foramen	Mandible, Right
	Mandible, Left
Mentalis muscle	Facial Muscle
Mesoappendix	Mesentery
Mesocolon	Mesentery
Metacarpal ligament	Hand Bursa and Ligament, Right
	Hand Bursa and Ligament, Left
Metacarpophalangeal ligament	Hand Bursa and Ligament, Right
	Hand Bursa and Ligament, Left
Metatarsal ligament	Foot Bursa and Ligament, Right
	Foot Bursa and Ligament, Left
Metatarsophalangeal (MTP) joint	Metatarsal-Phalangeal Joint, Right
	Metatarsal-Phalangeal Joint, Left
Metatarsophalangeal ligament	Foot Bursa and Ligament, Right
	Foot Bursa and Ligament, Left
Metathalamus	Thalamus
Midcarpal joint	Carpal Joint, Right
	Carpal Joint, Left
Middle cardiac nerve	Thoracic Sympathetic Nerve
Middle cerebral artery	Intracranial Artery
Middle cerebral vein	Intracranial Vein
Middle colic vein	Colic Vein
Middle genicular artery	Popliteal Artery, Right
	Popliteal Artery, Left
Middle hemorrhoidal vein	Hypogastric Vein, Right
	Hypogastric Vein, Left
Middle rectal artery	Internal Iliac Artery, Right
	Internal Iliac Artery, Left

Anatomical Term	ICD-10-PCS Value
Middle suprarenal artery	Abdominal Aorta
Middle temporal artery	Temporal Artery, Right
	Temporal Artery, Left
Middle turbinate	Nasal Turbinate
Mitral annulus	Mitral Valve
Molar gland	Buccal Mucosa
Musculocutaneous nerve	Brachial Plexus
Musculophrenic artery	Internal Mammary Artery, Right
	Internal Mammary Artery, Left
Musculospiral nerve	Radial Nerve
Myelencephalon	Medulla Oblongata
Myenteric (Auerbach's) plexus	Abdominal Sympathetic Nerve
Myometrium	Uterus
Nail bed	Finger Nail
	Toe Nail
Nail plate	Finger Nail
	Toe Nail
Nasal cavity	Nasal Mucosa and Soft Tissue
Nasal concha	Nasal Turbinate
Nasalis muscle	Facial Muscle
Nasolacrimal duct	Lacrimal Duct, Right
	Lacrimal Duct, Left
Navicular bone	Tarsal, Right
	Tarsal, Left
Neck of femur	Upper Femur, Right
	Upper Femur, Left
Neck of humerus (anatomical) (surgical)	Humeral Head, Right
	Humeral Head, Left
Nerve to the stapedius	Facial Nerve
Neurohypophysis	Pituitary Gland
Ninth cranial nerve	Glossopharyngeal Nerve
Nostril	Nasal Mucosa and Soft Tissue
Obturator artery	Internal Iliac Artery, Right
	Internal Iliac Artery, Left
Obturator lymph node	Lymphatic, Pelvis
Obturator muscle	Hip Muscle, Right
	Hip Muscle, Left
Obturator nerve	Lumbar Plexus
Obturator vein	Hypogastric Vein, Right
	Hypogastric Vein, Left
Obtuse margin	Heart, Left
Occipital artery	External Carotid Artery, Right
	External Carotid Artery, Left
Occipital lobe	Cerebral Hemisphere
Occipital lymph node	Lymphatic, Right Neck
	Lymphatic, Left Neck
Occipitofrontalis muscle	Facial Muscle

Anatomical Term	ICD-10-PCS Value
Odontoid process	Cervical Vertebra
Olecranon bursa	Elbow Bursa and Ligament, Right
	Elbow Bursa and Ligament, Left
Olecranon process	Ulna, Right
	Ulna, Left
Olfactory bulb	Olfactory Nerve
Ophthalmic artery	Intracranial Artery
Ophthalmic nerve	Trigeminal Nerve
Ophthalmic vein	Intracranial Vein
Optic chiasma	Optic Nerve
Optic disc	Retina, Right
	Retina, Left
Optic foramen	Sphenoid Bone
Orbicularis oculi muscle	Upper Eyelid, Right
	Upper Eyelid, Left
Orbicularis oris muscle	Facial Muscle
Orbital fascia	Subcutaneous Tissue and Fascia, Face
Orbital portion of ethmoid bone	Orbit, Right
	Orbit, Left
Orbital portion of frontal bone	Orbit, Right
	Orbit, Left
Orbital portion of lacrimal bone	Orbit, Right
	Orbit, Left
Orbital portion of maxilla	Orbit, Right
	Orbit, Left
Orbital portion of palatine bone	Orbit, Right
	Orbit, Left
Orbital portion of sphenoid bone	Orbit, Right
	Orbit, Left
Orbital portion of zygomatic bone	Orbit, Right
	Orbit, Left
Oropharynx	Pharynx
Otic ganglion	Head and Neck Sympathetic Nerve
Oval window	Middle Ear, Right
	Middle Ear, Left
Ovarian artery	Abdominal Aorta
Ovarian ligament	Uterine Supporting Structure
Oviduct	Fallopian Tube, Right
	Fallopian Tube, Left
Palatine gland	Buccal Mucosa
Palatine tonsil	Tonsils
Palatine uvula	Uvula
Palatoglossal muscle	Tongue, Palate, Pharynx Muscle
Palatopharyngeal muscle	Tongue, Palate, Pharynx Muscle
Palmar (volar) digital vein	Hand Vein, Right
	Hand Vein, Left

Anatomical Term	ICD-10-PCS Value
Palmar (volar) metacarpal vein	Hand Vein, Right
	Hand Vein, Left
Palmar cutaneous nerve	Median Nerve
	Radial Nerve
Palmar fascia (aponeurosis)	Subcutaneous Tissue and Fascia, Right Hand
	Subcutaneous Tissue and Fascia, Left Hand
Palmar interosseous muscle	Hand Muscle, Right
	Hand Muscle, Left
Palmar ulnocarpal ligament	Wrist Bursa and Ligament, Right
	Wrist Bursa and Ligament, Left
Palmaris longus muscle	Lower Arm and Wrist Muscle, Right
	Lower Arm and Wrist Muscle, Left
Pancreatic artery	Splenic Artery
Pancreatic plexus	Abdominal Sympathetic Nerve
Pancreatic vein	Splenic Vein
Pancreaticosplenic lymph node	Lymphatic, Aortic
Paraaortic lymph node	Lymphatic, Aortic
Pararectal lymph node	Lymphatic, Mesenteric
Parasternal lymph node	Lymphatic, Thorax
Paratracheal lymph node	Lymphatic, Thorax
Paraurethral (Skene's) gland	Vestibular Gland
Parietal lobe	Cerebral Hemisphere
Parotid lymph node	Lymphatic, Head
Parotid plexus	Facial Nerve
Pars flaccida	Tympanic Membrane, Right
	Tympanic Membrane, Left
Patellar ligament	Knee Bursa and Ligament, Right
	Knee Bursa and Ligament, Left
Patellar tendon	Knee Tendon, Right
	Knee Tendon, Left
Patellofemoral joint	Knee Joint, Right
	Knee Joint, Left
	Knee Joint, Femoral Surface, Right
	Knee Joint, Femoral Surface, Left
Pectineus muscle	Upper Leg Muscle, Right
	Upper Leg Muscle, Left
Pectoral (anterior) lymph node	Lymphatic, Right Axillary
	Lymphatic, Left Axillary
Pectoral fascia	Subcutaneous Tissue and Fascia, Chest
Pectoralis major muscle	Thorax Muscle, Right
	Thorax Muscle, Left
Pectoralis minor muscle	Thorax Muscle, Right
	Thorax Muscle, Left

Anatomical Term	ICD-10-PCS Value
Pelvic splanchnic nerve	Abdominal Sympathetic Nerve
	Sacral Sympathetic Nerve
Penile urethra	Urethra
Pericardiophrenic artery	Internal Mammary Artery, Right
	Internal Mammary Artery, Left
Perimetrium	Uterus
Peroneus brevis muscle	Lower Leg Muscle, Right
	Lower Leg Muscle, Left
Peroneus longus muscle	Lower Leg Muscle, Right
	Lower Leg Muscle, Left
Petrous part of temporal bone	Temporal Bone, Right
	Temporal Bone, Left
Pharyngeal constrictor muscle	Tongue, Palate, Pharynx Muscle
Pharyngeal plexus	Vagus Nerve
Pharyngeal recess	Nasopharynx
Pharyngeal tonsil	Adenoids
Pharyngotympanic tube	Eustachian Tube, Right
	Eustachian Tube, Left
Pia mater, intracranial	Cerebral Meninges
Pia mater, spinal	Spinal Meninges
Pinna	External Ear, Right
	External Ear, Left
	External Ear, Bilateral
Piriform recess (sinus)	Pharynx
Piriformis muscle	Hip Muscle, Right
	Hip Muscle, Left
Pisiform bone	Carpal, Right
	Carpal, Left
Pisohamate ligament	Hand Bursa and Ligament, Right
	Hand Bursa and Ligament, Left
Pisometacarpal ligament	Hand Bursa and Ligament, Right
	Hand Bursa and Ligament, Left
Plantar digital vein	Foot Vein, Right
	Foot Vein, Left
Plantar fascia (aponeurosis)	Subcutaneous Tissue and Fascia, Right Foot
	Subcutaneous Tissue and Fascia, Left Foot
Plantar metatarsal vein	Foot Vein, Right
	Foot Vein, Left
Plantar venous arch	Foot Vein, Right
	Foot Vein, Left
Platysma muscle	Neck Muscle, Right
	Neck Muscle, Left
Plica semilunaris	Conjunctiva, Right
	Conjunctiva, Left
Pneumogastric nerve	Vagus Nerve

Anatomical Term	ICD-10-PCS Value
Pneumotaxic center	Pons
Pontine tegmentum	Pons
Popliteal ligament	Knee Bursa and Ligament, Right
	Knee Bursa and Ligament, Left
Popliteal lymph node	Lymphatic, Right Lower Extremity
	Lymphatic, Left Lower Extremity
Popliteal vein	Femoral Vein, Right
	Femoral Vein, Left
Popliteus muscle	Lower Leg Muscle, Right
	Lower Leg Muscle, Left
Postauricular (mastoid) lymph node	Lymphatic, Right Neck
	Lymphatic, Left Neck
Postcava	Inferior Vena Cava
Posterior (subscapular) lymph node	Lymphatic, Right Axillary
	Lymphatic, Left Axillary
Posterior auricular artery	External Carotid Artery, Right
	External Carotid Artery, Left
Posterior auricular nerve	Facial Nerve
Posterior auricular vein	External Jugular Vein, Right
	External Jugular Vein, Left
Posterior cerebral artery	Intracranial Artery
Posterior chamber	Eye, Right
	Eye, Left
Posterior circumflex humeral artery	Axillary Artery, Right
	Axillary Artery, Left
Posterior communicating artery	Intracranial Artery
Posterior cruciate ligament (PCL)	Knee Bursa and Ligament, Right
	Knee Bursa and Ligament, Left
Posterior facial (retromandibular) vein	Face Vein, Right
	Face Vein, Left
Posterior femoral cutaneous nerve	Sacral Plexus
Posterior inferior cerebellar artery(PICA)	Intracranial Artery
Posterior interosseous nerve	Radial Nerve
Posterior labial nerve	Pudendal Nerve
Posterior scrotal nerve	Pudendal Nerve
Posterior spinal artery	Vertebral Artery, Right
	Vertebral Artery, Left
Posterior tibial recurrent artery	Anterior Tibial Artery, Right
	Anterior Tibial Artery, Left
Posterior ulnar recurrent artery	Ulnar Artery, Right
	Ulnar Artery, Left
Posterior vagal trunk	Vagus Nerve
Preauricular lymph node	Lymphatic, Head
Precava	Superior Vena Cava

Anatomical Term	ICD-10-PCS Value
Prepatellar bursa	Knee Bursa and Ligament, Right
	Knee Bursa and Ligament, Left
Pretracheal fascia	Subcutaneous Tissue and Fascia, Right Neck
	Subcutaneous Tissue and Fascia, Left Neck
Prevertebral fascia	Subcutaneous Tissue and Fascia, Right Neck
	Subcutaneous Tissue and Fascia, Left Neck
Princeps pollicis artery	Hand Artery, Right
	Hand Artery, Left
Procerus muscle	Facial Muscle
Profunda brachii	Brachial Artery, Right
	Brachial Artery, Left
Profunda femoris (deep femoral) vein	Femoral Vein, Right
	Femoral Vein, Left
Pronator quadratus muscle	Lower Arm and Wrist Muscle, Right
	Lower Arm and Wrist Muscle, Left
Pronator teres muscle	Lower Arm and Wrist Muscle, Right
	Lower Arm and Wrist Muscle, Left
Prostatic urethra	Urethra
Proximal radioulnar joint	Elbow Joint, Right
	Elbow Joint, Left
Psoas muscle	Hip Muscle, Right
	Hip Muscle, Left
Pterygoid muscle	Head Muscle
Pterygoid process	Sphenoid Bone
Pterygopalatine (sphenopalatine) ganglion	Head and Neck Sympathetic Nerve
Pubis	Pelvic Bone, Right
	Pelvic Bone, Left
Pubofemoral ligament	Hip Bursa and Ligament, Right
	Hip Bursa and Ligament, Left
Pudendal nerve	Sacral Plexus
Pulmoaortic canal	Pulmonary Artery, Left
Pulmonary annulus	Pulmonary Valve
Pulmonary plexus	Vagus Nerve
	Thoracic Sympathetic Nerve
Pulmonic valve	Pulmonary Valve
Pulvinar	Thalamus
Pyloric antrum	Stomach, Pylorus
Pyloric canal	Stomach, Pylorus
Pyloric sphincter	Stomach, Pylorus
Pyramidalis muscle	Abdomen Muscle, Right
	Abdomen Muscle, Left
Quadrangular cartilage	Nasal Septum
Quadrate lobe	Liver

Anatomical Term	ICD-10-PCS Value
Quadratus femoris muscle	Hip Muscle, Right
	Hip Muscle, Left
Quadratus lumborum muscle	Trunk Muscle, Right
	Trunk Muscle, Left
Quadratus plantae muscle	Foot Muscle, Right
	Foot Muscle, Left
Quadriceps (femoris)	Upper Leg Muscle, Right
	Upper Leg Muscle, Left
Radial collateral carpal ligament	Wrist Bursa and Ligament, Right
	Wrist Bursa and Ligament, Left
Radial collateral ligament	Elbow Bursa and Ligament, Right
	Elbow Bursa and Ligament, Left
Radial notch	Ulna, Right
	Ulna, Left
Radial recurrent artery	Radial Artery, Right
	Radial Artery, Left
Radial vein	Brachial Vein, Right
	Brachial Vein, Left
Radialis indicis	Hand Artery, Right
	Hand Artery, Left
Radiocarpal joint	Wrist Joint, Right
	Wrist Joint, Left
Radiocarpal ligament	Wrist Bursa and Ligament, Right
	Wrist Bursa and Ligament, Left
Radioulnar ligament	Wrist Bursa and Ligament, Right
	Wrist Bursa and Ligament, Left
Rectosigmoid junction	Sigmoid Colon
Rectus abdominis muscle	Abdomen Muscle, Right
	Abdomen Muscle, Left
Rectus femoris muscle	Upper Leg Muscle, Right
	Upper Leg Muscle, Left
Recurrent laryngeal nerve	Vagus Nerve
Renal calyx	Kidney, Right
	Kidney, Left
	Kidneys, Bilateral
	Kidney
Renal capsule	Kidney, Right
	Kidney, Left
	Kidneys, Bilateral
	Kidney
Renal cortex	Kidney, Right
	Kidney, Left
	Kidneys, Bilateral
	Kidney
Renal plexus	Abdominal Sympathetic Nerve

Anatomical Term	ICD-10-PCS Value
Renal segment	Kidney, Right
	Kidney, Left
	Kidneys, Bilateral
	Kidney
Renal segmental artery	Renal Artery, Right
	Renal Artery, Left
Retroperitoneal lymph node	Lymphatic, Aortic
Retroperitoneal space	Retroperitoneum
Retropharyngeal lymph node	Lymphatic, Right Neck
	Lymphatic, Left Neck
Retropubic space	Pelvic Cavity
Rhinopharynx	Nasopharynx
Rhomboid major muscle	Trunk Muscle, Right
	Trunk Muscle, Left
Rhomboid minor muscle	Trunk Muscle, Right
	Trunk Muscle, Left
Right ascending lumbar vein	Azygos Vein
Right atrioventricular valve	Tricuspid Valve
Right auricular appendix	Atrium, Right
Right colic vein	Colic Vein
Right coronary sulcus	Heart, Right
Right gastric artery	Gastric Artery
Right gastroepiploic vein	Superior Mesenteric Vein
Right inferior phrenic vein	Inferior Vena Cava
Right inferior pulmonary vein	Pulmonary Vein, Right
Right jugular trunk	Lymphatic, Right Neck
Right lateral ventricle	Cerebral Ventricle
Right lymphatic duct	Lymphatic, Right Neck
Right ovarian vein	Inferior Vena Cava
Right second lumbar vein	Inferior Vena Cava
Right subclavian trunk	Lymphatic, Right Neck
Right subcostal vein	Azygos Vein
Right superior pulmonary vein	Pulmonary Vein, Right
Right suprarenal vein	Inferior Vena Cava
Right testicular vein	Inferior Vena Cava
Rima glottidis	Larynx
Risorius muscle	Facial Muscle
Round ligament of uterus	Uterine Supporting Structure
Round window	Inner Ear, Right
	Inner Ear, Left
Sacral ganglion	Sacral Sympathetic Nerve
Sacral lymph node	Lymphatic, Pelvis
Sacral splanchnic nerve	Sacral Sympathetic Nerve
Sacrococcygeal ligament	Lower Spine Bursa and Ligament
Sacrococcygeal symphysis	Sacrococcygeal Joint
Sacroiliac ligament	Lower Spine Bursa and Ligament
Sacrospinous ligament	Lower Spine Bursa and Ligament
Sacrotuberous ligament	Lower Spine Bursa and Ligament

Anatomical Term	ICD-10-PCS Value
Salpingopharyngeus muscle	Tongue, Palate, Pharynx Muscle
Salpinx	Fallopian Tube, Right
	Fallopian Tube, Left
Saphenous nerve	Femoral Nerve
Sartorius muscle	Upper Leg Muscle, Right
	Upper Leg Muscle, Left
Scalene muscle	Neck Muscle, Right
	Neck Muscle, Left
Scaphoid bone	Carpal, Right
	Carpal, Left
Scapholunate ligament	Hand Bursa and Ligament, Right
	Hand Bursa and Ligament, Left
Scaphotrapezium ligament	Hand Bursa and Ligament, Right
	Hand Bursa and Ligament, Left
Scarpa's (vestibular) ganglion	Acoustic Nerve
Sebaceous gland	Skin
Second cranial nerve	Optic Nerve
Sella turcica	Sphenoid Bone
Semicircular canal	Inner Ear, Right
	Inner Ear, Left
Semimembranosus muscle	Upper Leg Muscle, Right
	Upper Leg Muscle, Left
Semitendinosus muscle	Upper Leg Muscle, Right
	Upper Leg Muscle, Left
Septal cartilage	Nasal Septum
Serratus anterior muscle	Thorax Muscle, Right
	Thorax Muscle, Left
Serratus posterior muscle	Trunk Muscle, Right
	Trunk Muscle, Left
Seventh cranial nerve	Facial Nerve
Short gastric artery	Splenic Artery
Sigmoid artery	Inferior Mesenteric Artery
Sigmoid flexure	Sigmoid Colon
Sigmoid vein	Inferior Mesenteric Vein
Sinoatrial node	Conduction Mechanism
Sinus venosus	Atrium, Right
Sixth cranial nerve	Abducens Nerve
Skene's (paraurethral) gland	Vestibular Gland
Small saphenous vein	Saphenous Vein, Right
	Saphenous Vein, Left
Solar (celiac) plexus	Abdominal Sympathetic Nerve
Soleus muscle	Lower Leg Muscle, Right
	Lower Leg Muscle, Left
Sphenomandibular ligament	Head and Neck Bursa and Ligament
Sphenopalatine (pterygopalatine) ganglion	Head and Neck Sympathetic Nerve
Spinal nerve, cervical	Cervical Nerve

Anatomical Term	ICD-10-PCS Value
Spinal nerve, lumbar	Lumbar Nerve
Spinal nerve, sacral	Sacral Nerve
Spinal nerve, thoracic	Thoracic Nerve
Spinous process	Cervical Vertebra
	Thoracic Vertebra
	Lumbar Vertebra
Spiral ganglion	Acoustic Nerve
Splenic flexure	Transverse Colon
Splenic plexus	Abdominal Sympathetic Nerve
Splenius capitis muscle	Head Muscle
Splenius cervicis muscle	Neck Muscle, Right
	Neck Muscle, Left
Stapes	Auditory Ossicle, Right
	Auditory Ossicle, Left
Stellate ganglion	Head and Neck Sympathetic Nerve
Stensen's duct	Parotid Duct, Right
	Parotid Duct, Left
Sternoclavicular ligament	Shoulder Bursa and Ligament, Right
	Shoulder Bursa and Ligament, Left
Sternocleidomastoid artery	Thyroid Artery, Right
	Thyroid Artery, Left
Sternocleidomastoid muscle	Neck Muscle, Right
	Neck Muscle, Left
Sternocostal ligament	Sternum Bursa and Ligament
	Rib(s) Bursa and Ligament
Styloglossus muscle	Tongue, Palate, Pharynx Muscle
Stylomandibular ligament	Head and Neck Bursa and Ligament
Stylopharyngeus muscle	Tongue, Palate, Pharynx Muscle
Subacromial bursa	Shoulder Bursa and Ligament, Right
	Shoulder Bursa and Ligament, Left
Subaortic (common iliac) lymph node	Lymphatic, Pelvis
Subarachnoid space, spinal	Spinal Canal
Subclavicular (apical) lymph node	Lymphatic, Right Axillary
	Lymphatic, Left Axillary
Subclavius muscle	Thorax Muscle, Right
	Thorax Muscle, Left
Subclavius nerve	Brachial Plexus
Subcostal artery	Upper Artery
Subcostal muscle	Thorax Muscle, Right
	Thorax Muscle, Left
Subcostal nerve	Thoracic Nerve
Subdural space, spinal	Spinal Canal
Submandibular ganglion	Facial Nerve
	Head and Neck Sympathetic Nerve

Anatomical Term	ICD-10-PCS Value
Submandibular gland	Submaxillary Gland, Right
	Submaxillary Gland, Left
Submandibular lymph node	Lymphatic, Head
Submaxillary ganglion	Head and Neck Sympathetic Nerve
Submaxillary lymph node	Lymphatic, Head
Submental artery	Face Artery
Submental lymph node	Lymphatic, Head
Submucous (Meissner's) plexus	Abdominal Sympathetic Nerve
Suboccipital nerve	Cervical Nerve
Suboccipital venous plexus	Vertebral Vein, Right
	Vertebral Vein, Left
Subparotid lymph node	Lymphatic, Head
Subscapular (posterior) lymph node	Lymphatic, Right Axillary
	Lymphatic, Left Axillary
Subscapular aponeurosis	Subcutaneous Tissue and Fascia, Right Upper Arm
	Subcutaneous Tissue and Fascia, Left Upper Arm
Subscapular artery	Axillary Artery, Right
	Axillary Artery, Left
Subscapularis muscle	Shoulder Muscle, Right
	Shoulder Muscle, Left
Substantia nigra	Basal Ganglia
Subtalar (talocalcaneal) joint	Tarsal Joint, Right
	Tarsal Joint, Left
Subtalar ligament	Foot Bursa and Ligament, Right
	Foot Bursa and Ligament, Left
Subthalamic nucleus	Basal Ganglia
Superficial circumflex iliac vein	Saphenous Vein, Right
	Saphenous Vein, Left
Superficial epigastric artery	Femoral Artery, Right
	Femoral Artery, Left
Superficial epigastric vein	Saphenous Vein, Right
	Saphenous Vein, Left
Superficial palmar arch	Hand Artery, Right
	Hand Artery, Left
Superficial palmar venous arch	Hand Vein, Right
	Hand Vein, Left
Superficial temporal artery	Temporal Artery, Right
	Temporal Artery, Left
Superficial transverse perineal muscle	Perineum Muscle
Superior cardiac nerve	Thoracic Sympathetic Nerve
Superior cerebellar vein	Intracranial Vein
Superior cerebral vein	Intracranial Vein
Superior clunic (cluneal) nerve	Lumbar Nerve
Superior epigastric artery	Internal Mammary Artery, Right
	Internal Mammary Artery, Left

Anatomical Term	ICD-10-PCS Value
Superior genicular artery	Popliteal Artery, Right
	Popliteal Artery, Left
Superior gluteal artery	Internal Iliac Artery, Right
	Internal Iliac Artery, Left
Superior gluteal nerve	Lumbar Plexus
Superior hypogastric plexus	Abdominal Sympathetic Nerve
Superior labial artery	Face Artery
Superior laryngeal artery	Thyroid Artery, Right
	Thyroid Artery, Left
Superior laryngeal nerve	Vagus Nerve
Superior longitudinal muscle	Tongue, Palate, Pharynx Muscle
Superior mesenteric ganglion	Abdominal Sympathetic Nerve
Superior mesenteric lymph node	Lymphatic, Mesenteric
Superior mesenteric plexus	Abdominal Sympathetic Nerve
Superior oblique muscle	Extraocular Muscle, Right
	Extraocular Muscle, Left
Superior olivary nucleus	Pons
Superior rectal artery	Inferior Mesenteric Artery
Superior rectal vein	Inferior Mesenteric Vein
Superior rectus muscle	Extraocular Muscle, Right
	Extraocular Muscle, Left
Superior tarsal plate	Upper Eyelid, Right
	Upper Eyelid, Left
Superior thoracic artery	Axillary Artery, Right
	Axillary Artery, Left
Superior thyroid artery	External Carotid Artery, Right
	External Carotid Artery, Left
	Thyroid Artery, Right
	Thyroid Artery, Left
Superior turbinate	Nasal Turbinate
Superior ulnar collateral artery	Brachial Artery, Right
	Brachial Artery, Left
Supraclavicular (Virchow's) lymph node	Lymphatic, Right Neck
	Lymphatic, Left Neck
Supraclavicular nerve	Cervical Plexus
Suprahyoid lymph node	Lymphatic, Head
Suprahyoid muscle	Neck Muscle, Right
	Neck Muscle, Left
Suprainguinal lymph node	Lymphatic, Pelvis
Supraorbital vein	Face Vein, Right
	Face Vein, Left
Suprarenal gland	Adrenal Gland, Left
	Adrenal Gland, Right
	Adrenal Glands, Bilateral
	Adrenal Gland
Suprarenal plexus	Abdominal Sympathetic Nerve

Anatomical Term	ICD-10-PCS Value
Suprascapular nerve	Brachial Plexus
Supraspinatus fascia	Subcutaneous Tissue and Fascia, Right Upper Arm
	Subcutaneous Tissue and Fascia, Left Upper Arm
Supraspinatus muscle	Shoulder Muscle, Right
	Shoulder Muscle, Left
Supraspinous ligament	Upper Spine Bursa and Ligament
	Lower Spine Bursa and Ligament
Suprasternal notch	Sternum
Supratrochlear lymph node	Lymphatic, Right Upper Extremity
	Lymphatic, Left Upper Extremity
Sural artery	Popliteal Artery, Right
	Popliteal Artery, Left
Sweat gland	Skin
Talocalcaneal (subtalar) joint	Tarsal Joint, Right
	Tarsal Joint, Left
Talocalcaneal ligament	Foot Bursa and Ligament, Right
	Foot Bursa and Ligament, Left
Talocalcaneonavicular joint	Tarsal Joint, Right
	Tarsal Joint, Left
Talocalcaneonavicular ligament	Foot Bursa and Ligament, Right
	Foot Bursa and Ligament, Left
Talocrural joint	Ankle Joint, Right
	Ankle Joint, Left
Talofibular ligament	Ankle Bursa and Ligament, Right
	Ankle Bursa and Ligament, Left
Talus bone	Tarsal, Right
	Tarsal, Left
Tarsometatarsal ligament	Foot Bursa and Ligament, Right
	Foot Bursa and Ligament, Left
Temporal lobe	Cerebral Hemisphere
Temporalis muscle	Head Muscle
Temporoparietalis muscle	Head Muscle
Tensor fasciae latae muscle	Hip Muscle, Right
	Hip Muscle, Left
Tensor veli palatini muscle	Tongue, Palate, Pharynx Muscle
Tenth cranial nerve	Vagus Nerve
Tentorium cerebelli	Dura Mater
Teres major muscle	Shoulder Muscle, Right
	Shoulder Muscle, Left
Teres minor muscle	Shoulder Muscle, Right
	Shoulder Muscle, Left
Testicular artery	Abdominal Aorta
Thenar muscle	Hand Muscle, Right
	Hand Muscle, Left
Third cranial nerve	Oculomotor Nerve

Anatomical Term	ICD-10-PCS Value
Third occipital nerve	Cervical Nerve
Third ventricle	Cerebral Ventricle
Thoracic aortic plexus	Thoracic Sympathetic Nerve
Thoracic esophagus	Esophagus, Middle
Thoracic facet joint	Thoracic Vertebral Joint
Thoracic ganglion	Thoracic Sympathetic Nerve
Thoracoacromial artery	Axillary Artery, Right
	Axillary Artery, Left
Thoracolumbar facet joint	Thoracolumbar Vertebral Joint
Thymus gland	Thymus
Thyroarytenoid muscle	Neck Muscle, Right
	Neck Muscle, Left
Thyrocervical trunk	Thyroid Artery, Right
	Thyroid Artery, Left
Thyroid cartilage	Larynx
Tibialis anterior muscle	Lower Leg Muscle, Right
	Lower Leg Muscle, Left
Tibialis posterior muscle	Lower Leg Muscle, Right
	Lower Leg Muscle, Left
Tibiofemoral joint	Knee Joint, Right
	Knee Joint, Left
	Knee Joint, Tibial Surface, Right
	Knee Joint, Tibial Surface, Left
Tongue, base of	Pharynx
Tracheobronchial lymph node	Lymphatic, Thorax
Tragus	External Ear, Right
	External Ear, Left
	External Ear, Bilateral
Transversalis fascia	Subcutaneous Tissue and Fascia, Trunk
Transverse (cutaneous) cervical nerve	Cervical Plexus
Transverse acetabular ligament	Hip Bursa and Ligament, Right
	Hip Bursa and Ligament, Left
Transverse facial artery	Temporal Artery, Right
	Temporal Artery, Left
Transverse foramen	Cervical Vertebra
Transverse humeral ligament	Shoulder Bursa and Ligament, Right
	Shoulder Bursa and Ligament, Left
Transverse ligament of atlas	Head and Neck Bursa and Ligament
Transverse process	Cervical Vertebra
	Thoracic Vertebra
	Lumbar Vertebra
Transverse scapular ligament	Shoulder Bursa and Ligament, Right
	Shoulder Bursa and Ligament, Left

Anatomical Term	ICD-10-PCS Value
Transverse thoracis muscle	Thorax Muscle, Right
	Thorax Muscle, Left
Transversospinalis muscle	Trunk Muscle, Right
	Trunk Muscle, Left
Transversus abdominis muscle	Abdomen Muscle, Right
	Abdomen Muscle, Left
Trapezium bone	Carpal, Right
	Carpal, Left
Trapezius muscle	Trunk Muscle, Right
	Trunk Muscle, Left
Trapezoid bone	Carpal, Right
	Carpal, Left
Triceps brachii muscle	Upper Arm Muscle, Right
	Upper Arm Muscle, Left
Tricuspid annulus	Tricuspid Valve
Trifacial nerve	Trigeminal Nerve
Trigone of bladder	Bladder
Triquetral bone	Carpal, Right
	Carpal, Left
Trochanteric bursa	Hip Bursa and Ligament, Right
	Hip Bursa and Ligament, Left
Twelfth cranial nerve	Hypoglossal Nerve
Tympanic cavity	Middle Ear, Right
	Middle Ear, Left
Tympanic nerve	Glossopharyngeal Nerve
Tympanic part of temporal bone	Temporal Bone, Right
	Temporal Bone, Left
Ulnar collateral carpal ligament	Wrist Bursa and Ligament, Right
	Wrist Bursa and Ligament, Left
Ulnar collateral ligament	Elbow Bursa and Ligament, Right
	Elbow Bursa and Ligament, Left
Ulnar notch	Radius, Right
	Radius, Left
Ulnar vein	Brachial Vein, Right
	Brachial Vein, Left
Umbilical artery	Internal Iliac Artery, Right
	Internal Iliac Artery, Left
	Lower Artery
Ureteral orifice	Ureter, Right
	Ureter, Left
	Ureters, Bilateral
	Ureter
Ureteropelvic junction (UPJ)	Kidney Pelvis, Right
	Kidney Pelvis, Left

Anatomical Term	ICD-10-PCS Value
Ureterovesical orifice	Ureter, Right
	Ureter, Left
	Ureters, Bilateral
	Ureter
Uterine Artery	Internal Iliac Artery, Right
	Internal Iliac Artery, Left
Uterine cornu	Uterus
Uterine tube	Fallopian Tube, Right
	Fallopian Tube, Left
Uterine vein	Hypogastric Vein, Right
	Hypogastric Vein, Left
Vaginal artery	Internal Iliac Artery, Right
	Internal Iliac Artery, Left
Vaginal vein	Hypogastric Vein, Right
	Hypogastric Vein, Left
Vastus intermedius muscle	Upper Leg Muscle, Right
	Upper Leg Muscle, Left
Vastus lateralis muscle	Upper Leg Muscle, Right
	Upper Leg Muscle, Left
Vastus medialis muscle	Upper Leg Muscle, Right
	Upper Leg Muscle, Left
Ventricular fold	Larynx
Vermiform appendix	Appendix
Vermilion border	Upper Lip
	Lower Lip
Vertebral arch	Cervical Vertebra
	Thoracic Vertebra
	Lumbar Vertebra
Vertebral body	Cervical Vertebra
	Thoracic Vertebra
	Lumbar Vertebra
Vertebral canal	Spinal Canal
Vertebral foramen	Cervical Vertebra
	Thoracic Vertebra
	Lumbar Vertebra
Vertebral lamina	Cervical Vertebra
	Thoracic Vertebra
	Lumbar Vertebra
Vertebral pedicle	Cervical Vertebra
	Thoracic Vertebra
	Lumbar Vertebra
Vesical vein	Hypogastric Vein, Right
	Hypogastric Vein, Left
Vestibular (Scarpa's) ganglion	Acoustic Nerve
Vestibular nerve	Acoustic Nerve
Vestibulocochlear nerve	Acoustic Nerve

Anatomical Term	ICD-10-PCS Value
Virchow's (supraclavicular) lymph node	Lymphatic, Right Neck
	Lymphatic, Left Neck
Vitreous body	Vitreous, Right
	Vitreous, Left
Vocal fold	Vocal Cord, Right
	Vocal Cord, Left
Volar (palmar) digital vein	Hand Vein, Right
	Hand Vein, Left
Volar (palmar) metacarpal vein	Hand Vein, Right
	Hand Vein, Left
Vomer bone	Nasal Septum
Vomer of nasal septum	Nasal Bone
Xiphoid process	Sternum
Zonule of Zinn	Lens, Right
	Lens, Left
Zygomatic process of frontal bone	Frontal Bone
Zygomatic process of temporal bone	Temporal Bone, Right
	Temporal Bone, Left
Zygomaticus muscle	Facial Muscle

This page intentionally left blank

Appendix C: Device Key

Device Term	ICD-10-PCS Value
3f® (Aortic) Bioprosthesis valve	Zooplastic Tissue in Heart and Great Vessels
AbioCor® Total Replacement Heart	Synthetic Substitute
Absolute Pro® Vascular (OTW) Self-Expanding Stent System	Intraluminal Device
Acculink™ (RX) Carotid Stent System	Intraluminal Device
Acellular Hydrated Dermis	Nonautologous Tissue Substitute
Acetabular cup	Liner in Lower Joints
Activa PC® neurostimulator	Stimulator Generator, Multiple Array for Insertion in Subcutaneous Tissue and Fascia
Activa RC® neurostimulator	Stimulator Generator, Multiple Array Rechargeable for Insertion in Subcutaneous Tissue and Fascia
Activa SC® neurostimulator	Stimulator Generator, Single Array for Insertion in Subcutaneous Tissue and Fascia
ACUITY™ Steerable Lead	Cardiac Lead, Pacemaker for Insertion in Heart and Great Vessels
	Cardiac Lead, Defibrillator for Insertion in Heart and Great Vessels
Advisa MRI™	Pacemaker, Dual Chamber for Insertion in Subcutaneous Tissue and Fascia
AFX® Endovascular AAA System	Intraluminal Device
AMPLATZER® Muscular VSD Occluder	Synthetic Substitute
AMS 800® Urinary Control System	Artificial Sphincter in Urinary System
AneuRx® AAA Advantage®	Intraluminal Device
Annuloplasty ring	Synthetic Substitute
Artificial anal sphincter (AAS)	Artificial Sphincter in Gastrointestinal System
Artificial bowel sphincter (neosphincter)	Artificial Sphincter in Gastrointestinal System
Artificial urinary sphincter (AUS)	Artificial Sphincter in Urinary System
Ascenda® Intrathecal Catheter	Infusion Device
Assurant (Cobalt)® stent	Intraluminal Device
AtriClip® LAA Exclusion System	Extraluminal Device
Attain Ability® lead	Cardiac Lead, Pacemaker for Insertion in Heart and Great Vessels
	Cardiac Lead, Defibrillator for Insertion in Heart and Great Vessels
Attain StarFix® (OTW) lead	Cardiac Lead, Pacemaker for Insertion in Heart and Great Vessels
	Cardiac Lead, Defibrillator for Insertion in Heart and Great Vessels

Device Term	ICD-10-PCS Value
Autograft	Autologous Tissue Substitute
Autologous artery graft	Autologous Arterial Tissue in Heart and Great Vessels
	Autologous Arterial Tissue in Upper Arteries
	Autologous Arterial Tissue in Lower Arteries
	Autologous Arterial Tissue in Upper Veins
	Autologous Arterial Tissue in Lower Veins
Autologous vein graft	Autologous Venous Tissue in Heart and Great Vessels
	Autologous Venous Tissue in Upper Arteries
	Autologous Venous Tissue in Lower Arteries
	Autologous Venous Tissue in Upper Veins
	Autologous Venous Tissue in Lower Veins
Axial Lumbar Interbody Fusion System	Interbody Fusion Device in Lower Joints
AxiaLIF® System	Interbody Fusion Device in Lower Joints
BAK/C® Interbody Cervical FusionSystem	Interbody Fusion Device in Upper Joints
Bard® Composix® (E/X)(LP) mesh	Synthetic Substitute
Bard® Composix® Kugel® patch	Synthetic Substitute
Bard® Dulex™ mesh	Synthetic Substitute
Bard® Ventralex™ hernia patch	Synthetic Substitute
Baroreflex Activation Therapy®(BAT®)	Stimulator Lead in Upper Arteries
	Stimulator Generator in Subcutaneous Tissue and Fascia
Berlin Heart® Ventricular Assist Device	Implantable Heart Assist System in Heart and Great Vessels
Bioactive embolization coil(s)	Intraluminal Device, Bioactive in Upper Arteries
Biventricular external heart assist system	Short-term External Heart Assist System in Heart and Great Vessels
Blood glucose monitoring system	Monitoring Device
Bone anchored hearing device	Hearing Device, Bone Conduction for Insertion in Ear, Nose, Sinus
	Hearing Device in Head and Facial Bones
Bone bank bone graft	Nonautologous Tissue Substitute
Bone screw(interlocking)(lag)(pedicle)(recessed)	Internal Fixation Device in Head and Facial Bones
	Internal Fixation Device in Upper Bones
	Internal Fixation Device in Lower Bones

Device Term	ICD-10-PCS Value
Bovine pericardial valve	Zooplastic Tissue in Heart and Great Vessels
Bovine pericardium graft	Zooplastic Tissue in Heart and Great Vessels
Brachytherapy seeds	Radioactive Element
BRYAN® Cervical Disc System	Synthetic Substitute
BVS 5000® Ventricular Assist Device	Short-term External Heart Assist System in Heart and Great Vessels
Cardiac contractility modulation lead	Cardiac Lead in Heart and Great Vessels
Cardiac event recorder	Monitoring Device
Cardiac resynchronization therapy(CRT) lead	Cardiac Lead, Pacemaker for Insertion in Heart and Great Vessels
	Cardiac Lead, Defibrillator for Insertion in Heart and Great Vessels
CardioMEMS® pressure sensor	Monitoring Device, Pressure Sensor for Insertion in Heart and Great Vessels
Carotid (artery) sinus (baroreceptor)lead	Stimulator Lead in Upper Arteries
Carotid WALLSTENT® Monorail®Endoprosthesis	Intraluminal Device
Centrimag® Blood Pump	Short-term External Heart Assist System in Heart and Great Vessels
Ceramic on ceramic bearing surface	Synthetic Substitute, Ceramic for Replacement in Lower Joints
Cesium-131 Collagen Implant	Radioactive Element, Cesium-131 Collagen Implant for Insertion in Central Nervous System and Cranial Nerves
Clamp and rod internal fixation system(CRIF)	Internal Fixation Device in Upper Bones
	Internal Fixation Device in Lower Bones
COALESCE® radiolucent interbody fusion device	Interbody Fusion Device, Radiolucent Porous in New Technology
CoAxia NeuroFlo™ catheter	Intraluminal Device
Cobalt/chromium head and polyethylene socket	Synthetic Substitute, Metal on Polyethylene for Replacement in Lower Joints
Cobalt/chromium head and socket	Synthetic Substitute, Metal for Replacement in Lower Joints
Cochlear implant (CI), multiple channel(electrode)	Hearing Device, Multiple Channel Cochlear Prosthesis for Insertion in Ear, Nose, Sinus
Cochlear implant (CI), single channel(electrode)	Hearing Device, Single Channel Cochlear Prosthesis for Insertion in Ear, Nose, Sinus
COGNIS® CRT-D	Cardiac Resynchronization Defibrillator Pulse Generator for Insertion in Subcutaneous Tissue and Fascia
COHERE® radiolucent interbody fusion device	Interbody Fusion Device, Radiolucent Porous in New Technology

Device Term	ICD-10-PCS Value
Colonic Z-Stent®	Intraluminal Device
Complete® (SE) stent	Intraluminal Device
Concerto® II CRT-D	Cardiac Resynchronization Defibrillator Pulse Generator for Insertion in Subcutaneous Tissue and Fascia
CONSERVE® PLUS Total Resurfacing Hip System	Resurfacing Device in Lower Joints
Consulta® CRT-D	Cardiac Resynchronization Defibrillator Pulse Generator for Insertion in Subcutaneous Tissue and Fascia
Consulta® CRT-P	Cardiac Resynchronization Pacemaker Pulse Generator for Insertion in Subcutaneous Tissue and Fascia
CONTAK RENEWAL® 3 RF (HE) CRT-D	Cardiac Resynchronization Defibrillator Pulse Generator for Insertion in Subcutaneous Tissue and Fascia
Contegra® Pulmonary Valved Conduit	Zooplastic Tissue in Heart and Great Vessels
Continuous Glucose Monitoring (CGM) device	Monitoring Device
Cook Biodesign® Fistula Plug(s)	Nonautologous Tissue Substitute
Cook Biodesign® Hernia Graft(s)	Nonautologous Tissue Substitute
Cook Biodesign® Layered Graft(s)	Nonautologous Tissue Substitute
Cook Zenapro™ Layered Graft(s)	Nonautologous Tissue Substitute
Cook Zenith® AAA Endovascular Graft	Intraluminal Device, Branched or Fenestrated, One or Two Arteries for Restriction in Lower Arteries
	Intraluminal Device, Branched or Fenestrated, Three or More Arteries for Restriction in Lower Arteries
	Intraluminal Device
CoreValve™ transcatheter aortic valve	Zooplastic Tissue in Heart and Great Vessels
Cormet™ Hip Resurfacing System	Resurfacing Device in Lower Joints
CoRoent® XL	Interbody Fusion Device in Lower Joints
Corox® (OTW) Bipolar Lead	Cardiac Lead, Pacemaker for Insertion in Heart and Great Vessels
	Cardiac Lead, Defibrillator for Insertion in Heart and Great Vessels
Cortical strip neurostimulator lead	Neurostimulator Lead in Central Nervous System and Cranial Nerves
Cultured epidermal cell autograft	Autologous Tissue Substitute
CYPHER® Stent	Intraluminal Device, Drug-eluting in Heart and Great Vessels
Cystostomy tube	Drainage Device
DBS™ lead	Neurostimulator Lead in Central Nervous System and Cranial Nerves

Device Term	ICD-10-PCS Value	Device Term	ICD-10-PCS Value
DeBakey® Left Ventricular Assist Device	Implantable Heart Assist System in Heart and Great Vessels	Endotracheal tube (cuffed) (double-lumen)	Intraluminal Device, Endotracheal Airway in Respiratory System
Deep brain neurostimulator lead	Neurostimulator Lead in Central Nervous System and Cranial Nerves	Endurant® Endovascular Stent Graft	Intraluminal Device
Delta frame external fixator	External Fixation Device, Hybrid for Insertion in Upper Bones	Endurant® II AAA stent graft system	Intraluminal Device
	External Fixation Device, Hybrid for Reposition in Upper Bones	EnRhythm®	Pacemaker, Dual Chamber for Insertion in Subcutaneous Tissue and Fascia
	External Fixation Device, Hybrid for Insertion in Lower Bones	Enterra® gastric neurostimulator	Stimulator Generator, Multiple Array for Insertion in Subcutaneous Tissue and Fascia
	External Fixation Device, Hybrid for Reposition in Lower Bones	Epic™ Stented Tissue Valve (aortic)	Zooplastic Tissue in Heart and Great Vessels
Delta III™ Reverse shoulder prosthesis	Synthetic Substitute, Reverse Ball and Socket for Replacement in Upper Joints	Epicel® cultured epidermal autograft	Autologous Tissue Substitute
Diaphragmatic pacemaker generator	Stimulator Generator in Subcutaneous Tissue and Fascia	Esophageal obturator airway (EOA)	Intraluminal Device, Airway in Gastrointestinal System
Direct Lateral Interbody Fusion (DLIF)device	Interbody Fusion Device in Lower Joints	Esteem® implantable hearing system	Hearing Device in Ear, Nose, Sinus
Driver stent (RX) (OTW)	Intraluminal Device	Evera™ (XT)(S)(DR/VR)	Defibrillator Generator for Insertion in Subcutaneous Tissue and Fascia
DuraHeart® Left Ventricular Assist System	Implantable Heart Assist System in Heart and Great Vessels	Everolimus-eluting coronary stent	Intraluminal Device, Drug-eluting in Heart and Great Vessels
Durata® Defibrillation Lead	Cardiac Lead, Defibrillator for Insertion in Heart and Great Vessels	Ex-PRESS™ mini glaucoma shunt	Synthetic Substitute
Dynesys® Dynamic Stabilization System	Spinal Stabilization Device, Pedicle-Based for Insertion in Upper Joints	EXCLUDER® AAA Endoprosthesis	Intraluminal Device, Branched or Fenestrated, One or Two Arteries for Restriction in Lower Arteries
	Spinal Stabilization Device, Pedicle-Based for Insertion in Lower Joints		Intraluminal Device, Branched or Fenestrated, Three or More Arteries for Restriction in Lower Arteries
E-Luminexx™ (Biliary)(Vascular) Stent	Intraluminal Device		Intraluminal Device
EDWARDS INTUITY Elite™ valve system	Zooplastic Tissue, Rapid Deployment Technique in New Technology	EXCLUDER® IBE Endoprosthesis	Intraluminal Device, Branched or Fenestrated, One or Two Arteries for Restriction in Lower Arteries
Electrical bone growth stimulator (EBGS)	Bone Growth Stimulator in Head and Facial Bones	Express® (LD) Premounted Stent System	Intraluminal Device
	Bone Growth Stimulator in Upper Bones	Express® Biliary SD Monorail® Premounted Stent System	Intraluminal Device
	Bone Growth Stimulator in Lower Bones	Express® SD Renal Monorail® Premounted Stent System	Intraluminal Device
Electrical muscle stimulation (EMS) lead	Stimulator Lead in Muscles	External fixator	External Fixation Device in Head and Facial Bones
Electronic muscle stimulator lead	Stimulator Lead in Muscles		External Fixation Device in Upper Bones
Embolization coil(s)	Intraluminal Device		External Fixation Device in Lower Bones
Endeavor® (III)(IV) (Sprint) Zotarolimus-eluting Coronary Stent System	Intraluminal Device, Drug-eluting in Heart and Great Vessels		External Fixation Device in Upper Joints
Endologix AFX® Endovascular AAA System	Intraluminal Device		External Fixation Device in Lower Joints
EndoSure® sensor	Monitoring Device, Pressure Sensor for Insertion in Heart and Great Vessels	EXtreme Lateral Interbody Fusion(XLIF) device	Interbody Fusion Device in Lower Joints
ENDOTAK RELIANCE® (G) Defibrillation Lead	Cardiac Lead, Defibrillator for Insertion in Heart and Great Vessels	Facet replacement spinal stabilization device	Spinal Stabilization Device, Facet Replacement for Insertion in Upper Joints
			Spinal Stabilization Device, Facet Replacement for Insertion in Lower Joints

Device Term	ICD-10-PCS Value
FLAIR® Endovascular Stent Graft	Intraluminal Device
Flexible Composite Mesh	Synthetic Substitute
Foley catheter	Drainage Device
Formula™ Balloon-Expandable Renal Stent System	Intraluminal Device
Freestyle® (Stentless) Aortic Root Bioprosthesis	Zooplastic Tissue in Heart and Great Vessels
Fusion screw(compression)(lag) (locking)	Internal Fixation Device in Upper Joints
	Internal Fixation Device in Lower Joints
GammaTile™	Radioactive Element, Cesium-131 Collagen Implant for Insertion in Central Nervous System and Cranial Nerves
Gastric electrical stimulation (GES) lead	Stimulator Lead in Gastrointestinal System
Gastric pacemaker lead	Stimulator Lead in Gastrointestinal System
GORE EXCLUDER® AAA Endoprosthesis	Intraluminal Device, Branched or Fenestrated, One or Two Arteries for Restriction in Lower Arteries
	Intraluminal Device, Branched or Fenestrated, Three or More Arteries for Restriction in Lower Arteries
	Intraluminal Device
GORE EXCLUDER® IBE Endoprosthesis	Intraluminal Device, Branched or Fenestrated, One or Two Arteries for Restriction in Lower Arteries
GORE TAG® Thoracic Endoprosthesis	Intraluminal Device
GORE® DUALMESH®	Synthetic Substitute
Guedel airway	Intraluminal Device, Airway in Mouth and Throat
Hancock® Bioprosthesis (aortic) (mitral) valve	Zooplastic Tissue in Heart and Great Vessels
Hancock® Bioprosthetic Valved Conduit	Zooplastic Tissue in Heart and Great Vessels
HeartMate 3™ LVAS	Implantable Heart Assist System in Heart and Great Vessels
HeartMate II® Left Ventricular AssistDevice (LVAD)	Implantable Heart Assist System in Heart and Great Vessels
HeartMate XVE® Left Ventricular Assist Device (LVAD)	Implantable Heart Assist System in Heart and Great Vessels
Herculink® (RX) Elite Renal Stent System	Intraluminal Device
Hip (joint) liner	Liner in Lower Joints
Holter valve ventricular shunt	Synthetic Substitute
Ilizarov external fixator	External Fixation Device, Ring for Insertion in Upper Bones
	External Fixation Device, Ring for Reposition in Upper Bones
	External Fixation Device, Ring for Insertion in Lower Bones
	External Fixation Device, Ring for Reposition in Lower Bones

Device Term	ICD-10-PCS Value
Ilizarov-Vecklich device	External Fixation Device, Limb Lengthening for Insertion in Upper Bones
	External Fixation Device, Limb Lengthening for Insertion in Lower Bones
Impella® heart pump	Short-term External Heart Assist System in Heart and Great Vessels
Implantable cardioverter-defibrillator (ICD)	Defibrillator Generator for Insertion in Subcutaneous Tissue and Fascia
Implantable drug infusion pump (anti-spasmodic)(chemotherapy)(pain)	Infusion Device, Pump in Subcutaneous Tissue and Fascia
Implantable glucose monitoring device	Monitoring Device
Implantable hemodynamic monitor (IHM)	Monitoring Device, Hemodynamic for Insertion in Subcutaneous Tissue and Fascia
Implantable hemodynamic monitoring system (IHMS)	Monitoring Device, Hemodynamic for Insertion in Subcutaneous Tissue and Fascia
Implantable Miniature Telescope™(IMT)	Synthetic Substitute, Intraocular Telescope for Replacement in Eye
Implanted (venous)(access) port	Vascular Access Device, Totally Implantable in Subcutaneous Tissue and Fascia
InDura®, intrathecal catheter (1P) (spinal)	Infusion Device
Injection reservoir, port	Vascular Access Device, Totally Implantable in Subcutaneous Tissue and Fascia
Injection reservoir, pump	Infusion Device, Pump in Subcutaneous Tissue and Fascia
Interbody fusion (spine) cage	Interbody Fusion Device in Upper Joints
	Interbody Fusion Device in Lower Joints
Interspinous process spinal stabilization device	Spinal Stabilization Device, Interspinous Process for Insertion in Upper Joints
	Spinal Stabilization Device, Interspinous Process for Insertion in Lower Joints
InterStim® Therapy lead	Neurostimulator Lead in Peripheral Nervous System
InterStim® Therapy neurostimulator	Stimulator Generator, Single Array for Insertion in Subcutaneous Tissue and Fascia
Intramedullary (IM) rod (nail)	Internal Fixation Device, Intramedullary in Upper Bones
	Internal Fixation Device, Intramedullary in Lower Bones
Intramedullary skeletal kinetic distractor (ISKD)	Internal Fixation Device, Intramedullary in Upper Bones
	Internal Fixation Device, Intramedullary in Lower Bones

Device Term	ICD-10-PCS Value
Intrauterine device (IUD)	Contraceptive Device in Female Reproductive System
INTUITY Elite® valve system,EDWARDS	Zooplastic Tissue, Rapid Deployment Technique in New Technology
Itrel® (3)(4) neurostimulator	Stimulator Generator, Single Array for Insertion in Subcutaneous Tissue and Fascia
Joint fixation plate	Internal Fixation Device in Upper Joints
	Internal Fixation Device in Lower Joints
Joint liner (insert)	Liner in Lower Joints
Joint spacer (antibiotic)	Spacer in Upper Joints
	Spacer in Lower Joints
Kappa®	Pacemaker, Dual Chamber for Insertion in Subcutaneous Tissue and Fascia
Kirschner wire (K-wire)	Internal Fixation Device in Head and Facial Bones
	Internal Fixation Device in Upper Bones
	Internal Fixation Device in Lower Bones
	Internal Fixation Device in Upper Joints
	Internal Fixation Device in Lower Joints
Knee (implant) insert	Liner in Lower Joints
Kuntscher nail	Internal Fixation Device, Intramedullary in Upper Bones
	Internal Fixation Device, Intramedullary in Lower Bones
LAP-BAND® adjustable gastric banding system	Extraluminal Device
LifeStent® (Flexstar)(XL) Vascular Stent System	Intraluminal Device
LIVIAN™ CRT-D	Cardiac Resynchronization Defibrillator Pulse Generator for Insertion in Subcutaneous Tissue and Fascia
Loop recorder, implantable	Monitoring Device
MAGEC® Spinal Bracing and Distraction System	Magnetically Controlled Growth Rod(s) in New Technology
Mark IV™ Breathing Pacemaker System	Stimulator Generator in Subcutaneous Tissue and Fascia
Maximo® II DR (VR)	Defibrillator Generator for Insertion in Subcutaneous Tissue and Fascia
Maximo® II DR CRT-D	Cardiac Resynchronization Defibrillator Pulse Generator for Insertion in Subcutaneous Tissue and Fascia
Medtronic Endurant® II AAA stent graft system	Intraluminal Device

Device Term	ICD-10-PCS Value
Melody® transcatheter pulmonary valve	Zooplastic Tissue in Heart and Great Vessels
Metal on metal bearing surface	Synthetic Substitute, Metal for Replacement in Lower Joints
Micro-Driver® stent (RX) (OTW)	Intraluminal Device
MicroMed HeartAssist™	Implantable Heart Assist System in Heart and Great Vessels
Micrus CERECYTE® microcoil	Intraluminal Device, Bioactive in Upper Arteries
MIRODERM™ Biologic Wound Matrix	Skin Substitute, Porcine Liver Derived in New Technology
MitraClip® valve repair system	Synthetic Substitute
Mitroflow® Aortic Pericardial HeartValve	Zooplastic Tissue in Heart and Great Vessels
Mosaic® Bioprosthesis (aortic) (mitral) valve	Zooplastic Tissue in Heart and Great Vessels
MULTI-LINK (VISION®)(MINI-VISION VISION®)(ULTRA™) Coronary Stent System	Intraluminal Device
nanoLOCK™ interbody fusion device	Interbody Fusion Device, Nanotextured Surface in New Technology
Nasopharyngeal airway (NPA)	Intraluminal Device, Airway in Ear, Nose, Sinus
Neuromuscular electrical stimulation (NEMS) lead	Stimulator Lead in Muscles
Neurostimulator generator, multiple channel	Stimulator Generator, Multiple Array for Insertion in Subcutaneous Tissue and Fascia
Neurostimulator generator, multiple channel rechargeable	Stimulator Generator, Multiple Array Rechargeable for Insertion in Subcutaneous Tissue and Fascia
Neurostimulator generator, single channel	Stimulator Generator, Single Array for Insertion in Subcutaneous Tissue and Fascia
Neurostimulator generator, single channel rechargeable	Stimulator Generator, Single Array Rechargeable for Insertion in Subcutaneous Tissue and Fascia
Neutralization plate	Internal Fixation Device in Head and Facial Bones
	Internal Fixation Device in Upper Bones
	Internal Fixation Device in Lower Bones
Nitinol framed polymer mesh	Synthetic Substitute
Non-tunneled central venous catheter	Infusion Device
Novacor® Left Ventricular Assist Device	Implantable Heart Assist System in Heart and Great Vessels
Novation® Ceramic AHS®(Articulation Hip System)	Synthetic Substitute, Ceramic for Replacement in Lower Joints
Omnilink Elite® Vascular Balloon Expandable Stent System	Intraluminal Device
Open Pivot™ (mechanical) valve	Synthetic Substitute
Open Pivot™ Aortic Valve Graft (AVG)	Synthetic Substitute

Device Term	ICD-10-PCS Value
Optimizer™ III implantable pulse generator	Contractility Modulation Device for Insertion in Subcutaneous Tissue and Fascia
Oropharyngeal airway (OPA)	Intraluminal Device, Airway in Mouth and Throat
Ovatio™ CRT-D	Cardiac Resynchronization Defibrillator Pulse Generator for Insertion in Subcutaneous Tissue and Fascia
OXINIUM™	Synthetic Substitute, Oxidized Zirconium on Polyethylene for Replacement in Lower Joints
Paclitaxel-eluting coronary stent	Intraluminal Device, Drug-eluting in Heart and Great Vessels
Paclitaxel-eluting peripheral stent	Intraluminal Device, Drug-eluting in Upper Arteries
	Intraluminal Device, Drug-eluting in Lower Arteries
Partially absorbable mesh	Synthetic Substitute
Pedicle-based dynamic stabilization device	Spinal Stabilization Device, Pedicle-Based for Insertion in Upper Joints
	Spinal Stabilization Device, Pedicle-Based for Insertion in Lower Joints
Perceval sutureless valve	Zooplastic Tissue, Rapid Deployment Technique in New Technology
Percutaneous endoscopic gastrojejunostomy (PEG/J) tube	Feeding Device in Gastrointestinal System
Percutaneous endoscopic gastrostomy (PEG) tube	Feeding Device in Gastrointestinal System
Percutaneous nephrostomy catheter	Drainage Device
Peripherally inserted central catheter (PICC)	Infusion Device
Pessary ring	Intraluminal Device, Pessary in Female Reproductive System
Phrenic nerve stimulator generator	Stimulator Generator in Subcutaneous Tissue and Fascia
Phrenic nerve stimulator lead	Diaphragmatic Pacemaker Lead in Respiratory System
PHYSIOMESH™ Flexible Composite Mesh	Synthetic Substitute
Pipeline™ Embolization device (PED)	Intraluminal Device
Polyethylene socket	Synthetic Substitute, Polyethylene for Replacement in Lower Joints
Polymethylmethacrylate (PMMA)	Synthetic Substitute
Polypropylene mesh	Synthetic Substitute
Porcine (bioprosthetic) valve	Zooplastic Tissue in Heart and Great Vessels
PRESTIGE® Cervical Disc	Synthetic Substitute
PrimeAdvanced® neurostimulator (SureScan®) (MRI Safe)	Stimulator Generator, Multiple Array for Insertion in Subcutaneous Tissue and Fascia
PROCEED™ Ventral Patch	Synthetic Substitute

Device Term	ICD-10-PCS Value
Prodisc-C™	Synthetic Substitute
Prodisc-L™	Synthetic Substitute
PROLENE® Polypropylene Hernia System (PHS)	Synthetic Substitute
Protecta™ XT CRT-D	Cardiac Resynchronization Defibrillator Pulse Generator for Insertion in Subcutaneous Tissue and Fascia
Protecta™ XT DR (XT VR)	Defibrillator Generator for Insertion in Subcutaneous Tissue and Fascia
Protege® RX Carotid Stent System	Intraluminal Device
Pump reservoir	Infusion Device, Pump in Subcutaneous Tissue and Fascia
REALIZE® Adjustable Gastric Band	Extraluminal Device
Rebound HRD® (Hernia Repair Device)	Synthetic Substitute
RestoreAdvanced® neurostimulator (SureScan®)(MRI Safe)	Stimulator Generator, Multiple Array Rechargeable for Insertion in Subcutaneous Tissue and Fascia
RestoreSensor® neurostimulator (SureScan®)(MRI Safe)	Stimulator Generator, Multiple Array Rechargeable for Insertion in Subcutaneous Tissue and Fascia
RestoreUltra® neurostimulator (SureScan®)(MRI Safe)	Stimulator Generator, Multiple Array Rechargeable for Insertion in Subcutaneous Tissue and Fascia
Reveal® (DX)(XT)	Monitoring Device
Reverse® Shoulder Prosthesis	Synthetic Substitute, Reverse Ball and Socket for Replacement in Upper Joints
Revo MRI™ SureScan® pacemaker	Pacemaker, Dual Chamber for Insertion in Subcutaneous Tissue and Fascia
Rheos® System device	Stimulator Generator in Subcutaneous Tissue and Fascia
Rheos® System lead	Stimulator Lead in Upper Arteries
RNS® System lead	Neurostimulator Lead in Central Nervous System and Cranial Nerves
RNS® system neurostimulator generator	Neurostimulator Generator in Head and Facial Bones
Sacral nerve modulation (SNM) lead	Stimulator Lead in Urinary System
Sacral neuromodulation lead	Stimulator Lead in Urinary System
SAPIEN® transcatheter aortic valve	Zooplastic Tissue in Heart and Great Vessels
Secura™ (DR) (VR)	Defibrillator Generator for Insertion in Subcutaneous Tissue and Fascia
Sheffield hybrid external fixator	External Fixation Device, Hybrid for Insertion in Upper Bones
	External Fixation Device, Hybrid for Reposition in Upper Bones
	External Fixation Device, Hybrid for Insertion in Lower Bones
	External Fixation Device, Hybrid for Reposition in Lower Bones

Device Term	ICD-10-PCS Value	Device Term	ICD-10-PCS Value
Sheffield ring external fixator	External Fixation Device, Ring for Insertion in Upper Bones	Talent® Stent Graft (abdominal) (thoracic)	Intraluminal Device
	External Fixation Device, Ring for Reposition in Upper Bones	Tandem Heart® System	Short-term External Heart Assist System in Heart and Great Vessels
	External Fixation Device, Ring for Insertion in Lower Bones	TAXUS® Liberte® Paclitaxel-eluting Coronary Stent System	Intraluminal Device, Drug-eluting in Heart and Great Vessels
	External Fixation Device, Ring for Reposition in Lower Bones	Therapeutic occlusion coil(s)	Intraluminal Device
Single lead pacemaker (atrium) (ventricle)	Pacemaker, Single Chamber for Insertion in Subcutaneous Tissue and Fascia	Thoracostomy tube	Drainage Device
		Thoratec® IVAD (Implantable VentricularAssist Device)	Implantable Heart Assist System in Heart and Great Vessels
Single lead rate responsive pacemaker (atrium) (ventricle)	Pacemaker, Single Chamber Rate Responsive for Insertion in Subcutaneous Tissue and Fascia	Thoratec Paracorporeal Ventricular Assist Device	Short-term External Heart Assist System in Heart and Great Vessels
		Tibial insert	Liner in Lower Joints
Sirolimus-eluting coronary stent	Intraluminal Device, Drug-eluting in Heart and Great Vessels	Tissue bank graft	Nonautologous Tissue Substitute
SJM Biocor® Stented Valve System	Zooplastic Tissue in Heart and Great Vessels	Tissue expander (inflatable) (injectable)	Tissue Expander in Skin and Breast
			Tissue Expander in Subcutaneous Tissue and Fascia
Spinal cord neurostimulator lead	Neurostimulator Lead in Central Nervous System and Cranial Nerves	Titanium Sternal Fixation System (TSFS)	Internal Fixation Device, Rigid Plate for Insertion in Upper Bones
Spinal growth rods, magnetically controlled	Magnetically Controlled Growth Rod(s) in New Technology		Internal Fixation Device, Rigid Plate for Reposition in Upper Bones
Spiration IBV™ Valve System	Intraluminal Device, Endobronchial Valve in Respiratory System	Total artificial (replacement) heart	Synthetic Substitute
Stent, intraluminal (cardiovascular) (gastrointestinal)(hepatobiliary) (urinary)	Intraluminal Device	Tracheostomy tube	Tracheostomy Device in Respiratory System
		Trifecta™ Valve (aortic)	Zooplastic Tissue in Heart and Great Vessels
Stented tissue valve	Zooplastic Tissue in Heart and Great Vessels	Tunneled central venous catheter	Vascular Access Device, Tunneled in Subcutaneous Tissue and Fascia
Stratos LV®	Cardiac Resynchronization Pacemaker Pulse Generator for Insertion in Subcutaneous Tissue and Fascia	Tunneled spinal (intrathecal) catheter	Infusion Device
		Two lead pacemaker	Pacemaker, Dual Chamber for Insertion in Subcutaneous Tissue and Fascia
Subcutaneous injection reservoir, port	Vascular Access Device, Totally Implantable in Subcutaneous Tissue and Fascia	Ultraflex™ Precision Colonic Stent System	Intraluminal Device
Subcutaneous injection reservoir, pump	Infusion Device, Pump in Subcutaneous Tissue and Fascia	ULTRAPRO® Hernia System (UHS)	Synthetic Substitute
Subdermal progesterone implant	Contraceptive Device in Subcutaneous Tissue and Fascia	ULTRAPRO® Partially Absorbable Lightweight Mesh	Synthetic Substitute
Sutureless valve, Perceval™	Zooplastic Tissue, Rapid Deployment Technique in New Technology	ULTRAPRO® Plug	Synthetic Substitute
		Ultrasonic osteogenic stimulator	Bone Growth Stimulator in Head and Facial Bones
SynCardia™ Total Artificial Heart	Synthetic Substitute		Bone Growth Stimulator in Upper Bones
Synchra™ CRT-P	Cardiac Resynchronization Pacemaker Pulse Generator for Insertion in Subcutaneous Tissue and Fascia		Bone Growth Stimulator in Lower Bones
SynchroMed® pump	Infusion Device, Pump in Subcutaneous Tissue and Fascia	Ultrasound bone healing system	Bone Growth Stimulator in Head and Facial Bones
Talent® Converter	Intraluminal Device		Bone Growth Stimulator in Upper Bones
Talent® Occluder	Intraluminal Device		Bone Growth Stimulator in Lower Bones

Device Term	ICD-10-PCS Value
Uniplanar external fixator	External Fixation Device, Monoplanar for Insertion in Upper Bones
	External Fixation Device, Monoplanar for Reposition in Upper Bones
	External Fixation Device, Monoplanar for Insertion in Lower Bones
	External Fixation Device, Monoplanar for Reposition in Lower Bones
Urinary incontinence stimulator lead	Stimulator Lead in Urinary System
Vaginal pessary	Intraluminal Device, Pessary in Female Reproductive System
Valiant® Thoracic Stent Graft	Intraluminal Device
Vectra® Vascular Access Graft	Vascular Access Device, Tunneled in Subcutaneous Tissue and Fascia
Ventrio™ Hernia Patch	Synthetic Substitute
Versa®	Pacemaker, Dual Chamber for Insertion in Subcutaneous Tissue and Fascia
Virtuoso® (II) (DR) (VR)	Defibrillator Generator for Insertion in Subcutaneous Tissue and Fascia
Viva™ (XT)(S)	Cardiac Resynchronization Defibrillator Pulse Generator for Insertion in Subcutaneous Tissue and Fascia
WALLSTENT® Endoprosthesis	Intraluminal Device
X-STOP® Spacer	Spinal Stabilization Device, Interspinous Process for Insertion in Upper Joints
	Spinal Stabilization Device, Interspinous Process for Insertion in Lower Joints

Device Term	ICD-10-PCS Value
Xact® Carotid Stent System	Intraluminal Device
Xenograft	Zooplastic Tissue in Heart and Great Vessels
XIENCE™ Everolimus Eluting Coronary Stent System	Intraluminal Device, Drug-eluting in Heart and Great Vessels
XLIF® System	Interbody Fusion Device in Lower Joints
Zenith® AAA Endovascular Graft	Intraluminal Device, Branched or Fenestrated, One or Two Arteries for Restriction in Lower Arteries
	Intraluminal Device, Branched or Fenestrated, Three or More Arteries for Restriction in Lower Arteries
	Intraluminal Device
Zenith Flex® AAA Endovascular Graft	Intraluminal Device
Zenith TX2® TAA Endovascular Graft	Intraluminal Device
Zenith® Renu™ AAA Ancillary Graft	Intraluminal Device
Zilver® PTX® (paclitaxel) Drug-Eluting Peripheral Stent	Intraluminal Device, Drug-eluting in Upper Arteries
	Intraluminal Device, Drug-eluting in Lower Arteries
Zimmer® NexGen® LPS Mobile Bearing Knee	Synthetic Substitute
Zimmer® NexGen® LPS-Flex Mobile Knee	Synthetic Substitute
Zotarolimus-eluting coronary stent	Intraluminal Device, Drug-eluting in Heart and Great Vessels

Appendix D: Device Aggregation Table

Specific Device	For Operation	In Body System	General Device
Autologous Arterial Tissue	All applicable	Heart and Great Vessels	**7** Autologous Tissue Substitute
		Lower Arteries	
		Lower Veins	
		Upper Arteries	
		Upper Veins	
Autologous Venous Tissue	All applicable	Heart and Great Vessels	**7** Autologous Tissue Substitute
		Lower Arteries	
		Lower Veins	
		Upper Arteries	
		Upper Veins	
Cardiac Lead, Defibrillator	Insertion	Heart and Great Vessels	**M** Cardiac Lead
Cardiac Lead, Pacemaker	Insertion	Heart and Great Vessels	**M** Cardiac Lead
Cardiac Resynchronization Defibrillator Pulse Generator	Insertion	Subcutaneous Tissue and Fascia	**P** Cardiac Rhythm Related Device
Cardiac Resynchronization Pacemaker Pulse Generator	Insertion	Subcutaneous Tissue and Fascia	**P** Cardiac Rhythm Related Device
Contractility Modulation Device	Insertion	Subcutaneous Tissue and Fascia	**P** Cardiac Rhythm Related Device
Defibrillator Generator	Insertion	Subcutaneous Tissue and Fascia	**P** Cardiac Rhythm Related Device
Epiretinal Visual Prosthesis	All applicable	Eye	**J** Synthetic Substitute
External Fixation Device, Hybrid	Insertion	Lower Bones	**5** External Fixation Device
		Upper Bones	
External Fixation Device, Hybrid	Reposition	Lower Bones	**5** External Fixation Device
		Upper Bones	
External Fixation Device, Limb Lengthening	Insertion	Lower Bones	**5** External Fixation Device
		Upper Bones	
External Fixation Device, Monoplanar	Insertion	Lower Bones	**5** External Fixation Device
		Upper Bones	
External Fixation Device, Monoplanar	Reposition	Lower Bones	**5** External Fixation Device
		Upper Bones	
External Fixation Device, Ring	Insertion	Lower Bones	**5** External Fixation Device
		Upper Bones	
External Fixation Device, Ring	Reposition	Lower Bones	**5** External Fixation Device
		Upper Bones	
Hearing Device, Bone Conduction	Insertion	Ear, Nose, Sinus	**S** Hearing Device
Hearing Device, Multiple Channel Cochlear Prosthesis	Insertion	Ear, Nose, Sinus	**S** Hearing Device
Hearing Device, Single Channel Cochlear Prosthesis	Insertion	Ear, Nose, Sinus	**S** Hearing Device
Internal Fixation Device, Intramedullary	All applicable	Lower Bones	**4** Internal Fixation Device
		Upper Bones	
Internal Fixation Device, Rigid Plate	Insertion	Upper Bones	**4** Internal Fixation Device
Internal Fixation Device, Rigid Plate	Reposition	Upper Bones	**4** Internal Fixation Device
Intraluminal Device, Airway	All applicable	Ear, Nose, Sinus Gastrointestinal System Mouth and Throat	**D** Intraluminal Device
Intraluminal Device, Bioactive	All applicable	Upper Arteries	**D** Intraluminal Device

Specific Device	For Operation	In Body System	General Device
Intraluminal Device, Branched or Fenestrated, One or Two Arteries	Restriction	Heart and Great Vessels	**D** Intraluminal Device
		Lower Arteries	
Intraluminal Device, Branched or Fenestrated, Three or More Arteries	Restriction	Heart and Great Vessels	**D** Intraluminal Device
		Lower Arteries	
Intraluminal Device, Drug-eluting	All applicable	Heart and Great Vessels	**D** Intraluminal Device
		Lower Arteries	
		Upper Arteries	
Intraluminal Device, Drug-eluting, Four or More	All applicable	Heart and Great Vessels	**D** Intraluminal Device
		Lower Arteries	
		Upper Arteries	
Intraluminal Device, Drug-eluting, Three	All applicable	Heart and Great Vessels	**D** Intraluminal Device
		Lower Arteries	
		Upper Arteries	
Intraluminal Device, Drug-eluting, Two	All applicable	Heart and Great Vessels	**D** Intraluminal Device
		Lower Arteries	
		Upper Arteries	
Intraluminal Device, Endobronchial Valve	All applicable	Respiratory System	**D** Intraluminal Device
Intraluminal Device, Endotracheal Airway	All applicable	Respiratory System	**D** Intraluminal Device
Intraluminal Device, Four or More	All applicable	Heart and Great Vessels	**D** Intraluminal Device
		Lower Arteries	
		Upper Arteries	
Intraluminal Device, Pessary	All applicable	Female Reproductive System	**D** Intraluminal Device
Intraluminal Device, Radioactive	All applicable	Heart and Great Vessels	**D** Intraluminal Device
Intraluminal Device, Three	All applicable	Heart and Great Vessels	**D** Intraluminal Device
		Lower Arteries	
		Upper Arteries	
Intraluminal Device, Two	All applicable	Heart and Great Vessels	**D** Intraluminal Device
		Lower Arteries	
		Upper Arteries	
Monitoring Device, Hemodynamic	Insertion	Subcutaneous Tissue and Fascia	**2** Monitoring Device
Monitoring Device, Pressure Sensor	Insertion	Heart and Great Vessels	**2** Monitoring Device
Pacemaker, Dual Chamber	Insertion	Subcutaneous Tissue and Fascia	**P** Cardiac Rhythm Related Device
Pacemaker, Single Chamber	Insertion	Subcutaneous Tissue and Fascia	**P** Cardiac Rhythm Related Device
Pacemaker, Single Chamber Rate Responsive	Insertion	Subcutaneous Tissue and Fascia	**P** Cardiac Rhythm Related Device
Spinal Stabilization Device, Facet Replacement	Insertion	Lower Joints	**4** Internal Fixation Device
		Upper Joints	
Spinal Stabilization Device, Interspinous Process	Insertion	Lower Joints	**4** Internal Fixation Device
		Upper Joints	
Spinal Stabilization Device, Pedicle-Based	Insertion	Lower Joints	**4** Internal Fixation Device
		Upper Joints	
Stimulator Generator, Multiple Array	Insertion	Subcutaneous Tissue and Fascia	**M** Stimulator Generator
Stimulator Generator, Multiple Array Rechargeable	Insertion	Subcutaneous Tissue and Fascia	**M** Stimulator Generator
Stimulator Generator, Single Array	Insertion	Subcutaneous Tissue and Fascia	**M** Stimulator Generator

Specific Device	For Operation	In Body System	General Device
Stimulator Generator, Single Array Rechargeable	Insertion	Subcutaneous Tissue and Fascia	**M** Stimulator Generator
Synthetic Substitute, Ceramic	Replacement	Lower Joints	**J** Synthetic Substitute
Synthetic Substitute, Ceramic on Polyethylene	Replacement	Lower Joints	**J** Synthetic Substitute
Synthetic Substitute, Intraocular Telescope	Replacement	Eye	**J** Synthetic Substitute
Synthetic Substitute, Metal	Replacement	Lower Joints	**J** Synthetic Substitute
Synthetic Substitute, Metal on Polyethylene	Replacement	Lower Joints	**J** Synthetic Substitute
Synthetic Substitute, Oxidized Zirconium on Polyethylene	Replacement	Lower Joints	**J** Synthetic Substitute
Synthetic Substitute, Polyethylene	Replacement	Lower Joints	**J** Synthetic Substitute
Synthetic Substitute, Reverse Ball and Socket	Replacement	Upper Joints	**J** Synthetic Substitute
Synthetic Substitute, Unicondylar	Replacement	Lower Joints	**J** Synthetic Substitute

This page intentionally left blank

Appendix E: Character Meaning

0: Medical and Surgical
0: Central Nervous System and Cranial Nerves

Operation-Character 3	Body Part-Character 4	Approach-Character 5	Device-Character 6	Qualifier-Character 7
1 Bypass	**0** Brain	**0** Open	**0** Drainage Device	**0** Nasopharynx
2 Change	**1** Cerebral Meninges	**3** Percutaneous	**2** Monitoring Device	**1** Mastoid Sinus
5 Destruction	**2** Dura Mater	**4** Percutaneous Endoscopic	**3** Infusion Device	**2** Atrium
7 Dilation	**3** Epidural Space, Intracranial	**X** External	**7** Autologous Tissue Substitute	**3** Blood Vessel
8 Division	**4** Subdural Space, Intracranial		**J** Synthetic Substitute	**4** Pleural Cavity
9 Drainage	**5** Subarachnoid Space, Intracranial		**K** Nonautologous Tissue Substitute	**5** Intestine
B Excision	**6** Cerebral Ventricle		**M** Neurostimulator Lead	**6** Peritoneal Cavity
C Extirpation	**7** Cerebral Hemisphere		**Y** Other Device	**7** Urinary Tract
D Extraction	**8** Basal Ganglia		**Z** No Device	**8** Bone Marrow
F Fragmentation	**9** Thalamus			**9** Fallopian Tube
H Insertion	**A** Hypothalamus			**B** Cerebral Cisterns
J Inspection	**B** Pons			**F** Olfactory Nerve
K Map	**C** Cerebellum			**G** Optic Nerve
N Release	**D** Medulla Oblongata			**H** Oculomotor Nerve
P Removal	**E** Cranial Nerve			**J** Trochlear Nerve
Q Repair	**F** Olfactory Nerve			**K** Trigeminal Nerve
R Replacement	**G** Optic Nerve			**L** Abducens Nerve
S Reposition	**H** Oculomotor Nerve			**M** Facial Nerve
T Resection	**J** Trochlear Nerve			**N** Acoustic Nerve
U Supplement	**K** Trigeminal Nerve			**P** Glossopharyngeal Nerve
W Revision	**L** Abducens Nerve			**Q** Vagus Nerve
X Transfer	**M** Facial Nerve			**R** Accessory Nerve
	N Acoustic Nerve			**S** Hypoglossal Nerve
	P Glossopharyngeal Nerve			**X** Diagnostic
	Q Vagus Nerve			**Z** No Qualifier
	R Accessory Nerve			
	S Hypoglossal Nerve			
	T Spinal Meninges			
	U Spinal Canal			
	V Spinal Cord			
	W Cervical Spinal Cord			
	X Thoracic Spinal Cord			
	Y Lumbar Spinal Cord			

0: Medical and Surgical
1: Peripheral Nervous System and Cranial Nerves

Operation-Character 3	Body Part-Character 4	Approach-Character 5	Device-Character 6	Qualifier-Character 7
2 Change	0 Cervical Plexus	0 Open	0 Drainage Device	1 Cervical Nerve
5 Destruction	1 Cervical Nerve	3 Percutaneous	2 Monitoring Device	2 Phrenic Nerve
8 Division	2 Phrenic Nerve	4 Percutaneous Endoscopic	7 Autologous Tissue Substitute	4 Ulnar Nerve
9 Drainage	3 Brachial Plexus	X External	J Synthetic Substitute	5 Median Nerve
B Excision	4 Ulnar Nerve		K Nonautologous Tissue Substitute	6 Radial Nerve
C Extirpation	5 Median Nerve		M Neurostimulator Lead	8 Thoracic Nerve
D Extraction	6 Radial Nerve		Y Other Device	B Lumbar Nerve
H Insertion	8 Thoracic Nerve		Z No Device	C Perineal Nerve
J Inspection	9 Lumbar Plexus			D Femoral Nerve
N Release	A Lumbosacral Plexus			F Sciatic Nerve
P Removal	B Lumbar Nerve			G Tibial Nerve
Q Repair	C Pudendal Nerve			H Peroneal Nerve
R Replacement	D Femoral Nerve			X Diagnostic
S Reposition	F Sciatic Nerve			Z No Qualifier
U Supplement	G Tibial Nerve			
W Revision	H Peroneal Nerve			
X Transfer	K Head and Neck Sympathetic Nerve			
	L Thoracic Sympathetic Nerve			
	M Abdominal Sympathetic Nerve			
	N Lumbar Sympathetic Nerve			
	P Sacral Sympathetic Nerve			
	Q Sacral Plexus			
	R Sacral Nerve			
	Y Peripheral Nerve			

0: Medical and Surgical
2: Heart and Great Vessels

Operation-Character 3	Body Part-Character 4	Approach-Character 5	Device-Character 6	Qualifier-Character 7
1 Bypass	**0** Coronary Artery, One Artery	**0** Open	**0** Monitoring Device, Pressure Sensor	**0** Allogeneic
4 Creation	**1** Coronary Artery, Two Arteries	**3** Percutaneous	**2** Monitoring Device	**1** Syngeneic
5 Destruction	**2** Coronary Artery, Three Arteries	**4** Percutaneous Endoscopic	**3** Infusion Device	**2** Zooplastic
7 Dilation	**3** Coronary Artery, Four or More Arteries	**X** External	**4** Intraluminal Device, Drug-eluting	**2** Common Atrioventricular Valve
8 Division	**4** Coronary Vein		**5** Intraluminal Device, Drug-Eluting, Two	**3** Coronary Artery
B Excision	**5** Atrial Septum		**6** Intraluminal Device, Drug-Eluting, Three	**4** Coronary Vein
C Extirpation	**6** Atrium, Right		**7** Intraluminal Device, Drug-Eluting, Four or More	**5** Coronary Circulation
F Fragmentation	**7** Atrium, Left		**7** Autologous Tissue Substitute	**6** Bifurcation
H Insertion	**8** Conduction Mechanism		**8** Zooplastic Tissue	**7** Atrium, Left
J Inspection	**9** Chordae Tendineae		**9** Autologous Venous Tissue	**8** Internal Mammary, Right
K Map	**A** Heart		**A** Autologous Arterial Tissue	**9** Internal Mammary, Left
L Occlusion	**B** Heart, Right		**C** Extraluminal Device	**A** Innominate Artery
N Release	**C** Heart, Left		**D** Intraluminal Device	**B** Subclavian
P Removal	**D** Papillary Muscle		**E** Intraluminal Device, Two	**C** Thoracic Artery
Q Repair	**F** Aortic Valve		**E** Intraluminal Device, Branched or Fenestrated, One or Two Arteries	**D** Carotid
R Replacement	**G** Mitral Valve		**F** Intraluminal Device, Three	**E** Atrioventricular Valve, Left
S Reposition	**H** Pulmonary Valve		**F** Intraluminal Device, Branched or Fenestrated, Three or More Arteries	**F** Abdominal Artery
T Resection	**J** Tricuspid Valve		**G** Intraluminal Device, Four or More	**G** Atrioventricular Valve, Right
U Supplement	**K** Ventricle, Right		**J** Cardiac Lead, Pacemaker	**H** Transapical
V Restriction	**L** Ventricle, Left		**J** Synthetic Substitute	**J** Truncal Valve
W Revision	**M** Ventricular Septum		**K** Cardiac Lead, Defibrillator	**K** Left Atrial Appendage
Y Transplantation	**N** Pericardium		**K** Nonautologous Tissue Substitute	**P** Pulmonary Trunk
	P Pulmonary Trunk		**M** Cardiac Lead	**Q** Pulmonary Artery, Right
	Q Pulmonary Artery, Right		**N** Intracardiac Pacemaker	**R** Pulmonary Artery, Left
	R Pulmonary Artery, Left		**Q** Implantable Heart Assist System	**S** Biventricular
	S Pulmonary Vein, Right		**R** Short-term External Heart Assist System	**S** Pulmonary Vein, Right
	T Pulmonary Vein, Left		**T** Intraluminal Device, Radioactive	**T** Pulmonary Vein, Left
	V Superior Vena Cava		**Z** No Device	**T** Ductus Arteriosus
	W Thoracic Aorta, Descending			**U** Pulmonary Vein, Confluence
	X Thoracic Aorta, Ascending/Arch			**W** Aorta
	Y Great Vessel			**X** Diagnostic
				Z No Qualifier

0: Medical and Surgical
3: Upper Arteries

Operation-Character 3	Body Part-Character 4	Approach-Character 5	Device-Character 6	Qualifier-Character 7
1 Bypass	0 Internal Mammary Artery, Right	0 Open	0 Drainage Device	0 Upper Arm Artery, Right
5 Destruction	1 Internal Mammary Artery, Left	3 Percutaneous	2 Monitoring Device	1 Upper Arm Artery, Left
7 Dilation	2 Innominate Artery	4 Percutaneous Endoscopic	3 Infusion Device	2 Upper Arm Artery, Bilateral
9 Drainage	3 Subclavian Artery, Right	X External	4 Intraluminal Device, Drugeluting	3 Lower Arm Artery, Right
B Excision	4 Subclavian Artery, Left		5 Intraluminal Device, Drugeluting, Two	4 Lower Arm Artery, Left
C Extirpation	5 Axillary Artery, Right		6 Intraluminal Device, Drugeluting, Three	5 Lower Arm Artery, Bilateral
H Insertion	6 Axillary Artery, Left		7 Autologous Tissue Substitute	6 Bifurcation
J Inspection	7 Brachial Artery, Right		7 Intraluminal Device, Drugeluting, Four or More	6 Upper Leg Artery, Right
L Occlusion	8 Brachial Artery, Left		9 Autologous Venous Tissue	7 Upper Leg Artery, Left
N Release	9 Ulnar Artery, Right		A Autologous Arterial Tissue	8 Upper Leg Artery, Bilateral
P Removal	A Ulnar Artery, Left		B Intraluminal Device, Bioactive	9 Lower Leg Artery, Right
Q Repair	B Radial Artery, Right		C Extraluminal Device	B Lower Leg Artery, Left
R Replacement	C Radial Artery, Left		D Intraluminal Device	C Lower Leg Artery, Bilateral
S Reposition	D Hand Artery, Right		E Intraluminal Device, Two	D Upper Arm Vein
U Supplement	F Hand Artery, Left		F Intraluminal Device, Three	F Lower Arm Vein
V Restriction	G Intracranial Artery		G Intraluminal Device, Four or More	G Intracranial Artery
W Revision	H Common Carotid Artery, Right		J Synthetic Substitute	J Extracranial Artery, Right
	J Common Carotid Artery, Left		K Nonautologous Tissue Substitute	K Extracranial Artery, Left
	K Internal Carotid Artery, Right		M Stimulator Lead	M Pulmonary Artery, Right
	L Internal Carotid Artery, Left		Y Other Device	N Pulmonary Artery, Left
	M External Carotid Artery, Right		Z No Device	V Superior Vena Cava
	N External Carotid Artery, Left			X Diagnostic
	P Vertebral Artery, Right			Z No Qualifier
	Q Vertebral Artery, Left			
	R Face Artery			
	S Temporal Artery, Right			
	T Temporal Artery, Left			
	U Thyroid Artery, Right			
	V Thyroid Artery, Left			
	Y Upper Artery			

0: Medical and Surgical
4: Lower Arteries

Operation-Character 3	Body Part-Character 4	Approach-Character 5	Device-Character 6	Qualifier-Character 7
1 Bypass	0 Abdominal Aorta	0 Open	0 Drainage Device	0 Abdominal Aorta
5 Destruction	1 Celiac Artery	3 Percutaneous	1 Radioactive Element	1 Celiac Artery
7 Dilation	2 Gastric Artery	4 Percutaneous Endoscopic	2 Monitoring Device	1 Drug-Coated Balloon
9 Drainage	3 Hepatic Artery	X External	3 Infusion Device	2 Mesenteric Artery
B Excision	4 Splenic Artery		4 Intraluminal Device, Drugeluting	3 Renal Artery, Right
C Extirpation	5 Superior Mesenteric Artery		5 Intraluminal Device, Drugeluting, Two	4 Renal Artery, Left
H Insertion	6 Colic Artery, Right		6 Intraluminal Device, Drugeluting, Three	5 Renal Artery, Bilateral
J Inspection	7 Colic Artery, Left		7 Autologous Tissue Substitute	6 Bifurcation
L Occlusion	8 Colic Artery, Middle		7 Intraluminal Device, Drugeluting, Four or More	6 Common Iliac Artery, Right
N Release	9 Renal Artery, Right		9 Autologous Venous Tissue	7 Common Iliac Artery, Left
P Removal	A Renal Artery, Left		A Autologous Arterial Tissue	8 Common Iliac Arteries, Bilateral
Q Repair	B Inferior Mesenteric Artery		C Extraluminal Device	9 Internal Iliac Artery, Right
R Replacement	C Common Iliac Artery, Right		D Intraluminal Device	B Internal Iliac Artery, Left
S Reposition	D Common Iliac Artery, Left		E Intraluminal Device, Branched or Fenestrated, One or Two Arteries	C Internal Iliac Arteries, Bilateral
U Supplement	E Internal Iliac Artery, Right		E Intraluminal Device, Two	D External Iliac Artery, Right
V Restriction	F Internal Iliac Artery, Left		F Intraluminal Device, Branched or Fenestrated, Three or More Arteries	F External Iliac Artery, Left
W Revision	H External Iliac Artery, Right		F Intraluminal Device, Three	G External Iliac Arteries, Bilateral
	J External Iliac Artery, Left		G Intraluminal Device, Four or More	H Femoral Artery, Right
	K Femoral Artery, Right		J Synthetic Substitute	J Femoral Artery, Left
	L Femoral Artery, Left		K Nonautologous Tissue Substitute	J Temporary
	M Popliteal Artery, Right		Y Other Device	K Femoral Arteries, Bilateral
	N Popliteal Artery, Left		Z No Device	L Popliteal Artery
	P Anterior Tibial Artery, Right			M Peroneal Artery
	Q Anterior Tibial Artery, Left			N Posterior Tibial Artery
	R Posterior Tibial Artery, Right			P Foot Artery
	S Posterior Tibial Artery, Left			Q Lower Extremity Artery
	T Peroneal Artery, Right			R Lower Artery
	U Peroneal Artery, Left			S Lower Extremity Vein
	V Foot Artery, Right			T Uterine Artery, Right
	W Foot Artery, Left			U Uterine Artery, Left
	Y Lower Artery			X Diagnostic
				Z No Qualifier

0: Medical and Surgical
5: Upper Veins

Operation-Character 3	Body Part-Character 4	Approach-Character 5	Device-Character 6	Qualifier-Character 7
1 Bypass	**0** Azygos Vein	**0** Open	**0** Drainage Device	**X** Diagnostic
5 Destruction	**1** Hemiazygos Vein	**3** Percutaneous	**2** Monitoring Device	**Y** Upper Vein
7 Dilation	**3** Innominate Vein, Right	**4** Percutaneous Endoscopic	**3** Infusion Device	**Z** No Qualifier
9 Drainage	**4** Innominate Vein, Left	**X** External	**7** Autologous Tissue Substitute	
B Excision	**5** Subclavian Vein, Right		**9** Autologous Venous Tissue	
C Extirpation	**6** Subclavian Vein, Left		**A** Autologous Arterial Tissue	
D Extraction	**7** Axillary Vein, Right		**C** Extraluminal Device	
H Insertion	**8** Axillary Vein, Left		**D** Intraluminal Device	
J Inspection	**9** Brachial Vein, Right		**J** Synthetic Substitute	
L Occlusion	**A** Brachial Vein, Left		**K** Nonautologous Tissue Substitute	
N Release	**B** Basilic Vein, Right		**M** Neurostimulator Lead	
P Removal	**C** Basilic Vein, Left		**Y** Other Device	
Q Repair	**D** Cephalic Vein, Right		**Z** No Device	
R Replacement	**F** Cephalic Vein, Left			
S Reposition	**G** Hand Vein, Right			
U Supplement	**H** Hand Vein, Left			
V Restriction	**L** Intracranial Vein			
W Revision	**M** Internal Jugular Vein, Right			
	N Internal Jugular Vein, Left			
	P External Jugular Vein, Right			
	Q External Jugular Vein, Left			
	R Vertebral Vein, Right			
	S Vertebral Vein, Left			
	T Face Vein, Right			
	V Face Vein, Left			
	Y Upper Vein			

0: Medical and Surgical
6: Lower Veins

Operation-Character 3	Body Part-Character 4	Approach-Character 5	Device-Character 6	Qualifier-Character 7
1 Bypass	**0** Inferior Vena Cava	**0** Open	**0** Drainage Device	**4** Hepatic Vein
5 Destruction	**1** Splenic Vein	**3** Percutaneous	**2** Monitoring Device	**5** Superior Mesenteric Vein
7 Dilation	**2** Gastric Vein	**4** Percutaneous Endoscopic	**3** Infusion Device	**6** Inferior Mesenteric Vein
9 Drainage	**3** Esophageal Vein	**X** External	**7** Autologous Tissue Substitute	**9** Renal Vein, Right
B Excision	**4** Hepatic Vein		**9** Autologous Venous Tissue	**B** Renal Vein, Left
C Extirpation	**5** Superior Mesenteric Vein		**A** Autologous Arterial Tissue	**C** Hemorrhoidal Plexus
D Extraction	**6** Inferior Mesenteric Vein		**C** Extraluminal Device	**P** Pulmonary Trunk
H Insertion	**7** Colic Vein		**D** Intraluminal Device	**Q** Pulmonary Artery, Right
J Inspection	**8** Portal Vein		**J** Synthetic Substitute	**R** Pulmonary Artery, Left
L Occlusion	**9** Renal Vein, Right		**K** Nonautologous Tissue Substitute	**T** Via Umbilical Vein
N Release	**B** Renal Vein, Left		**Y** Other Device	**X** Diagnostic
P Removal	**C** Common Iliac Vein, Right		**Z** No Device	**Y** Lower Vein
Q Repair	**D** Common Iliac Vein, Left			**Z** No Qualifier
R Replacement	**F** External Iliac Vein, Right			
S Reposition	**G** External Iliac Vein, Left			
U Supplement	**H** Hypogastric Vein, Right			
V Restriction	**J** Hypogastric Vein, Left			
W Revision	**M** Femoral Vein, Right			
	N Femoral Vein, Left			
	P Saphenous Vein, Right			
	Q Saphenous Vein, Left			
	T Foot Vein, Right			
	V Foot Vein, Left			
	Y Lower Vein			

0: Medical and Surgical
7: Lymphatic and Hemic Systems

Operation-Character 3	Body Part-Character 4	Approach-Character 5	Device-Character 6	Qualifier-Character 7
2 Change	**0** Lymphatic, Head	**0** Open	**0** Drainage Device	**0** Allogeneic
5 Destruction	**1** Lymphatic, Right Neck	**3** Percutaneous	**3** Infusion Device	**1** Syngeneic
9 Drainage	**2** Lymphatic, Left Neck	**4** Percutaneous Endoscopic	**7** Autologous Tissue Substitute	**2** Zooplastic
B Excision	**3** Lymphatic, Right Upper Extremity	**X** External	**C** Extraluminal Device	**X** Diagnostic
C Extirpation	**4** Lymphatic, Left Upper Extremity		**D** Intraluminal Device	**Z** No Qualifier
D Extraction	**5** Lymphatic, Right Axillary		**J** Synthetic Substitute	
H Insertion	**6** Lymphatic, Left Axillary		**K** Nonautologous Tissue Substitute	
J Inspection	**7** Lymphatic, Thorax		**Y** Other Device	
L Occlusion	**8** Lymphatic, Internal Mammary, Right		**Z** No Device	
N Release	**9** Lymphatic, Internal Mammary, Left			
P Removal	**B** Lymphatic, Mesenteric			
Q Repair	**C** Lymphatic, Pelvis			
S Reposition	**D** Lymphatic, Aortic			
T Resection	**F** Lymphatic, Right Lower Extremity			
U Supplement	**G** Lymphatic, Left Lower Extremity			
V Restriction	**H** Lymphatic, Right Inguinal			
W Revision	**J** Lymphatic, Left Inguinal			
Y Transplantation	**K** Thoracic Duct			
	L Cisterna Chyli			
	M Thymus			
	N Lymphatic			
	P Spleen			
	Q Bone Marrow, Sternum			
	R Bone Marrow, Iliac			
	S Bone Marrow, Vertebral			
	T Bone Marrow			

0: Medical and Surgical
8: Eye

Operation-Character 3	Body Part-Character 4	Approach-Character 5	Device-Character 6	Qualifier-Character 7
0 Alteration	**0** Eye, Right	**0** Open	**0** Drainage Device	**3** Nasal Cavity
1 Bypass	**1** Eye, Left	**3** Percutaneous	**0** Synthetic Substitute, Intraocular Telescope	**4** Sclera
2 Change	**2** Anterior Chamber, Right	**7** Via Natural or Artificial Opening	**1** Radioactive Element	**X** Diagnostic
5 Destruction	**3** Anterior Chamber, Left	**8** Via Natural or Artificial Opening Endoscopic	**3** Infusion Device	**Z** No Qualifier
7 Dilation	**4** Vitreous, Right	**X** External	**5** Epiretinal Visual Prosthesis	
9 Drainage	**5** Vitreous, Left		**7** Autologous Tissue Substitute	
B Excision	**6** Sclera, Right		**C** Extraluminal Device	
C Extirpation	**7** Sclera, Left		**D** Intraluminal Device	
D Extraction	**8** Cornea, Right		**J** Synthetic Substitute	
F Fragmentation	**9** Cornea, Left		**K** Nonautologous Tissue Substitute	
H Insertion	**A** Choroid, Right		**Y** Other Device	
J Inspection	**B** Choroid, Left		**Z** No Device	
L Occlusion	**C** Iris, Right			
M Reattachment	**D** Iris, Left			
N Release	**E** Retina, Right			
P Removal	**F** Retina, Left			
Q Repair	**G** Retinal Vessel, Right			
R Replacement	**H** Retinal Vessel, Left			
S Reposition	**J** Lens, Right			
T Resection	**K** Lens, Left			
U Supplement	**L** Extraocular Muscle, Right			
V Restriction	**M** Extraocular Muscle, Left			
W Revision	**N** Upper Eyelid, Right			
X Transfer	**P** Upper Eyelid, Left			
	Q Lower Eyelid, Right			
	R Lower Eyelid, Left			
	S Conjunctiva, Right			
	T Conjunctiva, Left			
	V Lacrimal Gland, Right			
	W Lacrimal Gland, Left			
	X Lacrimal Duct, Right			
	Y Lacrimal Duct, Left			

0: Medical and Surgical
9: Ear, Nose, Sinus

Operation-Character 3	Body Part-Character 4	Approach-Character 5	Device-Character 6	Qualifier-Character 7
0 Alteration	**0** External Ear, Right	**0** Open	**0** Drainage Device	**0** Endolymphatic
1 Bypass	**1** External Ear, Left	**3** Percutaneous	**4** Hearing Device, Bone Conduction	**X** Diagnostic
2 Change	**2** External Ear, Bilateral	**4** Percutaneous Endoscopic	**5** Hearing Device, Single Channel Cochlear Prosthesis	**Z** No Qualifier
5 Destruction	**3** External Auditory Canal, Right	**7** Via Natural or Artificial Opening	**6** Hearing Device, Multiple Channel Cochlear Prosthesis	
7 Dilation	**4** External Auditory Canal, Left	**8** Via Natural or Artificial Opening Endoscopic	**7** Autologous Tissue Substitute	
8 Division	**5** Middle Ear, Right	**X** External	**B** Intraluminal Device, Airway	
9 Drainage	**6** Middle Ear, Left		**D** Intraluminal Device	
B Excision	**7** Tympanic Membrane, Right		**J** Synthetic Substitute	
C Extirpation	**8** Tympanic Membrane, Left		**K** Nonautologous Tissue Substitute	
D Extraction	**9** Auditory Ossicle, Right		**S** Hearing Device	
H Insertion	**A** Auditory Ossicle, Left		**Y** Other Device	
J Inspection	**B** Mastoid Sinus, Right		**Z** No Device	
M Reattachment	**C** Mastoid Sinus, Left			
N Release	**D** Inner Ear, Right			
P Removal	**E** Inner Ear, Left			
Q Repair	**F** Eustachian Tube, Right			
R Replacement	**G** Eustachian Tube, Left			
S Reposition	**H** Ear, Right			
T Resection	**J** Ear, Left			
U Supplement	**K** Nasal Mucosa and Soft Tissue			
W Revision	**L** Nasal Turbinate			
	M Nasal Septum			
	N Nasopharynx			
	P Accessory Sinus			
	Q Maxillary Sinus, Right			
	R Maxillary Sinus, Left			
	S Frontal Sinus, Right			
	T Frontal Sinus, Left			
	U Ethmoid Sinus, Right			
	V Ethmoid Sinus, Left			
	W Sphenoid Sinus, Right			
	X Sphenoid Sinus, Left			
	Y Sinus			

0: Medical and Surgical
B: Respiratory System

Operation-Character 3	Body Part-Character 4	Approach-Character 5	Device-Character 6	Qualifier-Character 7
1 Bypass	**0** Tracheobronchial Tree	**0** Open	**0** Drainage Device	**0** Allogeneic
2 Change	**1** Trachea	**3** Percutaneous	**1** Radioactive Element	**1** Syngeneic
5 Destruction	**2** Carina	**4** Percutaneous Endoscopic	**2** Monitoring Device	**2** Zooplastic
7 Dilation	**3** Main Bronchus, Right	**7** Via Natural or Artificial Opening	**3** Infusion Device	**4** Cutaneous
9 Drainage	**4** Upper Lobe Bronchus, Right	**8** Via Natural or Artificial Opening Endoscopic	**7** Autologous Tissue Substitute	**6** Esophagus
B Excision	**5** Middle Lobe Bronchus, Right	**X** External	**C** Extraluminal Device	**X** Diagnostic
C Extirpation	**6** Lower Lobe Bronchus, Right		**D** Intraluminal Device	**Z** No Qualifier
D Extraction	**7** Main Bronchus, Left		**E** Intraluminal Device, Endotracheal Airway	
F Fragmentation	**8** Upper Lobe Bronchus, Left		**F** Tracheostomy Device	
H Insertion	**9** Lingula Bronchus		**G** Intraluminal Device, Endobronchial Valve	
J Inspection	**B** Lower Lobe Bronchus, Left		**J** Synthetic Substitute	
L Occlusion	**C** Upper Lung Lobe, Right		**K** Nonautologous Tissue Substitute	
M Reattachment	**D** Middle Lung Lobe, Right		**M** Diaphragmatic Pacemaker Lead	
N Release	**F** Lower Lung Lobe, Right		**Y** Other Device	
P Removal	**G** Upper Lung Lobe, Left		**Z** No Device	
Q Repair	**H** Lung Lingula			
R Replacement	**J** Lower Lung Lobe, Left			
S Reposition	**K** Lung, Right			
T Resection	**L** Lung, Left			
U Supplement	**M** Lungs, Bilateral			
V Restriction	**N** Pleura, Right			
W Revision	**P** Pleura, Left			
Y Transplantation	**Q** Pleura			
	T Diaphragm			

0: Medical and Surgical
C: Mouth and Throat

Operation-Character 3	Body Part-Character 4	Approach-Character 5	Device-Character 6	Qualifier-Character 7
0 Alteration	**0** Upper Lip	**0** Open	**0** Drainage Device	**0** Single
2 Change	**1** Lower Lip	**3** Percutaneous	**1** Radioactive Element	**1** Multiple
5 Destruction	**2** Hard Palate	**4** Percutaneous Endoscopic	**5** External Fixation Device	**2** All
7 Dilation	**3** Soft Palate	**7** Via Natural or Artificial Opening	**7** Autologous Tissue Substitute	**X** Diagnostic
9 Drainage	**4** Buccal Mucosa	**8** Via Natural or Artificial Opening Endoscopic	**B** Intraluminal Device, Airway	**Z** No Qualifier
B Excision	**5** Upper Gingiva	**X** External	**C** Extraluminal Device	
C Extirpation	**6** Lower Gingiva		**D** Intraluminal Device	
D Extraction	**7** Tongue		**J** Synthetic Substitute	
F Fragmentation	**8** Parotid Gland, Right		**K** Nonautologous Tissue Substitute	
H Insertion	**9** Parotid Gland, Left		**Y** Other Device	
J Inspection	**A** Salivary Gland		**Z** No Device	
L Occlusion	**B** Parotid Duct, Right			
M Reattachment	**C** Parotid Duct, Left			
N Release	**D** Sublingual Gland, Right			
P Removal	**F** Sublingual Gland, Left			
Q Repair	**G** Submaxillary Gland, Right			
R Replacement	**H** Submaxillary Gland, Left			
S Reposition	**J** Minor Salivary Gland			
T Resection	**M** Pharynx			
U Supplement	**N** Uvula			
V Restriction	**P** Tonsils			
W Revision	**Q** Adenoids			
X Transfer	**R** Epiglottis			
	S Larynx			
	T Vocal Cord, Right			
	V Vocal Cord, Left			
	W Upper Tooth			
	X Lower Tooth			
	Y Mouth and Throat			

0: Medical and Surgical
D: Gastrointestinal System

Operation-Character 3	Body Part-Character 4	Approach-Character 5	Device-Character 6	Qualifier-Character 7
1 Bypass	**0** Upper Intestinal Tract	**0** Open	**0** Drainage Device	**0** Allogeneic
2 Change	**1** Esophagus, Upper	**3** Percutaneous	**1** Radioactive Element	**1** Syngeneic
5 Destruction	**2** Esophagus, Middle	**4** Percutaneous Endoscopic	**2** Monitoring Device	**2** Zooplastic
7 Dilation	**3** Esophagus, Lower	**7** Via Natural or Artificial Opening	**3** Infusion Device	**3** Vertical
8 Division	**4** Esophagogastric Junction	**8** Via Natural or Artificial Opening Endoscopic	**7** Autologous Tissue Substitute	**4** Cutaneous
9 Drainage	**5** Esophagus	**X** External	**B** Intraluminal Device, Airway	**5** Esophagus
B Excision	**6** Stomach		**C** Extraluminal Device	**6** Stomach
C Extirpation	**7** Stomach, Pylorus		**D** Intraluminal Device	**9** Duodenum
D Extraction	**8** Small Intestine		**J** Synthetic Substitute	**A** Jejunum
F Fragmentation	**9** Duodenum		**K** Nonautologous Tissue Substitute	**B** Ileum
H Insertion	**A** Jejunum		**L** Artificial Sphincter	**H** Cecum
J Inspection	**B** Ileum		**M** Stimulator Lead	**K** Ascending Colon
L Occlusion	**C** Ileocecal Valve		**U** Feeding Device	**L** Transverse Colon
M Reattachment	**D** Lower Intestinal Tract		**Y** Other Device	**M** Descending Colon
N Release	**E** Large Intestine		**Z** No Device	**N** Sigmoid Colon
P Removal	**F** Large Intestine, Right			**P** Rectum
Q Repair	**G** Large Intestine, Left			**Q** Anus
R Replacement	**H** Cecum			**X** Diagnostic
S Reposition	**J** Appendix			**Z** No Qualifier
T Resection	**K** Ascending Colon			
U Supplement	**L** Transverse Colon			
V Restriction	**M** Descending Colon			
W Revision	**N** Sigmoid Colon			
X Transfer	**P** Rectum			
Y Transplantation	**Q** Anus			
	R Anal Sphincter			
	U Omentum			
	V Mesentery			
	W Peritoneum			

0: Medical and Surgical
F: Hepatobiliary System and Pancreas

Operation-Character 3	Body Part-Character 4	Approach-Character 5	Device-Character 6	Qualifier-Character 7
1 Bypass	0 Liver	0 Open	0 Drainage Device	0 Allogeneic
2 Change	1 Liver, Right Lobe	3 Percutaneous	1 Radioactive Element	1 Syngeneic
5 Destruction	2 Liver, Left Lobe	4 Percutaneous Endoscopic	2 Monitoring Device	2 Zooplastic
7 Dilation	4 Gallbladder	7 Via Natural or Artificial Opening	3 Infusion Device	3 Duodenum
8 Division	5 Hepatic Duct, Right	8 Via Natural or Artificial Opening Endoscopic	7 Autologous Tissue Substitute	4 Stomach
9 Drainage	6 Hepatic Duct, Left	X External	C Extraluminal Device	5 Hepatic Duct, Right
B Excision	7 Hepatic Duct, Common		D Intraluminal Device	6 Hepatic Duct, Left
C Extirpation	8 Cystic Duct		J Synthetic Substitute	7 Hepatic Duct, Caudate
F Fragmentation	9 Common Bile Duct		K Nonautologous Tissue Substitute	8 Cystic Duct
H Insertion	B Hepatobiliary Duct		Y Other Device	9 Common Bile Duct
J Inspection	C Ampulla of Vater		Z No Device	B Small Intestine
L Occlusion	D Pancreatic Duct			C Large Intestine
M Reattachment	F Pancreatic Duct, Accessory			X Diagnostic
N Release	G Pancreas			Z No Qualifier
P Removal				
Q Repair				
R Replacement				
S Reposition				
T Resection				
U Supplement				
V Restriction				
W Revision				
Y Transplantation				

0: Medical and Surgical
G: Endocrine System

Operation-Character 3	Body Part-Character 4	Approach-Character 5	Device-Character 6	Qualifier-Character 7
2 Change	**0** Pituitary Gland	**0** Open	**0** Drainage Device	**X** Diagnostic
5 Destruction	**1** Pineal Body	**3** Percutaneous	**2** Monitoring Device	**Z** No Qualifier
8 Division	**2** Adrenal Gland, Left	**4** Percutaneous Endoscopic	**3** Infusion Device	
9 Drainage	**3** Adrenal Gland, Right	**X** External	**Y** Other Device	
B Excision	**4** Adrenal Glands, Bilateral		**Z** No Device	
C Extirpation	**5** Adrenal Gland			
H Insertion	**6** Carotid Body, Left			
J Inspection	**7** Carotid Body, Right			
M Reattachment	**8** Carotid Bodies, Bilateral			
N Release	**9** Para-aortic Body			
P Removal	**B** Coccygeal Glomus			
Q Repair	**C** Glomus Jugulare			
S Reposition	**D** Aortic Body			
T Resection	**F** Paraganglion Extremity			
W Revision	**G** Thyroid Gland Lobe, Left			
	H Thyroid Gland Lobe, Right			
	J Thyroid Gland Isthmus			
	K Thyroid Gland			
	L Superior Parathyroid Gland, Right			
	M Superior Parathyroid Gland, Left			
	N Inferior Parathyroid Gland, Right			
	P Inferior Parathyroid Gland, Left			
	Q Parathyroid Glands, Multiple			
	R Parathyroid Gland			
	S Endocrine Gland			

0: Medical and Surgical
H: Skin and Breast

Operation-Character 3	Body Part-Character 4	Approach-Character 5	Device-Character 6	Qualifier-Character 7
0 Alteration	**0** Skin, Scalp	**0** Open	**0** Drainage Device	**3** Full Thickness
2 Change	**1** Skin, Face	**3** Percutaneous	**1** Radioactive Element	**4** Partial Thickness
5 Destruction	**2** Skin, Right Ear	**7** Via Natural or Artificial Opening	**7** Autologous Tissue Substitute	**5** Latissimus Dorsi Myocutaneous Flap
8 Division	**3** Skin, Left Ear	**8** Via Natural or Artificial Opening Endoscopic	**J** Synthetic Substitute	**6** Transverse Rectus Abdominis Myocutaneous Flap
9 Drainage	**4** Skin, Neck	**X** External	**K** Nonautologous Tissue Substitute	**7** Deep Inferior Epigastric Artery Perforator Flap
B Excision	**5** Skin, Chest		**N** Tissue Expander	**8** Superficial Inferior Epigastric Artery Flap
C Extirpation	**6** Skin, Back		**Y** Other Device	**9** Gluteal Artery Perforator Flap
D Extraction	**7** Skin, Abdomen		**Z** No Device	**D** Multiple
H Insertion	**8** Skin, Buttock			**X** Diagnostic
J Inspection	**9** Skin, Perineum			**Z** No Qualifier
M Reattachment	**A** Skin, Inguinal			
N Release	**B** Skin, Right Upper Arm			
P Removal	**C** Skin, Left Upper Arm			
Q Repair	**D** Skin, Right Lower Arm			
R Replacement	**E** Skin, Left Lower Arm			
S Reposition	**F** Skin, Right Hand			
T Resection	**G** Skin, Left Hand			
U Supplement	**H** Skin, Right Upper Leg			
W Revision	**J** Skin, Left Upper Leg			
X Transfer	**K** Skin, Right Lower Leg			
	L Skin, Left Lower Leg			
	M Skin, Right Foot			
	N Skin, Left Foot			
	P Skin			
	Q Finger Nail			
	R Toe Nail			
	S Hair			
	T Breast, Right			
	U Breast, Left			
	V Breast, Bilateral			
	W Nipple, Right			
	X Nipple, Left			
	Y Supernumerary Breast			

0: Medical and Surgical
J: Subcutaneous Tissue and Fascia

Operation-Character 3	Body Part-Character 4	Approach-Character 5	Device-Character 6	Qualifier-Character 7
0 Alteration	**0** Subcutaneous Tissue and Fascia, Scalp	**0** Open	**0** Drainage Device	**B** Skin and Subcutaneous Tissue
2 Change	**1** Subcutaneous Tissue and Fascia, Face	**3** Percutaneous	**0** Monitoring Device, Hemodynamic	**C** Skin, Subcutaneous Tissue and Fascia
5 Destruction	**4** Subcutaneous Tissue and Fascia, Right Neck	**X** External	**1** Radioactive Element	**X** Diagnostic
8 Division	**5** Subcutaneous Tissue and Fascia, Left Neck		**2** Monitoring Device	**Z** No Qualifier
9 Drainage	**6** Subcutaneous Tissue and Fascia, Chest		**3** Infusion Device	
B Excision	**7** Subcutaneous Tissue and Fascia, Back		**4** Pacemaker, Single Chamber	
C Extirpation	**8** Subcutaneous Tissue and Fascia, Abdomen		**5** Pacemaker, Single Chamber Rate Responsive	
D Extraction	**9** Subcutaneous Tissue and Fascia, Buttock		**6** Pacemaker, Dual Chamber	
H Insertion	**B** Subcutaneous Tissue and Fascia, Perineum		**7** Autologous Tissue Substitute	
J Inspection	**C** Subcutaneous Tissue and Fascia, Pelvic Region		**7** Cardiac Resynchronization Pacemaker Pulse Generator	
N Release	**D** Subcutaneous Tissue and Fascia, Right Upper Arm		**8** Defibrillator Generator	
P Removal	**F** Subcutaneous Tissue and Fascia, Left Upper Arm		**9** Cardiac Resynchronization Defibrillator Pulse Generator	
Q Repair	**G** Subcutaneous Tissue and Fascia, Right Lower Arm		**A** Contractility Modulation Device	
R Replacement	**H** Subcutaneous Tissue and Fascia, Left Lower Arm		**B** Stimulator Generator, Single Array	
U Supplement	**J** Subcutaneous Tissue and Fascia, Right Hand		**C** Stimulator Generator, Single Array Rechargeable	
W Revision	**K** Subcutaneous Tissue and Fascia, Left Hand		**D** Stimulator Generator, Multiple Array	
X Transfer	**L** Subcutaneous Tissue and Fascia, Right Upper Leg		**E** Stimulator Generator, Multiple Array Rechargeable	
	M Subcutaneous Tissue and Fascia, Left Upper Leg		**H** Contraceptive Device	
	N Subcutaneous Tissue and Fascia, Right Lower Leg		**J** Synthetic Substitute	
	P Subcutaneous Tissue and Fascia, Left Lower Leg		**K** Nonautologous Tissue Substitute	
	Q Subcutaneous Tissue and Fascia, Right Foot		**M** Stimulator Generator	
	R Subcutaneous Tissue and Fascia, Left Foot		**N** Tissue Expander	
	S Subcutaneous Tissue and Fascia, Head and Neck		**P** Cardiac Rhythm Related Device	
	T Subcutaneous Tissue and Fascia, Trunk		**V** Infusion Device, Pump	
	V Subcutaneous Tissue and Fascia, Upper Extremity		**W** Vascular Access Device, Totally Implantable	
	W Subcutaneous Tissue and Fascia, Lower Extremity		**X** Vascular Access Device, Tunneled	
			Y Other Device	
			Z No Device	

0: Medical and Surgical
K: Muscles

Operation-Character 3	Body Part-Character 4	Approach-Character 5	Device-Character 6	Qualifier-Character 7
2 Change	0 Head Muscle	0 Open	0 Drainage Device	0 Skin
5 Destruction	1 Facial Muscle	3 Percutaneous	7 Autologous Tissue Substitute	1 Subcutaneous Tissue
8 Division	2 Neck Muscle, Right	4 Percutaneous Endoscopic	J Synthetic Substitute	2 Skin and Subcutaneous Tissue
9 Drainage	3 Neck Muscle, Left	X External	K Nonautologous Tissue Substitute	5 Latissimus Dorsi Myocutaneous Flap
B Excision	4 Tongue, Palate, Pharynx Muscle		M Stimulator Lead	6 Transverse Rectus Abdominis Myocutaneous Flap
C Extirpation	5 Shoulder Muscle, Right		Y Other Device	7 Deep Inferior Epigastric Artery Perforator Flap
D Extraction	6 Shoulder Muscle, Left		Z No Device	8 Superficial Inferior Epigastric Artery Flap
H Insertion	7 Upper Arm Muscle, Right			9 Gluteal Artery Perforator Flap
J Inspection	8 Upper Arm Muscle, Left			X Diagnostic
M Reattachment	9 Lower Arm and Wrist Muscle, Right			Z No Qualifier
N Release	B Lower Arm and Wrist Muscle, Left			
P Removal	C Hand Muscle, Right			
Q Repair	D Hand Muscle, Left			
R Replacement	F Trunk Muscle, Right			
S Reposition	G Trunk Muscle, Left			
T Resection	H Thorax Muscle, Right			
U Supplement	J Thorax Muscle, Left			
W Revision	K Abdomen Muscle, Right			
X Transfer	L Abdomen Muscle, Left			
	M Perineum Muscle			
	N Hip Muscle, Right			
	P Hip Muscle, Left			
	Q Upper Leg Muscle, Right			
	R Upper Leg Muscle, Left			
	S Lower Leg Muscle, Right			
	T Lower Leg Muscle, Left			
	V Foot Muscle, Right			
	W Foot Muscle, Left			
	X Upper Muscle			
	Y Lower Muscle			

0: Medical and Surgical
L: Tendons

Operation-Character 3	Body Part-Character 4	Approach-Character 5	Device-Character 6	Qualifier-Character 7
2 Change	**0** Head and Neck Tendon	**0** Open	**0** Drainage Device	**X** Diagnostic
5 Destruction	**1** Shoulder Tendon, Right	**3** Percutaneous	**7** Autologous Tissue Substitute	**Z** No Qualifier
8 Division	**2** Shoulder Tendon, Left	**4** Percutaneous Endoscopic	**J** Synthetic Substitute	
9 Drainage	**3** Upper Arm Tendon, Right	**X** External	**K** Nonautologous Tissue Substitute	
B Excision	**4** Upper Arm Tendon, Left		**Y** Other Device	
C Extirpation	**5** Lower Arm and Wrist Tendon, Right		**Z** No Device	
D Extraction	**6** Lower Arm and Wrist Tendon, Left			
H Insertion	**7** Hand Tendon, Right			
J Inspection	**8** Hand Tendon, Left			
M Reattachment	**9** Trunk Tendon, Right			
N Release	**B** Trunk Tendon, Left			
P Removal	**C** Thorax Tendon, Right			
Q Repair	**D** Thorax Tendon, Left			
R Replacement	**F** Abdomen Tendon, Right			
S Reposition	**G** Abdomen Tendon, Left			
T Resection	**H** Perineum Tendon			
U Supplement	**J** Hip Tendon, Right			
W Revision	**K** Hip Tendon, Left			
X Transfer	**L** Upper Leg Tendon, Right			
	M Upper Leg Tendon, Left			
	N Lower Leg Tendon, Right			
	P Lower Leg Tendon, Left			
	Q Knee Tendon, Right			
	R Knee Tendon, Left			
	S Ankle Tendon, Right			
	T Ankle Tendon, Left			
	V Foot Tendon, Right			
	W Foot Tendon, Left			
	X Upper Tendon			
	Y Lower Tendon			

0: Medical and Surgical
M: Bursae and Ligaments

Operation-Character 3	Body Part-Character 4	Approach-Character 5	Device-Character 6	Qualifier-Character 7
2 Change	**0** Head and Neck Bursa and Ligament	**0** Open	**0** Drainage Device	**X** Diagnostic
5 Destruction	**1** Shoulder Bursa and Ligament, Right	**3** Percutaneous	**7** Autologous Tissue Substitute	**Z** No Qualifier
8 Division	**2** Shoulder Bursa and Ligament, Left	**4** Percutaneous Endoscopic	**J** Synthetic Substitute	
9 Drainage	**3** Elbow Bursa and Ligament, Right	**X** External	**K** Nonautologous Tissue Substitute	
B Excision	**4** Elbow Bursa and Ligament, Left		**Y** Other Device	
C Extirpation	**5** Wrist Bursa and Ligament, Right		**Z** No Device	
D Extraction	**6** Wrist Bursa and Ligament, Left			
H Insertion	**7** Hand Bursa and Ligament, Right			
J Inspection	**8** Hand Bursa and Ligament, Left			
M Reattachment	**9** Upper Extremity Bursa and Ligament, Right			
N Release	**B** Upper Extremity Bursa and Ligament, Left			
P Removal	**C** Upper Spine Bursa and Ligament			
Q Repair	**D** Lower Spine Bursa and Ligament			
R Replacement	**F** Sternum Bursa and Ligament			
S Reposition	**G** Rib(s) Bursa and Ligament			
T Resection	**H** Abdomen Bursa and Ligament, Right			
U Supplement	**J** Abdomen Bursa and Ligament, Left			
W Revision	**K** Perineum Bursa and Ligament			
X Transfer	**L** Hip Bursa and Ligament, Right			
	M Hip Bursa and Ligament, Left			
	N Knee Bursa and Ligament, Right			
	P Knee Bursa and Ligament, Left			
	Q Ankle Bursa and Ligament, Right			
	R Ankle Bursa and Ligament, Left			
	S Foot Bursa and Ligament, Right			
	T Foot Bursa and Ligament, Left			
	V Lower Extremity Bursa and Ligament, Right			
	W Lower Extremity Bursa and Ligament, Left			
	X Upper Bursa and Ligament			
	Y Lower Bursa and Ligament			

0: Medical and Surgical
N: Head and Facial Bones

Operation-Character 3	Body Part-Character 4	Approach-Character 5	Device-Character 6	Qualifier-Character 7
2 Change	**0** Skull	**0** Open	**0** Drainage Device	**X** Diagnostic
5 Destruction	**1** Frontal Bone	**3** Percutaneous	**4** Internal Fixation Device	**Z** No Qualifier
8 Division	**3** Parietal Bone, Right	**4** Percutaneous Endoscopic	**5** External Fixation Device	
9 Drainage	**4** Parietal Bone, Left	**X** External	**7** Autologous Tissue Substitute	
B Excision	**5** Temporal Bone, Right		**J** Synthetic Substitute	
C Extirpation	**6** Temporal Bone, Left		**K** Nonautologous Tissue Substitute	
D Extraction	**7** Occipital Bone		**M** Bone Growth Stimulator	
H Insertion	**B** Nasal Bone		**N** Neurostimulator Generator	
J Inspection	**C** Sphenoid Bone		**S** Hearing Device	
N Release	**F** Ethmoid Bone, Right		**Y** Other Device	
P Removal	**G** Ethmoid Bone, Left		**Z** No Device	
Q Repair	**H** Lacrimal Bone, Right			
R Replacement	**J** Lacrimal Bone, Left			
S Reposition	**K** Palatine Bone, Right			
T Resection	**L** Palatine Bone, Left			
U Supplement	**M** Zygomatic Bone, Right			
W Revision	**N** Zygomatic Bone, Left			
	P Orbit, Right			
	Q Orbit, Left			
	R Maxilla			
	T Mandible, Right			
	V Mandible, Left			
	W Facial Bone			
	X Hyoid Bone			

0: Medical and Surgical
P: Upper Bones

Operation-Character 3	Body Part-Character 4	Approach-Character 5	Device-Character 6	Qualifier-Character 7
2 Change	**0** Sternum	**0** Open	**0** Drainage Device	**X** Diagnostic
5 Destruction	**1** Ribs, 1 to 2	**3** Percutaneous	**0** Internal Fixation Device, Rigid Plate	**Z** No Qualifier
8 Division	**2** Ribs, 3 or More	**4** Percutaneous Endoscopic	**4** Internal Fixation Device	
9 Drainage	**3** Cervical Vertebra	**X** External	**5** External Fixation Device	
B Excision	**4** Thoracic Vertebra		**6** Internal Fixation Device, Intramedullary	
C Extirpation	**5** Scapula, Right		**7** Autologous Tissue Substitute	
D Extraction	**6** Scapula, Left		**8** External Fixation Device, Limb Lengthening	
H Insertion	**7** Glenoid Cavity, Right		**B** External Fixation Device, Monoplanar	
J Inspection	**8** Glenoid Cavity, Left		**C** External Fixation Device, Ring	
N Release	**9** Clavicle, Right		**D** External Fixation Device, Hybrid	
P Removal	**B** Clavicle, Left		**J** Synthetic Substitute	
Q Repair	**C** Humeral Head, Right		**K** Nonautologous Tissue Substitute	
R Replacement	**D** Humeral Head, Left		**M** Bone Growth Stimulator	
S Reposition	**F** Humeral Shaft, Right		**Y** Other Device	
T Resection	**G** Humeral Shaft, Left		**Z** No Device	
U Supplement	**H** Radius, Right			
W Revision	**J** Radius, Left			
	K Ulna, Right			
	L Ulna, Left			
	M Carpal, Right			
	N Carpal, Left			
	P Metacarpal, Right			
	Q Metacarpal, Left			
	R Thumb Phalanx, Right			
	S Thumb Phalanx, Left			
	T Finger Phalanx, Right			
	V Finger Phalanx, Left			
	Y Upper Bone			

0: Medical and Surgical
Q: Lower Bones

Operation-Character 3	Body Part-Character 4	Approach-Character 5	Device-Character 6	Qualifier-Character 7
2 Change	**0** Lumbar Vertebra	**0** Open	**0** Drainage Device	**2** Sesamoid Bone(s) 1st Toe
5 Destruction	**1** Sacrum	**3** Percutaneous	**4** Internal Fixation Device	**X** Diagnostic
8 Division	**2** Pelvic Bone, Right	**4** Percutaneous Endoscopic	**5** External Fixation Device	**Z** No Qualifier
9 Drainage	**3** Pelvic Bone, Left	**X** External	**6** Internal Fixation Device, Intramedullary	
B Excision	**4** Acetabulum, Right		**7** Autologous Tissue Substitute	
C Extirpation	**5** Acetabulum, Left		**8** External Fixation Device, Limb Lengthening	
D Extraction	**6** Upper Femur, Right		**B** External Fixation Device, Monoplanar	
H Insertion	**7** Upper Femur, Left		**C** External Fixation Device, Ring	
J Inspection	**8** Femoral Shaft, Right		**D** External Fixation Device, Hybrid	
N Release	**9** Femoral Shaft, Left		**J** Synthetic Substitute	
P Removal	**B** Lower Femur, Right		**K** Nonautologous Tissue Substitute	
Q Repair	**C** Lower Femur, Left		**M** Bone Growth Stimulator	
R Replacement	**D** Patella, Right		**Y** Other Device	
S Reposition	**F** Patella, Left		**Z** No Device	
T Resection	**G** Tibia, Right			
U Supplement	**H** Tibia, Left			
W Revision	**J** Fibula, Right			
	K Fibula, Left			
	L Tarsal, Right			
	M Tarsal, Left			
	N Metatarsal, Right			
	P Metatarsal, Left			
	Q Toe Phalanx, Right			
	R Toe Phalanx, Left			
	S Coccyx			
	Y Lower Bone			

0: Medical and Surgical
R: Upper Joints

Operation-Character 3	Body Part-Character 4	Approach-Character 5	Device-Character 6	Qualifier-Character 7
2 Change	0 Occipital-cervical Joint	0 Open	0 Drainage Device	0 Anterior Approach, Anterior Column
5 Destruction	1 Cervical Vertebral Joint	3 Percutaneous	0 Synthetic Substitute, Reverse Ball and Socket	1 Posterior Approach, Posterior Column
9 Drainage	2 Cervical Vertebral Joints, 2 or more	4 Percutaneous Endoscopic	3 Infusion Device	6 Humeral Surface
B Excision	3 Cervical Vertebral Disc	X External	4 Internal Fixation Device	7 Glenoid Surface
C Extirpation	4 Cervicothoracic Vertebral Joint		5 External Fixation Device	J Posterior Approach, Anterior Column
G Fusion	5 Cervicothoracic Vertebral Disc		7 Autologous Tissue Substitute	X Diagnostic
H Insertion	6 Thoracic Vertebral Joint		8 Spacer	Z No Qualifier
J Inspection	7 Thoracic Vertebral Joints, 2 to 7		A Interbody Fusion Device	
N Release	8 Thoracic Vertebral Joints, 8 or more		B Spinal Stabilization Device, Interspinous Process	
P Removal	9 Thoracic Vertebral Disc		C Spinal Stabilization Device, Pedicle-Based	
Q Repair	A Thoracolumbar Vertebral Joint		D Spinal Stabilization Device, Facet Replacement	
R Replacement	B Thoracolumbar Vertebral Disc		J Synthetic Substitute	
S Reposition	C Temporomandibular Joint, Right		K Nonautologous Tissue Substitute	
T Resection	D Temporomandibular Joint, Left		Y Other Device	
U Supplement	E Sternoclavicular Joint, Right		Z No Device	
W Revision	F Sternoclavicular Joint, Left			
	G Acromioclavicular Joint, Right			
	H Acromioclavicular Joint, Left			
	J Shoulder Joint, Right			
	K Shoulder Joint, Left			
	L Elbow Joint, Right			
	M Elbow Joint, Left			
	N Wrist Joint, Right			
	P Wrist Joint, Left			
	Q Carpal Joint, Right			
	R Carpal Joint, Left			
	S Carpometacarpal Joint, Right			
	T Carpometacarpal Joint, Left			
	U Metacarpophalangeal Joint, Right			
	V Metacarpophalangeal Joint, Left			
	W Finger Phalangeal Joint, Right			
	X Finger Phalangeal Joint, Left			
	Y Upper Joint			

0: Medical and Surgical
S: Lower Joints

Operation-Character 3	Body Part-Character 4	Approach-Character 5	Device-Character 6	Qualifier-Character 7
2 Change	0 Lumbar Vertebral Joint	0 Open	0 Drainage Device	0 Anterior Approach, Anterior Column
5 Destruction	1 Lumbar Vertebral Joints, 2 or more	3 Percutaneous	0 Synthetic Substitute, Polyethylene	1 Posterior Approach, Posterior Column
9 Drainage	2 Lumbar Vertebral Disc	4 Percutaneous Endoscopic	1 Synthetic Substitute, Metal	9 Cemented
B Excision	3 Lumbosacral Joint	X External	2 Synthetic Substitute, Metal on Polyethylene	A Uncemented
C Extirpation	4 Lumbosacral Disc		3 Infusion Device	C Patellar Surface
G Fusion	5 Sacrococcygeal Joint		3 Synthetic Substitute, Ceramic	J Posterior Approach, Anterior Column
H Insertion	6 Coccygeal Joint		4 Internal Fixation Device	X Diagnostic
J Inspection	7 Sacroiliac Joint, Right		4 Synthetic Substitute, Ceramic on Polyethylene	Z No Qualifier
N Release	8 Sacroiliac Joint, Left		5 External Fixation Device	
P Removal	9 Hip Joint, Right		6 Synthetic Substitute, Oxidized Zirconium on Polyethylene	
Q Repair	A Hip Joint, Acetabular Surface, Right		7 Autologous Tissue Substitute	
R Replacement	B Hip Joint, Left		8 Spacer	
S Reposition	C Knee Joint, Right		9 Liner	
T Resection	D Knee Joint, Left		A Interbody Fusion Device	
U Supplement	E Hip Joint, Acetabular Surface, Left		B Resurfacing Device	
W Revision	F Ankle Joint, Right		B Spinal Stabilization Device, Interspinous Process	
	G Ankle Joint, Left		C Spinal Stabilization Device, Pedicle-Based	
	H Tarsal Joint, Right		D Spinal Stabilization Device, Facet Replacement	
	J Tarsal Joint, Left		J Synthetic Substitute	
	K Tarsometatarsal Joint, Right		K Nonautologous Tissue Substitute	
	L Tarsometatarsal Joint, Left		L Synthetic Substitute, Unicondylar	
	M Metatarsal-Phalangeal Joint, Right		Y Other Device	
	N Metatarsal-Phalangeal Joint, Left		Z No Device	
	P Toe Phalangeal Joint, Right			
	Q Toe Phalangeal Joint, Left			
	R Hip Joint, Femoral Surface, Right			
	S Hip Joint, Femoral Surface, Left			
	T Knee Joint, Femoral Surface, Right			
	U Knee Joint, Femoral Surface, Left			
	V Knee Joint, Tibial Surface, Right			
	W Knee Joint, Tibial Surface, Left			
	Y Lower Joint			

0: Medical and Surgical
T: Urinary System

Operation-Character 3	Body Part-Character 4	Approach-Character 5	Device-Character 6	Qualifier-Character 7
1 Bypass	**0** Kidney, Right	**0** Open	**0** Drainage Device	**0** Allogeneic
2 Change	**1** Kidney, Left	**3** Percutaneous	**2** Monitoring Device	**1** Syngeneic
5 Destruction	**2** Kidneys, Bilateral	**4** Percutaneous Endoscopic	**3** Infusion Device	**2** Zooplastic
7 Dilation	**3** Kidney Pelvis, Right	**7** Via Natural or Artificial Opening	**7** Autologous Tissue Substitute	**3** Kidney Pelvis, Right
8 Division	**4** Kidney Pelvis, Left	**8** Via Natural or Artificial Opening Endoscopic	**C** Extraluminal Device	**4** Kidney Pelvis, Left
9 Drainage	**5** Kidney	**X** External	**D** Intraluminal Device	**6** Ureter, Right
B Excision	**6** Ureter, Right		**J** Synthetic Substitute	**7** Ureter, Left
C Extirpation	**7** Ureter, Left		**K** Nonautologous Tissue Substitute	**8** Colon
D Extraction	**8** Ureters, Bilateral		**L** Artificial Sphincter	**9** Colocutaneous
F Fragmentation	**9** Ureter		**M** Stimulator Lead	**A** Ileum
H Insertion	**B** Bladder		**Y** Other Device	**B** Bladder
J Inspection	**C** Bladder Neck		**Z** No Device	**C** Ileocutaneous
L Occlusion	**D** Urethra			**D** Cutaneous
M Reattachment				**X** Diagnostic
N Release				**Z** No Qualifier
P Removal				
Q Repair				
R Replacement				
S Reposition				
T Resection				
U Supplement				
V Restriction				
W Revision				
Y Transplantation				

0: Medical and Surgical
U: Female Reproductive System

Operation-Character 3	Body Part-Character 4	Approach-Character 5	Device-Character 6	Qualifier-Character 7
1 Bypass	**0** Ovary, Right	**0** Open	**0** Drainage Device	**0** Allogeneic
2 Change	**1** Ovary, Left	**3** Percutaneous	**1** Radioactive Element	**1** Syngeneic
5 Destruction	**2** Ovaries, Bilateral	**4** Percutaneous Endoscopic	**3** Infusion Device	**2** Zooplastic
7 Dilation	**3** Ovary	**7** Via Natural or Artificial Opening	**7** Autologous Tissue Substitute	**5** Fallopian Tube, Right
8 Division	**4** Uterine Supporting Structure	**8** Via Natural or Artificial Opening Endoscopic	**C** Extraluminal Device	**6** Fallopian Tube, Left
9 Drainage	**5** Fallopian Tube, Right	**F** Via Natural or Artificial Opening With Percutaneous Endoscopic Assistance	**D** Intraluminal Device	**9** Uterus
B Excision	**6** Fallopian Tube, Left	**X** External	**G** Intraluminal Device, Pessary	**X** Diagnostic
C Extirpation	**7** Fallopian Tubes, Bilateral		**H** Contraceptive Device	**Z** No Qualifier
D Extraction	**8** Fallopian Tube		**J** Synthetic Substitute	
F Fragmentation	**9** Uterus		**K** Nonautologous Tissue Substitute	
H Insertion	**B** Endometrium		**Y** Other Device	
J Inspection	**C** Cervix		**Z** No Device	
L Occlusion	**D** Uterus and Cervix			
M Reattachment	**F** Cul-de-sac			
N Release	**G** Vagina			
P Removal	**H** Vagina and Cul-de-sac			
Q Repair	**J** Clitoris			
S Reposition	**K** Hymen			
T Resection	**L** Vestibular Gland			
U Supplement	**M** Vulva			
V Restriction	**N** Ova			
W Revision				
Y Transplantation				

0: Medical and Surgical
V: Male Reproductive System

Operation-Character 3	Body Part-Character 4	Approach-Character 5	Device-Character 6	Qualifier-Character 7
1 Bypass	**0** Prostate	**0** Open	**0** Drainage Device	**J** Epididymis, Right
2 Change	**1** Seminal Vesicle, Right	**3** Percutaneous	**1** Radioactive Element	**K** Epididymis, Left
5 Destruction	**2** Seminal Vesicle, Left	**4** Percutaneous Endoscopic	**3** Infusion Device	**N** Vas Deferens, Right
7 Dilation	**3** Seminal Vesicles, Bilateral	**7** Via Natural or Artificial Opening	**7** Autologous Tissue Substitute	**P** Vas Deferens, Left
9 Drainage	**4** Prostate and Seminal Vesicles	**8** Via Natural or Artificial Opening Endoscopic	**C** Extraluminal Device	**X** Diagnostic
B Excision	**5** Scrotum	**X** External	**D** Intraluminal Device	**Z** No Qualifier
C Extirpation	**6** Tunica Vaginalis, Right		**J** Synthetic Substitute	
H Insertion	**7** Tunica Vaginalis, Left		**K** Nonautologous Tissue Substitute	
J Inspection	**8** Scrotum and Tunica Vaginalis		**Y** Other Device	
L Occlusion	**9** Testis, Right		**Z** No Device	
M Reattachment	**B** Testis, Left			
N Release	**C** Testes, Bilateral			
P Removal	**D** Testis			
Q Repair	**F** Spermatic Cord, Right			
R Replacement	**G** Spermatic Cord, Left			
S Reposition	**H** Spermatic Cords, Bilateral			
T Resection	**J** Epididymis, Right			
U Supplement	**K** Epididymis, Left			
W Revision	**L** Epididymis, Bilateral			
	M Epididymis and Spermatic Cord			
	N Vas Deferens, Right			
	P Vas Deferens, Left			
	Q Vas Deferens, Bilateral			
	R Vas Deferens			
	S Penis			
	T Prepuce			

0: Medical and Surgical
W: Anatomical Regions, General

Operation-Character 3	Body Part-Character 4	Approach-Character 5	Device-Character 6	Qualifier-Character 7
0 Alteration	**0** Head	**0** Open	**0** Drainage Device	**0** Allogeneic
1 Bypass	**1** Cranial Cavity	**3** Percutaneous	**1** Radioactive Element	**0** Vagina
2 Change	**2** Face	**4** Percutaneous Endoscopic	**3** Infusion Device	**1** Penis
3 Control	**3** Oral Cavity and Throat	**7** Via Natural or Artificial Opening	**7** Autologous Tissue Substitute	**1** Syngeneic
4 Creation	**4** Upper Jaw	**8** Via Natural or Artificial Opening Endoscopic	**J** Synthetic Substitute	**2** Stoma
8 Division	**5** Lower Jaw	**X** External	**K** Nonautologous Tissue Substitute	**4** Cutaneous
9 Drainage	**6** Neck		**Y** Other Device	**9** Pleural Cavity, Right
B Excision	**8** Chest Wall		**Z** No Device	**B** Pleural Cavity, Left
C Extirpation	**9** Pleural Cavity, Right			**G** Peritoneal Cavity
F Fragmentation	**B** Pleural Cavity, Left			**J** Pelvic Cavity
H Insertion	**C** Mediastinum			**X** Diagnostic
J Inspection	**D** Pericardial Cavity			**Y** Lower Vein
M Reattachment	**F** Abdominal Wall			**Z** No Qualifier
P Removal	**G** Peritoneal Cavity			
Q Repair	**H** Retroperitoneum			
U Supplement	**J** Pelvic Cavity			
W Revision	**K** Upper Back			
Y Transplantation	**L** Lower Back			
	M Perineum, Male			
	N Perineum, Female			
	P Gastrointestinal Tract			
	Q Respiratory Tract			
	R Genitourinary Tract			

0: Medical and Surgical
X: Anatomical Regions, Upper Extremities

Operation-Character 3	Body Part-Character 4	Approach-Character 5	Device-Character 6	Qualifier-Character 7
0 Alteration	**0** Forequarter, Right	**0** Open	**0** Drainage Device	**0** Allogeneic
2 Change	**1** Forequarter, Left	**3** Percutaneous	**1** Radioactive Element	**0** Complete
3 Control	**2** Shoulder Region, Right	**4** Percutaneous Endoscopic	**3** Infusion Device	**1** High
6 Detachment	**3** Shoulder Region, Left	**X** External	**7** Autologous Tissue Substitute	**1** Syngeneic
9 Drainage	**4** Axilla, Right		**J** Synthetic Substitute	**2** Mid
B Excision	**5** Axilla, Left		**K** Nonautologous Tissue Substitute	**3** Low
H Insertion	**6** Upper Extremity, Right		**Y** Other Device	**4** Complete 1st Ray
J Inspection	**7** Upper Extremity, Left		**Z** No Device	**5** Complete 2nd Ray
M Reattachment	**8** Upper Arm, Right			**6** Complete 3rd Ray
P Removal	**9** Upper Arm, Left			**7** Complete 4th Ray
Q Repair	**B** Elbow Region, Right			**8** Complete 5th Ray
R Replacement	**C** Elbow Region, Left			**9** Partial 1st Ray
U Supplement	**D** Lower Arm, Right			**B** Partial 2nd Ray
W Revision	**F** Lower Arm, Left			**C** Partial 3rd Ray
X Transfer	**G** Wrist Region, Right			**D** Partial 4th Ray
Y Transplantation	**H** Wrist Region, Left			**F** Partial 5th Ray
	J Hand, Right			**L** Thumb, Right
	K Hand, Left			**M** Thumb, Left
	L Thumb, Right			**N** Toe, Right
	M Thumb, Left			**P** Toe, Left
	N Index Finger, Right			**X** Diagnostic
	P Index Finger, Left			**Z** No Qualifier
	Q Middle Finger, Right			
	R Middle Finger, Left			
	S Ring Finger, Right			
	T Ring Finger, Left			
	V Little Finger, Right			
	W Little Finger, Left			

0: Medical and Surgical
Y: Anatomical Regions, Lower Extremities

Operation-Character 3	Body Part-Character 4	Approach-Character 5	Device-Character 6	Qualifier-Character 7
0 Alteration	**0** Buttock, Right	**0** Open	**0** Drainage Device	**0** Complete
2 Change	**1** Buttock, Left	**3** Percutaneous	**1** Radioactive Element	**1** High
3 Control	**2** Hindquarter, Right	**4** Percutaneous Endoscopic	**3** Infusion Device	**2** Mid
6 Detachment	**3** Hindquarter, Left	**X** External	**7** Autologous Tissue Substitute	**3** Low
9 Drainage	**4** Hindquarter, Bilateral		**J** Synthetic Substitute	**4** Complete 1st Ray
B Excision	**5** Inguinal Region, Right		**K** Nonautologous Tissue Substitute	**5** Complete 2nd Ray
H Insertion	**6** Inguinal Region, Left		**Y** Other Device	**6** Complete 3rd Ray
J Inspection	**7** Femoral Region, Right		**Z** No Device	**7** Complete 4th Ray
M Reattachment	**8** Femoral Region, Left			**8** Complete 5th Ray
P Removal	**9** Lower Extremity, Right			**9** Partial 1st Ray
Q Repair	**A** Inguinal Region, Bilateral			**B** Partial 2nd Ray
U Supplement	**B** Lower Extremity, Left			**C** Partial 3rd Ray
W Revision	**C** Upper Leg, Right			**D** Partial 4th Ray
	D Upper Leg, Left			**F** Partial 5th Ray
	E Femoral Region, Bilateral			**X** Diagnostic
	F Knee Region, Right			**Z** No Qualifier
	G Knee Region, Left			
	H Lower Leg, Right			
	J Lower Leg, Left			
	K Ankle Region, Right			
	L Ankle Region, Left			
	M Foot, Right			
	N Foot, Left			
	P 1st Toe, Right			
	Q 1st Toe, Left			
	R 2nd Toe, Right			
	S 2nd Toe, Left			
	T 3rd Toe, Right			
	U 3rd Toe, Left			
	V 4th Toe, Right			
	W 4th Toe, Left			
	X 5th Toe, Right			
	Y 5th Toe, Left			

1: Obstetrics
0: Pregnancy

Operation-Character 3	Body Part-Character 4	Approach-Character 5	Device-Character 6	Qualifier-Character 7
2 Change	**0** Products of Conception	**0** Open	**3** Monitoring Electrode	**0** Classical
9 Drainage	**1** Products of Conception, Retained	**3** Percutaneous	**Y** Other Device	**1** Low Cervical
A Abortion	**2** Products of Conception, Ectopic	**4** Percutaneous Endoscopic	**Z** No Device	**2** Extraperitoneal
D Extraction		**7** Via Natural or Artificial Opening		**3** Low Forceps
E Delivery		**8** Via Natural or Artificial Opening Endoscopic		**4** Mid Forceps
H Insertion		**X** External		**5** High Forceps
J Inspection				**6** Vacuum
P Removal				**7** Internal Version
Q Repair				**8** Other
S Reposition				**9** Fetal Blood
T Resection				**9** Manual
Y Transplantation				**A** Fetal Cerebrospinal Fluid
				B Fetal Fluid, Other
				C Amniotic Fluid,
				D Fluid, Other Therapeutic
				E Nervous System
				F Cardiovascular System
				G Lymphatics and Hemic
				H Eye
				J Ear, Nose and Sinus
				K Respiratory System
				L Mouth and Throat
				M Gastrointestinal System
				N Hepatobiliary and Pancreas
				P Endocrine System
				Q Skin
				R Musculoskeletal System
				S Urinary System
				T Female Reproductive System
				U Amniotic Fluid, Diagnostic
				V Male Reproductive System
				W Laminaria
				X Abortifacient
				Y Other Body System
				Z No Qualifier

2: Placement
W: Anatomical Regions

Operation-Character 3	Body Region-Character 4	Approach-Character 5	Device-Character 6	Qualifier-Character 7
0 Change	**0** Head	**X** External	**0** Traction Apparatus	**Z** No Qualifier
1 Compression	**1** Face		**1** Splint	
2 Dressing	**2** Neck		**2** Cast	
3 Immobilization	**3** Abdominal Wall		**3** Brace	
4 Packing	**4** Chest Wall		**4** Bandage	
5 Removal	**5** Back		**5** Packing Material	
6 Traction	**6** Inguinal Region, Right		**6** Pressure Dressing	
	7 Inguinal Region, Left		**7** Intermittent Pressure Device	
	8 Upper Extremity, Right		**9** Wire	
	9 Upper Extremity, Left		**Y** Other Device	
	A Upper Arm, Right		**Z** No Device	
	B Upper Arm, Left			
	C Lower Arm, Right			
	D Lower Arm, Left			
	E Hand, Right			
	F Hand, Left			
	G Thumb, Right			
	H Thumb, Left			
	J Finger, Right			
	K Finger, Left			
	L Lower Extremity, Right			
	M Lower Extremity, Left			
	N Upper Leg, Right			
	P Upper Leg, Left			
	Q Lower Leg, Right			
	R Lower Leg, Left			
	S Foot, Right			
	T Foot, Left			
	U Toe, Right			
	V Toe, Left			

2: Placement
Y: Anatomical Orifices

Operation-Character 3	Body Region-Character 4	Approach-Character 5	Device-Character 6	Qualifier-Character 7
0 Change	**0** Mouth and Pharynx	**X** External	**5** Packing Material	**Z** No Qualifier
4 Packing	**1** Nasal			
5 Removal	**2** Ear			
	3 Anorectal			
	4 Female Genital Tract			
	5 Urethra			

3: Administration
0: Circulatory

Operation-Character 3	Body System/ Region-Character 4	Approach-Character 5	Substance-Character 6	Qualifier-Character 7
2 Transfusion	**3** Peripheral Vein	**0** Open	**A** Stem Cells, Embryonic	**0** Autologous
	4 Central Vein	**3** Percutaneous	**B** 4-Factor Prothrombin Complex Concentrate	**1** Nonautologous
	5 Peripheral Artery	**7** Via Natural or Artificial Opening	**G** Bone Marrow	**2** Allogeneic, Related
	6 Central Artery		**H** Whole Blood	**3** Allogeneic, Unrelated
	7 Products of Conception, Circulatory		**J** Serum Albumin	**4** Allogeneic, Unspecified
	8 Vein		**K** Frozen Plasma	**Z** No Qualifier
			L Fresh Plasma	
			M Plasma Cryoprecipitate	
			N Red Blood Cells	
			P Frozen Red Cells	
			Q White Cells	
			R Platelets	
			S Globulin	
			T Fibrinogen	
			V Antihemophilic Factors	
			W Factor IX	
			X Stem Cells, Cord Blood	
			Y Stem Cells, Hematopoietic	

3: Administration
C: Indwelling Device

Operation-Character 3	Body System/ Region-Character 4	Approach-Character 5	Substance-Character 6	Qualifier-Character 7
1 Irrigation	**Z** None	**X** External	**8** Irrigating Substance	**Z** No Qualifier

3: Administration
E: Physiological Systems and Anatomical Regions

Operation-Character 3	Body System/ Region- Character 4	Approach-Character 5	Substance-Character 6	Qualifier-Character 7
0 Introduction	**0** Skin and Mucous Membranes	**0** Open	**0** Antineoplastic	**0** Autologous
1 Irrigation	**1** Subcutaneous Tissue	**3** Percutaneous	**1** Thrombolytic	**1** Nonautologous
	2 Muscle	**7** Via Natural or Artificial Opening	**2** Anti-infective	**2** High-dose Interleukin-2
	3 Peripheral Vein	**8** Via Natural or Artificial Opening Endoscopic	**3** Anti-inflammatory	**3** Low-dose Interleukin-2
	4 Central Vein	**X** External	**4** Serum, Toxoid and Vaccine	**4** Liquid Brachytherapy Radioisotope
	5 Peripheral Artery		**5** Adhesion Barrier	**5** Other Antineoplastic
	6 Central Artery		**6** Nutritional Substance	**6** Recombinant Human activated Protein C
	7 Coronary Artery		**7** Electrolytic and Water Balance Substance	**7** Other Thrombolytic
	8 Heart		**8** Irrigating Substance	**8** Oxazolidinones
	9 Nose		**9** Dialysate	**9** Other Anti-infective
	A Bone Marrow		**A** Stem Cells, Embryonic	**A** Anti-Infective Envelope
	B Ear		**B** Anesthetic Agent	**B** Recombinant Bone Morphogenetic Protein
	C Eye		**E** Stem Cells, Somatic	**C** Other Substance
	D Mouth and Pharynx		**F** Intracirculatory Anesthetic	**D** Nitric Oxide
	E Products of Conception		**G** Other Therapeutic Substance	**F** Other Gas
	F Respiratory Tract		**H** Radioactive Substance	**G** Insulin
	G Upper GI		**K** Other Diagnostic Substance	**H** Human B-type Natriuretic Peptide
	H Lower GI		**L** Sperm	**J** Other Hormone
	J Biliary and Pancreatic Tract		**M** Pigment	**K** Immunostimulator
	K Genitourinary Tract		**N** Analgesics, Hypnotics, Sedatives	**L** Immunosuppressive
	L Pleural Cavity		**P** Platelet Inhibitor	**M** Monoclonal Antibody
	M Peritoneal Cavity		**Q** Fertilized Ovum	**N** Blood Brain Barrier Disruption
	N Male Reproductive		**R** Antiarrhythmic	**P** Clofarabine
	P Female Reproductive		**S** Gas	**Q** Glucarpidase
	Q Cranial Cavity and Brain		**T** Destructive Agent	**Z** No Qualifier
	R Spinal Canal		**U** Pancreatic Islet Cells	
	S Epidural Space		**V** Hormone	
	T Peripheral Nerves and Plexi		**W** Immunotherapeutic	
	U Joints		**X** Vasopressor	
	V Bones			
	W Lymphatics			
	X Cranial Nerves			
	Y Pericardial Cavity			

4: Measurement and Monitoring
A: Physiological Systems

Operation-Character 3	Body System-Character 4	Approach-Character 5	Function/ Device-Character 6	Qualifier-Character 7
0 Measurement	**0** Central Nervous	**0** Open	**0** Acuity	**0** Central
1 Monitoring	**1** Peripheral Nervous	**3** Percutaneous	**1** Capacity	**1** Peripheral
	2 Cardiac	**7** Via Natural or Artificial Opening	**2** Conductivity	**2** Portal
	3 Arterial	**8** Via Natural or Artificial Opening Endoscopic	**3** Contractility	**3** Pulmonary
	4 Venous	**X** External	**4** Electrical Activity	**4** Stress
	5 Circulatory		**5** Flow	**5** Ambulatory
	6 Lymphatic		**6** Metabolism	**6** Right Heart
	7 Visual		**7** Mobility	**7** Left Heart
	8 Olfactory		**8** Motility	**8** Bilateral
	9 Respiratory		**9** Output	**9** Sensory
	B Gastrointestinal		**B** Pressure	**A** Guidance
	C Biliary		**C** Rate	**B** Motor
	D Urinary		**D** Resistance	**C** Coronary
	F Musculoskeletal		**F** Rhythm	**D** Intracranial
	G Skin and Breast		**G** Secretion	**F** Other Thoracic
	H Products of Conception, Cardiac		**H** Sound	**G** Intraoperative
	J Products of Conception, Nervous		**J** Pulse	**H** Indocyanine Green Dye
	Z None		**K** Temperature	**Z** No Qualifier
			L Volume	
			M Total Activity	
			N Sampling and Pressure	
			P Action Currents	
			Q Sleep	
			R Saturation	
			S Vascular Perfusion	

4: Measurement and Monitoring
B: Physiological Devices

Operation-Character 3	Body System-Character 4	Approach-Character 5	Function/ Device-Character 6	Qualifier-Character 7
0 Measurement	**0** Central Nervous	**X** External	**S** Pacemaker	**Z** No Qualifier
	1 Peripheral Nervous		**T** Defibrillator	
	2 Cardiac		**V** Stimulator	
	9 Respiratory			
	F Musculoskeletal			

5: Extracorporeal Assistance and Performance
A: Physiological Systems

Operation-Character 3	Body System-Character 4	Duration-Character 5	Function-Character 6	Qualifier-Character 7
0 Assistance	**2** Cardiac	**0** Single	**0** Filtration	**0** Balloon Pump
1 Performance	**5** Circulatory	**1** Intermittent	**1** Output	**1** Hyperbaric
2 Restoration	**9** Respiratory	**2** Continuous	**2** Oxygenation	**2** Manual
	C Biliary	**3** Less than 24 Consecutive Hours	**3** Pacing	**3** Membrane
	D Urinary	**4** 24-96 Consecutive Hours	**4** Rhythm	**4** Nonmechanical
		5 Greater than 96 Consecutive Hours	**5** Ventilation	**5** Pulsatile Compression
		6 Multiple		**6** Other Pump
				7 Continuous Positive Airway Pressure
				8 Intermittent Positive Airway Pressure
				9 Continuous Negative Airway Pressure
				B Intermittent Negative Airway Pressure
				C Supersaturated
				D Impeller Pump
				Z No Qualifier

6: Extracorporeal Therapies
A: Physiological Systems

Operation-Character 3	Body System-Character 4	Duration-Character 5	Qualifier-Character 6	Qualifier-Character 7
0 Atmospheric Control	**0** Skin	**0** Single	**B** Donor Organ	**0** Erythrocytes
1 Decompression	**1** Urinary	**1** Multiple	**Z** No Qualifier	**1** Leukocytes
2 Electromagnetic Therapy	**2** Central Nervous			**2** Platelets
3 Hyperthermia	**3** Musculoskeletal			**3** Plasma
4 Hypothermia	**5** Circulatory			**4** Head and Neck Vessels
5 Pheresis	**B** Respiratory System			**5** Heart
6 Phototherapy	**F** Hepatobiliary System and Pancreas			**6** Peripheral Vessels
7 Ultrasound Therapy	**T** Urinary System			**7** Other Vessels
8 Ultraviolet Light Therapy	**Z** None			**T** Stem Cells, Cord Blood
9 Shock Wave Therapy				**V** Stem Cells, Hematopoietic
B Perfusion				**Z** No Qualifier

7: Osteopathic
W: Anatomical Regions

Operation-Character 3	Body Region-Character 4	Approach-Character 5	Method-Character 6	Qualifier-Character 7
0 Treatment	**0** Head	**X** External	**0** Articulatory-Raising	**Z** None
	1 Cervical		**1** Fascial Release	
	2 Thoracic		**2** General Mobilization	
	3 Lumbar		**3** High Velocity-Low Amplitude	
	4 Sacrum		**4** Indirect	
	5 Pelvis		**5** Low Velocity-High Amplitude	
	6 Lower Extremities		**6** Lymphatic Pump	
	7 Upper Extremities		**7** Muscle Energy-Isometric	
	8 Rib Cage		**8** Muscle Energy-Isotonic	
	9 Abdomen		**9** Other Method	

8: Other Procedures
C: Indwelling Device

Operation-Character 3	Body Region-Character 4	Approach-Character 5	Method-Character 6	Qualifier-Character 7
0 Other Procedures	1 Nervous System	X External	6 Collection	J Cerebrospinal Fluid
	2 Circulatory System			K Blood
				L Other Fluid

8: Other Procedures
E: Physiological Systems and Anatomical Regions

Operation-Character 3	Body Region-Character 4	Approach-Character 5	Method-Character 6	Qualifier-Character 7
0 Other Procedures	1 Nervous System	0 Open	0 Acupuncture	0 Anesthesia
	2 Circulatory System	3 Percutaneous	1 Therapeutic Massage	1 In Vitro Fertilization
	9 Head and Neck Region	7 Via Natural or Artificial Opening	6 Collection	2 Breast Milk
	H Integumentary System and Breast	8 Via Natural or Artificial Opening Endoscopic	B Computer Assisted Procedure	3 Sperm
	K Musculoskeletal System	X External	C Robotic Assisted Procedure	4 Yoga Therapy
	U Female Reproductive System		D Near Infrared Spectroscopy	5 Meditation
	V Male Reproductive System		Y Other Method	6 Isolation
	W Trunk Region			7 Examination
	X Upper Extremity			8 Suture Removal
	Y Lower Extremity			9 Piercing
	Z None			C Prostate
				D Rectum
				F With Fluoroscopy
				G With Computerized Tomography
				H With Magnetic Resonance Imaging
				Z No Qualifier

9: Chiropractic
W: Anatomical Regions

Operation-Character 3	Body Region-Character 4	Approach-Character 5	Method-Character 6	Qualifier-Character 7
B Manipulation	**0** Head	**X** External	**B** Non-Manual	**Z** None
	1 Cervical		**C** Indirect Visceral	
	2 Thoracic		**D** Extra-Articular	
	3 Lumbar		**F** Direct Visceral	
	4 Sacrum		**G** Long Lever Specific Contact	
	5 Pelvis		**H** Short Lever Specific Contact	
	6 Lower Extremities		**J** Long and Short Lever Specific Contact	
	7 Upper Extremities		**K** Mechanically Assisted	
	8 Rib Cage		**L** Other Method	
	9 Abdomen			

B: Imaging
0: Central Nervous System

Type-Character 3	Body Part-Character 4	Contrast-Character 5	Qualifier-Character 6	Qualifier-Character 7
0 Plain Radiography	**0** Brain	**0** High Osmolar	**0** Unenhanced and Enhanced	**Z** None
1 Fluoroscopy	**7** Cisterna	**1** Low Osmolar	**Z** None	
2 Computerized Tomography (CT Scan)	**8** Cerebral Ventricle(s)	**Y** Other Contrast		
3 Magnetic Resonance Imaging (MRI)	**9** Sella Turcica/Pituitary Gland	**Z** None		
4 Ultrasonography	**B** Spinal Cord			
	C Acoustic Nerves			

B: Imaging
2: Heart

Type-Character 3	Body Part-Character 4	Contrast-Character 5	Qualifier-Character 6	Qualifier-Character 7
0 Plain Radiography	**0** Coronary Artery, Single	**0** High Osmolar	**0** Unenhanced and Enhanced	**0** Intraoperative
1 Fluoroscopy	**1** Coronary Arteries, Multiple	**1** Low Osmolar	**1** Laser	**3** Intravascular
2 Computerized Tomography (CT Scan)	**2** Coronary Artery Bypass Graft, Single	**Y** Other Contrast	**2** Intravascular Optical Coherence	**4** Transesophageal
3 Magnetic Resonance Imaging (MRI)	**3** Coronary Artery Bypass Grafts, Multiple	**Z** None	**Z** None	**Z** None
4 Ultrasonography	**4** Heart, Right			
	5 Heart, Left			
	6 Heart, Right and Left			
	7 Internal Mammary Bypass Graft, Right			
	8 Internal Mammary Bypass Graft, Left			
	B Heart with Aorta			
	C Pericardium			
	D Pediatric Heart			
	F Bypass Graft, Other			

B: Imaging
3: Upper Arteries

Type-Character 3	Body Part-Character 4	Contrast-Character 5	Qualifier-Character 6	Qualifier-Character 7
0 Plain Radiography	**0** Thoracic Aorta	**0** High Osmolar	**0** Unenhanced and Enhanced	**0** Intraoperative
1 Fluoroscopy	**1** Brachiocephalic-Subclavian Artery, Right	**1** Low Osmolar	**1** Laser	**3** Intravascular
2 Computerized Tomography (CT Scan)	**2** Subclavian Artery, Left	**Y** Other Contrast	**2** Intravascular Optical Coherence	**Z** None
3 Magnetic Resonance Imaging (MRI)	**3** Common Carotid Artery, Right	**Z** None	**Z** None	
4 Ultrasonography	**4** Common Carotid Artery, Left			
	5 Common Carotid Arteries, Bilateral			
	6 Internal Carotid Artery, Right			
	7 Internal Carotid Artery, Left			
	8 Internal Carotid Arteries, Bilateral			
	9 External Carotid Artery, Right			
	B External Carotid Artery, Left			
	C External Carotid Arteries, Bilateral			
	D Vertebral Artery, Right			
	F Vertebral Artery, Left			
	G Vertebral Arteries, Bilateral			
	H Upper Extremity Arteries, Right			
	J Upper Extremity Arteries, Left			
	K Upper Extremity Arteries, Bilateral			
	L Intercostal and Bronchial Arteries			
	M Spinal Arteries			
	N Upper Arteries, Other			
	P Thoraco-Abdominal Aorta			
	Q Cervico-Cerebral Arch			
	R Intracranial Arteries			
	S Pulmonary Artery, Right			
	T Pulmonary Artery, Left			
	U Pulmonary Trunk			
	V Ophthalmic Arteries			

B: Imaging
4: Lower Arteries

Type-Character 3	Body Part-Character 4	Contrast-Character 5	Qualifier-Character 6	Qualifier-Character 7
0 Plain Radiography	**0** Abdominal Aorta	**0** High Osmolar	**0** Unenhanced and Enhanced	**0** Intraoperative
1 Fluoroscopy	**1** Celiac Artery	**1** Low Osmolar	**1** Laser	**3** Intravascular
2 Computerized Tomography (CT Scan)	**2** Hepatic Artery	**Y** Other Contrast	**2** Intravascular Optical Coherence	**Z** None
3 Magnetic Resonance Imaging (MRI)	**3** Splenic Arteries	**Z** None	**Z** None	
4 Ultrasonography	**4** Superior Mesenteric Artery			
	5 Inferior Mesenteric Artery			
	6 Renal Artery, Right			
	7 Renal Artery, Left			
	8 Renal Arteries, Bilateral			
	9 Lumbar Arteries			
	B Intra-Abdominal Arteries, Other			
	C Pelvic Arteries			
	D Aorta and Bilateral Lower Extremity Arteries			
	F Lower Extremity Arteries, Right			
	G Lower Extremity Arteries, Left			
	H Lower Extremity Arteries, Bilateral			
	J Lower Arteries, Other			
	K Celiac and Mesenteric Arteries			
	L Femoral Artery			
	M Renal Artery Transplant			
	N Penile Arteries			

B: Imaging
5: Veins

Type-Character 3	Body Part-Character 4	Contrast-Character 5	Qualifier-Character 6	Qualifier-Character 7
0 Plain Radiography	**0** Epidural Veins	**0** High Osmolar	**0** Unenhanced and Enhanced	**3** Intravascular
1 Fluoroscopy	**1** Cerebral and Cerebellar Veins	**1** Low Osmolar	**2** Intravascular Optical Coherence	**A** Guidance
2 Computerized Tomography (CT Scan)	**2** Intracranial Sinuses	**Y** Other Contrast	**Z** None	**Z** None
3 Magnetic Resonance Imaging (MRI)	**3** Jugular Veins, Right	**Z** None		
4 Ultrasonography	**4** Jugular Veins, Left			
	5 Jugular Veins, Bilateral			
	6 Subclavian Vein, Right			
	7 Subclavian Vein, Left			
	8 Superior Vena Cava			
	9 Inferior Vena Cava			
	B Lower Extremity Veins, Right			
	C Lower Extremity Veins, Left			
	D Lower Extremity Veins, Bilateral			
	F Pelvic (Iliac) Veins, Right			
	G Pelvic (Iliac) Veins, Left			
	H Pelvic (Iliac) Veins, Bilateral			
	J Renal Vein, Right			
	K Renal Vein, Left			
	L Renal Veins, Bilateral			
	M Upper Extremity Veins, Right			
	N Upper Extremity Veins, Left			
	P Upper Extremity Veins, Bilateral			
	Q Pulmonary Vein, Right			
	R Pulmonary Vein, Left			
	S Pulmonary Veins, Bilateral			
	T Portal and Splanchnic Veins			
	V Veins, Other			
	W Dialysis Shunt/Fistula			

B: Imaging
7: Lymphatic System

Type-Character 3	Body Part-Character 4	Contrast-Character 5	Qualifier-Character 6	Qualifier-Character 7
0 Plain Radiography	**0** Abdominal/Retroperitoneal Lymphatics, Unilateral	**0** High Osmolar	**Z** None	**Z** None
	1 Abdominal/Retroperitoneal Lymphatics, Bilateral	**1** Low Osmolar		
	4 Lymphatics, Head and Neck	**Y** Other Contrast		
	5 Upper Extremity Lymphatics, Right			
	6 Upper Extremity Lymphatics, Left			
	7 Upper Extremity Lymphatics, Bilateral			
	8 Lower Extremity Lymphatics, Right			
	9 Lower Extremity Lymphatics, Left			
	B Lower Extremity Lymphatics, Bilateral			
	C Lymphatics, Pelvic			

B: Imaging
8: Eye

Type-Character 3	Body Part-Character 4	Contrast-Character 5	Qualifier-Character 6	Qualifier-Character 7
0 Plain Radiography	**0** Lacrimal Duct, Right	**0** High Osmolar	**0** Unenhanced and Enhanced	**Z** None
2 Computerized Tomography (CT Scan)	**1** Lacrimal Duct, Left	**1** Low Osmolar	**Z** None	
3 Magnetic Resonance Imaging (MRI)	**2** Lacrimal Ducts, Bilateral	**Y** Other Contrast		
4 Ultrasonography	**3** Optic Foramina, Right	**Z** None		
	4 Optic Foramina, Left			
	5 Eye, Right			
	6 Eye, Left			
	7 Eyes, Bilateral			

B: Imaging
9: Ear, Nose, Mouth and Throat

Type-Character 3	Body Part-Character 4	Contrast-Character 5	Qualifier-Character 6	Qualifier-Character 7
0 Plain Radiography	**0** Ear	**0** High Osmolar	**0** Unenhanced and Enhanced	**Z** None
1 Fluoroscopy	**2** Paranasal Sinuses	**1** Low Osmolar	**Z** None	
2 Computerized Tomography (CT Scan)	**4** Parotid Gland, Right	**Y** Other Contrast		
3 Magnetic Resonance Imaging (MRI)	**5** Parotid Gland, Left	**Z** None		
	6 Parotid Glands, Bilateral			
	7 Submandibular Gland, Right			
	8 Submandibular Gland, Left			
	9 Submandibular Glands, Bilateral			
	B Salivary Gland, Right			
	C Salivary Gland, Left			
	D Salivary Glands, Bilateral			
	F Nasopharynx/Oropharynx			
	G Pharynx and Epiglottis			
	H Mastoids			
	J Larynx			

B: Imaging
B: Respiratory System

Type-Character 3	Body Part-Character 4	Contrast-Character 5	Qualifier-Character 6	Qualifier-Character 7
0 Plain Radiography	**2** Lung, Right	**0** High Osmolar	**0** Unenhanced and Enhanced	**Z** None
1 Fluoroscopy	**3** Lung, Left	**1** Low Osmolar	**Z** None	
2 Computerized Tomography (CT Scan)	**4** Lungs, Bilateral	**Y** Other Contrast		
3 Magnetic Resonance Imaging (MRI)	**6** Diaphragm	**Z** None		
4 Ultrasonography	**7** Tracheobronchial Tree, Right			
	8 Tracheobronchial Tree, Left			
	9 Tracheobronchial Trees, Bilateral			
	B Pleura			
	C Mediastinum			
	D Upper Airways			
	F Trachea/Airways			
	G Lung Apices			

B: Imaging
D: Gastrointestinal System

Type-Character 3	Body Part-Character 4	Contrast-Character 5	Qualifier-Character 6	Qualifier-Character 7
1 Fluoroscopy	**1** Esophagus	**0** High Osmolar	**0** Unenhanced and Enhanced	**Z** None
2 Computerized Tomography (CT Scan)	**2** Stomach	**1** Low Osmolar	**Z** None	
4 Ultrasonography	**3** Small Bowel	**Y** Other Contrast		
	4 Colon	**Z** None		
	5 Upper GI			
	6 Upper GI and Small Bowel			
	7 Gastrointestinal Tract			
	8 Appendix			
	9 Duodenum			
	B Mouth/Oropharynx			
	C Rectum			

B: Imaging
F: Hepatobiliary System and Pancreas

Type-Character 3	Body Part-Character 4	Contrast-Character 5	Qualifier-Character 6	Qualifier-Character 7
0 Plain Radiography	**0** Bile Ducts	**0** High Osmolar	**0** Unenhanced and Enhanced	**Z** None
1 Fluoroscopy	**1** Biliary and Pancreatic Ducts	**1** Low Osmolar	**Z** None	
2 Computerized Tomography (CT Scan)	**2** Gallbladder	**Y** Other Contrast		
3 Magnetic Resonance Imaging (MRI)	**3** Gallbladder and Bile Ducts	**Z** None		
4 Ultrasonography	**4** Gallbladder, Bile Ducts and Pancreatic Ducts			
	5 Liver			
	6 Liver and Spleen			
	7 Pancreas			
	8 Pancreatic Ducts			
	C Hepatobiliary System, All			

B: Imaging
G: Endocrine System

Type-Character 3	Body Part-Character 4	Contrast-Character 5	Qualifier-Character 6	Qualifier-Character 7
2 Computerized Tomography (CT Scan)	**0** Adrenal Gland, Right	**0** High Osmolar	**0** Unenhanced and Enhanced	**Z** None
3 Magnetic Resonance Imaging (MRI)	**1** Adrenal Gland, Left	**1** Low Osmolar	**Z** None	
4 Ultrasonography	**2** Adrenal Glands, Bilateral	**Y** Other Contrast		
	3 Parathyroid Glands	**Z** None		
	4 Thyroid Gland			

B: Imaging
H: Skin, Subcutaneous Tissue and Breast

Type-Character 3	Body Part-Character 4	Contrast-Character 5	Qualifier-Character 6	Qualifier-Character 7
0 Plain Radiography	**0** Breast, Right	**0** High Osmolar	**0** Unenhanced and Enhanced	**Z** None
3 Magnetic Resonance Imaging (MRI)	**1** Breast, Left	**1** Low Osmolar	**Z** None	
4 Ultrasonography	**2** Breasts, Bilateral	**Y** Other Contrast		
	3 Single Mammary Duct, Right	**Z** None		
	4 Single Mammary Duct, Left			
	5 Multiple Mammary Ducts, Right			
	6 Multiple Mammary Ducts, Left			
	7 Extremity, Upper			
	8 Extremity, Lower			
	9 Abdominal Wall			
	B Chest Wall			
	C Head and Neck			
	D Subcutaneous Tissue, Head/Neck			
	F Subcutaneous Tissue, Upper Extremity			
	G Subcutaneous Tissue, Thorax			
	H Subcutaneous Tissue, Abdomen and Pelvis			
	J Subcutaneous Tissue, Lower Extremity			

B: Imaging
L: Connective Tissue

Type-Character 3	Body Part-Character 4	Contrast-Character 5	Qualifier-Character 6	Qualifier-Character 7
3 Magnetic Resonance Imaging (MRI)	**0** Connective Tissue, Upper Extremity	**Y** Other Contrast	**0** Unenhanced and Enhanced	**Z** None
4 Ultrasonography	**1** Connective Tissue, Lower Extremity	**Z** None	**Z** None	
	2 Tendons, Upper Extremity			
	3 Tendons, Lower Extremity			

B: Imaging
N: Skull and Facial Bones

Type-Character 3	Body Part-Character 4	Contrast-Character 5	Qualifier-Character 6	Qualifier-Character 7
0 Plain Radiography	**0** Skull	**0** High Osmolar	**Z** None	**Z** None
1 Fluoroscopy	**1** Orbit, Right	**1** Low Osmolar		
2 Computerized Tomography (CT Scan)	**2** Orbit, Left	**Y** Other Contrast		
3 Magnetic Resonance Imaging (MRI)	**3** Orbits, Bilateral	**Z** None		
	4 Nasal Bones			
	5 Facial Bones			
	6 Mandible			
	7 Temporomandibular Joint, Right			
	8 Temporomandibular Joint, Left			
	9 Temporomandibular Joints, Bilateral			
	B Zygomatic Arch, Right			
	C Zygomatic Arch, Left			
	D Zygomatic Arches, Bilateral			
	F Temporal Bones			
	G Tooth, Single			
	H Teeth, Multiple			
	J Teeth, All			

B: Imaging
P: Non-Axial Upper Bones

Type-Character 3	Body Part-Character 4	Contrast-Character 5	Qualifier-Character 6	Qualifier-Character 7
0 Plain Radiography	**0** Sternoclavicular Joint, Right	**0** High Osmolar	**0** Unenhanced and Enhanced	**1** Densitometry
1 Fluoroscopy	**1** Sternoclavicular Joint, Left	**1** Low Osmolar	**Z** None	**Z** None
2 Computerized Tomography (CT Scan)	**2** Sternoclavicular Joints, Bilateral	**Y** Other Contrast		
3 Magnetic Resonance Imaging (MRI)	**3** Acromioclavicular Joints, Bilateral	**Z** None		
4 Ultrasonography	**4** Clavicle, Right			
	5 Clavicle, Left			
	6 Scapula, Right			
	7 Scapula, Left			
	8 Shoulder, Right			
	9 Shoulder, Left			
	A Humerus, Right			
	B Humerus, Left			
	C Hand/Finger Joint, Right			
	D Hand/Finger Joint, Left			
	E Upper Arm, Right			
	F Upper Arm, Left			
	G Elbow, Right			
	H Elbow, Left			
	J Forearm, Right			
	K Forearm, Left			
	L Wrist, Right			
	M Wrist, Left			
	N Hand, Right			
	P Hand, Left			
	Q Hands and Wrists, Bilateral			
	R Finger(s), Right			
	S Finger(s), Left			
	T Upper Extremity, Right			
	U Upper Extremity, Left			
	V Upper Extremities, Bilateral			
	W Thorax			
	X Ribs, Right			
	Y Ribs, Left			

B: Imaging
Q: Non-Axial Lower Bones

Type-Character 3	Body Part-Character 4	Contrast-Character 5	Qualifier-Character 6	Qualifier-Character 7
0 Plain Radiography	**0** Hip, Right	**0** High Osmolar	**0** Unenhanced and Enhanced	**1** Densitometry
1 Fluoroscopy	**1** Hip, Left	**1** Low Osmolar	**Z** None	**Z** None
2 Computerized Tomography (CT Scan)	**2** Hips, Bilateral	**Y** Other Contrast		
3 Magnetic Resonance Imaging (MRI)	**3** Femur, Right	**Z** None		
4 Ultrasonography	**4** Femur, Left			
	7 Knee, Right			
	8 Knee, Left			
	9 Knees, Bilateral			
	B Tibia/Fibula, Right			
	C Tibia/Fibula, Left			
	D Lower Leg, Right			
	F Lower Leg, Left			
	G Ankle, Right			
	H Ankle, Left			
	J Calcaneus, Right			
	K Calcaneus, Left			
	L Foot, Right			
	M Foot, Left			
	P Toe(s), Right			
	Q Toe(s), Left			
	R Lower Extremity, Right			
	S Lower Extremity, Left			
	V Patella, Right			
	W Patella, Left			
	X Foot/Toe Joint, Right			
	Y Foot/Toe Joint, Left			

B: Imaging
R: Axial Skeleton, Except Skull and Facial Bones

Type-Character 3	Body Part-Character 4	Contrast-Character 5	Qualifier-Character 6	Qualifier-Character 7
0 Plain Radiography	**0** Cervical Spine	**0** High Osmolar	**0** Unenhanced and Enhanced	**1** Densitometry
1 Fluoroscopy	**1** Cervical Disc(s)	**1** Low Osmolar	**Z** None	**Z** None
2 Computerized Tomography (CT Scan)	**2** Thoracic Disc(s)	**Y** Other Contrast		
3 Magnetic Resonance Imaging (MRI)	**3** Lumbar Disc(s)	**Z** None		
4 Ultrasonography	**4** Cervical Facet Joint(s)			
	5 Thoracic Facet Joint(s)			
	6 Lumbar Facet Joint(s)			
	7 Thoracic Spine			
	8 Thoracolumbar Joint			
	9 Lumbar Spine			
	B Lumbosacral Joint			
	C Pelvis			
	D Sacroiliac Joints			
	F Sacrum and Coccyx			
	G Whole Spine			
	H Sternum			

B: Imaging
T: Urinary System

Type-Character 3	Body Part-Character 4	Contrast-Character 5	Qualifier-Character 6	Qualifier-Character 7
0 Plain Radiography	**0** Bladder	**0** High Osmolar	**0** Unenhanced and Enhanced	**Z** None
1 Fluoroscopy	**1** Kidney, Right	**1** Low Osmolar	**Z** None	
2 Computerized Tomography (CT Scan)	**2** Kidney, Left	**Y** Other Contrast		
3 Magnetic Resonance Imaging (MRI)	**3** Kidneys, Bilateral	**Z** None		
4 Ultrasonography	**4** Kidneys, Ureters and Bladder			
	5 Urethra			
	6 Ureter, Right			
	7 Ureter, Left			
	8 Ureters, Bilateral			
	9 Kidney Transplant			
	B Bladder and Urethra			
	C Ileal Diversion Loop			
	D Kidney, Ureter and Bladder, Right			
	F Kidney, Ureter and Bladder, Left			
	G Ileal Loop, Ureters and Kidneys			
	J Kidneys and Bladder			

B: Imaging
U: Female Reproductive System

Type-Character 3	Body Part-Character 4	Contrast-Character 5	Qualifier-Character 6	Qualifier-Character 7
0 Plain Radiography	**0** Fallopian Tube, Right	**0** High Osmolar	**0** Unenhanced and Enhanced	**Z** None
1 Fluoroscopy	**1** Fallopian Tube, Left	**1** Low Osmolar	**Z** None	
3 Magnetic Resonance Imaging (MRI)	**2** Fallopian Tubes, Bilateral	**Y** Other Contrast		
4 Ultrasonography	**3** Ovary, Right	**Z** None		
	4 Ovary, Left			
	5 Ovaries, Bilateral			
	6 Uterus			
	8 Uterus and Fallopian Tubes			
	9 Vagina			
	B Pregnant Uterus			
	C Uterus and Ovaries			

B: Imaging
V: Male Reproductive System

Type-Character 3	Body Part-Character 4	Contrast-Character 5	Qualifier-Character 6	Qualifier-Character 7
0 Plain Radiography	**0** Corpora Cavernosa	**0** High Osmolar	**0** Unenhanced and Enhanced	**Z** None
1 Fluoroscopy	**1** Epididymis, Right	**1** Low Osmolar	**Z** None	
2 Computerized Tomography (CT Scan)	**2** Epididymis, Left	**Y** Other Contrast		
3 Magnetic Resonance Imaging (MRI)	**3** Prostate	**Z** None		
4 Ultrasonography	**4** Scrotum			
	5 Testicle, Right			
	6 Testicle, Left			
	7 Testicles, Bilateral			
	8 Vasa Vasorum			
	9 Prostate and Seminal Vesicles			
	B Penis			

B: Imaging
W: Anatomical Regions

Type-Character 3	Body Part-Character 4	Contrast-Character 5	Qualifier-Character 6	Qualifier-Character 7
0 Plain Radiography	**0** Abdomen	**0** High Osmolar	**0** Unenhanced and Enhanced	**Z** None
1 Fluoroscopy	**1** Abdomen and Pelvis	**1** Low Osmolar	**Z** None	
2 Computerized Tomography (CT Scan)	**3** Chest	**Y** Other Contrast		
3 Magnetic Resonance Imaging (MRI)	**4** Chest and Abdomen	**Z** None		
4 Ultrasonography	**5** Chest, Abdomen and Pelvis			
	8 Head			
	9 Head and Neck			
	B Long Bones, All			
	C Lower Extremity			
	F Neck			
	G Pelvic Region			
	H Retroperitoneum			
	J Upper Extremity			
	K Whole Body			
	L Whole Skeleton			
	M Whole Body, Infant			
	P Brachial Plexus			

B: Imaging
Y: Fetus and Obstetrical

Type-Character 3	Body Part-Character 4	Contrast-Character 5	Qualifier-Character 6	Qualifier-Character 7
3 Magnetic Resonance Imaging (MRI)	0 Fetal Head	Y Other Contrast	0 Unenhanced and Enhanced	Z None
4 Ultrasonography	1 Fetal Heart	Z None	Z None	
	2 Fetal Thorax			
	3 Fetal Abdomen			
	4 Fetal Spine			
	5 Fetal Extremities			
	6 Whole Fetus			
	7 Fetal Umbilical Cord			
	8 Placenta			
	9 First Trimester, Single Fetus			
	B First Trimester, Multiple Gestation			
	C Second Trimester, Single Fetus			
	D Second Trimester, Multiple Gestation			
	F Third Trimester, Single Fetus			
	G Third Trimester, Multiple Gestation			

C: Nuclear Medicine
0: Central Nervous System

Type-Character 3	Body Part-Character 4	Radionuclide-Character 5	Qualifier-Character 6	Qualifier-Character 7
1 Planar Nuclear Medicine Imaging	0 Brain	1 Technetium 99m (Tc-99m)	Z None	Z None
2 Tomographic (Tomo) Nuclear Medicine Imaging	5 Cerebrospinal Fluid	B Carbon 11 (C-11)		
3 Positron Emission Tomographic (PET) Imaging	Y Central Nervous System	D Indium 111 (In-111)		
5 Nonimaging Nuclear Medicine Probe		F Iodine 123 (I-123)		
		K Fluorine 18 (F-18)		
		M Oxygen 15 (O-15)		
		S Thallium 201 (Tl-201)		
		V Xenon 133 (Xe-133)		
		Y Other Radionuclide		

C: Nuclear Medicine
2: Heart

Type-Character 3	Body Part-Character 4	Radionuclide-Character 5	Qualifier-Character 6	Qualifier-Character 7
1 Planar Nuclear Medicine Imaging	6 Heart, Right and Left	1 Technetium 99m (Tc-99m)	Z None	Z None
2 Tomographic (Tomo) Nuclear Medicine Imaging	G Myocardium	D Indium 111 (In-111)		
3 Positron Emission Tomographic (PET) Imaging	Y Heart	K Fluorine 18 (F-18)		
5 Nonimaging Nuclear Medicine Probe		M Oxygen 15 (O-15)		
		Q Rubidium 82 (Rb-82)		
		R Nitrogen 13 (N-13)		
		S Thallium 201 (Tl-201)		
		Y Other Radionuclide		
		Z None		

C: Nuclear Medicine
5: Veins

Type-Character 3	Body Part-Character 4	Radionuclide-Character 5	Qualifier-Character 6	Qualifier-Character 7
1 Planar Nuclear Medicine Imaging	**B** Lower Extremity Veins, Right	**1** Technetium 99m (Tc-99m)	**Z** None	**Z** None
	C Lower Extremity Veins, Left	**Y** Other Radionuclide		
	D Lower Extremity Veins, Bilateral			
	N Upper Extremity Veins, Right			
	P Upper Extremity Veins, Left			
	Q Upper Extremity Veins, Bilateral			
	R Central Veins			
	Y Veins			

C: Nuclear Medicine
7: Lymphatic and Hematologic System

Type-Character 3	Body Part-Character 4	Radionuclide-Character 5	Qualifier-Character 6	Qualifier-Character 7
1 Planar Nuclear Medicine Imaging	**0** Bone Marrow	**1** Technetium 99m (Tc-99m)	**Z** None	**Z** None
2 Tomographic (Tomo) Nuclear Medicine Imaging	**2** Spleen	**7** Cobalt 58 (Co-58)		
5 Nonimaging Nuclear Medicine Probe	**3** Blood	**C** Cobalt 57 (Co-57)		
6 Nonimaging Nuclear Medicine Assay	**5** Lymphatics, Head and Neck	**D** Indium 111 (In-111)		
	D Lymphatics, Pelvic	**H** Iodine 125 (I-125)		
	J Lymphatics, Head	**W** Chromium (Cr-51)		
	K Lymphatics, Neck	**Y** Other Radionuclide		
	L Lymphatics, Upper Chest			
	M Lymphatics, Trunk			
	N Lymphatics, Upper Extremity			
	P Lymphatics, Lower Extremity			
	Y Lymphatic and Hematologic System			

C: Nuclear Medicine
8: Eye

Type-Character 3	Body Part-Character 4	Radionuclide-Character 5	Qualifier-Character 6	Qualifier-Character 7
1 Planar Nuclear Medicine Imaging	**9** Lacrimal Ducts, Bilateral	**1** Technetium 99m (Tc-99m)	**Z** None	**Z** None
	Y Eye	**Y** Other Radionuclide		

C: Nuclear Medicine
9: Ear, Nose, Mouth and Throat

Type-Character 3	Body Part-Character 4	Radionuclide-Character 5	Qualifier-Character 6	Qualifier-Character 7
1 Planar Nuclear Medicine Imaging	**B** Salivary Glands, Bilateral	**1** Technetium 99m (Tc-99m)	**Z** None	**Z** None
	Y Ear, Nose, Mouth and Throat	**Y** Other Radionuclide		

C: Nuclear Medicine
B: Respiratory System

Type-Character 3	Body Part-Character 4	Radionuclide-Character 5	Qualifier-Character 6	Qualifier-Character 7
1 Planar Nuclear Medicine Imaging	**2** Lungs and Bronchi	**1** Technetium 99m (Tc-99m)	**Z** None	**Z** None
2 Tomographic (Tomo) Nuclear Medicine Imaging	**Y** Respiratory System	**9** Krypton (Kr-81m)		
3 Positron Emission Tomographic (PET) Imaging		**K** Fluorine 18 (F-18)		
		T Xenon 127 (Xe-127)		
		V Xenon 133 (Xe-133)		
		Y Other Radionuclide		

C: Nuclear Medicine
D: Gastrointestinal System

Type-Character 3	Body Part-Character 4	Radionuclide-Character 5	Qualifier-Character 6	Qualifier-Character 7
1 Planar Nuclear Medicine Imaging	**5** Upper Gastrointestinal Tract	**1** Technetium 99m (Tc-99m)	**Z** None	**Z** None
2 Tomographic (Tomo) Nuclear Medicine Imaging	**7** Gastrointestinal Tract	**D** Indium 111 (In-111)		
	Y Digestive System	**Y** Other Radionuclide		

C: Nuclear Medicine
F: Hepatobiliary System and Pancreas

Type-Character 3	Body Part-Character 4	Radionuclide-Character 5	Qualifier-Character 6	Qualifier-Character 7
1 Planar Nuclear Medicine Imaging	**4** Gallbladder	**1** Technetium 99m (Tc-99m)	**Z** None	**Z** None
2 Tomographic (Tomo) Nuclear Medicine Imaging	**5** Liver	**Y** Other Radionuclide		
	6 Liver and Spleen			
	C Hepatobiliary System, All			
	Y Hepatobiliary System and Pancreas			

C: Nuclear Medicine
G: Endocrine System

Type-Character 3	Body Part-Character 4	Radionuclide-Character 5	Qualifier-Character 6	Qualifier-Character 7
1 Planar Nuclear Medicine Imaging	**1** Parathyroid Glands	**1** Technetium 99m (Tc-99m)	**Z** None	**Z** None
2 Tomographic (Tomo) Nuclear Medicine Imaging	**2** Thyroid Gland	**F** Iodine 123 (I-123)		
4 Nonimaging Nuclear Medicine Uptake	**4** Adrenal Glands, Bilateral	**G** Iodine 131 (I-131)		
	Y Endocrine System	**S** Thallium 201 (Tl-201)		
		Y Other Radionuclide		

C: Nuclear Medicine
H: Skin, Subcutaneous Tissue and Breast

Type-Character 3	Body Part-Character 4	Radionuclide-Character 5	Qualifier-Character 6	Qualifier-Character 7
1 Planar Nuclear Medicine Imaging	**0** Breast, Right	**1** Technetium 99m (Tc-99m)	**Z** None	**Z** None
2 Tomographic (Tomo) Nuclear Medicine Imaging	**1** Breast, Left	**S** Thallium 201 (Tl-201)		
	2 Breasts, Bilateral	**Y** Other Radionuclide		
	Y Skin, Subcutaneous Tissue and Breast			

C: Nuclear Medicine
P: Musculoskeletal System

Type-Character 3	Body Part-Character 4	Radionuclide-Character 5	Qualifier-Character 6	Qualifier-Character 7
1 Planar Nuclear Medicine Imaging	**1** Skull	**1** Technetium 99m (Tc-99m)	**Z** None	**Z** None
2 Tomographic (Tomo) Nuclear Medicine Imaging	**2** Cervical Spine	**Y** Other Radionuclide		
5 Nonimaging Nuclear Medicine Probe	**3** Skull and Cervical Spine	**Z** None		
	4 Thorax			
	5 Spine			
	6 Pelvis			
	7 Spine and Pelvis			
	8 Upper Extremity, Right			
	9 Upper Extremity, Left			
	B Upper Extremities, Bilateral			
	C Lower Extremity, Right			
	D Lower Extremity, Left			
	F Lower Extremities, Bilateral			
	G Thoracic Spine			
	H Lumbar Spine			
	J Thoracolumbar Spine			
	N Upper Extremities			
	P Lower Extremities			
	Y Musculoskeletal System, Other			
	Z Musculoskeletal System, All			

C: Nuclear Medicine
T: Urinary System

Type-Character 3	Body Part-Character 4	Radionuclide-Character 5	Qualifier-Character 6	Qualifier-Character 7
1 Planar Nuclear Medicine Imaging	**3** Kidneys, Ureters and Bladder	**1** Technetium 99m (Tc-99m)	**Z** None	**Z** None
2 Tomographic (Tomo) Nuclear Medicine Imaging	**H** Bladder and Ureters	**F** Iodine 123 (I-123)		
6 Nonimaging Nuclear Medicine Assay	**Y** Urinary System	**G** Iodine 131 (I-131)		
		H Iodine 125 (I-125)		
		Y Other Radionuclide		

C: Nuclear Medicine
V: Male Reproductive System

Type-Character 3	Body Part-Character 4	Radionuclide-Character 5	Qualifier-Character 6	Qualifier-Character 7
1 Planar Nuclear Medicine Imaging	**9** Testicles, Bilateral	**1** Technetium 99m (Tc-99m)	**Z** None	**Z** None
	Y Male Reproductive System	**Y** Other Radionuclide		

C: Nuclear Medicine
W: Anatomical Regions

Type-Character 3	Body Part-Character 4	Radionuclide-Character 5	Qualifier-Character 6	Qualifier-Character 7
1 Planar Nuclear Medicine Imaging	**0** Abdomen	**1** Technetium 99m (Tc-99m)	**Z** None	**Z** None
2 Tomographic (Tomo) Nuclear Medicine Imaging	**1** Abdomen and Pelvis	**8** Samarium 153 (Sm-153)		
3 Positron Emission Tomographic (PET) Imaging	**3** Chest	**D** Indium 111 (In-111)		
5 Nonimaging Nuclear Medicine Probe	**4** Chest and Abdomen	**F** Iodine 123 (I-123)		
7 Systemic Nuclear Medicine Therapy	**6** Chest and Neck	**G** Iodine 131 (I-131)		
	B Head and Neck	**K** Fluorine 18 (F-18)		
	D Lower Extremity	**L** Gallium 67 (Ga-67)		
	G Thyroid	**N** Phosphorus 32 (P-32)		
	J Pelvic Region	**P** Strontium 89 (Sr-89)		
	M Upper Extremity	**S** Thallium 201 (Tl-201)		
	N Whole Body	**Y** Other Radionuclide		
	Y Anatomical Regions, Multiple	**Z** None		
	Z Anatomical Region, Other			

D: Radiation Therapy
0: Central and Peripheral Nervous System

Modality-Character 3	Treatment Site -Character 4	Modality Qualifier-Character 5	Isotope -Character 6	Qualifier-Character 7
0 Beam Radiation	**0** Brain	**0** Photons <1 MeV	**7** Cesium 137 (Cs-137)	**0** Intraoperative
1 Brachytherapy	**1** Brain Stem	**1** Photons 1 - 10 MeV	**8** Iridium 192 (Ir-192)	**Z** None
2 Stereotactic Radiosurgery	**6** Spinal Cord	**2** Photons >10 MeV	**9** Iodine 125 (I-125)	
Y Other Radiation	**7** Peripheral Nerve	**3** Electrons	**B** Palladium 103 (Pd-103)	
		4 Heavy Particles (Protons,Ions)	**C** Californium 252 (Cf-252)	
		5 Neutrons	**Y** Other Isotope	
		6 Neutron Capture	**Z** None	
		7 Contact Radiation		
		8 Hyperthermia		
		9 High Dose Rate (HDR)		
		B Low Dose Rate (LDR)		
		D Stereotactic Other Photon Radiosurgery		
		F Plaque Radiation		
		H Stereotactic Particulate Radiosurgery		
		J Stereotactic Gamma Beam Radiosurgery		
		K Laser Interstitial Thermal Therapy		

D: Radiation Therapy
7: Lymphatic and Hematologic System

Modality-Character 3	Treatment Site -Character 4	Modality Qualifier-Character 5	Isotope -Character 6	Qualifier-Character 7
0 Beam Radiation	**0** Bone Marrow	**0** Photons <1 MeV	**7** Cesium 137 (Cs-137)	**0** Intraoperative
1 Brachytherapy	**1** Thymus	**1** Photons 1 - 10 MeV	**8** Iridium 192 (Ir-192)	**Z** None
2 Stereotactic Radiosurgery	**2** Spleen	**2** Photons >10 MeV	**9** Iodine 125 (I-125)	
Y Other Radiation	**3** Lymphatics, Neck	**3** Electrons	**B** Palladium 103 (Pd-103)	
	4 Lymphatics, Axillary	**4** Heavy Particles (Protons,Ions)	**C** Californium 252 (Cf-252)	
	5 Lymphatics, Thorax	**5** Neutrons	**Y** Other Isotope	
	6 Lymphatics, Abdomen	**6** Neutron Capture	**Z** None	
	7 Lymphatics, Pelvis	**8** Hyperthermia		
	8 Lymphatics, Inguinal	**9** High Dose Rate (HDR)		
		B Low Dose Rate (LDR)		
		D Stereotactic Other Photon Radiosurgery		
		F Plaque Radiation		
		H Stereotactic Particulate Radiosurgery		
		J Stereotactic Gamma Beam Radiosurgery		

D: Radiation Therapy
8: Eye

Modality-Character 3	Treatment Site -Character 4	Modality Qualifier-Character 5	Isotope -Character 6	Qualifier-Character 7
0 Beam Radiation	**0** Eye	**0** Photons <1 MeV	**7** Cesium 137 (Cs-137)	**0** Intraoperative
1 Brachytherapy		**1** Photons 1 - 10 MeV	**8** Iridium 192 (Ir-192)	**Z** None
2 Stereotactic Radiosurgery		**2** Photons >10 MeV	**9** Iodine 125 (I-125)	
Y Other Radiation		**3** Electrons	**B** Palladium 103 (Pd-103)	
		4 Heavy Particles (Protons,Ions)	**C** Californium 252 (Cf-252)	
		5 Neutrons	**Y** Other Isotope	
		6 Neutron Capture	**Z** None	
		7 Contact Radiation		
		8 Hyperthermia		
		9 High Dose Rate (HDR)		
		B Low Dose Rate (LDR)		
		D Stereotactic Other Photon Radiosurgery		
		F Plaque Radiation		
		H Stereotactic Particulate Radiosurgery		
		J Stereotactic Gamma Beam Radiosurgery		

D: Radiation Therapy
9: Ear, Nose, Mouth and Throat

Modality-Character 3	Treatment Site -Character 4	Modality Qualifier-Character 5	Isotope -Character 6	Qualifier-Character 7
0 Beam Radiation	**0** Ear	**0** Photons <1 MeV	**7** Cesium 137 (Cs-137)	**0** Intraoperative
1 Brachytherapy	**1** Nose	**1** Photons 1 - 10 MeV	**8** Iridium 192 (Ir-192)	**Z** None
2 Stereotactic Radiosurgery	**3** Hypopharynx	**2** Photons >10 MeV	**9** Iodine 125 (I-125)	
Y Other Radiation	**4** Mouth	**3** Electrons	**B** Palladium 103 (Pd-103)	
	5 Tongue	**4** Heavy Particles (Protons,Ions)	**C** Californium 252 (Cf-252)	
	6 Salivary Glands	**5** Neutrons	**Y** Other Isotope	
	7 Sinuses	**6** Neutron Capture	**Z** None	
	8 Hard Palate	**7** Contact Radiation		
	9 Soft Palate	**8** Hyperthermia		
	B Larynx	**9** High Dose Rate (HDR)		
	C Pharynx	**B** Low Dose Rate (LDR)		
	D Nasopharynx	**C** Intraoperative Radiation Therapy (IORT)		
	F Oropharynx	**D** Stereotactic Other Photon Radiosurgery		
		F Plaque Radiation		
		H Stereotactic Particulate Radiosurgery		
		J Stereotactic Gamma Beam Radiosurgery		

D: Radiation Therapy
B: Respiratory System

Modality-Character 3	Treatment Site -Character 4	Modality Qualifier-Character 5	Isotope -Character 6	Qualifier-Character 7
0 Beam Radiation	**0** Trachea	**0** Photons <1 MeV	**7** Cesium 137 (Cs-137)	**0** Intraoperative
1 Brachytherapy	**1** Bronchus	**1** Photons 1 - 10 MeV	**8** Iridium 192 (Ir-192)	**Z** None
2 Stereotactic Radiosurgery	**2** Lung	**2** Photons >10 MeV	**9** Iodine 125 (I-125)	
Y Other Radiation	**5** Pleura	**3** Electrons	**B** Palladium 103 (Pd-103)	
	6 Mediastinum	**4** Heavy Particles (Protons,Ions)	**C** Californium 252 (Cf-252)	
	7 Chest Wall	**5** Neutrons	**Y** Other Isotope	
	8 Diaphragm	**6** Neutron Capture	**Z** None	
		7 Contact Radiation		
		8 Hyperthermia		
		9 High Dose Rate (HDR)		
		B Low Dose Rate (LDR)		
		D Stereotactic Other Photon Radiosurgery		
		F Plaque Radiation		
		H Stereotactic Particulate Radiosurgery		
		J Stereotactic Gamma Beam Radiosurgery		
		K Laser Interstitial Thermal Therapy		

D: Radiation Therapy
D: Gastrointestinal System

Modality-Character 3	Treatment Site -Character 4	Modality Qualifier-Character 5	Isotope -Character 6	Qualifier-Character 7
0 Beam Radiation	**0** Esophagus	**0** Photons <1 MeV	**7** Cesium 137 (Cs-137)	**0** Intraoperative
1 Brachytherapy	**1** Stomach	**1** Photons 1 - 10 MeV	**8** Iridium 192 (Ir-192)	**Z** None
2 Stereotactic Radiosurgery	**2** Duodenum	**2** Photons >10 MeV	**9** Iodine 125 (I-125)	
Y Other Radiation	**3** Jejunum	**3** Electrons	**B** Palladium 103 (Pd-103)	
	4 Ileum	**4** Heavy Particles (Protons,Ions)	**C** Californium 252 (Cf-252)	
	5 Colon	**5** Neutrons	**Y** Other Isotope	
	7 Rectum	**6** Neutron Capture	**Z** None	
	8 Anus	**7** Contact Radiation		
		8 Hyperthermia		
		9 High Dose Rate (HDR)		
		B Low Dose Rate (LDR)		
		C Intraoperative Radiation Therapy (IORT)		
		D Stereotactic Other Photon Radiosurgery		
		F Plaque Radiation		
		H Stereotactic Particulate Radiosurgery		
		J Stereotactic Gamma Beam Radiosurgery		
		K Laser Interstitial Thermal Therapy		

D: Radiation Therapy
F: Hepatobiliary System and Pancreas

Modality- Character 3	Treatment Site -Character 4	Modality Qualifier- Character 5	Isotope -Character 6	Qualifier-Character 7
0 Beam Radiation	**0** Liver	**0** Photons <1 MeV	**7** Cesium 137 (Cs-137)	**0** Intraoperative
1 Brachytherapy	**1** Gallbladder	**1** Photons 1 - 10 MeV	**8** Iridium 192 (Ir-192)	**Z** None
2 Stereotactic Radiosurgery	**2** Bile Ducts	**2** Photons >10 MeV	**9** Iodine 125 (I-125)	
Y Other Radiation	**3** Pancreas	**3** Electrons	**B** Palladium 103 (Pd-103)	
		4 Heavy Particles (Protons,Ions)	**C** Californium 252 (Cf-252)	
		5 Neutrons	**Y** Other Isotope	
		6 Neutron Capture	**Z** None	
		7 Contact Radiation		
		8 Hyperthermia		
		9 High Dose Rate (HDR)		
		B Low Dose Rate (LDR)		
		C Intraoperative Radiation Therapy (IORT)		
		D Stereotactic Other Photon Radiosurgery		
		F Plaque Radiation		
		H Stereotactic Particulate Radiosurgery		
		J Stereotactic Gamma Beam Radiosurgery		
		K Laser Interstitial Thermal Therapy		

D: Radiation Therapy
G: Endocrine System

Modality- Character 3	Treatment Site -Character 4	Modality Qualifier- Character 5	Isotope -Character 6	Qualifier-Character 7
0 Beam Radiation	**0** Pituitary Gland	**0** Photons <1 MeV	**7** Cesium 137 (Cs-137)	**0** Intraoperative
1 Brachytherapy	**1** Pineal Body	**1** Photons 1 - 10 MeV	**8** Iridium 192 (Ir-192)	**Z** None
2 Stereotactic Radiosurgery	**2** Adrenal Glands	**2** Photons >10 MeV	**9** Iodine 125 (I-125)	
Y Other Radiation	**4** Parathyroid Glands	**3** Electrons	**B** Palladium 103 (Pd-103)	
	5 Thyroid	**5** Neutrons	**C** Californium 252 (Cf-252)	
		6 Neutron Capture	**Y** Other Isotope	
		7 Contact Radiation	**Z** None	
		8 Hyperthermia		
		9 High Dose Rate (HDR)		
		B Low Dose Rate (LDR)		
		D Stereotactic Other Photon Radiosurgery		
		F Plaque Radiation		
		H Stereotactic Particulate Radiosurgery		
		J Stereotactic Gamma Beam Radiosurgery		
		K Laser Interstitial Thermal Therapy		

D: Radiation Therapy
H: Skin

Modality-Character 3	Treatment Site -Character 4	Modality Qualifier-Character 5	Isotope -Character 6	Qualifier-Character 7
0 Beam Radiation	**2** Skin, Face	**0** Photons <1 MeV	**Z** None	**0** Intraoperative
Y Other Radiation	**3** Skin, Neck	**1** Photons 1 - 10 MeV		**Z** None
	4 Skin, Arm	**2** Photons >10 MeV		
	5 Skin, Hand	**3** Electrons		
	6 Skin, Chest	**4** Heavy Particles (Protons,Ions)		
	7 Skin, Back	**5** Neutrons		
	8 Skin, Abdomen	**6** Neutron Capture		
	9 Skin, Buttock	**7** Contact Radiation		
	B Skin, Leg	**8** Hyperthermia		
	C Skin, Foot	**F** Plaque Radiation		

D: Radiation Therapy
M: Breast

Modality-Character 3	Treatment Site -Character 4	Modality Qualifier-Character 5	Isotope -Character 6	Qualifier-Character 7
0 Beam Radiation	**0** Breast, Left	**0** Photons <1 MeV	**7** Cesium 137 (Cs-137)	**0** Intraoperative
1 Brachytherapy	**1** Breast, Right	**1** Photons 1 - 10 MeV	**8** Iridium 192 (Ir-192)	**Z** None
2 Stereotactic Radiosurgery		**2** Photons >10 MeV	**9** Iodine 125 (I-125)	
Y Other Radiation		**3** Electrons	**B** Palladium 103 (Pd-103)	
		4 Heavy Particles (Protons,Ions)	**C** Californium 252 (Cf-252)	
		5 Neutrons	**Y** Other Isotope	
		6 Neutron Capture	**Z** None	
		7 Contact Radiation		
		8 Hyperthermia		
		9 High Dose Rate (HDR)		
		B Low Dose Rate (LDR)		
		D Stereotactic Other Photon Radiosurgery		
		F Plaque Radiation		
		H Stereotactic Particulate Radiosurgery		
		J Stereotactic Gamma Beam Radiosurgery		
		K Laser Interstitial Thermal Therapy		

D: Radiation Therapy
P: Musculoskeletal System

Modality-Character 3	Treatment Site -Character 4	Modality Qualifier-Character 5	Isotope -Character 6	Qualifier-Character 7
0 Beam Radiation	**0** Skull	**0** Photons <1 MeV	**Z** None	**0** Intraoperative
Y Other Radiation	**2** Maxilla	**1** Photons 1 - 10 MeV		**Z** None
	3 Mandible	**2** Photons >10 MeV		
	4 Sternum	**3** Electrons		
	5 Rib(s)	**4** Heavy Particles (Protons,Ions)		
	6 Humerus	**5** Neutrons		
	7 Radius/Ulna	**6** Neutron Capture		
	8 Pelvic Bones	**7** Contact Radiation		
	9 Femur	**8** Hyperthermia		
	B Tibia/Fibula	**F** Plaque Radiation		
	C Other Bone			

D: Radiation Therapy
T: Urinary System

Modality-Character 3	Treatment Site -Character 4	Modality Qualifier-Character 5	Isotope -Character 6	Qualifier-Character 7
0 Beam Radiation	**0** Kidney	**0** Photons <1 MeV	**7** Cesium 137 (Cs-137)	**0** Intraoperative
1 Brachytherapy	**1** Ureter	**1** Photons 1 - 10 MeV	**8** Iridium 192 (Ir-192)	**Z** None
2 Stereotactic Radiosurgery	**2** Bladder	**2** Photons >10 MeV	**9** Iodine 125 (I-125)	
Y Other Radiation	**3** Urethra	**3** Electrons	**B** Palladium 103 (Pd-103)	
		4 Heavy Particles (Protons,Ions)	**C** Californium 252 (Cf-252)	
		5 Neutrons	**Y** Other Isotope	
		6 Neutron Capture	**Z** None	
		7 Contact Radiation		
		8 Hyperthermia		
		9 High Dose Rate (HDR)		
		B Low Dose Rate (LDR)		
		C Intraoperative Radiation Therapy (IORT)		
		D Stereotactic Other Photon Radiosurgery		
		F Plaque Radiation		
		H Stereotactic Particulate Radiosurgery		
		J Stereotactic Gamma Beam Radiosurgery		

D: Radiation Therapy
U: Female Reproductive System

Modality-Character 3	Treatment Site -Character 4	Modality Qualifier-Character 5	Isotope -Character 6	Qualifier-Character 7
0 Beam Radiation	**0** Ovary	**0** Photons <1 MeV	**7** Cesium 137 (Cs-137)	**0** Intraoperative
1 Brachytherapy	**1** Cervix	**1** Photons 1 - 10 MeV	**8** Iridium 192 (Ir-192)	**Z** None
2 Stereotactic Radiosurgery	**2** Uterus	**2** Photons >10 MeV	**9** Iodine 125 (I-125)	
Y Other Radiation		**3** Electrons	**B** Palladium 103 (Pd-103)	
		4 Heavy Particles (Protons,Ions)	**C** Californium 252 (Cf-252)	
		5 Neutrons	**Y** Other Isotope	
		6 Neutron Capture	**Z** None	
		7 Contact Radiation		
		8 Hyperthermia		
		9 High Dose Rate (HDR)		
		B Low Dose Rate (LDR)		
		C Intraoperative Radiation Therapy (IORT)		
		D Stereotactic Other Photon Radiosurgery		
		F Plaque Radiation		
		H Stereotactic Particulate Radiosurgery		
		J Stereotactic Gamma Beam Radiosurgery		

D: Radiation Therapy
V: Male Reproductive System

Modality-Character 3	Treatment Site -Character 4	Modality Qualifier-Character 5	Isotope -Character 6	Qualifier-Character 7
0 Beam Radiation	**0** Prostate	**0** Photons <1 MeV	**7** Cesium 137 (Cs-137)	**0** Intraoperative
1 Brachytherapy	**1** Testis	**1** Photons 1 - 10 MeV	**8** Iridium 192 (Ir-192)	**Z** None
2 Stereotactic Radiosurgery		**2** Photons >10 MeV	**9** Iodine 125 (I-125)	
Y Other Radiation		**3** Electrons	**B** Palladium 103 (Pd-103)	
		4 Heavy Particles (Protons,Ions)	**C** Californium 252 (Cf-252)	
		5 Neutrons	**Y** Other Isotope	
		6 Neutron Capture	**Z** None	
		7 Contact Radiation		
		8 Hyperthermia		
		9 High Dose Rate (HDR)		
		B Low Dose Rate (LDR)		
		C Intraoperative Radiation Therapy (IORT)		
		D Stereotactic Other Photon Radiosurgery		
		F Plaque Radiation		
		H Stereotactic Particulate Radiosurgery		
		J Stereotactic Gamma Beam Radiosurgery		

D: Radiation Therapy
W: Anatomical Regions

Modality-Character 3	Treatment Site -Character 4	Modality Qualifier-Character 5	Isotope -Character 6	Qualifier-Character 7
0 Beam Radiation	**1** Head and Neck	**0** Photons <1 MeV	**7** Cesium 137 (Cs-137)	**0** Intraoperative
1 Brachytherapy	**2** Chest	**1** Photons 1 - 10 MeV	**8** Iridium 192 (Ir-192)	**Z** None
2 Stereotactic Radiosurgery	**3** Abdomen	**2** Photons >10 MeV	**9** Iodine 125 (I-125)	
Y Other Radiation	**4** Hemibody	**3** Electrons	**B** Palladium 103 (Pd-103)	
	5 Whole Body	**4** Heavy Particles (Protons,Ions)	**C** Californium 252 (Cf-252)	
	6 Pelvic Region	**5** Neutrons	**D** Iodine 131 (I-131)	
		6 Neutron Capture	**F** Phosphorus 32 (P-32)	
		7 Contact Radiation	**G** Strontium 89 (Sr-89)	
		8 Hyperthermia	**H** Strontium 90 (Sr-90)	
		9 High Dose Rate (HDR)	**Y** Other Isotope	
		B Low Dose Rate (LDR)	**Z** None	
		D Stereotactic Other Photon Radiosurgery		
		F Plaque Radiation		
		G Isotope Administration		
		H Stereotactic Particulate Radiosurgery		
		J Stereotactic Gamma Beam Radiosurgery		

F: Physical Rehabilitation and Diagnostic Audiology
0: Rehabilitation

Type-Character 3	Body System / Region- Character 4	Type Qualifier-Character 5	Equipment-Character 6	Qualifier- Character 7
0 Speech Assessment	**0** Neurological System - Head and Neck	**0** Bathing/Showering	**1** Audiometer	**Z** None
1 Motor and/or Nerve Function Assessment	**1** Neurological System - Upper Back / Upper Extremity	**0** Bathing/Showering Technique	**2** Sound Field / Booth	
2 Activities of Daily Living Assessment	**2** Neurological System - Lower Back / Lower Extremity	**0** Bathing/Showering Techniques	**4** Electroacoustic Immittance / Acoustic Reflex	
6 Speech Treatment	**3** Neurological System - Whole Body	**0** Cochlear Implant Rehabilitation	**5** Hearing Aid Selection / Fitting / Test	
7 Motor Treatment	**4** Circulatory System - Head and Neck	**0** Filtered Speech	**7** Electrophysiologic	
8 Activities of Daily Living Treatment	**5** Circulatory System - Upper Back / Upper Extremity	**0** Hearing and Related Disorders Counseling	**8** Vestibular / Balance	
9 Hearing Treatment	**6** Circulatory System - Lower Back / Lower Extremity	**0** Muscle Performance	**9** Cochlear Implant	
B Cochlear Implant Treatment	**7** Circulatory System - Whole Body	**0** Nonspoken Language	**B** Physical Agents	
C Vestibular Treatment	**8** Respiratory System - Head and Neck	**0** Range of Motion and Joint Mobility	**C** Mechanical	
D Device Fitting	**9** Respiratory System - Upper Back / Upper Extremity	**0** Tinnitus Masker	**D** Electrotherapeutic	
F Caregiver Training	**B** Respiratory System - Lower Back / Lower Extremity	**0** Vestibular	**E** Orthosis	
	C Respiratory System - Whole Body	**1** Dressing	**F** Assistive, Adaptive, Supportive or Protective	
	D Integumentary System - Head and Neck	**1** Dressing Techniques	**G** Aerobic Endurance and Conditioning	
	F Integumentary System - Upper Back / Upper Extremity	**1** Hearing and Related Disorders Prevention	**H** Mechanical or Electromechanical	
	G Integumentary System -Lower Back / Lower Extremity	**1** Integumentary Integrity	**J** Somatosensory	
	H Integumentary System - Whole Body	**1** Monaural Hearing Aid	**K** Audiovisual	
	J Musculoskeletal System - Head and Neck	**1** Muscle Performance	**L** Assistive Listening	
	K Musculoskeletal System - Upper Back / Upper Extremity	**1** Perceptual Processing	**M** Augmentative / Alternative Communication	
	L Musculoskeletal System - Lower Back / Lower Extremity	**1** Speech Threshold	**N** Biosensory Feedback	
	M Musculoskeletal System - Whole Body	**1** Speech-Language Pathology and Related Disorders Counseling	**P** Computer	
	N Genitourinary System	**2** Auditory Processing	**Q** Speech Analysis	
	Z None	**2** Binaural Hearing Aid	**S** Voice Analysis	
		2 Coordination/Dexterity	**T** Aerodynamic Function	
		2 Feeding and Eating	**U** Prosthesis	
		2 Feeding/Eating	**V** Speech Prosthesis	
		2 Grooming/Personal Hygiene	**W** Swallowing	
		2 Speech/Word Recognition	**X** Cerumen Management	
		2 Speech-Language Pathology and Related Disorders Prevention	**Y** Other Equipment	
		2 Visual Motor Integration	**Z** None	
		3 Aphasia		
		3 Augmentative/Alternative Communication System		
		3 Cerumen Management		
		3 Coordination/Dexterity		
		3 Feeding/Eating		

Type-Character 3	Body System / Region-Character 4	Type Qualifier-Character 5	Equipment-Character 6	Qualifier-Character 7
		3 Grooming/Personal Hygiene		
		3 Motor Function		
		3 Postural Control		
		3 Staggered Spondaic Word		
		4 Articulation/Phonology		
		4 Bed Mobility		
		4 Home Management		
		4 Motor Function		
		4 Sensorineural Acuity Level		
		4 Voice Prosthetic		
		4 Wheelchair Mobility		
		5 Assistive Listening Device		
		5 Aural Rehabilitation		
		5 Bed Mobility		
		5 Perceptual Processing		
		5 Range of Motion and Joint Integrity		
		5 Synthetic Sentence Identification		
		5 Transfer		
		5 Wound Management		
		6 Communicative/Cognitive Integration Skills		
		6 Dynamic Orthosis		
		6 Psychosocial Skills		
		6 Sensory Awareness/Processing/Integrity		
		6 Speech and/or Language Screening		
		6 Therapeutic Exercise		
		6 Wheelchair Mobility		
		7 Aerobic Capacity and Endurance		
		7 Facial Nerve Function		
		7 Fluency		
		7 Manual Therapy Techniques		
		7 Nonspoken Language		
		7 Static Orthosis		
		7 Therapeutic Exercise		
		7 Vocational Activities and Functional Community or Work Reintegration Skills		
		8 Airway Clearance Techniques		
		8 Anthropometric Characteristics		
		8 Motor Speech		
		8 Prosthesis		
		8 Receptive/Expressive Language		
		8 Transfer Training		
		9 Articulation/Phonology		
		9 Assistive, Adaptive, Supportive or Protective Devices		
		9 Cranial Nerve Integrity		
		9 Gait Training/Functional Ambulation		
		9 Orofacial Myofunctional		
		9 Somatosensory Evoked Potentials		
		9 Wound Management		
		B Bed Mobility		

Type-Character 3	Body System / Region-Character 4	Type Qualifier-Character 5	Equipment-Character 6	Qualifier-Character 7
		B Environmental, Home and Work Barriers		
		B Motor Speech		
		B Receptive/Expressive Language		
		B Vocational Activities and Functional Community or Work Reintegration Skills		
		C Aphasia		
		C Ergonomics and Body Mechanics		
		C Gait Training/Functional Ambulation		
		C Transfer		
		C Voice		
		D Application, Proper Use and Care of Devices		
		D Fluency		
		D Gait and/or Balance		
		D Neuromotor Development		
		D Swallowing Dysfunction		
		F Application, Proper Use and Care of Orthoses		
		F Pain		
		F Voice		
		F Wheelchair Mobility		
		G Application, Proper Use and Care of Prosthesis		
		G Communicative/Cognitive Integration Skills		
		G Reflex Integrity		
		G Ventilation, Respiration and Circulation		
		H Bedside Swallowing and Oral Function		
		H Home Management		
		H Vocational Activities and Functional Community or Work Reintegration Skills		
		J Communication Skills		
		J Instrumental Swallowing and Oral Function		
		K Orofacial Myofunctional		
		L Augmentative/Alternative Communication System		
		M Voice Prosthetic		
		N Non-invasive Instrumental Status		
		P Oral Peripheral Mechanism		
		Q Performance Intensity Phonetically Balanced Speech Discrimination		
		R Brief Tone Stimuli		
		S Distorted Speech		
		T Dichotic Stimuli		
		V Temporal Ordering of Stimuli		
		W Masking Patterns		
		X Other Specified Central Auditory Processing		

F: Physical Rehabilitation and Diagnostic Audiology
1: Diagnostic Audiology

Type-Character 3	Body System / Region-Character 4	Type Qualifier-Character 5	Equipment-Character 6	Qualifier-Character 7
3 Hearing Assessment	Z None	0 Bithermal, Binaural Caloric Irrigation	0 Occupational Hearing	Z None
4 Hearing Aid Assessment		0 Cochlear Implant	1 Audiometer	
5 Vestibular Assessment		0 Hearing Screening	2 Sound Field / Booth	
		1 Bithermal, Monaural Caloric Irrigation	3 Tympanometer	
		1 Ear Canal Probe Microphone	4 Electroacoustic Immittance / Acoustic Reflex	
		1 Pure Tone Audiometry, Air	5 Hearing Aid Selection / Fitting / Test	
		2 Monaural Hearing Aid	6 Otoacoustic Emission (OAE)	
		2 Pure Tone Audiometry, Air and Bone	7 Electrophysiologic	
		2 Unithermal Binaural Screen	8 Vestibular / Balance	
		3 Bekesy Audiometry	9 Cochlear Implant	
		3 Binaural Hearing Aid	K Audiovisual	
		3 Oscillating Tracking	L Assistive Listening	
		4 Assistive Listening System/Device Selection	P Computer	
		4 Conditioned Play Audiometry	Y Other Equipment	
		4 Sinusoidal Vertical Axis Rotational	Z None	
		5 Dix-Hallpike Dynamic		
		5 Select Picture Audiometry		
		5 Sensory Aids		
		6 Binaural Electroacoustic Hearing Aid Check		
		6 Computerized Dynamic Posturography		
		6 Visual Reinforcement Audiometry		
		7 Alternate Binaural or Monaural Loudness Balance		
		7 Ear Protector Attenuation		
		7 Tinnitus Masker		
		8 Monaural Electroacoustic Hearing Aid Check		
		8 Tone Decay		
		9 Short Increment Sensitivity Index		
		B Stenger		
		C Pure Tone Stenger		
		D Tympanometry		
		F Eustachian Tube Function		
		G Acoustic Reflex Patterns		
		H Acoustic Reflex Threshold		
		J Acoustic Reflex Decay		
		K Electrocochleography		
		L Auditory Evoked Potentials		
		M Evoked Otoacoustic Emissions, Screening		
		N Evoked Otoacoustic Emissions, Diagnostic		
		P Aural Rehabilitation Status		
		Q Auditory Processing		

G: Mental Health
Z: None

Type-Character 3	Qualifier-Character 4	Qualifier-Character 5	Qualifier-Character 6	Qualifier-Character 7
1 Psychological Tests	**0** Developmental	**Z** None	**Z** None	**Z** None
2 Crisis Intervention	**0** Educational			
3 Medication Management	**0** Interactive			
5 Individual Psychotherapy	**0** Unilateral-Single Seizure			
6 Counseling	**1** Behavioral			
7 Family Psychotherapy	**1** Personality and Behavioral			
B Electroconvulsive Therapy	**1** Unilateral-Multiple Seizure			
C Biofeedback	**1** Vocational			
F Hypnosis	**2** Bilateral-Single Seizure			
G Narcosynthesis	**2** Cognitive			
H Group Psychotherapy	**2** Intellectual and Psychoeducational			
J Light Therapy	**2** Other Family Psychotherapy			
	3 Bilateral-Multiple Seizure			
	3 Interpersonal			
	3 Neuropsychological			
	3 Other Counseling			
	4 Neurobehavioral and Cognitive Status			
	4 Other Electroconvulsive Therapy			
	4 Psychoanalysis			
	5 Psychodynamic			
	6 Supportive			
	8 Cognitive-Behavioral			
	9 Other Biofeedback			
	9 Psychophysiological			
	Z None			

H: Substance Abuse Treatment
Z: None

Type-Character 3	Qualifier-Character 4	Qualifier-Character 5	Qualifier-Character 6	Qualifier-Character 7
2 Detoxification Services	**0** Cognitive	**Z** None	**Z** None	**Z** None
3 Individual Counseling	**0** Nicotine Replacement			
4 Group Counseling	**1** Behavioral			
5 Individual Psychotherapy	**1** Methadone Maintenance			
6 Family Counseling	**2** Cognitive-Behavioral			
8 Medication Management	**2** Levo-alpha-acetylmethadol (LAAM)			
9 Pharmacotherapy	**3** 12-Step			
	3 Antabuse			
	3 Other Family Counseling			
	4 Interpersonal			
	4 Naltrexone			
	5 Interactive			
	5 Naloxone			
	5 Vocational			
	6 Clonidine			
	6 Psychoeducation			
	7 Bupropion			
	7 Motivational Enhancement			
	8 Confrontational			
	8 Psychiatric Medication			
	9 Continuing Care			
	9 Other Replacement Medication			
	9 Supportive			
	B Psychoanalysis			
	B Spiritual			
	C Pre/Post-Test Infectious Disease			
	C Psychodynamic			
	D Psychophysiological			
	Z None			

X: New Technology
2: Cardiovascular System

Operation-Character 3	Body Part-Character 4	Approach-Character 5	Device-Character 6	Qualifier-Character 7
A Assistance	**0** Coronary Artery, One Artery	**0** Open	**1** Cerebral Embolic Filtration, Dual Filter	**1** New Technology Group 1
C Extirpation	**1** Coronary Artery, Two Arteries	**3** Percutaneous	**3** Zooplastic Tissue, Rapid Deployment Technique	**2** New Technology Group 2
R Replacement	**2** Coronary Artery, Three Arteries	**4** Percutaneous Endoscopic	**6** Orbital Atherectomy Technology	
	3 Coronary Artery, Four or More Arteries			
	5 Innominate Artery and Left Common Carotid Artery			
	F Aortic Valve			

X: New Technology
H: Skin, Subcutaneous Tissue, Fascia and Breast

Operation-Character 3	Body Part-Character 4	Approach-Character 5	Device-Character 6	Qualifier-Character 7
R Replacement	**P** Skin	**X** External	**L** Skin Substitute, Porcine Liver Derived	**2** New Technology Group 2

X: New Technology
K: Muscles, Tendons, Bursae and Ligaments

Operation-Character 3	Body Part-Character 4	Approach-Character 5	Device-Character 6	Qualifier-Character 7
0 Introduction	**2** Muscle	**3** Percutaneous	**0** Concentrated Bone Marrow Aspirate	**3** New Technology Group 3

X: New Technology
N: Bones

Operation-Character 3	Body Part-Character 4	Approach-Character 5	Device-Character 6	Qualifier-Character 7
S Reposition	**0** Lumbar Vertebra	**0** Open	**3** Magnetically Controlled Growth Rod(s)	**2** New Technology Group 2
	3 Cervical Vertebra	**3** Percutaneous		
	4 Thoracic Vertebra			

X: New Technology
R: Joints

Operation-Character 3	Body Part-Character 4	Approach-Character 5	Device-Character 6	Qualifier-Character 7
2 Monitoring	**0** Occipital-cervical Joint	**0** Open	**2** Intraoperative Knee Replacement Sensor	**1** New Technology Group 1
G Fusion	**1** Cervical Vertebral Joint		**9** Interbody Fusion Device, Nanotextured Surface	**2** New Technology Group 2
	2 Cervical Vertebral Joints, 2 or more		**F** Interbody Fusion Device, Radiolucent Porous	**3** New Technology Group 3
	4 Cervicothoracic Vertebral Joint			
	6 Thoracic Vertebral Joint			
	7 Thoracic Vertebral Joints, 2 to 7			
	8 Thoracic Vertebral Joints, 8 or more			
	A Thoracolumbar Vertebral Joint			
	B Lumbar Vertebral Joint			
	C Lumbar Vertebral Joints, 2 or more			
	D Lumbosacral Joint			
	G Knee Joint, Right			
	H Knee Joint, Left			

X: New Technology
W: Anatomical Regions

Operation-Character 3	Body Part-Character 4	Approach-Character 5	Device-Character 6	Qualifier-Character 7
0 Introduction	**3** Peripheral Vein	**3** Percutaneous	**2** Ceftazidime-Avibactam Anti-infective	**1** New Technology Group 1
	4 Central Vein	**X** External	**3** Idarucizumab, Dabigatran Reversal Agent	**2** New Technology Group 2
	D Mouth and Pharynx		**4** Isavuconazole Antiinfective	**3** New Technology Group 3
			5 Blinatumomab Antineoplastic Immunotherapy	

Operation-Character 3	Body Part-Character 4	Approach-Character 5	Device-Character 6	Qualifier-Character 7
			7 Andexanet Alfa, Factor Xa Inhibitor Reversal Agent	
			8 Uridine Triacetate	
			9 Defibrotide Sodium Anticoagulant	
			A Bezlotoxumab Monoclonal Antibody	
			B Cytarabine and Daunorubicin Liposome Antineoplastic	
			C Engineered Autologous Chimeric Antigen Receptor	
			F Other New Technology Therapeutic Substance	
			T-cell Immunotherapy	

X: New Technology
W: Anatomical Regions

Operation-Character 3	Body Part-Character 4	Approach-Character 5	Device-Character 6	Qualifier-Character 7
0 Introduction	**V** Vein Graft	**X** External	**8** Endothelial Damage Inhibitor	**3** New Technology Group 3

This page intentionally left blank

Appendix F: Substance Key

Substance Term	ICD-10-PCS Value
AIGISRx® Antibacterial Envelope Antimicrobial Envelope	Anti-Infective Envelope
Axicabtagene Ciloeucel	Engineered Autologous Chimeric Antigen Receptor T-cell Immunotherapy
Bone Morphogenetic Protein 2 (BMP 2)	Recombinant Bone Morphogenetic Protein
CBMA (Concentrated Bone Marrow Aspirate)	Concentrated Bone Marrow Aspirate
Clolar®	Clofarabine
Defitelio®	Defibrotide Sodium Anticoagulant
DuraGraft® Endothelial Damage Inhibitor	Endothelial Damage Inhibitor
Factor Xa Inhibitor Reversal Agent, Andexanet Alfa	Andexanet Alfa, Factor Xa Inhibitor Reversal Agent
Kcentra®	4-Factor Prothrombin Complex Concentrate
Nesiritide®	Human B-type Natriuretic Peptide
rhBMP-2	Recombinant Bone Morphogenetic Protein
Seprafilm®	Adhesion Barrier
STELARA®	Other New Technology Therapeutic Substance
Tissue Plasminogen Activator (tPA)(r- tPA)	Other Thrombolytic
Ustekinumab	Other New Technology Therapeutic Substance
Vistogard®	Uridine Triacetate
Voraxaze®	Glucarpidase
VYXEOS™	Cytarabine and Daunorubicin Liposome Antineoplastic
ZINPLAVA™	Bezlotoxumab Monoclonal Antibody
Zyvox®	Oxazolidinones

This page intentionally left blank

Appendix G: Combination Clusters

Due to the nature of a specific procedure, the first code in the cluster needs to be reported with one or more of the additional codes listed for all codes to be considered valid. The example below is for insertion of a cardiac defibrillator lead into the right ventricle (highlighted code). The additional procedure describes the exact location of where the lead is inserted, which is required for correct reporting:

02HK0KZ

and   0JH609Z

You would need to review the first procedure in the combination/cluster to determine whether you need to report the additional code.

The CMS site also provides additional information on combinations/clusters.

02H60KZ and 0JH608Z	02H73KZ and 0JH638Z	02HA4RS and 02PA3RZ	02HK3KZ and 0JH808Z	02HL0KZ and 0JH809Z	02HL3MZ and 0JH80AZ	02WA0QZ and 02PA4RZ
02H60KZ and 0JH638Z	02H73KZ and 0JH808Z	02HA4RS and 02PA4RZ	02HK3KZ and 0JH809Z	02HL0KZ and 0JH838Z	02HL3MZ and 0JH83AZ	02WA0RZ and 02PA0RZ
02H60KZ and 0JH808Z	02H73KZ and 0JH838Z	02HA4RZ and 02PA0RZ	02HK3KZ and 0JH838Z	02HL0KZ and 0JH839Z	02HL4KZ and 0JH608Z	02WA0RZ and 02PA3RZ
02H60KZ and 0JH838Z	02H74KZ and 0JH608Z	02HA4RZ and 02PA3RZ	02HK3KZ and 0JH839Z	02HL0MZ and 0JH60AZ	02HL4KZ and 0JH609Z	02WA0RZ and 02PA4RZ
02H63KZ and 0JH608Z	02H74KZ and 0JH638Z	02HA4RZ and 02PA4RZ	02HK4KZ and 0JH608Z	02HL0MZ and 0JH63AZ	02HL4KZ and 0JH638Z	02WA3QZ and 02PA0RZ
02H63KZ and 0JH638Z	02H74KZ and 0JH808Z	02HK0KZ and 0JH608Z	02HK4KZ and 0JH609Z	02HL0MZ and 0JH80AZ	02HL4KZ and 0JH639Z	02WA3QZ and 02PA3RZ
02H63KZ and 0JH808Z	02H74KZ and 0JH838Z	02HK0KZ and 0JH609Z	02HK4KZ and 0JH638Z	02HL0MZ and 0JH83AZ	02HL4KZ and 0JH808Z	02WA3QZ and 02PA4RZ
02H63KZ and 0JH838Z	02HA0RS and 02PA0RZ	02HK0KZ and 0JH638Z	02HK4KZ and 0JH639Z	02HL3KZ and 0JH608Z	02HL4KZ and 0JH809Z	02WA3RZ and 02PA0RZ
02H64KZ and 0JH608Z	02HA0RS and 02PA3RZ	02HK0KZ and 0JH639Z	02HK4KZ and 0JH808Z	02HL3KZ and 0JH609Z	02HL4KZ and 0JH838Z	02WA3RZ and 02PA3RZ
02H64KZ and 0JH638Z	02HA0RS and 02PA4RZ	02HK0KZ and 0JH808Z	02HK4KZ and 0JH809Z	02HL3KZ and 0JH638Z	02HL4KZ and 0JH839Z	02WA3RZ and 02PA4RZ
02H64KZ and 0JH808Z	02HA0RZ and 02PA0RZ	02HK0KZ and 0JH809Z	02HK4KZ and 0JH838Z	02HL3KZ and 0JH639Z	02HL4MZ and 0JH60AZ	02WA4QZ and 02PA0RZ
02H64KZ and 0JH838Z	02HA0RZ and 02PA3RZ	02HK0KZ and 0JH838Z	02HK4KZ and 0JH839Z	02HL3KZ and 0JH808Z	02HL4MZ and 0JH63AZ	02WA4QZ and 02PA3RZ
02H70KZ and 0JH608Z	02HA0RZ and 02PA4RZ	02HK0KZ and 0JH839Z	02HL0KZ and 0JH608Z	02HL3KZ and 0JH809Z	02HL4MZ and 0JH80AZ	02WA4QZ and 02PA4RZ
02H70KZ and 0JH638Z	02HA3RS and 02PA0RZ	02HK3KZ and 0JH608Z	02HL0KZ and 0JH609Z	02HL3KZ and 0JH838Z	02HL4MZ and 0JH83AZ	02WA4RZ and 02PA0RZ
02H70KZ and 0JH808Z	02HA3RS and 02PA3RZ	02HK3KZ and 0JH609Z	02HL0KZ and 0JH638Z	02HL3KZ and 0JH839Z	02RK0JZ and 02RL0JZ	02WA4RZ and 02PA3RZ
02H70KZ and 0JH838Z	02HA3RS and 02PA4RZ	02HK3KZ and 0JH638Z	02HL0KZ and 0JH639Z	02HL3MZ and 0JH60AZ	02WA0QZ and 02PA0RZ	02WA4RZ and 02PA4RZ
02H73KZ and 0JH608Z	02HA4RS and 02PA0RZ	02HK3KZ and 0JH639Z	02HL0KZ and 0JH808Z	02HL3MZ and 0JH63AZ	02WA0QZ and 02PA3RZ	07BH0ZZ and 0UTM0ZZ

07BH0ZZ and 0UTMXZZ	0DQ80ZZ and 0WQFXZ2	0HRU37Z and 0JD93ZZ	0JH609Z and 02H43KZ	0JH60BZ and 00HU3MZ	0JH60CZ and 00HE4MZ	0JH60DZ and 00H00MZ
07BH4ZZ and 0UTM0ZZ	0DQ90ZZ and 0WQFXZ2	0HRU37Z and 0JDL3ZZ	0JH609Z and 02H43MZ	0JH60BZ and 00HU4MZ	0JH60CZ and 00HU0MZ	0JH60DZ and 00H03MZ
07BH4ZZ and 0UTMXZZ	0DQA0ZZ and 0WQFXZ2	0HRU37Z and 0JDM3ZZ	0JH609Z and 02H44KZ	0JH60BZ and 00HV0MZ	0JH60CZ and 00HU3MZ	0JH60DZ and 00H04MZ
07BJ0ZZ and 0UTM0ZZ	0DQB0ZZ and 0WQFXZ2	0HRV37Z and 0JD63ZZ	0JH609Z and 02H60KZ	0JH60BZ and 00HV3MZ	0JH60CZ and 00HU4MZ	0JH60DZ and 00H60MZ
07BJ0ZZ and 0UTMXZZ	0DQE0ZZ and 0WQFXZ2	0HRV37Z and 0JD73ZZ	0JH609Z and 02H63KZ	0JH60BZ and 00HV4MZ	0JH60CZ and 00HV0MZ	0JH60DZ and 00H63MZ
07BJ4ZZ and 0UTM0ZZ	0DQF0ZZ and 0WQFXZ2	0HRV37Z and 0JD83ZZ	0JH609Z and 02H64KZ	0JH60BZ and 01HY0MZ	0JH60CZ and 00HV3MZ	0JH60DZ and 00H64MZ
07BJ4ZZ and 0UTMXZZ	0DQG0ZZ and 0WQFXZ2	0HRV37Z and 0JD93ZZ	0JH609Z and 02H70KZ	0JH60BZ and 01HY3MZ	0JH60CZ and 00HV4MZ	0JH60DZ and 00HE0MZ
07T50ZZ and 07T60ZZ and 07T70ZZ and 07T80ZZ and 07T90ZZ and 0HTV0ZZ and 0KTH0ZZ and 0KTJ0ZZ	0DQH0ZZ and 0WQFXZ2	0HRV37Z and 0JDL3ZZ	0JH609Z and 02H73KZ	0JH60BZ and 01HY4MZ	0JH60CZ and 01HY0MZ	0JH60DZ and 00HE3MZ
	0DQK0ZZ and 0WQFXZ2	0HRV37Z and 0JDM3ZZ	0JH609Z and 02H74KZ	0JH60BZ and 05H00MZ	0JH60CZ and 01HY3MZ	0JH60DZ and 00HE4MZ
	0DQL0ZZ and 0WQFXZ2	0JH608Z and 02H40KZ	0JH609Z and 02HN0JZ	0JH60BZ and 05H03MZ	0JH60CZ and 01HY4MZ	0JH60DZ and 00HU0MZ
07T50ZZ and 07T60ZZ and 0HTV0ZZ	0DQM0ZZ and 0WQFXZ2	0JH608Z and 02H44KZ	0JH609Z and 02HN0KZ	0JH60BZ and 05H04MZ	0JH60CZ and 05H00MZ	0JH60DZ and 00HU3MZ
07T50ZZ and 07T60ZZ and 0HTV0ZZ and 0KTH0ZZ and 0KTJ0ZZ	0DQN0ZZ and 0WQFXZ2	0JH608Z and 02HN0JZ	0JH609Z and 02HN0MZ	0JH60BZ and 05H30MZ	0JH60CZ and 05H03MZ	0JH60DZ and 00HU4MZ
	0DT90ZZ and 0FTG0ZZ	0JH608Z and 02HN0KZ	0JH609Z and 02HN3JZ	0JH60BZ and 05H33MZ	0JH60CZ and 05H04MZ	0JH60DZ and 00HV0MZ
	0HRT37Z and 0JD63ZZ	0JH608Z and 02HN0MZ	0JH609Z and 02HN3KZ	0JH60BZ and 05H34MZ	0JH60CZ and 05H30MZ	0JH60DZ and 00HV3MZ
07T50ZZ and 07T70ZZ and 07T80ZZ and 0HTT0ZZ and 0KTH0ZZ	0HRT37Z and 0JD73ZZ	0JH608Z and 02HN3JZ	0JH609Z and 02HN3MZ	0JH60BZ and 05H40MZ	0JH60CZ and 05H33MZ	0JH60DZ and 00HV4MZ
	0HRT37Z and 0JD83ZZ	0JH608Z and 02HN3KZ	0JH609Z and 02HN4JZ	0JH60BZ and 05H43MZ	0JH60CZ and 05H34MZ	0JH60DZ and 01HY0MZ
07T50ZZ and 0HTT0ZZ	0HRT37Z and 0JD93ZZ	0JH608Z and 02HN3MZ	0JH609Z and 02HN4KZ	0JH60BZ and 05H44MZ	0JH60CZ and 05H40MZ	0JH60DZ and 01HY3MZ
07T50ZZ and 0HTT0ZZ and 0KTH0ZZ	0HRT37Z and 0JDL3ZZ	0JH608Z and 02HN4JZ	0JH609Z and 02HN4MZ	0JH60BZ and 0DH60MZ	0JH60CZ and 05H43MZ	0JH60DZ and 01HY4MZ
07T60ZZ and 07T70ZZ and 07T90ZZ and 0HTU0ZZ and 0KTJ0ZZ	0HRT37Z and 0JDM3ZZ	0JH608Z and 02HN4KZ	0JH60BZ and 00HE0MZ	0JH60BZ and 0DH63MZ	0JH60CZ and 05H44MZ	0JH60DZ and 05H00MZ
	0HRU37Z and 0JD63ZZ	0JH608Z and 02HN4MZ	0JH60BZ and 00HE3MZ	0JH60BZ and 0DH64MZ	0JH60CZ and 0DH60MZ	0JH60DZ and 05H03MZ
07T60ZZ and 0HTU0ZZ	0HRU37Z and 0JD73ZZ	0JH609Z and 02H40KZ	0JH60BZ and 00HE4MZ	0JH60CZ and 00HE0MZ	0JH60CZ and 0DH63MZ	0JH60DZ and 05H04MZ
07T60ZZ and 0HTU0ZZ and 0KTJ0ZZ	0HRU37Z and 0JD83ZZ	0JH609Z and 02H43JZ	0JH60BZ and 00HU0MZ	0JH60CZ and 00HE3MZ	0JH60CZ and 0DH64MZ	0JH60DZ and 05H30MZ

0JH60DZ and 05H33MZ	0JH60EZ and 00HV4MZ	0JH638Z and 02HN3KZ	0JH639Z and 02HN4JZ	0JH63BZ and 05H43MZ	0JH63CZ and 05H34MZ	0JH63DZ and 01HY0MZ
0JH60DZ and 05H34MZ	0JH60EZ and 01HY0MZ	0JH638Z and 02HN3MZ	0JH639Z and 02HN4KZ	0JH63BZ and 05H44MZ	0JH63CZ and 05H40MZ	0JH63DZ and 01HY3MZ
0JH60DZ and 05H40MZ	0JH60EZ and 01HY3MZ	0JH638Z and 02HN4JZ	0JH639Z and 02HN4MZ	0JH63BZ and 0DH60MZ	0JH63CZ and 05H43MZ	0JH63DZ and 01HY4MZ
0JH60DZ and 05H43MZ	0JH60EZ and 01HY4MZ	0JH638Z and 02HN4KZ	0JH63BZ and 00HE0MZ	0JH63BZ and 0DH63MZ	0JH63CZ and 05H44MZ	0JH63DZ and 05H00MZ
0JH60DZ and 05H44MZ	0JH60EZ and 05H00MZ	0JH638Z and 02HN4MZ	0JH63BZ and 00HE3MZ	0JH63BZ and 0DH64MZ	0JH63CZ and 0DH60MZ	0JH63DZ and 05H03MZ
0JH60DZ and 0DH60MZ	0JH60EZ and 05H03MZ	0JH639Z and 02H40KZ	0JH63BZ and 00HE4MZ	0JH63CZ and 00HE0MZ	0JH63CZ and 0DH63MZ	0JH63DZ and 05H04MZ
0JH60DZ and 0DH63MZ	0JH60EZ and 05H04MZ	0JH639Z and 02H43JZ	0JH63BZ and 00HU0MZ	0JH63CZ and 00HE3MZ	0JH63CZ and 0DH64MZ	0JH63DZ and 05H30MZ
0JH60DZ and 0DH64MZ	0JH60EZ and 05H30MZ	0JH639Z and 02H43KZ	0JH63BZ and 00HU3MZ	0JH63CZ and 00HE4MZ	0JH63DZ and 00H00MZ	0JH63DZ and 05H33MZ
0JH60EZ and 00H00MZ	0JH60EZ and 05H33MZ	0JH639Z and 02H43MZ	0JH63BZ and 00HU4MZ	0JH63CZ and 00HU0MZ	0JH63DZ and 00H03MZ	0JH63DZ and 05H34MZ
0JH60EZ and 00H03MZ	0JH60EZ and 05H34MZ	0JH639Z and 02H44KZ	0JH63BZ and 00HV0MZ	0JH63CZ and 00HU3MZ	0JH63DZ and 00H04MZ	0JH63DZ and 05H40MZ
0JH60EZ and 00H04MZ	0JH60EZ and 05H40MZ	0JH639Z and 02H60KZ	0JH63BZ and 00HV3MZ	0JH63CZ and 00HU4MZ	0JH63DZ and 00H60MZ	0JH63DZ and 05H43MZ
0JH60EZ and 00H60MZ	0JH60EZ and 05H43MZ	0JH639Z and 02H63KZ	0JH63BZ and 00HV4MZ	0JH63CZ and 00HV0MZ	0JH63DZ and 00H63MZ	0JH63DZ and 05H44MZ
0JH60EZ and 00H63MZ	0JH60EZ and 05H44MZ	0JH639Z and 02H64KZ	0JH63BZ and 01HY0MZ	0JH63CZ and 00HV3MZ	0JH63DZ and 00H64MZ	0JH63DZ and 0DH60MZ
0JH60EZ and 00H64MZ	0JH60EZ and 0DH60MZ	0JH639Z and 02H70KZ	0JH63BZ and 01HY3MZ	0JH63CZ and 00HV4MZ	0JH63DZ and 00HE0MZ	0JH63DZ and 0DH63MZ
0JH60EZ and 00HE0MZ	0JH60EZ and 0DH63MZ	0JH639Z and 02H73KZ	0JH63BZ and 01HY4MZ	0JH63CZ and 01HY0MZ	0JH63DZ and 00HE3MZ	0JH63DZ and 0DH64MZ
0JH60EZ and 00HE3MZ	0JH60EZ and 0DH64MZ	0JH639Z and 02H74KZ	0JH63BZ and 05H00MZ	0JH63CZ and 01HY3MZ	0JH63DZ and 00HE4MZ	0JH63EZ and 00H00MZ
0JH60EZ and 00HE4MZ	0JH638Z and 02H40KZ	0JH639Z and 02HN0JZ	0JH63BZ and 05H03MZ	0JH63CZ and 01HY4MZ	0JH63DZ and 00HU0MZ	0JH63EZ and 00H03MZ
0JH60EZ and 00HU0MZ	0JH638Z and 02H44KZ	0JH639Z and 02HN0KZ	0JH63BZ and 05H04MZ	0JH63CZ and 05H00MZ	0JH63DZ and 00HU3MZ	0JH63EZ and 00H04MZ
0JH60EZ and 00HU3MZ	0JH638Z and 02HN0JZ	0JH639Z and 02HN0MZ	0JH63BZ and 05H30MZ	0JH63CZ and 05H03MZ	0JH63DZ and 00HU4MZ	0JH63EZ and 00H60MZ
0JH60EZ and 00HU4MZ	0JH638Z and 02HN0KZ	0JH639Z and 02HN3JZ	0JH63BZ and 05H33MZ	0JH63CZ and 05H04MZ	0JH63DZ and 00HV0MZ	0JH63EZ and 00H63MZ
0JH60EZ and 00HV0MZ	0JH638Z and 02HN0MZ	0JH639Z and 02HN3KZ	0JH63BZ and 05H34MZ	0JH63CZ and 05H30MZ	0JH63DZ and 00HV3MZ	0JH63EZ and 00H64MZ
0JH60EZ and 00HV3MZ	0JH638Z and 02HN3JZ	0JH639Z and 02HN3MZ	0JH63BZ and 05H40MZ	0JH63CZ and 05H33MZ	0JH63DZ and 00HV4MZ	0JH63EZ and 00HE0MZ

0JH63EZ and 00HE3MZ	0JH63EZ and 0DH64MZ	0JH70BZ and 0DH60MZ	0JH70CZ and 05H43MZ	0JH70DZ and 01HY4MZ	0JH70EZ and 00HU0MZ	0JH73BZ and 00HE3MZ
0JH63EZ and 00HE4MZ	0JH70BZ and 00HE0MZ	0JH70BZ and 0DH63MZ	0JH70CZ and 05H44MZ	0JH70DZ and 05H00MZ	0JH70EZ and 00HU3MZ	0JH73BZ and 00HE4MZ
0JH63EZ and 00HU0MZ	0JH70BZ and 00HE3MZ	0JH70BZ and 0DH64MZ	0JH70CZ and 0DH60MZ	0JH70DZ and 05H03MZ	0JH70EZ and 00HU4MZ	0JH73BZ and 00HU0MZ
0JH63EZ and 00HU3MZ	0JH70BZ and 00HE4MZ	0JH70CZ and 00HE0MZ	0JH70CZ and 0DH63MZ	0JH70DZ and 05H04MZ	0JH70EZ and 00HV0MZ	0JH73BZ and 00HU3MZ
0JH63EZ and 00HU4MZ	0JH70BZ and 00HU0MZ	0JH70CZ and 00HE3MZ	0JH70CZ and 0DH64MZ	0JH70DZ and 05H30MZ	0JH70EZ and 00HV3MZ	0JH73BZ and 00HU4MZ
0JH63EZ and 00HV0MZ	0JH70BZ and 00HU3MZ	0JH70CZ and 00HE4MZ	0JH70DZ and 00H00MZ	0JH70DZ and 05H33MZ	0JH70EZ and 00HV4MZ	0JH73BZ and 00HV0MZ
0JH63EZ and 00HV3MZ	0JH70BZ and 00HU4MZ	0JH70CZ and 00HU0MZ	0JH70DZ and 00H03MZ	0JH70DZ and 05H34MZ	0JH70EZ and 01HY0MZ	0JH73BZ and 00HV3MZ
0JH63EZ and 00HV4MZ	0JH70BZ and 00HV0MZ	0JH70CZ and 00HU3MZ	0JH70DZ and 00H04MZ	0JH70DZ and 05H40MZ	0JH70EZ and 01HY3MZ	0JH73BZ and 00HV4MZ
0JH63EZ and 01HY0MZ	0JH70BZ and 00HV3MZ	0JH70CZ and 00HU4MZ	0JH70DZ and 00H60MZ	0JH70DZ and 05H43MZ	0JH70EZ and 01HY4MZ	0JH73BZ and 01HY0MZ
0JH63EZ and 01HY3MZ	0JH70BZ and 00HV4MZ	0JH70CZ and 00HV0MZ	0JH70DZ and 00H63MZ	0JH70DZ and 05H44MZ	0JH70EZ and 05H00MZ	0JH73BZ and 01HY3MZ
0JH63EZ and 01HY4MZ	0JH70BZ and 01HY0MZ	0JH70CZ and 00HV3MZ	0JH70DZ and 00H64MZ	0JH70DZ and 0DH60MZ	0JH70EZ and 05H03MZ	0JH73BZ and 01HY4MZ
0JH63EZ and 05H00MZ	0JH70BZ and 01HY3MZ	0JH70CZ and 00HV4MZ	0JH70DZ and 00HE0MZ	0JH70DZ and 0DH63MZ	0JH70EZ and 05H04MZ	0JH73BZ and 05H00MZ
0JH63EZ and 05H03MZ	0JH70BZ and 01HY4MZ	0JH70CZ and 01HY0MZ	0JH70DZ and 00HE3MZ	0JH70DZ and 0DH64MZ	0JH70EZ and 05H30MZ	0JH73BZ and 05H03MZ
0JH63EZ and 05H04MZ	0JH70BZ and 05H00MZ	0JH70CZ and 01HY3MZ	0JH70DZ and 00HE4MZ	0JH70EZ and 00H00MZ	0JH70EZ and 05H33MZ	0JH73BZ and 05H04MZ
0JH63EZ and 05H30MZ	0JH70BZ and 05H03MZ	0JH70CZ and 01HY4MZ	0JH70DZ and 00HU0MZ	0JH70EZ and 00H03MZ	0JH70EZ and 05H34MZ	0JH73BZ and 05H30MZ
0JH63EZ and 05H33MZ	0JH70BZ and 05H04MZ	0JH70CZ and 05H00MZ	0JH70DZ and 00HU3MZ	0JH70EZ and 00H04MZ	0JH70EZ and 05H40MZ	0JH73BZ and 05H33MZ
0JH63EZ and 05H34MZ	0JH70BZ and 05H30MZ	0JH70CZ and 05H03MZ	0JH70DZ and 00HU4MZ	0JH70EZ and 00H60MZ	0JH70EZ and 05H43MZ	0JH73BZ and 05H34MZ
0JH63EZ and 05H40MZ	0JH70BZ and 05H33MZ	0JH70CZ and 05H04MZ	0JH70DZ and 00HV0MZ	0JH70EZ and 00H63MZ	0JH70EZ and 05H44MZ	0JH73BZ and 05H40MZ
0JH63EZ and 05H43MZ	0JH70BZ and 05H34MZ	0JH70CZ and 05H30MZ	0JH70DZ and 00HV3MZ	0JH70EZ and 00H64MZ	0JH70EZ and 0DH60MZ	0JH73BZ and 05H43MZ
0JH63EZ and 05H44MZ	0JH70BZ and 05H40MZ	0JH70CZ and 05H33MZ	0JH70DZ and 00HV4MZ	0JH70EZ and 00HE0MZ	0JH70EZ and 0DH63MZ	0JH73BZ and 05H44MZ
0JH63EZ and 0DH60MZ	0JH70BZ and 05H43MZ	0JH70CZ and 05H34MZ	0JH70DZ and 01HY0MZ	0JH70EZ and 00HE3MZ	0JH70EZ and 0DH64MZ	0JH73BZ and 0DH60MZ
0JH63EZ and 0DH63MZ	0JH70BZ and 05H44MZ	0JH70CZ and 05H40MZ	0JH70DZ and 01HY3MZ	0JH70EZ and 00HE4MZ	0JH70EZ and 00HE0MZ	0JH73BZ and 0DH63MZ

0JH73BZ and 0DH64MZ	0JH73CZ and 0DH60MZ	0JH73DZ and 05H03MZ	0JH73EZ and 00HU4MZ	0JH808Z and 02HN0KZ	0JH809Z and 02HN3JZ	0JH80BZ and 05H33MZ
0JH73CZ and 00HE0MZ	0JH73CZ and 0DH63MZ	0JH73DZ and 05H04MZ	0JH73EZ and 00HV0MZ	0JH808Z and 02HN0MZ	0JH809Z and 02HN3KZ	0JH80BZ and 05H34MZ
0JH73CZ and 00HE3MZ	0JH73CZ and 0DH64MZ	0JH73DZ and 05H30MZ	0JH73EZ and 00HV3MZ	0JH808Z and 02HN3JZ	0JH809Z and 02HN3MZ	0JH80BZ and 05H40MZ
0JH73CZ and 00HE4MZ	0JH73DZ and 00H00MZ	0JH73DZ and 05H33MZ	0JH73EZ and 00HV4MZ	0JH808Z and 02HN3KZ	0JH809Z and 02HN4JZ	0JH80BZ and 05H43MZ
0JH73CZ and 00HU0MZ	0JH73DZ and 00H03MZ	0JH73DZ and 05H34MZ	0JH73EZ and 01HY0MZ	0JH808Z and 02HN3MZ	0JH809Z and 02HN4KZ	0JH80BZ and 05H44MZ
0JH73CZ and 00HU3MZ	0JH73DZ and 00H04MZ	0JH73DZ and 05H40MZ	0JH73EZ and 01HY3MZ	0JH808Z and 02HN4JZ	0JH809Z and 02HN4MZ	0JH80BZ and 0DH60MZ
0JH73CZ and 00HU4MZ	0JH73DZ and 00H60MZ	0JH73DZ and 05H43MZ	0JH73EZ and 01HY4MZ	0JH808Z and 02HN4KZ	0JH80BZ and 00HE0MZ	0JH80BZ and 0DH63MZ
0JH73CZ and 00HV0MZ	0JH73DZ and 00H63MZ	0JH73DZ and 05H44MZ	0JH73EZ and 05H00MZ	0JH808Z and 02HN4MZ	0JH80BZ and 00HE3MZ	0JH80BZ and 0DH64MZ
0JH73CZ and 00HV3MZ	0JH73DZ and 00H64MZ	0JH73DZ and 0DH60MZ	0JH73EZ and 05H03MZ	0JH809Z and 02H40KZ	0JH80BZ and 00HE4MZ	0JH80CZ and 00HE0MZ
0JH73CZ and 00HV4MZ	0JH73DZ and 00HE0MZ	0JH73DZ and 0DH63MZ	0JH73EZ and 05H04MZ	0JH809Z and 02H43JZ	0JH80BZ and 00HU0MZ	0JH80CZ and 00HE3MZ
0JH73CZ and 01HY0MZ	0JH73DZ and 00HE3MZ	0JH73DZ and 0DH64MZ	0JH73EZ and 05H30MZ	0JH809Z and 02H43KZ	0JH80BZ and 00HU3MZ	0JH80CZ and 00HE4MZ
0JH73CZ and 01HY3MZ	0JH73DZ and 00HE4MZ	0JH73EZ and 00H00MZ	0JH73EZ and 05H33MZ	0JH809Z and 02H43MZ	0JH80BZ and 00HU4MZ	0JH80CZ and 00HU0MZ
0JH73CZ and 01HY4MZ	0JH73DZ and 00HU0MZ	0JH73EZ and 00H03MZ	0JH73EZ and 05H34MZ	0JH809Z and 02H44KZ	0JH80BZ and 00HV0MZ	0JH80CZ and 00HU3MZ
0JH73CZ and 05H00MZ	0JH73DZ and 00HU3MZ	0JH73EZ and 00H04MZ	0JH73EZ and 05H40MZ	0JH809Z and 02H60KZ	0JH80BZ and 00HV3MZ	0JH80CZ and 00HU4MZ
0JH73CZ and 05H03MZ	0JH73DZ and 00HU4MZ	0JH73EZ and 00H60MZ	0JH73EZ and 05H43MZ	0JH809Z and 02H63KZ	0JH80BZ and 00HV4MZ	0JH80CZ and 00HV0MZ
0JH73CZ and 05H04MZ	0JH73DZ and 00HV0MZ	0JH73EZ and 00H63MZ	0JH73EZ and 05H44MZ	0JH809Z and 02H64KZ	0JH80BZ and 01HY0MZ	0JH80CZ and 00HV3MZ
0JH73CZ and 05H30MZ	0JH73DZ and 00HV3MZ	0JH73EZ and 00H64MZ	0JH73EZ and 0DH60MZ	0JH809Z and 02H70KZ	0JH80BZ and 01HY3MZ	0JH80CZ and 00HV4MZ
0JH73CZ and 05H33MZ	0JH73DZ and 00HV4MZ	0JH73EZ and 00HE0MZ	0JH73EZ and 0DH63MZ	0JH809Z and 02H73KZ	0JH80BZ and 01HY4MZ	0JH80CZ and 01HY0MZ
0JH73CZ and 05H34MZ	0JH73DZ and 01HY0MZ	0JH73EZ and 00HE3MZ	0JH73EZ and 0DH64MZ	0JH809Z and 02H74KZ	0JH80BZ and 05H00MZ	0JH80CZ and 01HY3MZ
0JH73CZ and 05H40MZ	0JH73DZ and 01HY3MZ	0JH73EZ and 00HE4MZ	0JH808Z and 02H40KZ	0JH809Z and 02HN0JZ	0JH80BZ and 05H03MZ	0JH80CZ and 01HY4MZ
0JH73CZ and 05H43MZ	0JH73DZ and 01HY4MZ	0JH73EZ and 00HU0MZ	0JH808Z and 02H44KZ	0JH809Z and 02HN0KZ	0JH80BZ and 05H04MZ	0JH80CZ and 05H00MZ
0JH73CZ and 05H44MZ	0JH73DZ and 05H00MZ	0JH73EZ and 00HU3MZ	0JH808Z and 02HN0JZ	0JH809Z and 02HN0MZ	0JH80BZ and 05H30MZ	0JH80CZ and 05H03MZ

0JH80CZ and 05H04MZ	0JH80DZ and 00HV0MZ	0JH80EZ and 00H63MZ	0JH80EZ and 05H44MZ	0JH839Z and 02H64KZ	0JH83BZ and 01HY0MZ	0JH83CZ and 00HV3MZ
0JH80CZ and 05H30MZ	0JH80DZ and 00HV3MZ	0JH80EZ and 00H64MZ	0JH80EZ and 0DH60MZ	0JH839Z and 02H70KZ	0JH83BZ and 01HY3MZ	0JH83CZ and 00HV4MZ
0JH80CZ and 05H33MZ	0JH80DZ and 00HV4MZ	0JH80EZ and 00HE0MZ	0JH80EZ and 0DH63MZ	0JH839Z and 02H73KZ	0JH83BZ and 01HY4MZ	0JH83CZ and 01HY0MZ
0JH80CZ and 05H34MZ	0JH80DZ and 01HY0MZ	0JH80EZ and 00HE3MZ	0JH80EZ and 0DH64MZ	0JH839Z and 02H74KZ	0JH83BZ and 05H00MZ	0JH83CZ and 01HY3MZ
0JH80CZ and 05H40MZ	0JH80DZ and 01HY3MZ	0JH80EZ and 00HE4MZ	0JH838Z and 02H40KZ	0JH839Z and 02HN0JZ	0JH83BZ and 05H03MZ	0JH83CZ and 01HY4MZ
0JH80CZ and 05H43MZ	0JH80DZ and 01HY4MZ	0JH80EZ and 00HU0MZ	0JH838Z and 02H44KZ	0JH839Z and 02HN0KZ	0JH83BZ and 05H04MZ	0JH83CZ and 05H00MZ
0JH80CZ and 05H44MZ	0JH80DZ and 05H00MZ	0JH80EZ and 00HU3MZ	0JH838Z and 02HN0JZ	0JH839Z and 02HN0MZ	0JH83BZ and 05H30MZ	0JH83CZ and 05H03MZ
0JH80CZ and 0DH60MZ	0JH80DZ and 05H03MZ	0JH80EZ and 00HU4MZ	0JH838Z and 02HN0KZ	0JH839Z and 02HN3JZ	0JH83BZ and 05H33MZ	0JH83CZ and 05H04MZ
0JH80CZ and 0DH63MZ	0JH80DZ and 05H04MZ	0JH80EZ and 00HV0MZ	0JH838Z and 02HN0MZ	0JH839Z and 02HN3KZ	0JH83BZ and 05H34MZ	0JH83CZ and 05H30MZ
0JH80CZ and 0DH64MZ	0JH80DZ and 05H30MZ	0JH80EZ and 00HV3MZ	0JH838Z and 02HN3JZ	0JH839Z and 02HN3MZ	0JH83BZ and 05H40MZ	0JH83CZ and 05H33MZ
0JH80DZ and 00H00MZ	0JH80DZ and 05H33MZ	0JH80EZ and 00HV4MZ	0JH838Z and 02HN3KZ	0JH839Z and 02HN4JZ	0JH83BZ and 05H43MZ	0JH83CZ and 05H34MZ
0JH80DZ and 00H03MZ	0JH80DZ and 05H34MZ	0JH80EZ and 01HY0MZ	0JH838Z and 02HN3MZ	0JH839Z and 02HN4KZ	0JH83BZ and 05H44MZ	0JH83CZ and 05H40MZ
0JH80DZ and 00H04MZ	0JH80DZ and 05H40MZ	0JH80EZ and 01HY3MZ	0JH838Z and 02HN4JZ	0JH839Z and 02HN4MZ	0JH83BZ and 0DH60MZ	0JH83CZ and 05H43MZ
0JH80DZ and 00H60MZ	0JH80DZ and 05H43MZ	0JH80EZ and 01HY4MZ	0JH838Z and 02HN4KZ	0JH83BZ and 00HE0MZ	0JH83BZ and 0DH63MZ	0JH83CZ and 05H44MZ
0JH80DZ and 00H63MZ	0JH80DZ and 05H44MZ	0JH80EZ and 05H00MZ	0JH838Z and 02HN4MZ	0JH83BZ and 00HE3MZ	0JH83BZ and 0DH64MZ	0JH83CZ and 0DH60MZ
0JH80DZ and 00H64MZ	0JH80DZ and 0DH60MZ	0JH80EZ and 05H03MZ	0JH839Z and 02H40KZ	0JH83BZ and 00HE4MZ	0JH83CZ and 00HE0MZ	0JH83CZ and 0DH63MZ
0JH80DZ and 00HE0MZ	0JH80DZ and 0DH63MZ	0JH80EZ and 05H04MZ	0JH839Z and 02H43JZ	0JH83BZ and 00HU0MZ	0JH83CZ and 00HE3MZ	0JH83CZ and 0DH64MZ
0JH80DZ and 00HE3MZ	0JH80DZ and 0DH64MZ	0JH80EZ and 05H30MZ	0JH839Z and 02H43KZ	0JH83BZ and 00HU3MZ	0JH83CZ and 00HE4MZ	0JH83DZ and 00H00MZ
0JH80DZ and 00HE4MZ	0JH80EZ and 00H00MZ	0JH80EZ and 05H33MZ	0JH839Z and 02H43MZ	0JH83BZ and 00HU4MZ	0JH83CZ and 00HU0MZ	0JH83DZ and 00H03MZ
0JH80DZ and 00HU0MZ	0JH80EZ and 00H03MZ	0JH80EZ and 05H34MZ	0JH839Z and 02H44KZ	0JH83BZ and 00HV0MZ	0JH83CZ and 00HU3MZ	0JH83DZ and 00H04MZ
0JH80DZ and 00HU3MZ	0JH80EZ and 00H04MZ	0JH80EZ and 05H40MZ	0JH839Z and 02H60KZ	0JH83BZ and 00HV3MZ	0JH83CZ and 00HU4MZ	0JH83DZ and 00H60MZ
0JH80DZ and 00HU4MZ	0JH80EZ and 00H60MZ	0JH80EZ and 05H43MZ	0JH839Z and 02H63KZ	0JH83BZ and 00HV4MZ	0JH83CZ and 00HV0MZ	0JH83DZ and 00H63MZ

0JH83DZ and 00H64MZ	0JH83DZ and 0DH60MZ	0JH83EZ and 05H30MZ	0SP908Z and 0SR901Z	0SP908Z and 0SRA0J9	0SP909Z and 0SR903A	0SP909Z and 0SRR01Z
0JH83DZ and 00HE0MZ	0JH83DZ and 0DH63MZ	0JH83EZ and 05H33MZ	0SP908Z and 0SR9029	0SP908Z and 0SRA0JA	0SP909Z and 0SR903Z	0SP909Z and 0SRR039
0JH83DZ and 00HE3MZ	0JH83DZ and 0DH64MZ	0JH83EZ and 05H34MZ	0SP908Z and 0SR902A	0SP908Z and 0SRA0JZ	0SP909Z and 0SR9049	0SP909Z and 0SRR03A
0JH83DZ and 00HE4MZ	0JH83EZ and 00H00MZ	0JH83EZ and 05H40MZ	0SP908Z and 0SR902Z	0SP908Z and 0SRR019	0SP909Z and 0SR904A	0SP909Z and 0SRR03Z
0JH83DZ and 00HU0MZ	0JH83EZ and 00H03MZ	0JH83EZ and 05H43MZ	0SP908Z and 0SR9039	0SP908Z and 0SRR01A	0SP909Z and 0SR904Z	0SP909Z and 0SRR0J9
0JH83DZ and 00HU3MZ	0JH83EZ and 00H04MZ	0JH83EZ and 05H44MZ	0SP908Z and 0SR903A	0SP908Z and 0SRR01Z	0SP909Z and 0SR90J9	0SP909Z and 0SRR0JA
0JH83DZ and 00HU4MZ	0JH83EZ and 00H60MZ	0JH83EZ and 0DH60MZ	0SP908Z and 0SR903Z	0SP908Z and 0SRR039	0SP909Z and 0SR90JA	0SP909Z and 0SRR0JZ
0JH83DZ and 00HV0MZ	0JH83EZ and 00H63MZ	0JH83EZ and 0DH63MZ	0SP908Z and 0SR9049	0SP908Z and 0SRR03A	0SP909Z and 0SR90JZ	0SP909Z and 0SU909Z
0JH83DZ and 00HV3MZ	0JH83EZ and 00H64MZ	0JH83EZ and 0DH64MZ	0SP908Z and 0SR904A	0SP908Z and 0SRR03Z	0SP909Z and 0SRA009	0SP909Z and 0SU909Z
0JH83DZ and 00HV4MZ	0JH83EZ and 00HE0MZ	0NH00NZ and 00H00MZ	0SP908Z and 0SR904Z	0SP908Z and 0SRR0J9	0SP909Z and 0SRA00A	0SP909Z and 0SUA09Z
0JH83DZ and 01HY0MZ	0JH83EZ and 00HE3MZ	0NH00NZ and 00H03MZ	0SP908Z and 0SR90J9	0SP908Z and 0SRR0JA	0SP909Z and 0SRA00Z	0SP909Z and 0SUA09Z
0JH83DZ and 01HY3MZ	0JH83EZ and 00HE4MZ	0NH00NZ and 00H04MZ	0SP908Z and 0SR90JA	0SP908Z and 0SRR0JZ	0SP909Z and 0SRA019	0SP909Z and 0SUR09Z
0JH83DZ and 01HY4MZ	0JH83EZ and 00HU0MZ	0NH00NZ and 00H60MZ	0SP908Z and 0SR90JZ	0SP908Z and 0SU909Z	0SP909Z and 0SRA01A	0SP909Z and 0SUR09Z
0JH83DZ and 05H00MZ	0JH83EZ and 00HU3MZ	0NH00NZ and 00H63MZ	0SP908Z and 0SRA009	0SP908Z and 0SUA09Z	0SP909Z and 0SRA01Z	0SP90BZ and 0SR9019
0JH83DZ and 05H03MZ	0JH83EZ and 00HU4MZ	0NH00NZ and 00H64MZ	0SP908Z and 0SRA00A	0SP908Z and 0SUR09Z	0SP909Z and 0SRA039	0SP90BZ and 0SR901A
0JH83DZ and 05H04MZ	0JH83EZ and 00HV0MZ	0PS33ZZ and 0PU33JZ	0SP908Z and 0SRA00Z	0SP909Z and 0SR9019	0SP909Z and 0SRA03A	0SP90BZ and 0SR901Z
0JH83DZ and 05H30MZ	0JH83EZ and 01HY0MZ	0PS43ZZ and 0PU43JZ	0SP908Z and 0SRA019	0SP909Z and 0SR901A	0SP909Z and 0SRA03Z	0SP90BZ and 0SR9029
0JH83DZ and 05H33MZ	0JH83EZ and 01HY3MZ	0QS03ZZ and 0QU03JZ	0SP908Z and 0SRA01A	0SP909Z and 0SR901Z	0SP909Z and 0SRA0J9	0SP90BZ and 0SR902A
0JH83DZ and 05H34MZ	0JH83EZ and 01HY4MZ	0QS13ZZ and 0QU13JZ	0SP908Z and 0SRA01Z	0SP909Z and 0SR9029	0SP909Z and 0SRA0JA	0SP90BZ and 0SR902Z
0JH83DZ and 05H40MZ	0JH83EZ and 05H00MZ	0QSS3ZZ and 0QUS3JZ	0SP908Z and 0SRA039	0SP909Z and 0SR902A	0SP909Z and 0SRA0JZ	0SP90BZ and 0SR9039
0JH83DZ and 05H43MZ	0JH83EZ and 05H03MZ	0SP908Z and 0SR9019	0SP908Z and 0SRA03A	0SP909Z and 0SR902Z	0SP909Z and 0SRR019	0SP90BZ and 0SR903A
0JH83DZ and 05H44MZ	0JH83EZ and 05H04MZ	0SP908Z and 0SR901A	0SP908Z and 0SRA03Z	0SP909Z and 0SR9039	0SP909Z and 0SRR01A	0SP90BZ and 0SR903Z

0SP90BZ and 0SR9049	0SP90BZ and 0SRR03A	0SP90JZ and 0SR90JZ	0SP948Z and 0SR9019	0SP948Z and 0SRA03A	0SP94JZ and 0SR902Z	0SP94JZ and 0SRR019
0SP90BZ and 0SR904A	0SP90BZ and 0SRR03Z	0SP90JZ and 0SRA009	0SP948Z and 0SR901A	0SP948Z and 0SRA03Z	0SP94JZ and 0SR9039	0SP94JZ and 0SRR01A
0SP90BZ and 0SR904Z	0SP90BZ and 0SRR0J9	0SP90JZ and 0SRA00A	0SP948Z and 0SR901Z	0SP948Z and 0SRA0J9	0SP94JZ and 0SR903A	0SP94JZ and 0SRR01Z
0SP90BZ and 0SR90J9	0SP90BZ and 0SRR0JA	0SP90JZ and 0SRA00Z	0SP948Z and 0SR9029	0SP948Z and 0SRA0JA	0SP94JZ and 0SR903Z	0SP94JZ and 0SRR039
0SP90BZ and 0SR90JA	0SP90BZ and 0SRR0JZ	0SP90JZ and 0SRA019	0SP948Z and 0SR902A	0SP948Z and 0SRA0JZ	0SP94JZ and 0SR9049	0SP94JZ and 0SRR03A
0SP90BZ and 0SR90JZ	0SP90BZ and 0SU909Z	0SP90JZ and 0SRA01A	0SP948Z and 0SR902Z	0SP948Z and 0SRR019	0SP94JZ and 0SR904A	0SP94JZ and 0SRR03Z
0SP90BZ and 0SRA009	0SP90BZ and 0SUA09Z	0SP90JZ and 0SRA01Z	0SP948Z and 0SR9039	0SP948Z and 0SRR01A	0SP94JZ and 0SR904Z	0SP94JZ and 0SRR0J9
0SP90BZ and 0SRA00A	0SP90BZ and 0SUR09Z	0SP90JZ and 0SRA039	0SP948Z and 0SR903A	0SP948Z and 0SRR01Z	0SP94JZ and 0SR90J9	0SP94JZ and 0SRR0JA
0SP90BZ and 0SRA00Z	0SP90JZ and 0SR9019	0SP90JZ and 0SRA03A	0SP948Z and 0SR903Z	0SP948Z and 0SRR039	0SP94JZ and 0SR90JA	0SP94JZ and 0SRR0JZ
0SP90BZ and 0SRA019	0SP90JZ and 0SR901A	0SP90JZ and 0SRA03Z	0SP948Z and 0SR9049	0SP948Z and 0SRR03A	0SP94JZ and 0SR90JZ	0SP94JZ and 0SU909Z
0SP90BZ and 0SRA01A	0SP90JZ and 0SR901Z	0SP90JZ and 0SRA0J9	0SP948Z and 0SR904A	0SP948Z and 0SRR03Z	0SP94JZ and 0SRA009	0SP94JZ and 0SUA09Z
0SP90BZ and 0SRA01Z	0SP90JZ and 0SR9029	0SP90JZ and 0SRA0JA	0SP948Z and 0SR904Z	0SP948Z and 0SRR0J9	0SP94JZ and 0SRA00A	0SP94JZ and 0SUR09Z
0SP90BZ and 0SRA039	0SP90JZ and 0SR902A	0SP90JZ and 0SRA0JZ	0SP948Z and 0SR90J9	0SP948Z and 0SRR0JA	0SP94JZ and 0SRA00Z	0SPA0JZ and 0SR9019
0SP90BZ and 0SRA03A	0SP90JZ and 0SR902Z	0SP90JZ and 0SRR019	0SP948Z and 0SR90JA	0SP948Z and 0SRR0JZ	0SP94JZ and 0SRA019	0SPA0JZ and 0SR901A
0SP90BZ and 0SRA03Z	0SP90JZ and 0SR9039	0SP90JZ and 0SRR01A	0SP948Z and 0SR90JZ	0SP948Z and 0SU909Z	0SP94JZ and 0SRA01A	0SPA0JZ and 0SR901Z
0SP90BZ and 0SRA0J9	0SP90JZ and 0SR903A	0SP90JZ and 0SRR01Z	0SP948Z and 0SRA009	0SP948Z and 0SUA09Z	0SP94JZ and 0SRA01Z	0SPA0JZ and 0SR9029
0SP90BZ and 0SRA0JA	0SP90JZ and 0SR903Z	0SP90JZ and 0SRR039	0SP948Z and 0SRA00A	0SP948Z and 0SUR09Z	0SP94JZ and 0SRA039	0SPA0JZ and 0SR902A
0SP90BZ and 0SRA0JZ	0SP90JZ and 0SR9049	0SP90JZ and 0SRR03A	0SP948Z and 0SRA00Z	0SP94JZ and 0SR9019	0SP94JZ and 0SRA03A	0SPA0JZ and 0SR902Z
0SP90BZ and 0SRR019	0SP90JZ and 0SR904A	0SP90JZ and 0SRR03Z	0SP948Z and 0SRA019	0SP94JZ and 0SR901A	0SP94JZ and 0SRA03Z	0SPA0JZ and 0SR9039
0SP90BZ and 0SRR01A	0SP90JZ and 0SR904Z	0SP90JZ and 0SRR0J9	0SP948Z and 0SRA01A	0SP94JZ and 0SR901Z	0SP94JZ and 0SRA0J9	0SPA0JZ and 0SR903A
0SP90BZ and 0SRR01Z	0SP90JZ and 0SR90J9	0SP90JZ and 0SRR0JA	0SP948Z and 0SRA01Z	0SP94JZ and 0SR9029	0SP94JZ and 0SRA0JA	0SPA0JZ and 0SR903Z
0SP90BZ and 0SRR039	0SP90JZ and 0SR90JA	0SP90JZ and 0SRR0JZ	0SP948Z and 0SRA039	0SP94JZ and 0SR902A	0SP94JZ and 0SRA0JZ	0SPA0JZ and 0SR9049

0SPA0JZ and 0SR904A	0SPA0JZ and 0SRR03Z	0SPA4JZ and 0SRA019	0SPB08Z and 0SRB01A
0SPA0JZ and 0SR904Z	0SPA0JZ and 0SRR0J9	0SPA4JZ and 0SRA01A	0SPB08Z and 0SRB01Z
0SPA0JZ and 0SR90J9	0SPA0JZ and 0SRR0JA	0SPA4JZ and 0SRA01Z	0SPB08Z and 0SRB029
0SPA0JZ and 0SR90JA	0SPA0JZ and 0SRR0JZ	0SPA4JZ and 0SRA039	0SPB08Z and 0SRB02A
0SPA0JZ and 0SR90JZ	0SPA4JZ and 0SR9019	0SPA4JZ and 0SRA03A	0SPB08Z and 0SRB02Z
0SPA0JZ and 0SRA009	0SPA4JZ and 0SR901A	0SPA4JZ and 0SRA03Z	0SPB08Z and 0SRB039
0SPA0JZ and 0SRA00A	0SPA4JZ and 0SR901Z	0SPA4JZ and 0SRA0J9	0SPB08Z and 0SRB03A
0SPA0JZ and 0SRA00Z	0SPA4JZ and 0SR9029	0SPA4JZ and 0SRA0JA	0SPB08Z and 0SRB03Z
0SPA0JZ and 0SRA019	0SPA4JZ and 0SR902A	0SPA4JZ and 0SRA0JZ	0SPB08Z and 0SRB049
0SPA0JZ and 0SRA01A	0SPA4JZ and 0SR902Z	0SPA4JZ and 0SRR019	0SPB08Z and 0SRB04A
0SPA0JZ and 0SRA01Z	0SPA4JZ and 0SR9039	0SPA4JZ and 0SRR01A	0SPB08Z and 0SRB04Z
0SPA0JZ and 0SRA039	0SPA4JZ and 0SR903A	0SPA4JZ and 0SRR01Z	0SPB08Z and 0SRB0J9
0SPA0JZ and 0SRA03A	0SPA4JZ and 0SR903Z	0SPA4JZ and 0SRR039	0SPB08Z and 0SRB0JA
0SPA0JZ and 0SRA03Z	0SPA4JZ and 0SR9049	0SPA4JZ and 0SRR03A	0SPB08Z and 0SRB0JZ
0SPA0JZ and 0SRA0J9	0SPA4JZ and 0SR904A	0SPA4JZ and 0SRR03Z	0SPB08Z and 0SRE009
0SPA0JZ and 0SRA0JA	0SPA4JZ and 0SR904Z	0SPA4JZ and 0SRR0J9	0SPB08Z and 0SRE00A
0SPA0JZ and 0SRA0JZ	0SPA4JZ and 0SR90J9	0SPA4JZ and 0SRR0JA	0SPB08Z and 0SRE00Z
0SPA0JZ and 0SRR019	0SPA4JZ and 0SR90JA	0SPA4JZ and 0SRR0JZ	0SPB08Z and 0SRE019
0SPA0JZ and 0SRR01A	0SPA4JZ and 0SR90JZ	0SPA4JZ and 0SU909Z	0SPB08Z and 0SRE01A
0SPA0JZ and 0SRR01Z	0SPA4JZ and 0SRA009	0SPA4JZ and 0SUA09Z	0SPB08Z and 0SRE01Z
0SPA0JZ and 0SRR039	0SPA4JZ and 0SRA00A	0SPA4JZ and 0SUR09Z	0SPB08Z and 0SRE039
0SPA0JZ and 0SRR03A	0SPA4JZ and 0SRA00Z	0SPB08Z and 0SRB019	0SPB08Z and 0SRE03A

0SPB08Z and 0SRE03Z	0SPB09Z and 0SRB039	0SPB09Z and 0SRS01A
0SPB08Z and 0SRE0J9	0SPB09Z and 0SRB03A	0SPB09Z and 0SRS01Z
0SPB08Z and 0SRE0JA	0SPB09Z and 0SRB03Z	0SPB09Z and 0SRS039
0SPB08Z and 0SRE0JZ	0SPB09Z and 0SRB049	0SPB09Z and 0SRS03A
0SPB08Z and 0SRS019	0SPB09Z and 0SRB04A	0SPB09Z and 0SRS03Z
0SPB08Z and 0SRS01A	0SPB09Z and 0SRB04Z	0SPB09Z and 0SRS0J9
0SPB08Z and 0SRS01Z	0SPB09Z and 0SRB0J9	0SPB09Z and 0SRS0JA
0SPB08Z and 0SRS039	0SPB09Z and 0SRB0JA	0SPB09Z and 0SRS0JZ
0SPB08Z and 0SRS03A	0SPB09Z and 0SRB0JZ	0SPB09Z and 0SUB09Z
0SPB08Z and 0SRS03Z	0SPB09Z and 0SRE009	0SPB09Z and 0SUB09Z
0SPB08Z and 0SRS0J9	0SPB09Z and 0SRE00A	0SPB09Z and 0SUE09Z
0SPB08Z and 0SRS0JA	0SPB09Z and 0SRE00Z	0SPB09Z and 0SUE09Z
0SPB08Z and 0SRS0JZ	0SPB09Z and 0SRE019	0SPB09Z and 0SUS09Z
0SPB08Z and 0SUB09Z	0SPB09Z and 0SRE01A	0SPB09Z and 0SUS09Z
0SPB08Z and 0SUE09Z	0SPB09Z and 0SRE01Z	0SPB0BZ and 0SRB019
0SPB08Z and 0SUS09Z	0SPB09Z and 0SRE039	0SPB0BZ and 0SRB01A
0SPB09Z and 0SRB019	0SPB09Z and 0SRE03A	0SPB0BZ and 0SRB01Z
0SPB09Z and 0SRB01A	0SPB09Z and 0SRE03Z	0SPB0BZ and 0SRB029
0SPB09Z and 0SRB01Z	0SPB09Z and 0SRE0J9	0SPB0BZ and 0SRB02A
0SPB09Z and 0SRB029	0SPB09Z and 0SRE0JA	0SPB0BZ and 0SRB02Z
0SPB09Z and 0SRB02A	0SPB09Z and 0SRE0JZ	0SPB0BZ and 0SRB039
0SPB09Z and 0SRB02Z	0SPB09Z and 0SRS019	0SPB0BZ and 0SRB03A

0SPB0BZ and 0SRB03Z	0SPB0BZ and 0SRS039	0SPB0JZ and 0SRB0JA	0SPB0JZ and 0SRS0JZ	0SPB48Z and 0SRE039	0SPB4JZ and 0SRB02A	0SPB4JZ and 0SRE0JZ
0SPB0BZ and 0SRB049	0SPB0BZ and 0SRS03A	0SPB0JZ and 0SRB0JZ	0SPB48Z and 0SRB019	0SPB48Z and 0SRE03A	0SPB4JZ and 0SRB02Z	0SPB4JZ and 0SRS019
0SPB0BZ and 0SRB04A	0SPB0BZ and 0SRS03Z	0SPB0JZ and 0SRE009	0SPB48Z and 0SRB01A	0SPB48Z and 0SRE03Z	0SPB4JZ and 0SRB039	0SPB4JZ and 0SRS01A
0SPB0BZ and 0SRB04Z	0SPB0BZ and 0SRS0J9	0SPB0JZ and 0SRE00A	0SPB48Z and 0SRB01Z	0SPB48Z and 0SRE0J9	0SPB4JZ and 0SRB03A	0SPB4JZ and 0SRS01Z
0SPB0BZ and 0SRB0J9	0SPB0BZ and 0SRS0JA	0SPB0JZ and 0SRE00Z	0SPB48Z and 0SRB029	0SPB48Z and 0SRE0JA	0SPB4JZ and 0SRB03Z	0SPB4JZ and 0SRS039
0SPB0BZ and 0SRB0JA	0SPB0BZ and 0SRS0JZ	0SPB0JZ and 0SRE019	0SPB48Z and 0SRB02A	0SPB48Z and 0SRE0JZ	0SPB4JZ and 0SRB049	0SPB4JZ and 0SRS03A
0SPB0BZ and 0SRB0JZ	0SPB0BZ and 0SUB09Z	0SPB0JZ and 0SRE01A	0SPB48Z and 0SRB02Z	0SPB48Z and 0SRS019	0SPB4JZ and 0SRB04A	0SPB4JZ and 0SRS03Z
0SPB0BZ and 0SRE009	0SPB0BZ and 0SUE09Z	0SPB0JZ and 0SRE01Z	0SPB48Z and 0SRB039	0SPB48Z and 0SRS01A	0SPB4JZ and 0SRB04Z	0SPB4JZ and 0SRS0J9
0SPB0BZ and 0SRE00A	0SPB0BZ and 0SUS09Z	0SPB0JZ and 0SRE039	0SPB48Z and 0SRB03A	0SPB48Z and 0SRS01Z	0SPB4JZ and 0SRB0J9	0SPB4JZ and 0SRS0JA
0SPB0BZ and 0SRE00Z	0SPB0JZ and 0SRB019	0SPB0JZ and 0SRE03A	0SPB48Z and 0SRB03Z	0SPB48Z and 0SRS039	0SPB4JZ and 0SRB0JA	0SPB4JZ and 0SRS0JZ
0SPB0BZ and 0SRE019	0SPB0JZ and 0SRB01A	0SPB0JZ and 0SRE03Z	0SPB48Z and 0SRB049	0SPB48Z and 0SRS03A	0SPB4JZ and 0SRB0JZ	0SPB4JZ and 0SUB09Z
0SPB0BZ and 0SRE01A	0SPB0JZ and 0SRB01Z	0SPB0JZ and 0SRE0J9	0SPB48Z and 0SRB04A	0SPB48Z and 0SRS03Z	0SPB4JZ and 0SRE009	0SPB4JZ and 0SUE09Z
0SPB0BZ and 0SRE01Z	0SPB0JZ and 0SRB029	0SPB0JZ and 0SRE0JA	0SPB48Z and 0SRB04Z	0SPB48Z and 0SRS0J9	0SPB4JZ and 0SRE00A	0SPB4JZ and 0SUS09Z
0SPB0BZ and 0SRE039	0SPB0JZ and 0SRB02A	0SPB0JZ and 0SRE0JZ	0SPB48Z and 0SRB0J9	0SPB48Z and 0SRS0JA	0SPB4JZ and 0SRE00Z	0SPC08Z and 0SRC0J9
0SPB0BZ and 0SRE03A	0SPB0JZ and 0SRB02Z	0SPB0JZ and 0SRS019	0SPB48Z and 0SRB0JA	0SPB48Z and 0SRS0JZ	0SPB4JZ and 0SRE019	0SPC08Z and 0SRC0JA
0SPB0BZ and 0SRE03Z	0SPB0JZ and 0SRB039	0SPB0JZ and 0SRS01A	0SPB48Z and 0SRB0JZ	0SPB48Z and 0SUB09Z	0SPB4JZ and 0SRE01A	0SPC08Z and 0SRC0JZ
0SPB0BZ and 0SRE0J9	0SPB0JZ and 0SRB03A	0SPB0JZ and 0SRS01Z	0SPB48Z and 0SRE009	0SPB48Z and 0SUE09Z	0SPB4JZ and 0SRE01Z	0SPC08Z and 0SRT0J9
0SPB0BZ and 0SRE0JA	0SPB0JZ and 0SRB03Z	0SPB0JZ and 0SRS039	0SPB48Z and 0SRE00A	0SPB48Z and 0SUS09Z	0SPB4JZ and 0SRE039	0SPC08Z and 0SRT0JA
0SPB0BZ and 0SRE0JZ	0SPB0JZ and 0SRB049	0SPB0JZ and 0SRS03A	0SPB48Z and 0SRE00Z	0SPB4JZ and 0SRB019	0SPB4JZ and 0SRE03A	0SPC08Z and 0SRT0JZ
0SPB0BZ and 0SRS019	0SPB0JZ and 0SRB04A	0SPB0JZ and 0SRS03Z	0SPB48Z and 0SRE019	0SPB4JZ and 0SRB01A	0SPB4JZ and 0SRE03Z	0SPC08Z and 0SRV0J9
0SPB0BZ and 0SRS01A	0SPB0JZ and 0SRB04Z	0SPB0JZ and 0SRS0J9	0SPB48Z and 0SRE01A	0SPB4JZ and 0SRB01Z	0SPB4JZ and 0SRE0J9	0SPC08Z and 0SRV0JA
0SPB0BZ and 0SRS01Z	0SPB0JZ and 0SRB0J9	0SPB0JZ and 0SRS0JA	0SPB48Z and 0SRE01Z	0SPB4JZ and 0SRB029	0SPB4JZ and 0SRE0JA	0SPC08Z and 0SRV0JZ

0SPC09Z and 0SRC0J9	0SPC0JZ and 0SRC0J9	0SPC48Z and 0SRC0JA	0SPC4JZ and 0SRT0JA	0SPD09Z and 0SRT0JA	0SPD0JZ and 0SRU0JZ	0SPD48Z and 0SRW0JZ
0SPC09Z and 0SRC0JA	0SPC0JZ and 0SRC0JA	0SPC48Z and 0SRC0JZ	0SPC4JZ and 0SRT0JZ	0SPD09Z and 0SRT0JZ	0SPD0JZ and 0SRW0J9	0SPD4JC and 0SRD0J9
0SPC09Z and 0SRC0JZ	0SPC0JZ and 0SRC0JZ	0SPC48Z and 0SRT0J9	0SPC4JZ and 0SRV0J9	0SPD09Z and 0SRV0J9	0SPD0JZ and 0SRW0JA	0SPD4JC and 0SRD0JA
0SPC09Z and 0SRC0L9	0SPC0JZ and 0SRC0L9	0SPC48Z and 0SRT0JA	0SPC4JZ and 0SRV0JA	0SPD09Z and 0SRV0JA	0SPD0JZ and 0SRW0JZ	0SPD4JC and 0SRD0JZ
0SPC09Z and 0SRC0LA	0SPC0JZ and 0SRC0LA	0SPC48Z and 0SRT0JZ	0SPC4JZ and 0SRV0JZ	0SPD09Z and 0SRV0JZ	0SPD38Z and 0SRD0J9	0SPD4JC and 0SRU0J9
0SPC09Z and 0SRC0LZ	0SPC0JZ and 0SRC0LZ	0SPC48Z and 0SRV0J9	0SPD08Z and 0SRD0J9	0SPD09Z and 0SUW09Z	0SPD38Z and 0SRD0JA	0SPD4JC and 0SRU0JA
0SPC09Z and 0SRT0J9	0SPC0JZ and 0SRT0J9	0SPC48Z and 0SRV0JA	0SPD08Z and 0SRD0JA	0SPD0JC and 0SRD0J9	0SPD38Z and 0SRD0JZ	0SPD4JC and 0SRW0J9
0SPC09Z and 0SRT0JA	0SPC0JZ and 0SRT0JA	0SPC48Z and 0SRV0JZ	0SPD08Z and 0SRD0JZ	0SPD0JC and 0SRD0JA	0SPD38Z and 0SRD0JZ	0SPD4JC and 0SRW0JA
0SPC09Z and 0SRT0JZ	0SPC0JZ and 0SRT0JZ	0SPC4JC and 0SRC0J9	0SPD08Z and 0SRU0J9	0SPD0JC and 0SRD0JZ	0SPD38Z and 0SRU0J9	0SPD4JC and 0SRW0JZ
0SPC09Z and 0SRV0J9	0SPC0JZ and 0SRV0J9	0SPC4JC and 0SRC0JA	0SPD08Z and 0SRU0JA	0SPD0JC and 0SRU0J9	0SPD38Z and 0SRU0JA	0SPD4JZ and 0SRD0J9
0SPC09Z and 0SRV0JA	0SPC0JZ and 0SRV0JA	0SPC4JC and 0SRC0JZ	0SPD08Z and 0SRU0JZ	0SPD0JC and 0SRU0JA	0SPD38Z and 0SRU0JZ	0SPD4JZ and 0SRD0JA
0SPC09Z and 0SRV0JZ	0SPC0JZ and 0SRV0JZ	0SPC4JC and 0SRT0J9	0SPD08Z and 0SRW0J9	0SPD0JC and 0SRU0JZ	0SPD38Z and 0SRW0J9	0SPD4JZ and 0SRD0JZ
0SPC09Z and 0SUV09Z	0SPC38Z and 0SRC0J9	0SPC4JC and 0SRT0JA	0SPD08Z and 0SRW0JA	0SPD0JC and 0SRW0J9	0SPD38Z and 0SRW0JA	0SPD4JZ and 0SRD0L9
0SPC0JC and 0SRC0J9	0SPC38Z and 0SRC0JA	0SPC4JC and 0SRV0J9	0SPD08Z and 0SRW0JZ	0SPD0JC and 0SRW0JA	0SPD38Z and 0SRW0JZ	0SPD4JZ and 0SRD0LA
0SPC0JC and 0SRC0JA	0SPC38Z and 0SRC0JZ	0SPC4JC and 0SRV0JA	0SPD09Z and 0SRD0J9	0SPD0JC and 0SRW0JZ	0SPD48Z and 0SRD0J9	0SPD4JZ and 0SRD0LZ
0SPC0JC and 0SRC0JZ	0SPC38Z and 0SRT0J9	0SPC4JZ and 0SRC0J9	0SPD09Z and 0SRD0JA	0SPD0JZ and 0SRD0J9	0SPD48Z and 0SRD0JA	0SPD4JZ and 0SRU0J9
0SPC0JC and 0SRT0J9	0SPC38Z and 0SRT0JA	0SPC4JZ and 0SRC0JA	0SPD09Z and 0SRD0JZ	0SPD0JZ and 0SRD0JA	0SPD48Z and 0SRD0JZ	0SPD4JZ and 0SRU0JA
0SPC0JC and 0SRT0JA	0SPC38Z and 0SRT0JZ	0SPC4JZ and 0SRC0JZ	0SPD09Z and 0SRD0L9	0SPD0JZ and 0SRD0JZ	0SPD48Z and 0SRU0J9	0SPD4JZ and 0SRU0JZ
0SPC0JC and 0SRT0JZ	0SPC38Z and 0SRV0J9	0SPC4JZ and 0SRC0L9	0SPD09Z and 0SRD0LA	0SPD0JZ and 0SRD0L9	0SPD48Z and 0SRU0JA	0SPD4JZ and 0SRW0J9
0SPC0JC and 0SRV0J9	0SPC38Z and 0SRV0JA	0SPC4JZ and 0SRC0LA	0SPD09Z and 0SRD0LZ	0SPD0JZ and 0SRD0LA	0SPD48Z and 0SRU0JZ	0SPD4JZ and 0SRW0JA
0SPC0JC and 0SRV0JA	0SPC38Z and 0SRV0JZ	0SPC4JZ and 0SRC0LZ	0SPD09Z and 0SRU0JA	0SPD0JZ and 0SRD0LZ	0SPD48Z and 0SRW0J9	0SPD4JZ and 0SRW0JZ
0SPC0JC and 0SRV0JZ	0SPC48Z and 0SRC0J9	0SPC4JZ and 0SRT0J9		0SPD0JZ and 0SRU0J9	0SPD48Z and 0SRW0JA	0SPE0JZ and 0SRB019
				0SPD0JZ and 0SRU0JA		

0SPE0JZ and 0SRB01A	0SPE0JZ and 0SRE03Z	0SPE4JZ and 0SRB049	0SPE4JZ and 0SRS03A	0SPR0JZ and 0SR90JZ	0SPR4JZ and 0SR9019	0SPR4JZ and 0SRA03A
0SPE0JZ and 0SRB01Z	0SPE0JZ and 0SRE0J9	0SPE4JZ and 0SRB04A	0SPE4JZ and 0SRS03Z	0SPR0JZ and 0SRA009	0SPR4JZ and 0SR901A	0SPR4JZ and 0SRA03Z
0SPE0JZ and 0SRB029	0SPE0JZ and 0SRE0JA	0SPE4JZ and 0SRB04Z	0SPE4JZ and 0SRS0J9	0SPR0JZ and 0SRA00A	0SPR4JZ and 0SR901Z	0SPR4JZ and 0SRA0J9
0SPE0JZ and 0SRB02A	0SPE0JZ and 0SRE0JZ	0SPE4JZ and 0SRB0J9	0SPE4JZ and 0SRS0JA	0SPR0JZ and 0SRA00Z	0SPR4JZ and 0SR9029	0SPR4JZ and 0SRA0JA
0SPE0JZ and 0SRB02Z	0SPE0JZ and 0SRS019	0SPE4JZ and 0SRB0JA	0SPE4JZ and 0SRS0JZ	0SPR0JZ and 0SRA019	0SPR4JZ and 0SR902A	0SPR4JZ and 0SRA0JZ
0SPE0JZ and 0SRB039	0SPE0JZ and 0SRS01A	0SPE4JZ and 0SRB0JZ	0SPE4JZ and 0SUB09Z	0SPR0JZ and 0SRA01A	0SPR4JZ and 0SR902Z	0SPR4JZ and 0SRR019
0SPE0JZ and 0SRB03A	0SPE0JZ and 0SRS01Z	0SPE4JZ and 0SRE009	0SPE4JZ and 0SUE09Z	0SPR0JZ and 0SRA01Z	0SPR4JZ and 0SR9039	0SPR4JZ and 0SRR01A
0SPE0JZ and 0SRB03Z	0SPE0JZ and 0SRS039	0SPE4JZ and 0SRE00A	0SPE4JZ and 0SUS09Z	0SPR0JZ and 0SRA039	0SPR4JZ and 0SR903A	0SPR4JZ and 0SRR01Z
0SPE0JZ and 0SRB049	0SPE0JZ and 0SRS03A	0SPE4JZ and 0SRE00Z	0SPR0JZ and 0SR9019	0SPR0JZ and 0SRA03A	0SPR4JZ and 0SR903Z	0SPR4JZ and 0SRR039
0SPE0JZ and 0SRB04A	0SPE0JZ and 0SRS03Z	0SPE4JZ and 0SRE019	0SPR0JZ and 0SR901A	0SPR0JZ and 0SRA03Z	0SPR4JZ and 0SR9049	0SPR4JZ and 0SRR03A
0SPE0JZ and 0SRB04Z	0SPE0JZ and 0SRS0J9	0SPE4JZ and 0SRE01A	0SPR0JZ and 0SR901Z	0SPR0JZ and 0SRA0J9	0SPR4JZ and 0SR904A	0SPR4JZ and 0SRR03Z
0SPE0JZ and 0SRB0J9	0SPE0JZ and 0SRS0JA	0SPE4JZ and 0SRE01Z	0SPR0JZ and 0SR9029	0SPR0JZ and 0SRA0JA	0SPR4JZ and 0SR904Z	0SPR4JZ and 0SRR0J9
0SPE0JZ and 0SRB0JA	0SPE0JZ and 0SRS0JZ	0SPE4JZ and 0SRE039	0SPR0JZ and 0SR902A	0SPR0JZ and 0SRA0JZ	0SPR4JZ and 0SR90J9	0SPR4JZ and 0SRR0JA
0SPE0JZ and 0SRB0JZ	0SPE4JZ and 0SRB019	0SPE4JZ and 0SRE03A	0SPR0JZ and 0SR902Z	0SPR0JZ and 0SRR019	0SPR4JZ and 0SR90JA	0SPR4JZ and 0SRR0JZ
0SPE0JZ and 0SRE009	0SPE4JZ and 0SRB01A	0SPE4JZ and 0SRE03Z	0SPR0JZ and 0SR9039	0SPR0JZ and 0SRR01A	0SPR4JZ and 0SR90JZ	0SPR4JZ and 0SU909Z
0SPE0JZ and 0SRE00A	0SPE4JZ and 0SRB01Z	0SPE4JZ and 0SRE0J9	0SPR0JZ and 0SR903A	0SPR0JZ and 0SRR01Z	0SPR4JZ and 0SRA009	0SPR4JZ and 0SUA09Z
0SPE0JZ and 0SRE00Z	0SPE4JZ and 0SRB029	0SPE4JZ and 0SRE0JA	0SPR0JZ and 0SR903Z	0SPR0JZ and 0SRR039	0SPR4JZ and 0SRA00A	0SPR4JZ and 0SUR09Z
0SPE0JZ and 0SRE019	0SPE4JZ and 0SRB02A	0SPE4JZ and 0SRE0JZ	0SPR0JZ and 0SR9049	0SPR0JZ and 0SRR03A	0SPR4JZ and 0SRA00Z	0SPS0JZ and 0SRB019
0SPE0JZ and 0SRE01A	0SPE4JZ and 0SRB02Z	0SPE4JZ and 0SRS019	0SPR0JZ and 0SR904A	0SPR0JZ and 0SRR03Z	0SPR4JZ and 0SRA019	0SPS0JZ and 0SRB01A
0SPE0JZ and 0SRE01Z	0SPE4JZ and 0SRB039	0SPE4JZ and 0SRS01A	0SPR0JZ and 0SR904Z	0SPR0JZ and 0SRR0J9	0SPR4JZ and 0SRA01A	0SPS0JZ and 0SRB01Z
0SPE0JZ and 0SRE039	0SPE4JZ and 0SRB03A	0SPE4JZ and 0SRS01Z	0SPR0JZ and 0SR90J9	0SPR0JZ and 0SRR0JA	0SPR4JZ and 0SRA01Z	0SPS0JZ and 0SRB029
0SPE0JZ and 0SRE03A	0SPE4JZ and 0SRB03Z	0SPE4JZ and 0SRS039	0SPR0JZ and 0SR90JA	0SPR0JZ and 0SRR0JZ	0SPR4JZ and 0SRA039	0SPS0JZ and 0SRB02A

0SPS0JZ and 0SRB02Z

0SPS0JZ and 0SRB039

0SPS0JZ and 0SRB03A

0SPS0JZ and 0SRB03Z

0SPS0JZ and 0SRB049

0SPS0JZ and 0SRB04A

0SPS0JZ and 0SRB04Z

0SPS0JZ and 0SRB0J9

0SPS0JZ and 0SRB0JA

0SPS0JZ and 0SRB0JZ

0SPS0JZ and 0SRE009

0SPS0JZ and 0SRE00A

0SPS0JZ and 0SRE00Z

0SPS0JZ and 0SRE019

0SPS0JZ and 0SRE01A

0SPS0JZ and 0SRE01Z

0SPS0JZ and 0SRE039

0SPS0JZ and 0SRE03A

0SPS0JZ and 0SRE03Z

0SPS0JZ and 0SRE0J9

0SPS0JZ and 0SRE0JA

0SPS0JZ and 0SRE0JZ

0SPS0JZ and 0SRS019

0SPS0JZ and 0SRS01A

0SPS0JZ and 0SRS01Z

0SPS0JZ and 0SRS039

0SPS0JZ and 0SRS03A

0SPS0JZ and 0SRS03Z

0SPS0JZ and 0SRS0J9

0SPS0JZ and 0SRS0JA

0SPS0JZ and 0SRS0JZ

0SPS4JZ and 0SRB019

0SPS4JZ and 0SRB01A

0SPS4JZ and 0SRB01Z

0SPS4JZ and 0SRB029

0SPS4JZ and 0SRB02A

0SPS4JZ and 0SRB02Z

0SPS4JZ and 0SRB039

0SPS4JZ and 0SRB03A

0SPS4JZ and 0SRB03Z

0SPS4JZ and 0SRB049

0SPS4JZ and 0SRB04A

0SPS4JZ and 0SRB04Z

0SPS4JZ and 0SRB0J9

0SPS4JZ and 0SRB0JA

0SPS4JZ and 0SRB0JZ

0SPS4JZ and 0SRE009

0SPS4JZ and 0SRE00A

0SPS4JZ and 0SRE00Z

0SPS4JZ and 0SRE019

0SPS4JZ and 0SRE01A

0SPS4JZ and 0SRE01Z

0SPS4JZ and 0SRE039

0SPS4JZ and 0SRE03A

0SPS4JZ and 0SRE03Z

0SPS4JZ and 0SRE0J9

0SPS4JZ and 0SRE0JA

0SPS4JZ and 0SRE0JZ

0SPS4JZ and 0SRS019

0SPS4JZ and 0SRS01A

0SPS4JZ and 0SRS01Z

0SPS4JZ and 0SRS039

0SPS4JZ and 0SRS03A

0SPS4JZ and 0SRS03Z

0SPS4JZ and 0SRS0J9

0SPS4JZ and 0SRS0JA

0SPS4JZ and 0SRS0JZ

0SPS4JZ and 0SUB09Z

0SPS4JZ and 0SUE09Z

0SPS4JZ and 0SUS09Z

0SPT0JZ and 0SRC0J9

0SPT0JZ and 0SRC0JA

0SPT0JZ and 0SRC0JZ

0SPT0JZ and 0SRT0J9

0SPT0JZ and 0SRT0JA

0SPT0JZ and 0SRT0JZ

0SPT0JZ and 0SRV0J9

0SPT0JZ and 0SRV0JA

0SPT0JZ and 0SRV0JZ

0SPT4JZ and 0SRC0J9

0SPT4JZ and 0SRC0JA

0SPT4JZ and 0SRC0JZ

0SPT4JZ and 0SRT0J9

0SPT4JZ and 0SRT0JA

0SPT4JZ and 0SRV0J9

0SPT4JZ and 0SRV0JA

0SPU0JZ and 0SRD0J9

0SPU0JZ and 0SRD0JA

0SPU0JZ and 0SRD0JZ

0SPU0JZ and 0SRU0J9

0SPU0JZ and 0SRU0JA

0SPU0JZ and 0SRU0JZ

0SPU0JZ and 0SRW0J9

0SPU0JZ and 0SRW0JA

0SPU0JZ and 0SRW0JZ

0SPU4JZ and 0SRD0J9

0SPU4JZ and 0SRD0JA

0SPU4JZ and 0SRD0JZ

0SPU4JZ and 0SRU0J9

0SPU4JZ and 0SRU0JA

0SPU4JZ and 0SRV0JZ

0SPU4JZ and 0SRW0J9

0SPU4JZ and 0SRW0JA

0SPU4JZ and 0SRW0JZ

0SPV0JZ and 0SRC0J9

0SPV0JZ and 0SRC0JA

0SPV0JZ and 0SRC0JZ

0SPV0JZ and 0SRT0J9

0SPV0JZ and 0SRT0JA

0SPV0JZ and 0SRV0J9

0SPV0JZ and 0SRV0JA

0SPV0JZ and 0SRV0JZ

0SPV4JZ and 0SRC0J9

0SPV4JZ and 0SRC0JA

0SPV4JZ and 0SRC0JZ

0SPV4JZ and 0SRT0J9

0SPV4JZ and 0SRT0JA

0SPV4JZ and 0SRV0J9

0SPV4JZ and 0SRV0JZ

0SPW0JZ and 0SRD0J9

0SPW0JZ and 0SRD0JA

0SPW0JZ and 0SRD0JZ

0SPW0JZ and 0SRU0J9

0SPW0JZ and 0SRU0JA

0SPW0JZ and 0SRU0JZ

0SPW0JZ and 0SRW0J9

0SPW0JZ and 0SRW0JA

0SPW0JZ and 0SRW0JZ

0SPW4JZ and 0SRD0J9

0SPW4JZ and 0SRD0JA

0SPW4JZ and 0SRD0JZ

0SPW4JZ and 0SRU0J9

0SPW4JZ and 0SRU0JA

0SPW4JZ and 0SRW0J9

0SPW4JZ and 0SRW0JA

0SPW4JZ and 0SRW0JZ

0TQB0ZZ and 0WQFXZ2

0TQB0ZZ and 0WQFXZZ

0TQB3ZZ and 0WQFXZ2

0TQB3ZZ and 0WQFXZZ

0TQB4ZZ and 0WQFXZ2

0TQB4ZZ and 0WQFXZZ

0TTB0ZZ
and 0TTD0ZZ
and 0UT20ZZ
and 0UT70ZZ
and 0UT90ZZ
and 0UTC0ZZ
and 0UTG0ZZ

0TY00Z0 and 0FYG0Z0

0TY00Z0 and 0FYG0Z1

0TY00Z0 and 0FYG0Z2

0TY00Z1 and 0FYG0Z0

0TY00Z1 and 0FYG0Z1

0TY00Z1 and 0FYG0Z2

0TY00Z2 and 0FYG0Z0

0TY00Z2 and 0FYG0Z1

0TY00Z2 and 0FYG0Z2

0TY10Z0
and 0FYG0Z0

0TY10Z0
and 0FYG0Z1

0TY10Z0
and 0FYG0Z2

0TY10Z1
and 0FYG0Z0

0TY10Z1
and 0FYG0Z1

0TY10Z1
and 0FYG0Z2

0TY10Z2
and 0FYG0Z0

0TY10Z2
and 0FYG0Z1

0TY10Z2
and 0FYG0Z2

0UT40ZZ
and 0UT90ZZ
and 0UTC0ZZ

0UT44ZZ
and 0UT94ZZ
and 0UTC4ZZ

0UT44ZZ
and 0UT9FZZ
and 0UTC4ZZ

0UT47ZZ
and 0UT97ZZ
and 0UTC7ZZ

0UT47ZZ
and 0UT97ZZ
and 0UTC8ZZ

0UT47ZZ
and 0UT98ZZ
and 0UTC7ZZ

0UT47ZZ
and 0UT98ZZ
and 0UTC8ZZ

0UT48ZZ
and 0UT97ZZ
and 0UTC7ZZ

0UT48ZZ
and 0UT97ZZ
and 0UTC8ZZ

0UT48ZZ
and 0UT98ZZ
and 0UTC7ZZ

0UT48ZZ
and 0UT98ZZ
and 0UTC8ZZ

0VT00ZZ
and 0VT30ZZ

0VT00ZZ
and 0VT34ZZ

0VT04ZZ
and 0VT30ZZ

0VT04ZZ
and 0VT34ZZ

0VT07ZZ
and 0VT30ZZ

0VT07ZZ
and 0VT34ZZ

0VT08ZZ
and 0VT30ZZ

0VT08ZZ
and 0VT34ZZ

One of
0RG7070
0RG70A0
0RG70J0
0RG70K0
0RG70Z0
0RG7370
0RG73A0
0RG73J0
0RG73K0
0RG73Z0
0RG7470
0RG74A0
0RG74J0
0RG74K0
0RG74Z0

---

with one of
0SG1070
0SG10A0
0SG10J0
0SG10K0
0SG10Z0
0SG1370
0SG13A0
0SG13J0
0SG13K0
0SG13Z0
0SG1470
0SG14A0
0SG14J0
0SG14K0
0SG14Z0

One of
0RG7071
0RG707J
0RG70AJ
0RG70J1
0RG70JJ
0RG70K1
0RG70KJ
0RG70Z1
0RG70ZJ
0RG7371

0RG737J
0RG73AJ
0RG73J1
0RG73JJ
0RG73K1
0RG73KJ
0RG73Z1
0RG73ZJ
0RG7471
0RG747J
0RG74AJ
0RG74J1
0RG74JJ
0RG74K1
0RG74KJ
0RG74Z1
0RG74ZJ
XRG7092

with one of
0SG1071
0SG107J
0SG10AJ
0SG10J1
0SG10JJ
0SG10K1
0SG10KJ
0SG10Z1

0SG10ZJ
0SG1371
0SG137J
0SG13AJ
0SG13J1
0SG13JJ
0SG13K1
0SG13KJ
0SG13Z1
0SG13ZJ
0SG1471
0SG147J
0SG14AJ
0SG14J1
0SG14JJ
0SG14K1
0SG14KJ
0SG14Z1
0SG14ZJ
XRGC092

Appendix H: Non-OR Not Affecting MS-DRG Assignment

00160ZB	005D3ZZ	008F3ZZ	00920ZX	00990ZX	009H0ZX	00B83ZX	00BM3ZX	00C14ZZ	00CP4ZZ	00DR4ZZ
00163ZB	005D4ZZ	008F4ZZ	00920ZZ	00990ZZ	009H0ZZ	00B84ZX	00BM3ZZ	00C20ZZ	00CQ0ZZ	00DS0ZZ
0016470	005F0ZZ	008G0ZZ	009230Z	009930Z	009H30Z	00B93ZX	00BM4ZX	00C23ZZ	00CQ3ZZ	00DS3ZZ
0016471	005F3ZZ	008G3ZZ	00923ZX	00993ZX	009H3ZX	00B94ZX	00BM4ZZ	00C24ZZ	00CQ4ZZ	00DS4ZZ
0016472	005F4ZZ	008G4ZZ	00923ZZ	00993ZZ	009H3ZZ	00BA3ZX	00BN0ZX	00C30ZZ	00CR0ZZ	00DT0ZZ
0016473	005G0ZZ	008H0ZZ	009240Z	009940Z	009H40Z	00BA4ZX	00BN0ZZ	00C33ZZ	00CR3ZZ	00DT3ZZ
0016474	005G3ZZ	008H3ZZ	00924ZX	00994ZX	009H4ZX	00BA4ZZ	00BN3ZX	00C34ZZ	00CR4ZZ	00DT4ZZ
0016475	005G4ZZ	008H4ZZ	00924ZZ	00994ZZ	009H4ZZ	00BB0ZX	00BN3ZZ	00C40ZZ	00CS0ZZ	00F30ZZ
0016476	005H0ZZ	008J0ZZ	009300Z	009A00Z	009J00Z	00BB0ZZ	00BN4ZX	00C43ZZ	00CS3ZZ	00F33ZZ
0016477	005H3ZZ	008J3ZZ	00930ZX	009A0ZX	009J0ZX	00BB3ZX	00BN4ZZ	00C44ZZ	00CS4ZZ	00F34ZZ
0016478	005H4ZZ	008J4ZZ	00930ZZ	009A0ZZ	009J0ZZ	00BB3ZZ	00BP0ZX	00C50ZZ	00CT0ZZ	00F3XZZ
001647B	005J0ZZ	008K0ZZ	009330Z	009A30Z	009J30Z	00BB4ZX	00BP0ZZ	00C53ZZ	00CT3ZZ	00F40ZZ
00164J0	005J3ZZ	008K3ZZ	00933ZX	009A3ZX	009J3ZX	00BB4ZZ	00BP3ZX	00C54ZZ	00CT4ZZ	00F43ZZ
00164J1	005J4ZZ	008K4ZZ	00933ZZ	009A3ZZ	009J3ZZ	00BC0ZX	00BP3ZZ	00C60ZZ	00CU0ZZ	00F44ZZ
00164J2	005K0ZZ	008L0ZZ	009340Z	009A40Z	009J40Z	00BC0ZZ	00BP4ZX	00C63ZZ	00CU3ZZ	00F4XZZ
00164J3	005K3ZZ	008L3ZZ	00934ZX	009A4ZX	009J4ZX	00BC3ZX	00BP4ZZ	00C64ZZ	00CU4ZZ	00F50ZZ
00164J4	005K4ZZ	008L4ZZ	00934ZZ	009A4ZZ	009J4ZZ	00BC3ZZ	00BQ0ZX	00C70ZZ	00CW0ZZ	00F5XZZ
00164J5	005L0ZZ	008M0ZZ	009400Z	009B00Z	009K00Z	00BC4ZX	00BQ0ZZ	00C73ZZ	00CW3ZZ	00F6XZZ
00164J6	005L3ZZ	008M3ZZ	00940ZX	009B0ZX	009K0ZX	00BC4ZZ	00BQ3ZX	00C74ZZ	00CW4ZZ	00H004Z
00164J7	005L4ZZ	008M4ZZ	00940ZZ	009B0ZZ	009K0ZZ	00BD0ZX	00BQ3ZZ	00C80ZZ	00CX0ZZ	00H00YZ
00164J8	005M0ZZ	008N0ZZ	009430Z	009B30Z	009K30Z	00BD0ZZ	00BQ4ZX	00C83ZZ	00CX3ZZ	00H03YZ
00164JB	005M3ZZ	008N3ZZ	00943ZX	009B3ZX	009K3ZX	00BD3ZX	00BQ4ZZ	00C84ZZ	00CX4ZZ	00H04YZ
00164K0	005M4ZZ	008N4ZZ	00943ZZ	009B3ZZ	009K3ZZ	00BD3ZZ	00BR0ZX	00C90ZZ	00CY0ZZ	00H60YZ
00164K1	005N0ZZ	008P0ZZ	009440Z	009B40Z	009K40Z	00BD4ZX	00BR0ZZ	00C93ZZ	00CY3ZZ	00H63YZ
00164K2	005N3ZZ	008P3ZZ	00944ZX	009B4ZX	009K4ZX	00BD4ZZ	00BR3ZX	00C94ZZ	00CY4ZZ	00H64YZ
00164K3	005N4ZZ	008P4ZZ	00944ZZ	009B4ZZ	009K4ZZ	00BF0ZX	00BR3ZZ	00CA0ZZ	00D10ZZ	00HE0YZ
00164K4	005P0ZZ	008Q0ZZ	009500Z	009C00Z	009L00Z	00BF0ZZ	00BR4ZX	00CA3ZZ	00D13ZZ	00HE3YZ
00164K5	005P3ZZ	008Q3ZZ	00950ZX	009C0ZX	009L0ZX	00BF3ZX	00BR4ZZ	00CA4ZZ	00D14ZZ	00HE4YZ
00164K6	005P4ZZ	008Q4ZZ	00950ZZ	009C0ZZ	009L0ZZ	00BF3ZZ	00BS0ZX	00CB0ZZ	00D20ZZ	00HU03Z
00164K7	005Q0ZZ	008R0ZZ	009530Z	009C30Z	009L30Z	00BF4ZX	00BS0ZZ	00CB3ZZ	00D23ZZ	00HU0YZ
00164K8	005Q3ZZ	008R3ZZ	00953ZX	009C3ZX	009L3ZX	00BF4ZZ	00BS3ZX	00CB4ZZ	00D24ZZ	00HU33Z
00164KB	005Q4ZZ	008R4ZZ	00953ZZ	009C3ZZ	009L3ZZ	00BG0ZX	00BS3ZZ	00CC0ZZ	00DF0ZZ	00HU3YZ
00164ZB	005R0ZZ	008S0ZZ	009540Z	009C40Z	009L40Z	00BG0ZZ	00BS4ZX	00CC3ZZ	00DF3ZZ	00HU43Z
0020X0Z	005R3ZZ	008S3ZZ	00954ZX	009C4ZX	009L4ZX	00BG3ZX	00BS4ZZ	00CC4ZZ	00DF4ZZ	00HU4YZ
0020XYZ	005R4ZZ	008S4ZZ	00954ZZ	009C4ZZ	009L4ZZ	00BG3ZZ	00BT0ZX	00CD0ZZ	00DG0ZZ	00HV03Z
002EX0Z	005S0ZZ	008W0ZZ	009600Z	009D00Z	009M3ZX	00BG4ZX	00BT0ZZ	00CD3ZZ	00DG3ZZ	00HV0YZ
002EXYZ	005S3ZZ	008W3ZZ	00960ZX	009D0ZX	009M4ZX	00BG4ZZ	00BT3ZX	00CD4ZZ	00DG4ZZ	00HV33Z
002UX0Z	005S4ZZ	008W4ZZ	00960ZZ	009D0ZZ	009N3ZX	00BH0ZX	00BT3ZZ	00CF0ZZ	00DH0ZZ	00HV3YZ
002UXYZ	005T0ZZ	008X0ZZ	009630Z	009D30Z	009N4ZX	00BH0ZZ	00BT4ZX	00CF3ZZ	00DH3ZZ	00HV43Z
00523ZZ	005T3ZZ	008X3ZZ	00963ZX	009D3ZX	009P3ZX	00BH3ZX	00BT4ZZ	00CF4ZZ	00DH4ZZ	00HV4YZ
00524ZZ	005T4ZZ	008X4ZZ	00963ZZ	009D3ZZ	009P4ZX	00BH3ZZ	00BW0ZX	00CG0ZZ	00DJ0ZZ	00JE3ZZ
00560ZZ	005W0ZZ	008Y0ZZ	009640Z	009D40Z	009Q3ZX	00BH4ZX	00BW0ZZ	00CG3ZZ	00DJ3ZZ	00N10ZZ
00563ZZ	005W3ZZ	008Y3ZZ	00964ZX	009D4ZX	009Q4ZX	00BH4ZZ	00BW3ZX	00CG4ZZ	00DJ4ZZ	00N13ZZ
00564ZZ	005W4ZZ	008Y4ZZ	00964ZZ	009D4ZZ	009R3ZX	00BJ0ZX	00BW3ZZ	00CH0ZZ	00DK0ZZ	00N14ZZ
00570ZZ	005X0ZZ	009000Z	009700Z	009F00Z	009R4ZX	00BJ0ZZ	00BW4ZX	00CH3ZZ	00DK3ZZ	00N20ZZ
00573ZZ	005X3ZZ	00900ZX	00970ZX	009F0ZX	009S3ZX	00BJ3ZX	00BW4ZZ	00CH4ZZ	00DK4ZZ	00N23ZZ
00574ZZ	005X4ZZ	00900ZZ	00970ZZ	009F0ZZ	009S4ZX	00BJ3ZZ	00BX0ZX	00CJ0ZZ	00DL0ZZ	00N24ZZ
00580ZZ	005Y0ZZ	009030Z	009730Z	009F30Z	009U30Z	00BJ4ZX	00BX0ZZ	00CJ3ZZ	00DL3ZZ	00N60ZZ
00583ZZ	005Y3ZZ	00903ZX	00973ZX	009F3ZX	009U3ZX	00BJ4ZZ	00BX3ZX	00CJ4ZZ	00DL4ZZ	00N63ZZ
00584ZZ	005Y4ZZ	00903ZZ	00973ZZ	009F3ZZ	009U3ZZ	00BK0ZX	00BX3ZZ	00CK0ZZ	00DM0ZZ	00N64ZZ
00590ZZ	00760ZZ	009040Z	009740Z	009F40Z	009U40Z	00BK0ZZ	00BX4ZX	00CK3ZZ	00DM3ZZ	00N70ZZ
00593ZZ	00763ZZ	00904ZX	00974ZX	009F4ZX	009U4ZX	00BK3ZX	00BX4ZZ	00CK4ZZ	00DM4ZZ	00N73ZZ
00594ZZ	00764ZZ	00904ZZ	00974ZZ	009F4ZZ	009U4ZZ	00BK3ZZ	00BY0ZX	00CL0ZZ	00DN0ZZ	00N74ZZ
005A0ZZ	00800ZZ	009100Z	009800Z	009G00Z	00B03ZX	00BK4ZX	00BY0ZZ	00CL3ZZ	00DN3ZZ	00N80ZZ
005A3ZZ	00803ZZ	00910ZX	00980ZX	009G0ZX	00B04ZX	00BK4ZZ	00BY3ZX	00CL4ZZ	00DN4ZZ	00N83ZZ
005A4ZZ	00804ZZ	00910ZZ	00980ZZ	009G0ZZ	00B13ZX	00BL0ZX	00BY3ZZ	00CM0ZZ	00DP0ZZ	00N84ZZ
005B0ZZ	00870ZZ	009130Z	009830Z	009G30Z	00B14ZX	00BL0ZZ	00BY4ZX	00CM3ZZ	00DP3ZZ	00N90ZZ
005B3ZZ	00873ZZ	00913ZX	00983ZX	009G3ZX	00B23ZX	00BL3ZX	00BY4ZZ	00CM4ZZ	00DP4ZZ	00N93ZZ
005B4ZZ	00874ZZ	00913ZZ	00983ZZ	009G3ZZ	00B24ZX	00BL3ZZ	00C00ZZ	00CN0ZZ	00DQ0ZZ	00N94ZZ
005C0ZZ	00880ZZ	009140Z	009840Z	009G40Z	00B63ZX	00BL4ZX	00C03ZZ	00CN3ZZ	00DQ3ZZ	00NA0ZZ
005C3ZZ	00883ZZ	00914ZX	00984ZX	009G4ZX	00B64ZX	00BL4ZZ	00C04ZZ	00CN4ZZ	00DQ4ZZ	00NA3ZZ
005C4ZZ	00884ZZ	00914ZZ	00984ZZ	009G4ZZ	00B73ZX	00BM0ZX	00C10ZZ	00CP0ZZ	00DR0ZZ	00NA4ZZ
005D0ZZ	008F0ZZ	009200Z	009900Z	009H00Z	00B74ZX	00BM0ZZ	00C13ZZ	00CP3ZZ	00DR3ZZ	00NB0ZZ

00NB3ZZ	00P033Z	00PU0MZ	00Q94ZZ	00RM4JZ	00UG0KZ	00UP3KZ	00W0X3Z	00WU4JZ	00XG0ZJ	00XQ0ZS
00NB4ZZ	00P037Z	00PU0YZ	00QA0ZZ	00RM4KZ	00UG37Z	00UP47Z	00W0X7Z	00WU4MZ	00XG0ZK	00XQ4ZF
00NC0ZZ	00P03JZ	00PU30Z	00QA3ZZ	00RN07Z	00UG3JZ	00UP4JZ	00W0XJZ	00WU4YZ	00XG0ZL	00XQ4ZG
00NC3ZZ	00P03KZ	00PU33Z	00QA4ZZ	00RN0JZ	00UG3KZ	00UP4KZ	00W0XKZ	00WUX0Z	00XG0ZM	00XQ4ZH
00NC4ZZ	00P03MZ	00PU3JZ	00QB0ZZ	00RN0KZ	00UG47Z	00UQ07Z	00W0XMZ	00WUX2Z	00XG0ZN	00XQ4ZJ
00ND0ZZ	00P03YZ	00PU3MZ	00QB3ZZ	00RN47Z	00UG4JZ	00UQ0JZ	00W600Z	00WUX3Z	00XG0ZP	00XQ4ZK
00ND3ZZ	00P040Z	00PU3YZ	00QB4ZZ	00RN4JZ	00UG4KZ	00UQ0KZ	00W602Z	00WUXJZ	00XG0ZQ	00XQ4ZL
00ND4ZZ	00P042Z	00PU40Z	00QC0ZZ	00RN4KZ	00UH07Z	00UQ37Z	00W603Z	00WUXMZ	00XG0ZR	00XQ4ZM
00NF0ZZ	00P043Z	00PU42Z	00R107Z	00RP07Z	00UH0JZ	00UQ3JZ	00W60JZ	00WV00Z	00XG0ZS	00XQ4ZN
00NF3ZZ	00P047Z	00PU43Z	00R10JZ	00RP0JZ	00UH0KZ	00UQ3KZ	00W60MZ	00WV02Z	00XG4ZF	00XQ4ZP
00NF4ZZ	00P04JZ	00PU4JZ	00R10KZ	00RP0KZ	00UH37Z	00UQ47Z	00W60YZ	00WV03Z	00XG4ZG	00XQ4ZQ
00NG0ZZ	00P04KZ	00PU4MZ	00R147Z	00RP47Z	00UH3JZ	00UQ4JZ	00W630Z	00WV07Z	00XG4ZH	00XQ4ZR
00NG3ZZ	00P04MZ	00PU4YZ	00R14JZ	00RP4JZ	00UH3KZ	00UQ4KZ	00W632Z	00WV0JZ	00XG4ZJ	00XQ4ZS
00NG4ZZ	00P04YZ	00PUX0Z	00R14KZ	00RP4KZ	00UH47Z	00UR07Z	00W633Z	00WV0KZ	00XG4ZK	00XR0ZF
00NH0ZZ	00P0X0Z	00PUX2Z	00R207Z	00RQ07Z	00UH4JZ	00UR0JZ	00W63JZ	00WV0MZ	00XG4ZL	00XR0ZG
00NH3ZZ	00P0X2Z	00PUX3Z	00R20JZ	00RQ0JZ	00UH4KZ	00UR0KZ	00W63MZ	00WV0YZ	00XG4ZM	00XR0ZH
00NH4ZZ	00P0X3Z	00PUXMZ	00R20KZ	00RQ0KZ	00UJ07Z	00UR37Z	00W63YZ	00WV30Z	00XG4ZN	00XR0ZJ
00NJ0ZZ	00P0XMZ	00PV00Z	00R247Z	00RQ47Z	00UJ0JZ	00UR3JZ	00W640Z	00WV32Z	00XG4ZP	00XR0ZK
00NJ3ZZ	00P600Z	00PV02Z	00R24JZ	00RQ4JZ	00UJ0KZ	00UR3KZ	00W642Z	00WV33Z	00XG4ZQ	00XR0ZL
00NJ4ZZ	00P602Z	00PV03Z	00R24KZ	00RQ4KZ	00UJ37Z	00UR47Z	00W643Z	00WV37Z	00XG4ZR	00XR0ZM
00NK0ZZ	00P603Z	00PV07Z	00R607Z	00RR07Z	00UJ3JZ	00UR4JZ	00W64JZ	00WV3JZ	00XG4ZS	00XR0ZN
00NK3ZZ	00P60JZ	00PV0JZ	00R60JZ	00RR0JZ	00UJ3KZ	00UR4KZ	00W64MZ	00WV3KZ	00XH0ZF	00XR0ZP
00NK4ZZ	00P60MZ	00PV0KZ	00R60KZ	00RR0KZ	00UJ47Z	00US07Z	00W64YZ	00WV3MZ	00XH0ZG	00XR0ZQ
00NL0ZZ	00P60YZ	00PV0MZ	00R647Z	00RR47Z	00UJ4JZ	00US0JZ	00W6X0Z	00WV3YZ	00XH0ZH	00XR0ZR
00NL3ZZ	00P630Z	00PV0YZ	00R64JZ	00RR4JZ	00UJ4KZ	00US0KZ	00W6X2Z	00WV40Z	00XH0ZJ	00XR0ZS
00NL4ZZ	00P632Z	00PV0YZ	00R64KZ	00RR4KZ	00UK07Z	00US37Z	00W6X3Z	00WV42Z	00XH0ZK	00XR4ZF
00NM0ZZ	00P633Z	00PV30Z	00RF07Z	00RS07Z	00UK0JZ	00US3JZ	00W6XJZ	00WV43Z	00XH0ZL	00XR4ZG
00NM3ZZ	00P63JZ	00PV32Z	00RF0JZ	00RS0JZ	00UK0KZ	00US3KZ	00W6XMZ	00WV47Z	00XH0ZM	00XR4ZH
00NM4ZZ	00P63MZ	00PV33Z	00RF0KZ	00RS0KZ	00UK37Z	00US47Z	00WE00Z	00WV4JZ	00XH0ZN	00XR4ZJ
00NN0ZZ	00P63YZ	00PV37Z	00RF47Z	00RS47Z	00UK3JZ	00US4JZ	00WE02Z	00WV4KZ	00XH0ZP	00XR4ZK
00NN3ZZ	00P63JZ	00PV3JZ	00RF4JZ	00RS4JZ	00UK3KZ	00US4KZ	00WE03Z	00WV4MZ	00XH0ZQ	00XR4ZL
00NN4ZZ	00P642Z	00PV3KZ	00RF4KZ	00RS4KZ	00UK47Z	00UT07Z	00WE07Z	00WV4YZ	00XH0ZR	00XR4ZM
00NP0ZZ	00P643Z	00PV3MZ	00RG07Z	00RT07Z	00UK4JZ	00UT0JZ	00WE0MZ	00WVX0Z	00XH0ZS	00XR4ZN
00NP3ZZ	00P64JZ	00PV3YZ	00RG0JZ	00RT0JZ	00UK4KZ	00UT0KZ	00WE0YZ	00WVX2Z	00XH4ZF	00XR4ZP
00NP4ZZ	00P64MZ	00PV40Z	00RG0KZ	00RT0KZ	00UL07Z	00UT37Z	00WE30Z	00WVX3Z	00XH4ZG	00XR4ZQ
00NQ0ZZ	00P64YZ	00PV42Z	00RG47Z	00RT47Z	00UL0JZ	00UT3JZ	00WE32Z	00WVX7Z	00XH4ZH	00XR4ZR
00NQ3ZZ	00P6X0Z	00PV43Z	00RG4JZ	00RT4JZ	00UL0KZ	00UT3KZ	00WE33Z	00WVXJZ	00XH4ZJ	00XR4ZS
00NQ4ZZ	00P6X2Z	00PV47Z	00RG4KZ	00RT4KZ	00UL37Z	00UT47Z	00WE37Z	00WVXKZ	00XH4ZK	00XS0ZF
00NR0ZZ	00P6X3Z	00PV4JZ	00RH07Z	00U20JZ	00UL3JZ	00UT4JZ	00WE3MZ	00WVXMZ	00XH4ZL	00XS0ZG
00NR3ZZ	00P6XMZ	00PV4KZ	00RH0JZ	00U20KZ	00UL3KZ	00UT4KZ	00WE3YZ	00XF0ZF	00XH4ZM	00XS0ZH
00NR4ZZ	00PE00Z	00PV4MZ	00RH0KZ	00U237Z	00UL47Z	00WE00Z	00WE40Z	00XF0ZG	00XH4ZN	00XS0ZJ
00NS0ZZ	00PE02Z	00PV4YZ	00RH47Z	00U23JZ	00UL4JZ	00W002Z	00WE42Z	00XF0ZH	00XH4ZP	00XS0ZK
00NS3ZZ	00PE03Z	00PVX0Z	00RH4JZ	00U23KZ	00UL4KZ	00W003Z	00WE43Z	00XF0ZJ	00XH4ZQ	00XS0ZL
00NS4ZZ	00PE07Z	00PVX2Z	00RH4KZ	00U247Z	00UM07Z	00W007Z	00WE47Z	00XF0ZK	00XH4ZR	00XS0ZM
00NT0ZZ	00PE0MZ	00PVX3Z	00RJ07Z	00U24JZ	00UM0JZ	00W00JZ	00WE4MZ	00XF0ZL	00XH4ZS	00XS0ZN
00NT3ZZ	00PE0YZ	00PVXMZ	00RJ0JZ	00U24KZ	00UM0KZ	00W00KZ	00WE4YZ	00XF0ZM	00XJ0ZF	00XS0ZP
00NT4ZZ	00PE30Z	00Q00ZZ	00RJ0KZ	00U607Z	00UM37Z	00W00MZ	00WEX0Z	00XF0ZN	00XJ0ZG	00XS0ZQ
00NW0ZZ	00PE32Z	00Q03ZZ	00RJ47Z	00U60JZ	00UM3JZ	00W00YZ	00WEX2Z	00XF0ZP	00XJ0ZH	00XS0ZR
00NW3ZZ	00PE33Z	00Q04ZZ	00RJ4JZ	00U60KZ	00UM3KZ	00W030Z	00WEX3Z	00XF0ZQ	00XJ0ZJ	00XS0ZS
00NW4ZZ	00PE37Z	00Q10ZZ	00RJ4KZ	00U637Z	00UM47Z	00W032Z	00WEX7Z	00XF0ZR	00XJ0ZK	00XS4ZF
00NX0ZZ	00PE3MZ	00Q13ZZ	00RK07Z	00U63JZ	00UM4JZ	00W033Z	00WEXMZ	00XF0ZS	00XJ0ZL	00XS4ZG
00NX3ZZ	00PE3YZ	00Q14ZZ	00RK0JZ	00U63KZ	00UM4KZ	00W037Z	00WU00Z	00XF4ZF	00XJ0ZM	00XS4ZH
00NX4ZZ	00PE40Z	00Q20ZZ	00RK0KZ	00U647Z	00UN07Z	00W03JZ	00WU02Z	00XF4ZG	00XJ0ZN	00XS4ZJ
00NY0ZZ	00PE42Z	00Q23ZZ	00RK47Z	00U64JZ	00UN0JZ	00W03KZ	00WU03Z	00XF4ZH	00XJ0ZP	00XS4ZK
00NY3ZZ	00PE43Z	00Q24ZZ	00RK4JZ	00U64KZ	00UN0KZ	00W03MZ	00WU0JZ	00XF4ZJ	00XJ0ZQ	00XS4ZL
00NY4ZZ	00PE47Z	00Q60ZZ	00RK4KZ	00UF07Z	00UN37Z	00W03YZ	00WU0MZ	00XF4ZK	00XJ0ZR	00XS4ZM
00P000Z	00PE4MZ	00Q63ZZ	00RL07Z	00UF0JZ	00UN3JZ	00W040Z	00WU0YZ	00XF4ZL	00XJ0ZS	00XS4ZN
00P002Z	00PE4YZ	00Q64ZZ	00RL0JZ	00UF0KZ	00UN3KZ	00W042Z	00WU30Z	00XF4ZM	00XJ4ZF	00XS4ZP
00P003Z	00PEX0Z	00Q70ZZ	00RL0KZ	00UF37Z	00UN47Z	00W043Z	00WU32Z	00XF4ZN	00XJ4ZG	00XS4ZQ
00P007Z	00PEX2Z	00Q73ZZ	00RL47Z	00UF3JZ	00UN4JZ	00W047Z	00WU33Z	00XF4ZP	00XJ4ZH	00XS4ZR
00P00JZ	00PEX3Z	00Q74ZZ	00RL4JZ	00UF3KZ	00UN4KZ	00W04JZ	00WU3JZ	00XF4ZQ	00XJ4ZJ	00XS4ZS
00P00KZ	00PEXMZ	00Q80ZZ	00RL4KZ	00UF47Z	00UP07Z	00W04KZ	00WU3MZ	00XF4ZR	00XJ4ZK	012YX0Z
00P00MZ	00PU00Z	00Q83ZZ	00RM07Z	00UF4JZ	00UP0JZ	00W04MZ	00WU3YZ	00XF4ZS	00XJ4ZL	012YXYZ
00P00YZ	00PU02Z	00Q84ZZ	00RM0JZ	00UF4KZ	00UP0KZ	00W04YZ	00WU40Z	00XG0ZF	00XJ4ZM	01500ZZ
00P030Z	00PU03Z	00Q90ZZ	00RM0KZ	00UG07Z	00UP37Z	00W0X0Z	00WU42Z	00XG0ZG	00XJ4ZN	01503ZZ
00P032Z	00PU0JZ	00Q93ZZ	00RM47Z	00UG0JZ	00UP3JZ	00W0X2Z	00WU43Z	00XG0ZH	00XQ0ZR	01504ZZ

01510ZZ	01800ZZ	018R0ZZ	019800Z	019G30Z	019Q40Z	01DB0ZZ	01N50ZZ	01PY47Z	01QP0ZZ	01RF47Z
01513ZZ	01803ZZ	018R3ZZ	01980ZX	019G3ZX	019Q4ZX	01DB3ZZ	01N53ZZ	01PY4MZ	01QP3ZZ	01RF4JZ
01514ZZ	01804ZZ	018R4ZZ	01980ZZ	019G3ZZ	019Q4ZZ	01DB4ZZ	01N54ZZ	01PY4YZ	01QP4ZZ	01RF4KZ
01520ZZ	01810ZZ	019000Z	019830Z	019G40Z	019R00Z	01DC0ZZ	01N60ZZ	01PYX0Z	01QQ0ZZ	01RG07Z
01523ZZ	01813ZZ	01900ZX	019830ZX	019G4ZX	019R0ZX	01DC3ZZ	01N63ZZ	01PYX2Z	01QQ3ZZ	01RG0JZ
01524ZZ	01814ZZ	01900ZZ	01983ZZ	019G4ZZ	019R0ZZ	01DC4ZZ	01N64ZZ	01PYXMZ	01QQ4ZZ	01RG0KZ
01530ZZ	01820ZZ	019030Z	019840Z	019H00Z	019R30Z	01DD0ZZ	01N80ZZ	01Q00ZZ	01QR0ZZ	01RG47Z
01533ZZ	01823ZZ	01903ZX	01984ZX	019H0ZX	019R3ZX	01DD3ZZ	01N83ZZ	01Q03ZZ	01QR3ZZ	01RG4JZ
01534ZZ	01824ZZ	01903ZZ	01984ZZ	019H0ZZ	019R3ZZ	01DD4ZZ	01N84ZZ	01Q04ZZ	01QR4ZZ	01RG4KZ
01540ZZ	01830ZZ	019040Z	019900Z	019H30Z	019R40Z	01DF0ZZ	01N90ZZ	01Q10ZZ	01R107Z	01RH07Z
01543ZZ	01833ZZ	01904ZX	01990ZX	019H3ZX	019R4ZX	01DF3ZZ	01N93ZZ	01Q13ZZ	01R10JZ	01RH0JZ
01544ZZ	01834ZZ	01904ZZ	01990ZZ	019H3ZZ	019R4ZZ	01DF4ZZ	01N94ZZ	01Q14ZZ	01R10KZ	01RH0KZ
01550ZZ	01840ZZ	019100Z	019930Z	019H40Z	01B00ZX	01DG0ZZ	01NA0ZZ	01Q20ZZ	01R147Z	01RH47Z
01553ZZ	01843ZZ	01910ZX	01993ZX	019H4ZX	01B00ZZ	01DG3ZZ	01NA3ZZ	01Q23ZZ	01R14JZ	01RH4JZ
01554ZZ	01844ZZ	01910ZZ	01993ZZ	019H4ZZ	01B03ZX	01DG4ZZ	01NA4ZZ	01Q24ZZ	01R14KZ	01RH4KZ
01560ZZ	01850ZZ	019130Z	019940Z	019K00Z	01B03ZZ	01DH0ZZ	01NB0ZZ	01Q30ZZ	01R207Z	01RR07Z
01563ZZ	01853ZZ	01913ZX	01994ZX	019K0ZX	01B04ZX	01DH3ZZ	01NB3ZZ	01Q33ZZ	01R20JZ	01RR0JZ
01564ZZ	01854ZZ	01913ZZ	01994ZZ	019K0ZZ	01B04ZZ	01DH4ZZ	01NB4ZZ	01Q34ZZ	01R20KZ	01RR0KZ
01580ZZ	01860ZZ	019140Z	019A00Z	019K30Z	01B10ZX	01DK0ZZ	01NC0ZZ	01Q40ZZ	01R247Z	01RR47Z
01583ZZ	01863ZZ	01914ZX	019A0ZX	019K3ZX	01B10ZZ	01DK3ZZ	01NC3ZZ	01Q43ZZ	01R24JZ	01RR4JZ
01584ZZ	01864ZZ	01914ZZ	019A0ZZ	019K3ZZ	01B13ZX	01DK4ZZ	01NC4ZZ	01Q44ZZ	01R24KZ	01RR4KZ
01590ZZ	01880ZZ	019200Z	019A30Z	019K40Z	01B13ZZ	01DL0ZZ	01ND0ZZ	01Q50ZZ	01R407Z	01S00ZZ
01593ZZ	01883ZZ	01920ZX	019A3ZX	019K4ZX	01B14ZX	01DL3ZZ	01ND3ZZ	01Q53ZZ	01R40JZ	01S03ZZ
01594ZZ	01884ZZ	01920ZZ	019A3ZZ	019K4ZZ	01B14ZZ	01DL4ZZ	01ND4ZZ	01Q54ZZ	01R40KZ	01S04ZZ
015A0ZZ	01890ZZ	019230Z	019A40Z	019L00Z	01B20ZX	01DM0ZZ	01NF0ZZ	01Q60ZZ	01R447Z	01S10ZZ
015A3ZZ	01893ZZ	01923ZX	019A4ZX	019L0ZX	01B20ZZ	01DM3ZZ	01NF3ZZ	01Q63ZZ	01R44JZ	01S13ZZ
015A4ZZ	01894ZZ	01923ZZ	019A4ZZ	019L0ZZ	01B23ZX	01DM4ZZ	01NF4ZZ	01Q64ZZ	01R44KZ	01S14ZZ
015B0ZZ	018A0ZZ	019240Z	019B00Z	019L30Z	01B23ZZ	01DN0ZZ	01NG0ZZ	01Q80ZZ	01R507Z	01S20ZZ
015B3ZZ	018A3ZZ	01924ZX	019B0ZX	019L3ZX	01B24ZX	01DN3ZZ	01NG3ZZ	01Q83ZZ	01R50JZ	01S23ZZ
015B4ZZ	018A4ZZ	01924ZZ	019B0ZZ	019L3ZZ	01B24ZZ	01DN4ZZ	01NG4ZZ	01Q84ZZ	01R50KZ	01S24ZZ
015C0ZZ	018B0ZZ	019300Z	019B30Z	019L40Z	01B30ZX	01DP0ZZ	01NH0ZZ	01Q90ZZ	01R547Z	01S30ZZ
015C3ZZ	018B3ZZ	01930ZX	019B3ZX	019L4ZX	01B30ZZ	01DP3ZZ	01NH3ZZ	01Q93ZZ	01R54JZ	01S33ZZ
015C4ZZ	018B4ZZ	01930ZZ	019B3ZZ	019L4ZZ	01B33ZX	01DP4ZZ	01NH4ZZ	01Q94ZZ	01R54KZ	01S34ZZ
015D0ZZ	018C0ZZ	019330Z	019B40Z	019M00Z	01B33ZZ	01DQ0ZZ	01NK0ZZ	01QA0ZZ	01R607Z	01S40ZZ
015D3ZZ	018C3ZZ	01933ZX	019B4ZX	019M0ZX	01B34ZX	01DQ3ZZ	01NK3ZZ	01QA3ZZ	01R60JZ	01S43ZZ
015D4ZZ	018C4ZZ	01933ZZ	019B4ZZ	019M0ZZ	01B34ZZ	01DQ4ZZ	01NK4ZZ	01QA4ZZ	01R60KZ	01S44ZZ
015F0ZZ	018D0ZZ	019340Z	019C00Z	019M30Z	01B43ZX	01DR0ZZ	01NL0ZZ	01QB0ZZ	01R647Z	01S50ZZ
015F3ZZ	018D3ZZ	01934ZX	019C0ZX	019M3ZX	01B44ZX	01DR3ZZ	01NL3ZZ	01QB3ZZ	01R64JZ	01S53ZZ
015F4ZZ	018D4ZZ	01934ZZ	019C0ZZ	019M3ZZ	01B53ZX	01DR4ZZ	01NL4ZZ	01QB4ZZ	01R64KZ	01S54ZZ
015G0ZZ	018F0ZZ	019400Z	019C30Z	019M40Z	01B54ZX	01HY02Z	01NM0ZZ	01QC0ZZ	01R807Z	01S60ZZ
015G3ZZ	018F3ZZ	01940ZX	019C3ZX	019M4ZX	01B63ZX	01HY0MZ	01NM3ZZ	01QC3ZZ	01R80JZ	01S63ZZ
015G4ZZ	018F4ZZ	01940ZZ	019C3ZZ	019M4ZZ	01B64ZX	01HY0YZ	01NM4ZZ	01QC4ZZ	01R80KZ	01S64ZZ
015H0ZZ	018G0ZZ	019430Z	019C40Z	019N00Z	01B83ZX	01HY32Z	01NN0ZZ	01QD0ZZ	01R847Z	01S80ZZ
015H3ZZ	018G3ZZ	01943ZX	019C4ZX	019N0ZX	01B84ZX	01HY3MZ	01NN3ZZ	01QD3ZZ	01R84JZ	01S83ZZ
015H4ZZ	018G4ZZ	01943ZZ	019C4ZZ	019N0ZZ	01B93ZX	01HY3YZ	01NN4ZZ	01QD4ZZ	01R84KZ	01S84ZZ
015K0ZZ	018H0ZZ	019440Z	019D00Z	019N30Z	01B94ZX	01HY42Z	01NP0ZZ	01QF0ZZ	01RB07Z	01S90ZZ
015K3ZZ	018H3ZZ	01944ZX	019D0ZX	019N3ZX	01BA3ZX	01HY4MZ	01NP3ZZ	01QF3ZZ	01RB0JZ	01S93ZZ
015K4ZZ	018H4ZZ	01944ZZ	019D0ZZ	019N3ZZ	01BA4ZX	01HY4YZ	01NP4ZZ	01QF4ZZ	01RB0KZ	01S94ZZ
015L0ZZ	018K0ZZ	019500Z	019D30Z	019N40Z	01BB3ZX	01JY0ZZ	01NQ0ZZ	01QG0ZZ	01RB47Z	01SA0ZZ
015L3ZZ	018K3ZZ	01950ZX	019D3ZX	019N4ZX	01BB4ZX	01JY3ZZ	01NQ3ZZ	01QG3ZZ	01RB4JZ	01SA3ZZ
015L4ZZ	018K4ZZ	01950ZZ	019D3ZZ	019N4ZZ	01BC3ZX	01JY4ZZ	01NQ4ZZ	01QG4ZZ	01RB4KZ	01SA4ZZ
015M0ZZ	018L0ZZ	019530Z	019D40Z	019P00Z	01BC4ZX	01NR0ZZ	01QH0ZZ	01RC07Z	01SB0ZZ
015M3ZZ	018L3ZZ	01953ZX	019D4ZX	019P0ZX	01BD3ZX	01NR3ZZ	01QH3ZZ	01RC0JZ	01SB3ZZ
015M4ZZ	018L4ZZ	01953ZZ	019D4ZZ	019P0ZZ	01BD4ZX	01NR4ZZ	01QH4ZZ	01RC0KZ	01SB4ZZ
015N0ZZ	018M0ZZ	019540Z	019F00Z	019P30Z	01BF3ZX	01PY00Z	01QK0ZZ	01RC47Z	01SC0ZZ
015N3ZZ	018M3ZZ	01954ZX	019F0ZX	019P3ZX	01BF4ZX	01PY02Z	01QK3ZZ	01RC4JZ	01SC3ZZ
015N4ZZ	018M4ZZ	01954ZZ	019F0ZZ	019P3ZZ	01BG3ZX	01PY07Z	01QK4ZZ	01RC4KZ	01SC4ZZ
015P0ZZ	018N0ZZ	019600Z	019F30Z	019P40Z	01BG4ZX	01PY0MZ	01QL0ZZ	01RD07Z	01SD0ZZ
015P3ZZ	018N3ZZ	01960ZX	019F3ZX	019P4ZX	01BH3ZX	01PY0YZ	01QL3ZZ	01RD0JZ	01SD3ZZ
015P4ZZ	018N4ZZ	01960ZZ	019F3ZZ	019P4ZZ	01BH4ZX	01PY30Z	01QL4ZZ	01RD0KZ	01SD4ZZ
015Q0ZZ	018P0ZZ	019630Z	019F40Z	019Q00Z	01BQ3ZX	01PY32Z	01QM0ZZ	01RD47Z	01SF0ZZ
015Q3ZZ	018P3ZZ	01963ZX	019F4ZX	019Q0ZX	01BQ4ZX	01PY37Z	01QM3ZZ	01RD4JZ	01SF3ZZ
015Q4ZZ	018P4ZZ	01963ZZ	019F4ZZ	019Q0ZZ	01BR3ZX	01PY3MZ	01QM4ZZ	01RD4KZ	01SF4ZZ
015R0ZZ	018Q0ZZ	019640Z	019G00Z	019Q30Z	01BR4ZX	01PY3YZ	01QN0ZZ	01RF07Z	01SG0ZZ
015R3ZZ	018Q3ZZ	01964ZX	019G0ZX	019Q3ZX	01DA3ZX	01PY40Z	01QN3ZZ	01RF0JZ	01SG3ZZ
015R4ZZ	018Q4ZZ	01964ZZ	019G0ZZ	019Q3ZZ	01DA4ZZ	01PY42Z	01QN4ZZ	01RF0KZ	01SG4ZZ

01SH0ZZ	01UB4JZ	02134AC	021709P	021K08P	021L0ZC	021Q08A	021R4KA	025T0ZZ	02704G6	0272046
01SH3ZZ	01UB4KZ	02134AF	021709Q	021K08Q	021L0ZF	021Q08B	021R4KB	025T3ZZ	02704GZ	027204Z
01SH4ZZ	01UC0JZ	02134AW	021709R	021K08R	021L0ZP	021Q08D	021R4KD	025T4ZZ	02704T6	0272056
01SQ0ZZ	01UC0KZ	02134D4	021709S	021K09P	021L0ZQ	021Q09A	021R4ZA	025V0ZZ	02704TZ	027205Z
01SQ3ZZ	01UC3JZ	02134J3	021709T	021K09Q	021L0ZR	021Q09B	021R4ZB	025V3ZZ	02704Z6	0272066
01SQ4ZZ	01UC3KZ	02134J8	021709U	021K09R	021L0ZW	021Q09D	021R4ZD	025V4ZZ	02704ZZ	027206Z
01SR0ZZ	01UC4JZ	02134J9	02170AP	021K0AP	021L48P	021Q0AA	021V08P	025W0ZZ	0271046	0272076
01SR3ZZ	01UC4KZ	02134JC	02170AQ	021K0AQ	021L48Q	021Q0AB	021V08Q	025W3ZZ	027104Z	027207Z
01SR4ZZ	01UD0JZ	02134JF	02170AR	021K0AR	021L48R	021Q0AD	021V08R	025W4ZZ	0271056	02720D6
01U107Z	01UD0KZ	02134JW	02170AS	021K0JP	021L49P	021Q0JA	021V08S	025X0ZZ	027105Z	02720DZ
01U10JZ	01UD3JZ	02134K3	02170AT	021K0JQ	021L49Q	021Q0JB	021V08T	025X3ZZ	0271066	02720E6
01U10KZ	01UD3KZ	02134K8	02170AU	021K0JR	021L49R	021Q0JD	021V08U	025X4ZZ	027106Z	02720EZ
01U137Z	01UD4JZ	02134K9	02170JP	021K0KP	021L4AP	021Q0KA	021V09P	0270046	0271076	02720F6
01U13JZ	01UD4KZ	02134KC	02170JQ	021K0KQ	021L4AQ	021Q0KB	021V09Q	027004Z	027107Z	02720FZ
01U13KZ	01UF0JZ	02134KF	02170JR	021K0KR	021L4AR	021Q0KD	021V09R	0270056	02710D6	02720G6
01U147Z	01UF0KZ	02134KW	02170JS	021K0Z5	021L4JP	021Q0ZA	021V09S	027005Z	02710DZ	02720GZ
01U14JZ	01UF3JZ	02134Z3	02170JT	021K0Z8	021L4JQ	021Q0ZB	021V09T	0270066	02710E6	02720T6
01U14KZ	01UF3KZ	02134Z8	02170JU	021K0Z9	021L4JR	021Q0ZD	021V09U	027006Z	02710EZ	02720TZ
01U207Z	01UF4JZ	02134Z9	02170KP	021K0ZC	021L4KP	021Q48A	021V0AP	0270076	02710F6	02720Z6
01U20JZ	01UF4KZ	02134ZC	02170KQ	021K0ZF	021L4KQ	021Q48B	021V0AQ	027007Z	02710FZ	02720ZZ
01U20KZ	01UG0JZ	02134ZF	02170KR	021K0ZP	021L4KR	021Q48D	021V0AR	02700D6	02710G6	0272346
01U237Z	01UG0KZ	021608P	02170KS	021K0ZQ	021L4Z5	021Q49A	021V0AS	02700DZ	02710GZ	027234Z
01U23JZ	01UG3JZ	021608Q	02170KT	021K0ZR	021L4Z8	021Q49B	021V0AT	02700E6	02710T6	0272356
01U23KZ	01UG3KZ	021608R	02170KU	021K0ZW	021L4Z9	021Q49D	021V0AU	02700EZ	02710TZ	027235Z
01U247Z	01UG4JZ	021609P	02170ZP	021K48P	021L4ZC	021Q4AA	021V0JP	02700F6	02710Z6	0272366
01U24JZ	01UG4KZ	021609Q	02170ZQ	021K48Q	021L4ZF	021Q4AB	021V0JQ	02700FZ	02710ZZ	027236Z
01U24KZ	01UH0JZ	021609R	02170ZR	021K48R	021L4ZP	021Q4AD	021V0JR	02700G6	0271346	0272376
01U407Z	01UH0KZ	02160AP	02170ZS	021K49P	021L4ZQ	021Q4JA	021V0JS	02700GZ	027134Z	027237Z
01U40JZ	01UH3JZ	02160AQ	02170ZT	021K49Q	021L4ZR	021Q4JB	021V0JT	02700T6	0271356	02723D6
01U40KZ	01UH3KZ	02160AR	02170ZU	021K49R	021L4ZW	021Q4JD	021V0JU	02700TZ	027135Z	02723DZ
01U437Z	01UH4JZ	02160JP	021748P	021K4AP	021P08A	021Q4KA	021W0JG	02700Z6	0271366	02723E6
01U43JZ	01UH4KZ	02160JQ	021748Q	021K4AQ	021P08B	021Q4KB	021W0JH	02700ZZ	027136Z	02723EZ
01U43KZ	01UR0JZ	02160JR	021748R	021K4AR	021P08D	021Q4KD	021W0KG	0270346	0271376	02723F6
01U447Z	01UR0KZ	02160KP	021748S	021K4JP	021P09A	021Q4ZA	021W0KH	027034Z	027137Z	02723FZ
01U44JZ	01UR3JZ	02160KQ	021748T	021K4JQ	021P09B	021Q4ZB	025G3ZZ	0270356	02713D6	02723G6
01U44KZ	01UR3KZ	02160KR	021748U	021K4JR	021P09D	021Q4ZD	025G4ZZ	027035Z	02713DZ	02723GZ
01U507Z	01UR4JZ	02160Z7	021749P	021K4KP	021P0AA	021R08A	025H0ZZ	0270366	02713E6	02723T6
01U50JZ	01UR4KZ	02160ZP	021749Q	021K4KQ	021P0AB	021R08B	025H3ZZ	027036Z	02713EZ	02723TZ
01U50KZ	01WY0YZ	02160ZQ	021749R	021K4KR	021P0AD	021R08D	025H4ZZ	0270376	02713F6	02723Z6
01U537Z	01WY3YZ	02160ZR	021749S	021K4Z5	021P0JA	021R09A	025J0ZZ	027037Z	02713FZ	02723ZZ
01U53JZ	01WY4YZ	02163Z7	021749T	021K4Z8	021P0JB	021R09B	025J3ZZ	02703D6	02713G6	0272446
01U53KZ	01WYX0Z	021648P	021749U	021K4Z9	021P0JD	021R09D	025J4ZZ	02703DZ	02713GZ	027244Z
01U547Z	01WYX2Z	021648Q	02174AP	021K4ZC	021P0KA	021R0AA	025K0ZZ	02703E6	02713T6	0272456
01U54JZ	01WYX7Z	021648R	02174AQ	021K4ZF	021P0KB	021R0AB	025K3ZZ	02703EZ	02713TZ	027245Z
01U54KZ	01WYXMZ	021649P	02174AR	021K4ZP	021P0KD	021R0AD	025K4ZZ	02703F6	02713Z6	0272466
01U607Z	02130Z9	021649Q	02174AS	021K4ZQ	021P0ZA	021R0JA	025L0ZZ	02703FZ	02713ZZ	027246Z
01U60JZ	02130ZC	021649R	02174AT	021K4ZR	021P0ZB	021R0JB	025L3ZZ	02703G6	0271446	0272476
01U60KZ	02130ZF	02164AP	02174AU	021K4ZW	021P0ZD	021R0JD	025L4ZZ	02703GZ	027144Z	027247Z
01U637Z	0213344	02164AQ	02174JP	021L08P	021P48A	021R0KA	025M0ZZ	02703T6	0271446	02724D6
01U63JZ	02133D4	02164AR	02174JQ	021L08Q	021P48B	021R0KB	025M3ZZ	02703TZ	027145Z	02724DZ
01U63KZ	0213444	02164JP	02174JR	021L08R	021P48D	021R0KD	025M4ZZ	02703Z6	0271466	02724E6
01U647Z	0213483	02164JQ	02174JS	021L09P	021P49A	021R0ZA	025N0ZZ	02703ZZ	027146Z	02724EZ
01U64JZ	0213488	02164JR	02174JT	021L09Q	021P49B	021R0ZB	025N3ZZ	0270446	0271476	02724F6
01U64KZ	0213489	02164KP	02174JU	021L09R	021P49D	021R0ZD	025N4ZZ	027044Z	027147Z	02724FZ
01U807Z	021348C	02164KQ	02174KP	021L0AP	021P4AA	021R48A	025P0ZZ	0270456	02714D6	02724G6
01U80JZ	021348F	02164KR	02174KQ	021L0AQ	021P4AB	021R48B	025P3ZZ	027045Z	02714DZ	02724GZ
01U80KZ	021348W	02164Z7	02174KR	021L0AR	021P4AD	021R48D	025P4ZZ	0270466	02714E6	02724T6
01U837Z	0213493	02164ZP	02174KS	021L0JP	021P4JA	021R49A	025Q0ZZ	027046Z	02714EZ	02724TZ
01U83JZ	0213498	02164ZQ	02174KT	021L0JQ	021P4JB	021R49B	025Q3ZZ	0270476	02714F6	02724Z6
01U83KZ	0213499	02164ZR	02174KU	021L0JR	021P4JD	021R49D	025Q4ZZ	027047Z	02714FZ	02724ZZ
01U84JZ	021349C	021708P	02174ZP	021L0KP	021P4KA	021R4AA	025R0ZZ	02704D6	02714G6	0273046
01U84KZ	021349F	021708Q	02174ZQ	021L0KQ	021P4KB	021R4AB	025R3ZZ	02704DZ	02714GZ	027304Z
01UB0JZ	021349W	021708R	02174ZR	021L0KR	021P4KD	021R4AD	025R4ZZ	02704E6	02714T6	0273056
01UB0KZ	02134A3	021708S	02174ZS	021L0Z5	021P4ZA	021R4JA	025S0ZZ	02704EZ	02714TZ	027305Z
01UB3JZ	02134A8	021708T	02174ZT	021L0Z8	021P4ZB	021R4JB	025S3ZZ	02704F6	02714Z6	0273066
01UB3KZ	02134A9	021708U	02174ZU	021L0Z9	021P4ZD	021R4JD	025S4ZZ	02704FZ	02714ZZ	027306Z

0273076	027G34Z	027R34T	02B40ZX	02BJ3ZZ	02H44YZ	02HP33Z	02HT4DZ	02LH3DZ	02LV4DZ	02NR0ZZ
027307Z	027G3DZ	027R34Z	02B40ZZ	02BJ4ZX	02H60YZ	02HP3DZ	02HT4YZ	02LH3ZZ	02LV4ZZ	02NR3ZZ
02730D6	027G3ZZ	027R3DT	02B43ZX	02BJ4ZZ	02H632Z	02HP3YZ	02HV00Z	02LH4CZ	02LW3DJ	02NR4ZZ
02730DZ	027G44Z	027R3DZ	02B43ZZ	02BK0ZX	02H633Z	02HP40Z	02HV02Z	02LH4DZ	02N00ZZ	02NS0ZZ
02730E6	027G4DZ	027R3ZT	02B44ZX	02BK0ZZ	02H63YZ	02HP42Z	02HV03Z	02LH4ZZ	02N03ZZ	02NS3ZZ
02730EZ	027G4ZZ	027R3ZZ	02B44ZZ	02BK3ZX	02H64YZ	02HP43Z	02HV0DZ	02LP0CZ	02N04ZZ	02NS4ZZ
02730F6	027H04Z	027R44T	02B50ZX	02BK3ZZ	02H70YZ	02HP4DZ	02HV0YZ	02LP0DZ	02N10ZZ	02NT0ZZ
02730FZ	027H0DZ	027R44Z	02B50ZZ	02BK4ZX	02H732Z	02HP4YZ	02HV30Z	02LP0ZZ	02N13ZZ	02NT3ZZ
02730G6	027H0ZZ	027R4DT	02B53ZX	02BK4ZZ	02H733Z	02HQ00Z	02HV32Z	02LP3CZ	02N14ZZ	02NT4ZZ
02730GZ	027H34Z	027R4DZ	02B53ZZ	02BL0ZX	02H73YZ	02HQ02Z	02HV33Z	02LP3DZ	02N20ZZ	02NV0ZZ
02730T6	027H3DZ	027R4ZT	02B54ZX	02BL0ZZ	02H74YZ	02HQ03Z	02HV3DZ	02LP3ZZ	02N23ZZ	02NV3ZZ
02730TZ	027H3ZZ	027R4ZZ	02B54ZZ	02BL3ZX	02HA0RJ	02HQ0DZ	02HV3YZ	02LP4CZ	02N24ZZ	02NV4ZZ
02730Z6	027H44Z	027S04Z	02B60ZX	02BL3ZZ	02HA0YZ	02HQ0YZ	02HV40Z	02LP4DZ	02N30ZZ	02NW0ZZ
02730ZZ	027H4DZ	027S0DZ	02B60ZZ	02BL4ZX	02HA3RJ	02HQ30Z	02HV42Z	02LP4ZZ	02N33ZZ	02NW3ZZ
0273346	027H4ZZ	027S0ZZ	02B63ZX	02BL4ZZ	02HA3YZ	02HQ32Z	02HV43Z	02LQ0CZ	02N34ZZ	02NW4ZZ
027334Z	027J04Z	027S34Z	02B63ZZ	02BM0ZX	02HA4RJ	02HQ33Z	02HV4DZ	02LQ0DZ	02N40ZZ	02NX0ZZ
0273356	027J0DZ	027S3DZ	02B64ZX	02BM0ZZ	02HA4YZ	02HQ3DZ	02HV4YZ	02LQ0ZZ	02N43ZZ	02NX3ZZ
027335Z	027J0ZZ	027S3ZZ	02B64ZZ	02BM3ZX	02HK0YZ	02HQ3YZ	02HW00Z	02LQ3CZ	02N44ZZ	02NX4ZZ
0273366	027J34Z	027S44Z	02B70ZK	02BM3ZZ	02HK33Z	02HQ40Z	02HW02Z	02LQ3DZ	02N50ZZ	02PA02Z
027336Z	027J3DZ	027S4DZ	02B70ZX	02BM4ZX	02HK3YZ	02HQ42Z	02HW03Z	02LQ3ZZ	02N53ZZ	02PA03Z
0273376	027J3ZZ	027S4ZZ	02B70ZZ	02BM4ZZ	02HK4YZ	02HQ43Z	02HW0DZ	02LQ4CZ	02N54ZZ	02PA07Z
027337Z	027J44Z	027T04Z	02B73ZK	02BN0ZX	02HL0NZ	02HQ4DZ	02HW0YZ	02LQ4DZ	02N60ZZ	02PA08Z
02733D6	027J4DZ	027T0DZ	02B73ZX	02BN0ZZ	02HL0YZ	02HQ4YZ	02HW30Z	02LQ4ZZ	02N63ZZ	02PA0CZ
02733DZ	027J4ZZ	027T0ZZ	02B73ZZ	02BN3ZX	02HL30Z	02HR00Z	02HW32Z	02LR0CT	02N64ZZ	02PA0DZ
02733E6	027K04Z	027T34Z	02B74ZK	02BN3ZZ	02HL32Z	02HR02Z	02HW33Z	02LR0CZ	02N70ZZ	02PA0JZ
02733EZ	027K0DZ	027T3DZ	02B74ZX	02BN4ZX	02HL33Z	02HR03Z	02HW3DZ	02LR0DT	02N73ZZ	02PA0KZ
02733F6	027K0ZZ	027T3ZZ	02B74ZZ	02BN4ZZ	02HL3DZ	02HR0DZ	02HW3YZ	02LR0DZ	02N74ZZ	02PA0MZ
02733FZ	027K34Z	027T44Z	02B80ZX	02BP0ZX	02HL3JZ	02HR0YZ	02HW40Z	02LR0ZT	02N80ZZ	02PA0NZ
02733G6	027K3DZ	027T4DZ	02B80ZZ	02BP0ZZ	02HL3KZ	02HR30Z	02HW42Z	02LR0ZZ	02N83ZZ	02PA0QZ
02733GZ	027K3ZZ	027T4ZZ	02B83ZX	02BP3ZX	02HL3MZ	02HR32Z	02HW43Z	02LR3CT	02N84ZZ	02PA0RS
02733T6	027K44Z	027V04Z	02B83ZZ	02BP3ZZ	02HL3NZ	02HR33Z	02HW4DZ	02LR3CZ	02N90ZZ	02PA0RZ
02733TZ	027K4DZ	027V0DZ	02B84ZX	02BP4ZX	02HL3YZ	02HR3DZ	02HW4YZ	02LR3DT	02N93ZZ	02PA0YZ
02733Z6	027K4ZZ	027V0ZZ	02B84ZZ	02BP4ZZ	02HL40Z	02HR3YZ	02HX00Z	02LR3DZ	02N94ZZ	02PA32Z
02733ZZ	027L04Z	027V34Z	02B90ZX	02BQ0ZX	02HL42Z	02HR40Z	02HX02Z	02LR3ZT	02ND0ZZ	02PA33Z
0273446	027L0DZ	027V3DZ	02B90ZZ	02BQ0ZZ	02HL43Z	02HR42Z	02HX03Z	02LR3ZZ	02ND3ZZ	02PA37Z
027344Z	027L0ZZ	027V3ZZ	02B93ZX	02BQ3ZX	02HL4DZ	02HR43Z	02HX0DZ	02LR4CT	02ND4ZZ	02PA38Z
0273456	027L34Z	027V44Z	02B93ZZ	02BQ3ZZ	02HL4JZ	02HR4DZ	02HX30Z	02LR4CZ	02NF0ZZ	02PA3CZ
027345Z	027L3DZ	027V4DZ	02B94ZX	02BQ4ZX	02HL4KZ	02HR4YZ	02HX32Z	02LR4DT	02NF3ZZ	02PA3DZ
0273466	027L3ZZ	027V4ZZ	02B94ZZ	02BQ4ZZ	02HL4MZ	02HS00Z	02HX33Z	02LR4DZ	02NF4ZZ	02PA3JZ
027346Z	027L44Z	027W04Z	02BD0ZX	02BR0ZX	02HL4NZ	02HS02Z	02HX3DZ	02LR4ZT	02NG0ZZ	02PA3KZ
0273476	027L4DZ	027W0DZ	02BD0ZZ	02BR0ZZ	02HL4YZ	02HS03Z	02HX40Z	02LR4ZZ	02NG3ZZ	02PA3MZ
027347Z	027L4ZZ	027W0ZZ	02BD3ZX	02BR3ZX	02HN00Z	02HS0DZ	02HX42Z	02LS0CZ	02NG4ZZ	02PA3NZ
02734D6	027P04Z	027W34Z	02BD3ZZ	02BR3ZZ	02HN02Z	02HS0YZ	02HX43Z	02LS0DZ	02NH0ZZ	02PA3QZ
02734DZ	027P0DZ	027W3DZ	02BD4ZX	02BR4ZX	02HN0JZ	02HS30Z	02HX4DZ	02LS0ZZ	02NH3ZZ	02PA3RS
02734E6	027P0ZZ	027W3ZZ	02BD4ZZ	02BR4ZZ	02HN0KZ	02HS32Z	02JA0ZZ	02LS3CZ	02NH4ZZ	02PA3RZ
02734EZ	027P34Z	027W44Z	02BF0ZX	02BS0ZX	02HN0MZ	02HS33Z	02JA3ZZ	02LS3DZ	02NJ0ZZ	02PA3YZ
02734F6	027P3DZ	027W4DZ	02BF0ZZ	02BS0ZZ	02HN0YZ	02HS3DZ	02JA4ZZ	02LS3ZZ	02NJ3ZZ	02PA42Z
02734FZ	027P3ZZ	027W4ZZ	02BF3ZX	02BS3ZX	02HN30Z	02HS3YZ	02JY0ZZ	02LS4CZ	02NJ4ZZ	02PA43Z
02734G6	027P44Z	027X04Z	02BF3ZZ	02BS3ZZ	02HN3JZ	02HS40Z	02JY3ZZ	02LS4DZ	02NK0ZZ	02PA47Z
02734GZ	027P4DZ	027X0DZ	02BF4ZX	02BS4ZX	02HN3KZ	02HS42Z	02JY4ZZ	02LS4ZZ	02NK3ZZ	02PA48Z
02734T6	027P4ZZ	027X0ZZ	02BF4ZZ	02BS4ZZ	02HN3MZ	02HS43Z	02K80ZZ	02LT0CZ	02NK4ZZ	02PA4CZ
02734TZ	027Q04Z	027X34Z	02BG0ZX	02BT0ZX	02HN3YZ	02HS4DZ	02K83ZZ	02LT0DZ	02NL0ZZ	02PA4DZ
02734Z6	027Q0DZ	027X3DZ	02BG0ZZ	02BT0ZZ	02HN40Z	02HS4YZ	02K84ZZ	02LT0ZZ	02NL3ZZ	02PA4JZ
02734ZZ	027Q0ZZ	027X3ZZ	02BG3ZX	02BT3ZX	02HN42Z	02HT00Z	02L70CK	02LT3CZ	02NL4ZZ	02PA4KZ
027F04Z	027Q34Z	027X44Z	02BG3ZZ	02BT3ZZ	02HN4JZ	02HT02Z	02L70DK	02LT3DZ	02NM0ZZ	02PA4MZ
027F0DZ	027Q3DZ	027X4DZ	02BG4ZX	02BT4ZX	02HN4KZ	02HT03Z	02L70ZK	02LT3ZZ	02NM3ZZ	02PA4NZ
027F0ZZ	027Q3ZZ	027X4ZZ	02BG4ZZ	02BT4ZZ	02HN4MZ	02HT0DZ	02L73CK	02LT4CZ	02NM4ZZ	02PA4QZ
027F34Z	027Q44Z	02880ZZ	02BH0ZX	02BV0ZX	02HN4YZ	02HT0YZ	02L73DK	02LT4DZ	02NN0ZZ	02PA4RS
027F3DZ	027Q4DZ	02883ZZ	02BH0ZZ	02BV0ZZ	02HP00Z	02HT30Z	02L73ZK	02LT4ZZ	02NN3ZZ	02PA4RZ
027F3ZZ	027Q4ZZ	02884ZZ	02BH3ZX	02BV3ZX	02HP02Z	02HT32Z	02L74CK	02LH0CZ	02NN4ZZ	02PA4YZ
027F44Z	027R04T	02890ZZ	02BH3ZZ	02BV3ZZ	02HP03Z	02HT33Z	02L74DK	02LH0DZ	02NP0ZZ	02PAX2Z
027F4DZ	027R04Z	02893ZZ	02BH4ZX	02FNXZZ	02HP0DZ	02HT3DZ	02L74ZK	02LH0ZZ	02NP3ZZ	02PAX3Z
027F4ZZ	027R0DT	02894ZZ	02BH4ZZ	02H40YZ	02HP0YZ	02HT3YZ	02LH0CZ	02LV0CZ	02NP4ZZ	02PAXDZ
027G04Z	027R0DZ	028D0ZZ	02BJ0ZX	02H432Z	02HP30Z	02HT40Z	02LH0DZ	02LV0DZ	02NQ0ZZ	02PAXMZ
027G0DZ	027R0ZT	028D3ZZ	02BJ0ZZ	02H433Z	02HP32Z	02HT42Z	02LH0ZZ	02LV0ZZ	02NQ3ZZ	02PY02Z
027G0ZZ	027R0ZZ	028D4ZZ	02BJ3ZX	02H43YZ	02HP32Z	02HT43Z	02LH3CZ	02LV4CZ	02NQ4ZZ	02PY03Z

02PY07Z	02QC4ZZ	02R548Z	02U63KZ	02UF3JZ	02UJ48Z	02UQ08Z	02UW3KZ	02VS3DZ	02WYXJZ	03140KF
02PY08Z	02QD0ZZ	02R54JZ	02U647Z	02UF3KJ	02UJ4JG	02UQ0JZ	02UW47Z	02VS3ZZ	02WYXKZ	03140KJ
02PY0CZ	02QD3ZZ	02R54KZ	02U648Z	02UF3KZ	02UJ4JZ	02UQ0KZ	02UW48Z	02VS4CZ	0314093	03140KK
02PY0DZ	02QD4ZZ	02R607Z	02U64JZ	02UF47J	02UJ4KG	02UQ37Z	02UW4JZ	02VS4DZ	0314094	03140KM
02PY0JZ	02QF0ZJ	02R608Z	02U64KZ	02UF47Z	02UK07Z	02UQ38Z	02UW4KZ	02VS4ZZ	0314095	03140KN
02PY0KZ	02QF0ZZ	02R60JZ	02U707Z	02UF48J	02UK08Z	02UQ3JZ	02UX07Z	02VT0CZ	0314096	03140Z0
02PY0YZ	02QF3ZJ	02R60KZ	02U708Z	02UF48Z	02UK0JZ	02UQ3KZ	02UX08Z	02VT0DZ	0314097	03140Z1
02PY32Z	02QF3ZZ	02R647Z	02U70JZ	02UF4JJ	02UK0KZ	02UQ47Z	02UX0JZ	02VT0ZZ	0314098	03140Z2
02PY33Z	02QF4ZJ	02RJ37H	02U70KZ	02UF4JZ	02UK37Z	02UQ48Z	02UX0KZ	02VT3CZ	0314099	03140Z3
02PY37Z	02QF4ZZ	02RJ37Z	02U737Z	02UF4KJ	02UK38Z	02UQ4JZ	02UX37Z	02VT3DZ	031409B	03140Z4
02PY38Z	02QG0ZE	02RJ38H	02U738Z	02UF4KZ	02UK3JZ	02UQ4KZ	02UX38Z	02VT3ZZ	031409C	03140Z5
02PY3CZ	02QG0ZZ	02RJ38Z	02U73JZ	02UG07E	02UK3KZ	02UR07Z	02UX3JZ	02VT4CZ	031409D	03140Z6
02PY3DZ	02QG3ZE	02RJ3JH	02U73KZ	02UG07Z	02UK47Z	02UR08Z	02UX3KZ	02VT4DZ	031409F	03140Z7
02PY3JZ	02QG3ZZ	02RJ3JZ	02U747Z	02UG08E	02UK48Z	02UR0JZ	02UX47Z	02VT4ZZ	031409J	03140Z8
02PY3KZ	02QG4ZE	02RJ3KH	02U748Z	02UG08Z	02UK4JZ	02UR0KZ	02UX48Z	02VV0CZ	031409K	03140Z9
02PY3YZ	02QG4ZZ	02RJ3KZ	02U74JZ	02UG0JE	02UK4KZ	02UR37Z	02UX4JZ	02VV0DZ	031409M	03140ZB
02PY42Z	02QH0ZZ	02S00ZZ	02U74KZ	02UG0JZ	02UL07Z	02UR38Z	02UX4KZ	02VV0ZZ	031409N	03140ZC
02PY43Z	02QH3ZZ	02S10ZZ	02U907Z	02UG0KE	02UL08Z	02UR3JZ	02VA0CZ	02VV3CZ	03140A0	03140ZD
02PY47Z	02QH4ZZ	02SP0ZZ	02U908Z	02UG0KZ	02UL0JZ	02UR3KZ	02VA0ZZ	02VV3DZ	03140A1	03140ZF
02PY48Z	02QJ0ZG	02SQ0ZZ	02U90JZ	02UG37E	02UL0KZ	02UR47Z	02VA3CZ	02VV3ZZ	03140A2	03140ZJ
02PY4CZ	02QJ0ZZ	02SR0ZZ	02U90KZ	02UG37Z	02UL37Z	02UR48Z	02VA3ZZ	02VV4CZ	03140A3	03140ZK
02PY4DZ	02QJ3ZG	02SS0ZZ	02U937Z	02UG38E	02UL38Z	02UR4JZ	02VA4CZ	02VV4DZ	03140A4	03140ZM
02PY4JZ	02QJ3ZZ	02ST0ZZ	02U938Z	02UG38Z	02UL3JZ	02UR4KZ	02VA4ZZ	02WA0RS	03140A5	03140ZN
02PY4KZ	02QJ4ZG	02SV0ZZ	02U93JZ	02UG3JE	02UL3KZ	02US07Z	02VG0ZZ	02WA0YZ	03140A6	0315090
02PY4YZ	02QJ4ZZ	02SW0ZZ	02U93KZ	02UG3JZ	02UL47Z	02US08Z	02VG3ZZ	02WA3RS	03140A7	0315091
02PYX2Z	02QK0ZZ	02SX0ZZ	02U947Z	02UG3KE	02UL48Z	02US0JZ	02VG4ZZ	02WA3YZ	03140A8	0315092
02PYX3Z	02QK3ZZ	02T50ZZ	02U948Z	02UG3KZ	02UL4JZ	02US0KZ	02VP0CZ	02WA4RS	03140A9	0315093
02PYXDZ	02QK4ZZ	02T53ZZ	02U94JZ	02UG47E	02UL4KZ	02US37Z	02VP0DZ	02WA4YZ	03140AB	0315094
02Q00ZZ	02QL0ZZ	02T54ZZ	02U94KZ	02UG47Z	02UM07Z	02US38Z	02VP0ZZ	02WAX2Z	03140AC	0315095
02Q03ZZ	02QL3ZZ	02T80ZZ	02UA07Z	02UG48E	02UM08Z	02US3JZ	02VP3CZ	02WAX3Z	03140AD	0315096
02Q04ZZ	02QL4ZZ	02T83ZZ	02UA08Z	02UG48Z	02UM0JZ	02US3KZ	02VP3DZ	02WAX7Z	03140AF	0315097
02Q10ZZ	02QM0ZZ	02T84ZZ	02UA0JZ	02UG4JE	02UM0KZ	02US47Z	02VP3ZZ	02WAX8Z	03140AJ	0315098
02Q13ZZ	02QM3ZZ	02T90ZZ	02UA0KZ	02UG4JZ	02UM37Z	02US48Z	02VP4CZ	02WAXCZ	03140AK	0315099
02Q14ZZ	02QM4ZZ	02T93ZZ	02UA37Z	02UG4KE	02UM38Z	02US4JZ	02VP4DZ	02WAXDZ	03140AM	031509B
02Q20ZZ	02QN0ZZ	02T94ZZ	02UA38Z	02UG4KZ	02UM3JZ	02US4KZ	02VP4ZZ	02WAXJZ	03140AN	031509C
02Q23ZZ	02QN3ZZ	02TD0ZZ	02UA3JZ	02UH07Z	02UM3KZ	02UT07Z	02VQ0CZ	02WAXKZ	03140J0	031509D
02Q24ZZ	02QN4ZZ	02TD3ZZ	02UA3KZ	02UH08Z	02UM47Z	02UT08Z	02VQ0DZ	02WAXMZ	03140J1	031509F
02Q30ZZ	02QP0ZZ	02TD4ZZ	02UA47Z	02UH0JZ	02UM48Z	02UT0JZ	02VQ0ZZ	02WAXNZ	03140J2	031509J
02Q33ZZ	02QP3ZZ	02TH0ZZ	02UA48Z	02UH0KZ	02UM4JZ	02UT0KZ	02VQ3CZ	02WAXQZ	03140J3	031509K
02Q34ZZ	02QP4ZZ	02TH3ZZ	02UA4JZ	02UH37Z	02UM4KZ	02UT37Z	02VQ3DZ	02WAXRS	03140J4	031509V
02Q40ZZ	02QQ0ZZ	02TH4ZZ	02UA4KZ	02UH38Z	02UN07Z	02UT38Z	02VQ3ZZ	02WAXRZ	03140J5	03150A0
02Q43ZZ	02QQ3ZZ	02TM0ZZ	02UD07Z	02UH3JZ	02UN08Z	02UT3JZ	02VQ4CZ	02WF37Z	03140J6	03150A1
02Q44ZZ	02QQ4ZZ	02TM3ZZ	02UD08Z	02UH3KZ	02UN0JZ	02UT3KZ	02VQ4DZ	02WF38Z	03140J7	03150A2
02Q50ZZ	02QR0ZZ	02TM4ZZ	02UD0JZ	02UH47Z	02UN0KZ	02UT47Z	02VQ4ZZ	02WF3JZ	03140J8	03150A3
02Q53ZZ	02QR3ZZ	02TN0ZZ	02UD0KZ	02UH48Z	02UN37Z	02UT48Z	02VR0CT	02WF3KZ	03140J9	03150A4
02Q54ZZ	02QR4ZZ	02TN3ZZ	02UD37Z	02UH4JZ	02UN38Z	02UT4JZ	02VR0CZ	02WG37Z	03140JB	03150A5
02Q60ZZ	02QS0ZZ	02TN4ZZ	02UD38Z	02UH4KZ	02UN3JZ	02UT4KZ	02VR0DT	02WG38Z	03140JC	03150A6
02Q63ZZ	02QS3ZZ	02U507Z	02UD3JZ	02UJ07G	02UN3KZ	02UV07Z	02VR0DZ	02WG3JZ	03140JD	03150A7
02Q64ZZ	02QS4ZZ	02U508Z	02UD3KZ	02UJ07Z	02UN47Z	02UV08Z	02VR0ZT	02WG3KZ	03140JF	03150A8
02Q70ZZ	02QT0ZZ	02U50JZ	02UD47Z	02UJ08G	02UN48Z	02UV0JZ	02VR0ZZ	02WH37Z	03140JJ	03150A9
02Q73ZZ	02QT3ZZ	02U50KZ	02UD48Z	02UJ08Z	02UN4JZ	02UV0KZ	02VR3CT	02WH38Z	03140JK	03150AB
02Q74ZZ	02QT4ZZ	02U537Z	02UD4JZ	02UJ0JG	02UN4KZ	02UV37Z	02VR3CZ	02WH3JZ	03140JM	03150AC
02Q80ZZ	02QV0ZZ	02U538Z	02UD4KZ	02UJ0JZ	02UP07Z	02UV38Z	02VR3DT	02WH3KZ	03140JN	03150AD
02Q83ZZ	02QV3ZZ	02U53JZ	02UF07J	02UJ0KG	02UP08Z	02UV3JZ	02VR3DZ	02WJ37Z	03140K0	03150AF
02Q84ZZ	02QV4ZZ	02U53KZ	02UF07Z	02UJ0KZ	02UP0JZ	02UV3KZ	02VR3ZT	02WJ38Z	03140K1	03150AJ
02Q90ZZ	02QW0ZZ	02U547Z	02UF08J	02UJ37G	02UP0KZ	02UV47Z	02VR3ZZ	02WJ3JZ	03140K2	03150AK
02Q93ZZ	02QW3ZZ	02U548Z	02UF08Z	02UJ37Z	02UP37Z	02UV48Z	02VR4CT	02WJ3KZ	03140K3	03150AV
02Q94ZZ	02QW4ZZ	02U54JZ	02UF0JJ	02UJ38G	02UP38Z	02UV4JZ	02VR4CZ	02WY0YZ	03140K4	03150J0
02QA0ZZ	02QX0ZZ	02U54KZ	02UF0JZ	02UJ38Z	02UP3JZ	02UV4KZ	02VR4DT	02WY3YZ	03140K5	03150J1
02QA3ZZ	02QX3ZZ	02U607Z	02UF0KJ	02UJ3JG	02UP3KZ	02UW07Z	02VR4DZ	02WY4YZ	03140K6	03150J2
02QA4ZZ	02QX4ZZ	02U608Z	02UF0KZ	02UJ3JZ	02UP47Z	02UW08Z	02VR4ZT	02WYX2Z	03140K7	03150J3
02QB0ZZ	02R507Z	02U60JZ	02UF37J	02UJ3KG	02UP48Z	02UW0JZ	02VR4ZZ	02WYX3Z	03140K8	03150J4
02QB3ZZ	02R508Z	02U60KZ	02UF37Z	02UJ3KZ	02UP4JZ	02UW0KZ	02VS0CZ	02WYX7Z	03140K9	03150J5
02QB4ZZ	02R50JZ	02U637Z	02UF38J	02UJ47G	02UP4KZ	02UW37Z	02VS0DZ	02WYX8Z	03140KB	03150J6
02QC0ZZ	02R50KZ	02U638Z	02UF38Z	02UJ47Z	02UQ07Z	02UW38Z	02VS0ZZ	02WYXCZ	03140KC	03150J7
02QC3ZZ	02R547Z	02U63JZ	02UF3JJ	02UJ48G	02UQ07Z	02UW3JZ	02VS3CZ	02WYXDZ	03140KD	03150J8

03150J9	03160A7	03170A0	031B09F	031L0AJ	03714D6	0373056	03740G6	03753D6	0376456	03794D6
03150JB	03160A8	03170A3	031B0A3	031L0AK	03714DZ	037305Z	03740GZ	03753DZ	037645Z	03794DZ
03150JC	03160A9	03170AD	031B0AF	031L0JJ	03714E6	0373066	03740Z6	03753E6	0376466	03794E6
03150JD	03160AB	03170AF	031B0J3	031L0JK	03714EZ	037306Z	03740ZZ	03753EZ	0376476	03794EZ
03150JF	03160AC	03170AV	031B0JF	031L0KJ	03714F6	0373076	0374346	03753F6	0376476	03794F6
03150JJ	03160AD	03170J0	031B0K3	031L0KK	03714FZ	037307Z	03743434Z	03753FZ	037647Z	03794FZ
03150JK	03160AF	03170J3	031B0KF	031L0ZJ	03714G6	03730D6	0374356	03753G6	03764D6	03794G6
03150JV	03160AJ	03170JD	031B0Z3	031L0ZK	03714GZ	03730DZ	037435Z	03753GZ	03764DZ	03794GZ
03150K0	03160AK	03170JF	031B0ZF	031M09J	03714Z6	03730E6	0374366	03753Z6	03764E6	03794Z6
03150K1	03160AV	03170JV	031C094	031M09K	03714ZZ	03730EZ	037436Z	03753ZZ	03764EZ	03794ZZ
03150K2	03160J0	03170K0	031C09F	031M0AJ	0372046	03730F6	0374376	0375446	03764F6	037A046
03150K3	03160J1	03170K3	031C0A4	031M0AK	037204Z	03730FZ	037437Z	037544Z	03764FZ	037A04Z
03150K4	03160J2	03170KD	031C0AF	031M0JJ	0372056	03730G6	0374446	0375456	03764G6	037A056
03150K5	03160J3	03170KF	031C0J4	031M0JK	037205Z	03730GZ	037444Z	037545Z	03764GZ	037A05Z
03150K6	03160J4	03170KV	031C0JF	031M0KJ	0372066	03730Z6	0374456	0375466	03764Z6	037A066
03150K7	03160J5	03170Z0	031C0K4	031M0KK	037206Z	03730ZZ	037445Z	037546Z	03764ZZ	037A06Z
03150K8	03160J6	03170Z3	031C0KF	031M0ZK	0372076	0373346	0374466	0375476	0377046	037A076
03150K9	03160J7	03170ZD	031C0Z4	031N09J	037207Z	037334Z	037446Z	037547Z	0377704Z	037A07Z
03150KB	03160J8	03170ZF	031C0ZF	031N0AJ	03720D6	0373356	0374476	03754D6	0377056	037A0D6
03150KC	03160J9	03170ZV	031G09G	031N0JJ	03720DZ	037335Z	037447Z	03754DZ	037705Z	037A0DZ
03150KD	03160JB	0318091	031G0AG	031N0KJ	03720E6	0373366	03754446	03754E6	0377066	037A0E6
03150KF	03160JC	0318094	031G0JG	031N0ZJ	03720EZ	037336Z	03754444Z	03754EZ	037706Z	037A0EZ
03150KJ	03160JD	031809D	031G0KG	0371046	03720F6	0373376	0374456	03754F6	0377076	037A0F6
03150KK	03160JF	031809F	031G0ZG	037104Z	03720FZ	037337Z	037445Z	03754FZ	037707Z	037A0FZ
03150KV	03160JJ	031809V	031H09G	0371056	03720G6	03733D6	0374466	03754G6	03770D6	037A0G6
03150Z0	03160JK	03180A1	031H09J	037105Z	03720GZ	03733DZ	037446Z	03754GZ	03770DZ	037A0GZ
03150Z1	03160JV	03180A4	031H09K	0371066	03720Z6	03733E6	0374476	03754Z6	03770E6	037A0Z6
03150Z2	03160K0	03180AD	031H0AG	037106Z	03720ZZ	03733EZ	037447Z	03754ZZ	03770EZ	037A0ZZ
03150Z3	03160K1	03180AF	031H0AJ	0371076	0372346	03733F6	03744D6	0376046	03770F6	037A346
03150Z4	03160K2	03180AV	031H0AK	037107Z	037234Z	03733FZ	03744DZ	037604Z	03770FZ	037A34Z
03150Z5	03160K3	03180J1	031H0JG	03710D6	0372356	03733G6	03744E6	0376056	03770G6	037A356
03150Z6	03160K4	03180J4	031H0JJ	03710DZ	037235Z	03733GZ	03744EZ	037605Z	03770GZ	037A35Z
03150Z7	03160K5	03180JD	031H0JK	03710E6	0372366	03733Z6	03744F6	0376066	03770Z6	037A366
03150Z8	03160K6	03180JF	031H0KG	03710EZ	037236Z	03733ZZ	03744FZ	037606Z	03770ZZ	037A36Z
03150Z9	03160K7	03180JV	031H0KJ	03710F6	0372376	0373446	03744G6	0376076	0377346	037A376
03150ZB	03160K8	03180K1	031H0KK	03710FZ	037237Z	037344Z	03744GZ	037607Z	037734Z	037A37Z
03150ZC	03160K9	03180K4	031H0ZG	03710G6	03723D6	0373456	03744Z6	03760D6	0377356	037A3D6
03150ZD	03160KB	03180KD	031H0ZJ	03710GZ	03723DZ	037345Z	03744ZZ	03760DZ	037735Z	037A3DZ
03150ZF	03160KC	03180KF	031H0ZK	03710Z6	03723E6	0373466	03744ZZ	03760E6	0377366	037A3E6
03150ZJ	03160KD	03180KV	031J09G	03710ZZ	03723EZ	037346Z	03744ZZ	03760EZ	037736Z	037A3EZ
03150ZK	03160KF	03180Z1	031J09J	0371346	03723F6	0373476	0375046	03760F6	0377376	037A3F6
03150ZV	03160KJ	03180Z4	031J09K	037134Z	03723FZ	037347Z	037504Z	03760FZ	037737Z	037A3FZ
0316090	03160KK	03180ZD	031J0AG	0371356	03723G6	03734D6	0375056	03760G6	03773D6	037A3G6
0316091	03160KV	03180ZF	031J0AJ	037135Z	03723GZ	03734DZ	037505Z	03760GZ	03773DZ	037A3GZ
0316092	03160Z0	03180ZV	031J0AK	0371366	03723Z6	03734E6	0375066	03760Z6	0379366	037A3Z6
0316093	03160Z1	0319093	031J0JG	037136Z	03723ZZ	03734EZ	037506Z	03760ZZ	037936Z	037A3ZZ
0316094	03160Z2	031909F	031J0JJ	0371376	0372446	03734F6	0375076	0376346	0379376	037A446
0316095	03160Z3	03190A3	031J0JK	037137Z	037244Z	03734FZ	037507Z	037634Z	037937Z	037A44Z
0316096	03160Z4	03190AF	031J0KG	03713D6	0372456	03734G6	03750D6	0376356	03793D6	037A456
0316097	03160Z5	03190J3	031J0KJ	03713DZ	037245Z	03734GZ	03750DZ	037635Z	03793DZ	037A45Z
0316098	03160Z6	03190JF	031J0KK	03713E6	0372466	03734Z6	03750E6	0376366	03793E6	037A466
0316099	03160Z7	03190K3	031J0ZG	03713EZ	037246Z	03734ZZ	03750EZ	037636Z	03793EZ	037A46Z
031609B	03160Z8	03190KF	031J0ZJ	03713F6	0372476	0374046	03750F6	0376376	03793F6	037A476
031609C	03160Z9	03190Z3	031J0ZK	03713FZ	037247Z	037404Z	03750FZ	037637Z	03793FZ	037A47Z
031609D	03160ZB	03190ZF	031K09J	03713G6	03724D6	0374056	03750G6	03763D6	03793G6	037A4D6
031609F	03160ZC	031A094	031K09K	03713GZ	03724DZ	037405Z	03750GZ	03763DZ	03793GZ	037A4DZ
031609J	03160ZD	031A09F	031K0AJ	03713Z6	03724E6	0374066	03750Z6	03763E6	03793Z6	037A4E6
031609K	03160ZF	031A0A4	031K0AK	03713ZZ	03724EZ	037406Z	03750ZZ	03763EZ	03793ZZ	037A4EZ
031609V	03160ZJ	031A0AF	031K0JJ	0371446	03724F6	0374076	0375346	03763F6	0379446	037A4F6
03160A0	03160ZK	031A0J4	031K0JK	037144Z	03724FZ	037407Z	037534Z	03763FZ	037944Z	037A4FZ
03160A1	03160ZV	031A0JF	031K0KJ	0371456	03724G6	03740D6	0375356	03763G6	0379456	037A4G6
03160A2	0317090	031A0K4	031K0KK	037145Z	03724GZ	03740DZ	037535Z	03763GZ	037945Z	037A4GZ
03160A3	0317093	031A0KF	031K0ZJ	0371466	03724Z6	03740E6	0375366	03763Z6	0379466	037A4Z6
03160A4	031709D	031A0Z4	031K0ZK	037146Z	03724ZZ	03740EZ	037536Z	03763ZZ	037946Z	037A4ZZ
03160A5	031709F	031A0ZF	031L09J	0371476	0373046	03740F6	0375376	0376446	0379476	037B046
03160A6	031709V	031B093	031L09K	037147Z	037304Z	03740FZ	037537Z	037644Z	037947Z	037B04Z

037B056	037C0G6	037D3D6	037F456	037G4G6	037L076	037M346	037N3F6	037R46Z	037S4ZZ	037U0EZ
037B05Z	037C0GZ	037D3DZ	037F45Z	037G4GZ	037L07Z	037M34Z	037N3FZ	037R476	037T046	037U0F6
037B066	037C0Z6	037D3E6	037F466	037G4Z6	037L0D6	037M356	037N3G6	037R47Z	037T04Z	037U0FZ
037B06Z	037C0ZZ	037D3EZ	037F46Z	037G4ZZ	037L0DZ	037M35Z	037N3GZ	037R4D6	037T056	037U0G6
037B076	037C346	037D3F6	037F476	037H046	037L0E6	037M366	037N3Z6	037R4DZ	037T05Z	037U0GZ
037B07Z	037C34Z	037D3FZ	037F47Z	037H04Z	037L0EZ	037M36Z	037N3ZZ	037R4E6	037T066	037U0Z6
037B0D6	037C356	037D3G6	037F4D6	037H056	037L0F6	037M376	037N446	037R4EZ	037T06Z	037U0ZZ
037B0DZ	037C35Z	037D3GZ	037F4DZ	037H05Z	037L0FZ	037M37Z	037N44Z	037R4F6	037T076	037U346
037B0E6	037C366	037D3Z6	037F4E6	037H066	037L0G6	037M3D6	037N456	037R4FZ	037T07Z	037U34Z
037B0EZ	037C36Z	037D3ZZ	037F4EZ	037H06Z	037L0GZ	037M3DZ	037N45Z	037R4G6	037T0D6	037U356
037B0F6	037C376	037D446	037F4F6	037H076	037L0Z6	037M3E6	037N466	037R4GZ	037T0DZ	037U35Z
037B0FZ	037C37Z	037D44Z	037F4FZ	037H07Z	037L0ZZ	037M3EZ	037N46Z	037R4Z6	037T0E6	037U366
037B0G6	037C3D6	037D456	037F4G6	037H0D6	037L346	037M3F6	037N476	037R4ZZ	037T0EZ	037U36Z
037B0GZ	037C3DZ	037D45Z	037F4GZ	037H0DZ	037L34Z	037M3FZ	037N47Z	037S046	037T0F6	037U376
037B0Z6	037C3E6	037D466	037F4Z6	037H0E6	037L356	037M3G6	037N4D6	037S04Z	037T0FZ	037U37Z
037B0ZZ	037C3EZ	037D46Z	037F4ZZ	037H0EZ	037L35Z	037M3GZ	037N4DZ	037S056	037T0G6	037U3D6
037B346	037C3F6	037D476	037G046	037H0F6	037L366	037M3Z6	037N4E6	037S05Z	037T0GZ	037U3DZ
037B34Z	037C3FZ	037D47Z	037G04Z	037H0FZ	037L36Z	037M3ZZ	037N4EZ	037S066	037T0Z6	037U3E6
037B356	037C3G6	037D4D6	037G056	037H0D6	037L376	037M446	037N4F6	037S06Z	037T0ZZ	037U3EZ
037B35Z	037C3GZ	037D4DZ	037G05Z	037K0F6	037L37Z	037M44Z	037N4FZ	037S076	037T346	037U3F6
037B366	037C3Z6	037D4E6	037G066	037K0FZ	037L3D6	037M456	037N4G6	037S07Z	037T34Z	037U3FZ
037B36Z	037C3ZZ	037D4EZ	037G06Z	037K0G6	037L3DZ	037M45Z	037N4GZ	037S0D6	037T356	037U3G6
037B376	037C446	037D4F6	037G076	037K0GZ	037L3E6	037M466	037N4Z6	037S0DZ	037T35Z	037U3GZ
037B37Z	037C44Z	037D4FZ	037G07Z	037K0Z6	037L3EZ	037M46Z	037N4ZZ	037S0E6	037T366	037U3Z6
037B3D6	037C456	037D4G6	037G0D6	037K0ZZ	037L3F6	037M476	037P046	037S0EZ	037T36Z	037U3ZZ
037B3DZ	037C45Z	037D4GZ	037G0DZ	037K346	037L3FZ	037M47Z	037P04Z	037S0F6	037T376	037U446
037B3E6	037C466	037D4Z6	037G0E6	037K34Z	037L3G6	037M4D6	037P056	037S0FZ	037T37Z	037U44Z
037B3EZ	037C46Z	037D4ZZ	037G0EZ	037K356	037L3GZ	037M4DZ	037P05Z	037S0G6	037T3D6	037U456
037B3F6	037C476	037F046	037G0F6	037K35Z	037L3Z6	037M4E6	037P066	037S0GZ	037T3DZ	037U45Z
037B3FZ	037C47Z	037F04Z	037G0FZ	037K366	037L3ZZ	037M4EZ	037P06Z	037S0Z6	037T3E6	037U466
037B3G6	037C4D6	037F056	037G0G6	037K36Z	037L446	037M4F6	037P076	037S0ZZ	037T3EZ	037U46Z
037B3GZ	037C4DZ	037F05Z	037G0GZ	037K376	037L44Z	037M4FZ	037P07Z	037S346	037T3F6	037U476
037B3Z6	037C4E6	037F066	037G0Z6	037K37Z	037L456	037M4G6	037P0D6	037S34Z	037T3FZ	037U47Z
037B3ZZ	037C4EZ	037F06Z	037G0ZZ	037K3D6	037L45Z	037M4GZ	037R0D6	037S356	037T3G6	037U4D6
037B446	037C4F6	037F076	037G346	037K3DZ	037L466	037M4Z6	037R0DZ	037S35Z	037T3GZ	037U4DZ
037B44Z	037C4FZ	037F07Z	037G34Z	037K3E6	037L46Z	037M4ZZ	037R0E6	037S366	037T3Z6	037U4E6
037B456	037C4G6	037F0D6	037G356	037K3EZ	037L476	037N046	037R0EZ	037S36Z	037T3ZZ	037U4EZ
037B45Z	037C4GZ	037F0DZ	037G35Z	037K3F6	037L47Z	037N04Z	037R0F6	037S376	037T446	037U4F6
037B466	037C4Z6	037F0E6	037G366	037K3FZ	037L4D6	037N056	037R0FZ	037S37Z	037T44Z	037U4FZ
037B46Z	037C4ZZ	037F0EZ	037G36Z	037K3G6	037L4DZ	037N05Z	037R0G6	037S3D6	037T456	037U4G6
037B476	037D046	037F0F6	037G376	037K3GZ	037L4E6	037N066	037R0GZ	037S3DZ	037T45Z	037U4GZ
037B47Z	037D04Z	037F0FZ	037G37Z	037K3Z6	037L4EZ	037N06Z	037R0Z6	037S3E6	037T466	037U4Z6
037B4D6	037D056	037F0G6	037G3D6	037K3ZZ	037L4F6	037N076	037R0ZZ	037S3EZ	037T46Z	037U4ZZ
037B4DZ	037D05Z	037F0GZ	037G3DZ	037K446	037L4FZ	037N07Z	037R346	037S3F6	037T476	037V046
037B4E6	037D066	037F0Z6	037G3E6	037K44Z	037L4G6	037N0D6	037R34Z	037S3FZ	037T47Z	037V04Z
037B4EZ	037D06Z	037F0ZZ	037G3EZ	037K456	037L4GZ	037N0DZ	037R356	037S3G6	037T4D6	037V056
037B4F6	037D076	037F346	037G3F6	037K45Z	037L4Z6	037N0E6	037R35Z	037S3GZ	037T4DZ	037V05Z
037B4FZ	037D07Z	037F34Z	037G3FZ	037K466	037L4ZZ	037N0EZ	037R366	037S3Z6	037T4E6	037V066
037B4G6	037D0D6	037F356	037G3G6	037K46Z	037M046	037N0F6	037R36Z	037S3ZZ	037T4EZ	037V06Z
037B4GZ	037D0DZ	037F35Z	037G3GZ	037K47Z	037M04Z	037N0FZ	037R376	037S446	037T4F6	037V076
037B4Z6	037D0E6	037F366	037G3Z6	037K4D6	037M056	037N0G6	037R37Z	037S44Z	037T4FZ	037V07Z
037B4ZZ	037D0EZ	037F36Z	037G3ZZ	037K4DZ	037M05Z	037N0GZ	037R3D6	037S456	037T4G6	037V0D6
037C046	037D0F6	037F376	037G446	037K4E6	037M066	037N0Z6	037R3DZ	037S45Z	037T4GZ	037V0DZ
037C04Z	037D0FZ	037F37Z	037G44Z	037K4EZ	037M06Z	037N0ZZ	037R3E6	037S466	037T4Z6	037V0E6
037C056	037D0G6	037F3D6	037G456	037K4F6	037M076	037N346	037R3EZ	037S46Z	037T4ZZ	037V0EZ
037C05Z	037D0GZ	037F3DZ	037G45Z	037K4FZ	037M07Z	037N34Z	037R3F6	037S476	037U046	037V0F6
037C066	037D0Z6	037F3E6	037G466	037K4G6	037M0D6	037N356	037R3FZ	037S47Z	037U04Z	037V0FZ
037C06Z	037D0ZZ	037F3EZ	037G46Z	037K4GZ	037M0DZ	037N35Z	037R3G6	037S4D6	037U056	037V0G6
037C076	037D346	037F3F6	037G476	037K4Z6	037M0E6	037N366	037R3GZ	037S4DZ	037U05Z	037V0GZ
037C07Z	037D34Z	037F3FZ	037G47Z	037K4ZZ	037M0EZ	037N36Z	037R3Z6	037S4E6	037U066	037V0Z6
037C0D6	037D356	037F3G6	037G4D6	037L046	037M0F6	037N376	037R3ZZ	037S4EZ	037U06Z	037V0ZZ
037C0DZ	037D35Z	037F3GZ	037G4DZ	037L04Z	037M0FZ	037N37Z	037R446	037S4F6	037U076	037V346
037C0E6	037D366	037F3Z6	037G4E6	037L056	037M0G6	037N3D6	037R44Z	037S4FZ	037U07Z	037V34Z
037C0EZ	037D36Z	037F3ZZ	037G4EZ	037L05Z	037M0GZ	037N3DZ	037R456	037S4G6	037U0D6	037V356
037C0F6	037D376	037F446	037G4F6	037L066	037M0Z6	037N3E6	037R45Z	037S4GZ	037U0DZ	037V35Z
037C0FZ	037D37Z	037F44Z	037G4FZ	037L06Z	037M0ZZ	037N3EZ	037R466	037S4Z6	037U0E6	037V366

037V36Z	037Y3ZZ	03950ZZ	039C3ZZ	039L4ZZ	039U0ZZ	03B64ZZ	03C74Z6	03CK4Z6	03CY4Z6	03HF43Z
037V376	037Y446	039530Z	039C40Z	039M00Z	039U30Z	03B70ZX	03C74ZZ	03CK4ZZ	03CY4ZZ	03HG03Z
037V37Z	037Y44Z	03953ZX	039C4ZX	039M0ZX	039U3ZX	03B70ZZ	03C80Z6	03CL0Z6	03H003Z	03HG33Z
037V3D6	037Y456	03953ZZ	039C4ZZ	039M0ZZ	039U3ZZ	03B73ZX	03C80ZZ	03CL0ZZ	03H00DZ	03HG43Z
037V3DZ	037Y45Z	039540Z	039D00Z	039M30Z	039U40Z	03B73ZZ	03C83Z6	03CL3Z6	03H033Z	03HH03Z
037V3E6	037Y466	03954ZX	039D0ZX	039M3ZX	039U4ZX	03B74ZX	03C83ZZ	03CL3ZZ	03H03DZ	03HH33Z
037V3EZ	037Y46Z	03954ZZ	039D0ZZ	039M3ZZ	039U4ZZ	03B74ZZ	03C84Z6	03CL4Z6	03H043Z	03HH43Z
037V3F6	037Y476	039600Z	039D30Z	039M40Z	039V00Z	03B80ZX	03C84ZZ	03CL4ZZ	03H04DZ	03HJ03Z
037V3FZ	037Y47Z	03960ZX	039D3ZX	039M4ZX	039V0ZX	03B80ZZ	03C90Z6	03CM0Z6	03H103Z	03HJ33Z
037V3G6	037Y4D6	03960ZZ	039D3ZZ	039M4ZZ	039V0ZZ	03B83ZX	03C90ZZ	03CM0ZZ	03H10DZ	03HJ43Z
037V3GZ	037Y4DZ	039630Z	039D40Z	039N00Z	039V30Z	03B83ZZ	03C93Z6	03CM3Z6	03H133Z	03HK03Z
037V3Z6	037Y4E6	03963ZX	039D4ZX	039N0ZX	039V3ZX	03B84ZX	03C93ZZ	03CM3ZZ	03H13DZ	03HK33Z
037V3ZZ	037Y4EZ	03963ZZ	039D4ZZ	039N0ZZ	039V3ZZ	03B84ZZ	03C94Z6	03CM4Z6	03H143Z	03HK43Z
037V446	037Y4F6	039640Z	039F00Z	039N30Z	039V40Z	03B90ZX	03C94ZZ	03CM4ZZ	03H14DZ	03HL03Z
037V44Z	037Y4FZ	03964ZX	039F0ZX	039N3ZX	039V4ZX	03B90ZZ	03CA0Z6	03CN0Z6	03H203Z	03HL33Z
037V456	037Y4G6	03964ZZ	039F0ZZ	039N3ZZ	039V4ZZ	03B93ZX	03CA0ZZ	03CN0ZZ	03H20DZ	03HL43Z
037V45Z	037Y4GZ	039700Z	039F30Z	039N40Z	039Y00Z	03B93ZZ	03CA3Z6	03CN3Z6	03H233Z	03HM03Z
037V466	037Y4Z6	03970ZX	039F3ZX	039N4ZX	039Y0ZX	03B94ZX	03CA3ZZ	03CN3ZZ	03H23DZ	03HM33Z
037V46Z	037Y4ZZ	03970ZZ	039F3ZZ	039N4ZZ	039Y0ZZ	03B94ZZ	03CA4Z6	03CN4Z6	03H243Z	03HM43Z
037V476	039000Z	039730Z	039F40Z	039P00Z	039Y30Z	03BA0ZX	03CA4ZZ	03CN4ZZ	03H24DZ	03HN03Z
037V47Z	03900ZX	03973ZX	039F4ZX	039P0ZX	039Y3ZX	03BA0ZZ	03CB0Z6	03CP0Z6	03H303Z	03HN33Z
037V4D6	03900ZZ	03973ZZ	039F4ZZ	039P0ZZ	039Y3ZZ	03BA3ZX	03CB0ZZ	03CP0ZZ	03H30DZ	03HN43Z
037V4DZ	039030Z	039740Z	039G00Z	039P30Z	039Y40Z	03BA3ZZ	03CB3Z6	03CP3Z6	03H333Z	03HP03Z
037V4E6	03903ZX	03974ZX	039G0ZX	039P3ZX	039Y4ZX	03BA4ZX	03CB3ZZ	03CP3ZZ	03H33DZ	03HP33Z
037V4EZ	03903ZZ	03974ZZ	039G0ZZ	039P3ZZ	039Y4ZZ	03BA4ZZ	03CB4Z6	03CP4Z6	03H343Z	03HP43Z
037V4F6	039040Z	039800Z	039G30Z	039P40Z	03B00ZX	03BB0ZX	03CB4ZZ	03CP4ZZ	03H34DZ	03HQ03Z
037V4FZ	03904ZX	03980ZX	039G3ZX	039P4ZX	03B00ZZ	03BB0ZZ	03CC0Z6	03CQ0Z6	03H403Z	03HQ33Z
037V4G6	03904ZZ	03980ZZ	039G3ZZ	039P4ZZ	03B03ZX	03BB3ZX	03CC0ZZ	03CQ0ZZ	03H40DZ	03HQ43Z
037V4GZ	039100Z	039830Z	039G40Z	039Q00Z	03B03ZZ	03BB3ZZ	03CC3Z6	03CQ3Z6	03H433Z	03HR03Z
037V4Z6	03910ZX	03983ZX	039G4ZX	039Q0ZX	03B04ZX	03BB4ZX	03CC3ZZ	03CQ3ZZ	03H43DZ	03HR33Z
037V4ZZ	03910ZZ	03983ZZ	039G4ZZ	039Q0ZZ	03B04ZZ	03BB4ZZ	03CC4Z6	03CQ4Z6	03H443Z	03HR43Z
037Y046	039130Z	039840Z	039H00Z	039Q30Z	03B10ZX	03BC0ZX	03CC4ZZ	03CQ4ZZ	03H44DZ	03HS03Z
037Y04Z	03913ZX	03984ZX	039H0ZX	039Q3ZX	03B10ZZ	03BC0ZZ	03CD0Z6	03CR0Z6	03H503Z	03HS33Z
037Y056	03913ZZ	03984ZZ	039H0ZZ	039Q3ZZ	03B13ZX	03BC3ZX	03CD0ZZ	03CR0ZZ	03H50DZ	03HS43Z
037Y05Z	039140Z	039900Z	039H30Z	039Q40Z	03B13ZZ	03BC3ZZ	03CD3Z6	03CR3Z6	03H533Z	03HT03Z
037Y066	03914ZX	03990ZX	039H3ZX	039Q4ZX	03B14ZX	03C23ZZ	03CD3ZZ	03CR3ZZ	03H53DZ	03HT33Z
037Y06Z	03914ZZ	03990ZZ	039H3ZZ	039Q4ZZ	03B14ZZ	03C24Z6	03CD4Z6	03CR4Z6	03H543Z	03HT43Z
037Y076	039200Z	039930Z	039H40Z	039R00Z	03B20ZX	03C24ZZ	03CD4ZZ	03CR4ZZ	03H54DZ	03HU03Z
037Y07Z	03920ZX	03993ZX	039H4ZX	039R0ZX	03B20ZZ	03C30Z6	03CF0Z6	03CS0Z6	03H603Z	03HU33Z
037Y0D6	03920ZZ	03993ZZ	039H4ZZ	039R0ZZ	03B23ZX	03C30ZZ	03CF0ZZ	03CS0ZZ	03H60DZ	03HU43Z
037Y0DZ	039230Z	039940Z	039J00Z	039R30Z	03B23ZZ	03C33Z6	03CF3Z6	03CS3Z6	03H633Z	03HV03Z
037Y0E6	03923ZX	03994ZX	039J0ZX	039R3ZX	03B24ZX	03C33ZZ	03CF3ZZ	03CS3ZZ	03H63DZ	03HV33Z
037Y0EZ	03923ZZ	03994ZZ	039J0ZZ	039R3ZZ	03B24ZZ	03C34Z6	03CF4Z6	03CS4Z6	03H643Z	03HV43Z
037Y0F6	039240Z	039A00Z	039J30Z	039R40Z	03B30ZX	03C34ZZ	03CF4ZZ	03CS4ZZ	03H703Z	03HY03Z
037Y0FZ	03924ZX	039A0ZX	039J3ZX	039R4ZX	03B30ZZ	03C40Z6	03CG0Z6	03CT0Z6	03H733Z	03HY0YZ
037Y0G6	03924ZZ	039A0ZZ	039J3ZZ	039R4ZZ	03B33ZX	03C40ZZ	03CG0ZZ	03CT0ZZ	03H743Z	03HY32Z
037Y0GZ	039300Z	039A30Z	039J40Z	039S00Z	03B33ZZ	03C43Z6	03CG3Z6	03CT3Z6	03H803Z	03HY33Z
037Y0Z6	03930ZX	039A3ZX	039J4ZX	039S0ZX	03B34ZX	03C43ZZ	03CG3ZZ	03CT3ZZ	03H833Z	03HY3YZ
037Y0ZZ	03930ZZ	039A3ZZ	039J4ZZ	039S0ZZ	03B34ZZ	03C44Z6	03CG4Z6	03CT4Z6	03H843Z	03HY43Z
037Y346	039330Z	039A40Z	039K00Z	039S30Z	03B40ZX	03C44ZZ	03CG4ZZ	03CT4ZZ	03H903Z	03HY4YZ
037Y34Z	03933ZX	039A4ZX	039K0ZX	039S3ZX	03B40ZZ	03C50Z6	03CH0Z6	03CU0Z6	03H933Z	03JY3ZZ
037Y356	03933ZZ	039A4ZZ	039K0ZZ	039S3ZZ	03B43ZX	03C50ZZ	03CH0ZZ	03CU0ZZ	03H943Z	03JY4ZZ
037Y35Z	039340Z	039B00Z	039K30Z	039S40Z	03B43ZZ	03C53Z6	03CH3Z6	03CU3Z6	03HA03Z	03JYXZZ
037Y366	03934ZX	039B0ZX	039K3ZX	039S4ZX	03B44ZX	03C53ZZ	03CH3ZZ	03CU3ZZ	03HA33Z	03L00ZZ
037Y36Z	03934ZZ	039B0ZZ	039K3ZZ	039S4ZZ	03B44ZZ	03C54Z6	03CH4Z6	03CU4Z6	03HA43Z	03L03CZ
037Y376	039400Z	039B30Z	039K40Z	039T00Z	03B50ZX	03C54ZZ	03CH4ZZ	03CU4ZZ	03HB03Z	03L03DZ
037Y37Z	03940ZX	039B3ZX	039K4ZX	039T0ZX	03B50ZZ	03C60Z6	03CJ0Z6	03CV0Z6	03HB33Z	03L03ZZ
037Y3D6	03940ZZ	039B3ZZ	039K4ZZ	039T0ZZ	03B53ZX	03C60ZZ	03CJ0ZZ	03CV0ZZ	03HB43Z	03L04CZ
037Y3DZ	039430Z	039B40Z	039L00Z	039T30Z	03B53ZZ	03C63Z6	03CJ3Z6	03CV3Z6	03HC03Z	03L04DZ
037Y3E6	03943ZX	039B4ZX	039L0ZX	039T3ZX	03B54ZX	03C63ZZ	03CJ3ZZ	03CV3ZZ	03HC33Z	03L04ZZ
037Y3EZ	03943ZZ	039B4ZZ	039L0ZZ	039T3ZZ	03B54ZZ	03C64Z6	03CJ4Z6	03CV4Z6	03HC43Z	03L10CZ
037Y3F6	039440Z	039C00Z	039L30Z	039T40Z	03B60ZX	03C64ZZ	03CJ4ZZ	03CV4ZZ	03HD03Z	03L10DZ
037Y3FZ	03944ZX	039C0ZX	039L3ZX	039T4ZX	03B60ZZ	03C70Z6	03CK0Z6	03CY0Z6	03HD33Z	03L13CZ
037Y3G6	03944ZZ	039C0ZZ	039L3ZZ	039T4ZZ	03B63ZX	03C70ZZ	03CK0ZZ	03CY0ZZ	03HD43Z	03L13DZ
037Y3GZ	039500Z	039C30Z	039L40Z	039U00Z	03B63ZZ	03C73Z6	03CK3Z6	03CY3Z6	03HF03Z	03L13ZZ
037Y3Z6	03950ZX	039C3ZX	039L4ZX	039U0ZX	03B64ZX	03C73ZZ	03CK3ZZ	03CY3ZZ	03HF33Z	

03L14CZ	03L90CZ	03LH0BZ	03LY3CZ	03NM0ZZ	03Q03ZZ	03QP3ZZ	03R70JZ	03SU3ZZ	03U63JZ	03UD4JZ
03L14DZ	03L90DZ	03LH0CZ	03LY3DZ	03NM3ZZ	03Q04ZZ	03QP4ZZ	03R70KZ	03SU4ZZ	03U63KZ	03UD4KZ
03L14ZZ	03L90ZZ	03LH0DZ	03LY3ZZ	03NM4ZZ	03Q10ZZ	03QQ0ZZ	03R747Z	03SV0ZZ	03U647Z	03UF07Z
03L20CZ	03L93CZ	03LH0ZZ	03LY4CZ	03NN0ZZ	03Q13ZZ	03QQ3ZZ	03R74JZ	03SV3ZZ	03U64JZ	03UF0JZ
03L20DZ	03L93DZ	03LH3BZ	03LY4DZ	03NN3ZZ	03Q14ZZ	03QQ4ZZ	03R74KZ	03SV4ZZ	03U64KZ	03UF0KZ
03L20ZZ	03L93ZZ	03LH3CZ	03LY4ZZ	03NN4ZZ	03Q20ZZ	03QR0ZZ	03R807Z	03SY0ZZ	03U707Z	03UF37Z
03L23CZ	03L94CZ	03LH3DZ	03N00ZZ	03NP0ZZ	03Q23ZZ	03QR3ZZ	03R80JZ	03SY3ZZ	03U70JZ	03UF3JZ
03L23DZ	03L94DZ	03LH3ZZ	03N03ZZ	03NP3ZZ	03Q24ZZ	03QR4ZZ	03R80KZ	03SY4ZZ	03U70KZ	03UF3KZ
03L23ZZ	03L94ZZ	03LH4BZ	03N04ZZ	03NP4ZZ	03Q30ZZ	03QS0ZZ	03R847Z	03U007Z	03U737Z	03UF47Z
03L24CZ	03LA0CZ	03LH4CZ	03N10ZZ	03NQ0ZZ	03Q33ZZ	03QS3ZZ	03R84JZ	03U00JZ	03U73JZ	03UF4JZ
03L24DZ	03LA0DZ	03LH4DZ	03N13ZZ	03NQ3ZZ	03Q34ZZ	03QS4ZZ	03R84KZ	03U00KZ	03U73KZ	03UF4KZ
03L24ZZ	03LA0ZZ	03LH4ZZ	03N14ZZ	03NQ4ZZ	03Q40ZZ	03QT0ZZ	03R907Z	03U037Z	03U747Z	03UG07Z
03L30CZ	03LA3CZ	03LJ0BZ	03N20ZZ	03NR0ZZ	03Q43ZZ	03QT3ZZ	03R90JZ	03U03JZ	03U74JZ	03UG0JZ
03L30DZ	03LA3DZ	03LJ0CZ	03N23ZZ	03NR3ZZ	03Q44ZZ	03QT4ZZ	03R90KZ	03U03KZ	03U74KZ	03UG0KZ
03L30ZZ	03LA3ZZ	03LJ0DZ	03N24ZZ	03NR4ZZ	03Q50ZZ	03QU0ZZ	03R947Z	03U047Z	03U807Z	03UG37Z
03L33CZ	03LA4CZ	03LJ0ZZ	03N30ZZ	03NS0ZZ	03Q53ZZ	03QU3ZZ	03R94JZ	03U04JZ	03U80JZ	03UG3JZ
03L33DZ	03LA4DZ	03LJ3BZ	03N33ZZ	03NS3ZZ	03Q54ZZ	03QU4ZZ	03R94KZ	03U04KZ	03U80KZ	03UG3KZ
03L33ZZ	03LA4ZZ	03LJ3CZ	03N34ZZ	03NS4ZZ	03Q60ZZ	03QV0ZZ	03RA07Z	03U107Z	03U837Z	03UG47Z
03L34CZ	03LB0CZ	03LJ3DZ	03N40ZZ	03NT0ZZ	03Q63ZZ	03QV3ZZ	03RA0JZ	03U10JZ	03U83JZ	03UG4JZ
03L34DZ	03LB0DZ	03LJ3ZZ	03N43ZZ	03NT3ZZ	03Q64ZZ	03QV4ZZ	03RA0KZ	03U10KZ	03U83KZ	03UG4KZ
03L34ZZ	03LB0ZZ	03LJ4BZ	03N44ZZ	03NT4ZZ	03Q70ZZ	03QY0ZZ	03RA47Z	03U137Z	03U847Z	03UH07Z
03L40CZ	03LB3CZ	03LJ4CZ	03N50ZZ	03NU0ZZ	03Q73ZZ	03QY3ZZ	03RA4JZ	03U13JZ	03U84JZ	03UH0JZ
03L40DZ	03LB3DZ	03LJ4DZ	03N53ZZ	03NU3ZZ	03Q74ZZ	03QY4ZZ	03RA4KZ	03U13KZ	03U84KZ	03UH0KZ
03L40ZZ	03LB3ZZ	03LJ4ZZ	03N54ZZ	03NU4ZZ	03Q80ZZ	03R007Z	03RB07Z	03U147Z	03U907Z	03UH37Z
03L43CZ	03LB4CZ	03LK0BZ	03N60ZZ	03NV0ZZ	03Q83ZZ	03R00JZ	03RB0JZ	03U14JZ	03U90JZ	03UH3JZ
03L43DZ	03LB4DZ	03LK0CZ	03N63ZZ	03NV3ZZ	03Q84ZZ	03R00KZ	03RB0KZ	03U14KZ	03U90KZ	03UH3KZ
03L43ZZ	03LB4ZZ	03LK0DZ	03N64ZZ	03NV4ZZ	03Q90ZZ	03R047Z	03RB47Z	03U207Z	03U937Z	03UH47Z
03L44CZ	03LC0CZ	03LK0ZZ	03N70ZZ	03NY0ZZ	03Q93ZZ	03R04JZ	03RB4JZ	03U20JZ	03U93JZ	03UH4JZ
03L44DZ	03LC0DZ	03LK3BZ	03N73ZZ	03NY3ZZ	03Q94ZZ	03R04KZ	03RB4KZ	03U20KZ	03U93KZ	03UH4KZ
03L44ZZ	03LC0ZZ	03LK3CZ	03N74ZZ	03NY4ZZ	03QA0ZZ	03R107Z	03RC07Z	03U237Z	03U947Z	03UJ07Z
03L50CZ	03LC3CZ	03LK3DZ	03N80ZZ	03PY00Z	03QA3ZZ	03R10JZ	03RC0JZ	03U23JZ	03U94JZ	03UJ0JZ
03L50DZ	03LC3DZ	03LK3ZZ	03N83ZZ	03PY02Z	03QA4ZZ	03R10KZ	03RC0KZ	03U23KZ	03U94KZ	03UJ0KZ
03L50ZZ	03LC3ZZ	03LK4BZ	03N84ZZ	03PY03Z	03QB0ZZ	03R147Z	03RC47Z	03U247Z	03UA07Z	03UJ37Z
03L53CZ	03LC4CZ	03LK4CZ	03N90ZZ	03PY07Z	03QB3ZZ	03R14JZ	03RC4JZ	03U24JZ	03UA0JZ	03UJ3JZ
03L53DZ	03LC4DZ	03LK4DZ	03N93ZZ	03PY0CZ	03QB4ZZ	03R14KZ	03RC4KZ	03U24KZ	03UA0KZ	03UJ3KZ
03L53ZZ	03LC4ZZ	03LK4ZZ	03N94ZZ	03PY0DZ	03QC0ZZ	03R207Z	03SJ0ZZ	03U307Z	03UA37Z	03UJ47Z
03L54CZ	03LD0CZ	03LL0BZ	03NA0ZZ	03PY0JZ	03QC3ZZ	03R20JZ	03SJ3ZZ	03U30JZ	03UA3JZ	03UJ4JZ
03L54DZ	03LD0DZ	03LL0CZ	03NA3ZZ	03PY0KZ	03QC4ZZ	03R20KZ	03SJ4ZZ	03U30KZ	03UA3KZ	03UJ4KZ
03L54ZZ	03LD0ZZ	03LL0DZ	03NA4ZZ	03PY0MZ	03QD0ZZ	03R247Z	03SK0ZZ	03U337Z	03UA47Z	03UK07Z
03L60CZ	03LD3CZ	03LL0ZZ	03NB0ZZ	03PY0YZ	03QD3ZZ	03R24JZ	03SK3ZZ	03U33JZ	03UA4JZ	03UK0JZ
03L60DZ	03LD3DZ	03LL3BZ	03NB3ZZ	03PY30Z	03QD4ZZ	03R24KZ	03SK4ZZ	03U33KZ	03UA4KZ	03UK0KZ
03L60ZZ	03LD3ZZ	03LL3CZ	03NB4ZZ	03PY32Z	03QF0ZZ	03R307Z	03SL0ZZ	03U347Z	03UB07Z	03UK37Z
03L63CZ	03LD4CZ	03LL3DZ	03NC0ZZ	03PY33Z	03QF3ZZ	03R30JZ	03SL3ZZ	03U34JZ	03UB0JZ	03UK3JZ
03L63DZ	03LD4DZ	03LL3ZZ	03NC3ZZ	03PY37Z	03QF4ZZ	03R30KZ	03SL4ZZ	03U34KZ	03UB0KZ	03UK3KZ
03L63ZZ	03LD4ZZ	03LL4BZ	03NC4ZZ	03PY3CZ	03QG0ZZ	03R347Z	03SM0ZZ	03U407Z	03UB37Z	03UK47Z
03L64CZ	03LF0CZ	03LL4CZ	03ND0ZZ	03PY3DZ	03QG3ZZ	03R34JZ	03SM3ZZ	03U40JZ	03UB3JZ	03UK4JZ
03L64DZ	03LF0DZ	03LL4DZ	03ND3ZZ	03PY3JZ	03QG4ZZ	03R34KZ	03SM4ZZ	03U40KZ	03UB3KZ	03UK4KZ
03L64ZZ	03LF0ZZ	03LL4ZZ	03ND4ZZ	03PY3KZ	03QH0ZZ	03R407Z	03SN0ZZ	03U437Z	03UB47Z	03UL07Z
03L70CZ	03LF3CZ	03LM0BZ	03NF0ZZ	03PY3MZ	03QH3ZZ	03R40JZ	03SN3ZZ	03U43JZ	03UB4JZ	03UL0JZ
03L70DZ	03LF3DZ	03LM0CZ	03NF3ZZ	03PY3YZ	03QH4ZZ	03R40KZ	03SN4ZZ	03U43KZ	03UB4KZ	03UL0KZ
03L70ZZ	03LF3ZZ	03LM0DZ	03NF4ZZ	03PY40Z	03QJ0ZZ	03R447Z	03SP0ZZ	03U447Z	03UC07Z	03UL37Z
03L73CZ	03LF4CZ	03LM0ZZ	03NG0ZZ	03PY42Z	03QJ3ZZ	03R44JZ	03SP3ZZ	03U44JZ	03UC0JZ	03UL3JZ
03L73DZ	03LF4DZ	03LM3BZ	03NG3ZZ	03PY43Z	03QJ4ZZ	03R44KZ	03SP4ZZ	03U44KZ	03UC0KZ	03UL3KZ
03L73ZZ	03LF4ZZ	03LM3CZ	03NG4ZZ	03PY47Z	03QK0ZZ	03R507Z	03SQ0ZZ	03U507Z	03UC37Z	03UL47Z
03L74CZ	03LG0BZ	03LV0CZ	03NH0ZZ	03PY4CZ	03QK3ZZ	03R50JZ	03SQ3ZZ	03U50JZ	03UC3JZ	03UL4JZ
03L74DZ	03LG0CZ	03LV0DZ	03NH3ZZ	03PY4DZ	03QK4ZZ	03R50KZ	03SQ4ZZ	03U50KZ	03UC3KZ	03UL4KZ
03L74ZZ	03LG0DZ	03LV0ZZ	03NH4ZZ	03PY4JZ	03QL0ZZ	03R547Z	03SR0ZZ	03U537Z	03UC47Z	03UM07Z
03L80CZ	03LG0ZZ	03LV3CZ	03NJ0ZZ	03PY4KZ	03QL3ZZ	03R54JZ	03SR3ZZ	03U53JZ	03UC4JZ	03UM0JZ
03L80DZ	03LG3BZ	03LV3DZ	03NJ3ZZ	03PY4MZ	03QL4ZZ	03R54KZ	03SR4ZZ	03U53KZ	03UC4KZ	03UM0KZ
03L80ZZ	03LG3CZ	03LV3ZZ	03NJ4ZZ	03PY4YZ	03QM0ZZ	03R607Z	03SS0ZZ	03U547Z	03UD07Z	03UM37Z
03L83CZ	03LG3DZ	03LV4CZ	03NK0ZZ	03PYX0Z	03QM3ZZ	03R60JZ	03SS3ZZ	03U54JZ	03UD0JZ	03UM3JZ
03L83DZ	03LG3ZZ	03LV4DZ	03NK3ZZ	03PYX2Z	03QM4ZZ	03R60KZ	03SS4ZZ	03U54KZ	03UD0KZ	03UM3KZ
03L83ZZ	03LG4BZ	03LV4ZZ	03NK4ZZ	03PYX3Z	03QN0ZZ	03R647Z	03ST0ZZ	03U607Z	03UD37Z	03UM47Z
03L84CZ	03LG4CZ	03LY0CZ	03NL0ZZ	03PYXDZ	03QN3ZZ	03R64JZ	03ST3ZZ	03U60JZ	03UD3JZ	03UM4JZ
03L84DZ	03LG4DZ	03LY0DZ	03NL3ZZ	03PYXMZ	03QN4ZZ	03R64KZ	03ST4ZZ	03U60KZ	03UD3KZ	03UM4KZ
03L84ZZ	03LG4ZZ	03LY0ZZ	03NL4ZZ	03Q00ZZ	03QP0ZZ	03R707Z	03SU0ZZ	03U637Z	03UD47Z	03UN07Z

03UN0JZ	03UV3JZ	03VM3DZ	03VT4CZ	03WYXJZ	04100K3	04104A9	041C4K2	041D0A8	041D0ZG	041D4K0
03UN0KZ	03UV3KZ	03VM3ZZ	03VT4DZ	03WYXKZ	04100K4	04104AB	041C4K3	041D0A9	041D0ZH	041D4K1
03UN37Z	03UV47Z	03VM4BZ	03VT4ZZ	03WYXMZ	04100K5	04104AC	041C4K4	041D0AB	041D0ZJ	041D4K2
03UN3JZ	03UV4JZ	03VM4CZ	03VU0CZ	0410090	04100K6	04104AD	041C4K5	041D0AC	041D0ZK	041D4K3
03UN3KZ	03UV4KZ	03VM4DZ	03VU0DZ	0410091	04100K7	0413093	041C4K6	041D0AD	041D0ZQ	041D4K4
03UN47Z	03UY07Z	03VM4ZZ	03VU0ZZ	0410092	04100K8	0413094	041C4K7	041D0AF	041D0ZR	041D4K5
03UN4JZ	03UY0JZ	03VN0BZ	03VU3CZ	0410093	04100K9	0413095	041C4K8	041D0AG	041D490	041D4K6
03UN4KZ	03UY0KZ	03VN0CZ	03VU3DZ	0410094	04100KB	04130A3	041C4K9	041D0AH	041D491	041D4K7
03UP07Z	03UY37Z	03VN0DZ	03VU3ZZ	0410095	04100KC	04130A4	041C4KB	041D0AJ	041D492	041D4K8
03UP0JZ	03UY3JZ	03VN0ZZ	03VU4CZ	0410096	04100KD	04130A5	041C4KC	041D0AK	041D493	041D4K9
03UP0KZ	03UY3KZ	03VN3BZ	03VU4DZ	0410097	04100KF	04130J3	041C4KD	041D0AQ	041D494	041D4KB
03UP37Z	03UY47Z	03VN3CZ	03VU4ZZ	0410098	04100KG	04130J4	041C4KF	041D0AR	041D495	041D4KC
03UP3JZ	03UY4JZ	03VN3DZ	03VV0CZ	0410099	04100KH	04130J5	041C4KG	041D0J0	041D496	041D4KD
03UP3KZ	03UY4KZ	03VN3ZZ	03VV0DZ	041009B	04100KJ	04130K3	041C4KH	041D0J1	041D497	041D4KF
03UP47Z	03V00CZ	03VN4BZ	03VV0ZZ	041009C	04100KK	04130K4	041C4KJ	041D0J2	041D498	041D4KG
03UP4JZ	03V00DZ	03VN4CZ	03VV3CZ	041009D	04100KQ	04130K5	041C4KK	041D0J3	041D499	041D4KH
03UP4KZ	03V00ZZ	03VN4DZ	03VV3DZ	041009F	04100KR	04130Z3	041C4KQ	041D0J4	041D49B	041D4KJ
03UQ07Z	03V03CZ	03VN4ZZ	03VV3ZZ	041009G	04100Z0	04130Z4	041C4KR	041D0J5	041D49C	041D4KK
03UQ0JZ	03V03DZ	03VP0BZ	03VV4CZ	041009H	04100Z1	04130Z5	041C4Z0	041D0J6	041D49D	041D4KQ
03UQ0KZ	03V03ZZ	03VP0CZ	03VV4DZ	041009J	04100Z2	0413493	041C4Z1	041D0J7	041D49F	041D4KR
03UQ37Z	03V04CZ	03VP0DZ	03VV4ZZ	041009K	04100Z3	0413494	041C4Z2	041D0J8	041D49G	041D4Z0
03UQ3JZ	03V04DZ	03VP0ZZ	03VY0CZ	041009Q	04100Z4	0413495	041C4Z3	041D0J9	041D49H	041D4Z1
03UQ3KZ	03V04ZZ	03VP3BZ	03VY0DZ	041009R	04100Z5	04134A3	041C4Z4	041D0JB	041D49J	041D4Z2
03UQ47Z	03V10CZ	03VP3CZ	03VY0ZZ	04100A0	04100Z6	04134A4	041C4Z5	041D0JC	041D49K	041D4Z3
03UQ4JZ	03V10DZ	03VP3DZ	03VY3CZ	04100A1	04100Z7	04134A5	041C4Z6	041D0JD	041D49Q	041D4Z4
03UQ4KZ	03V10ZZ	03VP3ZZ	03VY3DZ	04100A2	04100Z8	04134J3	041C4Z7	041D0JF	041D49R	041D4Z5
03UR07Z	03V13CZ	03VP4BZ	03VY3ZZ	04100A3	04100Z9	04134J4	041C4Z8	041D0JG	041D4A0	041D4Z6
03UR0JZ	03V13DZ	03VP4CZ	03VY4CZ	04100A4	04100ZB	04134J5	041C4Z9	041D0JH	041D4A1	041D4Z7
03UR0KZ	03V13ZZ	03VP4DZ	03VY4DZ	04100A5	04100ZC	04134K3	041C4ZB	041D0JJ	041D4A2	041D4Z8
03UR37Z	03V14CZ	03VP4ZZ	03VY4ZZ	04100A6	04100ZD	04134K4	041C4ZC	041D0JK	041D4A3	041D4Z9
03UR3JZ	03V14DZ	03VQ0BZ	03WY00Z	04100A7	04100ZF	04134K5	041C4ZD	041D0JQ	041D4A4	041D4ZB
03UR3KZ	03V14ZZ	03VQ0CZ	03WY02Z	04100A8	04100ZG	04134Z3	041C4ZF	041D0JR	041D4A5	041D4ZC
03UR47Z	03V20CZ	03VQ0DZ	03WY03Z	04100A9	04100ZH	04134Z4	041C4ZG	041D0K0	041D4A6	041D4ZD
03UR4JZ	03V20DZ	03VQ0ZZ	03WY07Z	04100AB	04100ZJ	04134Z5	041C4ZH	041D0K1	041D4A7	041D4ZF
03UR4KZ	03V20ZZ	03VQ3BZ	03WY0CZ	04100AC	04100ZK	041C4AB	041C4ZJ	041D0K2	041D4A8	041D4ZG
03US07Z	03V23CZ	03VQ3CZ	03WY0DZ	04100AD	04100ZQ	041C4AC	041C4ZK	041D0K3	041D4A9	041D4ZH
03US0JZ	03V23DZ	03VQ3DZ	03WY0JZ	04100AF	04100ZR	041C4AD	041C4ZQ	041D0K4	041D4AB	041D4ZJ
03US0KZ	03V23ZZ	03VQ3ZZ	03WY0KZ	04100AG	0410490	041C4AF	041C4ZR	041D0K5	041D4AC	041D4ZK
03US37Z	03V24CZ	03VQ4BZ	03WY0MZ	04100AH	0410491	041C4AG	041D090	041D0K6	041D4AD	041D4ZQ
03US3JZ	03V24DZ	03VQ4CZ	03WY0YZ	04100AJ	0410492	041C4AH	041D091	041D0K7	041D4AF	041D4ZR
03US3KZ	03V24ZZ	03VQ4DZ	03WY30Z	04100AK	0410493	041C4AJ	041D092	041D0K8	041D4AG	041E099
03US47Z	03V30CZ	03VQ4ZZ	03WY32Z	04100AQ	0410494	041C4AK	041D093	041D0K9	041D4AH	041E09B
03US4JZ	03V30DZ	03VR0CZ	03WY33Z	04100AR	0410495	041C4AQ	041D094	041D0KB	041D4AJ	041E09C
03US4KZ	03V30ZZ	03VR0DZ	03WY37Z	04100J0	0410496	041C4AR	041D095	041D0KC	041D4AK	041E09D
03UT07Z	03V33CZ	03VR0ZZ	03WY3CZ	04100J1	0410497	041C4J0	041D096	041D0KD	041D4AQ	041E09F
03UT0JZ	03V33DZ	03VR3CZ	03WY3DZ	04100J2	0410498	041C4J1	041D097	041D0KF	041D4AR	041E09G
03UT0KZ	03V33ZZ	03VR3DZ	03WY3JZ	04100J3	0410499	041C4J2	041D098	041D0KG	041D4J0	041E09H
03UT37Z	03V34CZ	03VR3ZZ	03WY3KZ	04100J4	041049B	041C4J3	041D099	041D0KH	041D4J1	041E09J
03UT3JZ	03VL0BZ	03VR4CZ	03WY3MZ	04100J5	041049C	041C4J4	041D09B	041D0KJ	041D4J2	041E09K
03UT3KZ	03VL0CZ	03VR4DZ	03WY3YZ	04100J6	041049D	041C4J5	041D09C	041D0KK	041D4J3	041E09P
03UT47Z	03VL0DZ	03VR4ZZ	03WY40Z	04100J7	041049F	041C4J6	041D09D	041D0KQ	041D4J4	041E09Q
03UT4JZ	03VL0ZZ	03VS0CZ	03WY42Z	04100J8	041049G	041C4J7	041D09F	041D0KR	041D4J5	041E0A9
03UT4KZ	03VL3BZ	03VS0DZ	03WY43Z	04100J9	041049H	041C4J8	041D09G	041D0Z0	041D4J6	041E0AB
03UU07Z	03VL3CZ	03VS0ZZ	03WY47Z	04100JB	041049J	041C4J9	041D09H	041D0Z1	041D4J7	041E0AC
03UU0JZ	03VL3DZ	03VS3CZ	03WY4CZ	04100JC	041049K	041C4JB	041D09J	041D0Z2	041D4J8	041E0AD
03UU0KZ	03VL3ZZ	03VS3DZ	03WY4DZ	04100JD	041049Q	041C4JC	041D09K	041D0Z3	041D4J9	041E0AF
03UU37Z	03VL4BZ	03VS3ZZ	03WY4JZ	04100JF	041049R	041C4JD	041D09Q	041D0Z4	041D4JB	041E0AG
03UU3JZ	03VL4CZ	03VS4CZ	03WY4KZ	04100JG	04104A0	041C4JF	041D09R	041D0Z5	041D4JC	041E0AH
03UU3KZ	03VL4DZ	03VS4DZ	03WY4MZ	04100JH	04104A1	041C4JG	041D0A0	041D0Z6	041D4JD	041E0AJ
03UU47Z	03VL4ZZ	03VS4ZZ	03WY4YZ	04100JJ	04104A2	041C4JH	041D0A1	041D0Z7	041D4JF	041E0AK
03UU4JZ	03VM0BZ	03VT0CZ	03WYX0Z	04100JK	04104A3	041C4JJ	041D0A2	041D0Z8	041D4JG	041E0AP
03UU4KZ	03VM0CZ	03VT0DZ	03WYX2Z	04100JQ	04104A4	041C4JK	041D0A3	041D0Z9	041D4JH	041E0AQ
03UV07Z	03VM0DZ	03VT0ZZ	03WYX3Z	04100JR	04104A5	041C4JQ	041D0A4	041D0ZB	041D4JJ	041E0J9
03UV0JZ	03VM0ZZ	03VT3CZ	03WYX7Z	04100K0	04104A6	041C4JR	041D0A5	041D0ZC	041D4JK	041E0JB
03UV0KZ	03VM3BZ	03VT3DZ	03WYXCZ	04100K1	04104A7	041C4K0	041D0A6	041D0ZD	041D4JQ	041E0JC
03UV37Z	03VM3CZ	03VT3ZZ	03WYXDZ	04100K2	04104A8	041C4K1	041D0A7	041D0ZF	041D4JR	041E0JD

041E0JF	041E4KF	041F0ZF	041H09F	041K4AM	041L0KQ	041M0JL	041N49M	041U0ZP	041W4AP	045K0ZZ
041E0JG	041E4KG	041F0ZG	041H09G	041K4AN	041L0KS	041M0JM	041N49P	041U0ZQ	041W4AQ	045K3ZZ
041E0JH	041E4KH	041F0ZH	041H09H	041K4AP	041L0ZH	041M0JP	041N49Q	041U0ZS	041W4AS	045K4ZZ
041E0JJ	041E4KJ	041F0ZJ	041H09J	041K4AQ	041L0ZJ	041M0JQ	041N49S	041U49P	041W4JP	045L0ZZ
041E0JK	041E4KK	041F0ZK	041H09K	041K4AS	041L0ZK	041M0JS	041N4AL	041U49Q	041W4JQ	045L3ZZ
041E0JP	041E4KP	041F0ZP	041H09P	041K4JH	041L0ZL	041M0KL	041N4AM	041U49S	041W4JS	045L4ZZ
041E0JQ	041E4KQ	041F0ZQ	041H09Q	041K4JJ	041L0ZM	041M0KM	041N4AP	041U4AP	041W4KP	045M0ZZ
041E0K9	041E4Z9	041F499	041H0A9	041K4JK	041L0ZN	041M0KP	041N4AQ	041U4AQ	041W4KQ	045M3ZZ
041E0KB	041E4ZB	041F49B	041H0AB	041K4JL	041L0ZP	041M0KQ	041N4AS	041U4AS	041W4KS	045M4ZZ
041E0KC	041E4ZC	041F49C	041H0AC	041K4JM	041L0ZQ	041M0KS	041N4JL	041U4JP	041W4ZP	045N0ZZ
041E0KD	041E4ZD	041F49D	041H0AD	041K4JN	041L0ZS	041M0ZL	041N4JM	041U4JQ	041W4ZQ	045N3ZZ
041E0KF	041E4ZF	041F49F	041H0AF	041K4JP	041L49H	041M0ZM	041N4JP	041U4JS	041W4ZS	045N4ZZ
041E0KG	041E4ZG	041F49G	041H0AG	041K4JQ	041L49J	041M0ZP	041N4JQ	041U4KP	04500ZZ	045P0ZZ
041E0KH	041E4ZH	041F49H	041H0AH	041K4JS	041L49K	041M0ZQ	041N4JS	041U4KQ	04503ZZ	045P3ZZ
041E0KJ	041E4ZJ	041F49J	041H0AJ	041K4KH	041L49L	041M0ZS	041N4KL	041U4KS	04504ZZ	045P4ZZ
041E0KK	041E4ZK	041F49K	041H0AK	041K4KJ	041L49M	041M49L	041N4KM	041U4ZP	04510ZZ	045Q0ZZ
041E0KP	041E4ZP	041F49P	041H0AP	041K4KK	041L49N	041M49M	041N4KP	041U4ZQ	04513ZZ	045Q3ZZ
041E0KQ	041E4ZQ	041F49Q	041H0AQ	041K4KL	041L49P	041M49P	041N4KQ	041U4ZS	04514ZZ	045Q4ZZ
041E0Z9	041F099	041F4A9	041H0J9	041K4KM	041L49Q	041M49Q	041N4KS	041V09P	04520ZZ	045R0ZZ
041E0ZB	041F09B	041F4AB	041H0JB	041K4KN	041L49S	041M49S	041N4ZL	041V09Q	04523ZZ	045R3ZZ
041E0ZC	041F09C	041F4AC	041H0JC	041K4KP	041L4AH	041M4AL	041N4ZM	041V09S	04524ZZ	045R4ZZ
041E0ZD	041F09D	041F4AD	041H0JD	041K4KQ	041L4AJ	041M4AM	041N4ZP	041V0AP	04530ZZ	045S0ZZ
041E0ZF	041F09F	041F4AF	041H0JF	041K4KS	041L4AK	041M4AP	041N4ZQ	041V0AQ	04533ZZ	045S3ZZ
041E0ZG	041F09G	041F4AG	041H0JG	041K4ZH	041L4AL	041M4AQ	041N4ZS	041V0AS	04534ZZ	045S4ZZ
041E0ZH	041F09H	041F4AH	041H0JH	041K4ZJ	041L4AM	041M4AS	041N4ZL	041V0JP	04540ZZ	045T0ZZ
041E0ZJ	041F09J	041F4AJ	041H0JJ	041K4ZK	041L4AN	041M4JL	041N4JM	041V0JQ	04543ZZ	045T3ZZ
041E0ZK	041F09K	041F4AK	041H0JK	041K4ZL	041L4AP	041M4JM	041N4JP	041V0JS	04544ZZ	045T4ZZ
041E0ZP	041F09P	041F4AP	041H0JP	041K4ZM	041L4AQ	041M4JP	041N4JQ	041V0KP	04550ZZ	0470041
041E0ZQ	041F09Q	041F4AQ	041H0JQ	041K4ZN	041L4AS	041M4JQ	041N4JS	041V0KQ	04553ZZ	04700D1
041E499	041F0A9	041F4J9	041H0K9	041K4ZP	041L4JH	041M4JS	041N4KL	041V0KS	04554ZZ	04700Z1
041E49B	041F0AB	041F4JB	041H0KB	041K4ZQ	041L4JJ	041M4KL	041N4KM	041V0ZP	04560ZZ	0470341
041E49C	041F0AC	041F4JC	041H0KC	041K4ZS	041L4JK	041M4KM	041N4KP	041V0ZQ	04563ZZ	04703D1
041E49D	041F0AD	041F4JD	041H0KD	041L09H	041L4JL	041M4KP	041N4KQ	041V0ZS	04564ZZ	04703Z1
041E49F	041F0AF	041F4JF	041H0KF	041L09J	041L4JM	041M4KQ	041N4KS	041V49P	04570ZZ	0470441
041E49G	041F0AG	041F4JG	041H0KG	041L09K	041L4JN	041M4KS	041N4ZL	041V49Q	04573ZZ	04704D1
041E49H	041F0AH	041F4JH	041H0KH	041L09L	041L4JP	041M4ZL	041N4ZM	041V49S	04574ZZ	04704Z1
041E49J	041F0AJ	041F4JJ	041H0KJ	041L09M	041L4JQ	041M4ZM	041N4ZP	041V4AP	04580ZZ	0471041
041E49K	041F0AK	041F4JK	041H0KK	041L09N	041L4JS	041M4ZP	041N4ZQ	041V4AQ	04583ZZ	04710D1
041E49P	041F0AP	041F4JP	041H0KP	041L09P	041L4KH	041M4ZQ	041N4ZS	041V4AS	04584ZZ	04710Z1
041E49Q	041F0AQ	041F4JQ	041H0KQ	041L09Q	041L4KJ	041M4ZS	041N09L	041V4JP	04590ZZ	0471341
041E4A9	041F0J9	041F4K9	041H0Z9	041L09S	041L4KK	041N09L	041N09M	041V4JQ	04593ZZ	04713D1
041E4AB	041F0JB	041F4KB	041H0ZB	041L0AH	041L4KL	041N09M	041N09P	041V4JS	04594ZZ	04713E6
041E4AC	041F0JC	041F4KC	041H0ZC	041L0AJ	041L4KM	041N09P	041N09Q	041V4KP	045A0ZZ	04713EZ
041E4AD	041F0JD	041F4KD	041H0ZD	041L0AK	041L4KN	041N09Q	041N09S	041V4KQ	045A3ZZ	04713F6
041E4AF	041F0JF	041F4KF	041K0ZH	041L0AL	041L4KP	041N09S	041N0AL	041V4KS	045A4ZZ	04713FZ
041E4AG	041F0JG	041F4KG	041K0ZJ	041L0AM	041L4KQ	041N0AL	041N0AM	041V4ZP	045B0ZZ	04713G6
041E4AH	041F0JH	041F4KH	041K0ZK	041L0AN	041L4KS	041N0AM	041N0AP	041V4ZQ	045B3ZZ	04713GZ
041E4AJ	041F0JJ	041F4KJ	041K0ZL	041L0AP	041L4ZH	041N0AP	041N0AQ	041V4ZS	045B4ZZ	04713Z1
041E4AK	041F0JK	041F4KK	041K0ZM	041L0AQ	041L4ZJ	041N0AQ	041N0AS	041W09P	045C0ZZ	04713Z6
041E4AP	041F0JP	041F4KP	041K0ZN	041L0AS	041L4ZK	041N0AS	041N0JL	041W09Q	045C3ZZ	04713ZZ
041E4AQ	041F0JQ	041F4KQ	041K0ZP	041L0JH	041L4ZL	041N0JL	041N0JM	041W09S	045C4ZZ	0471441
041E4J9	041F0K9	041F4Z9	041K0ZQ	041L0JJ	041L4ZM	041N0JM	041N0JP	041W0AP	045D0ZZ	0471446
041E4JB	041F0KB	041F4ZB	041K0ZS	041L0JK	041L4ZN	041N0JP	041N0JQ	041W0AQ	045D3ZZ	047144Z
041E4JC	041F0KC	041F4ZC	041K49H	041L0JL	041L4ZP	041N0JQ	041N0JS	041W0AS	045D4ZZ	0471456
041E4JD	041F0KD	041F4ZD	041K49J	041L0JM	041L4ZQ	041N0JS	041N0KL	041W0JP	045E0ZZ	047145Z
041E4JF	041F0KF	041F4ZF	041K49K	041L0JN	041L4ZS	041N0KL	041N0KM	041W0JQ	045E3ZZ	0471466
041E4JG	041F0KG	041F4ZG	041K49L	041L0JP	041M09L	041N0KM	041N0KP	041W0JS	045E4ZZ	047146Z
041E4JH	041F0KH	041F4ZH	041K49M	041L0JQ	041M09M	041N0KP	041N0KQ	041W0KP	045F0ZZ	0471476
041E4JJ	041F0KJ	041F4ZJ	041K49N	041L0JS	041M09P	041N0KQ	041N0KS	041W0KQ	045F3ZZ	047147Z
041E4JK	041F0KK	041F4ZK	041K49P	041L0KH	041M09Q	041N0KS	041N0ZL	041W0KS	045F4ZZ	04714D1
041E4JP	041F0KP	041F4ZP	041K49Q	041L0KJ	041M09S	041N0ZL	041N0ZM	041W0ZP	045H0ZZ	04714D6
041E4JQ	041F0KQ	041F4ZQ	041K49S	041L0KK	041M0AL	041N0ZM	041N0ZP	041W0ZQ	045H3ZZ	04714DZ
041E4K9	041F0Z9	041H099	041K4AH	041L0KL	041M0AM	041N0ZP	041N0ZQ	041W0ZS	045H4ZZ	04714E6
041E4KB	041F0ZB	041H09B	041K4AJ	041L0KM	041M0AP	041N0ZQ	041N0ZS	041W49P	045J0ZZ	04714EZ
041E4KC	041F0ZC	041H09C	041K4AK	041L0KN	041M0AQ	041N0ZS	041N49L	041W49Q	045J3ZZ	04714F6
041E4KD	041F0ZD	041H09D	041K4AL	041L0KP	041M0AS	041N49L	041U0KS	041W49S	045J4ZZ	04714FZ

04714G6	04724Z6	0474046	04760D1	04773F6	04783GZ	04793ZZ	047B4D1	047C4E6	047D4FZ	047E4Z1
04714GZ	04724ZZ	047404Z	04760Z1	04773FZ	04783Z1	0479441	047B4D6	047C4EZ	047D4G6	047E4Z6
04714Z1	0473041	0474056	0476341	04773G6	04783Z6	0479446	047B4DZ	047C4F6	047D4GZ	047E4ZZ
04714Z6	0473046	047405Z	04763D1	04773GZ	04783ZZ	0479944Z	047B4E6	047C4FZ	047D4Z1	047F041
04714ZZ	047304Z	0474066	04763FZ	04773Z1	0478441	0479456	047B4EZ	047C4G6	047D4Z6	047F046
0472041	0473056	047406Z	04763G6	04773Z6	0478446	047945Z	047B4F6	047C4GZ	047D4ZZ	047F04Z
0472046	047305Z	0474076	04763GZ	04773ZZ	047844Z	0479466	047B4FZ	047C4Z1	047E041	047F056
047204Z	0473066	047407Z	04763Z1	0477441	0478456	0479476	047B4G6	047C4Z6	047E046	047F05Z
0472056	047306Z	04740D1	04763Z6	0477446	047845Z	047947Z	047B4GZ	047C4ZZ	047E04Z	047F066
047205Z	0473076	04740D6	04763ZZ	047744Z	0478466	04794D1	047B4Z1	047D041	047E056	047F06Z
0472066	047307Z	04740DZ	0476441	0477456	047846Z	04794D6	047B4Z6	047D046	047E05Z	047F076
047206Z	04730D1	04740E6	0476446	047745Z	0478476	04794DZ	047B4ZZ	047D04Z	047E066	047F07Z
0472076	04730D6	04740EZ	047644Z	0477466	047847Z	04794E6	047C041	047D056	047E06Z	047F0D1
047207Z	04730DZ	04740F6	0476456	047746Z	04784D1	04794EZ	047C046	047D05Z	047E076	047F0D6
04720D1	04730E6	04740FZ	047645Z	0477476	04784D6	04794F6	047C04Z	047D066	047E07Z	047F0DZ
04720D6	04730EZ	04740G6	0476466	047747Z	04784DZ	04794FZ	047C056	047D06Z	047E0D1	047F0E6
04720DZ	04730F6	04740GZ	047646Z	04774D1	04784E6	04794G6	047C05Z	047D076	047E0D6	047F0EZ
04720E6	04730FZ	04740Z1	0476476	04774D6	04784EZ	04794GZ	047C066	047D07Z	047E0DZ	047F0F6
04720EZ	04730G6	04740Z6	047647Z	04774DZ	04784F6	04794Z1	047C06Z	047D0D1	047E0E6	047F0FZ
04720F6	04730GZ	04740ZZ	04764D1	04774E6	04784FZ	04794Z6	047C076	047D0D6	047E0EZ	047F0G6
04720FZ	04730Z1	0474341	04764D6	04774EZ	04784G6	04794ZZ	047C07Z	047D0DZ	047E0F6	047F0GZ
04720G6	04730Z6	0474346	04764DZ	04774F6	04784GZ	047A041	047C0D1	047D0E6	047E0FZ	047F0Z1
04720GZ	04730ZZ	047434Z	04764E6	04774FZ	04784Z1	047A046	047C0D6	047D0EZ	047E0G6	047F0Z6
04720Z1	0473341	0474356	04764EZ	04774G6	04784Z6	047A04Z	047C0DZ	047D0F6	047E0GZ	047F0ZZ
04720Z6	0473346	047435Z	04764F6	04774GZ	04784ZZ	047A056	047C0E6	047D0FZ	047E0Z1	047F341
04720ZZ	047334Z	0474366	04764FZ	04774Z1	0479041	047A05Z	047C0EZ	047D0G6	047E0Z6	047F346
0472341	0473356	047436Z	04764G6	04774Z6	0479046	047A066	047C0F6	047D0GZ	047E0ZZ	047F34Z
0472346	047335Z	0474376	04764GZ	04774ZZ	047904Z	047A06Z	047C0FZ	047D0Z1	047E341	047F356
047234Z	0473366	047437Z	04764Z1	0478041	0479056	047A076	047C0G6	047D0Z6	047E346	047F35Z
0472356	047336Z	04743D1	04764Z6	0478046	047905Z	047A07Z	047C0GZ	047D0ZZ	047E34Z	047F366
047235Z	0473376	04743D6	04764ZZ	047804Z	0479066	047A0D1	047C0Z1	047D341	047E356	047F3D1
0472366	047337Z	04743DZ	0477041	0478056	047906Z	047A0D6	047C0Z6	047D346	047E35Z	047F3Z1
047236Z	04733D1	04743E6	0477046	047805Z	0479076	047A0DZ	047C0ZZ	047D34Z	047E366	047F441
0472376	04733D6	04743EZ	047704Z	0478066	047907Z	047A0E6	047C341	047D356	047E36Z	047F4D1
047237Z	04733DZ	04743F6	0477056	047806Z	04790D1	047A0EZ	047C346	047D35Z	047E376	047F4Z1
04723D1	04733E6	04743FZ	047705Z	0478076	04790D6	047A0F6	047C34Z	047D366	047E37Z	047H041
04723D6	04733EZ	04743G6	0477066	047807Z	04790DZ	047A0FZ	047C356	047D36Z	047E3D1	047H0D1
04723DZ	04733F6	04743GZ	047706Z	04780D1	04790E6	047A0G6	047C35Z	047D376	047E3D6	047H0Z1
04723E6	04733FZ	04743Z1	0477076	04780D6	04790EZ	047A0GZ	047C366	047D37Z	047E3DZ	047H341
04723EZ	04733G6	04743Z6	047707Z	04780DZ	04790F6	047A0Z1	047C36Z	047D3D1	047E3E6	047H3D1
04723F6	04733GZ	04743ZZ	04770D1	04780E6	04790FZ	047A0Z6	047C376	047D3D6	047E3EZ	047H3Z1
04723FZ	04733Z1	0474441	04770D6	04780EZ	04790G6	047A0ZZ	047C37Z	047D3DZ	047E3F6	047H441
04723G6	04733Z6	0474446	04770DZ	04780F6	04790GZ	047A341	047C3D1	047D3E6	047E3FZ	047H4D1
04723GZ	04733ZZ	047444Z	04770E6	04780FZ	04790Z1	047A346	047C3D6	047D3EZ	047E3G6	047H4Z1
04723Z1	0473441	0474456	04770EZ	04780G6	04790Z6	047A34Z	047C3DZ	047D3F6	047E3GZ	047J041
04723Z6	0473446	047445Z	04770F6	04780GZ	04790ZZ	047A3D1	047C3E6	047D3FZ	047E3Z1	047J06Z
04723ZZ	047344Z	0474466	04770FZ	04780Z1	0479341	047A3Z1	047C3EZ	047D3G6	047E3Z6	047J076
0472441	0473456	047446Z	04770G6	04780Z6	0479346	047A441	047C3F6	047D3GZ	047E3ZZ	047J07Z
0472446	047345Z	0474476	04770GZ	04780ZZ	047934Z	047A4D1	047C3FZ	047D3Z1	047E441	047J0D1
047244Z	0473466	047447Z	04770Z1	0478341	0479356	047A4Z1	047C3G6	047D3Z6	047E446	047J0D6
0472456	047346Z	04744D1	04770Z6	0478346	047935Z	047B041	047C3GZ	047D3ZZ	047E44Z	047J0DZ
047245Z	0473476	04744D6	04770ZZ	047834Z	0479366	047B0D1	047C3Z1	047D441	047E456	047J0E6
0472466	047347Z	04744DZ	0477341	0478356	047936Z	047B0Z1	047C3Z6	047D446	047E45Z	047J0EZ
047246Z	04734D1	04744E6	0477346	047835Z	0479376	047B341	047C3ZZ	047D44Z	047E466	047J0F6
0472476	04734D6	04744EZ	047734Z	0478366	047937Z	047B3D1	047C441	047D456	047E46Z	047J0FZ
047247Z	04734DZ	04744Z1	0477356	047836Z	04793D1	047B3Z1	047C446	047D45Z	047E476	047J0G6
04724D1	04734E6	0475041	047735Z	0478376	04793D6	047B3ZZ	047C44Z	047D466	047E47Z	047J0GZ
04724D6	04734EZ	04750D1	0477366	047837Z	04793DZ	047B441	047C456	047D46Z	047E4D1	047J0Z1
04724DZ	04734F6	04750Z1	047736Z	04783D1	04793E6	047B446	047C45Z	047D476	047E4D6	047J0Z6
04724E6	04734FZ	0475341	0477376	04783D6	04793EZ	047B44Z	047C466	047D47Z	047E4DZ	047J0ZZ
04724EZ	04734G6	04753D1	047737Z	04783DZ	04793F6	047B456	047C46Z	047D4D1	047E4E6	047J341
04724F6	04734GZ	04753Z1	04773D1	04783E6	04793FZ	047B45Z	047C476	047D4D6	047E4EZ	047J346
04724FZ	04734Z1	0475441	04773D6	04783EZ	04793G6	047B466	047C47Z	047D4DZ	047E4F6	047J34Z
04724G6	04734Z6	04754D1	04773DZ	04783F6	04793GZ	047B46Z	047C4D1	047D4E6	047E4FZ	047J356
04724GZ	04734ZZ	04754Z1	04773E6	04783FZ	04793Z1	047B476	047C4D6	047D4EZ	047E4G6	047J35Z
04724Z1	0474041	0476041	04773EZ	04783G6	04793Z6	047B47Z	047C4DZ	047D4F6	047E4GZ	047J366

047J36Z	047K3D1	047L3E6	047Q076	047R0D6	047S0EZ	047T0G6	047U0Z6	047V346	047W35Z	047Y376
047J376	047K3D6	047L3EZ	047Q07Z	047R0DZ	047S0F6	047T0GZ	047U0ZZ	047V34Z	047W366	047Y37Z
047J37Z	047K3DZ	047L3F6	047Q0D1	047R0E6	047S0FZ	047T0Z1	047U341	047V356	047W36Z	047Y3D1
047J3D1	047K3E6	047L3FZ	047Q0D6	047R0EZ	047S0G6	047T0Z6	047U346	047V35Z	047W376	047Y3D6
047J3D6	047K3EZ	047L3G6	047Q0DZ	047R0F6	047S0GZ	047T0ZZ	047U34Z	047V366	047W37Z	047Y3DZ
047J3DZ	047K3F6	047L3GZ	047Q0E6	047R0FZ	047S0Z1	047T341	047U356	047V376	047W3D1	047Y3E6
047J3E6	047K3FZ	047P041	047Q0EZ	047R0G6	047S0Z6	047T346	047U35Z	047V37Z	047W3D6	047Y3EZ
047J3EZ	047K3G6	047P0D1	047Q0F6	047R0GZ	047S0ZZ	047T34Z	047U366	047V3D1	047W3DZ	047Y3F6
047J3F6	047K3GZ	047P0E6	047Q0FZ	047R0Z1	047S341	047T356	047U36Z	047V3D6	047W3E6	047Y3FZ
047J3FZ	047K3Z1	047P0EZ	047Q0G6	047R0Z6	047S346	047T35Z	047U376	047V3DZ	047W3EZ	047Y3G6
047J3G6	047K3Z6	047P0F6	047Q0GZ	047R0ZZ	047S34Z	047T366	047U37Z	047V3E6	047W3F6	047Y3GZ
047J3GZ	047K3ZZ	047P0FZ	047Q0Z1	047R341	047S356	047T36Z	047U3D1	047V3EZ	047W3FZ	047Y3Z1
047J3Z1	047K441	047P0G6	047Q0Z6	047R346	047S35Z	047T376	047U3D6	047V3F6	047W3G6	047Y3Z6
047J3Z6	047K446	047P0GZ	047Q0ZZ	047R34Z	047S366	047T37Z	047U3DZ	047V3FZ	047W3GZ	047Y3ZZ
047J3ZZ	047K44Z	047P0Z1	047Q341	047R356	047S36Z	047T3D1	047U3E6	047V3G6	047W3Z1	047Y441
047J441	047K456	047P0Z6	047Q346	047R35Z	047S376	047T3D6	047U3EZ	047V3GZ	047W3Z6	047Y446
047J446	047K45Z	047P0ZZ	047Q34Z	047R366	047S37Z	047T3DZ	047U3F6	047V3Z1	047W3ZZ	047Y44Z
047J44Z	047K466	047P341	047Q356	047R36Z	047S3D1	047T3E6	047U3FZ	047V3Z6	047W441	047Y456
047J456	047K46Z	047P346	047Q35Z	047R376	047S3D6	047T3EZ	047U3G6	047V3ZZ	047W446	047Y45Z
047J45Z	047K476	047P34Z	047Q366	047R37Z	047S3DZ	047T3F6	047U3GZ	047V441	047W44Z	047Y466
047J466	047K47Z	047P356	047Q36Z	047R3D1	047S3E6	047T3FZ	047U3Z1	047V446	047W456	047Y46Z
047J46Z	047K4D1	047P35Z	047Q376	047R3D6	047S3EZ	047T3G6	047U3Z6	047V44Z	047W45Z	047Y476
047J476	047K4D6	047P366	047Q37Z	047R3DZ	047S3F6	047T3GZ	047U3ZZ	047V456	047W466	047Y47Z
047J47Z	047K4DZ	047P36Z	047Q3D1	047R3E6	047S3FZ	047T3Z1	047U441	047V45Z	047W46Z	047Y4D1
047J4D1	047K4E6	047P376	047Q3D6	047R3EZ	047S3G6	047T3Z6	047U446	047V466	047W476	047Y4D6
047J4D6	047K4EZ	047P37Z	047Q3DZ	047R3F6	047S3GZ	047T3ZZ	047U44Z	047V46Z	047W47Z	047Y4DZ
047J4DZ	047K4F6	047P3D1	047Q3E6	047R3FZ	047S3Z1	047T441	047U456	047V476	047W4D1	047Y4E6
047J4E6	047K4FZ	047P3D6	047Q3EZ	047R3G6	047S3Z6	047T446	047U45Z	047V47Z	047W4D6	047Y4EZ
047J4EZ	047K4G6	047P3DZ	047Q3F6	047R3GZ	047S3ZZ	047T44Z	047U466	047V4D1	047W4DZ	047Y4F6
047J4F6	047K4GZ	047P3E6	047Q3FZ	047R3Z1	047S441	047T456	047U46Z	047V4D6	047W4E6	047Y4FZ
047J4FZ	047K4Z1	047P3EZ	047Q3G6	047R3Z6	047S446	047T45Z	047U476	047V4DZ	047W4EZ	047Y4G6
047J4G6	047K4Z6	047P3F6	047Q3GZ	047R3ZZ	047S44Z	047T466	047U47Z	047V4E6	047W4F6	047Y4GZ
047J4GZ	047K4ZZ	047P3FZ	047Q3Z1	047R441	047S456	047T46Z	047U4D1	047V4EZ	047W4FZ	047Y4Z1
047J4Z1	047L041	047P3G6	047Q3Z6	047R446	047S45Z	047T476	047U4D6	047V4F6	047W4G6	047Y4Z6
047J4Z6	047L046	047P3GZ	047Q3ZZ	047R44Z	047S466	047T47Z	047U4DZ	047V4FZ	047W4GZ	047Y4ZZ
047J4ZZ	047L04Z	047P3Z1	047Q441	047R456	047S46Z	047T4D1	047U4E6	047V4G6	047W4Z1	049000Z
047K041	047L056	047P3Z6	047Q446	047R45Z	047S476	047T4D6	047U4EZ	047V4GZ	047W4Z6	04900ZX
047K046	047L05Z	047P3ZZ	047Q44Z	047R466	047S47Z	047T4DZ	047U4F6	047V4Z1	047W4ZZ	04900ZZ
047K04Z	047L066	047P441	047Q456	047R46Z	047S4D1	047T4E6	047U4FZ	047V4Z6	047Y041	049030Z
047K056	047L06Z	047P446	047Q45Z	047R476	047S4D6	047T4EZ	047U4G6	047V4ZZ	047Y046	04903ZX
047K05Z	047L076	047P44Z	047Q466	047R47Z	047S4DZ	047T4F6	047U4GZ	047W041	047Y04Z	04903ZZ
047K066	047L07Z	047P456	047Q46Z	047R4D1	047S4E6	047T4FZ	047U4Z1	047W046	047Y056	049040Z
047K06Z	047L0D1	047P45Z	047Q476	047R4D6	047S4EZ	047T4G6	047U4Z6	047W04Z	047Y05Z	04904ZX
047K076	047L0D6	047P466	047Q47Z	047R4DZ	047S4F6	047T4GZ	047U4ZZ	047W056	047Y066	04904ZZ
047K07Z	047L0DZ	047P46Z	047Q4D1	047R4E6	047S4FZ	047T4Z1	047V041	047W05Z	047Y06Z	049100Z
047K0D1	047L0E6	047P476	047Q4D6	047R4EZ	047S4G6	047T4Z6	047V046	047W066	047Y076	04910ZX
047K0D6	047L0EZ	047P47Z	047Q4DZ	047R4F6	047S4GZ	047T4ZZ	047V04Z	047W06Z	047Y07Z	04910ZZ
047K0DZ	047L0F6	047P4D1	047Q4E6	047R4FZ	047S4Z1	047U041	047V056	047W076	047Y0D1	049130Z
047K0E6	047L0FZ	047P4D6	047Q4EZ	047R4G6	047S4Z6	047U046	047V05Z	047W07Z	047Y0D6	04913ZX
047K0EZ	047L0G6	047P4DZ	047Q4F6	047R4GZ	047S4ZZ	047U04Z	047V066	047W0D1	047Y0DZ	04913ZZ
047K0F6	047L0GZ	047P4E6	047Q4FZ	047R4Z1	047T041	047U056	047V06Z	047W0D6	047Y0E6	049140Z
047K0FZ	047L0Z1	047P4EZ	047Q4G6	047R4Z6	047T046	047U05Z	047V076	047W0DZ	047Y0EZ	04914ZX
047K0G6	047L0Z6	047P4F6	047Q4GZ	047R4ZZ	047T04Z	047U066	047V07Z	047W0E6	047Y0F6	04914ZZ
047K0GZ	047L0ZZ	047P4FZ	047Q4Z1	047S041	047T056	047U06Z	047V0D1	047W0EZ	047Y0FZ	049200Z
047K0Z1	047L341	047P4G6	047Q4Z6	047S046	047T05Z	047U076	047V0D6	047W0F6	047Y0G6	04920ZX
047K0Z6	047L346	047P4GZ	047Q4ZZ	047S04Z	047T066	047U07Z	047V0DZ	047W0FZ	047Y0GZ	04920ZZ
047K0ZZ	047L34Z	047P4Z1	047R041	047S056	047T06Z	047U0D1	047V0E6	047W0G6	047Y0Z1	049230Z
047K341	047L356	047P4Z6	047R046	047S05Z	047T076	047U0D6	047V0EZ	047W0GZ	047Y0Z6	04923ZX
047K346	047L35Z	047P4ZZ	047R04Z	047S066	047T07Z	047U0DZ	047V0F6	047W0Z1	047Y0ZZ	04923ZZ
047K34Z	047L366	047Q041	047R056	047S06Z	047T0D1	047U0E6	047V0FZ	047W0Z6	047Y341	049240Z
047K356	047L36Z	047Q046	047R05Z	047S076	047T0D6	047U0EZ	047V0G6	047W0ZZ	047Y346	04924ZX
047K35Z	047L376	047Q04Z	047R066	047S07Z	047T0DZ	047U0F6	047V0GZ	047W341	047Y34Z	04924ZZ
047K366	047L37Z	047Q056	047R06Z	047S0D1	047T0E6	047U0FZ	047V0Z1	047W346	047Y356	049300Z
047K36Z	047L3D1	047Q05Z	047R076	047S0D6	047T0EZ	047U0G6	047V0Z6	047W34Z	047Y35Z	04930ZX
047K376	047L3D6	047Q066	047R07Z	047S0DZ	047T0F6	047U0GZ	047V0ZZ	047W356	047Y366	04930ZZ
047K37Z	047L3DZ	047Q06Z	047R0D1	047S0E6	047T0FZ	047U0Z1	047V341	047W356	047Y36Z	049330Z

04933ZX	049A4ZX	049K0ZX	049S3ZX	04B24ZX	04CA0ZZ	04CN0ZZ	04HC03Z	04HQ03Z	04L04DZ	04L80DZ
04933ZZ	049A4ZZ	049K0ZZ	049S3ZZ	04B24ZZ	04CA3Z6	04CN3Z6	04HC0DZ	04HQ0DZ	04L04ZZ	04L80ZZ
049340Z	049B00Z	049K30Z	049S40Z	04B30ZX	04CA3ZZ	04CN3ZZ	04HC33Z	04HQ33Z	04L10CZ	04L83CZ
04934ZX	049B0ZX	049K3ZX	049S4ZX	04B30ZZ	04CA4Z6	04CN4Z6	04HC3DZ	04HQ3DZ	04L10DZ	04L83DZ
04934ZZ	049B0ZZ	049K3ZZ	049S4ZZ	04B33ZX	04CA4ZZ	04CN4ZZ	04HC43Z	04HQ43Z	04L10ZZ	04L83ZZ
049400Z	049B30Z	049K4ZX	049T00Z	04B33ZZ	04CB0Z6	04CP0Z6	04HC4DZ	04HQ4DZ	04L13CZ	04L84CZ
04940ZX	049B3ZX	049K4ZZ	049T0ZX	04C00ZZ	04CB0ZZ	04CP0ZZ	04HD03Z	04HR03Z	04L13DZ	04L84DZ
04940ZZ	049B3ZZ	049L00Z	049T0ZZ	04C03Z6	04CB3Z6	04CP3Z6	04HD0DZ	04HR0DZ	04L13ZZ	04L84ZZ
049430Z	049B40Z	049L0ZX	049T30Z	04C03ZZ	04CB3ZZ	04CP3ZZ	04HD33Z	04HR33Z	04L14CZ	04L90CZ
04943ZX	049B4ZX	049L0ZZ	049T3ZX	04C04Z6	04CB4Z6	04CP4Z6	04HD3DZ	04HR3DZ	04L14DZ	04L90DZ
04943ZZ	049B4ZZ	049L30Z	049T3ZZ	04C04ZZ	04CB4ZZ	04CP4ZZ	04HD43Z	04HR43Z	04L14ZZ	04L90ZZ
049440Z	049C00Z	049L3ZX	049T40Z	04C10Z6	04CC0Z6	04CQ0Z6	04HD4DZ	04HR4DZ	04L20CZ	04L93CZ
04944ZX	049C0ZX	049L3ZZ	049T4ZX	04C10ZZ	04CC0ZZ	04CQ0ZZ	04HE03Z	04HS03Z	04L20DZ	04L93DZ
04944ZZ	049C0ZZ	049L40Z	049T4ZZ	04C13Z6	04CC3Z6	04CQ3Z6	04HE0DZ	04HS0DZ	04L20ZZ	04L93ZZ
049500Z	049C30Z	049L4ZX	049U00Z	04C13ZZ	04CC3ZZ	04CQ3ZZ	04HE33Z	04HS33Z	04L23CZ	04L94CZ
04950ZX	049C3ZX	049L4ZZ	049U0ZX	04C14Z6	04CC4Z6	04CQ4Z6	04HE3DZ	04HS3DZ	04L23DZ	04L94DZ
04950ZZ	049C3ZZ	049M00Z	049U0ZZ	04C14ZZ	04CC4ZZ	04CQ4ZZ	04HE43Z	04HS43Z	04L23ZZ	04L94ZZ
049530Z	049C40Z	049M0ZX	049U30Z	04C20Z6	04CD0Z6	04CR0Z6	04HE4DZ	04HS4DZ	04L24CZ	04LA0CZ
04953ZX	049C4ZX	049M0ZZ	049U3ZX	04C20ZZ	04CD0ZZ	04CR0ZZ	04HF03Z	04HT03Z	04L24DZ	04LA0DZ
04953ZZ	049C4ZZ	049M30Z	049U3ZZ	04C23Z6	04CD3Z6	04CR3Z6	04HF0DZ	04HT0DZ	04L24ZZ	04LA0ZZ
049540Z	049D00Z	049M3ZX	049U40Z	04C23ZZ	04CD3ZZ	04CR3ZZ	04HF33Z	04HT33Z	04L30CZ	04LA3CZ
04954ZX	049D0ZX	049M3ZZ	049U4ZX	04C24Z6	04CD4Z6	04CR4Z6	04HF3DZ	04HT3DZ	04L30DZ	04LA3DZ
04954ZZ	049D0ZZ	049M40Z	049U4ZZ	04C24ZZ	04CD4ZZ	04CR4ZZ	04HF43Z	04HT43Z	04L30ZZ	04LA3ZZ
049600Z	049D30Z	049M4ZX	049V00Z	04C30Z6	04CE0Z6	04CS0Z6	04HF4DZ	04HT4DZ	04L33CZ	04LA4CZ
04960ZX	049D3ZX	049M4ZZ	049V0ZX	04C30ZZ	04CE0ZZ	04CS0ZZ	04HH03Z	04HU03Z	04L33DZ	04LA4DZ
04960ZZ	049D3ZZ	049N00Z	049V0ZZ	04C33Z6	04CE3Z6	04CS3Z6	04HH0DZ	04HU0DZ	04L33ZZ	04LA4ZZ
049630Z	049D40Z	049N0ZX	049V30Z	04C33ZZ	04CE3ZZ	04H002Z	04HH33Z	04HU33Z	04L34CZ	04LB0CZ
04963ZX	049D4ZX	049N0ZZ	049V3ZX	04C34Z6	04CE4Z6	04H003Z	04HH3DZ	04HU3DZ	04L34DZ	04LB0DZ
04963ZZ	049D4ZZ	049N30Z	049V3ZZ	04C34ZZ	04CE4ZZ	04H032Z	04HH43Z	04HU43Z	04L34ZZ	04LB0ZZ
049640Z	049E00Z	049N3ZX	049V40Z	04C40Z6	04CF0Z6	04H033Z	04HH4DZ	04HU4DZ	04L40CZ	04LB3CZ
04964ZX	049E0ZX	049N3ZZ	049V4ZX	04C40ZZ	04CF0ZZ	04H042Z	04HJ03Z	04HV03Z	04L40DZ	04LB3DZ
04964ZZ	049E0ZZ	049N40Z	049V4ZZ	04C43Z6	04CF3Z6	04H043Z	04HJ0DZ	04HV0DZ	04L40ZZ	04LB3ZZ
049700Z	049E30Z	049N4ZX	049W00Z	04C43ZZ	04CF3ZZ	04H103Z	04HJ33Z	04HV33Z	04L43CZ	04LB4CZ
04970ZX	049E3ZX	049N4ZZ	049W0ZX	04C44Z6	04CF4Z6	04H133Z	04HJ3DZ	04HV3DZ	04L43DZ	04LB4DZ
04970ZZ	049E3ZZ	049P00Z	049W0ZZ	04C44ZZ	04CF4ZZ	04H143Z	04HJ43Z	04HV43Z	04L43ZZ	04LB4ZZ
049730Z	049E40Z	049P0ZX	049W30Z	04C50Z6	04CH0Z6	04H203Z	04HJ4DZ	04HV4DZ	04L44CZ	04LC0CZ
04973ZX	049E4ZX	049P0ZZ	049W3ZX	04C50ZZ	04CH0ZZ	04H233Z	04HK03Z	04HW03Z	04L44DZ	04LC0DZ
04973ZZ	049E4ZZ	049P30Z	049W3ZZ	04C53Z6	04CH3Z6	04H243Z	04HK0DZ	04HW0DZ	04L44ZZ	04LC0ZZ
049740Z	049F00Z	049P3ZX	049W40Z	04C53ZZ	04CH3ZZ	04H303Z	04HK33Z	04HW33Z	04L50CZ	04LC3CZ
04974ZX	049F0ZX	049P3ZZ	049W4ZX	04C54Z6	04CH4Z6	04H333Z	04HK3DZ	04HW3DZ	04L50DZ	04LC3DZ
04974ZZ	049F0ZZ	049P40Z	049W4ZZ	04C54ZZ	04CH4ZZ	04H343Z	04HK43Z	04HW43Z	04L50ZZ	04LC3ZZ
049800Z	049F30Z	049P4ZX	049Y00Z	04C60Z6	04CJ0Z6	04H403Z	04HK4DZ	04HW4DZ	04L53CZ	04LC4CZ
04980ZX	049F3ZX	049P4ZZ	049Y0ZX	04C60ZZ	04CJ0ZZ	04H433Z	04HL03Z	04HY02Z	04L53DZ	04LC4DZ
04980ZZ	049F3ZZ	049Q00Z	049Y0ZZ	04C63Z6	04CJ3Z6	04H443Z	04HL0DZ	04HY03Z	04L53ZZ	04LC4ZZ
049830Z	049F40Z	049Q0ZX	049Y30Z	04C63ZZ	04CJ3ZZ	04H503Z	04HL33Z	04HY0DZ	04L54CZ	04LD0CZ
04983ZX	049F4ZX	049Q0ZZ	049Y3ZX	04C64Z6	04CJ4Z6	04H533Z	04HL3DZ	04HY0YZ	04L54DZ	04LD0DZ
04983ZZ	049F4ZZ	049Q30Z	049Y3ZZ	04C64ZZ	04CJ4ZZ	04H543Z	04HL43Z	04HY32Z	04L54ZZ	04LD0ZZ
049840Z	049H00Z	049Q3ZX	049Y40Z	04C70Z6	04CK0Z6	04H603Z	04HL4DZ	04HY33Z	04L60CZ	04LD3CZ
04984ZX	049H0ZX	049Q3ZZ	049Y4ZX	04C70ZZ	04CK0ZZ	04H633Z	04HM03Z	04HY3DZ	04L60DZ	04LD3DZ
04984ZZ	049H0ZZ	049Q40Z	049Y4ZZ	04C73Z6	04CK3Z6	04H643Z	04HM0DZ	04HY3YZ	04L60ZZ	04LT4DZ
049900Z	049H30Z	049Q4ZX	04B00ZX	04C73ZZ	04CK3ZZ	04H703Z	04HM33Z	04HY42Z	04L63CZ	04LT4ZZ
04990ZX	049H3ZX	049Q4ZZ	04B00ZZ	04C74Z6	04CK4Z6	04H733Z	04HM3DZ	04HY43Z	04L63DZ	04LU0CZ
04990ZZ	049H3ZZ	049R00Z	04B03ZX	04C74ZZ	04CK4ZZ	04H743Z	04HM43Z	04HY4DZ	04L63ZZ	04LU0DZ
049930Z	049H40Z	049R0ZX	04B03ZZ	04C80Z6	04CL0Z6	04H803Z	04HM4DZ	04HY4YZ	04L64CZ	04LU0ZZ
04993ZX	049H4ZX	049R0ZZ	04B04ZX	04C80ZZ	04CL0ZZ	04H833Z	04HN03Z	04JY0ZZ	04L64DZ	04LU3CZ
04993ZZ	049H4ZZ	049R30Z	04B04ZZ	04C83Z6	04CL3Z6	04H843Z	04HN0DZ	04JY3ZZ	04L64ZZ	04LU3DZ
049940Z	049J00Z	049R3ZX	04B10ZX	04C83ZZ	04CL3ZZ	04H903Z	04HN33Z	04JY4ZZ	04L70CZ	04LU3ZZ
04994ZX	049J0ZX	049R3ZZ	04B10ZZ	04C84Z6	04CL4Z6	04H933Z	04HN3DZ	04JYXZZ	04L70DZ	04LU4CZ
04994ZZ	049J0ZZ	049R40Z	04B13ZX	04C84ZZ	04CL4ZZ	04H943Z	04HN43Z	04L00CZ	04L70ZZ	04LU4DZ
049A00Z	049J30Z	049R4ZX	04B13ZZ	04C90Z6	04CM0Z6	04HA03Z	04HN4DZ	04L00DZ	04L73CZ	04LU4ZZ
049A0ZX	049J3ZX	049R4ZZ	04B14ZX	04C90ZZ	04CM0ZZ	04HA33Z	04HP03Z	04L00ZZ	04L73DZ	04LV0CZ
049A0ZZ	049J3ZZ	049S00Z	04B14ZZ	04C93Z6	04CM3Z6	04HA43Z	04HP0DZ	04L03CZ	04L73ZZ	04LV0DZ
049A30Z	049J40Z	049S0ZX	04B20ZX	04C93ZZ	04CM3ZZ	04HB03Z	04HP33Z	04L03DJ	04L74CZ	04LV0ZZ
049A3ZX	049J4ZX	049S0ZZ	04B20ZZ	04C94Z6	04CM4Z6	04HB33Z	04HP3DZ	04L03DZ	04L74DZ	04LV3CZ
049A3ZZ	049J4ZZ	049S30Z	04B23ZX	04C94ZZ	04CM4ZZ	04HB43Z	04HP43Z	04L03ZZ	04L74ZZ	04LV3DZ
049A40Z	049K00Z	049S30Z	04B23ZZ	04CA0Z6	04CN0Z6	04HB4DZ	04HP4DZ	04L04CZ	04L80CZ	04LV3ZZ

04LV4CZ	04NF0ZZ	04PY40Z	04QJ3ZZ	04RR4KZ	04S94ZZ	04U00KZ	04U73KZ	04V10ZZ	04V83ZZ	04VF0ZZ
04LV4DZ	04NF3ZZ	04PY42Z	04QJ4ZZ	04RS07Z	04SA0ZZ	04U037Z	04U747Z	04V13CZ	04V84CZ	04VF3CZ
04LV4ZZ	04NF4ZZ	04PY43Z	04QK0ZZ	04RS0JZ	04SA3ZZ	04U03JZ	04U74JZ	04V13DZ	04V84DZ	04VF3DZ
04LW0CZ	04NH0ZZ	04PY47Z	04QK3ZZ	04RS0KZ	04SA4ZZ	04U03KZ	04U74KZ	04V13ZZ	04V84ZZ	04VF3ZZ
04LW0DZ	04NH3ZZ	04PY4CZ	04QK4ZZ	04RS47Z	04SB0ZZ	04U047Z	04U807Z	04V14CZ	04V90CZ	04VF4CZ
04LW0ZZ	04NH4ZZ	04PY4DZ	04QL0ZZ	04RS4JZ	04SB3ZZ	04U04JZ	04U80JZ	04V14DZ	04V90DZ	04VF4DZ
04LW3CZ	04NJ0ZZ	04PY4JZ	04QL3ZZ	04RS4KZ	04SB4ZZ	04U04KZ	04U80KZ	04V14ZZ	04V90ZZ	04VF4ZZ
04LW3DZ	04NJ3ZZ	04PY4KZ	04QL4ZZ	04RT07Z	04SC0ZZ	04U107Z	04U837Z	04V20CZ	04V93CZ	04VH0CZ
04LW3ZZ	04NJ4ZZ	04PY4YZ	04QM0ZZ	04RT0JZ	04SC3ZZ	04U10JZ	04U83JZ	04V20DZ	04V93DZ	04VH0DZ
04LW4CZ	04NK0ZZ	04PYX0Z	04QM3ZZ	04RT0KZ	04SC4ZZ	04U10KZ	04U83KZ	04V20ZZ	04V93ZZ	04VH3CZ
04LW4DZ	04NK3ZZ	04PYX1Z	04QM4ZZ	04RT47Z	04SD0ZZ	04U137Z	04U847Z	04V23CZ	04V94CZ	04VH3DZ
04LW4ZZ	04NK4ZZ	04PYX2Z	04QN0ZZ	04RT4JZ	04SD3ZZ	04U13JZ	04U84JZ	04V23DZ	04V94DZ	04VH3ZZ
04LY0CZ	04NL0ZZ	04PYX3Z	04QN3ZZ	04RT4KZ	04SD4ZZ	04U13KZ	04U84KZ	04V23ZZ	04V94ZZ	04VH4CZ
04LY0DZ	04NL3ZZ	04PYXDZ	04QN4ZZ	04RU07Z	04SE0ZZ	04U147Z	04U907Z	04V24CZ	04VA0CZ	04VH4DZ
04LY0ZZ	04NL4ZZ	04Q00ZZ	04QP0ZZ	04RU0JZ	04SE3ZZ	04U14JZ	04U90JZ	04V24DZ	04VA0DZ	04VH4ZZ
04LY3CZ	04NM0ZZ	04Q03ZZ	04QP3ZZ	04RU0KZ	04SE4ZZ	04U14KZ	04U90KZ	04V24ZZ	04VA0ZZ	04VJ0CZ
04LY3DZ	04NM3ZZ	04Q04ZZ	04QP4ZZ	04RU47Z	04SF0ZZ	04U207Z	04U937Z	04V30CZ	04VA3CZ	04VJ0DZ
04LY3ZZ	04NM4ZZ	04Q10ZZ	04QQ0ZZ	04RU4JZ	04SF3ZZ	04U20JZ	04U93JZ	04V30DZ	04VA3DZ	04VJ0ZZ
04LY4CZ	04NN0ZZ	04Q13ZZ	04QQ3ZZ	04RU4KZ	04SF4ZZ	04U20KZ	04U93KZ	04V30ZZ	04VA3ZZ	04VJ3CZ
04LY4DZ	04NN3ZZ	04Q14ZZ	04QQ4ZZ	04RV07Z	04SH0ZZ	04U237Z	04U947Z	04V33CZ	04VA4CZ	04VJ3DZ
04LY4ZZ	04NN4ZZ	04Q20ZZ	04QR0ZZ	04RV0JZ	04SH3ZZ	04U23JZ	04U94JZ	04V33DZ	04VA4DZ	04VJ3ZZ
04N00ZZ	04NP0ZZ	04Q23ZZ	04QR3ZZ	04RV0KZ	04SH4ZZ	04U23KZ	04U94KZ	04V33ZZ	04VA4ZZ	04VJ4CZ
04N03ZZ	04NP3ZZ	04Q24ZZ	04QR4ZZ	04RV47Z	04SJ0ZZ	04U247Z	04UA07Z	04V34CZ	04VB0CZ	04VJ4DZ
04N04ZZ	04NP4ZZ	04Q30ZZ	04QS0ZZ	04RV4JZ	04SJ3ZZ	04U24JZ	04UA0JZ	04V34DZ	04VB0DZ	04VJ4ZZ
04N10ZZ	04NQ0ZZ	04Q33ZZ	04QS3ZZ	04RV4KZ	04SJ4ZZ	04U24KZ	04UA0KZ	04V34ZZ	04VB0ZZ	04VK0CZ
04N13ZZ	04NQ3ZZ	04Q34ZZ	04QS4ZZ	04RW07Z	04SK0ZZ	04U307Z	04UA37Z	04V40CZ	04VB3CZ	04VK0DZ
04N14ZZ	04NQ4ZZ	04Q40ZZ	04QT0ZZ	04RW0JZ	04SK3ZZ	04U30JZ	04UA3JZ	04V40DZ	04VB3DZ	04VK0ZZ
04N20ZZ	04NR0ZZ	04Q43ZZ	04QT3ZZ	04RW0KZ	04SK4ZZ	04U30KZ	04UA3KZ	04V40ZZ	04VB3ZZ	04VK3CZ
04N23ZZ	04NR3ZZ	04Q44ZZ	04QT4ZZ	04RW47Z	04SL0ZZ	04U337Z	04UA47Z	04V43CZ	04VB4CZ	04VK3DZ
04N24ZZ	04NR4ZZ	04Q50ZZ	04QU0ZZ	04RW4JZ	04SL3ZZ	04U33JZ	04UA4JZ	04V43DZ	04VB4DZ	04VK3ZZ
04N30ZZ	04NS0ZZ	04Q53ZZ	04QU3ZZ	04RW4KZ	04SL4ZZ	04U33KZ	04UA4KZ	04V43ZZ	04VB4ZZ	04VK4CZ
04N33ZZ	04NS3ZZ	04Q54ZZ	04QU4ZZ	04RY07Z	04SM0ZZ	04U347Z	04UB07Z	04V44CZ	04VC0CZ	04VK4DZ
04N34ZZ	04NS4ZZ	04Q60ZZ	04QV0ZZ	04RY0JZ	04SM3ZZ	04U34JZ	04UB0JZ	04V44DZ	04VC0DZ	04VK4ZZ
04N40ZZ	04NT0ZZ	04Q63ZZ	04QV3ZZ	04RY0KZ	04SM4ZZ	04U34KZ	04UB0KZ	04V44ZZ	04VC0EZ	04VL0CZ
04N43ZZ	04NT3ZZ	04Q64ZZ	04QV4ZZ	04RY47Z	04SN0ZZ	04U407Z	04UB37Z	04V50CZ	04VC0ZZ	04VL0DZ
04N44ZZ	04NT4ZZ	04Q70ZZ	04QW0ZZ	04RY4JZ	04SN3ZZ	04U40JZ	04UB3JZ	04V50DZ	04VC3CZ	04VL0ZZ
04N50ZZ	04NU0ZZ	04Q73ZZ	04QW3ZZ	04RY4KZ	04SN4ZZ	04U40KZ	04UB3KZ	04V50ZZ	04VC3DZ	04VL3CZ
04N53ZZ	04NU3ZZ	04Q74ZZ	04QW4ZZ	04S00ZZ	04SP0ZZ	04U437Z	04UB47Z	04V53CZ	04VC3EZ	04VL3DZ
04N54ZZ	04NU4ZZ	04Q80ZZ	04QY0ZZ	04S03ZZ	04SP3ZZ	04U43JZ	04UB4JZ	04V53DZ	04VC3ZZ	04VL3ZZ
04N60ZZ	04NV0ZZ	04Q83ZZ	04QY3ZZ	04S04ZZ	04SP4ZZ	04U43KZ	04UB4KZ	04V53ZZ	04VC4CZ	04VL4CZ
04N63ZZ	04NV3ZZ	04Q84ZZ	04QY4ZZ	04S10ZZ	04SQ0ZZ	04U447Z	04UC07Z	04V54CZ	04VC4DZ	04VL4DZ
04N64ZZ	04NV4ZZ	04Q90ZZ	04R007Z	04S13ZZ	04SQ3ZZ	04U44JZ	04UC0JZ	04V54DZ	04VC4EZ	04VL4ZZ
04N70ZZ	04NW0ZZ	04Q93ZZ	04R00JZ	04S14ZZ	04SQ4ZZ	04U44KZ	04UC0KZ	04V54ZZ	04VC4ZZ	04VM0CZ
04N73ZZ	04NW3ZZ	04Q94ZZ	04R00KZ	04S20ZZ	04SR0ZZ	04U507Z	04UC37Z	04V60CZ	04VD0CZ	04VM0DZ
04N74ZZ	04NW4ZZ	04QA0ZZ	04R047Z	04S23ZZ	04SR3ZZ	04U50JZ	04UC3JZ	04V60DZ	04VD0DZ	04VM0ZZ
04N80ZZ	04NY0ZZ	04QA3ZZ	04R04JZ	04S24ZZ	04SR4ZZ	04U50KZ	04UC3KZ	04V60ZZ	04VD0EZ	04VM3CZ
04N83ZZ	04NY3ZZ	04QA4ZZ	04R04KZ	04S30ZZ	04SS0ZZ	04U537Z	04UC47Z	04V63CZ	04VD0ZZ	04VM3DZ
04N84ZZ	04NY4ZZ	04QB0ZZ	04R107Z	04S33ZZ	04SS3ZZ	04U53JZ	04UC4JZ	04V63DZ	04VD3CZ	04VM3ZZ
04N90ZZ	04PY00Z	04QB3ZZ	04R10JZ	04S34ZZ	04SS4ZZ	04U53KZ	04UC4KZ	04V63ZZ	04VD3DZ	04VM4CZ
04N93ZZ	04PY02Z	04QB4ZZ	04R10KZ	04S40ZZ	04ST0ZZ	04U547Z	04UD07Z	04V64CZ	04VD3EZ	04VM4DZ
04N94ZZ	04PY03Z	04QC0ZZ	04R147Z	04S43ZZ	04ST3ZZ	04U54JZ	04UD0JZ	04V64DZ	04VD3ZZ	04VM4ZZ
04NA0ZZ	04PY07Z	04QC3ZZ	04R14JZ	04S44ZZ	04ST4ZZ	04U54KZ	04UD0KZ	04V64ZZ	04VD4CZ	04VN0CZ
04NA3ZZ	04PY0CZ	04QC4ZZ	04R14KZ	04S50ZZ	04SU0ZZ	04U607Z	04UD37Z	04V70CZ	04VD4DZ	04VN0DZ
04NA4ZZ	04PY0DZ	04QD0ZZ	04R207Z	04S53ZZ	04SU3ZZ	04U60JZ	04UD3JZ	04V70DZ	04VD4EZ	04VN0ZZ
04NB0ZZ	04PY0JZ	04QD3ZZ	04R20JZ	04S54ZZ	04SU4ZZ	04U60KZ	04UD3KZ	04V70ZZ	04VD4ZZ	04VN3CZ
04NB3ZZ	04PY0KZ	04QD4ZZ	04R20KZ	04S60ZZ	04SV0ZZ	04U637Z	04UD47Z	04V73CZ	04VE0CZ	04VN3DZ
04NB4ZZ	04PY0YZ	04QE0ZZ	04R247Z	04S63ZZ	04SV3ZZ	04U63JZ	04UD4JZ	04V73DZ	04VE0DZ	04VN3ZZ
04NC0ZZ	04PY30Z	04QE3ZZ	04R24JZ	04S64ZZ	04SV4ZZ	04U63KZ	04UD4KZ	04V73ZZ	04VE0ZZ	04VN4CZ
04NC3ZZ	04PY32Z	04QE4ZZ	04R24KZ	04S70ZZ	04SW0ZZ	04U647Z	04UE07Z	04V74CZ	04VE3CZ	04VN4DZ
04NC4ZZ	04PY33Z	04QF0ZZ	04R307Z	04S73ZZ	04SW3ZZ	04U64JZ	04UE0JZ	04V74DZ	04VE3DZ	04VN4ZZ
04ND0ZZ	04PY37Z	04QF3ZZ	04R30JZ	04S74ZZ	04SW4ZZ	04U64KZ	04UE0KZ	04V74ZZ	04VE3ZZ	04VP0CZ
04ND3ZZ	04PY3CZ	04QF4ZZ	04R30KZ	04S80ZZ	04SY0ZZ	04U707Z	04UE37Z	04V80CZ	04VE4CZ	04VP0DZ
04ND4ZZ	04PY3DZ	04QH0ZZ	04R347Z	04S83ZZ	04SY3ZZ	04U70JZ	04UE3JZ	04V80DZ	04VE4DZ	04VP0ZZ
04NE0ZZ	04PY3JZ	04QH3ZZ	04R34JZ	04S84ZZ	04SY4ZZ	04U70KZ	04UE3KZ	04V80ZZ	04VE4ZZ	04VP3CZ
04NE3ZZ	04PY3KZ	04QH4ZZ	04R34KZ	04S90ZZ	04U007Z	04U737Z	04V10CZ	04V83CZ	04VF0CZ	04VP3DZ
04NE4ZZ	04PY3YZ	04QJ0ZZ	04R407Z	04S93ZZ	04U00JZ	04U73JZ	04V10DZ	04V83DZ	04VF0DZ	

04VP3ZZ	04VW4ZZ	05114JY	05700ZZ	057C0ZZ	057S0ZZ	05954ZX	059D0ZX	059P3ZX	05B10ZZ	05BD0ZZ
04VP4CZ	04VY0CZ	05114KY	05703DZ	057C3DZ	057S3DZ	05954ZZ	059D0ZZ	059P3ZZ	05B13ZX	05BD3ZX
04VP4DZ	04VY0DZ	05114ZY	05703ZZ	057C3ZZ	057S3ZZ	059600Z	059D30Z	059P40Z	05B13ZZ	05BD3ZZ
04VP4ZZ	04VY0ZZ	051307Y	05704DZ	057C4DZ	057S4DZ	05960ZX	059D3ZX	059P4ZX	05B14ZX	05BD4ZX
04VQ0CZ	04VY3CZ	051309Y	05704ZZ	057C4ZZ	057S4ZZ	05960ZZ	059D3ZZ	059P4ZZ	05B14ZZ	05BD4ZZ
04VQ0DZ	04VY3DZ	05130AY	05710DZ	057D0DZ	057T0DZ	059630Z	059D40Z	059Q00Z	05B30ZX	05BF0ZX
04VQ0ZZ	04VY3ZZ	05130JY	05710ZZ	057D0ZZ	057T0ZZ	05963ZX	059D4ZX	059Q0ZX	05B30ZZ	05BF0ZZ
04VQ3CZ	04VY4CZ	05130KY	05713DZ	057D3DZ	057T3DZ	05963ZZ	059D4ZZ	059Q0ZZ	05B33ZX	05BF3ZX
04VQ3DZ	04VY4DZ	05580ZZ	05713ZZ	057D3ZZ	057T3ZZ	059640Z	059F00Z	059Q30Z	05B33ZZ	05BF3ZZ
04VQ3ZZ	04VY4ZZ	05583ZZ	05714DZ	057D4DZ	057T4DZ	05964ZX	059F0ZX	059Q3ZX	05B34ZX	05BF4ZX
04VQ4CZ	04WY00Z	05584ZZ	05714ZZ	057D4ZZ	057T4ZZ	05964ZZ	059F0ZZ	059Q3ZZ	05B34ZZ	05BF4ZZ
04VQ4DZ	04WY02Z	05590ZZ	05730DZ	057F0DZ	057V0DZ	059700Z	059F30Z	059Q40Z	05B40ZX	05BG0ZX
04VQ4ZZ	04WY03Z	05593ZZ	05730ZZ	057F0ZZ	057V0ZZ	05970ZX	059F3ZX	059Q4ZX	05B40ZZ	05BG0ZZ
04VR0CZ	04WY07Z	05594ZZ	05733DZ	057F3DZ	057V3DZ	05970ZZ	059F3ZZ	059Q4ZZ	05B43ZX	05BG3ZX
04VR0DZ	04WY0CZ	055A0ZZ	05733ZZ	057F3ZZ	057V3ZZ	059730Z	059F40Z	059R00Z	05B43ZZ	05BG3ZZ
04VR0ZZ	04WY0DZ	055A3ZZ	05734DZ	057F4DZ	057V4DZ	05973ZX	059F4ZX	059R0ZX	05B44ZX	05BG4ZX
04VR3CZ	04WY0JZ	055A4ZZ	05734ZZ	057F4ZZ	057V4ZZ	05973ZZ	059F4ZZ	059R0ZZ	05B44ZZ	05BG4ZZ
04VR3DZ	04WY0KZ	055B0ZZ	05740DZ	057G0DZ	057Y0DZ	059740Z	059G00Z	059R30Z	05B50ZX	05BH0ZX
04VR3ZZ	04WY0YZ	055B3ZZ	05740ZZ	057G0ZZ	057Y0ZZ	05974ZX	059G0ZX	059R3ZX	05B50ZZ	05BH0ZZ
04VR4CZ	04WY30Z	055B4ZZ	05743DZ	057G3DZ	057Y3DZ	05974ZZ	059G0ZZ	059R3ZZ	05B53ZX	05BH3ZX
04VR4DZ	04WY32Z	055C0ZZ	05743ZZ	057G3ZZ	057Y3ZZ	059800Z	059G30Z	059R40Z	05B53ZZ	05BH3ZZ
04VR4ZZ	04WY33Z	055C3ZZ	05744DZ	057G4DZ	057Y4DZ	05980ZX	059G3ZX	059R4ZX	05B54ZX	05BH4ZX
04VS0CZ	04WY37Z	055C4ZZ	05744ZZ	057G4ZZ	057Y4ZZ	05980ZZ	059G3ZZ	059R4ZZ	05B54ZZ	05BH4ZZ
04VS0DZ	04WY3CZ	055D0ZZ	05750DZ	057H0DZ	059000Z	059830Z	059G40Z	059S00Z	05B60ZX	05BL0ZX
04VS0ZZ	04WY3DZ	055D3ZZ	05750ZZ	057H0ZZ	05900ZX	05983ZX	059G4ZX	059S0ZX	05B60ZZ	05BL0ZZ
04VS3CZ	04WY3JZ	055D4ZZ	05753DZ	057H3DZ	05900ZZ	05983ZZ	059G4ZZ	059S0ZZ	05B63ZX	05CT3ZZ
04VS3DZ	04WY3KZ	055F0ZZ	05753ZZ	057H3ZZ	059030Z	059840Z	059H00Z	059S30Z	05B63ZZ	05CT4ZZ
04VS3ZZ	04WY3YZ	055F3ZZ	05754DZ	057H4DZ	05903ZX	05984ZX	059H0ZX	059S3ZX	05B64ZX	05CV0ZZ
04VS4CZ	04WY40Z	055F4ZZ	05754ZZ	057H4ZZ	05903ZZ	05984ZZ	059H0ZZ	059S3ZZ	05B64ZZ	05CV3ZZ
04VS4DZ	04WY42Z	055G0ZZ	05760DZ	057L0DZ	059040Z	059900Z	059H30Z	059S40Z	05B70ZX	05CV4ZZ
04VS4ZZ	04WY43Z	055G3ZZ	05760ZZ	057L0ZZ	05904ZX	05990ZX	059H3ZX	059S4ZX	05B70ZZ	05CY0ZZ
04VT0CZ	04WY47Z	055G4ZZ	05763DZ	057L3DZ	05904ZZ	05990ZZ	059H3ZZ	059S4ZZ	05B73ZX	05CY3ZZ
04VT0DZ	04WY4CZ	055H0ZZ	05763ZZ	057L3ZZ	059100Z	059930Z	059H40Z	059T00Z	05B73ZZ	05CY4ZZ
04VT0ZZ	04WY4DZ	055H3ZZ	05764DZ	057L4DZ	05910ZX	05993ZX	059H4ZX	059T0ZX	05B74ZX	05D90ZZ
04VT3CZ	04WY4JZ	055H4ZZ	05764ZZ	057L4ZZ	05910ZZ	05993ZZ	059H4ZZ	059T0ZZ	05B74ZZ	05D93ZZ
04VT3DZ	04WY4KZ	055L0ZZ	05770DZ	057M0DZ	059130Z	059940Z	059L00Z	059T30Z	05B80ZX	05DA0ZZ
04VT3ZZ	04WY4YZ	055L3ZZ	05770ZZ	057M0ZZ	05913ZX	05994ZX	059L0ZX	059T3ZX	05B80ZZ	05DA3ZZ
04VT4CZ	04WYX0Z	055L4ZZ	05773DZ	057M3DZ	05913ZZ	05994ZZ	059L0ZZ	059T3ZZ	05B83ZX	05DB0ZZ
04VT4DZ	04WYX2Z	055M0ZZ	05773ZZ	057M3ZZ	059140Z	059A00Z	059L30Z	059T40Z	05B83ZZ	05DB3ZZ
04VT4ZZ	04WYX3Z	055M3ZZ	05774DZ	057M4DZ	05914ZX	059A0ZX	059L3ZX	059T4ZX	05B84ZX	05DC0ZZ
04VU0CZ	04WYX7Z	055M4ZZ	05774ZZ	057M4ZZ	05914ZZ	059A0ZZ	059L3ZZ	059T4ZZ	05B84ZZ	05DC3ZZ
04VU0DZ	04WYXCZ	055N0ZZ	05780DZ	057N0DZ	059300Z	059A30Z	059L40Z	059V00Z	05B90ZX	05DD0ZZ
04VU0ZZ	04WYXDZ	055N3ZZ	05780ZZ	057N0ZZ	05930ZX	059A3ZX	059L4ZX	059V0ZX	05B90ZZ	05DD3ZZ
04VU3CZ	04WYXJZ	055N4ZZ	05783DZ	057N3DZ	05930ZZ	059A3ZZ	059L4ZZ	059V0ZZ	05B93ZX	05DF0ZZ
04VU3DZ	04WYXKZ	055P0ZZ	05783ZZ	057N3ZZ	059330Z	059A40Z	059M00Z	059V30Z	05B93ZZ	05DF3ZZ
04VU3ZZ	051007Y	055P3ZZ	05784DZ	057N4DZ	05933ZX	059A4ZX	059M0ZX	059V3ZX	05B94ZX	05DG0ZZ
04VU4CZ	051009Y	055P4ZZ	05784ZZ	057N4ZZ	05933ZZ	059A4ZZ	059M0ZZ	059V3ZZ	05B94ZZ	05DG3ZZ
04VU4DZ	05100AY	055Q0ZZ	05790DZ	057P0DZ	059340Z	059B00Z	059M30Z	059V40Z	05BA0ZX	05DH0ZZ
04VU4ZZ	05100JY	055Q3ZZ	05790ZZ	057P0ZZ	05934ZX	059B0ZX	059M3ZX	059V4ZX	05BA0ZZ	05DH3ZZ
04VV0CZ	05100KY	055Q4ZZ	05793DZ	057P3DZ	05934ZZ	059B0ZZ	059M3ZZ	059V4ZZ	05BA3ZX	05DY0ZZ
04VV0DZ	05100ZY	055R0ZZ	05793ZZ	057P3ZZ	059400Z	059B30Z	059M40Z	059Y00Z	05BA3ZZ	05DY3ZZ
04VV0ZZ	051047Y	055R3ZZ	05794DZ	057P4DZ	05940ZX	059B3ZX	059M4ZX	059Y0ZX	05BA4ZX	05H002Z
04VV3CZ	051049Y	055R4ZZ	05794ZZ	057P4ZZ	05940ZZ	059B3ZZ	059M4ZZ	059Y0ZZ	05BA4ZZ	05H003Z
04VV3DZ	05104AY	055S0ZZ	057A0DZ	057Q0DZ	059430Z	059B40Z	059N00Z	059Y30Z	05BB0ZX	05H00DZ
04VV3ZZ	05104JY	055S3ZZ	057A0ZZ	057Q0ZZ	05943ZX	059B4ZX	059N0ZX	059Y3ZX	05BB0ZZ	05H00MZ
04VV4CZ	05104KY	055S4ZZ	057A3DZ	057Q3DZ	05943ZZ	059B4ZZ	059N0ZZ	059Y3ZZ	05BB3ZX	05H032Z
04VV4DZ	05104ZY	055T0ZZ	057A3ZZ	057Q3ZZ	059440Z	059C00Z	059N30Z	059Y40Z	05BB3ZZ	05H033Z
04VV4ZZ	051107Y	055T3ZZ	057A4DZ	057Q4DZ	05944ZX	059C0ZX	059N3ZX	059Y4ZX	05BB4ZX	05H03DZ
04VW0CZ	051109Y	055T4ZZ	057A4ZZ	057Q4ZZ	05944ZZ	059C0ZZ	059N3ZZ	059Y4ZZ	05BB4ZZ	05H03MZ
04VW0DZ	05110AY	055V0ZZ	057B0DZ	057R0DZ	059500Z	059C30Z	059N40Z	05B00ZX	05BC0ZX	05H042Z
04VW0ZZ	05110JY	055V3ZZ	057B0ZZ	057R0ZZ	05950ZX	059C3ZX	059N4ZX	05B00ZZ	05BC0ZZ	05H043Z
04VW3CZ	05110KY	055V4ZZ	057B3DZ	057R3DZ	05950ZZ	059C3ZZ	059N4ZZ	05B03ZX	05BC3ZX	05H04DZ
04VW3DZ	05110ZY	055Y0ZZ	057B3ZZ	057R3ZZ	059530Z	059C40Z	059P00Z	05B03ZZ	05BC3ZZ	05H04MZ
04VW3ZZ	051147Y	055Y3ZZ	057B4DZ	057R4DZ	05953ZX	059C4ZX	059P0ZX	05B04ZX	05BC4ZX	05H103Z
04VW4CZ	051149Y	055Y4ZZ	057B4ZZ	057R4ZZ	05953ZZ	059C4ZZ	059P0ZZ	05B04ZZ	05BC4ZZ	05H10DZ
04VW4DZ	05114AY	05700DZ	057C0DZ	057S0DZ	059540Z	059D00Z	059P30Z	05B10ZX	05BD0ZX	05H133Z

05H13DZ	05HC3DZ	05HS3DZ	05L44ZZ	05LS4ZZ	05ND4ZZ	05PY32Z	05QH0ZZ	05SD3ZZ	05U34JZ	05UB0JZ
05H143Z	05HC43Z	05HS43Z	05L50CZ	05LT0CZ	05NF0ZZ	05PY33Z	05QH3ZZ	05SD4ZZ	05U34KZ	05UB0KZ
05H14DZ	05HC4DZ	05HS4DZ	05L50DZ	05LT0DZ	05NF3ZZ	05PY37Z	05QH4ZZ	05SF0ZZ	05U407Z	05UB37Z
05H303Z	05HD03Z	05HT03Z	05L50ZZ	05LT0ZZ	05NF4ZZ	05PY3CZ	05QL0ZZ	05SF3ZZ	05U40JZ	05UB3JZ
05H30DZ	05HD0DZ	05HT0DZ	05L53CZ	05LT3CZ	05NG0ZZ	05PY3DZ	05QL3ZZ	05SF4ZZ	05U40KZ	05UB3KZ
05H30MZ	05HD33Z	05HT33Z	05L53DZ	05LT3DZ	05NG3ZZ	05PY3JZ	05QL4ZZ	05SG0ZZ	05U437Z	05UB47Z
05H333Z	05HD3DZ	05HT3DZ	05L53ZZ	05LT3ZZ	05NG4ZZ	05PY3KZ	05QM0ZZ	05SG3ZZ	05U43JZ	05UB4JZ
05H33DZ	05HD43Z	05HT43Z	05L54CZ	05LT4CZ	05NH0ZZ	05PY3YZ	05QM3ZZ	05SG4ZZ	05U43KZ	05UB4KZ
05H33MZ	05HD4DZ	05HT4DZ	05L54DZ	05LT4DZ	05NH3ZZ	05PY40Z	05QM4ZZ	05SH0ZZ	05U447Z	05UC07Z
05H343Z	05HF03Z	05HV03Z	05L54ZZ	05LT4ZZ	05NH4ZZ	05PY42Z	05QN0ZZ	05SH3ZZ	05U44JZ	05UC0JZ
05H34DZ	05HF0DZ	05HV0DZ	05L60CZ	05LV0CZ	05NL0ZZ	05PY43Z	05QN3ZZ	05SH4ZZ	05U44KZ	05UC0KZ
05H34MZ	05HF33Z	05HV33Z	05L60DZ	05LV0DZ	05NL3ZZ	05PY47Z	05QN4ZZ	05SL0ZZ	05U507Z	05UC37Z
05H403Z	05HF3DZ	05HV3DZ	05L60ZZ	05LV0ZZ	05NL4ZZ	05PY4CZ	05QP0ZZ	05SL3ZZ	05U50JZ	05UC3JZ
05H40DZ	05HF43Z	05HV43Z	05L63CZ	05LV3CZ	05NM0ZZ	05PY4DZ	05QP3ZZ	05SL4ZZ	05U50KZ	05UC3KZ
05H40MZ	05HF4DZ	05HV4DZ	05L63DZ	05LV3DZ	05NM3ZZ	05PY4JZ	05QP4ZZ	05SM0ZZ	05U537Z	05UC47Z
05H433Z	05HG03Z	05HY02Z	05L63ZZ	05LV3ZZ	05NM4ZZ	05PY4KZ	05QQ0ZZ	05SM3ZZ	05U53JZ	05UC4JZ
05H43DZ	05HG0DZ	05HY03Z	05L64CZ	05LV4CZ	05NN0ZZ	05PY4YZ	05QQ3ZZ	05SM4ZZ	05U53KZ	05UC4KZ
05H43MZ	05HG33Z	05HY0DZ	05L64DZ	05LV4DZ	05NN3ZZ	05PYX0Z	05QQ4ZZ	05SN0ZZ	05U547Z	05UD07Z
05H443Z	05HG3DZ	05HY0YZ	05L64ZZ	05LV4ZZ	05NN4ZZ	05PYX2Z	05QR0ZZ	05SN3ZZ	05U54JZ	05UD0JZ
05H44DZ	05HG43Z	05HY32Z	05L70CZ	05LY0CZ	05NP0ZZ	05PYX3Z	05QR3ZZ	05SN4ZZ	05U54KZ	05UD0KZ
05H44MZ	05HG4DZ	05HY33Z	05L70DZ	05LY0DZ	05NP3ZZ	05PYXDZ	05QR4ZZ	05SP0ZZ	05U607Z	05UD37Z
05H503Z	05HH03Z	05HY3DZ	05L70ZZ	05LY0ZZ	05NP4ZZ	05Q00ZZ	05QS0ZZ	05SP3ZZ	05U60JZ	05UD3JZ
05H50DZ	05HH0DZ	05HY3YZ	05LN0CZ	05LY3CZ	05NQ0ZZ	05Q03ZZ	05QS3ZZ	05SP4ZZ	05U60KZ	05UD3KZ
05H533Z	05HH33Z	05HY42Z	05LN0DZ	05LY3DZ	05NQ3ZZ	05Q04ZZ	05QS4ZZ	05SQ0ZZ	05U637Z	05UD47Z
05H53DZ	05HH3DZ	05HY43Z	05LN0ZZ	05LY3ZZ	05NQ4ZZ	05Q10ZZ	05QT0ZZ	05SQ3ZZ	05U63JZ	05UD4JZ
05H543Z	05HH43Z	05HY4DZ	05LN3CZ	05LY4CZ	05NR0ZZ	05Q13ZZ	05QT3ZZ	05SQ4ZZ	05U63KZ	05UD4KZ
05H54DZ	05HH4DZ	05HY4YZ	05LN3ZZ	05LY4DZ	05NR3ZZ	05Q14ZZ	05QT4ZZ	05SR0ZZ	05U647Z	05UF07Z
05H603Z	05HL03Z	05JY0ZZ	05LN4CZ	05LY4ZZ	05NR4ZZ	05Q30ZZ	05QV0ZZ	05SR3ZZ	05U64JZ	05UF0JZ
05H60DZ	05HL0DZ	05JY3ZZ	05LN4DZ	05N00ZZ	05NS0ZZ	05Q33ZZ	05QV3ZZ	05SR4ZZ	05U64KZ	05UF0KZ
05H633Z	05HL33Z	05JY4ZZ	05LN4ZZ	05N03ZZ	05NS3ZZ	05Q34ZZ	05QV4ZZ	05SS0ZZ	05U707Z	05UF37Z
05H63DZ	05HL3DZ	05JYXZZ	05LP0CZ	05N04ZZ	05NS4ZZ	05Q40ZZ	05QY0ZZ	05SS3ZZ	05U70JZ	05UF3JZ
05H643Z	05HL43Z	05L00CZ	05LP0DZ	05N10ZZ	05NT0ZZ	05Q43ZZ	05QY3ZZ	05SS4ZZ	05U70KZ	05UF3KZ
05H64DZ	05HL4DZ	05L00DZ	05LP0ZZ	05N13ZZ	05NT3ZZ	05Q44ZZ	05QY4ZZ	05ST0ZZ	05U737Z	05UF47Z
05H703Z	05HM03Z	05L00ZZ	05LP3CZ	05N14ZZ	05NT4ZZ	05Q50ZZ	05R007Z	05ST3ZZ	05U73JZ	05UF4JZ
05H70DZ	05HM0DZ	05L03CZ	05LP3DZ	05N30ZZ	05NV0ZZ	05Q53ZZ	05R00JZ	05ST4ZZ	05U73KZ	05UF4KZ
05H733Z	05HM33Z	05L03DZ	05LP3ZZ	05N33ZZ	05NV3ZZ	05Q54ZZ	05R00KZ	05SV0ZZ	05U747Z	05UG07Z
05H73DZ	05HM3DZ	05L03ZZ	05LP4CZ	05N34ZZ	05NV4ZZ	05Q60ZZ	05R047Z	05SV3ZZ	05U74JZ	05UG0JZ
05H743Z	05HM43Z	05L04CZ	05LP4DZ	05N40ZZ	05NY0ZZ	05Q63ZZ	05R04JZ	05SV4ZZ	05U74KZ	05UG0KZ
05H74DZ	05HM4DZ	05L04DZ	05LP4ZZ	05N43ZZ	05NY3ZZ	05Q64ZZ	05R04KZ	05SY0ZZ	05U807Z	05UG37Z
05H803Z	05HN03Z	05L04ZZ	05LQ0CZ	05N44ZZ	05NY4ZZ	05Q70ZZ	05S43ZZ	05SY3ZZ	05U80JZ	05UG3JZ
05H80DZ	05HN0DZ	05L10CZ	05LQ0DZ	05N50ZZ	05P002Z	05Q73ZZ	05S44ZZ	05SY4ZZ	05U80KZ	05UG3KZ
05H833Z	05HN33Z	05L10DZ	05LQ0ZZ	05N53ZZ	05P00MZ	05Q74ZZ	05S50ZZ	05U007Z	05U837Z	05UG47Z
05H83DZ	05HN3DZ	05L10ZZ	05LQ3CZ	05N54ZZ	05P032Z	05Q80ZZ	05S53ZZ	05U00JZ	05U83JZ	05UG4JZ
05H843Z	05HN43Z	05L13CZ	05LQ3DZ	05N60ZZ	05P03MZ	05Q83ZZ	05S54ZZ	05U00KZ	05U83KZ	05UG4KZ
05H84DZ	05HN4DZ	05L13DZ	05LQ3ZZ	05N63ZZ	05P042Z	05Q84ZZ	05S60ZZ	05U037Z	05U847Z	05UH07Z
05H903Z	05HP03Z	05L13ZZ	05LQ4CZ	05N64ZZ	05P04MZ	05Q90ZZ	05S63ZZ	05U03JZ	05U84JZ	05UH0JZ
05H90DZ	05HP0DZ	05L14CZ	05LQ4DZ	05N70ZZ	05P0X2Z	05Q93ZZ	05S64ZZ	05U03KZ	05U84KZ	05UH0KZ
05H933Z	05HP33Z	05L14DZ	05LQ4ZZ	05N73ZZ	05P0XMZ	05Q94ZZ	05S70ZZ	05U047Z	05U907Z	05UH37Z
05H93DZ	05HP3DZ	05L14ZZ	05LR0CZ	05N74ZZ	05P30MZ	05QA0ZZ	05S73ZZ	05U04JZ	05U90JZ	05UH3JZ
05H943Z	05HP43Z	05L30CZ	05LR0DZ	05N80ZZ	05P33MZ	05QA3ZZ	05S74ZZ	05U04KZ	05U90KZ	05UH3KZ
05H94DZ	05HP4DZ	05L30DZ	05LR0ZZ	05N83ZZ	05P34MZ	05QA4ZZ	05S80ZZ	05U107Z	05U937Z	05UH47Z
05HA03Z	05HQ03Z	05L30ZZ	05LR3CZ	05N84ZZ	05P3XMZ	05QB0ZZ	05S83ZZ	05U10JZ	05U93JZ	05UH4JZ
05HA0DZ	05HQ0DZ	05L33CZ	05LR3DZ	05N90ZZ	05P40MZ	05QB3ZZ	05S84ZZ	05U10KZ	05U93KZ	05UH4KZ
05HA33Z	05HQ33Z	05L33DZ	05LR3ZZ	05N93ZZ	05P43MZ	05QB4ZZ	05S90ZZ	05U137Z	05U947Z	05UL07Z
05HA3DZ	05HQ3DZ	05L33ZZ	05LR4CZ	05N94ZZ	05P44MZ	05QC0ZZ	05S93ZZ	05U13JZ	05U94JZ	05UL0JZ
05HA43Z	05HQ43Z	05L34CZ	05LR4DZ	05NA0ZZ	05P4XMZ	05QC3ZZ	05S94ZZ	05U13KZ	05U94KZ	05UL0KZ
05HA4DZ	05HQ4DZ	05L34DZ	05LR4ZZ	05NA3ZZ	05PY00Z	05QC4ZZ	05SA0ZZ	05U147Z	05UA07Z	05UL37Z
05HB03Z	05HR03Z	05L34ZZ	05LS0CZ	05NA4ZZ	05PY02Z	05QD0ZZ	05SA3ZZ	05U14JZ	05UA0JZ	05UL3JZ
05HB0DZ	05HR0DZ	05L40CZ	05LS0DZ	05NB0ZZ	05PY03Z	05QD3ZZ	05SA4ZZ	05U14KZ	05UA0KZ	05UL3KZ
05HB33Z	05HR33Z	05L40DZ	05LS0ZZ	05NB3ZZ	05PY07Z	05QD4ZZ	05SB0ZZ	05U307Z	05UA37Z	05UL47Z
05HB3DZ	05HR3DZ	05L40ZZ	05LS3CZ	05NB4ZZ	05PY0CZ	05QF0ZZ	05SB3ZZ	05U30JZ	05UA3JZ	05UL4JZ
05HB43Z	05HR43Z	05L43CZ	05LS3DZ	05NC0ZZ	05PY0DZ	05QF3ZZ	05SB4ZZ	05U30KZ	05UA3KZ	05UL4KZ
05HB4DZ	05HR4DZ	05L43DZ	05LS3ZZ	05NC3ZZ	05PY0JZ	05QF4ZZ	05SC0ZZ	05U337Z	05UA47Z	05UM07Z
05HC03Z	05HS03Z	05L43ZZ	05LS4CZ	05NC4ZZ	05PY0KZ	05QG0ZZ	05SC3ZZ	05U33JZ	05UA4JZ	05UM0JZ
05HC0DZ	05HS0DZ	05L44CZ	05LS4CZ	05ND0ZZ	05PY0YZ	05QG3ZZ	05SC4ZZ	05U33KZ	05UA4KZ	05UM0KZ
05HC33Z	05HS33Z	05L44DZ	05LS4DZ	05ND3ZZ	05PY30Z	05QG4ZZ	05SD0ZZ	05U347Z	05UB07Z	05UM37Z

05UM3JZ	05UV4JZ	05WY00Z	06100Z6	06114AB	061649Y	06194KY	061H0KY	061Q4KY	065F3ZZ	06750ZZ
05UM3KZ	05UV4KZ	05WY02Z	06100ZP	06114AY	06164AY	06194ZY	061H0ZY	061Q4ZY	065F4ZZ	06753DZ
05UM47Z	05UY07Z	05WY03Z	06100ZQ	06114J9	06164JY	061B07Y	061H47Y	061T07Y	065G0ZZ	06753ZZ
05UM4JZ	05UY0JZ	05WY07Z	06100ZR	06114JB	06164KY	061B09Y	061H49Y	061T09Y	065G3ZZ	06754DZ
05UM4KZ	05UY0KZ	05WY0CZ	06100ZY	06114JY	06164ZY	061B0AY	061H4AY	061T0AY	065G4ZZ	06754ZZ
05UN07Z	05UY37Z	05WY0DZ	0610475	06114K9	061707Y	061B0JY	061H4JY	061T0JY	065H0ZZ	06760DZ
05UN0JZ	05UY3JZ	05WY0JZ	0610476	06114KB	061709Y	061B0KY	061H4KY	061T0KY	065H3ZZ	06760ZZ
05UN0KZ	05UY3KZ	05WY0YZ	061047P	06114KY	06170AY	061B0ZY	061H4ZY	061T0ZY	065H4ZZ	06763DZ
05UN37Z	05UY4JZ	05WY30Z	061047Q	06114Z9	06170JY	061B47Y	061J07Y	061T47Y	065J0ZZ	06763ZZ
05UN3JZ	05UY4KZ	05WY32Z	061047R	06114ZB	06170KY	061B49Y	061J09Y	061T49Y	065J3ZZ	06764DZ
05UN3KZ	05V00CZ	05WY33Z	061047Y	06114ZY	06170ZY	061B4AY	061J0AY	061T4AY	065J4ZZ	06764ZZ
05UN47Z	05V00DZ	05WY37Z	0610495	061207Y	061747Y	061B4JY	061J0JY	061T4JY	065M0ZZ	06770DZ
05UN4JZ	05V00ZZ	05WY3CZ	0610496	061209Y	061749Y	061B4KY	061J0KY	061T4KY	065M3ZZ	06770ZZ
05UN4KZ	05V03CZ	05WY3DZ	061049P	06120AY	06174AY	061B4ZY	061J0ZY	061T4ZY	065M4ZZ	06773DZ
05UP07Z	05V03DZ	05WY3JZ	061049Q	06120JY	06174JY	061C07Y	061J47Y	061V07Y	065N0ZZ	06773ZZ
05UP0JZ	05V03ZZ	05WY3KZ	061049R	06120KY	06174KY	061C09Y	061J49Y	061V09Y	065N3ZZ	06774DZ
05UP0KZ	05V04CZ	05WY3YZ	061049Y	06120ZY	06174ZY	061C0AY	061J4AY	061V0AY	065N4ZZ	06774ZZ
05UP37Z	05V04DZ	05WY40Z	06104A5	061247Y	0618079	061C0JY	061J4JY	061V0JY	065P0ZZ	06780DZ
05UP3JZ	05V04ZZ	05WY42Z	06104A6	061249Y	061807B	061C0KY	061J4KY	061V0KY	065P3ZZ	06780ZZ
05UP3KZ	05V10CZ	05WY43Z	06104AP	06124AY	061807Y	061C0ZY	061J4ZY	061V0ZY	065P4ZZ	06783DZ
05UP47Z	05V10DZ	05WY47Z	06104AQ	06124JY	0618099	061C47Y	061M07Y	061V47Y	065Q0ZZ	06783ZZ
05UP4JZ	05V10ZZ	05WY4CZ	06104AR	06124KY	061809B	061C49Y	061M09Y	061V49Y	065Q3ZZ	06784DZ
05UP4KZ	05V13CZ	05WY4DZ	06104AY	06124ZY	061809Y	061C4AY	061M0AY	061V4AY	065Q4ZZ	06784ZZ
05UQ07Z	05V13DZ	05WY4JZ	06104J5	061307Y	06180A9	061C4JY	061M0JY	061V4JY	065T0ZZ	06790DZ
05UQ0JZ	05V13ZZ	05WY4KZ	06104J6	061309Y	06180AB	061C4KY	061M0KY	061V4KY	065T3ZZ	06790ZZ
05UQ0KZ	05V14CZ	05WY4YZ	06104JP	06130AY	06180AY	061C4ZY	061M0ZY	061V4ZY	065T4ZZ	06793DZ
05UQ37Z	05V14DZ	05WYX0Z	06104JQ	06130JY	06180J9	061D07Y	061M47Y	06500ZZ	065V0ZZ	06793ZZ
05UQ3JZ	05V14ZZ	05WYX2Z	06104JR	06130KY	06180JB	061D09Y	061M49Y	06503ZZ	065V3ZZ	06794DZ
05UQ3KZ	05V30CZ	05WYX3Z	06104JY	06130ZY	06180JY	061D0AY	061M4AY	06504ZZ	065V4ZZ	06794ZZ
05UQ47Z	05V30DZ	05WYX7Z	06104K5	061347Y	06180K9	061D0JY	061M4JY	06510ZZ	065Y0ZC	067B0DZ
05UQ4JZ	05V30ZZ	05WYXCZ	06104K6	061349Y	06180KB	061D0KY	061M4KY	06513ZZ	065Y0ZZ	067B0ZZ
05UQ4KZ	05V33CZ	05WYXDZ	06104KP	06134AY	06180KY	061D0ZY	061M4ZY	06514ZZ	065Y3ZC	067B3DZ
05UR07Z	05V33DZ	05WYXJZ	06104KQ	06134JY	06180Z9	061D47Y	061N07Y	06520ZZ	065Y3ZZ	067B3ZZ
05UR0JZ	05V33ZZ	05WYXKZ	06104KR	06134KY	06180ZB	061D49Y	061N09Y	06523ZZ	065Y4ZC	067B4DZ
05UR0KZ	05V34CZ	06104KY	06134ZY	06180ZY	061D4AY	061N0AY	06524ZZ	065Y4ZZ	067B4ZZ
05UR37Z	05V34DZ	0610075	06104Z5	061407Y	06183J4	061D4JY	061N0JY	06530ZZ	06700DZ	067C0DZ
05UR3JZ	05V34ZZ	0610076	06104Z6	061409Y	06183JY	061D4KY	061N0KY	06533ZZ	06700ZZ	067C0ZZ
05UR3KZ	05V40CZ	061007P	06104ZP	06140AY	0618479	061D4ZY	061N0ZY	06534ZZ	06703DZ	067C3DZ
05UR47Z	05V40DZ	061007Q	06104ZQ	06140JY	061847B	061F07Y	061N47Y	06540ZZ	06703ZZ	067C3ZZ
05UR4JZ	05V40ZZ	061007R	06104ZR	06140KY	061847Y	061F09Y	061N49Y	06543ZZ	06704DZ	067C4DZ
05UR4KZ	05V43CZ	061007Y	06104ZY	06140ZY	0618499	061F0AY	061N4AY	06544ZZ	06704ZZ	067C4ZZ
05US07Z	05V43DZ	0610095	0611079	061447Y	061849B	061F0JY	061N4JY	06550ZZ	06710DZ	067D0DZ
05US0JZ	05V43ZZ	0610096	061107B	061449Y	061849Y	061F0KY	061N4KY	06553ZZ	06710ZZ	067D0ZZ
05US0KZ	05V44CZ	061009P	061107Y	06144AY	06184A9	061F0ZY	061N4ZY	06554ZZ	06713DZ	067D3DZ
05US37Z	05V44DZ	061009Q	0611099	06144JY	06184AB	061F47Y	061P07Y	06560ZZ	06713ZZ	067D3ZZ
05US3JZ	05V44ZZ	061009R	061109B	06144KY	06184AY	061F49Y	061P09Y	06563ZZ	06714DZ	067D4DZ
05US3KZ	05V50CZ	061009Y	061109Y	06144ZY	06184J4	061F4AY	061P0AY	06564ZZ	06714ZZ	067D4ZZ
05US47Z	05V50DZ	06100A5	06110A9	061507Y	06184J9	061F4JY	061P0JY	06570ZZ	06720DZ	067F0DZ
05US4JZ	05V50ZZ	06100A6	06110AB	061509Y	06184JB	061F4KY	061P0KY	06573ZZ	06720ZZ	067F0ZZ
05US4KZ	05V53CZ	06100AP	06110AY	06150AY	06184JY	061F4ZY	061P0ZY	06574ZZ	06723DZ	067F3DZ
05UT07Z	05V53DZ	06100AQ	06110J9	06150JY	06184K9	061G07Y	061P47Y	06580ZZ	06723ZZ	067F3ZZ
05UT0JZ	05V53ZZ	06100AR	06110JB	06150KY	06184KB	061G09Y	061P49Y	06583ZZ	06724DZ	067F4DZ
05UT0KZ	05V54CZ	06100AY	06110JY	06150ZY	06184KY	061G0AY	061P4AY	06584ZZ	06724ZZ	067F4ZZ
05UT37Z	05V54DZ	06100J5	06110K9	061547Y	06184Z9	061G0JY	061P4JY	06590ZZ	06730DZ	067G0DZ
05UT3JZ	05W04MZ	06100J6	06110KB	061549Y	06184ZB	061G0KY	061P4KY	06593ZZ	06730ZZ	067G0ZZ
05UT3KZ	05W0X2Z	06100JP	06110KY	06154AY	06184ZY	061G0ZY	061P4ZY	06594ZZ	06733DZ	067G3DZ
05UT47Z	05W0XMZ	06100JQ	06110Z9	06154JY	061907Y	061G47Y	061Q07Y	065B0ZZ	06733ZZ	067G3ZZ
05UT4JZ	05W30MZ	06100JR	06110ZB	06154KY	061909Y	061G49Y	061Q09Y	065B3ZZ	06734DZ	067G4DZ
05UT4KZ	05W33MZ	06100JY	06110ZY	06154ZY	06190AY	061G4AY	061Q0AY	065B4ZZ	06734ZZ	067G4ZZ
05UV07Z	05W34MZ	06100K5	0611479	061607Y	06190JY	061G4JY	061Q0JY	065C0ZZ	06740DZ	067H0DZ
05UV0JZ	05W3XMZ	06100K6	061147B	061609Y	06190KY	061G4KY	061Q0KY	065C3ZZ	06740ZZ	067H0ZZ
05UV0KZ	05W40MZ	06100KP	061147Y	06160AY	06190ZY	061G4ZY	061Q0ZY	065C4ZZ	06743DZ	067H3DZ
05UV37Z	05W43MZ	06100KQ	0611499	06160JY	061947Y	061H07Y	061Q47Y	065D0ZZ	06743ZZ	067H3ZZ
05UV3JZ	05W44MZ	06100KR	061149B	06160KY	061949Y	061H09Y	061Q49Y	065D3ZZ	06744DZ	067H4DZ
05UV3KZ	05W4XMZ	06100KY	061149Y	06160ZY	06194AY	061H0AY	061Q4AY	065D4ZZ	06744ZZ	067H4ZZ
05UV47Z		06100Z5	06114A9	061647Y	06194JY	061H0JY	061Q4JY	065F0ZZ	06750DZ	067J0DZ

067J0ZZ	06923ZZ	069G0ZZ	06CQ0ZZ	06H50DZ	06HJ0DZ	06L10CZ	06LN3ZZ	06N24ZZ	06PY03Z	06QD3ZZ
067J3DZ	069240Z	069G30Z	06CQ3ZZ	06H533Z	06HJ33Z	06L10DZ	06LN4CZ	06N30ZZ	06PY07Z	06QD4ZZ
067J3ZZ	06924ZZ	069G3ZZ	06CQ4ZZ	06H53DZ	06HJ3DZ	06L10ZZ	06LN4DZ	06N33ZZ	06PY0CZ	06QF0ZZ
067J4DZ	069330Z	069G40Z	06CT0ZZ	06H543Z	06HJ43Z	06L13CZ	06LN4ZZ	06N34ZZ	06PY0DZ	06QF3ZZ
067J4ZZ	06933ZZ	069G4ZZ	06CT3ZZ	06H54DZ	06HJ4DZ	06L13DZ	06LP0CZ	06N40ZZ	06PY0JZ	06QF4ZZ
067M0DZ	069400Z	069H00Z	06CT4ZZ	06H603Z	06HM03Z	06L13ZZ	06LP0DZ	06N43ZZ	06PY0KZ	06QG0ZZ
067M0ZZ	06940ZZ	069H0ZZ	06CV0ZZ	06H60DZ	06HM0DZ	06L14CZ	06LP0ZZ	06N44ZZ	06PY0YZ	06QG3ZZ
067M3DZ	069430Z	069H30Z	06CV3ZZ	06H633Z	06HM33Z	06L14DZ	06LP3CZ	06N50ZZ	06PY30Z	06QG4ZZ
067M3ZZ	06943ZZ	069H3ZZ	06CV4ZZ	06H63DZ	06HM3DZ	06L14ZZ	06LP3DZ	06N53ZZ	06PY32Z	06QH0ZZ
067M4DZ	069440Z	069H40Z	06CY0ZZ	06H643Z	06HM43Z	06L20CZ	06LP3ZZ	06N54ZZ	06PY33Z	06QH3ZZ
067M4ZZ	06944ZZ	069H4ZZ	06CY3ZZ	06H64DZ	06HM4DZ	06L20DZ	06LP4CZ	06N60ZZ	06PY37Z	06QH4ZZ
067N0DZ	069500Z	069J00Z	06CY4ZZ	06H703Z	06HN03Z	06L20ZZ	06LP4DZ	06N63ZZ	06PY3CZ	06QJ0ZZ
067N0ZZ	06950ZZ	069J0ZZ	06DM0ZZ	06H70DZ	06HN0DZ	06L23CZ	06LP4ZZ	06N64ZZ	06PY3DZ	06QJ3ZZ
067N3DZ	069530Z	069J30Z	06DM3ZZ	06H733Z	06HN33Z	06L23DZ	06LQ0CZ	06N70ZZ	06PY3JZ	06QJ4ZZ
067N3ZZ	06953ZZ	069J3ZZ	06DM4ZZ	06H73DZ	06HN3DZ	06L23ZZ	06LQ0DZ	06N73ZZ	06PY3KZ	06QM0ZZ
067N4DZ	069540Z	069J40Z	06DN0ZZ	06H743Z	06HN43Z	06L24CZ	06LQ0ZZ	06N74ZZ	06PY3YZ	06QM3ZZ
067N4ZZ	06954ZZ	069J4ZZ	06DN3ZZ	06H74DZ	06HN4DZ	06L24DZ	06LQ3CZ	06N80ZZ	06PY40Z	06QM4ZZ
067P0DZ	069600Z	069M00Z	06DN4ZZ	06H803Z	06HP03Z	06L24ZZ	06LQ3DZ	06N83ZZ	06PY42Z	06QN0ZZ
067P0ZZ	06960ZZ	069M0ZZ	06DP0ZZ	06H80DZ	06HP0DZ	06L30CZ	06LQ3ZZ	06N84ZZ	06PY43Z	06QN3ZZ
067P3DZ	069630Z	069M30Z	06DP3ZZ	06H833Z	06HP33Z	06L30DZ	06LQ4CZ	06N90ZZ	06PY47Z	06QN4ZZ
067P3ZZ	06963ZZ	069M3ZZ	06DP4ZZ	06H83DZ	06HP3DZ	06L33CZ	06LQ4DZ	06N93ZZ	06PY4CZ	06QP0ZZ
067P4DZ	069640Z	069M40Z	06DQ0ZZ	06H843Z	06HP43Z	06L33DZ	06LQ4ZZ	06N94ZZ	06PY4DZ	06QP3ZZ
067P4ZZ	06964ZZ	069M4ZZ	06DQ3ZZ	06H84DZ	06HP4DZ	06L33ZZ	06LT0CZ	06NB0ZZ	06PY4JZ	06QP4ZZ
067Q0DZ	069700Z	069N00Z	06DQ4ZZ	06H903Z	06HQ03Z	06L34CZ	06LT0DZ	06NB3ZZ	06PY4KZ	06QQ0ZZ
067Q0ZZ	06970ZZ	069N0ZZ	06DT0ZZ	06H90DZ	06HQ0DZ	06L34DZ	06LT0ZZ	06NB4ZZ	06PY4YZ	06QQ3ZZ
067Q3DZ	069730Z	069N30Z	06DT3ZZ	06H933Z	06HQ33Z	06L34ZZ	06LT3CZ	06NC0ZZ	06PYX0Z	06QQ4ZZ
067Q3ZZ	06973ZZ	069N3ZZ	06DT4ZZ	06H93DZ	06HQ3DZ	06L37CZ	06LT3DZ	06NC3ZZ	06PYX2Z	06QT0ZZ
067Q4DZ	069740Z	069N40Z	06DV0ZZ	06H943Z	06HQ43Z	06L37DZ	06LT3ZZ	06NC4ZZ	06PYX3Z	06QT3ZZ
067Q4ZZ	06974ZZ	069N4ZZ	06DV3ZZ	06H94DZ	06HQ4DZ	06L37ZZ	06LT4CZ	06ND0ZZ	06PYXDZ	06QT4ZZ
067T0DZ	069800Z	069P00Z	06DV4ZZ	06HB03Z	06HT03Z	06L38CZ	06LT4DZ	06ND3ZZ	06Q00ZZ	06QV0ZZ
067T0ZZ	06980ZZ	069P0ZZ	06DY0ZZ	06HB0DZ	06HT0DZ	06L38DZ	06LT4ZZ	06ND4ZZ	06Q03ZZ	06QV3ZZ
067T3DZ	069830Z	069P30Z	06DY3ZZ	06HB33Z	06HT33Z	06L38ZZ	06LV0CZ	06NF0ZZ	06Q04ZZ	06QV4ZZ
067T3ZZ	06983ZZ	069P3ZZ	06DY4ZZ	06HB3DZ	06HT3DZ	06LG4DZ	06LV0DZ	06NF3ZZ	06Q10ZZ	06QY0ZZ
067T4DZ	069840Z	069P40Z	06H003T	06HB43Z	06HT43Z	06LG4ZZ	06LV0ZZ	06NF4ZZ	06Q13ZZ	06QY3ZZ
067T4ZZ	06984ZZ	069P4ZZ	06H003Z	06HB4DZ	06HT4DZ	06LH0CZ	06LV3CZ	06NG0ZZ	06Q14ZZ	06QY4ZZ
067V0DZ	069900Z	069Q00Z	06H00DZ	06HC03Z	06HV03Z	06LH0DZ	06LV3DZ	06NG3ZZ	06Q20ZZ	06R007Z
067V0ZZ	06990ZZ	069Q0ZZ	06H033T	06HC0DZ	06HV0DZ	06LH0ZZ	06LV3ZZ	06NG4ZZ	06Q23ZZ	06R00JZ
067V3DZ	069930Z	069Q30Z	06H033Z	06HC33Z	06HV33Z	06LH3CZ	06LV4CZ	06NH0ZZ	06Q24ZZ	06R00KZ
067V3ZZ	06993ZZ	069Q3ZZ	06H03DZ	06HC3DZ	06HV3DZ	06LH3DZ	06LV4DZ	06NH3ZZ	06Q30ZZ	06R047Z
067V4DZ	069940Z	069Q40Z	06H043Z	06HC43Z	06HV43Z	06LH3ZZ	06LV4ZZ	06NH4ZZ	06Q33ZZ	06R04JZ
067V4ZZ	06994ZZ	069Q4ZZ	06H04DZ	06HC4DZ	06HV4DZ	06LH4CZ	06LY0CC	06NJ0ZZ	06Q34ZZ	06R04KZ
067Y0DZ	069B00Z	069T00Z	06H103Z	06HD03Z	06HY02Z	06LH4DZ	06LY0CZ	06NJ3ZZ	06Q40ZZ	06R107Z
067Y0ZZ	069B0ZZ	069T0ZZ	06H10DZ	06HD0DZ	06HY03Z	06LH4ZZ	06LY0DC	06NJ4ZZ	06Q43ZZ	06R10JZ
067Y3DZ	069B30Z	069T30Z	06H133Z	06HD33Z	06HY0DZ	06LJ0CZ	06LY0DZ	06NM0ZZ	06Q44ZZ	06R10KZ
067Y3ZZ	069B3ZZ	069T3ZZ	06H13DZ	06HD3DZ	06HY0YZ	06LJ0DZ	06LY0ZC	06NM3ZZ	06Q50ZZ	06R147Z
067Y4DZ	069B40Z	069T40Z	06H143Z	06HD43Z	06HY32Z	06LJ0ZZ	06LY0ZZ	06NM4ZZ	06Q53ZZ	06R14JZ
067Y4ZZ	069B4ZZ	069T4ZZ	06H14DZ	06HD4DZ	06HY33Z	06LJ3CZ	06LY3CC	06NN0ZZ	06Q54ZZ	06R14KZ
069000Z	069C00Z	069V00Z	06H203Z	06HF03Z	06HY3DZ	06LJ3DZ	06LY3CZ	06NN3ZZ	06Q60ZZ	06R207Z
06900ZX	069C0ZZ	069V0DZ	06H20DZ	06HF0DZ	06HY3YZ	06LJ3ZZ	06LY3DC	06NN4ZZ	06Q63ZZ	06R20JZ
06900ZZ	069C30Z	069V30Z	06H233Z	06HF33Z	06HY42Z	06LJ4CZ	06LY3DZ	06NP0ZZ	06Q64ZZ	06R20KZ
069030Z	069C3ZZ	069V3ZZ	06H23DZ	06HF3DZ	06HY43Z	06LJ4DZ	06LY3ZC	06NP3ZZ	06Q70ZZ	06R247Z
06903ZX	069C40Z	069V40Z	06H243Z	06HF43Z	06HY4DZ	06LJ4ZZ	06LY3ZZ	06NP4Z	06Q73ZZ	06R24JZ
06903ZZ	069C4ZZ	069V4ZZ	06H24DZ	06HF4DZ	06HY4YZ	06LM0CZ	06LY4CC	06NQ0ZZ	06Q74ZZ	06R24KZ
069040Z	069D00Z	069Y00Z	06H303Z	06HG03Z	06JY0ZZ	06LM0DZ	06LY4CZ	06NQ3ZZ	06Q80ZZ	06R307Z
06904ZX	069D0ZZ	069Y0ZZ	06H30DZ	06HG0DZ	06JY3ZZ	06LM0ZZ	06LY4DC	06NQ4ZZ	06Q83ZZ	06R30JZ
06904ZZ	069D30Z	069Y30Z	06H333Z	06HG33Z	06JY4ZZ	06LM3CZ	06LY4DZ	06NT0ZZ	06Q84ZZ	06R30KZ
069100Z	069D3ZZ	069Y3ZZ	06H33DZ	06HG3DZ	06JYXZZ	06LM3DZ	06LY4ZC	06NT3ZZ	06Q90ZZ	06R347Z
06910ZX	069D40Z	069Y40Z	06H343Z	06HG43Z	06L00CZ	06LM3ZZ	06LY4ZZ	06NT4ZZ	06Q93ZZ	06R34JZ
06910ZZ	069D4ZZ	069Y4ZZ	06H34DZ	06HG4DZ	06L00DZ	06LM4CZ	06N00ZZ	06NV0ZZ	06Q94ZZ	06R34KZ
069130Z	069F00Z	06CM4ZZ	06H403Z	06HH03Z	06L00ZZ	06LM4DZ	06N03ZZ	06NV3ZZ	06QB0ZZ	06R407Z
06913ZZ	069F0ZZ	06CN0ZZ	06H40DZ	06HH0DZ	06L03CZ	06LM4ZZ	06N04ZZ	06NV4ZZ	06QB3ZZ	06R40JZ
069140Z	069F30Z	06CN3ZZ	06H433Z	06HH33Z	06L03DZ	06LN0CZ	06N10ZZ	06NY0ZZ	06QB4ZZ	06R40KZ
06914ZZ	069F3ZZ	06CN4ZZ	06H43DZ	06HH3DZ	06L03ZZ	06LN0DZ	06N13ZZ	06NY3ZZ	06QC0ZZ	06R447Z
069200Z	069F40Z	06CP0ZZ	06H443Z	06HH43Z	06L04CZ	06LN0ZZ	06N14ZZ	06NY4ZZ	06QC3ZZ	06R44JZ
06920ZZ	069F4ZZ	06CP3ZZ	06H44DZ	06HH4DZ	06L04DZ	06LN3CZ	06N20ZZ	06PY00Z	06QC4ZZ	06R44KZ
069230Z	069G00Z	06CP4ZZ	06H503Z	06HJ03Z	06L04ZZ	06LN3DZ	06N23ZZ	06PY02Z	06QD0ZZ	06R507Z

06R50JZ	06U13KZ	06U84KZ	06UJ0KZ	06UY3JZ	06WY3KZ	075C4ZZ	07930ZZ	07984ZZ	079G0ZZ	07B80ZZ
06R50KZ	06U147Z	06U907Z	06UJ37Z	06UY3KZ	06WY3YZ	075D0ZZ	079330Z	079880Z	079G30Z	07B83ZX
06R547Z	06U14JZ	06U90JZ	06UJ3JZ	06UY47Z	06WY40Z	075D3ZZ	07933ZX	07988ZX	079G3ZX	07B83ZZ
06R54JZ	06U14KZ	06U90KZ	06UJ3KZ	06UY4JZ	06WY42Z	075D4ZZ	07933ZZ	07988ZZ	079G3ZZ	07B84ZX
06R54KZ	06U207Z	06U937Z	06UJ47Z	06UY4KZ	06WY43Z	075F0ZZ	079340Z	079900Z	079G40Z	07B84ZZ
06R607Z	06U20JZ	06U93JZ	06UJ4JZ	06V00CZ	06WY47Z	075F3ZZ	07934ZX	07990ZX	079G4ZX	07B90ZX
06R60JZ	06U20KZ	06U93KZ	06UJ4KZ	06V00DZ	06WY4CZ	075F4ZZ	07934ZZ	07990ZZ	079G4ZZ	07B90ZZ
06R60KZ	06U237Z	06U947Z	06UM07Z	06V00ZZ	06WY4DZ	075G0ZZ	079380Z	079930Z	079G80Z	07B93ZX
06R647Z	06U23JZ	06U94JZ	06UM0JZ	06V03CZ	06WY4JZ	075G3ZZ	07938ZX	07993ZX	079G8ZX	07B93ZZ
06R64JZ	06U23KZ	06U94KZ	06UM0KZ	06V03DZ	06WY4KZ	075G4ZZ	07938ZZ	07993ZZ	079G8ZZ	07B94ZX
06R64KZ	06U247Z	06UB07Z	06UM37Z	06V03ZZ	06WY4YZ	075H0ZZ	079400Z	079940Z	079H00Z	07B94ZZ
06R707Z	06U24JZ	06UB0JZ	06UM3JZ	06V04CZ	06WYX0Z	075H3ZZ	07940ZX	07994ZX	079H0ZX	07BB0ZX
06R70JZ	06U24KZ	06UB0KZ	06UM3KZ	06V04DZ	06WYX2Z	075H4ZZ	07940ZZ	07994ZZ	079H0ZZ	07BB0ZZ
06R70KZ	06U307Z	06UB37Z	06UM47Z	06V04ZZ	06WYX3Z	075J0ZZ	079430Z	079980Z	079H30Z	07BB3ZX
06R747Z	06U30JZ	06UB3JZ	06UM4JZ	06V10CZ	06WYX7Z	075J3ZZ	07943ZX	07998ZX	079H3ZX	07BB3ZZ
06R74JZ	06U30KZ	06UB3KZ	06UM4KZ	06V10DZ	06WYXCZ	075J4ZZ	07943ZZ	07998ZZ	079H3ZZ	07BB4ZX
06R74KZ	06U337Z	06UB47Z	06UN07Z	06V10ZZ	06WYXDZ	075K0ZZ	079440Z	079B00Z	079H40Z	07BB4ZZ
06R807Z	06U33JZ	06UB4JZ	06UN0JZ	06V13CZ	06WYXJZ	075K3ZZ	07944ZX	079B0ZX	079H4ZX	07BC0ZX
06R80JZ	06U33KZ	06UB4KZ	06UN0KZ	06V13DZ	06WYXKZ	075K4ZZ	07944ZZ	079B0ZZ	079H4ZZ	07BC0ZZ
06R80KZ	06U347Z	06UC07Z	06UN37Z	06V13ZZ	072KX0Z	075L0ZZ	079480Z	079B30Z	079H80Z	07BC3ZX
06R847Z	06U34JZ	06UC0JZ	06UN3JZ	06V14CZ	072KXYZ	075L3ZZ	07948ZX	079B3ZX	079H8ZX	07BC3ZZ
06R84JZ	06U34KZ	06UC0KZ	06UN3KZ	06V14DZ	072LX0Z	075L4ZZ	07948ZZ	079B3ZZ	079H8ZZ	07BC4ZX
06R84KZ	06U407Z	06UC37Z	06UN47Z	06V14ZZ	072LXYZ	075M0ZZ	079500Z	079B40Z	079J00Z	07BC4ZZ
06R907Z	06U40JZ	06UC3JZ	06UN4JZ	06V20CZ	072MX0Z	075M3ZZ	07950ZX	079B4ZX	079J0ZX	07BD0ZX
06R90JZ	06U40KZ	06UC3KZ	06UN4KZ	06V20DZ	072MXYZ	075M4ZZ	07950ZZ	079B4ZZ	079J0ZZ	07BD0ZZ
06R90KZ	06U437Z	06UC47Z	06UP07Z	06V20ZZ	072NX0Z	075P0ZZ	079530Z	079B80Z	079J30Z	07BD3ZX
06R947Z	06U43JZ	06UC4JZ	06UP0JZ	06V23CZ	072NXYZ	075P3ZZ	07953ZX	079B8ZX	079J3ZX	07BD3ZZ
06R94JZ	06U43KZ	06UC4KZ	06UP0KZ	06V23DZ	072PX0Z	075P4ZZ	07953ZZ	079B8ZZ	079J3ZZ	07BD4ZX
06R94KZ	06U447Z	06UD07Z	06UP37Z	06V23ZZ	072PXYZ	079000Z	079540Z	079C00Z	079J40Z	07BD4ZZ
06RB07Z	06U44JZ	06UD0JZ	06UP3JZ	06V24CZ	072TX0Z	07900ZX	07954ZX	079C0ZX	079J4ZX	07BF0ZX
06SJ4ZZ	06U44KZ	06UD0KZ	06UP3KZ	06V24DZ	072TXYZ	07900ZZ	07954ZZ	079C0ZZ	079J4ZZ	07BF0ZZ
06SM0ZZ	06U507Z	06UD37Z	06UP47Z	06V24ZZ	07500ZZ	079030Z	079580Z	079C30Z	079J80Z	07BF3ZX
06SM3ZZ	06U50JZ	06UD3JZ	06UP4JZ	06V30CZ	07503ZZ	07903ZX	07958ZX	079C3ZX	079J8ZX	07BF3ZZ
06SM4ZZ	06U50KZ	06UD3KZ	06UP4KZ	06V30DZ	07504ZZ	07903ZZ	07958ZZ	079C3ZZ	079J8ZZ	07BF4ZX
06SN0ZZ	06U537Z	06UD47Z	06UQ07Z	06V30ZZ	07510ZZ	079040Z	079600Z	079C40Z	079K00Z	07BF4ZZ
06SN3ZZ	06U53JZ	06UD4JZ	06UQ0JZ	06V33CZ	07513ZZ	07904ZX	07960ZX	079C4ZX	079K0ZX	07BG0ZX
06SN4ZZ	06U53KZ	06UD4KZ	06UQ0KZ	06V33DZ	07514ZZ	07904ZZ	07960ZZ	079C4ZZ	079K30Z	07BG0ZZ
06SP0ZZ	06U547Z	06UF07Z	06UQ37Z	06V33ZZ	07520ZZ	079080Z	079630Z	079C80Z	079K3ZZ	07BG3ZX
06SP3ZZ	06U54JZ	06UF0JZ	06UQ3JZ	06V34CZ	07523ZZ	07908ZX	07963ZX	079C8ZX	079K80Z	07BG3ZZ
06SP4ZZ	06U54KZ	06UF0KZ	06UQ3KZ	06V34DZ	07524ZZ	07908ZZ	07963ZZ	079C8ZZ	079K8ZX	07BG4ZX
06SQ0ZZ	06U607Z	06UF37Z	06UQ47Z	06V34ZZ	07530ZZ	079100Z	079640Z	079D00Z	079K8ZZ	07BG4ZZ
06SQ3ZZ	06U60JZ	06UF3JZ	06UQ4JZ	06V40CZ	07533ZZ	07910ZX	07964ZX	079D0ZX	079L30Z	07BH0ZX
06SQ4ZZ	06U60KZ	06UF3KZ	06UQ4KZ	06V40DZ	07534ZZ	07910ZZ	07964ZZ	079D0ZZ	079L3ZZ	07BH0ZZ
06ST0ZZ	06U637Z	06UF47Z	06US47Z	06V40ZZ	07540ZZ	079130Z	079680Z	079D30Z	079L80Z	07BH3ZX
06ST3ZZ	06U63JZ	06UF4JZ	06UT07Z	06V43CZ	07543ZZ	07913ZX	07968ZX	079D3ZX	079L8ZX	07BH3ZZ
06ST4ZZ	06U63KZ	06UF4KZ	06UT0JZ	06V43DZ	07544ZZ	07913ZZ	07968ZZ	079D3ZZ	079P30Z	07BH4ZX
06SV0ZZ	06U647Z	06UG07Z	06UT0KZ	06V43ZZ	07550ZZ	079140Z	079700Z	079D40Z	079P3ZX	07BH4ZZ
06SV3ZZ	06U64JZ	06UG0JZ	06UT37Z	06V44CZ	07553ZZ	07914ZX	07970ZX	079D4ZX	079P3ZZ	07BJ0ZX
06SV4ZZ	06U64KZ	06UG0KZ	06UT3JZ	06V44DZ	07554ZZ	07914ZZ	07970ZZ	079D4ZZ	079P40Z	07BJ0ZZ
06SY0ZZ	06U707Z	06UG37Z	06UT3KZ	06V44ZZ	07560ZZ	079180Z	079730Z	079D80Z	079P4ZX	07BJ3ZX
06SY3ZZ	06U70JZ	06UG3JZ	06UT47Z	06V50CZ	07563ZZ	07918ZX	07973ZX	079D8ZX	079P4ZZ	07BJ3ZZ
06SY4ZZ	06U70KZ	06UG3KZ	06UT4JZ	06WY02Z	07564ZZ	07918ZZ	07973ZZ	079D8ZZ	079T00Z	07BJ4ZX
06U007Z	06U737Z	06UG47Z	06UT4KZ	06WY03Z	07570ZZ	079200Z	079740Z	079F00Z	079T0ZX	07BJ4ZZ
06U00JZ	06U73JZ	06UG4JZ	06UV07Z	06WY07Z	07573ZZ	07920ZX	07974ZX	079F0ZX	079T0ZZ	07BK0ZX
06U00KZ	06U73KZ	06UG4KZ	06UV0JZ	06WY0CZ	07574ZZ	07920ZZ	07974ZZ	079F0ZZ	079T30Z	07BK0ZZ
06U037Z	06U747Z	06UH07Z	06UV0KZ	06WY0DZ	07580ZZ	079230Z	079780Z	079F30Z	079T3ZX	07BK3ZX
06U03JZ	06U74JZ	06UH0JZ	06UV37Z	06WY0JZ	07583ZZ	07923ZX	07978ZX	079F3ZX	079T3ZZ	07BK3ZZ
06U03KZ	06U74KZ	06UH0KZ	06UV3JZ	06WY0KZ	07584ZZ	07923ZZ	07978ZZ	079F3ZZ	079T40Z	07BK4ZX
06U047Z	06U807Z	06UH37Z	06UV3KZ	06WY0YZ	07590ZZ	079240Z	079800Z	079F40Z	079T4ZX	07BK4ZZ
06U04JZ	06U80JZ	06UH3JZ	06UV47Z	06WY30Z	07593ZZ	07924ZX	07980ZX	079F4ZX	079T4ZZ	07BL0ZX
06U04KZ	06U80KZ	06UH3KZ	06UV4JZ	06WY32Z	07594ZZ	07924ZZ	07980ZZ	079F4ZZ		07BL0ZZ
06U107Z	06U837Z	06UH47Z	06UV4KZ	06WY33Z	075B0ZZ	079280Z	079830Z	079F80Z		07BL3ZX
06U10JZ	06U83JZ	06UH4JZ	06UY07Z	06WY37Z	075B3ZZ	07928ZX	07983ZX	079F8ZX		07BL3ZZ
06U10KZ	06U83KZ	06UH4KZ	06UY0JZ	06WY3CZ	075B4ZZ	07928ZZ	07983ZZ	079F8ZZ		07BL4ZX
06U137Z	06U847Z	06UJ07Z	06UY0KZ	06WY3DZ	075C0ZZ	079300Z	079840Z	079G00Z		07BL4ZZ
06U13JZ	06U84JZ	06UJ0JZ	06UY37Z	06WY3JZ	075C3ZZ	07930ZX	07984ZX	079G0ZZ		07BM0ZX

07BM0ZZ	07CL3ZZ	07DM4ZX	07L00CZ	07LL3DZ	07NP3ZZ	07PMX3Z	07Q58ZZ	07U30JZ	07UG0JZ	07V40DZ
07BM3ZX	07CL4ZZ	07DP3ZX	07L00DZ	07LL3ZZ	07NP4ZZ	07PN00Z	07Q60ZZ	07U30KZ	07UG0KZ	07V40ZZ
07BM3ZZ	07CM0ZZ	07DP4ZX	07L00ZZ	07LL4CZ	07PK00Z	07PN03Z	07Q63ZZ	07U347Z	07UG47Z	07V43CZ
07BM4ZX	07CM3ZZ	07DQ0ZX	07L03CZ	07LL4DZ	07PK03Z	07PN07Z	07Q64ZZ	07U34JZ	07UG4JZ	07V43DZ
07BM4ZZ	07CM4ZZ	07DQ0ZZ	07L03DZ	07LL4ZZ	07PK07Z	07PN0CZ	07Q68ZZ	07U34KZ	07UG4KZ	07V43ZZ
07BP0ZX	07CP0ZZ	07DQ3ZX	07L03ZZ	07N00ZZ	07PK0CZ	07PN0DZ	07Q70ZZ	07U407Z	07UH07Z	07V44CZ
07BP0ZZ	07CP3ZZ	07DQ3ZZ	07L04CZ	07N03ZZ	07PK0DZ	07PN0JZ	07Q73ZZ	07U40JZ	07UH0JZ	07V44DZ
07BP3ZX	07CP4ZZ	07DR0ZX	07L04DZ	07N04ZZ	07PK0JZ	07PN0KZ	07Q74ZZ	07U40KZ	07UH0KZ	07V44ZZ
07BP3ZZ	07D03ZX	07DR0ZZ	07L04ZZ	07N10ZZ	07PK0KZ	07PN0YZ	07Q78ZZ	07U447Z	07UH47Z	07V50CZ
07BP4ZX	07D04ZX	07DR3ZX	07L10CZ	07N13ZZ	07PK0YZ	07PN30Z	07Q80ZZ	07U44JZ	07UH4JZ	07V50DZ
07BP4ZZ	07D08ZX	07DR3ZZ	07L10DZ	07N14ZZ	07PK30Z	07PN33Z	07Q83ZZ	07U44KZ	07UH4KZ	07V50ZZ
07C00ZZ	07D13ZX	07DS0ZX	07L10ZZ	07N20ZZ	07PK33Z	07PN37Z	07Q84ZZ	07U507Z	07UJ07Z	07V53CZ
07C03ZZ	07D14ZX	07DS0ZZ	07L13CZ	07N23ZZ	07PK37Z	07PN3CZ	07Q88ZZ	07U50JZ	07UJ0JZ	07V53DZ
07C04ZZ	07D18ZX	07DS3ZX	07L13DZ	07N24ZZ	07PK3CZ	07PN3DZ	07Q90ZZ	07U50KZ	07UJ0KZ	07V53ZZ
07C10ZZ	07D23ZX	07DS3ZZ	07L13ZZ	07N30ZZ	07PK3DZ	07PN3JZ	07Q93ZZ	07U547Z	07UJ47Z	07V54CZ
07C13ZZ	07D24ZX	07HK03Z	07L14CZ	07N33ZZ	07PK3JZ	07PN3KZ	07Q94ZZ	07U54JZ	07UJ4JZ	07V54DZ
07C14ZZ	07D28ZX	07HK0YZ	07L14DZ	07N34ZZ	07PK3KZ	07PN3YZ	07Q98ZZ	07U54KZ	07UJ4KZ	07V54ZZ
07C20ZZ	07D33ZX	07HK33Z	07L14ZZ	07N40ZZ	07PK3YZ	07PN40Z	07QB0ZZ	07U607Z	07UK07Z	07V60CZ
07C23ZZ	07D34ZX	07HK3YZ	07L20CZ	07N43ZZ	07PK40Z	07PN43Z	07QB3ZZ	07U60JZ	07UK0JZ	07V60DZ
07C24ZZ	07D38ZX	07HK43Z	07L20DZ	07N44ZZ	07PK43Z	07PN47Z	07QB4ZZ	07U60KZ	07UK0KZ	07V60ZZ
07C30ZZ	07D43ZX	07HK4YZ	07L20ZZ	07N50ZZ	07PK47Z	07PN4CZ	07QB8ZZ	07U647Z	07UK47Z	07V63CZ
07C33ZZ	07D44ZX	07HL03Z	07L23CZ	07N53ZZ	07PK4CZ	07PN4DZ	07QC0ZZ	07U64JZ	07UK4JZ	07V63DZ
07C34ZZ	07D48ZX	07HL0YZ	07L23DZ	07N54ZZ	07PK4DZ	07PN4JZ	07QC3ZZ	07U64KZ	07UK4KZ	07V63ZZ
07C40ZZ	07D53ZX	07HL33Z	07L23ZZ	07N60ZZ	07PK4JZ	07PN4KZ	07QC4ZZ	07U707Z	07UL07Z	07V64CZ
07C43ZZ	07D54ZX	07HL3YZ	07L24CZ	07N63ZZ	07PK4KZ	07PN4YZ	07QC8ZZ	07U70JZ	07UL0JZ	07V64DZ
07C44ZZ	07D58ZX	07HL43Z	07L24DZ	07N64ZZ	07PK4YZ	07PNX0Z	07QD0ZZ	07U70KZ	07UL0KZ	07V64ZZ
07C50ZZ	07D63ZX	07HL4YZ	07L24ZZ	07N70ZZ	07PKX0Z	07PNX3Z	07QD3ZZ	07U747Z	07UL47Z	07V70CZ
07C53ZZ	07D64ZX	07HM03Z	07L30CZ	07N73ZZ	07PKX3Z	07PNXDZ	07QD4ZZ	07U74JZ	07UL4JZ	07V70DZ
07C54ZZ	07D68ZX	07HM0YZ	07L30DZ	07N74ZZ	07PKXDZ	07PP00Z	07QD8ZZ	07U74KZ	07UL4KZ	07V70ZZ
07C60ZZ	07D73ZX	07HM33Z	07L30ZZ	07N80ZZ	07PL00Z	07PP03Z	07QF0ZZ	07U807Z	07V00CZ	07V73CZ
07C63ZZ	07D74ZX	07HM3YZ	07L33CZ	07N83ZZ	07PL03Z	07PP0YZ	07QF3ZZ	07U80JZ	07V00DZ	07V73DZ
07C64ZZ	07D78ZX	07HM43Z	07L33DZ	07N84ZZ	07PL07Z	07PP30Z	07QF4ZZ	07U80KZ	07V00ZZ	07V73ZZ
07C70ZZ	07D83ZX	07HM4YZ	07L33ZZ	07N90ZZ	07PL0CZ	07PP33Z	07QF8ZZ	07U847Z	07V03CZ	07V74CZ
07C73ZZ	07D84ZX	07HN03Z	07L34CZ	07N93ZZ	07PL0DZ	07PP3YZ	07QG0ZZ	07U84JZ	07V03DZ	07V74DZ
07C74ZZ	07D88ZX	07HN0YZ	07LG4ZZ	07N94ZZ	07PL0JZ	07PP40Z	07QG3ZZ	07U84KZ	07V03ZZ	07V74ZZ
07C80ZZ	07D93ZX	07HN33Z	07LH0CZ	07NB0ZZ	07PL0KZ	07PP43Z	07QG4ZZ	07U907Z	07V04CZ	07V80CZ
07C83ZZ	07D94ZX	07HN3YZ	07LH0DZ	07NB3ZZ	07PL0YZ	07PP4YZ	07QG8ZZ	07U90JZ	07V04DZ	07V80DZ
07C84ZZ	07D98ZX	07HN43Z	07LH0ZZ	07NB4ZZ	07PL30Z	07PPX0Z	07QH0ZZ	07U90KZ	07V04ZZ	07V80ZZ
07C90ZZ	07DB3ZX	07HN4YZ	07LH3CZ	07NC0ZZ	07PL33Z	07PPX3Z	07QH3ZZ	07U947Z	07V10CZ	07V83CZ
07C93ZZ	07DB4ZX	07HP03Z	07LH3DZ	07NC3ZZ	07PL37Z	07PT00Z	07QH4ZZ	07U94JZ	07V10DZ	07V83DZ
07C94ZZ	07DB8ZX	07HP0YZ	07LH3ZZ	07NC4ZZ	07PL3CZ	07PT30Z	07QH8ZZ	07U94KZ	07V10ZZ	07V83ZZ
07CB0ZZ	07DC3ZX	07HP33Z	07LH4CZ	07ND0ZZ	07PL3DZ	07PT40Z	07QJ0ZZ	07UB07Z	07V13CZ	07V84CZ
07CB3ZZ	07DC4ZX	07HP3YZ	07LH4DZ	07ND3ZZ	07PL3JZ	07PTX0Z	07QJ8ZZ	07UB0JZ	07V13DZ	07V84DZ
07CB4ZZ	07DC8ZX	07HP43Z	07LH4ZZ	07ND4ZZ	07PL3KZ	07Q00ZZ	07QK8ZZ	07UB0KZ	07V13ZZ	07V84ZZ
07CC0ZZ	07DD3ZX	07HP4YZ	07LJ0CZ	07NF0ZZ	07PL3YZ	07Q03ZZ	07QL8ZZ	07UB47Z	07V14CZ	07V90CZ
07CC3ZZ	07DD4ZX	07JK0ZZ	07LJ0DZ	07NF3ZZ	07PL40Z	07Q04ZZ	07TP0ZZ	07UB4JZ	07V14DZ	07V90DZ
07CC4ZZ	07DD8ZX	07JK3ZZ	07LJ0ZZ	07NF4ZZ	07PL43Z	07Q08ZZ	07TP4ZZ	07UB4KZ	07V14ZZ	07V90ZZ
07CD0ZZ	07DF3ZX	07JK4ZZ	07LJ3CZ	07NG0ZZ	07PL47Z	07Q10ZZ	07U007Z	07UC07Z	07V20CZ	07V93CZ
07CD3ZZ	07DF4ZX	07JL0ZZ	07LJ3DZ	07NG3ZZ	07PL4CZ	07Q13ZZ	07U00JZ	07UC0JZ	07V20DZ	07V93DZ
07CD4ZZ	07DF8ZX	07JL3ZZ	07LJ3ZZ	07NG4ZZ	07PL4DZ	07Q14ZZ	07U00KZ	07UC0KZ	07V20ZZ	07V93ZZ
07CF0ZZ	07DG3ZX	07JL4ZZ	07LJ4CZ	07NH0ZZ	07PL4JZ	07Q18ZZ	07U047Z	07UC47Z	07V23CZ	07V94CZ
07CF3ZZ	07DG4ZX	07JM0ZZ	07LJ4DZ	07NH3ZZ	07PL4KZ	07Q20ZZ	07U04JZ	07UC4JZ	07V23DZ	07V94DZ
07CF4ZZ	07DG8ZX	07JM3ZZ	07LJ4ZZ	07NH4ZZ	07PL4YZ	07Q23ZZ	07U04KZ	07UC4KZ	07V23ZZ	07V94ZZ
07CG0ZZ	07DH3ZX	07JM4ZZ	07LK0CZ	07NJ0ZZ	07PLX0Z	07Q24ZZ	07U107Z	07UD07Z	07V24CZ	07VB0CZ
07CG3ZZ	07DH4ZX	07JN0ZZ	07LK0DZ	07NJ3ZZ	07PLX3Z	07Q28ZZ	07U10JZ	07UD0JZ	07V24DZ	07WK0YZ
07CG4ZZ	07DH8ZX	07JN3ZZ	07LK0ZZ	07NJ4ZZ	07PLXDZ	07Q30ZZ	07U10KZ	07UD0KZ	07V24ZZ	07WK3YZ
07CH0ZZ	07DJ3ZX	07JN4ZZ	07LK3CZ	07NK0ZZ	07PM00Z	07Q33ZZ	07U147Z	07UD47Z	07V30CZ	07WK4YZ
07CH3ZZ	07DJ4ZX	07JN8ZZ	07LK3DZ	07NK3ZZ	07PM03Z	07Q34ZZ	07U14JZ	07UD4JZ	07V30DZ	07WKX0Z
07CH4ZZ	07DJ8ZX	07JNXZZ	07LK3ZZ	07NK4ZZ	07PM0YZ	07Q38ZZ	07U14KZ	07UD4KZ	07V30ZZ	07WKX3Z
07CJ0ZZ	07DK3ZX	07JP0ZZ	07LK4CZ	07NL0ZZ	07PM30Z	07Q40ZZ	07U207Z	07UF07Z	07V33CZ	07WKX7Z
07CJ3ZZ	07DK4ZX	07JP3ZZ	07LK4DZ	07NL3ZZ	07PM33Z	07Q43ZZ	07U20JZ	07UF0JZ	07V33DZ	07WKXCZ
07CJ4ZZ	07DK8ZX	07JP4ZZ	07LK4ZZ	07NL4ZZ	07PM3YZ	07Q44ZZ	07U20KZ	07UF0KZ	07V33ZZ	07WKXDZ
07CK0ZZ	07DL3ZX	07JPXZZ	07LL0CZ	07NM0ZZ	07PM40Z	07Q48ZZ	07U247Z	07UF47Z	07V34CZ	07WKXJZ
07CK3ZZ	07DL4ZX	07JT0ZZ	07LL0DZ	07NM3ZZ	07PM43Z	07Q50ZZ	07U24JZ	07UF4JZ	07V34DZ	07WKXKZ
07CK4ZZ	07DL8ZX	07JT3ZZ	07LL0ZZ	07NM4ZZ	07PM4YZ	07Q53ZZ	07U24KZ	07UF4KZ	07V34ZZ	07WL0YZ
07CL0ZZ	07DM3ZX	07JT4ZZ	07LL3CZ	07NP0ZZ	07PMX0Z	07Q54ZZ	07U307Z	07UG07Z	07V40CZ	07WL3YZ

07WL4YZ	080N0JZ	0820XYZ	087Y3ZZ	089J3ZX	089W0ZX	08BE3ZZ	08NF3ZZ	08P08CZ	08PL30Z	08QY8ZZ
07WLX0Z	080N0KZ	0821X0Z	087Y7DZ	089J3ZZ	089W0ZZ	08BF3ZX	08NG3ZZ	08P08DZ	08PL37Z	08R007Z
07WLX3Z	080N0ZZ	0821XYZ	087Y7ZZ	089K30Z	089W30Z	08BF3ZZ	08NH3ZZ	08P08JZ	08PL3JZ	08R00JZ
07WLX7Z	080N37Z	0850XZZ	087Y8DZ	089K3ZX	089W3ZX	08BJ3ZX	08NJ3ZZ	08P08KZ	08PL3KZ	08R00KZ
07WLXCZ	080N3JZ	0851XZZ	087Y8ZZ	089K3ZZ	089W3ZZ	08BJ3ZZ	08NK3ZZ	08P08YZ	08PL3YZ	08R037Z
07WLXDZ	080N3KZ	08523ZZ	0890X0Z	089L00Z	089X00Z	08BK3ZX	08NL0ZZ	08P0X0Z	08PM00Z	08R03JZ
07WLXJZ	080N3ZZ	08533ZZ	0890XZX	089L0ZX	089X0ZX	08BK3ZZ	08NL3ZZ	08P0X1Z	08PM07Z	08R03KZ
07WLXKZ	080NX7Z	08543ZZ	0890XZZ	089L0ZZ	089X0ZZ	08BL0ZX	08NM0ZZ	08P0X3Z	08PM0JZ	08R107Z
07WM0YZ	080NXJZ	08553ZZ	0891X0Z	089L30Z	089X30Z	08BL0ZZ	08NM3ZZ	08P0X7Z	08PM0KZ	08R10JZ
07WM3YZ	080NXKZ	0856XZZ	0891XZX	089L3ZX	089X3ZX	08C2XZZ	08NN0ZZ	08P0XCZ	08PM0YZ	08R10KZ
07WM4YZ	080NXZZ	0857XZZ	0891XZZ	089L3ZZ	089X3ZZ	08C3XZZ	08NN3ZZ	08P0XDZ	08PM30Z	08R137Z
07WMX0Z	080P07Z	0858XZZ	089230Z	089M00Z	089X70Z	08C6XZZ	08NNXZZ	08P0XJZ	08PM37Z	08R13JZ
07WMX3Z	080P0JZ	0859XZZ	08923ZX	089M0ZX	089X7ZX	08C7XZZ	08NP0ZZ	08P0XKZ	08PM3JZ	08R13KZ
07WN00Z	080P0KZ	085A0ZZ	08923ZZ	089M0ZZ	089X7ZZ	08CN0ZZ	08NP3ZZ	08P100Z	08PM3KZ	08R437Z
07WN03Z	080P0ZZ	085A3ZZ	089330Z	089M30Z	089X80Z	08CN3ZZ	08NPXZZ	08P101Z	08PM3YZ	08R43JZ
07WN07Z	080P37Z	085B0ZZ	08933ZX	089M3ZX	089X8ZX	08CNXZZ	08NQ0ZZ	08P103Z	08Q0XZZ	08R43KZ
07WN0CZ	080P3JZ	085B3ZZ	08933ZZ	089M3ZZ	089X8ZZ	08CP0ZZ	08NQ3ZZ	08P107Z	08Q1XZZ	08R537Z
07WN0DZ	080P3KZ	085C3ZZ	089430Z	089N00Z	089Y00Z	08CP3ZZ	08NQXZZ	08P10CZ	08Q23ZZ	08R53JZ
07WN0JZ	080P3ZZ	085D3ZZ	08943ZX	089N0ZX	089Y0ZX	08CPXZZ	08NR0ZZ	08P10DZ	08Q33ZZ	08R53KZ
07WN0KZ	080PX7Z	085E3ZZ	08943ZZ	089N0ZZ	089Y0ZZ	08CQ0ZZ	08NR3ZZ	08P10JZ	08Q43ZZ	08R6X7Z
07WN0YZ	080PXJZ	085F3ZZ	089530Z	089N30Z	089Y30Z	08CQ3ZZ	08NRXZZ	08P10KZ	08Q53ZZ	08R6XJZ
07WN30Z	080PXKZ	085G3ZZ	08953ZX	089N3ZX	089Y3ZX	08CQXZZ	08NSXZZ	08P10YZ	08Q6XZZ	08R6XKZ
07WN33Z	080PXZZ	085H3ZZ	08953ZZ	089N3ZZ	089Y3ZZ	08CR0ZZ	08NTXZZ	08P130Z	08Q7XZZ	08R7X7Z
07WN37Z	080Q07Z	085J3ZZ	0896X0Z	089NX0Z	089Y70Z	08CR3ZZ	08NV0ZZ	08P131Z	08Q8XZZ	08R7XJZ
07WN3CZ	080Q0JZ	085K3ZZ	0896XZX	089NXZX	089Y7ZX	08CRXZZ	08NV3ZZ	08P133Z	08Q9XZZ	08R7XKZ
07WN3DZ	080Q0KZ	085L0ZZ	0896XZZ	089NXZZ	089Y7ZZ	08F4XZZ	08NW0ZZ	08P137Z	08QA0ZZ	08R837Z
07WN3JZ	080Q0ZZ	085L3ZZ	0897X0Z	089P00Z	089Y80Z	08F5XZZ	08NW3ZZ	08P13CZ	08QA3ZZ	08R83JZ
07WN3KZ	080Q37Z	085M0ZZ	0897XZX	089P0ZX	089Y8ZX	08H00YZ	08NX0ZZ	08P13DZ	08QB0ZZ	08R83KZ
07WN3YZ	080Q3JZ	085M3ZZ	0897XZZ	089P0ZZ	089Y8ZZ	08H03YZ	08NX3ZZ	08P13JZ	08QB3ZZ	08R8X7Z
07WN40Z	080Q3KZ	085N0ZZ	0898X0Z	089P30Z	08B00ZX	08H07YZ	08NX7ZZ	08P13KZ	08QC3ZZ	08R8XJZ
07WN43Z	080Q3ZZ	085N3ZZ	0898XZX	089P3ZX	08B00ZZ	08H08YZ	08NX8ZZ	08P13YZ	08QD3ZZ	08R8XKZ
07WN47Z	080QX7Z	085NXZZ	0898XZZ	089P3ZZ	08B03ZX	08H10YZ	08NY0ZZ	08P170Z	08QE3ZZ	08R937Z
07WN4CZ	080QXJZ	085P0ZZ	0899X0Z	089PX0Z	08B03ZZ	08H13YZ	08NY3ZZ	08P171Z	08QF3ZZ	08R93JZ
07WN4DZ	080QXKZ	085P3ZZ	0899XZX	089PXZX	08B0XZX	08H17YZ	08NY7ZZ	08P173Z	08QG3ZZ	08R93KZ
07WN4JZ	080QXZZ	085PXZZ	0899XZZ	089PXZZ	08B0XZZ	08H18YZ	08NY8ZZ	08P177Z	08QH3ZZ	08R9X7Z
07WN4KZ	080R07Z	085Q0ZZ	089A00Z	089Q00Z	08B10ZX	08J0XZZ	08P000Z	08P17CZ	08QJ3ZZ	08R9XJZ
07WN4YZ	080R0JZ	085Q3ZZ	089A0ZX	089Q0ZX	08B10ZZ	08J1XZZ	08P001Z	08P17DZ	08QK3ZZ	08R9XKZ
07WNX0Z	080R0KZ	085QXZZ	089A0ZZ	089Q0ZZ	08B13ZX	08JJXZZ	08P003Z	08P17JZ	08QL0ZZ	08RA07Z
07WNX3Z	080R0ZZ	085R0ZZ	089A30Z	089Q30Z	08B13ZZ	08JKXZZ	08P007Z	08P17KZ	08QL3ZZ	08RA0JZ
07WNX7Z	080R37Z	085R3ZZ	089A3ZX	089Q3ZX	08B1XZX	08JLXZZ	08P00CZ	08P17YZ	08QM0ZZ	08RA0KZ
07WNXCZ	080R3JZ	085RXZZ	089A3ZZ	089Q3ZZ	08B1XZZ	08JMXZZ	08P00DZ	08P180Z	08QM3ZZ	08RA37Z
07WNXDZ	080R3KZ	085SXZZ	089B00Z	089QX0Z	08B43ZX	08LY7DZ	08P00JZ	08P181Z	08QN0ZZ	08RA3JZ
07WNXJZ	080R3ZZ	085TXZZ	089B0ZX	089QXZX	08B43ZZ	08LY7ZZ	08P00KZ	08P183Z	08QN3ZZ	08RA3KZ
07WNXKZ	080RX7Z	085V0ZZ	089B0ZZ	089QXZZ	08B53ZX	08LY8DZ	08P00YZ	08P187Z	08QNXZZ	08RB07Z
07WP00Z	080RXJZ	085V3ZZ	089B30Z	089R00Z	08B53ZZ	08LY8ZZ	08P030Z	08P18CZ	08QP0ZZ	08RB0JZ
07WP03Z	080RXKZ	085W0ZZ	089B3ZX	089R0ZX	08B6XZX	08MNXZZ	08P031Z	08P18DZ	08QP3ZZ	08RB0KZ
07WP0YZ	080RXZZ	085W3ZZ	089B3ZZ	089R0ZZ	08B6XZZ	08MPXZZ	08P033Z	08P18JZ	08QPXZZ	08RB37Z
07WP30Z	08123J4	085X0ZZ	089C30Z	089R30Z	08B7XZX	08MQXZZ	08P037Z	08P18KZ	08QQ0ZZ	08RB3JZ
07WP33Z	08123K4	085X3ZZ	089C3ZX	089R3ZX	08B7XZZ	08MRXZZ	08P03CZ	08P18YZ	08QQ3ZZ	08RB3KZ
07WP3YZ	08123Z4	085X7ZZ	089C3ZZ	089R3ZZ	08B8XZX	08N0XZZ	08P03DZ	08P1X0Z	08QQXZZ	08RC37Z
07WP40Z	08133J4	085X8ZZ	089D30Z	089RX0Z	08B8XZZ	08N1XZZ	08P03JZ	08P1X1Z	08QR0ZZ	08RC3JZ
07WP43Z	08133K4	085Y0ZZ	089D3ZX	089RXZX	08B9XZX	08N23ZZ	08P03KZ	08P1X3Z	08QR3ZZ	08RC3KZ
07WP4YZ	08133Z4	085Y3ZZ	089D3ZZ	089RXZZ	08B9XZZ	08N33ZZ	08P03YZ	08P1X7Z	08QRXZZ	08RD37Z
07WPX0Z	081X0J3	085Y7ZZ	089E30Z	089SX0Z	08BA0ZX	08N43ZZ	08P070Z	08P1XCZ	08QSXZZ	08RD3JZ
07WPX3Z	081X0K3	085Y8ZZ	089E3ZX	089SXZX	08BA0ZZ	08N53ZZ	08P071Z	08P1XDZ	08QTXZZ	08RD3KZ
07WT00Z	081X0Z3	087X0DZ	089E3ZZ	089SXZZ	08BA3ZX	08N6XZZ	08P073Z	08P1XJZ	08QV0ZZ	08RG37Z
07WT30Z	081X3J3	087X0ZZ	089F30Z	089TX0Z	08BA3ZZ	08N7XZZ	08P077Z	08P1XKZ	08QV3ZZ	08RG3JZ
07WT40Z	081X3K3	087X3DZ	089F3ZX	089TXZX	08BB0ZX	08N8XZZ	08P07CZ	08PJ3JZ	08QW0ZZ	08RG3KZ
07WTX0Z	081X3Z3	087X3ZZ	089F3ZZ	089TXZZ	08BB0ZZ	08N9XZZ	08P07DZ	08PJ3YZ	08QW3ZZ	08RH37Z
07YM0Z0	081Y0J3	087X7DZ	089G30Z	089V00Z	08BB3ZX	08NA0ZZ	08P07JZ	08PK3JZ	08QX0ZZ	08RH3JZ
07YM0Z1	081Y0K3	087X7ZZ	089G3ZX	089V0ZX	08BB3ZZ	08NA3ZZ	08P07KZ	08PK3YZ	08QX3ZZ	08RH3KZ
07YM0Z2	081Y0Z3	087X8DZ	089G3ZZ	089V0ZZ	08BC3ZZ	08NB0ZZ	08P07YZ	08PL00Z	08QX7ZZ	08RJ30Z
07YP0Z0	081Y3J3	087X8ZZ	089H30Z	089V30Z	08BC3ZZ	08NB3ZZ	08P080Z	08PL07Z	08QX8ZZ	08RJ37Z
07YP0Z1	081Y3K3	087Y0DZ	089H3ZX	089V3ZX	08BD3ZX	08NC3ZZ	08P081Z	08PL0JZ	08QY0ZZ	08RJ3JZ
07YP0Z2	081Y3Z3	087Y0ZZ	089H3ZZ	089V3ZZ	08BD3ZZ	08ND3ZZ	08P083Z	08PL0KZ	08QY3ZZ	08RJ3KZ
080N07Z	0820X0Z	087Y3DZ	089J30Z	089W00Z	08BE3ZZ	08NE3ZZ	08P087Z	08PL0YZ	08QY7ZZ	08RK30Z

08RK37Z	08UD07Z	08UQX7Z	08W037Z	08W1XJZ	09020KZ	095S8ZZ	09940ZZ	099C8ZX	099L8ZZ	099S7ZX
08RK3JZ	08UD0JZ	08UQXJZ	08W03CZ	08W1XKZ	09020ZZ	095T8ZZ	099430Z	099C8ZZ	099M00Z	099S7ZZ
08RK3KZ	08UD0KZ	08UQXKZ	08W03DZ	08WJ3JZ	090237Z	095U8ZZ	09943ZX	099D70Z	099M0ZX	099S80Z
08RN07Z	08UD37Z	08UR07Z	08W03DZ	08WJ3YZ	09023JZ	095V8ZZ	09943ZZ	099D7ZX	099M0ZZ	099S8ZX
08RN0JZ	08UD3JZ	08UR0JZ	08W03KZ	08WJXJZ	09023ZZ	095W8ZZ	099440Z	099D7ZZ	099M30Z	099S8ZZ
08RN0KZ	08UD3KZ	08UR0KZ	08W03YZ	08WK3JZ	090247Z	095X8ZZ	09944ZX	099D80Z	099M3ZX	099T30Z
08RN37Z	08UE07Z	08UR37Z	08W070Z	08WK3YZ	09024JZ	097F0DZ	09944ZZ	099D8ZX	099M3ZZ	099T3ZZ
08RN3JZ	08UE0JZ	08UR3JZ	08W073Z	08WKXJZ	092HX0Z	097F0ZZ	099470Z	099D8ZZ	099M40Z	099T40Z
08RN3KZ	08UE0KZ	08UR3KZ	08W077Z	092HXYZ		097F3ZZ	09947ZX	099E70Z	099M4ZX	099T4ZX
08RNX7Z	08UE37Z	08URX7Z	08W07CZ	08WL00Z	092JX0Z	097F4ZZ	09947ZZ	099E7ZX	099M4ZZ	099T4ZZ
08RNXJZ	08UE3JZ	08URXJZ	08W07DZ	08WL07Z	092JXYZ	097F7DZ	099480Z	099E7ZZ	099M70Z	099T70Z
08RNXKZ	08UE3KZ	08URXKZ	08W07JZ	08WL0JZ	092KX0Z	097F7ZZ	09948ZX	099E80Z	099M7ZX	099T7ZX
08RP07Z	08UF07Z	08UX07Z	08W07KZ	08WL0KZ	092KXYZ	097F8DZ	09948ZZ	099E8ZX	099M7ZZ	099T7ZZ
08RP0JZ	08UF0JZ	08UX0JZ	08W07YZ	08WL0YZ	092YX0Z	097F8ZZ	0994X0Z	099E8ZZ	099M80Z	099T80Z
08RP0KZ	08UF0KZ	08UX0KZ	08W080Z	08WL30Z	092YXYZ	097G0DZ	0994XZX	099F00Z	099M8ZX	099T8ZX
08RP37Z	08UF37Z	08UX37Z	08W083Z	08WL37Z	09500ZZ	097G0ZZ	0994XZZ	099F0ZZ	099M8ZZ	099T8ZZ
08RP3JZ	08UF3JZ	08UX3JZ	08W087Z	08WL3JZ	09503ZZ	097G3ZZ	09950ZZ	099F30Z	099N0ZX	099U30Z
08RP3KZ	08UF3KZ	08UX3KZ	08W08CZ	08WL3KZ	09504ZZ	097G4ZZ	099570Z	099F3ZZ	099N30Z	099U3ZX
08RPX7Z	08UG07Z	08UX77Z	08W08DZ	08WL3YZ	0950XZZ	097G7DZ	09957ZX	099F40Z	099N3ZX	099U3ZZ
08RPXJZ	08UG0JZ	08UX7JZ	08W08JZ	08WM00Z	09510ZZ	097G7ZZ	09957ZZ	099F4ZZ	099N3ZZ	099U40Z
08RPXKZ	08UG0KZ	08UX7KZ	08W08KZ	08WM07Z	09513ZZ	097G8DZ	099580Z	099F70Z	099N4ZX	099U4ZX
08RQ07Z	08UG37Z	08UX87Z	08W08YZ	08WM0JZ	09514ZZ	097G8ZZ	09958ZX	099F7ZZ	099N7ZX	099U4ZZ
08RQ0JZ	08UG3JZ	08UX8JZ	08W0X0Z	08WM0KZ	0951XZZ	099000Z	09958ZZ	099F80Z	099N8ZX	099U70Z
08RQ0KZ	08UG3KZ	08UX8KZ	08W0X3Z	08WM0YZ	09530ZZ	09900ZX	09960ZZ	099F8ZZ	099P30Z	099U7ZX
08RQ37Z	08UH07Z	08UY07Z	08W0X7Z	08WM30Z	09533ZZ	09900ZZ	099670Z	099G00Z	099P3ZX	099U7ZZ
08RQ3JZ	08UH0JZ	08UY0JZ	08W0XCZ	08WM37Z	09534ZZ	099030Z	09967ZX	099G0ZZ	099P3ZZ	099U80Z
08RQ3KZ	08UH0KZ	08UY0KZ	08W0XDZ	08WM3KZ	09537ZZ	09903ZX	09967ZZ	099G30Z	099P40Z	099U8ZX
08RQX7Z	08UH37Z	08UY37Z	08W0XJZ	08WM3YZ	09538ZZ	09903ZZ	099680Z	099G3ZZ	099P4ZX	099U8ZZ
08RQXJZ	08UH3JZ	08UY3JZ	08W0XKZ	08XL0ZZ	0953XZZ	099040Z	09968ZX	099G40Z	099P4ZZ	099V30Z
08RQXKZ	08UH3KZ	08UY3KZ	08W100Z	08XL3ZZ	09540ZZ	09904ZX	09968ZZ	099G4ZZ	099P70Z	099V3ZX
08RR07Z	08UL07Z	08UY77Z	08W103Z	08XM0ZZ	09543ZZ	09904ZZ	09970ZZ	099G70Z	099P7ZX	099V3ZZ
08RR0JZ	08UL0JZ	08UY7JZ	08W107Z	08XM3ZZ	09544ZZ	0990X0Z	09973ZZ	099G7ZZ	099P7ZZ	099V40Z
08RR0KZ	08UL0KZ	08UY7KZ	08W10CZ	090007Z	09547ZZ	0990XZX	09974ZZ	099G80Z	099P80Z	099V4ZX
08RR37Z	08UL37Z	08UY87Z	08W10DZ	09000JZ	09548ZZ	0990XZZ	09977ZZ	099G8ZZ	099P8ZX	099V4ZZ
08RR3JZ	08UL3JZ	08UY8JZ	08W10JZ	09000KZ	0954XZZ	099100Z	09978ZZ	099K00Z	099P8ZZ	099V70Z
08RR3KZ	08UL3KZ	08UY8KZ	08W10KZ	09000ZZ	09558ZZ	09910ZX	09980ZZ	099K0ZX	099Q30Z	099V7ZX
08U107Z	08UM07Z	08VX0CZ	08W10YZ	090037Z	09568ZZ	09910ZZ	09983ZZ	099K0ZZ	099Q3ZX	099V7ZZ
08U10JZ	08UM0JZ	08VX0DZ	08W130Z	09003JZ	09598ZZ	099130Z	09984ZZ	099K30Z	099Q3ZZ	099V80Z
08U10KZ	08UM0KZ	08VX0ZZ	08W133Z	09003KZ	095A8ZZ	09913ZX	09987ZZ	099K3ZX	099Q40Z	099V8ZX
08U137Z	08UM37Z	08VX3CZ	08W137Z	09003ZZ	095B8ZZ	09913ZZ	09988ZZ	099K3ZZ	099Q4ZX	099V8ZZ
08U13JZ	08UM3JZ	08VX3DZ	08W13CZ	090047Z	095C8ZZ	099140Z	099970Z	099K40Z	099Q4ZZ	099W30Z
08U13KZ	08UM3KZ	08VX3ZZ	08W13DZ	09004JZ	095D8ZZ	09914ZX	09997ZX	099K4ZX	099Q70Z	099W3ZX
08U807Z	08UN07Z	08VX7DZ	08W13JZ	09004KZ	095E8ZZ	09914ZZ	09997ZZ	099K4ZZ	099Q7ZX	099W3ZZ
08U80JZ	08UN0JZ	08VX7ZZ	08W13KZ	09004ZZ	095F0ZZ	0991X0Z	099980Z	099K70Z	099Q7ZZ	099W40Z
08U80KZ	08UN0KZ	08VX8DZ	08W13YZ	0900X7Z	095F3ZZ	0991XZX	09998ZX	099K7ZX	099Q80Z	099W4ZX
08U837Z	08UN37Z	08VX8ZZ	08W170Z	0900XKZ	095F4ZZ	0991XZZ	09998ZZ	099K7ZZ	099Q8ZX	099W4ZZ
08U83JZ	08UN3JZ	08VY0CZ	08W173Z	0900XZZ	095F7ZZ	099300Z	099A70Z	099K80Z	099Q8ZZ	099W70Z
08U83KZ	08UN3KZ	08VY0DZ	08W177Z	090107Z	095F8ZZ	09930ZX	099A7ZX	099K8ZX	099R30Z	099W7ZX
08U8X7Z	08UNX7Z	08VY0ZZ	08W17CZ	09010JZ	095G0ZZ	09930ZZ	099A7ZZ	099K8ZZ	099R3ZX	099W7ZZ
08U8XJZ	08UNXJZ	08VY3CZ	08W17DZ	09010KZ	095G3ZZ	099330Z	099A80Z	099KX0Z	099R3ZZ	099W80Z
08U8XKZ	08UNXKZ	08VY3DZ	08W17JZ	09010ZZ	095G4ZZ	09933ZX	099A8ZX	099KXZX	099R40Z	099W8ZX
08U907Z	08UP07Z	08VY3ZZ	08W17KZ	090137Z	095G7ZZ	09933ZZ	099A8ZZ	099KXZZ	099R4ZX	099W8ZZ
08U90JZ	08UP0JZ	08VY7DZ	08W17YZ	09013JZ	095G8ZZ	099340Z	099B30Z	099L00Z	099R4ZZ	099X30Z
08U90KZ	08UP0KZ	08VY7ZZ	08W180Z	09013KZ	095K0ZZ	09934ZX	099B3ZZ	099L0ZX	099R70Z	099X3ZX
08U937Z	08UP37Z	08VY8DZ	08W183Z	09013ZZ	095K3ZZ	09934ZZ	099B70Z	099L0ZZ	099R7ZX	099X3ZZ
08U93JZ	08UP3JZ	08VY8ZZ	08W187Z	090147Z	095K4ZZ	099370Z	099B7ZX	099L30Z	099R7ZZ	099X40Z
08U93KZ	08UP3KZ	08W000Z	08W18CZ	09014JZ	095K8ZZ	09937ZX	099B7ZZ	099L3ZX	099R80Z	099X4ZX
08U9X7Z	08UPX7Z	08W003Z	08W18DZ	09014KZ	095KXZZ	09937ZZ	099B80Z	099L3ZZ	099R8ZX	099X4ZZ
08U9XJZ	08UPXJZ	08W007Z	08W18JZ	09014ZZ	095M0ZZ	099380Z	099B8ZX	099L40Z	099R8ZZ	099X70Z
08U9XKZ	08UPXKZ	08W00CZ	08W18KZ	0901X7Z	095M3ZZ	09938ZX	099B8ZZ	099L4ZX	099S30Z	099X7ZX
08UC07Z	08UQ07Z	08W00DZ	08W18YZ	0901XJZ	095M4ZZ	09938ZZ	099C30Z	099L4ZZ	099S3ZX	099X7ZZ
08UC0JZ	08UQ0JZ	08W00JZ	08W1X0Z	0901XKZ	095M8ZZ	0993X0Z	099C3ZZ	099L70Z	099S3ZZ	099X80Z
08UC0KZ	08UQ0KZ	08W00KZ	08W1X3Z	0901XZZ	095P8ZZ	0993XZX	099C70Z	099L7ZX	099S40Z	099X8ZX
08UC37Z	08UQ37Z	08W00YZ	08W1X7Z	090207Z	095Q8ZZ	0993XZZ	099C7ZZ	099L7ZZ	099S4ZX	099X8ZZ
08UC3JZ	08UQ3JZ	08W030Z	08W1XCZ	09020JZ	095R8ZZ	099400Z	099C80Z	099L80Z	099S4ZZ	09B00ZX
08UC3KZ	08UQ3KZ	08W033Z	08W1XDZ			09940ZX		099L8ZX	099S70Z	

09B00ZZ	09BG0ZZ	09BU8ZX	09CB4ZZ	09CV8ZZ	09HD34Z	09JH4ZZ	09NC3ZZ	09NW4ZZ	09PJ3YZ	09PY8YZ
09B03ZX	09BG3ZX	09BU8ZZ	09CB8ZZ	09CW0ZZ	09HD35Z	09JH7ZZ	09NC4ZZ	09NW8ZZ	09PJ40Z	09PYX0Z
09B03ZZ	09BG3ZZ	09BV0ZX	09CC0ZZ	09CW3ZZ	09HD36Z	09JH8ZZ	09NC8ZZ	09NX0ZZ	09PJ47Z	09Q00ZZ
09B04ZX	09BG4ZX	09BV0ZZ	09CC3ZZ	09CW4ZZ	09HD3SZ	09JHXZZ	09ND0ZZ	09NX3ZZ	09PJ4DZ	09Q03ZZ
09B04ZZ	09BG4ZZ	09BV3ZX	09CC4ZZ	09CW8ZZ	09HD44Z	09JJ0ZZ	09ND8ZZ	09NX4ZZ	09PJ4JZ	09Q04ZZ
09B0XZX	09BG7ZX	09BV3ZZ	09CC8ZZ	09CX0ZZ	09HD45Z	09JJ3ZZ	09NE0ZZ	09NX8ZZ	09PJ4KZ	09Q0XZZ
09B0XZZ	09BG7ZZ	09BV4ZX	09CD0ZZ	09CX3ZZ	09HD46Z	09JJ4ZZ	09NE8ZZ	09P700Z	09PJ4YZ	09Q10ZZ
09B10ZX	09BG8ZX	09BV4ZZ	09CD8ZZ	09CX4ZZ	09HD4SZ	09JJ7ZZ	09NF0ZZ	09P770Z	09PJ70Z	09Q13ZZ
09B10ZZ	09BG8ZZ	09BV8ZX	09CE0ZZ	09CX8ZZ	09HE04Z	09JJ8ZZ	09NF3ZZ	09P780Z	09PJ77Z	09Q14ZZ
09B13ZX	09BK0ZX	09BV8ZZ	09CE8ZZ	09D70ZZ	09HE05Z	09JJXZZ	09NF4ZZ	09P7X0Z	09PJ7DZ	09Q1XZZ
09B13ZZ	09BK0ZZ	09BW0ZX	09CF0ZZ	09D73ZZ	09HE06Z	09JK0ZZ	09NF7ZZ	09P800Z	09PJ7JZ	09Q20ZZ
09B14ZX	09BK3ZX	09BW0ZZ	09CF3ZZ	09D74ZZ	09HE0SZ	09JK3ZZ	09NF8ZZ	09P870Z	09PJ7KZ	09Q23ZZ
09B14ZZ	09BK3ZZ	09BW3ZX	09CF4ZZ	09D77ZZ	09HE34Z	09JK4ZZ	09NG0ZZ	09P880Z	09PJ7YZ	09Q24ZZ
09B1XZX	09BK4ZX	09BW3ZZ	09CF7ZZ	09D78ZZ	09HE35Z	09JK8ZZ	09NG3ZZ	09P8X0Z	09PJ80Z	09Q2XZZ
09B1XZZ	09BK4ZZ	09BW4ZX	09CF8ZZ	09D80ZZ	09HE36Z	09JKXZZ	09NG4ZZ	09PD0SZ	09PJ87Z	09Q30ZZ
09B30ZX	09BK8ZX	09BW4ZZ	09CG0ZZ	09D83ZZ	09HE3SZ	09JY0ZZ	09NG7ZZ	09PD7SZ	09PJ8DZ	09Q33ZZ
09B30ZZ	09BK8ZZ	09BW8ZX	09CG3ZZ	09D84ZZ	09HE44Z	09JY3ZZ	09NG8ZZ	09PD8SZ	09PJ8JZ	09Q34ZZ
09B33ZX	09BKXZX	09BW8ZZ	09CG4ZZ	09D87ZZ	09HE45Z	09JY4ZZ	09NK0ZZ	09PE0SZ	09PJ8KZ	09Q37ZZ
09B33ZZ	09BKXZZ	09BX0ZX	09CG7ZZ	09D88ZZ	09HE46Z	09JY8ZZ	09NK3ZZ	09PE7SZ	09PJ8YZ	09Q38ZZ
09B34ZX	09BL0ZX	09BX0ZZ	09CG8ZZ	09D90ZZ	09HE4SZ	09JYXZZ	09NK4ZZ	09PE8SZ	09PJX0Z	09Q3XZZ
09B34ZZ	09BL3ZX	09BX3ZX	09CK0ZZ	09DA0ZZ	09HH0YZ	09M0XZZ	09NK8ZZ	09PH00Z	09PJX7Z	09Q40ZZ
09B37ZX	09BL4ZX	09BX3ZZ	09CK3ZZ	09DB0ZZ	09HH3YZ	09M1XZZ	09NKXZZ	09PH07Z	09PJXDZ	09Q43ZZ
09B37ZZ	09BL7ZX	09BX4ZX	09CK4ZZ	09DB3ZZ	09HH4YZ	09MKXZZ	09NL0ZZ	09PH0DZ	09PJXJZ	09Q44ZZ
09B38ZX	09BL8ZX	09BX4ZZ	09CK8ZZ	09DB4ZZ	09HH7YZ	09N00ZZ	09NL3ZZ	09PH0JZ	09PJXKZ	09Q47ZZ
09B38ZZ	09BM0ZX	09BX8ZX	09CKXZZ	09DC0ZZ	09HH8YZ	09N03ZZ	09NL4ZZ	09PH0KZ	09PK00Z	09Q48ZZ
09B3XZX	09BM3ZX	09BX8ZZ	09CL0ZZ	09DC3ZZ	09HJ0YZ	09N04ZZ	09NL7ZZ	09PH0YZ	09PK07Z	09Q4XZZ
09B3XZZ	09BM4ZX	09C00ZZ	09CL3ZZ	09DC4ZZ	09HJ3YZ	09N0XZZ	09NL8ZZ	09PH30Z	09PK0DZ	09Q50ZZ
09B40ZX	09BM8ZX	09C03ZZ	09CL4ZZ	09DL0ZZ	09HJ4YZ	09N10ZZ	09NM0ZZ	09PH37Z	09PK0JZ	09Q58ZZ
09B40ZZ	09BM8ZZ	09C04ZZ	09CL7ZZ	09DL3ZZ	09HJ7YZ	09N13ZZ	09NM3ZZ	09PH3DZ	09PK0KZ	09Q60ZZ
09B43ZX	09BN0ZX	09C0XZZ	09CL8ZZ	09DL4ZZ	09HJ8YZ	09N14ZZ	09NM4ZZ	09PH3JZ	09PK0YZ	09Q68ZZ
09B43ZZ	09BN3ZX	09C10ZZ	09CM0ZZ	09DL7ZZ	09HK0YZ	09N1XZZ	09NM8ZZ	09PH3KZ	09PK30Z	09Q70ZZ
09B44ZX	09BN4ZX	09C13ZZ	09CM3ZZ	09DL8ZZ	09HK3YZ	09N30ZZ	09NN0ZZ	09PH3YZ	09PK37Z	09Q73ZZ
09B44ZZ	09BN7ZX	09C14ZZ	09CM4ZZ	09DM0ZZ	09HK4YZ	09N33ZZ	09NN3ZZ	09PH40Z	09PK3DZ	09Q74ZZ
09B47ZX	09BN8ZX	09C1XZZ	09CM8ZZ	09DM3ZZ	09HK7YZ	09N34ZZ	09NN4ZZ	09PH47Z	09PK3JZ	09Q77ZZ
09B47ZZ	09BP3ZX	09C30ZZ	09CN0ZZ	09DM4ZZ	09HK8YZ	09N37ZZ	09NN7ZZ	09PH4DZ	09PK3KZ	09Q78ZZ
09B48ZX	09BP4ZX	09C33ZZ	09CN3ZZ	09DP0ZZ	09HN7BZ	09N38ZZ	09NN8ZZ	09PH4JZ	09PK3YZ	09Q80ZZ
09B48ZZ	09BP8ZX	09C34ZZ	09CN4ZZ	09DP3ZZ	09HN8BZ	09N3XZZ	09NP0ZZ	09PH4KZ	09PK40Z	09Q83ZZ
09B4XZX	09BP8ZZ	09C37ZZ	09CN7ZZ	09DP4ZZ	09HY0YZ	09N40ZZ	09NP3ZZ	09PH4YZ	09PK47Z	09Q84ZZ
09B4XZZ	09BQ3ZX	09C38ZZ	09CN8ZZ	09DQ0ZZ	09HY3YZ	09N43ZZ	09NP4ZZ	09PH70Z	09PK4DZ	09Q87ZZ
09B58ZX	09BQ4ZX	09C3XZZ	09CP0ZZ	09DQ3ZZ	09HY4YZ	09N44ZZ	09NP8ZZ	09PH77Z	09PK4JZ	09Q88ZZ
09B58ZZ	09BQ8ZX	09C40ZZ	09CP3ZZ	09DQ4ZZ	09HY7YZ	09N47ZZ	09NQ0ZZ	09PH7DZ	09PK4KZ	09Q90ZZ
09B68ZX	09BQ8ZZ	09C43ZZ	09CP4ZZ	09DR0ZZ	09HY8YZ	09N48ZZ	09NQ3ZZ	09PH7JZ	09PK4YZ	09Q98ZZ
09B68ZZ	09BR3ZX	09C44ZZ	09CP8ZZ	09DR3ZZ	09J70ZZ	09N4XZZ	09NQ4ZZ	09PH7KZ	09PK70Z	09QA0ZZ
09B98ZX	09BR4ZX	09C47ZZ	09CQ0ZZ	09DR4ZZ	09J73ZZ	09N50ZZ	09NQ8ZZ	09PH7YZ	09PK77Z	09QA8ZZ
09B98ZZ	09BR8ZX	09C48ZZ	09CQ3ZZ	09DS0ZZ	09J74ZZ	09N58ZZ	09NR0ZZ	09PH80Z	09PK7DZ	09QB0ZZ
09BA8ZX	09BR8ZZ	09C4XZZ	09CQ4ZZ	09DS3ZZ	09J77ZZ	09N60ZZ	09NR3ZZ	09PH87Z	09PK7JZ	09QB3ZZ
09BA8ZZ	09BS3ZX	09C50ZZ	09CQ8ZZ	09DS4ZZ	09J78ZZ	09N68ZZ	09NR4ZZ	09PH8DZ	09PK7KZ	09QB4ZZ
09BB8ZX	09BS3ZZ	09C58ZZ	09CR0ZZ	09DT0ZZ	09J7XZZ	09N70ZZ	09NR8ZZ	09PH8JZ	09PK7YZ	09QB8ZZ
09BB8ZZ	09BS4ZX	09C60ZZ	09CR3ZZ	09DT3ZZ	09J80ZZ	09N73ZZ	09NS0ZZ	09PH8KZ	09PK80Z	09QC0ZZ
09BC8ZX	09BS4ZZ	09C68ZZ	09CR4ZZ	09DT4ZZ	09J83ZZ	09N74ZZ	09NS3ZZ	09PH8YZ	09PK87Z	09QC3ZZ
09BC8ZZ	09BS8ZX	09C70ZZ	09CR8ZZ	09DU0ZZ	09J84ZZ	09N77ZZ	09NS4ZZ	09PHX0Z	09PK8DZ	09QC4ZZ
09BD8ZX	09BS8ZZ	09C73ZZ	09CS0ZZ	09DU3ZZ	09J87ZZ	09N78ZZ	09NS8ZZ	09PHX7Z	09PK8JZ	09QC8ZZ
09BD8ZZ	09BT0ZX	09C74ZZ	09CS3ZZ	09DU4ZZ	09J88ZZ	09N80ZZ	09NT0ZZ	09PHXDZ	09PK8KZ	09QD0ZZ
09BE8ZX	09BT0ZZ	09C77ZZ	09CS4ZZ	09DV0ZZ	09J8XZZ	09N83ZZ	09NT3ZZ	09PHXJZ	09PK8YZ	09QD8ZZ
09BE8ZZ	09BT3ZX	09C78ZZ	09CS8ZZ	09DV3ZZ	09JD0ZZ	09N84ZZ	09NT4ZZ	09PHXKZ	09PKX0Z	09QE0ZZ
09BF0ZX	09BT3ZZ	09C80ZZ	09CT0ZZ	09DV4ZZ	09JD3ZZ	09N87ZZ	09NT8ZZ	09PJ00Z	09PKX7Z	09QE8ZZ
09BF0ZZ	09BT4ZX	09C83ZZ	09CT3ZZ	09DW0ZZ	09JD4ZZ	09N88ZZ	09NU0ZZ	09PJ07Z	09PKXDZ	09QF0ZZ
09BF3ZX	09BT4ZZ	09C84ZZ	09CT4ZZ	09DW3ZZ	09JD8ZZ	09N90ZZ	09NU3ZZ	09PJ0DZ	09PKXJZ	09QF3ZZ
09BF3ZZ	09BT8ZX	09C87ZZ	09CT8ZZ	09DW4ZZ	09JDXZZ	09N98ZZ	09NU4ZZ	09PJ0JZ	09PKXKZ	09QF4ZZ
09BF4ZX	09BT8ZZ	09C88ZZ	09CU0ZZ	09DX0ZZ	09JE0ZZ	09NA0ZZ	09NU8ZZ	09PJ0KZ	09PY00Z	09QF7ZZ
09BF4ZZ	09BU0ZX	09C90ZZ	09CU3ZZ	09DX3ZZ	09JE3ZZ	09NA8ZZ	09NV0ZZ	09PJ0YZ	09PY0YZ	09QF8ZZ
09BF7ZX	09BU0ZZ	09C98ZZ	09CU4ZZ	09DX4ZZ	09JE4ZZ	09NB0ZZ	09NV3ZZ	09PJ30Z	09PY30Z	09QFXZZ
09BF7ZZ	09BU3ZX	09CA0ZZ	09CU8ZZ	09HD04Z	09JE8ZZ	09NB3ZZ	09NV4ZZ	09PJ37Z	09PY3YZ	09QG0ZZ
09BF8ZX	09BU3ZZ	09CA8ZZ	09CV0ZZ	09HD05Z	09JEXZZ	09NB4ZZ	09NV8ZZ	09PJ3DZ	09PY40Z	09QG3ZZ
09BF8ZZ	09BU4ZX	09CB0ZZ	09CV3ZZ	09HD06Z	09JH0ZZ	09NB8ZZ	09NW0ZZ	09PJ3JZ	09PY4YZ	09QG4ZZ
09BG0ZX	09BU4ZZ	09CB3ZZ	09CV4ZZ	09HD0SZ	09JH3ZZ	09NC0ZZ	09NW3ZZ	09PJ3KZ	09PY7YZ	09QG7ZZ

09QG8ZZ	09R1X7Z	09RM07Z	09UL7KZ	09WE8SZ	09WJX0Z	0B2QX0Z	0B5F4ZZ	0B734DZ	0B7B0DZ	0B947ZZ
09QGXZZ	09R1XJZ	09RM0JZ	09UL87Z	09WH00Z	09WJX7Z	0B2QXYZ	0B5F7ZZ	0B734ZZ	0B7B0ZZ	0B9480Z
09QK0ZZ	09R1XKZ	09RM0KZ	09UL8JZ	09WH07Z	09WJXDZ	0B2TX0Z	0B5F8ZZ	0B737DZ	0B7B3DZ	0B948ZX
09QK3ZZ	09R207Z	09RM37Z	09UL8KZ	09WH0DZ	09WJXJZ	0B2TXYZ	0B5G0ZZ	0B737ZZ	0B7B3ZZ	0B948ZZ
09QK4ZZ	09R20JZ	09RM3JZ	09UM07Z	09WH0JZ	09WJXKZ	0B510ZZ	0B5G3ZZ	0B738DZ	0B7B4DZ	0B9500Z
09QK8ZZ	09R20KZ	09RM3KZ	09UM0JZ	09WH0KZ	09WK00Z	0B513ZZ	0B5G4ZZ	0B738ZZ	0B7B4ZZ	0B950ZX
09QKXZZ	09R2X7Z	09RM47Z	09UM0KZ	09WH0YZ	09WK07Z	0B514ZZ	0B5G7ZZ	0B740DZ	0B7B7DZ	0B950ZZ
09QL0ZZ	09R2XJZ	09RM4JZ	09UM37Z	09WH30Z	09WK0DZ	0B517ZZ	0B5G8ZZ	0B740ZZ	0B7B7ZZ	0B9530Z
09QL3ZZ	09R2XKZ	09SF0ZZ	09UM3JZ	09WH37Z	09WK0JZ	0B518ZZ	0B5H0ZZ	0B743DZ	0B7B8DZ	0B953ZX
09QL4ZZ	09R507Z	09SF4ZZ	09UM3KZ	09WH3DZ	09WK0KZ	0B520ZZ	0B5H3ZZ	0B743ZZ	0B7B8ZZ	0B953ZZ
09QL7ZZ	09R50JZ	09SF7ZZ	09UM47Z	09WH3JZ	09WK0YZ	0B523ZZ	0B5H4ZZ	0B744DZ	0B9100Z	0B9540Z
09QL8ZZ	09R50KZ	09SF8ZZ	09UM4JZ	09WH3KZ	09WK30Z	0B524ZZ	0B5H7ZZ	0B744ZZ	0B910ZX	0B954ZX
09QM0ZZ	09R607Z	09SG0ZZ	09UM4KZ	09WH3YZ	09WK37Z	0B527ZZ	0B5H8ZZ	0B747DZ	0B910ZZ	0B954ZZ
09QM3ZZ	09R60JZ	09SG4ZZ	09UM87Z	09WH40Z	09WK3DZ	0B528ZZ	0B5J0ZZ	0B747ZZ	0B9130Z	0B9570Z
09QM4ZZ	09R60KZ	09SG7ZZ	09UM8JZ	09WH47Z	09WK3JZ	0B530ZZ	0B5J3ZZ	0B748DZ	0B913ZX	0B957ZX
09QM8ZZ	09R707Z	09SG8ZZ	09UM8KZ	09WH4DZ	09WK3KZ	0B533ZZ	0B5J4ZZ	0B748ZZ	0B913ZZ	0B957ZZ
09QN0ZZ	09R70JZ	09T58ZZ	09UN07Z	09WH4JZ	09WK3YZ	0B534ZZ	0B5J7ZZ	0B750DZ	0B9140Z	0B9580Z
09QN3ZZ	09R70KZ	09T68ZZ	09UN0JZ	09WH4KZ	09WK40Z	0B537ZZ	0B5J8ZZ	0B750ZZ	0B914ZX	0B958ZX
09QN4ZZ	09R777Z	09T98ZZ	09UN0KZ	09WH4YZ	09WK47Z	0B538ZZ	0B5K0ZZ	0B753DZ	0B914ZZ	0B958ZZ
09QN7ZZ	09R77JZ	09TA8ZZ	09UN77Z	09WH70Z	09WK4DZ	0B540ZZ	0B5K3ZZ	0B753ZZ	0B9170Z	0B9600Z
09QN8ZZ	09R77KZ	09TB8ZZ	09UN7JZ	09WH77Z	09WK4JZ	0B543ZZ	0B5K4ZZ	0B754DZ	0B917ZX	0B960ZX
09QP0ZZ	09R787Z	09TC8ZZ	09UN7KZ	09WH7DZ	09WK4KZ	0B544ZZ	0B5K7ZZ	0B754ZZ	0B917ZZ	0B960ZZ
09QP3ZZ	09R78JZ	09TD8ZZ	09UN87Z	09WH7JZ	09WK4YZ	0B547ZZ	0B5K8ZZ	0B757DZ	0B9180Z	0B9630Z
09QP4ZZ	09R78KZ	09TE8ZZ	09UN8JZ	09WH7KZ	09WK70Z	0B548ZZ	0B5L0ZZ	0B757ZZ	0B918ZX	0B963ZX
09QP8ZZ	09R807Z	09TF0ZZ	09UN8KZ	09WH7YZ	09WK77Z	0B550ZZ	0B5L3ZZ	0B758DZ	0B918ZZ	0B963ZZ
09QQ0ZZ	09R80JZ	09TF4ZZ	09W707Z	09WH80Z	09WK7DZ	0B553ZZ	0B5L4ZZ	0B758ZZ	0B9200Z	0B9640Z
09QQ3ZZ	09R80KZ	09TF7ZZ	09W70JZ	09WH87Z	09WK7JZ	0B554ZZ	0B5L7ZZ	0B760DZ	0B920ZX	0B964ZX
09QQ4ZZ	09R877Z	09TF8ZZ	09W70KZ	09WH8DZ	09WK7KZ	0B557ZZ	0B5L8ZZ	0B760ZZ	0B920ZZ	0B9670Z
09QQ8ZZ	09R87JZ	09TG0ZZ	09W777Z	09WH8JZ	09WK7YZ	0B558ZZ	0B5M0ZZ	0B763DZ	0B9230Z	0B967ZX
09QR0ZZ	09R87KZ	09TG4ZZ	09W77JZ	09WH8KZ	09WK80Z	0B560ZZ	0B5M3ZZ	0B763ZZ	0B923ZX	0B967ZZ
09QR3ZZ	09R887Z	09TG7ZZ	09W77KZ	09WH8YZ	09WK87Z	0B563ZZ	0B5M4ZZ	0B764DZ	0B923ZZ	0B9680Z
09QR4ZZ	09R88JZ	09TG8ZZ	09W787Z	09WHX0Z	09WK8DZ	0B564ZZ	0B5M7ZZ	0B764ZZ	0B9240Z	0B968ZX
09QR8ZZ	09R88KZ	09TK8ZZ	09W78JZ	09WHX7Z	09WK8JZ	0B567ZZ	0B5M8ZZ	0B767DZ	0B924ZX	0B968ZZ
09QS0ZZ	09R907Z	09TM8ZZ	09W78KZ	09WHXDZ	09WK8KZ	0B568ZZ	0B5N0ZZ	0B767ZZ	0B924ZZ	0B9700Z
09QS3ZZ	09R90JZ	09TP8ZZ	09W807Z	09WHXJZ	09WK8YZ	0B570ZZ	0B5N3ZZ	0B768DZ	0B9270Z	0B970ZX
09QS4ZZ	09R90KZ	09TQ8ZZ	09W80JZ	09WHXKZ	09WKX0Z	0B573ZZ	0B5N4ZZ	0B768ZZ	0B927ZX	0B970ZZ
09QS8ZZ	09RA07Z	09TR8ZZ	09W80KZ	09WJ00Z	09WKX7Z	0B574ZZ	0B5P0ZZ	0B770DZ	0B927ZZ	0B9730Z
09QT0ZZ	09RA0JZ	09TS8ZZ	09W877Z	09WJ07Z	09WKXDZ	0B577ZZ	0B5P3ZZ	0B770ZZ	0B9280Z	0B973ZX
09QT3ZZ	09RA0KZ	09TT8ZZ	09W87JZ	09WJ0DZ	09WKXJZ	0B578ZZ	0B5P4ZZ	0B773DZ	0B928ZX	0B973ZZ
09QT4ZZ	09RD07Z	09TU8ZZ	09W87KZ	09WJ0JZ	09WKXKZ	0B580ZZ	0B5T0ZZ	0B773ZZ	0B928ZZ	0B9740Z
09QT8ZZ	09RD0JZ	09TV8ZZ	09W887Z	09WJ0KZ	09WY00Z	0B583ZZ	0B5T3ZZ	0B774DZ	0B9300Z	0B974ZX
09QU0ZZ	09RD0KZ	09TW8ZZ	09W88JZ	09WJ0YZ	09WY0YZ	0B584ZZ	0B5T4ZZ	0B774ZZ	0B930ZX	0B974ZZ
09QU3ZZ	09RE07Z	09TX8ZZ	09W88KZ	09WJ30Z	09WY30Z	0B587ZZ	0B710DZ	0B777DZ	0B930ZZ	0B9770Z
09QU4ZZ	09RE0JZ	09U587Z	09W907Z	09WJ37Z	09WY3YZ	0B588ZZ	0B710ZZ	0B777ZZ	0B9330Z	0B977ZX
09QU8ZZ	09RE0KZ	09U58JZ	09W90JZ	09WJ3DZ	09WY40Z	0B590ZZ	0B713DZ	0B778DZ	0B933ZX	0B977ZZ
09QV0ZZ	09RK0JZ	09U58KZ	09W90KZ	09WJ3JZ	09WY4YZ	0B593ZZ	0B713ZZ	0B778ZZ	0B933ZZ	0B9780Z
09QV3ZZ	09RK0KZ	09U687Z	09W977Z	09WJ3KZ	09WY7YZ	0B594ZZ	0B714DZ	0B780DZ	0B9340Z	0B978ZX
09QV4ZZ	09RKX7Z	09U68JZ	09W97JZ	09WJ3YZ	09WY9YZ	0B597ZZ	0B714ZZ	0B780ZZ	0B934ZX	0B978ZZ
09QV8ZZ	09RKXJZ	09U68KZ	09W97KZ	09WJ40Z	09WYX0Z	0B598ZZ	0B717DZ	0B783DZ	0B934ZZ	0B9800Z
09QW0ZZ	09RKXKZ	09U987Z	09W987Z	09WJ47Z	0B110D6	0B5B0ZZ	0B717ZZ	0B783ZZ	0B9370Z	0B980ZX
09QW3ZZ	09RL07Z	09U98JZ	09W98JZ	09WJ4DZ	0B110F4	0B5B3ZZ	0B718DZ	0B784DZ	0B937ZX	0B980ZZ
09QW4ZZ	09RL0JZ	09U98KZ	09W98KZ	09WJ4JZ	0B110Z4	0B5B4ZZ	0B718ZZ	0B784ZZ	0B937ZZ	0B9830Z
09QW8ZZ	09RL0KZ	09UA87Z	09WA07Z	09WJ4KZ	0B113F4	0B5B7ZZ	0B720DZ	0B787DZ	0B9380Z	0B983ZX
09QX0ZZ	09RL37Z	09UA8JZ	09WA0JZ	09WJ4YZ	0B113Z4	0B5B8ZZ	0B720ZZ	0B787ZZ	0B938ZX	0B983ZZ
09QX3ZZ	09RL3JZ	09UA8KZ	09WA0KZ	09WJ70Z	0B114F4	0B5C0ZZ	0B723DZ	0B788DZ	0B938ZZ	0B9840Z
09QX4ZZ	09RL3KZ	09UD87Z	09WA77Z	09WJ77Z	0B114Z4	0B5C3ZZ	0B723ZZ	0B788ZZ	0B9400Z	0B984ZX
09QX8ZZ	09RL47Z	09UD8JZ	09WA7JZ	09WJ7DZ	0B20X0Z	0B5C4ZZ	0B724DZ	0B790DZ	0B940ZX	0B984ZZ
09R007Z	09RL4JZ	09UD8KZ	09WA7KZ	09WJ7JZ	0B20XYZ	0B5C7ZZ	0B724ZZ	0B790ZZ	0B940ZZ	0B9870Z
09R00JZ	09RL4KZ	09UE87Z	09WA87Z	09WJ7KZ	0B21X0Z	0B5C8ZZ	0B727DZ	0B793DZ	0B9430Z	0B987ZX
09R00KZ	09RL77Z	09UE8JZ	09WA8JZ	09WJ7YZ	0B21XEZ	0B5D0ZZ	0B727ZZ	0B793ZZ	0B943ZX	0B987ZZ
09R0X7Z	09RL7JZ	09UE8KZ	09WA8KZ	09WJ80Z	0B21XFZ	0B5D3ZZ	0B728DZ	0B794DZ	0B943ZZ	0B9880Z
09R0XJZ	09RL7KZ	09UK87Z	09WD0SZ	09WJ87Z	0B21XYZ	0B5D4ZZ	0B728ZZ	0B794ZZ	0B9440Z	0B988ZX
09R0XKZ	09RL87Z	09UK8JZ	09WD7SZ	09WJ8DZ	0B2KX0Z	0B5D7ZZ	0B730DZ	0B797DZ	0B944ZX	0B988ZZ
09R107Z	09RL8JZ	09UK8KZ	09WD8SZ	09WJ8JZ	0B2KXYZ	0B5D8ZZ	0B730ZZ	0B797ZZ	0B944ZZ	0B9900Z
09R10JZ	09RL8KZ	09UL77Z	09WE0SZ	09WJ8KZ	0B2LX0Z	0B5F0ZZ	0B733DZ	0B798DZ	0B9470Z	0B990ZX
09R10KZ		09UL7JZ	09WE7SZ	09WJ8YZ	0B2LXYZ	0B5F3ZZ	0B733ZZ	0B798ZZ	0B947ZX	

0B990ZZ	0B9F4ZZ	0B9K8ZZ	0BB13ZX	0BB94ZZ	0BCK7ZZ	0BDP0ZZ	0BH002Z	0BH83GZ	0BHT4MZ	0BL30CZ
0B9930Z	0B9F70Z	0B9L00Z	0BB13ZZ	0BB97ZX	0BCK8ZZ	0BDP3ZX	0BH003Z	0BH84GZ	0BHT4YZ	0BL30DZ
0B993ZX	0B9F7ZX	0B9L0ZX	0BB14ZX	0BB98ZX	0BCL0ZZ	0BDP3ZX	0BH00DZ	0BH87GZ	0BHT7YZ	0BL30ZZ
0B993ZZ	0B9F7ZZ	0B9L0ZX	0BB14ZZ	0BB98ZZ	0BCL3ZZ	0BDP4ZX	0BH00YZ	0BH88GZ	0BHT8YZ	0BL33CZ
0B9940Z	0B9F80Z	0B9L30Z	0BB17ZX	0BBB3ZX	0BCL4ZZ	0BDP4ZZ	0BH031Z	0BH90GZ	0BJ00ZZ	0BL33DZ
0B994ZX	0B9F8ZX	0B9L3ZX	0BB17ZZ	0BBB4ZX	0BCL7ZZ	0BF10ZZ	0BH032Z	0BH93GZ	0BJ03ZZ	0BL33ZZ
0B994ZZ	0B9F8ZZ	0B9L3ZZ	0BB18ZX	0BBB4ZZ	0BCL8ZZ	0BF13ZZ	0BH033Z	0BH94GZ	0BJ04ZZ	0BL34CZ
0B9970Z	0B9G00Z	0B9L40Z	0BB18ZZ	0BBB7ZX	0BCM0ZZ	0BF14ZZ	0BH03DZ	0BH97GZ	0BJ07ZZ	0BL34DZ
0B997ZX	0B9G0ZX	0B9L4ZX	0BB20ZX	0BBB8ZX	0BCM3ZZ	0BF17ZZ	0BH03YZ	0BH98GZ	0BJ08ZZ	0BL34ZZ
0B997ZZ	0B9G0ZZ	0B9L4ZZ	0BB20ZZ	0BBB8ZZ	0BCM4ZZ	0BF18ZZ	0BH041Z	0BHB0GZ	0BJ0XZZ	0BL37DZ
0B9980Z	0B9G30Z	0B9L70Z	0BB23ZX	0BBC3ZX	0BCM7ZZ	0BF1XZZ	0BH042Z	0BHB3GZ	0BJ10ZZ	0BL37ZZ
0B998ZX	0B9G3ZX	0B9L7ZX	0BB23ZZ	0BBC8ZZ	0BCM8ZZ	0BF20ZZ	0BH043Z	0BHB4GZ	0BJ13ZZ	0BL38DZ
0B998ZZ	0B9G3ZZ	0B9L7ZZ	0BB24ZX	0BBD3ZX	0BCN0ZZ	0BF23ZZ	0BH04DZ	0BHB7GZ	0BJ14ZZ	0BL38ZZ
0B9B00Z	0B9G40Z	0B9L80Z	0BB24ZZ	0BBD8ZZ	0BCN3ZZ	0BF24ZZ	0BH04YZ	0BHB8GZ	0BJ17ZZ	0BL40CZ
0B9B0ZX	0B9G4ZX	0B9L8ZX	0BB27ZX	0BBF3ZX	0BCN4ZZ	0BF27ZZ	0BH071Z	0BHK01Z	0BJ18ZZ	0BL40DZ
0B9B0ZZ	0B9G4ZZ	0B9L8ZZ	0BB27ZZ	0BBF8ZZ	0BCP0ZZ	0BF28ZZ	0BH072Z	0BHK02Z	0BJ1XZZ	0BL40ZZ
0B9B30Z	0B9G70Z	0B9M00Z	0BB28ZX	0BBG3ZX	0BCP3ZZ	0BF2XZZ	0BH073Z	0BHK03Z	0BJK0ZZ	0BL43CZ
0B9B3ZX	0B9G7ZX	0B9M0ZX	0BB28ZZ	0BBG8ZZ	0BCP4ZZ	0BF30ZZ	0BH07DZ	0BHK0YZ	0BJK3ZZ	0BL43DZ
0B9B3ZZ	0B9G7ZZ	0B9M0ZZ	0BB30ZX	0BBH3ZX	0BCT0ZZ	0BF33ZZ	0BH07YZ	0BHK31Z	0BJK4ZZ	0BL43ZZ
0B9B40Z	0B9G80Z	0B9M30Z	0BB30ZZ	0BBH8ZZ	0BCT3ZZ	0BF34ZZ	0BH081Z	0BHK33Z	0BJK8ZZ	0BL44CZ
0B9B4ZX	0B9G8ZX	0B9M3ZX	0BB33ZX	0BBJ3ZX	0BCT4ZZ	0BF37ZZ	0BH082Z	0BHK3YZ	0BJKXZZ	0BL44DZ
0B9B4ZZ	0B9G8ZZ	0B9M3ZZ	0BB33ZZ	0BBJ8ZZ	0BD14ZX	0BF38ZZ	0BH083Z	0BHK41Z	0BJL0ZZ	0BL44ZZ
0B9B70Z	0B9H00Z	0B9M40Z	0BB34ZX	0BBK3ZX	0BD18ZX	0BF3XZZ	0BH08DZ	0BHK42Z	0BJL3ZZ	0BL47DZ
0B9B7ZX	0B9H0ZX	0B9M4ZX	0BB34ZZ	0BBK8ZZ	0BD24ZX	0BF40ZZ	0BH08YZ	0BHK43Z	0BJL4ZZ	0BL47ZZ
0B9B7ZZ	0B9H0ZZ	0B9M4ZZ	0BB37ZX	0BBL3ZX	0BD28ZX	0BF43ZZ	0BH102Z	0BHK4YZ	0BJL7ZZ	0BL48DZ
0B9B80Z	0B9H30Z	0B9M70Z	0BB37ZZ	0BBL8ZZ	0BD34ZX	0BF44ZZ	0BH10DZ	0BHK71Z	0BJL8ZZ	0BL48ZZ
0B9B8ZX	0B9H3ZX	0B9M7ZX	0BB38ZX	0BBM3ZX	0BD38ZX	0BF47ZZ	0BH10YZ	0BHK72Z	0BJLXZZ	0BL50CZ
0B9B8ZZ	0B9H3ZZ	0B9M7ZZ	0BB38ZZ	0BBM4ZZ	0BD44ZX	0BF48ZZ	0BH13DZ	0BHK73Z	0BJQ0ZZ	0BL50DZ
0B9C00Z	0B9H40Z	0B9M80Z	0BB40ZX	0BBM8ZZ	0BD48ZX	0BF4XZZ	0BH13EZ	0BHK7YZ	0BJQ3ZZ	0BL50ZZ
0B9C0ZX	0B9H4ZX	0B9M8ZX	0BB40ZZ	0BBN0ZX	0BD54ZX	0BF50ZZ	0BH13YZ	0BHK81Z	0BJQ4ZZ	0BL53CZ
0B9C0ZZ	0B9H4ZZ	0B9M8ZZ	0BB43ZX	0BBN3ZX	0BD58ZX	0BF53ZZ	0BH14DZ	0BHK82Z	0BJQ7ZZ	0BL53DZ
0B9C30Z	0B9H70Z	0B9N00Z	0BB43ZZ	0BBN8ZX	0BD64ZX	0BF54ZZ	0BH14YZ	0BHK83Z	0BJQ8ZZ	0BL53ZZ
0B9C3ZX	0B9H7ZX	0B9N0ZX	0BB44ZX	0BBN8ZZ	0BD68ZX	0BF57ZZ	0BH172Z	0BHK8YZ	0BJQXZZ	0BL54CZ
0B9C3ZZ	0B9H7ZZ	0B9N0ZZ	0BB44ZZ	0BBP0ZX	0BD74ZX	0BF58ZZ	0BH17DZ	0BHL01Z	0BJT0ZZ	0BL54DZ
0B9C40Z	0B9H80Z	0B9N30Z	0BB47ZX	0BBP3ZX	0BD78ZX	0BF5XZZ	0BH17EZ	0BHL02Z	0BJT3ZZ	0BL54ZZ
0B9C4ZX	0B9H8ZX	0B9N3ZX	0BB47ZZ	0BBP8ZX	0BD84ZX	0BF60ZZ	0BH17YZ	0BHL03Z	0BJT4ZZ	0BL57DZ
0B9C4ZZ	0B9H8ZZ	0B9N3ZZ	0BB48ZX	0BBP8ZZ	0BD88ZX	0BF63ZZ	0BH182Z	0BHL0YZ	0BJT7ZZ	0BL57ZZ
0B9C70Z	0B9J00Z	0B9N40Z	0BB48ZZ	0BBT0ZX	0BD94ZX	0BF64ZZ	0BH18DZ	0BHL31Z	0BJT8ZZ	0BL58DZ
0B9C7ZX	0B9J0ZX	0B9N4ZX	0BB50ZX	0BBT0ZZ	0BD98ZX	0BF67ZZ	0BH18EZ	0BHL32Z	0BJTXZZ	0BL58ZZ
0B9C7ZZ	0B9J0ZZ	0B9N4ZZ	0BB50ZZ	0BBT3ZX	0BDB4ZX	0BF68ZZ	0BH18YZ	0BHL33Z	0BL10CZ	0BL60CZ
0B9C80Z	0B9J30Z	0B9N80Z	0BB53ZX	0BBT3ZZ	0BDB8ZX	0BF6XZZ	0BH30GZ	0BHL3YZ	0BL10DZ	0BL60DZ
0B9C8ZX	0B9J3ZX	0B9N8ZX	0BB54ZX	0BBT4ZX	0BDC4ZX	0BF70ZZ	0BH33GZ	0BHL41Z	0BL10ZZ	0BL63CZ
0B9C8ZZ	0B9J3ZZ	0B9N8ZZ	0BB54ZZ	0BBT4ZZ	0BDC8ZX	0BF73ZZ	0BH34GZ	0BHL42Z	0BL13CZ	0BL63DZ
0B9D00Z	0B9J40Z	0B9P00Z	0BB57ZX	0BC17ZZ	0BDD4ZX	0BF74ZZ	0BH37GZ	0BHL43Z	0BL13DZ	0BL63ZZ
0B9D0ZX	0B9J4ZX	0B9P0ZX	0BB58ZX	0BC18ZZ	0BDD8ZX	0BF77ZZ	0BH38GZ	0BHL4YZ	0BL13ZZ	0BL64CZ
0B9D0ZZ	0B9J4ZZ	0B9P0ZZ	0BB58ZZ	0BC27ZZ	0BDF4ZX	0BF78ZZ	0BH40GZ	0BHL71Z	0BL14CZ	0BL64DZ
0B9D30Z	0B9J70Z	0B9P30Z	0BB63ZX	0BC28ZZ	0BDF8ZX	0BF7XZZ	0BH43GZ	0BHL72Z	0BL14DZ	0BL64ZZ
0B9D3ZX	0B9J7ZX	0B9P3ZX	0BB64ZX	0BC37ZZ	0BDG4ZX	0BF80ZZ	0BH44GZ	0BHL73Z	0BL14ZZ	0BL67DZ
0B9D3ZZ	0B9J7ZZ	0B9P3ZZ	0BB64ZZ	0BC38ZZ	0BDG8ZX	0BF83ZZ	0BH47GZ	0BHL7YZ	0BL17DZ	0BL67ZZ
0B9D40Z	0B9J80Z	0B9P40Z	0BB67ZX	0BC47ZZ	0BDH4ZX	0BF84ZZ	0BH48GZ	0BHL81Z	0BL17ZZ	0BL68DZ
0B9D4ZX	0B9J8ZX	0B9P4ZX	0BB68ZX	0BC48ZZ	0BDH8ZX	0BF87ZZ	0BH50GZ	0BHL82Z	0BL18DZ	0BL68ZZ
0B9D4ZZ	0B9J8ZZ	0B9P4ZZ	0BB68ZZ	0BC57ZZ	0BDJ4ZX	0BF88ZZ	0BH53GZ	0BHL83Z	0BL18ZZ	0BL70CZ
0B9D70Z	0B9K00Z	0B9P80Z	0BB73ZX	0BC58ZZ	0BDJ8ZX	0BF8XZZ	0BH54GZ	0BHL8YZ	0BL20CZ	0BL70DZ
0B9D7ZX	0B9K0ZX	0B9P8ZX	0BB74ZX	0BC67ZZ	0BDK4ZX	0BF90ZZ	0BH57GZ	0BHQ0YZ	0BL20DZ	0BL70ZZ
0B9D7ZZ	0B9K0ZZ	0B9P8ZZ	0BB74ZZ	0BC68ZZ	0BDK8ZX	0BF93ZZ	0BH58GZ	0BHQ3YZ	0BL20ZZ	0BL73CZ
0B9D80Z	0B9K30Z	0B9T00Z	0BB77ZX	0BC77ZZ	0BDL4ZX	0BF94ZZ	0BH60GZ	0BHQ4YZ	0BL23CZ	0BL73DZ
0B9D8ZX	0B9K3ZX	0B9T0ZX	0BB78ZX	0BC78ZZ	0BDL8ZX	0BF97ZZ	0BH63GZ	0BHQ7YZ	0BL23DZ	0BL73ZZ
0B9D8ZZ	0B9K3ZZ	0B9T0ZZ	0BB78ZZ	0BC87ZZ	0BDM4ZX	0BF98ZZ	0BH64GZ	0BHQ8YZ	0BL23ZZ	0BL74CZ
0B9F00Z	0B9K40Z	0B9T30Z	0BB83ZX	0BC88ZZ	0BDM8ZX	0BF9XZZ	0BH67GZ	0BHT02Z	0BL24CZ	0BL74DZ
0B9F0ZX	0B9K4ZX	0B9T3ZX	0BB84ZX	0BC97ZZ	0BDN0ZX	0BFB0ZZ	0BH68GZ	0BHT0MZ	0BL24DZ	0BL74ZZ
0B9F0ZZ	0B9K4ZZ	0B9T3ZZ	0BB84ZZ	0BC98ZZ	0BDN0ZZ	0BFB3ZZ	0BH70GZ	0BHT0YZ	0BL24ZZ	0BL77DZ
0B9F30Z	0B9K70Z	0B9T40Z	0BB87ZX	0BCB7ZZ	0BDN3ZX	0BFB4ZZ	0BH73GZ	0BHT32Z	0BL27DZ	0BL77ZZ
0B9F3ZX	0B9K7ZX	0B9T4ZX	0BB88ZX	0BCB8ZZ	0BDN3ZZ	0BFB7ZZ	0BH74GZ	0BHT3MZ	0BL27ZZ	0BL78DZ
0B9F3ZZ	0B9K7ZZ	0B9T4ZZ	0BB88ZZ	0BCK0ZZ	0BDN4ZX	0BFB8ZZ	0BH77GZ	0BHT3YZ	0BL28DZ	0BL78ZZ
0B9F40Z	0B9K80Z	0BB10ZX	0BB93ZX	0BCK3ZZ	0BDN4ZZ	0BFBXZZ	0BH78GZ	0BHT42Z	0BL28ZZ	0BL80CZ
0B9F4ZX	0B9K8ZX	0BB10ZZ	0BB94ZX	0BCK4ZZ	0BDP0ZZ	0BH001Z	0BH80GZ			

0BL80DZ	0BN28ZZ	0BNJ0ZZ	0BP07JZ	0BPK0YZ	0BPT3YZ	0BR94JZ	0BU34JZ	0BUB8JZ	0BV54CZ	0BVB4DZ
0BL80ZZ	0BN30ZZ	0BNJ3ZZ	0BP07KZ	0BPK30Z	0BPT4YZ	0BR94KZ	0BU34KZ	0BUB8KZ	0BV54DZ	0BVB4ZZ
0BL83CZ	0BN33ZZ	0BNJ4ZZ	0BP07YZ	0BPK31Z	0BPT70Z	0BRB07Z	0BU387Z	0BUT07Z	0BV54ZZ	0BVB7DZ
0BL83DZ	0BN34ZZ	0BNJ7ZZ	0BP080Z	0BPK32Z	0BPT72Z	0BRB0JZ	0BU38JZ	0BUT0JZ	0BV57DZ	0BVB7ZZ
0BL83ZZ	0BN37ZZ	0BNJ8ZZ	0BP081Z	0BPK33Z	0BPT7YZ	0BRB0KZ	0BU38KZ	0BUT0KZ	0BV57ZZ	0BVB8DZ
0BL84CZ	0BN38ZZ	0BNK0ZZ	0BP082Z	0BPK3YZ	0BPT80Z	0BRB47Z	0BU407Z	0BUT47Z	0BV58DZ	0BVB8ZZ
0BL84DZ	0BN40ZZ	0BNK3ZZ	0BP083Z	0BPK40Z	0BPT82Z	0BRB4JZ	0BU40JZ	0BUT4JZ	0BV58ZZ	0BW000Z
0BL84ZZ	0BN43ZZ	0BNK4ZZ	0BP087Z	0BPK41Z	0BPT8YZ	0BRB4KZ	0BU40KZ	0BUT4KZ	0BV60CZ	0BW002Z
0BL87DZ	0BN44ZZ	0BNK7ZZ	0BP08CZ	0BPK42Z	0BPTX0Z	0BRT07Z	0BU447Z	0BV10CZ	0BV60DZ	0BW003Z
0BL87ZZ	0BN47ZZ	0BNK8ZZ	0BP08DZ	0BPK43Z	0BPTX2Z	0BRT0JZ	0BU44JZ	0BV10DZ	0BV60ZZ	0BW007Z
0BL88DZ	0BN48ZZ	0BNL0ZZ	0BP08JZ	0BPK4YZ	0BPTXMZ	0BRT0KZ	0BU44KZ	0BV10ZZ	0BV63CZ	0BW00CZ
0BL88ZZ	0BN50ZZ	0BNL3ZZ	0BP08KZ	0BPK70Z	0BQT0ZZ	0BRT47Z	0BU487Z	0BV13CZ	0BV63DZ	0BW00DZ
0BL90CZ	0BN53ZZ	0BNL4ZZ	0BP08YZ	0BPK71Z	0BQT3ZZ	0BRT4JZ	0BU48JZ	0BV13DZ	0BV63ZZ	0BW00JZ
0BL90DZ	0BN54ZZ	0BNL7ZZ	0BP0X0Z	0BPK72Z	0BQT4ZZ	0BRT4KZ	0BU48KZ	0BV13ZZ	0BV64CZ	0BW00KZ
0BL90ZZ	0BN57ZZ	0BNL8ZZ	0BP0X1Z	0BPK73Z	0BR107Z	0BST0ZZ	0BU507Z	0BV14CZ	0BV64DZ	0BW00YZ
0BL93CZ	0BN58ZZ	0BNM0ZZ	0BP0X2Z	0BPK7YZ	0BR10JZ	0BT64ZZ	0BU50JZ	0BV14DZ	0BV64ZZ	0BW030Z
0BL93DZ	0BN60ZZ	0BNM3ZZ	0BP0X3Z	0BPK80Z	0BR10KZ	0BT70ZZ	0BU50KZ	0BV14ZZ	0BV67DZ	0BW032Z
0BL93ZZ	0BN63ZZ	0BNM4ZZ	0BP0XDZ	0BPK81Z	0BR147Z	0BT74ZZ	0BU547Z	0BV17DZ	0BV67ZZ	0BW033Z
0BL94CZ	0BN64ZZ	0BNM7ZZ	0BP100Z	0BPK82Z	0BR14JZ	0BT80ZZ	0BU54JZ	0BV17ZZ	0BV68DZ	0BW037Z
0BL94DZ	0BN67ZZ	0BNM8ZZ	0BP102Z	0BPK83Z	0BR14KZ	0BT84ZZ	0BU54KZ	0BV18DZ	0BV68ZZ	0BW03CZ
0BL94ZZ	0BN68ZZ	0BNN0ZZ	0BP107Z	0BPK8YZ	0BR207Z	0BT90ZZ	0BU587Z	0BV18ZZ	0BV70CZ	0BW03DZ
0BL97DZ	0BN70ZZ	0BNN3ZZ	0BP10CZ	0BPKX0Z	0BR20JZ	0BT94ZZ	0BU58JZ	0BV20CZ	0BV70DZ	0BW03JZ
0BL97ZZ	0BN73ZZ	0BNN4ZZ	0BP10DZ	0BPKX1Z	0BR20KZ	0BTB0ZZ	0BU58KZ	0BV20DZ	0BV70ZZ	0BW03KZ
0BL98DZ	0BN74ZZ	0BNP0ZZ	0BP10FZ	0BPKX2Z	0BR247Z	0BTB4ZZ	0BU607Z	0BV20ZZ	0BV73CZ	0BW03YZ
0BL98ZZ	0BN77ZZ	0BNP3ZZ	0BP10JZ	0BPKX3Z	0BR24JZ	0BTC0ZZ	0BU60JZ	0BV23CZ	0BV73DZ	0BW040Z
0BLB0CZ	0BN78ZZ	0BNP4ZZ	0BP10KZ	0BPL00Z	0BR24KZ	0BTC4ZZ	0BU60KZ	0BV23DZ	0BV73ZZ	0BW042Z
0BLB0DZ	0BN80ZZ	0BNT0ZZ	0BP130Z	0BPL01Z	0BR307Z	0BTD0ZZ	0BU647Z	0BV23ZZ	0BV74CZ	0BW043Z
0BLB0ZZ	0BN83ZZ	0BNT3ZZ	0BP132Z	0BPL0YZ	0BR30JZ	0BTD4ZZ	0BU64JZ	0BV24CZ	0BV74DZ	0BW047Z
0BLB3CZ	0BN84ZZ	0BNT4ZZ	0BP137Z	0BPL3YZ	0BR30KZ	0BTF0ZZ	0BU64KZ	0BV24DZ	0BV74ZZ	0BW04CZ
0BLB3DZ	0BN87ZZ	0BP000Z	0BP13CZ	0BPL4YZ	0BR347Z	0BTF4ZZ	0BU687Z	0BV24ZZ	0BV77DZ	0BW04DZ
0BLB3ZZ	0BN88ZZ	0BP001Z	0BP13DZ	0BPL70Z	0BR34JZ	0BTG0ZZ	0BU68JZ	0BV27DZ	0BV77ZZ	0BW04JZ
0BLB4CZ	0BN90ZZ	0BP002Z	0BP13FZ	0BPL72Z	0BR34KZ	0BTG4ZZ	0BU68KZ	0BV27ZZ	0BV78DZ	0BW04KZ
0BLB4DZ	0BN93ZZ	0BP003Z	0BP13JZ	0BPL73Z	0BR407Z	0BTH0ZZ	0BU707Z	0BV28DZ	0BV78ZZ	0BW04YZ
0BLB4ZZ	0BN94ZZ	0BP007Z	0BP13KZ	0BPL7YZ	0BR40JZ	0BTH4ZZ	0BU70JZ	0BV28ZZ	0BV80CZ	0BW070Z
0BLB7DZ	0BN97ZZ	0BP00CZ	0BP140Z	0BPL80Z	0BR40KZ	0BTJ0ZZ	0BU70KZ	0BV30CZ	0BV80DZ	0BW072Z
0BLB7ZZ	0BN98ZZ	0BP00DZ	0BP142Z	0BPL82Z	0BR447Z	0BTJ4ZZ	0BU747Z	0BV30DZ	0BV80ZZ	0BW073Z
0BLB8DZ	0BNB0ZZ	0BP00JZ	0BP147Z	0BPL83Z	0BR44JZ	0BTK0ZZ	0BU74JZ	0BV30ZZ	0BV83CZ	0BW077Z
0BLB8ZZ	0BNB3ZZ	0BP00KZ	0BP14CZ	0BPL8YZ	0BR44KZ	0BTK4ZZ	0BU74KZ	0BV33CZ	0BV83DZ	0BW07CZ
0BM10ZZ	0BNB4ZZ	0BP00YZ	0BP14DZ	0BPLX0Z	0BR507Z	0BTL0ZZ	0BU787Z	0BV33DZ	0BV83ZZ	0BW07DZ
0BM20ZZ	0BNB7ZZ	0BP030Z	0BP14FZ	0BPLX1Z	0BR50JZ	0BTL4ZZ	0BU78JZ	0BV33ZZ	0BV84CZ	0BW07JZ
0BM30ZZ	0BNB8ZZ	0BP031Z	0BP14JZ	0BPLX2Z	0BR50KZ	0BTM0ZZ	0BU78KZ	0BV34CZ	0BV84DZ	0BW07KZ
0BM40ZZ	0BNC0ZZ	0BP032Z	0BP14KZ	0BPLX3Z	0BR547Z	0BTM4ZZ	0BU807Z	0BV34DZ	0BV84ZZ	0BW07YZ
0BM50ZZ	0BNC3ZZ	0BP033Z	0BP170Z	0BPQ00Z	0BR54JZ	0BTT0ZZ	0BU80JZ	0BV34ZZ	0BV87DZ	0BW080Z
0BM60ZZ	0BNC4ZZ	0BP037Z	0BP172Z	0BPQ01Z	0BR54KZ	0BTT4ZZ	0BU80KZ	0BV37DZ	0BV87ZZ	0BW082Z
0BM70ZZ	0BNC7ZZ	0BP03CZ	0BP177Z	0BPQ02Z	0BR607Z	0BU107Z	0BU847Z	0BV37ZZ	0BV88DZ	0BW083Z
0BM80ZZ	0BNC8ZZ	0BP03DZ	0BP17CZ	0BPQ0YZ	0BR60JZ	0BU10JZ	0BU84JZ	0BV38DZ	0BV88ZZ	0BW087Z
0BM90ZZ	0BND0ZZ	0BP03JZ	0BP17DZ	0BPQ30Z	0BR60KZ	0BU10KZ	0BU84KZ	0BV38ZZ	0BV90CZ	0BW08CZ
0BMB0ZZ	0BND3ZZ	0BP03KZ	0BP17FZ	0BPQ31Z	0BR647Z	0BU147Z	0BU887Z	0BV40CZ	0BV90DZ	0BW08DZ
0BMC0ZZ	0BND4ZZ	0BP03YZ	0BP17JZ	0BPQ32Z	0BR64JZ	0BU14JZ	0BU88JZ	0BV40DZ	0BV90ZZ	0BW08JZ
0BMD0ZZ	0BND7ZZ	0BP040Z	0BP17KZ	0BPQ3YZ	0BR64KZ	0BU14KZ	0BU88KZ	0BV40ZZ	0BV93CZ	0BW08KZ
0BMF0ZZ	0BND8ZZ	0BP041Z	0BP180Z	0BPQ40Z	0BR707Z	0BU187Z	0BU907Z	0BV43CZ	0BV93DZ	0BW08YZ
0BMG0ZZ	0BNF0ZZ	0BP042Z	0BP182Z	0BPQ41Z	0BR70JZ	0BU18JZ	0BU90JZ	0BV43DZ	0BV93ZZ	0BW0X0Z
0BMH0ZZ	0BNF3ZZ	0BP043Z	0BP187Z	0BPQ42Z	0BR70KZ	0BU18KZ	0BU90KZ	0BV43ZZ	0BV94CZ	0BW0X2Z
0BMJ0ZZ	0BNF4ZZ	0BP047Z	0BP18CZ	0BPQ4YZ	0BR747Z	0BU207Z	0BU947Z	0BV44CZ	0BV94DZ	0BW0X3Z
0BMK0ZZ	0BNF7ZZ	0BP04CZ	0BP18DZ	0BPQ70Z	0BR74JZ	0BU20JZ	0BU94JZ	0BV44DZ	0BV94ZZ	0BW0X7Z
0BML0ZZ	0BNF8ZZ	0BP04DZ	0BP18FZ	0BPQ71Z	0BR74KZ	0BU20KZ	0BU94KZ	0BV44ZZ	0BV97DZ	0BW0XCZ
0BMT0ZZ	0BNG0ZZ	0BP04JZ	0BP18JZ	0BPQ72Z	0BR807Z	0BU247Z	0BU987Z	0BV47DZ	0BV97ZZ	0BW0XDZ
0BN10ZZ	0BNG3ZZ	0BP04KZ	0BP18KZ	0BPQ7YZ	0BR80JZ	0BU24JZ	0BU98JZ	0BV47ZZ	0BV98DZ	0BW0XJZ
0BN13ZZ	0BNG4ZZ	0BP04YZ	0BP1X0Z	0BPQ80Z	0BR80KZ	0BU24KZ	0BU98KZ	0BV48DZ	0BV98ZZ	0BW0XKZ
0BN14ZZ	0BNG7ZZ	0BP070Z	0BP1X2Z	0BPQ81Z	0BR847Z	0BU287Z	0BUB07Z	0BV48ZZ	0BVB0CZ	0BW100Z
0BN17ZZ	0BNG8ZZ	0BP071Z	0BP1XDZ	0BPQ82Z	0BR84JZ	0BU28JZ	0BUB0JZ	0BV50CZ	0BVB0DZ	0BW102Z
0BN18ZZ	0BNH0ZZ	0BP072Z	0BP1XFZ	0BPQ8YZ	0BR84KZ	0BU28KZ	0BUB0KZ	0BV50DZ	0BVB0ZZ	0BW107Z
0BN20ZZ	0BNH3ZZ	0BP073Z	0BPK00Z	0BPQX0Z	0BR907Z	0BU307Z	0BUB47Z	0BV50ZZ	0BVB3CZ	0BW10CZ
0BN23ZZ	0BNH4ZZ	0BP077Z	0BPK01Z	0BPQX1Z	0BR90JZ	0BU30JZ	0BUB4JZ	0BV53CZ	0BVB3DZ	0BW10DZ
0BN24ZZ	0BNH7ZZ	0BP07CZ	0BPK02Z	0BPQX2Z	0BR90KZ	0BU30KZ	0BUB4KZ	0BV53DZ	0BVB3ZZ	0BW10FZ
0BN27ZZ	0BNH8ZZ	0BP07DZ	0BPK03Z	0BPT0YZ	0BR947Z	0BU347Z	0BUB87Z	0BV53ZZ	0BVB4CZ	0BW10JZ

0BW10KZ	0BWL03Z	0BWT80Z	0C540ZZ	0C5XXZ2	0C993ZX	0C9T7ZX	0CBM4ZX	0CCH0ZZ	0CFB0ZZ	0CM00ZZ
0BW130Z	0BWL0YZ	0BWT82Z	0C543ZZ	0C7B0DZ	0C993ZZ	0C9T8ZX	0CBM7ZX	0CCH3ZZ	0CFB3ZZ	0CM10ZZ
0BW132Z	0BWL30Z	0BWT87Z	0C54XZZ	0C7B0ZZ	0C9B00Z	0C9V30Z	0CBM8ZX	0CCJ0ZZ	0CFB7ZZ	0CM30ZZ
0BW137Z	0BWL32Z	0BWT8JZ	0C550ZZ	0C7B3DZ	0C9B0ZZ	0C9V3ZX	0CBR3ZX	0CCJ3ZZ	0CFBXZZ	0CM70ZZ
0BW13CZ	0BWL33Z	0BWT8KZ	0C553ZZ	0C7B3ZZ	0C9B30Z	0C9V3ZZ	0CBR4ZX	0CCM0ZZ	0CFC0ZZ	0CMN0ZZ
0BW13DZ	0BWL3YZ	0BWT8MZ	0C55XZZ	0C7B7DZ	0C9B3ZX	0C9V4ZX	0CBR7ZX	0CCM3ZZ	0CFC3ZZ	0CMW0Z0
0BW13FZ	0BWL40Z	0BWT8YZ	0C560ZZ	0C7B7ZZ	0C9B3ZZ	0C9V7ZX	0CBR8ZX	0CCM4ZZ	0CFC7ZZ	0CMW0Z1
0BW13JZ	0BWL42Z	0BWTX0Z	0C563ZZ	0C7C0DZ	0C9C00Z	0C9V8ZX	0CBS3ZX	0CCM7ZZ	0CFCXZZ	0CMW0Z2
0BW13KZ	0BWL43Z	0BWTX2Z	0C56XZZ	0C7C0ZZ	0C9C0ZZ	0C9W000	0CBS4ZX	0CCM8ZZ	0CH701Z	0CMWXZ0
0BW140Z	0BWL4YZ	0BWTX7Z	0C570ZZ	0C7C3DZ	0C9C30Z	0C9W001	0CBS7ZX	0CCN0ZZ	0CH731Z	0CMWXZ1
0BW142Z	0BWL70Z	0BWTXJZ	0C573ZZ	0C7C3ZZ	0C9C3ZX	0C9W002	0CBS8ZX	0CCN3ZZ	0CH7X1Z	0CMWXZ2
0BW147Z	0BWL72Z	0BWTXKZ	0C57XZZ	0C7C7DZ	0C9C3ZZ	0C9W0Z0	0CBT3ZX	0CCNXZZ	0CHA0YZ	0CMX0Z0
0BW14CZ	0BWL73Z	0BWTXMZ	0C580ZZ	0C7C7ZZ	0C9D00Z	0C9W0Z1	0CBT4ZX	0CCP0ZZ	0CHA3YZ	0CMX0Z1
0BW14DZ	0BWL7YZ	0BYC0Z0	0C583ZZ	0C7M7DZ	0C9D0ZZ	0C9W0Z2	0CBT7ZX	0CCP3ZZ	0CHA7YZ	0CMX0Z2
0BW14FZ	0BWL80Z	0BYC0Z1	0C590ZZ	0C7M7ZZ	0C9D30Z	0C9WX00	0CBT8ZX	0CCPXZZ	0CHA8YZ	0CMXXZ0
0BW14JZ	0BWL82Z	0BYC0Z2	0C593ZZ	0C7M8DZ	0C9D3ZX	0C9WX01	0CBV3ZX	0CCQ0ZZ	0CHS0YZ	0CMXXZ1
0BW14KZ	0BWL83Z	0BYD0Z0	0C5B0ZZ	0C7M8ZZ	0C9D3ZZ	0C9WX02	0CBV4ZX	0CCQ3ZZ	0CHS3YZ	0CMXXZ2
0BW170Z	0BWL8YZ	0BYD0Z1	0C5B3ZZ	0C900ZX	0C9F00Z	0C9WXZ0	0CBV7ZX	0CCQXZZ	0CHS7YZ	0CN00ZZ
0BW172Z	0BWLX0Z	0BYD0Z2	0C5C0ZZ	0C9030Z	0C9F0ZZ	0C9WXZ1	0CBV8ZX	0CCR0ZZ	0CHS8YZ	0CN03ZZ
0BW177Z	0BWLX2Z	0BYF0Z0	0C5C3ZZ	0C903ZX	0C9F30Z	0C9WXZ2	0CBW0Z0	0CCR3ZZ	0CHY0YZ	0CN0XZZ
0BW17CZ	0BWLX3Z	0BYF0Z1	0C5D0ZZ	0C903ZZ	0C9F3ZX	0C9X000	0CBW0Z1	0CCR4ZZ	0CHY3YZ	0CN10ZZ
0BW17DZ	0BWQ00Z	0BYF0Z2	0C5D3ZZ	0C90XZZ	0C9F3ZZ	0C9X001	0CBW0Z2	0CCR7ZZ	0CHY7BZ	0CN13ZZ
0BW17FZ	0BWQ02Z	0BYG0Z0	0C5F0ZZ	0C910ZX	0C9G00Z	0C9X002	0CBWXZ0	0CCR8ZZ	0CHY7YZ	0CN1XZZ
0BW17JZ	0BWQ0YZ	0BYG0Z1	0C5F3ZZ	0C9130Z	0C9G0ZZ	0C9X0Z0	0CBWXZ1	0CCS0ZZ	0CHY8BZ	0CN20ZZ
0BW17KZ	0BWQ30Z	0BYG0Z2	0C5G0ZZ	0C913ZX	0C9G30Z	0C9X0Z1	0CBWXZ2	0CCS3ZZ	0CHY8YZ	0CN23ZZ
0BW180Z	0BWQ32Z	0BYH0Z0	0C5G3ZZ	0C913ZZ	0C9G3ZX	0C9X0Z2	0CBX0Z0	0CCS4ZZ	0CJA0ZZ	0CN2XZZ
0BW182Z	0BWQ3YZ	0BYH0Z1	0C5H0ZZ	0C91XZX	0C9G3ZZ	0C9XX00	0CBX0Z1	0CCS7ZZ	0CJA3ZZ	0CN30ZZ
0BW187Z	0BWQ40Z	0BYH0Z2	0C5H3ZZ	0C9230Z	0C9H00Z	0C9XX01	0CBX0Z2	0CCS8ZZ	0CJAXZZ	0CN33ZZ
0BW18CZ	0BWQ42Z	0BYJ0Z0	0C5J0ZZ	0C923ZZ	0C9H0ZZ	0C9XX02	0CBXXZ0	0CCT0ZZ	0CJS0ZZ	0CN3XZZ
0BW18DZ	0BWQ4YZ	0BYJ0Z1	0C5J3ZZ	0C9330Z	0C9H30Z	0C9XXZ0	0CBXXZ1	0CCT3ZZ	0CJS3ZZ	0CN40ZZ
0BW18FZ	0BWQ70Z	0BYJ0Z2	0C5M0ZZ	0C933ZZ	0C9H3ZX	0C9XXZ1	0CBXXZ2	0CCT4ZZ	0CJS4ZZ	0CN43ZZ
0BW18JZ	0BWQ72Z	0BYK0Z0	0C5M3ZZ	0C940ZX	0C9H3ZZ	0C9XXZ2	0CC0XZZ	0CCT7ZZ	0CJS7ZZ	0CN4XZZ
0BW18KZ	0BWQ7YZ	0BYK0Z1	0C5M4ZZ	0C9430Z	0C9J00Z	0CB00ZX	0CC13ZZ	0CCT8ZZ	0CJS8ZZ	0CN50ZZ
0BW1X0Z	0BWQ80Z	0BYK0Z2	0C5M7ZZ	0C943ZX	0C9J0ZZ	0CB03ZX	0CC1XZZ	0CCV0ZZ	0CJSXZZ	0CN53ZZ
0BW1X2Z	0BWQ82Z	0BYL0Z0	0C5M8ZZ	0C943ZZ	0C9J30Z	0CB0XZX	0CC20ZZ	0CCV3ZZ	0CJY0ZZ	0CN5XZZ
0BW1X7Z	0BWQ8YZ	0BYL0Z1	0C5N0ZZ	0C94XZX	0C9J3ZX	0CB10ZX	0CC23ZZ	0CCV4ZZ	0CJY3ZZ	0CN60ZZ
0BW1XCZ	0BWQX0Z	0BYL0Z2	0C5N3ZZ	0C9500Z	0C9J3ZZ	0CB13ZX	0CC2XZZ	0CCV7ZZ	0CJY4ZZ	0CN63ZZ
0BW1XDZ	0BWQX2Z	0BYM0Z0	0C5NXZZ	0C950ZX	0C9M0ZX	0CB1XZX	0CC30ZZ	0CCV8ZZ	0CJY7ZZ	0CN6XZZ
0BW1XFZ	0BWT00Z	0BYM0Z1	0C5P0ZZ	0C950ZZ	0C9M30Z	0CB40ZX	0CC33ZZ	0CCW0Z0	0CJY8ZZ	0CN70ZZ
0BW1XJZ	0BWT02Z	0BYM0Z2	0C5P3ZZ	0C9530Z	0C9M3ZX	0CB43ZX	0CC3XZZ	0CCW0Z1	0CJYXZZ	0CN73ZZ
0BW1XKZ	0BWT07Z	0C00X7Z	0C5PXZZ	0C953ZX	0C9M3ZZ	0CB4XZX	0CC40ZZ	0CCW0Z2	0CLB0CZ	0CN7XZZ
0BWK00Z	0BWT0JZ	0C00XJZ	0C5Q0ZZ	0C953ZZ	0C9M4ZX	0CB50ZX	0CC43ZZ	0CCWXZ0	0CLB0DZ	0CN80ZZ
0BWK02Z	0BWT0KZ	0C00XKZ	0C5Q3ZZ	0C95X0Z	0C9M7ZX	0CB50ZZ	0CC4XZZ	0CCWXZ1	0CLB0ZZ	0CN83ZZ
0BWK03Z	0BWT0MZ	0C00XZZ	0C5QXZZ	0C95XZX	0C9M8ZX	0CB53ZX	0CC50ZZ	0CCWXZ2	0CLB3CZ	0CN90ZZ
0BWK0YZ	0BWT0YZ	0C01X7Z	0C5R0ZZ	0C95XZZ	0C9N30Z	0CB53ZZ	0CC53ZZ	0CCX0Z0	0CLB3DZ	0CN93ZZ
0BWK30Z	0BWT30Z	0C01X1Z	0C5R3ZZ	0C9600Z	0C9N3ZZ	0CB5XZX	0CC5XZZ	0CCX0Z1	0CLB3ZZ	0CNB0ZZ
0BWK32Z	0BWT32Z	0C01XKZ	0C5R4ZZ	0C960ZX	0C9P30Z	0CB5XZZ	0CC60ZZ	0CCX0Z2	0CLB4CZ	0CNB3ZZ
0BWK33Z	0BWT37Z	0C01XZZ	0C5R7ZZ	0C960ZZ	0C9P3ZZ	0CB60ZX	0CC63ZZ	0CCXXZ0	0CLB4DZ	0CNC0ZZ
0BWK3YZ	0BWT3JZ	0C2AX0Z	0C5R8ZZ	0C9630Z	0C9Q30Z	0CB60ZZ	0CC6XZZ	0CCXXZ1	0CLB4ZZ	0CNC3ZZ
0BWK40Z	0BWT3KZ	0C2AXYZ	0C5S0ZZ	0C963ZX	0C9Q3ZZ	0CB63ZX	0CC70ZZ	0CCXXZ2	0CLB7DZ	0CND0ZZ
0BWK42Z	0BWT3MZ	0C2SX0Z	0C5S3ZZ	0C963ZZ	0C9R30Z	0CB63ZZ	0CC73ZZ	0CDT0ZZ	0CLB7ZZ	0CND3ZZ
0BWK43Z	0BWT3YZ	0C2SXYZ	0C5S4ZZ	0C96X0Z	0C9R3ZX	0CB6XZX	0CC7XZZ	0CDT3ZZ	0CLB8DZ	0CNF0ZZ
0BWK4YZ	0BWT40Z	0C2YX0Z	0C5S7ZZ	0C96XZX	0C9R3ZZ	0CB6XZZ	0CC80ZZ	0CDT4ZZ	0CLB8ZZ	0CNF3ZZ
0BWK70Z	0BWT42Z	0C2YXYZ	0C5S8ZZ	0C96XZZ	0C9R4ZX	0CB73ZX	0CC83ZZ	0CDT7ZZ	0CLC0CZ	0CNG0ZZ
0BWK72Z	0BWT47Z	0C500ZZ	0C5T0ZZ	0C9730Z	0C9R7ZX	0CB7XZX	0CC90ZZ	0CDT8ZZ	0CLC0DZ	0CNG3ZZ
0BWK73Z	0BWT4JZ	0C503ZZ	0C5W0Z0	0C973ZX	0C9R8ZX	0CB83ZX	0CC93ZZ	0CDV0ZZ	0CLC0ZZ	0CNH0ZZ
0BWK7YZ	0BWT4KZ	0C50XZZ	0C5W0Z1	0C973ZZ	0C9S30Z	0CB93ZX	0CCB0ZZ	0CDV3ZZ	0CLC3CZ	0CNH3ZZ
0BWK80Z	0BWT4MZ	0C510ZZ	0C5W0Z2	0C97XZX	0C9S3ZX	0CBB3ZX	0CCB3ZZ	0CDV4ZZ	0CLC3DZ	0CNJ0ZZ
0BWK82Z	0BWT4YZ	0C513ZZ	0C5WXZ0	0C9800Z	0C9S3ZZ	0CBC3ZX	0CCC0ZZ	0CDV7ZZ	0CLC3ZZ	0CNJ3ZZ
0BWK83Z	0BWT70Z	0C51XZZ	0C5WXZ1	0C980ZZ	0C9S4ZX	0CBD3ZX	0CCC3ZZ	0CDV8ZZ	0CLC4CZ	0CNM0ZZ
0BWK8YZ	0BWT72Z	0C520ZZ	0C5WXZ2	0C9830Z	0C9S7ZX	0CBF3ZX	0CCD0ZZ	0CDWXZ0	0CLC4DZ	0CNM3ZZ
0BWKX0Z	0BWT77Z	0C523ZZ	0C5X0Z0	0C983ZX	0C9S8ZX	0CBG3ZX	0CCD3ZZ	0CDWXZ1	0CLC4ZZ	0CNM4ZZ
0BWKX2Z	0BWT7JZ	0C52XZZ	0C5X0Z1	0C983ZZ	0C9T30Z	0CBH3ZX	0CCF0ZZ	0CDWXZ2	0CLC7DZ	0CNM7ZZ
0BWKX3Z	0BWT7KZ	0C530ZZ	0C5X0Z2	0C9900Z	0C9T3ZX	0CBJ3ZX	0CCF3ZZ	0CDXXZ0	0CLC7ZZ	0CNM8ZZ
0BWL00Z	0BWT7MZ	0C533ZZ	0C5XXZ0	0C990ZZ	0C9T3ZZ	0CBM0ZX	0CCG0ZZ	0CDXXZ1	0CLC8DZ	0CNN0ZZ
0BWL02Z	0BWT7YZ	0C53XZZ	0C5XXZ1	0C9930Z	0C9T4ZX	0CBM3ZX	0CCG3ZZ	0CDXXZ2	0CLC8ZZ	0CNN3ZZ

0CNNXZZ	0CPS87Z	0CQ73ZZ	0CR007Z	0CRWXJ2	0CU10KZ	0CUM7KZ	0CVC7ZZ	0CWY8DZ	0D11876	0D158JB
0CNP0ZZ	0CPS8DZ	0CQ7XZZ	0CR00JZ	0CRWXK0	0CU137Z	0CUM87Z	0CVC8DZ	0CWY8JZ	0D11879	0D158K4
0CNP3ZZ	0CPS8JZ	0CQ80ZZ	0CR00KZ	0CRWXK1	0CU13JZ	0CUM8JZ	0CVC8ZZ	0CWY8KZ	0D1187A	0D158K6
0CNPXZZ	0CPS8KZ	0CQ83ZZ	0CR037Z	0CRWXK2	0CU13KZ	0CUM8KZ	0CWA00Z	0CWY8YZ	0D1187B	0D158K9
0CNQ0ZZ	0CPS8YZ	0CQ90ZZ	0CR03JZ	0CRX070	0CU1X7Z	0CUN07Z	0CWA0CZ	0CWYX0Z	0D118J4	0D158KA
0CNQ3ZZ	0CPSX0Z	0CQ93ZZ	0CR03KZ	0CRX071	0CU1XJZ	0CUN0JZ	0CWA0YZ	0CWYX1Z	0D118J6	0D158KB
0CNQXZZ	0CPSX7Z	0CQB0ZZ	0CR0X7Z	0CRX072	0CU1XKZ	0CUN0KZ	0CWA30Z	0CWYX7Z	0D118J9	0D158Z4
0CNR0ZZ	0CPSXDZ	0CQB3ZZ	0CR0XJZ	0CRX0J0	0CU207Z	0CUN37Z	0CWA3CZ	0CWYXDZ	0D118JA	0D158Z6
0CNR3ZZ	0CPSXJZ	0CQC0ZZ	0CR0XKZ	0CRX0J1	0CU20JZ	0CUN3JZ	0CWA3YZ	0CWYXJZ	0D118JB	0D158Z9
0CNR4ZZ	0CPSXKZ	0CQC3ZZ	0CR107Z	0CRX0J2	0CU20KZ	0CUN3KZ	0CWA7YZ	0CWYXKZ	0D118K4	0D158ZA
0CNR7ZZ	0CPY00Z	0CQD0ZZ	0CR10JZ	0CRX0K0	0CU237Z	0CUNX7Z	0CWA8YZ	0CX00ZZ	0D118K6	0D158ZB
0CNR8ZZ	0CPY01Z	0CQD3ZZ	0CR10KZ	0CRX0K1	0CU23JZ	0CUNXJZ	0CWAX0Z	0CX0XZZ	0D118K9	0D16074
0CNS0ZZ	0CPY07Z	0CQF0ZZ	0CR137Z	0CRX0K2	0CU23KZ	0CUNXKZ	0CWAXCZ	0CX10ZZ	0D118KA	0D16079
0CNS3ZZ	0CPY0DZ	0CQF3ZZ	0CR13JZ	0CRXX70	0CU2X7Z	0CUR07Z	0CWS00Z	0CX1XZZ	0D118KB	0D1607A
0CNS4ZZ	0CPY0JZ	0CQG0ZZ	0CR13KZ	0CRXX71	0CU2XJZ	0CUR0JZ	0CWS07Z	0CX30ZZ	0D118Z4	0D1607B
0CNS7ZZ	0CPY0KZ	0CQG3ZZ	0CR1X7Z	0CRXX72	0CU2XKZ	0CUR0KZ	0CWS0DZ	0CX3XZZ	0D118Z6	0D1607L
0CNS8ZZ	0CPY0YZ	0CQH0ZZ	0CR1XJZ	0CRXXJ0	0CU307Z	0CUR77Z	0CWS0JZ	0CX40ZZ	0D118Z9	0D160J4
0CNT0ZZ	0CPY30Z	0CQH3ZZ	0CR1XKZ	0CRXXJ1	0CU30JZ	0CUR7JZ	0CWS0KZ	0CX4XZZ	0D118ZA	0D160J9
0CNT3ZZ	0CPY31Z	0CQJ0ZZ	0CR207Z	0CRXXJ2	0CU30KZ	0CUR7KZ	0CWS0YZ	0CX50ZZ	0D118ZB	0D160JA
0CNT4ZZ	0CPY37Z	0CQJ3ZZ	0CR20JZ	0CRXXK0	0CU337Z	0CUR87Z	0CWS30Z	0CX5XZZ	0D12074	0D160JB
0CNT7ZZ	0CPY3DZ	0CQM0ZZ	0CR20KZ	0CRXXK1	0CU33JZ	0CUR8JZ	0CWS37Z	0CX60ZZ	0D12076	0D160JL
0CNT8ZZ	0CPY3JZ	0CQM3ZZ	0CR237Z	0CRXXK2	0CU33KZ	0CUR8KZ	0CWS3DZ	0CX6XZZ	0D12079	0D160K4
0CNV0ZZ	0CPY3KZ	0CQM4ZZ	0CR23JZ	0CU3X7Z	0CWS3JZ	0CX70ZZ	0D1207A	0D160K9			
0CNV3ZZ	0CPY3YZ	0CQM7ZZ	0CR23KZ	0CSW050	0CU3XJZ	0CUS07Z	0CWS3KZ	0CX70ZZ	0D1207A	0D160K9
0CNV4ZZ	0CPY70Z	0CQM8ZZ	0CR2X7Z	0CSW051	0CU3XKZ	0CUS0JZ	0CWS3YZ	0CX7XZZ	0D1207B	0D160KA
0CNV7ZZ	0CPY71Z	0CQN0ZZ	0CR2XJZ	0CSW052	0CU407Z	0CUS0KZ	0CWS70Z	0D11074	0D120J4	0D160KB
0CNV8ZZ	0CPY77Z	0CQN3ZZ	0CR2XKZ	0CSW0Z0	0CU40JZ	0CUS77Z	0CWS77Z	0D11076	0D120J6	0D160KL
0CNW0Z0	0CPY7DZ	0CQNXZZ	0CR307Z	0CSW0Z1	0CU40KZ	0CUS7JZ	0CWS7DZ	0D11079	0D150K4	0D160Z4
0CNW0Z1	0CPY7JZ	0CQP0ZZ	0CR30JZ	0CSW0Z2	0CU437Z	0CUS7KZ	0CWS7JZ	0D1107A	0D150K6	0D160Z9
0CNW0Z2	0CPY7KZ	0CQP3ZZ	0CR30KZ	0CSWX50	0CU43JZ	0CUS87Z	0CWS7KZ	0D1107B	0D150K9	0D160ZA
0CNWXZ0	0CPY7YZ	0CQPXZZ	0CR337Z	0CSWX51	0CU43KZ	0CUS8JZ	0CWS7YZ	0D110J4	0D150KA	0D160ZB
0CNWXZ1	0CPY80Z	0CQQ0ZZ	0CR33JZ	0CSWX52	0CU4X7Z	0CUS8KZ	0CWS80Z	0D110J6	0D150KB	0D160ZL
0CNWXZ2	0CPY81Z	0CQQ3ZZ	0CR33KZ	0CSWXZ0	0CU4XJZ	0CUT07Z	0CWS87Z	0D110J9	0D150Z4	0D163J4
0CNX0Z0	0CPY87Z	0CQQXZZ	0CR3X7Z	0CSWXZ1	0CU4XKZ	0CUT0JZ	0CWS8DZ	0D110JA	0D150Z6	0D16474
0CNX0Z1	0CPY8DZ	0CQR0ZZ	0CR3XJZ	0CSWXZ2	0CU507Z	0CUT0KZ	0CWS8JZ	0D110JB	0D150Z9	0D16479
0CNX0Z2	0CPY8JZ	0CQR3ZZ	0CR3XKZ	0CSX050	0CU50JZ	0CUT77Z	0CWS8KZ	0D110K4	0D150ZA	0D1647A
0CNXXZ0	0CPY8KZ	0CQR4ZZ	0CR407Z	0CSX051	0CU50KZ	0CUT7JZ	0CWS8YZ	0D110K6	0D150ZB	0D1647B
0CNXXZ1	0CPY8YZ	0CQR7ZZ	0CR40JZ	0CSX052	0CU537Z	0CUT7KZ	0CWSX0Z	0D110K9	0D153J4	0D1647L
0CNXXZ2	0CPYX0Z	0CQR8ZZ	0CR40KZ	0CSX0Z0	0CU53JZ	0CUT87Z	0CWSX7Z	0D110KA	0D15474	0D164J4
0CPA00Z	0CPYX1Z	0CQS0ZZ	0CR437Z	0CSX0Z1	0CU53KZ	0CUT8JZ	0CWSXDZ	0D110KB	0D15476	0D164J9
0CPA0CZ	0CPYX7Z	0CQS3ZZ	0CR43JZ	0CSX0Z2	0CU5X7Z	0CUT8KZ	0CWSXJZ	0D110Z4	0D15479	0D164JA
0CPA0YZ	0CPYXDZ	0CQS4ZZ	0CR43KZ	0CSXX50	0CU5XJZ	0CUV07Z	0CWSXKZ	0D110Z6	0D1547A	0D164JB
0CPA30Z	0CPYXJZ	0CQS7ZZ	0CR4X7Z	0CSXX51	0CU5XKZ	0CUV0JZ	0CWY00Z	0D110Z9	0D1547B	0D164JL
0CPA3CZ	0CPYXKZ	0CQS8ZZ	0CR4XJZ	0CSXXZ0	0CU607Z	0CUV0KZ	0CWY01Z	0D110ZA	0D154J4	0D164K4
0CPA3YZ	0CQ00ZZ	0CQT0ZZ	0CR4XKZ	0CSXXZ1	0CU60JZ	0CUV77Z	0CWY07Z	0D110ZB	0D154J6	0D164K9
0CPA7YZ	0CQ03ZZ	0CQT3ZZ	0CR507Z	0CSXXZ2	0CU60KZ	0CUV7JZ	0CWY0DZ	0D113J4	0D154J9	0D164KA
0CPA8YZ	0CQ0XZZ	0CQT4ZZ	0CR50JZ	0CTV4ZZ	0CU637Z	0CUV7KZ	0CWY0JZ	0D11474	0D154JA	0D164KB
0CPS00Z	0CQ10ZZ	0CQT7ZZ	0CR50KZ	0CTV7ZZ	0CU63JZ	0CUV87Z	0CWY0KZ	0D11476	0D154JB	0D164KL
0CPS07Z	0CQ13ZZ	0CQT8ZZ	0CR537Z	0CTV8ZZ	0CU63KZ	0CUV8JZ	0CWY0YZ	0D11479	0D154K4	0D164Z4
0CPS0DZ	0CQ1XZZ	0CQV0ZZ	0CR53JZ	0CTW0Z0	0CU6X7Z	0CUV8KZ	0CWY30Z	0D1147A	0D154K6	0D164Z9
0CPS0JZ	0CQ20ZZ	0CQV3ZZ	0CR53KZ	0CTW0Z1	0CU6XJZ	0CVB0CZ	0CWY31Z	0D1147B	0D154K9	0D164ZA
0CPS0KZ	0CQ23ZZ	0CQV4ZZ	0CR5X7Z	0CTW0Z2	0CU6XKZ	0CVB0DZ	0CWY37Z	0D114J4	0D154KA	0D164ZB
0CPS0YZ	0CQ2XZZ	0CQV7ZZ	0CR5X7Z	0CTX0Z0	0CU707Z	0CVB0ZZ	0CWY3DZ	0D114J6	0D154KB	0D164ZL
0CPS30Z	0CQ30ZZ	0CQV8ZZ	0CRW070	0CTX0Z1	0CU70JZ	0CVB3CZ	0CWY3JZ	0D114J9	0D154Z4	0D16874
0CPS37Z	0CQ33ZZ	0CQW0Z0	0CRW071	0CTX0Z2	0CU70KZ	0CVB3DZ	0CWY3KZ	0D114JA	0D154Z6	0D16879
0CPS3DZ	0CQ3XZZ	0CQW0Z1	0CRW072	0CU007Z	0CU737Z	0CVB3ZZ	0CWY3YZ	0D114JB	0D154Z9	0D1687A
0CPS3JZ	0CQ40ZZ	0CQW0Z2	0CRW0J0	0CU00JZ	0CU73JZ	0CVB7DZ	0CWY70Z	0D114K4	0D154ZA	0D1687B
0CPS3KZ	0CQ43ZZ	0CQWXZ0	0CRW0J1	0CU00KZ	0CU73KZ	0CVB7ZZ	0CWY71Z	0D114K6	0D154ZB	0D1687L
0CPS3YZ	0CQ4XZZ	0CQWXZ1	0CRW0J2	0CU037Z	0CU7X7Z	0CVB8DZ	0CWY77Z	0D114K9	0D15874	0D168J4
0CPS70Z	0CQ50ZZ	0CQWXZ2	0CRW0K0	0CU03JZ	0CU7XJZ	0CVB8ZZ	0CWY7DZ	0D114KA	0D15876	0D168J9
0CPS77Z	0CQ53ZZ	0CQX0Z0	0CRW0K1	0CU03KZ	0CU7XKZ	0CVC0CZ	0CWY7JZ	0D114KB	0D15879	0D168JA
0CPS7DZ	0CQ5XZZ	0CQX0Z1	0CRW0K2	0CU0X7Z	0CUM07Z	0CVC0DZ	0CWY7KZ	0D114Z4	0D1587A	0D168JB
0CPS7JZ	0CQ60ZZ	0CQX0Z2	0CRWX70	0CU0XJZ	0CUM0JZ	0CVC0ZZ	0CWY7YZ	0D114Z6	0D1587B	0D168JL
0CPS7KZ	0CQ63ZZ	0CQXXZ0	0CRWX71	0CU0XKZ	0CUM0KZ	0CVC3CZ	0CWY80Z	0D114Z9	0D158J4	0D168K4
0CPS7YZ	0CQ6XZZ	0CQXXZ1	0CRWX72	0CU107Z	0CUM77Z	0CVC3DZ	0CWY81Z	0D114ZA	0D158J6	0D168K9
0CPS80Z	0CQ70ZZ	0CQXXZ2	0CRWXJ1	0CU10JZ	0CUM7JZ	0CVC7DZ	0CWY87Z	0D114ZB	0D158J9	0D168KA
								0D11874	0D158JA	0D168KB

0D168KL	0D1A4ZK	0D1B0KH	0D1H8ZN	0D1K8KM	0D1L8ZL	0D1N474	0D5H4ZZ	0D783DZ	0D7F8DZ	0D7P4DZ
0D168Z4	0D1A4ZL	0D1B0KK	0D1H8ZP	0D1K8KN	0D1L8ZM	0D1N47N	0D5H8ZZ	0D783ZZ	0D7F8ZZ	0D7P4ZZ
0D168Z9	0D1A4ZM	0D1B0KL	0D1K074	0D1K8KP	0D1L8ZN	0D1N47P	0D5K4ZZ	0D784DZ	0D7G0DZ	0D7P7DZ
0D168ZA	0D1A4ZN	0D1B0KM	0D1K07K	0D1K8Z4	0D1L8ZP	0D1N4J4	0D5K8ZZ	0D784ZZ	0D7G0ZZ	0D7P7ZZ
0D168ZB	0D1A4ZP	0D1B0KN	0D1K07L	0D1K8ZK	0D1M074	0D1N4JN	0D5L4ZZ	0D787DZ	0D7G3DZ	0D7P8DZ
0D168ZL	0D1A4ZQ	0D1B0KP	0D1K07M	0D1K8ZL	0D1M07M	0D1N4JP	0D5L8ZZ	0D787ZZ	0D7G3ZZ	0D7Q0DZ
0D19074	0D1A874	0D1B0KQ	0D1K07N	0D1K8ZM	0D1M07N	0D1N4K4	0D5M4ZZ	0D788DZ	0D7G4DZ	0D7Q0ZZ
0D19079	0D1A87A	0D1B0Z4	0D1K07P	0D1K8ZN	0D1M07P	0D1N4KN	0D5M8ZZ	0D788ZZ	0D7G4ZZ	0D7Q3DZ
0D1907A	0D1A87B	0D1B0ZB	0D1K0J4	0D1K8ZP	0D1M0J4	0D1N4KP	0D5N4ZZ	0D790DZ	0D7G7DZ	0D7Q3ZZ
0D1907B	0D1A87H	0D1B0ZH	0D1K0JK	0D1L074	0D1M0JM	0D1N4Z4	0D5N8ZZ	0D790ZZ	0D7G7ZZ	0D7Q4DZ
0D1907L	0D1A87K	0D1B0ZK	0D1K0JL	0D1L07L	0D1M0JN	0D1N4ZN	0D5P0ZZ	0D793DZ	0D7G8DZ	0D7Q4ZZ
0D190J4	0D1A87L	0D1B0ZL	0D1K0JM	0D1L07M	0D1M0JP	0D1N4ZP	0D5P3ZZ	0D793ZZ	0D7G8ZZ	0D7Q7DZ
0D190J9	0D1A87M	0D1B0ZM	0D1K0JN	0D1L07N	0D1M0K4	0D1N874	0D5P4ZZ	0D794DZ	0D7H0DZ	0D7Q7ZZ
0D190JA	0D1A87N	0D1B0ZN	0D1K0JP	0D1L07P	0D1M0KM	0D1N87N	0D5P7ZZ	0D794ZZ	0D7H0ZZ	0D7Q8DZ
0D190JB	0D1A87P	0D1B0ZP	0D1K0K4	0D1L0J4	0D1M0KN	0D1N87P	0D5P8ZZ	0D797DZ	0D7H3DZ	0D7Q8ZZ
0D190JL	0D1A87Q	0D1B0ZQ	0D1K0KK	0D1L0JL	0D1M0KP	0D1N8J4	0D5Q4ZZ	0D797ZZ	0D7H3ZZ	0D840ZZ
0D190K4	0D1A8J4	0D1B3J4	0D1K0KL	0D1L0JM	0D1M0Z4	0D1N8JN	0D5Q8ZZ	0D798DZ	0D7H4DZ	0D843ZZ
0D190K9	0D1A8JA	0D1B474	0D1K0KM	0D1L0JN	0D1M0ZM	0D1N8JP	0D5R4ZZ	0D798ZZ	0D7H4ZZ	0D844ZZ
0D190KA	0D1A8JB	0D1B47B	0D1K0KN	0D1L0JP	0D1M0ZN	0D1N8K4	0D5U0ZZ	0D7A0DZ	0D7H7DZ	0D847ZZ
0D190KB	0D1A8JH	0D1B47H	0D1K0KP	0D1L0K4	0D1M0ZP	0D1N8KN	0D5U3ZZ	0D7A0ZZ	0D7H7ZZ	0D848ZZ
0D190KL	0D1A8JK	0D1B47K	0D1K0Z4	0D1L0KL	0D1M3J4	0D1N8KP	0D5U4ZZ	0D7A3DZ	0D7H8DZ	0D870ZZ
0D190Z4	0D1A8JL	0D1B47L	0D1K0ZK	0D1L0KM	0D1M474	0D1N8Z4	0D717DZ	0D7A3ZZ	0D7H8ZZ	0D873ZZ
0D190Z9	0D1A8JM	0D1B47M	0D1K0ZL	0D1L0KN	0D1M47M	0D1N8ZN	0D717ZZ	0D7A4DZ	0D7K0DZ	0D874ZZ
0D190ZA	0D1A8JN	0D1B47N	0D1K0ZM	0D1L0KP	0D1M47N	0D1N8ZP	0D718DZ	0D7A4ZZ	0D7K0ZZ	0D877ZZ
0D190ZB	0D1A8JP	0D1B47P	0D1K0ZN	0D1L0Z4	0D1M47P	0D20X0Z	0D718ZZ	0D7A7DZ	0D7K3DZ	0D878ZZ
0D190ZL	0D1A8JQ	0D1B47Q	0D1K0ZP	0D1L0ZL	0D1M4J4	0D20XUZ	0D727DZ	0D7A7ZZ	0D7K3ZZ	0D8R0ZZ
0D193J4	0D1A8K4	0D1B4J4	0D1K3J4	0D1L0ZM	0D1M4JM	0D20XYZ	0D727ZZ	0D7A8DZ	0D7K4DZ	0D8R3ZZ
0D19474	0D1A8KA	0D1B4JB	0D1K474	0D1L0ZN	0D1M4JN	0D2DX0Z	0D728DZ	0D7A8ZZ	0D7K4ZZ	0D9100Z
0D19479	0D1A8KB	0D1B4JH	0D1K47K	0D1L0ZP	0D1M4JP	0D2DXUZ	0D728ZZ	0D7B0DZ	0D7K7DZ	0D910ZX
0D1947A	0D1A8KH	0D1B4JK	0D1K47L	0D1L3J4	0D1M4K4	0D2DXYZ	0D737DZ	0D7B0ZZ	0D7K7ZZ	0D910ZZ
0D1947B	0D1A8KK	0D1B4JL	0D1K47M	0D1L474	0D1M4KM	0D2UX0Z	0D737ZZ	0D7B3DZ	0D7K8DZ	0D9130Z
0D1947L	0D1A8KL	0D1B4JM	0D1K47N	0D1L47L	0D1M4KN	0D2UXYZ	0D738DZ	0D7B3ZZ	0D7K8ZZ	0D913ZX
0D194J4	0D1A8KM	0D1B4JN	0D1K47P	0D1L47M	0D1M4KP	0D2VX0Z	0D738ZZ	0D7B4DZ	0D7L0DZ	0D913ZZ
0D194J9	0D1A8KN	0D1B4JP	0D1K4J4	0D1L47N	0D1M4Z4	0D2VXYZ	0D747DZ	0D7B4ZZ	0D7L0ZZ	0D9140Z
0D194JA	0D1A8KP	0D1B4JQ	0D1K4JK	0D1L47P	0D1M4ZM	0D2WX0Z	0D747ZZ	0D7B7DZ	0D7L3DZ	0D914ZX
0D194JB	0D1A8KQ	0D1B4K4	0D1K4JL	0D1L4J4	0D1M4ZN	0D2WXYZ	0D748DZ	0D7B7ZZ	0D7L3ZZ	0D914ZZ
0D194JL	0D1A8Z4	0D1B4KB	0D1K4JM	0D1L4JL	0D1M4ZP	0D510ZZ	0D748ZZ	0D7B8DZ	0D7L4DZ	0D9170Z
0D194K4	0D1A8ZA	0D1B4KH	0D1K4JN	0D1L4JM	0D1M874	0D513ZZ	0D753ZZ	0D7B8ZZ	0D7L4ZZ	0D917ZX
0D194K9	0D1A8ZB	0D1B4KK	0D1K4JP	0D1L4JN	0D1M87M	0D514ZZ	0D754DZ	0D7C0DZ	0D7L7DZ	0D917ZZ
0D194KA	0D1A8ZH	0D1B4KL	0D1K4K4	0D1L4JP	0D1M87N	0D517ZZ	0D754ZZ	0D7C0ZZ	0D7L7ZZ	0D9180Z
0D194KB	0D1A8ZK	0D1B4KM	0D1K4KK	0D1L4K4	0D1M87P	0D518ZZ	0D757DZ	0D7C3DZ	0D7L8DZ	0D918ZX
0D194KL	0D1A8ZL	0D1B4KN	0D1K4KL	0D1L4KL	0D1M8J4	0D520ZZ	0D757ZZ	0D7C3ZZ	0D7L8ZZ	0D918ZZ
0D194Z4	0D1A8ZM	0D1B4KP	0D1K4KM	0D1L4KM	0D1M8JM	0D523ZZ	0D758DZ	0D7C4DZ	0D7M0DZ	0D9200Z
0D194Z9	0D1A8ZN	0D1B4KQ	0D1K4KN	0D1L4KN	0D1M8JN	0D524ZZ	0D758ZZ	0D7C4ZZ	0D7M0ZZ	0D920ZX
0D1A4JB	0D1A8ZP	0D1B4Z4	0D1K4KP	0D1L4KP	0D1M8JP	0D527ZZ	0D760DZ	0D7C7DZ	0D7M3DZ	0D920ZZ
0D1A4JH	0D1A8ZQ	0D1B4ZB	0D1K4Z4	0D1L4Z4	0D1M8K4	0D528ZZ	0D760ZZ	0D7C7ZZ	0D7M3ZZ	0D9230Z
0D1A4JK	0D1B074	0D1B4ZH	0D1K4ZK	0D1L4ZL	0D1M8KM	0D530ZZ	0D763DZ	0D7C8DZ	0D7M4DZ	0D923ZX
0D1A4JL	0D1B07B	0D1B4ZK	0D1K4ZL	0D1L4ZM	0D1M8KN	0D533ZZ	0D763ZZ	0D7C8ZZ	0D7M4ZZ	0D923ZZ
0D1A4JM	0D1B07H	0D1B4ZL	0D1K4ZM	0D1L4ZN	0D1M8KP	0D534ZZ	0D764DZ	0D7E0DZ	0D7M7DZ	0D9240Z
0D1A4JN	0D1B07K	0D1B4ZM	0D1K4ZN	0D1L4ZP	0D1M8Z4	0D538ZZ	0D764ZZ	0D7E0ZZ	0D7M7ZZ	0D924ZX
0D1A4JP	0D1B07L	0D1B4ZN	0D1K4ZP	0D1L874	0D1M8ZM	0D544ZZ	0D767DZ	0D7E3DZ	0D7M8DZ	0D924ZZ
0D1A4JQ	0D1B07M	0D1B4ZP	0D1K874	0D1L87L	0D1M8ZN	0D548ZZ	0D767ZZ	0D7E3ZZ	0D7M8ZZ	0D9270Z
0D1A4K4	0D1B07N	0D1B4ZQ	0D1K87K	0D1L87M	0D1M8ZP	0D554ZZ	0D768DZ	0D7E4DZ	0D7N0DZ	0D927ZX
0D1A4KA	0D1B07P	0D1B874	0D1K87L	0D1L87N	0D1N074	0D558ZZ	0D768ZZ	0D7E4ZZ	0D7N0ZZ	0D927ZZ
0D1A4KB	0D1B07Q	0D1B87B	0D1K87M	0D1L87P	0D1N07N	0D564ZZ	0D770DZ	0D7E7DZ	0D7N3DZ	0D9280Z
0D1A4KH	0D1B0J4	0D1B87H	0D1K87N	0D1L8J4	0D1N07P	0D568ZZ	0D770ZZ	0D7E7ZZ	0D7N3ZZ	0D928ZX
0D1A4KK	0D1B0JB	0D1B87K	0D1K87P	0D1L8JL	0D1N0J4	0D574ZZ	0D773DZ	0D7E8DZ	0D7N4DZ	0D928ZZ
0D1A4KL	0D1B0JH	0D1B87L	0D1K8J4	0D1L8JM	0D1N0JN	0D578ZZ	0D773ZZ	0D7E8ZZ	0D7N4ZZ	0D9300Z
0D1A4KM	0D1B0JK	0D1B87M	0D1K8JK	0D1L8JN	0D1N0JP	0D594ZZ	0D774DZ	0D7F0DZ	0D7N7DZ	0D930ZX
0D1A4KN	0D1B0JL	0D1B87N	0D1K8JL	0D1L8JP	0D1N0K4	0D598ZZ	0D774ZZ	0D7F0ZZ	0D7N7ZZ	0D930ZZ
0D1A4KP	0D1B0JM	0D1B87P	0D1K8JM	0D1L8K4	0D1N0KN	0D5E4ZZ	0D777DZ	0D7F3DZ	0D7N8DZ	0D9330Z
0D1A4KQ	0D1B0JN	0D1B87Q	0D1K8JN	0D1L8KL	0D1N0KP	0D5E8ZZ	0D777ZZ	0D7F3ZZ	0D7N8ZZ	0D933ZX
0D1A4Z4	0D1B0JP	0D1B8J4	0D1K8JP	0D1L8KM	0D1N0Z4	0D5F4ZZ	0D778DZ	0D7F4DZ	0D7P0DZ	0D933ZZ
0D1A4ZA	0D1B0JQ	0D1B8JB	0D1K8K4	0D1L8KN	0D1N0ZN	0D5F8ZZ	0D778ZZ	0D7F4ZZ	0D7P0ZZ	0D9340Z
0D1A4ZB	0D1B0K4	0D1B8JH	0D1K8KK	0D1L8KP	0D1N0ZP	0D5G4ZZ	0D780DZ	0D7F7DZ	0D7P3DZ	0D934ZX
0D1A4ZH	0D1B0KB	0D1B8JK	0D1K8KL	0D1L8Z4	0D1N3J4	0D5G8ZZ	0D780ZZ	0D7F7ZZ	0D7P3ZZ	

0D934ZZ	0D978ZZ	0D9C3ZZ	0D9H7ZZ	0D9N0ZZ	0D9V0ZZ	0DB60Z3	0DBK8ZZ	0DC53ZZ	0DCK4ZZ	0DD94ZX
0D9370Z	0D9800Z	0D9C40Z	0D9H80Z	0D9N30Z	0D9V30Z	0DB60ZX	0DBL3ZX	0DC54ZZ	0DCK7ZZ	0DD98ZX
0D937ZX	0D980ZX	0D9C4ZX	0D9H8ZX	0D9N3ZX	0D9V3ZX	0DB60ZZ	0DBL4ZX	0DC57ZZ	0DCK8ZZ	0DDA3ZX
0D937ZZ	0D980ZZ	0D9C4ZZ	0D9H8ZZ	0D9N3ZZ	0D9V3ZZ	0DB63Z3	0DBL7ZX	0DC58ZZ	0DCL0ZZ	0DDA4ZX
0D9380Z	0D9830Z	0D9C70Z	0D9J00Z	0D9N40Z	0D9V40Z	0DB63ZX	0DBL8ZX	0DC60ZZ	0DCL3ZZ	0DDA8ZX
0D938ZX	0D983ZX	0D9C7ZX	0D9J0ZX	0D9N4ZX	0D9V4ZX	0DB63ZZ	0DBL8ZZ	0DC63ZZ	0DCL4ZZ	0DDB3ZX
0D938ZZ	0D983ZZ	0D9C7ZZ	0D9J0ZZ	0D9N4ZZ	0D9V4ZZ	0DB64Z3	0DBLFZZ	0DC64ZZ	0DCL7ZZ	0DDB4ZX
0D9400Z	0D9840Z	0D9C80Z	0D9J30Z	0D9N70Z	0D9W00Z	0DB64ZX	0DBM3ZX	0DC67ZZ	0DCL8ZZ	0DDB8ZX
0D940ZX	0D984ZX	0D9C8ZX	0D9J3ZX	0D9N7ZX	0D9W0ZX	0DB64ZZ	0DBM4ZX	0DC68ZZ	0DCM0ZZ	0DDC3ZX
0D940ZZ	0D984ZZ	0D9C8ZZ	0D9J3ZZ	0D9N7ZZ	0D9W0ZZ	0DB67Z3	0DBM7ZX	0DC70ZZ	0DCM3ZZ	0DDC4ZX
0D9430Z	0D9870Z	0D9E00Z	0D9J40Z	0D9N80Z	0D9W30Z	0DB67ZX	0DBM8ZX	0DC73ZZ	0DCM4ZZ	0DDC8ZX
0D943ZX	0D987ZX	0D9E0ZX	0D9J4ZX	0D9N8ZX	0D9W3ZX	0DB68ZX	0DBM8ZZ	0DC74ZZ	0DCM7ZZ	0DDE3ZX
0D943ZZ	0D987ZZ	0D9E0ZZ	0D9J4ZZ	0D9N8ZZ	0D9W3ZZ	0DB68ZZ	0DBMFZZ	0DC77ZZ	0DCM8ZZ	0DDE4ZX
0D9440Z	0D9880Z	0D9E30Z	0D9J70Z	0D9P00Z	0D9W40Z	0DB73ZX	0DBN3ZX	0DC78ZZ	0DCN0ZZ	0DDE8ZX
0D944ZX	0D988ZX	0D9E3ZX	0D9J7ZX	0D9P0ZX	0D9W4ZX	0DB74ZX	0DBN4ZX	0DC80ZZ	0DCN3ZZ	0DDF3ZX
0D944ZZ	0D988ZZ	0D9E3ZZ	0D9J7ZZ	0D9P0ZZ	0D9W4ZZ	0DB74ZZ	0DBN7ZX	0DC83ZZ	0DCN4ZZ	0DDF4ZX
0D9470Z	0D9900Z	0D9E40Z	0D9J80Z	0D9P30Z	0DB10ZX	0DB77ZX	0DBN8ZX	0DC84ZZ	0DCN7ZZ	0DDF8ZX
0D947ZX	0D990ZX	0D9E4ZX	0D9J8ZX	0D9P3ZX	0DB10ZZ	0DB78ZX	0DBN8ZZ	0DC87ZZ	0DCN8ZZ	0DDG3ZX
0D947ZZ	0D990ZZ	0D9E4ZZ	0D9J8ZZ	0D9P3ZZ	0DB13ZX	0DB78ZZ	0DBNFZZ	0DC88ZZ	0DCP0ZZ	0DDG4ZX
0D9480Z	0D9930Z	0D9E70Z	0D9K00Z	0D9P40Z	0DB13ZZ	0DB83ZX	0DBP3ZX	0DC90ZZ	0DCP3ZZ	0DDG8ZX
0D948ZX	0D993ZX	0D9E7ZX	0D9K0ZX	0D9P4ZX	0DB14ZX	0DB84ZX	0DBP4ZX	0DC93ZZ	0DCP4ZZ	0DDH3ZX
0D948ZZ	0D993ZZ	0D9E7ZZ	0D9K0ZZ	0D9P4ZZ	0DB14ZZ	0DB87ZX	0DBP7ZX	0DC94ZZ	0DCP7ZZ	0DDH4ZX
0D9500Z	0D9940Z	0D9E80Z	0D9K30Z	0D9P70Z	0DB17ZX	0DB88ZX	0DBP8ZX	0DC97ZZ	0DCP8ZZ	0DDH8ZX
0D950ZX	0D994ZX	0D9E8ZX	0D9K3ZX	0D9P7ZX	0DB17ZZ	0DB93ZX	0DBP8ZZ	0DC98ZZ	0DCQ0ZZ	0DDJ3ZX
0D950ZZ	0D994ZZ	0D9E8ZZ	0D9K3ZZ	0D9P7ZZ	0DB18ZX	0DB94ZX	0DBQ0ZX	0DCA0ZZ	0DCQ3ZZ	0DDJ4ZX
0D9530Z	0D9970Z	0D9F00Z	0D9K40Z	0D9P80Z	0DB18ZZ	0DB94ZZ	0DBQ3ZX	0DCA3ZZ	0DCQ4ZZ	0DDJ8ZX
0D953ZX	0D997ZX	0D9F0ZX	0D9K4ZX	0D9P8ZX	0DB20ZX	0DB97ZX	0DBQ4ZX	0DCA7ZZ	0DCQ7ZZ	0DDK3ZX
0D953ZZ	0D997ZZ	0D9F0ZZ	0D9K4ZZ	0D9P8ZZ	0DB20ZZ	0DB98ZX	0DBQ7ZX	0DCA8ZZ	0DCQ8ZZ	0DDK4ZX
0D9540Z	0D9980Z	0D9F30Z	0D9K70Z	0D9Q00Z	0DB23ZX	0DB98ZZ	0DBQ8ZX	0DCB0ZZ	0DCQXZZ	0DDK8ZX
0D954ZX	0D998ZX	0D9F3ZX	0D9K7ZX	0D9Q0ZX	0DB23ZZ	0DBA3ZX	0DBQXZZ	0DCB3ZZ	0DCR0ZZ	0DDL3ZX
0D954ZZ	0D998ZZ	0D9F3ZZ	0D9K7ZZ	0D9Q0ZZ	0DB24ZX	0DBA4ZX	0DBR0ZX	0DCB4ZZ	0DCR3ZZ	0DDL4ZX
0D9570Z	0D9A00Z	0D9F40Z	0D9K80Z	0D9Q30Z	0DB24ZZ	0DBA7ZX	0DBR3ZX	0DCB7ZZ	0DCR4ZZ	0DDL8ZX
0D957ZX	0D9A0ZX	0D9F4ZX	0D9K8ZX	0D9Q3ZX	0DB27ZX	0DBA8ZX	0DBR4ZX	0DCB8ZZ	0DCU0ZZ	0DDM3ZX
0D957ZZ	0D9A0ZZ	0D9F4ZZ	0D9K8ZZ	0D9Q3ZZ	0DB27ZZ	0DBB3ZX	0DBU0ZX	0DCC0ZZ	0DCU3ZZ	0DDM4ZX
0D9580Z	0D9A30Z	0D9F70Z	0D9L00Z	0D9Q40Z	0DB28ZX	0DBB4ZX	0DBU0ZZ	0DCC3ZZ	0DCU4ZZ	0DDM8ZX
0D958ZX	0D9A3ZX	0D9F7ZX	0D9L0ZX	0D9Q4ZX	0DB28ZZ	0DBB7ZX	0DBU3ZX	0DCC4ZZ	0DCV0ZZ	0DDN3ZX
0D958ZZ	0D9A3ZZ	0D9F7ZZ	0D9L0ZZ	0D9Q4ZZ	0DB30ZX	0DBB8ZX	0DBU3ZZ	0DCC7ZZ	0DCV3ZZ	0DDN4ZX
0D9600Z	0D9A40Z	0D9F80Z	0D9L30Z	0D9Q70Z	0DB30ZZ	0DBC3ZX	0DBU4ZX	0DCC8ZZ	0DCV4ZZ	0DDN8ZX
0D960ZX	0D9A4ZX	0D9F8ZX	0D9L3ZX	0D9Q7ZX	0DB33ZX	0DBC4ZX	0DBU4ZZ	0DCE0ZZ	0DCW0ZZ	0DDP3ZX
0D960ZZ	0D9A4ZZ	0D9F8ZZ	0D9L3ZZ	0D9Q7ZZ	0DB33ZZ	0DBC7ZX	0DBV3ZX	0DCE3ZZ	0DCW3ZZ	0DDP4ZX
0D9630Z	0D9A70Z	0D9G00Z	0D9L40Z	0D9Q80Z	0DB34ZX	0DBC8ZX	0DBV4ZX	0DCE4ZZ	0DCW4ZZ	0DDP8ZX
0D963ZX	0D9A7ZX	0D9G0ZX	0D9L4ZX	0D9Q8ZX	0DB34ZZ	0DBE3ZX	0DBW3ZX	0DCE7ZZ	0DD13ZX	0DDQ3ZX
0D963ZZ	0D9A7ZZ	0D9G0ZZ	0D9L4ZZ	0D9Q8ZZ	0DB37ZX	0DBE4ZX	0DBW3ZZ	0DCE8ZZ	0DD14ZX	0DDQ4ZX
0D9640Z	0D9A80Z	0D9G30Z	0D9L70Z	0D9QX0Z	0DB37ZZ	0DBE7ZX	0DBW4ZX	0DCF0ZZ	0DD18ZX	0DDQ8ZX
0D964ZX	0D9A8ZX	0D9G3ZX	0D9L7ZX	0D9QXZX	0DB38ZX	0DBE8ZX	0DBW4ZZ	0DCF3ZZ	0DD23ZX	0DDQXZX
0D964ZZ	0D9A8ZZ	0D9G3ZZ	0D9L7ZZ	0D9QXZZ	0DB38ZZ	0DBE8ZZ	0DC10ZZ	0DCF4ZZ	0DD24ZX	0DF50ZZ
0D9670Z	0D9B00Z	0D9G40Z	0D9L80Z	0D9R00Z	0DB40ZX	0DBF3ZX	0DC13ZZ	0DCF7ZZ	0DD28ZX	0DF53ZZ
0D967ZX	0D9B0ZX	0D9G4ZX	0D9L8ZX	0D9R0ZX	0DB40ZZ	0DBF4ZX	0DC14ZZ	0DCF8ZZ	0DD33ZX	0DF54ZZ
0D967ZZ	0D9B0ZZ	0D9G4ZZ	0D9L8ZZ	0D9R0ZZ	0DB43ZX	0DBF7ZX	0DC17ZZ	0DCG0ZZ	0DD34ZX	0DF57ZZ
0D9680Z	0D9B30Z	0D9G70Z	0D9M00Z	0D9R30Z	0DB43ZZ	0DBF8ZX	0DC18ZZ	0DCG3ZZ	0DD38ZX	0DF58ZZ
0D968ZX	0D9B3ZX	0D9G7ZX	0D9M0ZX	0D9R3ZX	0DB44ZX	0DBF8ZZ	0DC20ZZ	0DCG4ZZ	0DD43ZX	0DF5XZZ
0D968ZZ	0D9B3ZZ	0D9G7ZZ	0D9M0ZZ	0D9R3ZZ	0DB44ZZ	0DBG3ZX	0DC23ZZ	0DCG7ZZ	0DD44ZX	0DF60ZZ
0D9700Z	0D9B40Z	0D9G80Z	0D9M30Z	0D9R40Z	0DB47ZX	0DBG4ZX	0DC24ZZ	0DCG8ZZ	0DD48ZX	0DF63ZZ
0D970ZX	0D9B4ZX	0D9G8ZX	0D9M3ZX	0D9R4ZX	0DB47ZZ	0DBG7ZX	0DC27ZZ	0DCH0ZZ	0DD53ZX	0DF64ZZ
0D970ZZ	0D9B4ZZ	0D9G8ZZ	0D9M3ZZ	0D9R4ZZ	0DB48ZX	0DBG8ZX	0DC28ZZ	0DCH3ZZ	0DD54ZX	0DF67ZZ
0D9730Z	0D9B70Z	0D9H00Z	0D9M40Z	0D9U00Z	0DB48ZZ	0DBG8ZZ	0DC30ZZ	0DCH4ZZ	0DD58ZX	0DF68ZZ
0D973ZX	0D9B7ZX	0D9H0ZX	0D9M4ZX	0D9U0ZX	0DB50ZX	0DBGFZZ	0DC33ZZ	0DCH7ZZ	0DD63ZX	0DF6XZZ
0D973ZZ	0D9B7ZZ	0D9H0ZZ	0D9M4ZZ	0D9U0ZZ	0DB50ZZ	0DBH3ZX	0DC34ZZ	0DCH8ZZ	0DD64ZX	0DF80ZZ
0D9740Z	0D9B80Z	0D9H30Z	0D9M70Z	0D9U30Z	0DB53ZX	0DBH4ZX	0DC37ZZ	0DCJ0ZZ	0DD68ZX	0DF83ZZ
0D974ZX	0D9B8ZX	0D9H3ZX	0D9M7ZX	0D9U3ZX	0DB53ZZ	0DBH7ZX	0DC38ZZ	0DCJ3ZZ	0DD73ZX	0DF84ZZ
0D974ZZ	0D9B8ZZ	0D9H3ZZ	0D9M7ZZ	0D9U3ZZ	0DB54ZX	0DBH8ZX	0DC40ZZ	0DCJ4ZZ	0DD74ZX	0DF87ZZ
0D9770Z	0D9C00Z	0D9H40Z	0D9M80Z	0D9U40Z	0DB54ZZ	0DBH8ZZ	0DC43ZZ	0DCJ7ZZ	0DD78ZX	0DF88ZZ
0D977ZX	0D9C0ZX	0D9H4ZX	0D9M8ZX	0D9U4ZX	0DB57ZX	0DBK3ZX	0DC44ZZ	0DCJ8ZZ	0DD83ZX	0DF8XZZ
0D977ZZ	0D9C0ZZ	0D9H4ZZ	0D9M8ZZ	0D9U4ZZ	0DB57ZZ	0DBK4ZX	0DC47ZZ	0DCK0ZZ	0DD84ZX	0DF90ZZ
0D9780Z	0D9C30Z	0D9H70Z	0D9N00Z	0D9V00Z	0DB58ZX	0DBK7ZX	0DC48ZZ	0DCK3ZZ	0DD88ZX	0DF93ZZ
0D978ZX	0D9C3ZX	0D9H7ZX	0D9N0ZX	0D9V0ZX	0DB58ZZ	0DBK8ZX	0DC50ZZ	0DCK3ZZ	0DD93ZX	0DF94ZZ

0DF97ZZ	0DFN7ZZ	0DH64DZ	0DHA72Z	0DJ63ZZ	0DL43DZ	0DNA3ZZ	0DNQ4ZZ	0DP0X0Z	0DP673Z	0DPD87Z
0DF98ZZ	0DFN8ZZ	0DH64MZ	0DHA73Z	0DJ64ZZ	0DL43ZZ	0DNA4ZZ	0DNQ7ZZ	0DP0X2Z	0DP677Z	0DPD8CZ
0DF9XZZ	0DFNXZZ	0DH64UZ	0DHA7DZ	0DJ67ZZ	0DL44CZ	0DNA8ZZ	0DNQ8ZZ	0DP0X3Z	0DP67CZ	0DPD8DZ
0DFA0ZZ	0DFP0ZZ	0DH64YZ	0DHA7UZ	0DJ68ZZ	0DL44DZ	0DNB0ZZ	0DNQXZZ	0DP0XDZ	0DP67DZ	0DPD8JZ
0DFA3ZZ	0DFP3ZZ	0DH672Z	0DHA82Z	0DJ6XZZ	0DL44ZZ	0DNB3ZZ	0DNR0ZZ	0DP0XUZ	0DP67JZ	0DPD8KZ
0DFA4ZZ	0DFP4ZZ	0DH673Z	0DHA83Z	0DJD0ZZ	0DL47DZ	0DNB4ZZ	0DNR3ZZ	0DP501Z	0DP67KZ	0DPD8UZ
0DFA7ZZ	0DFP7ZZ	0DH67DZ	0DHA8DZ	0DJD3ZZ	0DL47ZZ	0DNB7ZZ	0DNR4ZZ	0DP502Z	0DP67UZ	0DPD8YZ
0DFA8ZZ	0DFP8ZZ	0DH67UZ	0DHA8UZ	0DJD4ZZ	0DL48DZ	0DNB8ZZ	0DNU0ZZ	0DP503Z	0DP67YZ	0DPDX0Z
0DFAXZZ	0DFPXZZ	0DH67YZ	0DHB02Z	0DJD7ZZ	0DL48ZZ	0DNC0ZZ	0DNU3ZZ	0DP50UZ	0DP680Z	0DPDX2Z
0DFB0ZZ	0DFQ0ZZ	0DH682Z	0DHB03Z	0DJD8ZZ	0DL50CZ	0DNC3ZZ	0DNU4ZZ	0DP50YZ	0DP682Z	0DPDX3Z
0DFB3ZZ	0DFQ3ZZ	0DH683Z	0DHB0DZ	0DJDXZZ	0DL50DZ	0DNC4ZZ	0DNV0ZZ	0DP531Z	0DP683Z	0DPDXDZ
0DFB4ZZ	0DFQ4ZZ	0DH68DZ	0DHB0UZ	0DJU0ZZ	0DL50ZZ	0DNC7ZZ	0DNV3ZZ	0DP532Z	0DP687Z	0DPDXUZ
0DFB7ZZ	0DFQ7ZZ	0DH68UZ	0DHB32Z	0DJU3ZZ	0DL53CZ	0DNC8ZZ	0DNV4ZZ	0DP533Z	0DP68CZ	0DPP01Z
0DFB8ZZ	0DFQ8ZZ	0DH68YZ	0DHB33Z	0DJU4ZZ	0DL53DZ	0DNE0ZZ	0DNW0ZZ	0DP53UZ	0DP68DZ	0DPP31Z
0DFBXZZ	0DFQXZZ	0DH802Z	0DHB3DZ	0DJUXZZ	0DL53ZZ	0DNE3ZZ	0DNW3ZZ	0DP53YZ	0DP68JZ	0DPP41Z
0DFE0ZZ	0DH00YZ	0DH803Z	0DHB3UZ	0DJV0ZZ	0DL54CZ	0DNE4ZZ	0DNW4ZZ	0DP541Z	0DP68KZ	0DPP71Z
0DFE3ZZ	0DH03YZ	0DH80DZ	0DHB42Z	0DJV3ZZ	0DL54DZ	0DNE7ZZ	0DP000Z	0DP542Z	0DP68UZ	0DPP81Z
0DFE4ZZ	0DH04YZ	0DH80UZ	0DHB43Z	0DJV4ZZ	0DL54ZZ	0DNE8ZZ	0DP002Z	0DP543Z	0DP68YZ	0DPPX1Z
0DFE7ZZ	0DH07YZ	0DH832Z	0DHB4DZ	0DJVXZZ	0DL57DZ	0DNF0ZZ	0DP003Z	0DP54UZ	0DP6X0Z	0DPQ0LZ
0DFE8ZZ	0DH08YZ	0DH833Z	0DHB4UZ	0DJW0ZZ	0DL57ZZ	0DNF3ZZ	0DP007Z	0DP54YZ	0DP6X2Z	0DPQ3LZ
0DFEXZZ	0DH501Z	0DH83DZ	0DHB72Z	0DJW3ZZ	0DL58DZ	0DNF4ZZ	0DP00CZ	0DP571Z	0DP6X3Z	0DPQ4LZ
0DFF0ZZ	0DH502Z	0DH83UZ	0DHB73Z	0DJW4ZZ	0DL58ZZ	0DNF7ZZ	0DP00DZ	0DP57DZ	0DP6XDZ	0DPQ7LZ
0DFF3ZZ	0DH503Z	0DH842Z	0DHB7DZ	0DJWXZZ	0DL60CZ	0DNF8ZZ	0DP00JZ	0DP57YZ	0DP6XUZ	0DPQ8LZ
0DFF4ZZ	0DH50DZ	0DH843Z	0DHB7UZ	0DL10CZ	0DL60DZ	0DNG0ZZ	0DP00KZ	0DP581Z	0DPD00Z	0DPR0MZ
0DFF7ZZ	0DH50UZ	0DH84DZ	0DHB82Z	0DL10DZ	0DL60ZZ	0DNG3ZZ	0DP00UZ	0DP58DZ	0DPD02Z	0DPR3MZ
0DFF8ZZ	0DH50YZ	0DH84UZ	0DHB83Z	0DL10ZZ	0DL63CZ	0DNG4ZZ	0DP00YZ	0DP58YZ	0DPD03Z	0DPR4MZ
0DFFXZZ	0DH531Z	0DH872Z	0DHB8DZ	0DL13CZ	0DL63DZ	0DNG7ZZ	0DP030Z	0DP5X1Z	0DPD07Z	0DPU00Z
0DFG0ZZ	0DH532Z	0DH873Z	0DHB8UZ	0DL13DZ	0DL63ZZ	0DNG8ZZ	0DP032Z	0DP5X2Z	0DPD0CZ	0DPU01Z
0DFG3ZZ	0DH533Z	0DH87DZ	0DHD0YZ	0DL13ZZ	0DL64CZ	0DNH0ZZ	0DP033Z	0DP5X3Z	0DPD0DZ	0DPU07Z
0DFG4ZZ	0DH53DZ	0DH87UZ	0DHD3YZ	0DL14CZ	0DL64DZ	0DNH3ZZ	0DP037Z	0DP5XDZ	0DPD0JZ	0DPU0JZ
0DFG7ZZ	0DH53UZ	0DH882Z	0DHD4YZ	0DL14DZ	0DL64ZZ	0DNH4ZZ	0DP03CZ	0DP5XUZ	0DPD0KZ	0DPU0KZ
0DFG8ZZ	0DH53YZ	0DH883Z	0DHD7YZ	0DL14ZZ	0DL67DZ	0DNH7ZZ	0DP03DZ	0DP600Z	0DPD0UZ	0DPU30Z
0DFGXZZ	0DH541Z	0DH88DZ	0DHD8YZ	0DL17DZ	0DL67ZZ	0DNH8ZZ	0DP03JZ	0DP602Z	0DPD0YZ	0DPU31Z
0DFH0ZZ	0DH542Z	0DH88UZ	0DHE0DZ	0DL17ZZ	0DL68DZ	0DNJ0ZZ	0DP03KZ	0DP603Z	0DPD30Z	0DPU37Z
0DFH3ZZ	0DH543Z	0DH902Z	0DHE3DZ	0DL18DZ	0DL68ZZ	0DNJ3ZZ	0DP03UZ	0DP607Z	0DPD32Z	0DPU3JZ
0DFH4ZZ	0DH54DZ	0DH903Z	0DHE4DZ	0DL18ZZ	0DL70CZ	0DNJ4ZZ	0DP03YZ	0DP60CZ	0DPD33Z	0DPU3KZ
0DFH7ZZ	0DH54UZ	0DH90DZ	0DHE7DZ	0DL20CZ	0DN43ZZ	0DNJ7ZZ	0DP040Z	0DP60DZ	0DPD37Z	0DPU40Z
0DFH8ZZ	0DH54YZ	0DH90UZ	0DHE8DZ	0DL20DZ	0DN44ZZ	0DNJ8ZZ	0DP042Z	0DP60JZ	0DPD3CZ	0DPU41Z
0DFHXZZ	0DH571Z	0DH932Z	0DHP01Z	0DL20ZZ	0DN47ZZ	0DNK0ZZ	0DP043Z	0DP60KZ	0DPD3DZ	0DPU47Z
0DFJ0ZZ	0DH572Z	0DH933Z	0DHP0DZ	0DL23CZ	0DN48ZZ	0DNK3ZZ	0DP047Z	0DP60MZ	0DPD3JZ	0DPU4JZ
0DFJ3ZZ	0DH573Z	0DH93DZ	0DHP31Z	0DL23DZ	0DN50ZZ	0DNK4ZZ	0DP04CZ	0DP60UZ	0DPD3KZ	0DPU4KZ
0DFJ4ZZ	0DH57BZ	0DH93UZ	0DHP3DZ	0DL23ZZ	0DN53ZZ	0DNK7ZZ	0DP04DZ	0DP60YZ	0DPD3UZ	0DPV00Z
0DFJ7ZZ	0DH57DZ	0DH942Z	0DHP41Z	0DL24CZ	0DN54ZZ	0DNK8ZZ	0DP04JZ	0DP630Z	0DPD3YZ	0DPV01Z
0DFJ8ZZ	0DH57UZ	0DH943Z	0DHP4DZ	0DL24DZ	0DN57ZZ	0DNL0ZZ	0DP04KZ	0DP632Z	0DPD40Z	0DPV07Z
0DFJXZZ	0DH57YZ	0DH94DZ	0DHP71Z	0DL24ZZ	0DN58ZZ	0DNL3ZZ	0DP04UZ	0DP633Z	0DPD42Z	0DPV0JZ
0DFK0ZZ	0DH581Z	0DH94UZ	0DHP7DZ	0DL27DZ	0DN60ZZ	0DNL4ZZ	0DP04YZ	0DP637Z	0DPD43Z	0DPV0KZ
0DFK3ZZ	0DH582Z	0DH972Z	0DHP81Z	0DL27ZZ	0DN63ZZ	0DNL7ZZ	0DP070Z	0DP63CZ	0DPD47Z	0DPV30Z
0DFK4ZZ	0DH583Z	0DH973Z	0DHP8DZ	0DL28DZ	0DN64ZZ	0DNL8ZZ	0DP072Z	0DP63DZ	0DPD4CZ	0DPV31Z
0DFK7ZZ	0DH58BZ	0DH97DZ	0DHQ0DZ	0DL28ZZ	0DN67ZZ	0DNM0ZZ	0DP073Z	0DP63JZ	0DPD4DZ	0DPV37Z
0DFK8ZZ	0DH58DZ	0DH97UZ	0DHQ0LZ	0DL30CZ	0DN68ZZ	0DNM3ZZ	0DP077Z	0DP63KZ	0DPD4JZ	0DPV3JZ
0DFKXZZ	0DH58UZ	0DH982Z	0DHQ3DZ	0DL30DZ	0DN70ZZ	0DNM4ZZ	0DP07CZ	0DP63MZ	0DPD4KZ	0DPV3KZ
0DFL0ZZ	0DH58YZ	0DH983Z	0DHQ3LZ	0DL30ZZ	0DN73ZZ	0DNM7ZZ	0DP07DZ	0DP63UZ	0DPD4UZ	0DPV40Z
0DFL3ZZ	0DH602Z	0DH98DZ	0DHQ4DZ	0DL33CZ	0DN74ZZ	0DNM8ZZ	0DP07JZ	0DP63YZ	0DPD4YZ	0DPV41Z
0DFL4ZZ	0DH603Z	0DH98UZ	0DHQ4LZ	0DL33DZ	0DN77ZZ	0DNN0ZZ	0DP07KZ	0DP640Z	0DPD70Z	0DPV47Z
0DFL7ZZ	0DH60DZ	0DHA02Z	0DHQ7DZ	0DL33ZZ	0DN78ZZ	0DNN3ZZ	0DP07UZ	0DP642Z	0DPD72Z	0DPV4JZ
0DFL8ZZ	0DH60MZ	0DHA03Z	0DHQ8DZ	0DL34CZ	0DN80ZZ	0DNN4ZZ	0DP07YZ	0DP643Z	0DPD73Z	0DPV4KZ
0DFLXZZ	0DH60UZ	0DHA0DZ	0DHR0MZ	0DL34DZ	0DN83ZZ	0DNN7ZZ	0DP080Z	0DP647Z	0DPD77Z	0DPW00Z
0DFM0ZZ	0DH60YZ	0DHA0UZ	0DHR3MZ	0DL34ZZ	0DN84ZZ	0DNN8ZZ	0DP082Z	0DP64CZ	0DPD7CZ	0DPW01Z
0DFM3ZZ	0DH632Z	0DHA32Z	0DHR4MZ	0DL37DZ	0DN87ZZ	0DNP0ZZ	0DP083Z	0DP64DZ	0DPD7DZ	0DPW07Z
0DFM4ZZ	0DH633Z	0DHA33Z	0DJ00ZZ	0DL37ZZ	0DN88ZZ	0DNP3ZZ	0DP087Z	0DP64JZ	0DPD7JZ	0DPW0JZ
0DFM7ZZ	0DH63DZ	0DHA3DZ	0DJ03ZZ	0DL38DZ	0DN90ZZ	0DNP4ZZ	0DP08CZ	0DP64KZ	0DPD7KZ	0DPW0KZ
0DFM8ZZ	0DH63MZ	0DHA3UZ	0DJ04ZZ	0DL38ZZ	0DN93ZZ	0DNP7ZZ	0DP08DZ	0DP64MZ	0DPD7UZ	0DPW30Z
0DFMXZZ	0DH63UZ	0DHA42Z	0DJ07ZZ	0DL40CZ	0DN94ZZ	0DNP8ZZ	0DP08JZ	0DP64UZ	0DPD7YZ	0DPW31Z
0DFN0ZZ	0DH63YZ	0DHA43Z	0DJ08ZZ	0DL40DZ	0DN97ZZ	0DNQ0ZZ	0DP08KZ	0DP64YZ	0DPD80Z	0DPW37Z
0DFN3ZZ	0DH642Z	0DHA4DZ	0DJ0XZZ	0DL40ZZ	0DN98ZZ	0DNQ3ZZ	0DP08UZ	0DP670Z	0DPD82Z	0DPW3JZ
0DFN4ZZ	0DH643Z	0DHA4UZ	0DJ60ZZ	0DL43CZ	0DNA0ZZ	0DNQ3ZZ	0DP08YZ	0DP672Z	0DPD83Z	0DQU0ZZ

0DQU3ZZ	0DSAXZZ	0DT64ZZ	0DU647Z	0DUB87Z	0DUK47Z	0DUQ87Z	0DV37ZZ	0DW00YZ	0DW60MZ	0DWD00Z
0DQU4ZZ	0DSB0ZZ	0DT67ZZ	0DU64JZ	0DUB8JZ	0DUK4JZ	0DUQ8JZ	0DV38DZ	0DW030Z	0DW60UZ	0DWD02Z
0DQV3ZZ	0DSB4ZZ	0DT68ZZ	0DU64KZ	0DUB8KZ	0DUK4KZ	0DUQ8KZ	0DV38ZZ	0DW032Z	0DW60YZ	0DWD03Z
0DQV4ZZ	0DSB7ZZ	0DT70ZZ	0DU677Z	0DUC07Z	0DUK77Z	0DUQX7Z	0DV40CZ	0DW033Z	0DW630Z	0DWD07Z
0DQW0ZZ	0DSB8ZZ	0DT74ZZ	0DU67JZ	0DUC0JZ	0DUK7JZ	0DUQXJZ	0DV40DZ	0DW037Z	0DW632Z	0DWD0CZ
0DQW3ZZ	0DSBXZZ	0DT77ZZ	0DU67KZ	0DUC0KZ	0DUK7KZ	0DUQXKZ	0DV40ZZ	0DW03CZ	0DW633Z	0DWD0DZ
0DQW4ZZ	0DSE0ZZ	0DT78ZZ	0DU687Z	0DUC47Z	0DUK87Z	0DUR07Z	0DV43CZ	0DW03DZ	0DW637Z	0DWD0JZ
0DR507Z	0DSE4ZZ	0DT80ZZ	0DU68JZ	0DUC4JZ	0DUK8JZ	0DUR0JZ	0DV43DZ	0DW03JZ	0DW63CZ	0DWD0KZ
0DR50JZ	0DSE7ZZ	0DT84ZZ	0DU68KZ	0DUC4KZ	0DUK8KZ	0DUR0KZ	0DV43ZZ	0DW03KZ	0DW63DZ	0DWD0UZ
0DR50KZ	0DSE8ZZ	0DT87ZZ	0DU707Z	0DUC77Z	0DUL07Z	0DUR47Z	0DV44CZ	0DW03UZ	0DW63JZ	0DWD0YZ
0DR547Z	0DSH0ZZ	0DT88ZZ	0DU70JZ	0DUC7JZ	0DUL0JZ	0DUR4JZ	0DV44DZ	0DW03YZ	0DW63KZ	0DWD30Z
0DR54JZ	0DSH4ZZ	0DT90ZZ	0DU70KZ	0DUC7KZ	0DUL0KZ	0DUR4KZ	0DV44ZZ	0DW040Z	0DW63MZ	0DWD32Z
0DR54KZ	0DSH7ZZ	0DT94ZZ	0DU747Z	0DUC87Z	0DUL47Z	0DUU07Z	0DV47DZ	0DW042Z	0DW63UZ	0DWD33Z
0DR577Z	0DSH8ZZ	0DT97ZZ	0DU74JZ	0DUC8JZ	0DUL4JZ	0DUU0JZ	0DV47ZZ	0DW043Z	0DW63YZ	0DWD37Z
0DR57JZ	0DSHXZZ	0DT98ZZ	0DU74KZ	0DUC8KZ	0DUL4KZ	0DUU0KZ	0DV48DZ	0DW047Z	0DW640Z	0DWD3CZ
0DR57KZ	0DSK0ZZ	0DTA0ZZ	0DU777Z	0DUE07Z	0DUL77Z	0DUU47Z	0DV48ZZ	0DW04CZ	0DW642Z	0DWD3DZ
0DR587Z	0DSK4ZZ	0DTA4ZZ	0DU77JZ	0DUE0JZ	0DUL7JZ	0DUU4JZ	0DV50CZ	0DW04DZ	0DW643Z	0DWD3JZ
0DR58JZ	0DSK7ZZ	0DTA7ZZ	0DU77KZ	0DUE0KZ	0DUL7KZ	0DUU4KZ	0DV67DZ	0DW04JZ	0DW647Z	0DWD3KZ
0DR58KZ	0DSK8ZZ	0DTA8ZZ	0DU787Z	0DUE47Z	0DUL87Z	0DUV07Z	0DV68DZ	0DW04KZ	0DW64CZ	0DWD3UZ
0DRR07Z	0DSKXZZ	0DTB0ZZ	0DU78JZ	0DUE4JZ	0DUL8JZ	0DUV0JZ	0DVN3DZ	0DW04UZ	0DW64DZ	0DWD3YZ
0DRR0JZ	0DSL0ZZ	0DTB4ZZ	0DU78KZ	0DUE4KZ	0DUL8KZ	0DUV0KZ	0DVN3ZZ	0DW04YZ	0DW64JZ	0DWD40Z
0DRR0KZ	0DSL4ZZ	0DTB7ZZ	0DU807Z	0DUE77Z	0DUM07Z	0DUV47Z	0DVN4CZ	0DW070Z	0DW64KZ	0DWD42Z
0DRR47Z	0DSL7ZZ	0DTB8ZZ	0DU80JZ	0DUE7JZ	0DUM0JZ	0DUV4JZ	0DVN4DZ	0DW072Z	0DW64MZ	0DWD43Z
0DRR4JZ	0DSL8ZZ	0DTC0ZZ	0DU80KZ	0DUE7KZ	0DUM0KZ	0DUV4KZ	0DVN4ZZ	0DW073Z	0DW64UZ	0DWD47Z
0DRR4KZ	0DSLXZZ	0DTC4ZZ	0DU847Z	0DUE87Z	0DUM47Z	0DUW07Z	0DVN7DZ	0DW077Z	0DW64YZ	0DWD4CZ
0DRU07Z	0DSM0ZZ	0DTC7ZZ	0DU84JZ	0DUE8JZ	0DUM4JZ	0DUW0JZ	0DVN7ZZ	0DW07CZ	0DW670Z	0DWD4DZ
0DRU0JZ	0DSM4ZZ	0DTC8ZZ	0DU84KZ	0DUE8KZ	0DUM4KZ	0DUW0KZ	0DVN8DZ	0DW07DZ	0DW672Z	0DWD4JZ
0DRU0KZ	0DSM7ZZ	0DTE0ZZ	0DU877Z	0DUF07Z	0DUM77Z	0DUW47Z	0DVN8ZZ	0DW07JZ	0DW673Z	0DWD4KZ
0DRU47Z	0DSM8ZZ	0DTE4ZZ	0DU87JZ	0DUF0JZ	0DUM7JZ	0DUW4JZ	0DVP0CZ	0DW07KZ	0DW677Z	0DWD4UZ
0DRU4JZ	0DSMXZZ	0DTE7ZZ	0DU87KZ	0DUF0KZ	0DUM7KZ	0DUW4KZ	0DVP0DZ	0DW07UZ	0DW67CZ	0DWD4YZ
0DRU4KZ	0DSN0ZZ	0DTE8ZZ	0DU887Z	0DUF47Z	0DUM87Z	0DV10CZ	0DVP0ZZ	0DW07YZ	0DW67DZ	0DWD70Z
0DRV07Z	0DSN4ZZ	0DTF0ZZ	0DU88JZ	0DUF4JZ	0DUM8JZ	0DV10DZ	0DVP3CZ	0DW080Z	0DW67JZ	0DWD72Z
0DRV0JZ	0DSN7ZZ	0DTF4ZZ	0DU88KZ	0DUF4KZ	0DUM8KZ	0DV10ZZ	0DVP3DZ	0DW082Z	0DW67KZ	0DWD73Z
0DRV0KZ	0DSN8ZZ	0DTF7ZZ	0DU907Z	0DUF77Z	0DUN07Z	0DV13CZ	0DVP3ZZ	0DW083Z	0DW67UZ	0DWD77Z
0DRV47Z	0DSNXZZ	0DTF8ZZ	0DU90JZ	0DUF7JZ	0DUN0JZ	0DV13DZ	0DVP4CZ	0DW087Z	0DW67YZ	0DWD7CZ
0DRV4JZ	0DSP0ZZ	0DTG0ZZ	0DU90KZ	0DUF7KZ	0DUN0KZ	0DV13ZZ	0DVP4DZ	0DW08CZ	0DW680Z	0DWD7DZ
0DRV4KZ	0DSP4ZZ	0DTG4ZZ	0DU947Z	0DUF87Z	0DUN47Z	0DV14CZ	0DVP4ZZ	0DW08DZ	0DW682Z	0DWD7JZ
0DRW07Z	0DSP7ZZ	0DTG7ZZ	0DU94JZ	0DUF8JZ	0DUN4JZ	0DV14DZ	0DVP7DZ	0DW08JZ	0DW683Z	0DWD7KZ
0DRW0JZ	0DSP8ZZ	0DTG8ZZ	0DU94KZ	0DUF8KZ	0DUN4KZ	0DV14ZZ	0DVP7ZZ	0DW08KZ	0DW687Z	0DWD7UZ
0DRW0KZ	0DSPXZZ	0DTGFZZ	0DU977Z	0DUG07Z	0DUN77Z	0DV17DZ	0DVP8DZ	0DW08UZ	0DW68CZ	0DWD7YZ
0DRW47Z	0DSQ0ZZ	0DTH0ZZ	0DU97JZ	0DUG0JZ	0DUN7JZ	0DV17ZZ	0DVP8ZZ	0DW08YZ	0DW68DZ	0DWD80Z
0DRW4JZ	0DSQ4ZZ	0DTH4ZZ	0DU97KZ	0DUG0KZ	0DUN7KZ	0DV18DZ	0DVQ0CZ	0DW0X0Z	0DW68JZ	0DWD82Z
0DRW4KZ	0DSQ7ZZ	0DTH7ZZ	0DU987Z	0DUG47Z	0DUN87Z	0DV18ZZ	0DVQ0DZ	0DW0X2Z	0DW68KZ	0DWD83Z
0DS50ZZ	0DSQ8ZZ	0DTH8ZZ	0DU98JZ	0DUG4JZ	0DUN8JZ	0DV20CZ	0DVQ0ZZ	0DW0X3Z	0DW68UZ	0DWD87Z
0DS54ZZ	0DSQXZZ	0DTJ0ZZ	0DU98KZ	0DUG4KZ	0DUN8KZ	0DV20DZ	0DVQ3CZ	0DW0X7Z	0DW68YZ	0DWD8CZ
0DS57ZZ	0DT10ZZ	0DTJ4ZZ	0DUA07Z	0DUG77Z	0DUP07Z	0DV20ZZ	0DVQ3DZ	0DW0XCZ	0DW6X0Z	0DWD8DZ
0DS58ZZ	0DT14ZZ	0DTJ7ZZ	0DUA0JZ	0DUG7JZ	0DUP0JZ	0DV23CZ	0DVQ3DZ	0DW0XDZ	0DW6X2Z	0DWD8JZ
0DS5XZZ	0DT17ZZ	0DTJ8ZZ	0DUA0KZ	0DUG7KZ	0DUP0KZ	0DV23DZ	0DVQ3ZZ	0DW0XJZ	0DW6X3Z	0DWD8KZ
0DS60ZZ	0DT18ZZ	0DTK0ZZ	0DUA47Z	0DUG87Z	0DUP47Z	0DV23ZZ	0DVQ4CZ	0DW0XKZ	0DW6X7Z	0DWD8UZ
0DS64ZZ	0DT20ZZ	0DTK4ZZ	0DUA4JZ	0DUG8JZ	0DUP4JZ	0DV24CZ	0DVQ4DZ	0DW0XUZ	0DW6XCZ	0DWD8YZ
0DS67ZZ	0DT24ZZ	0DTLFZZ	0DUA4KZ	0DUG8KZ	0DUP4KZ	0DV24DZ	0DVQ4ZZ	0DW50YZ	0DW6XDZ	0DWDX0Z
0DS68ZZ	0DT27ZZ	0DTMFZZ	0DUA77Z	0DUH07Z	0DUP77Z	0DV24ZZ	0DVQ7DZ	0DW53YZ	0DW6XJZ	0DWDX2Z
0DS6XZZ	0DT28ZZ	0DTNFZZ	0DUA7JZ	0DUH0JZ	0DUP7JZ	0DV27DZ	0DVQ7ZZ	0DW54YZ	0DW6XKZ	0DWDX3Z
0DS80ZZ	0DT30ZZ	0DTU0ZZ	0DUA7KZ	0DUH0KZ	0DUP7KZ	0DV27ZZ	0DVQ8DZ	0DW57DZ	0DW6XUZ	0DWDX7Z
0DS84ZZ	0DT34ZZ	0DTU4ZZ	0DUA87Z	0DUH47Z	0DUP87Z	0DV28DZ	0DVQ8ZZ	0DW57YZ	0DW807Z	0DWDXCZ
0DS87ZZ	0DT37ZZ	0DU54JZ	0DUA8JZ	0DUH4JZ	0DUP8JZ	0DV28ZZ	0DVQXCZ	0DW58DZ	0DW80JZ	0DWDXDZ
0DS88ZZ	0DT38ZZ	0DU54KZ	0DUA8KZ	0DUH4KZ	0DUP8KZ	0DV30CZ	0DVQXDZ	0DW58YZ	0DW80KZ	0DWDXJZ
0DS90ZZ	0DT40ZZ	0DU577Z	0DUB07Z	0DUH77Z	0DUQ07Z	0DV30DZ	0DVQXZZ	0DW5XDZ	0DW847Z	0DWDXKZ
0DS94ZZ	0DT44ZZ	0DU57JZ	0DUB0JZ	0DUH7JZ	0DUQ0JZ	0DV30ZZ	0DW000Z	0DW600Z	0DW84JZ	0DWDXUZ
0DS97ZZ	0DT47ZZ	0DU57KZ	0DUB0KZ	0DUH7KZ	0DUQ0KZ	0DV33CZ	0DW002Z	0DW602Z	0DW84KZ	0DWE07Z
0DS98ZZ	0DT48ZZ	0DU587Z	0DUB47Z	0DUH87Z	0DUQ47Z	0DV33DZ	0DW003Z	0DW603Z	0DW877Z	0DWE0JZ
0DS9XZZ	0DT50ZZ	0DU58JZ	0DUB4JZ	0DUH8JZ	0DUQ4JZ	0DV33ZZ	0DW007Z	0DW607Z	0DW87JZ	0DWE0KZ
0DSA0ZZ	0DT54ZZ	0DU58KZ	0DUB4KZ	0DUH8KZ	0DUQ4KZ	0DV34CZ	0DW00CZ	0DW60CZ	0DW87KZ	0DWE47Z
0DSA4ZZ	0DT57ZZ	0DU607Z	0DUB77Z	0DUK07Z	0DUQ77Z	0DV34DZ	0DW00DZ	0DW60DZ	0DW887Z	0DWE4JZ
0DSA7ZZ	0DT58ZZ	0DU60JZ	0DUB7JZ	0DUK0JZ	0DUQ7JZ	0DV34ZZ	0DW00JZ	0DW60JZ	0DW88JZ	0DWE4KZ
0DSA8ZZ	0DT60ZZ	0DU60KZ	0DUB7KZ	0DUK0KZ	0DUQ7KZ	0DV37DZ	0DW00KZ	0DW60KZ	0DW88KZ	0DWE77Z

0DWE7JZ	0DYE0Z2	0F174D9	0F1F0Z3	0F594ZZ	0F794DZ	0F9400Z	0F9870Z	0F9G00Z	0FBC8ZZ	0FFDXZZ
0DWE7KZ	0F140D3	0F174DB	0F1F0ZB	0F597ZZ	0F794ZZ	0F940ZX	0F987ZX	0F9G0ZX	0FBD3ZX	0FFFXZZ
0DWE87Z	0F140D4	0F174Z3	0F1F0ZC	0F598ZZ	0F797DZ	0F940ZZ	0F987ZZ	0F9G0ZZ	0FBD4ZX	0FH003Z
0DWE8JZ	0F140D5	0F174Z4	0F1F4D3	0F5C0ZZ	0F797ZZ	0F9430Z	0F9880Z	0F9G30Z	0FBD4ZX	0FH00YZ
0DWE8KZ	0F140D6	0F174Z5	0F1F4DB	0F5C3ZZ	0F798DZ	0F943ZX	0F988ZX	0F9G3ZX	0FBD7ZX	0FH033Z
0DWQ0LZ	0F140D7	0F174Z6	0F1F4DC	0F5C4ZZ	0F798ZZ	0F943ZZ	0F988ZZ	0F9G3ZX	0FBD8ZZ	0FH03YZ
0DWQ3LZ	0F140D8	0F174Z7	0F1F4Z3	0F5C7ZZ	0F7C0DZ	0F9440Z	0F9900Z	0F9G40Z	0FBF3ZX	0FH043Z
0DWQ4LZ	0F140D9	0F174Z8	0F1F4Z8	0F5C8ZZ	0F7C0ZZ	0F944ZX	0F990ZX	0F9G4ZX	0FBF4ZX	0FH04YZ
0DWQ7LZ	0F140DB	0F174Z9	0F1F4ZC	0F5D0ZZ	0F7C3DZ	0F944ZZ	0F990ZZ	0F9G4ZZ	0FBF4ZZ	0FH103Z
0DWQ8LZ	0F140Z3	0F174ZB	0F1G0D3	0F5D3ZZ	0F7C3ZZ	0F9480Z	0F9930Z	0F9G80Z	0FBF7ZX	0FH133Z
0DWR0MZ	0F140Z4	0F184DB	0F1G0DB	0F5D4ZZ	0F7C4DZ	0F948ZX	0F993ZX	0F9G8ZX	0FBF8ZX	0FH143Z
0DWR3MZ	0F140Z5	0F184Z3	0F1G0DC	0F5D7ZZ	0F7C4ZZ	0F948ZZ	0F993ZZ	0F9G8ZZ	0FBF8ZZ	0FH203Z
0DWR4MZ	0F140Z6	0F184Z4	0F1G0Z3	0F5D8ZZ	0F7C7DZ	0F9500Z	0F9940Z	0FB00ZX	0FBF8ZZ	0FH233Z
0DWU00Z	0F140Z7	0F184Z5	0F1G0ZB	0F5F0ZZ	0F7C7ZZ	0F950ZX	0F994ZX	0FB00ZZ	0FBG3ZX	0FH243Z
0DWU07Z	0F140Z8	0F184Z6	0F1G0ZC	0F5F3ZZ	0F7C8DZ	0F950ZZ	0F994ZZ	0FB03ZX	0FBG4ZX	0FH403Z
0DWU0JZ	0F140Z9	0F184Z7	0F1G4D3	0F5F4ZZ	0F7C8ZZ	0F9530Z	0F9970Z	0FB03ZZ	0FBG8ZX	0FH40YZ
0DWU0KZ	0F140ZB	0F184Z8	0F1G4DB	0F5F7ZZ	0F7D0DZ	0F953ZX	0F997ZX	0FB04ZX	0FBG8ZZ	0FH433Z
0DWU30Z	0F144D3	0F184Z9	0F1G4DC	0F5F8ZZ	0F7D0ZZ	0F953ZZ	0F997ZZ	0FB04ZZ	0FC48ZZ	0FH443Z
0DWU37Z	0F144D4	0F184ZB	0F1G4Z3	0F5G0ZZ	0F7D3DZ	0F9540Z	0F9980Z	0FB10ZX	0FC53ZZ	0FH44YZ
0DWU3JZ	0F144D5	0F190D3	0F1G4ZB	0F5G3ZZ	0F7D3ZZ	0F954ZX	0F998ZX	0FB10ZZ	0FC54ZZ	0FHB03Z
0DWU3KZ	0F144D6	0F190D4	0F1G4ZC	0F5G4ZZ	0F7D4DZ	0F954ZZ	0F998ZZ	0FB13ZX	0FC57ZZ	0FHB0YZ
0DWU40Z	0F144D7	0F190D5	0F20X0Z	0F5G8ZZ	0F7D4ZZ	0F9570Z	0F9C00Z	0FB13ZZ	0FC58ZZ	0FHB33Z
0DWU47Z	0F144D8	0F190D6	0F20XYZ	0F750DZ	0F7D7DZ	0F957ZX	0F9C0ZX	0FB23ZX	0FC63ZZ	0FHB3YZ
0DWU4JZ	0F144D9	0F190D7	0F24X0Z	0F750ZZ	0F7D7ZZ	0F957ZZ	0F9C0ZZ	0FB43ZX	0FC64ZZ	0FHB43Z
0DWU4KZ	0F144DB	0F190D8	0F24XYZ	0F753DZ	0F7D8DZ	0F9580Z	0F9C30Z	0FB44ZX	0FC67ZZ	0FHB4DZ
0DWV00Z	0F144Z3	0F190D9	0F2BX0Z	0F753ZZ	0F7D8ZZ	0F958ZX	0F9C3ZX	0FB48ZX	0FC68ZZ	0FHB4YZ
0DWV07Z	0F144Z4	0F190DB	0F2BXYZ	0F754DZ	0F7F0ZZ	0F958ZZ	0F9C3ZZ	0FB48ZZ	0FC70ZZ	0FHB72Z
0DWV0JZ	0F144Z5	0F190Z3	0F2DX0Z	0F754ZZ	0F7F0ZZ	0F9600Z	0F9C40Z	0FB53ZX	0FC73ZZ	0FHB73Z
0DWV0KZ	0F144Z6	0F190Z4	0F2DXYZ	0F757DZ	0F7F3DZ	0F960ZX	0F9C4ZX	0FB54ZX	0FC74ZZ	0FHB7YZ
0DWV30Z	0F144Z7	0F190Z5	0F2GX0Z	0F757ZZ	0F7F3ZZ	0F960ZZ	0F9C4ZZ	0FB54ZZ	0FC77ZZ	0FHB82Z
0DWV37Z	0F144Z8	0F190Z6	0F2GXYZ	0F758DZ	0F7F4DZ	0F9630Z	0F9C70Z	0FB57ZX	0FC78ZZ	0FHB83Z
0DWV3JZ	0F144Z9	0F190Z7	0F500ZZ	0F758ZZ	0F7F4ZZ	0F963ZX	0F9C7ZX	0FB58ZX	0FC83ZZ	0FHB8DZ
0DWV3KZ	0F144ZB	0F190Z8	0F503ZZ	0F760DZ	0F7F7DZ	0F963ZZ	0F9C7ZZ	0FB58ZZ	0FC84ZZ	0FHB8YZ
0DWV40Z	0F150D3	0F190Z9	0F504ZZ	0F760ZZ	0F7F7ZZ	0F9640Z	0F9C80Z	0FB63ZX	0FC87ZZ	0FHD03Z
0DWV47Z	0F150D4	0F190ZB	0F510ZZ	0F763DZ	0F7F8DZ	0F964ZX	0F9C8ZX	0FB64ZX	0FC88ZZ	0FHD0YZ
0DWV4JZ	0F150D5	0F194D3	0F513ZZ	0F763ZZ	0F7F8ZZ	0F964ZZ	0F9C8ZZ	0FB64ZZ	0FC93ZZ	0FHD33Z
0DWV4KZ	0F150D6	0F194D4	0F514ZZ	0F764DZ	0F8G0ZZ	0F9670Z	0F9D00Z	0FB67ZX	0FC94ZZ	0FHD3YZ
0DWW00Z	0F150D7	0F194D5	0F520ZZ	0F764ZZ	0F8G3ZZ	0F967ZX	0F9D0ZX	0FB68ZX	0FC97ZZ	0FHD43Z
0DWW07Z	0F150D8	0F194D6	0F523ZZ	0F767DZ	0F8G4ZZ	0F967ZZ	0F9D0ZZ	0FB68ZZ	0FC98ZZ	0FHD4DZ
0DWW0JZ	0F150D9	0F194D7	0F524ZZ	0F767ZZ	0F9000Z	0F9680Z	0F9D30Z	0FB70ZX	0FCC4ZZ	0FHD4YZ
0DWW0KZ	0F150DB	0F194D8	0F540ZZ	0F768DZ	0F900ZX	0F968ZX	0F9D3ZX	0FB70ZZ	0FCC8ZZ	0FHD72Z
0DWW30Z	0F150Z3	0F194D9	0F543ZZ	0F768ZZ	0F900ZZ	0F968ZZ	0F9D3ZZ	0FB73ZX	0FCD3ZZ	0FHD73Z
0DWW37Z	0F150Z4	0F194DB	0F544ZZ	0F770DZ	0F9030Z	0F9700Z	0F9D40Z	0FB73ZZ	0FCD4ZZ	0FHD7YZ
0DWW3JZ	0F150Z5	0F194Z3	0F548ZZ	0F770ZZ	0F903ZX	0F970ZX	0F9D4ZX	0FB74ZX	0FCD8ZZ	0FHD82Z
0DWW3KZ	0F170D3	0F194Z4	0F550ZZ	0F773DZ	0F903ZZ	0F970ZZ	0F9D4ZZ	0FB74ZZ	0FCF3ZZ	0FHD83Z
0DWW40Z	0F170D4	0F194Z5	0F553ZZ	0F773ZZ	0F9040Z	0F9730Z	0F9D70Z	0FB77ZX	0FCF4ZZ	0FHD8DZ
0DWW47Z	0F170D5	0F194Z6	0F554ZZ	0F774DZ	0F904ZX	0F973ZX	0F9D7ZX	0FB77ZZ	0FCF8ZZ	0FHD8YZ
0DWW4JZ	0F170D6	0F194Z7	0F557ZZ	0F774ZZ	0F904ZZ	0F973ZZ	0F9D7ZZ	0FB78ZX	0FCG8ZZ	0FHG03Z
0DWW4KZ	0F170D7	0F194Z8	0F558ZZ	0F777DZ	0F9100Z	0F9740Z	0F9D80Z	0FB78ZZ	0FF48ZZ	0FHG0YZ
0DX60Z5	0F170D8	0F194Z9	0F560ZZ	0F777ZZ	0F910ZX	0F974ZX	0F9D8ZX	0FB83ZX	0FF4XZZ	0FHG33Z
0DX64Z5	0F170D9	0F194ZB	0F563ZZ	0F778DZ	0F910ZZ	0F974ZZ	0F9D8ZZ	0FB84ZX	0FF58ZZ	0FHG3YZ
0DX80Z5	0F170DB	0F1D0D3	0F564ZZ	0F778ZZ	0F9130Z	0F9770Z	0F9F00Z	0FB84ZZ	0FF5XZZ	0FHG43Z
0DX84Z5	0F170Z3	0F1D0DB	0F567ZZ	0F780DZ	0F913ZX	0F977ZX	0F9F0ZX	0FB87ZX	0FF68ZZ	0FHG4YZ
0DXE0Z5	0F170Z4	0F1D0DC	0F568ZZ	0F780ZZ	0F913ZZ	0F977ZZ	0F9F0ZZ	0FB88ZX	0FF6XZZ	0FJ0XZZ
0DXE4Z5	0F170Z5	0F1D0Z3	0F570ZZ	0F783DZ	0F9140Z	0F9780Z	0F9F30Z	0FB88ZZ	0FF70ZZ	0FJ40ZZ
0DY50Z0	0F170Z6	0F1D0ZB	0F573ZZ	0F783ZZ	0F914ZX	0F978ZX	0F9F3ZX	0FB93ZX	0FF73ZZ	0FJ43ZZ
0DY50Z1	0F170Z7	0F1D0ZC	0F574ZZ	0F784DZ	0F914ZZ	0F978ZZ	0F9F3ZZ	0FB94ZX	0FF74ZZ	0FJ44ZZ
0DY50Z2	0F170Z8	0F1D4D3	0F577ZZ	0F784ZZ	0F9200Z	0F9800Z	0F9F40Z	0FB94ZZ	0FF77ZZ	0FJ48ZZ
0DY60Z0	0F170Z9	0F1D4DB	0F578ZZ	0F787DZ	0F920ZX	0F980ZX	0F9F4ZX	0FB97ZX	0FF78ZZ	0FJ4XZZ
0DY60Z1	0F170ZB	0F1D4DC	0F580ZZ	0F787ZZ	0F920ZZ	0F980ZZ	0F9F4ZZ	0FB98ZX	0FF7XZZ	0FJB0ZZ
0DY60Z2	0F174D3	0F1D4Z3	0F583ZZ	0F788DZ	0F9230Z	0F9830Z	0F9F70Z	0FB98ZZ	0FF88ZZ	0FJB3ZZ
0DY80Z0	0F174D4	0F1D4ZB	0F584ZZ	0F788ZZ	0F923ZX	0F983ZX	0F9F7ZX	0FBC3ZX	0FF8XZZ	0FJB4ZZ
0DY80Z1	0F174D5	0F1D4ZC	0F587ZZ	0F790DZ	0F923ZZ	0F983ZZ	0F9F7ZZ	0FBC4ZX	0FF98ZZ	0FJB7ZZ
0DY80Z2	0F174D6	0F1F0D3	0F588ZZ	0F790ZZ	0F9240Z	0F9840Z	0F9F80Z	0FBC4ZZ	0FF9XZZ	0FJB8ZZ
0DYE0Z0	0F174D7	0F1F0DB	0F590ZZ	0F793DZ	0F924ZX	0F984ZX	0F9F8ZX	0FBC7ZX	0FFC8ZZ	0FJD0ZZ
0DYE0Z1	0F174D8	0F1F0DC	0F593ZZ	0F793ZZ	0F924ZZ	0F984ZZ	0F9F8ZZ	0FBC8ZX	0FFCXZZ	

0FJD3ZZ	0FL93ZZ	0FMC4ZZ	0FP003Z	0FPB77Z	0FPGX0Z	0FT64ZZ	0FU80JZ	0FV54DZ	0FVC4ZZ	0FWB02Z
0FJD4ZZ	0FL94CZ	0FMD0ZZ	0FP00YZ	0FPB7CZ	0FPGX2Z	0FT67ZZ	0FU80KZ	0FV54ZZ	0FVC7DZ	0FWB03Z
0FJD7ZZ	0FL94DZ	0FMD4ZZ	0FP030Z	0FPB7DZ	0FPGX3Z	0FT68ZZ	0FU837Z	0FV57DZ	0FVC7ZZ	0FWB07Z
0FJD8ZZ	0FL94ZZ	0FMF0ZZ	0FP032Z	0FPB7JZ	0FQ48ZZ	0FT70ZZ	0FU83JZ	0FV57ZZ	0FVC8DZ	0FWB0CZ
0FJG0ZZ	0FL97DZ	0FMG0ZZ	0FP033Z	0FPB7KZ	0FQ70ZZ	0FT74ZZ	0FU83KZ	0FV58DZ	0FVC8ZZ	0FWB0DZ
0FJG3ZZ	0FL97ZZ	0FMG4ZZ	0FP03YZ	0FPB7YZ	0FQ73ZZ	0FT77ZZ	0FU847Z	0FV58ZZ	0FVD0CZ	0FWB0JZ
0FJG4ZZ	0FL98DZ	0FN00ZZ	0FP040Z	0FPB80Z	0FQ74ZZ	0FT78ZZ	0FU84JZ	0FV60CZ	0FVD0DZ	0FWB0KZ
0FJG8ZZ	0FL98ZZ	0FN03ZZ	0FP042Z	0FPB81Z	0FQ77ZZ	0FT80ZZ	0FU84KZ	0FV60DZ	0FVD0ZZ	0FWB0YZ
0FJGXZZ	0FLC0CZ	0FN04ZZ	0FP043Z	0FPB82Z	0FQ78ZZ	0FT84ZZ	0FU887Z	0FV60ZZ	0FVD3CZ	0FWB30Z
0FL50CZ	0FLC0DZ	0FN10ZZ	0FP04YZ	0FPB83Z	0FQG8ZZ	0FT87ZZ	0FU88JZ	0FV63CZ	0FVD3DZ	0FWB32Z
0FL50DZ	0FLC0ZZ	0FN13ZZ	0FP0X0Z	0FPB87Z	0FR587Z	0FT88ZZ	0FU88KZ	0FV63DZ	0FVD3ZZ	0FWB33Z
0FL50ZZ	0FLC3CZ	0FN14ZZ	0FP0X2Z	0FPB8CZ	0FR58JZ	0FT90ZZ	0FU907Z	0FV63ZZ	0FVD4CZ	0FWB37Z
0FL53CZ	0FLC3DZ	0FN20ZZ	0FP0X3Z	0FPB8DZ	0FR58KZ	0FT94ZZ	0FU90JZ	0FV64CZ	0FVD4DZ	0FWB3CZ
0FL53DZ	0FLC3ZZ	0FN23ZZ	0FP400Z	0FPB8JZ	0FR687Z	0FT97ZZ	0FU90KZ	0FV64DZ	0FVD4ZZ	0FWB3DZ
0FL53ZZ	0FLC4CZ	0FN24ZZ	0FP402Z	0FPB8KZ	0FR68JZ	0FT98ZZ	0FU937Z	0FV64ZZ	0FVD7DZ	0FWB3JZ
0FL54CZ	0FLC4DZ	0FN40ZZ	0FP403Z	0FPB8YZ	0FR68KZ	0FTC0ZZ	0FU93JZ	0FV67DZ	0FVD7ZZ	0FWB3KZ
0FL54DZ	0FLC4ZZ	0FN43ZZ	0FP40DZ	0FPBX0Z	0FR707Z	0FTC4ZZ	0FU93KZ	0FV67ZZ	0FVD8DZ	0FWB3YZ
0FL54ZZ	0FLC7DZ	0FN44ZZ	0FP40YZ	0FPBX1Z	0FR70JZ	0FTC7ZZ	0FU947Z	0FV68DZ	0FVD8ZZ	0FWB40Z
0FL57DZ	0FLC7ZZ	0FN48ZZ	0FP430Z	0FPBX2Z	0FR70KZ	0FTC8ZZ	0FU94JZ	0FV68ZZ	0FVF0CZ	0FWB42Z
0FL57ZZ	0FLC8DZ	0FN50ZZ	0FP432Z	0FPBX3Z	0FR747Z	0FTD0ZZ	0FU94KZ	0FV70CZ	0FVF0DZ	0FWB43Z
0FL58DZ	0FLC8ZZ	0FN53ZZ	0FP433Z	0FPBXDZ	0FR74JZ	0FTD4ZZ	0FU987Z	0FV70DZ	0FVF0ZZ	0FWB47Z
0FL58ZZ	0FLD0CZ	0FN54ZZ	0FP43DZ	0FPD00Z	0FR74KZ	0FTD7ZZ	0FU98JZ	0FV70ZZ	0FVF3CZ	0FWB4CZ
0FL60CZ	0FLD0DZ	0FN57ZZ	0FP43YZ	0FPD01Z	0FR787Z	0FTD8ZZ	0FU98KZ	0FV73CZ	0FVF3DZ	0FWB4DZ
0FL60DZ	0FLD0ZZ	0FN58ZZ	0FP440Z	0FPD02Z	0FR78JZ	0FTF0ZZ	0FUC07Z	0FV73DZ	0FVF3ZZ	0FWB4JZ
0FL60ZZ	0FLD3CZ	0FN60ZZ	0FP442Z	0FPD03Z	0FR78KZ	0FTF4ZZ	0FUC0JZ	0FV73ZZ	0FVF4CZ	0FWB4KZ
0FL63CZ	0FLD3DZ	0FN63ZZ	0FP443Z	0FPD07Z	0FR887Z	0FTF7ZZ	0FUC0KZ	0FV74CZ	0FVF4DZ	0FWB4YZ
0FL63DZ	0FLD3ZZ	0FN64ZZ	0FP44DZ	0FPD0CZ	0FR88JZ	0FTF8ZZ	0FUC37Z	0FV74DZ	0FVF4ZZ	0FWB70Z
0FL63ZZ	0FLD4CZ	0FN67ZZ	0FP44YZ	0FPD0DZ	0FR88KZ	0FTG0ZZ	0FUC3JZ	0FV74ZZ	0FVF7DZ	0FWB72Z
0FL64CZ	0FLD4DZ	0FN68ZZ	0FP4X0Z	0FPD0JZ	0FR987Z	0FTG4ZZ	0FUC3KZ	0FV77DZ	0FVF7ZZ	0FWB73Z
0FL64DZ	0FLD4ZZ	0FN70ZZ	0FP4X2Z	0FPD0KZ	0FR98JZ	0FU507Z	0FUC47Z	0FV77ZZ	0FVF8DZ	0FWB77Z
0FL64ZZ	0FLD7DZ	0FN73ZZ	0FP4X3Z	0FPD0YZ	0FR98KZ	0FU50JZ	0FUC4JZ	0FV78DZ	0FVF8ZZ	0FWB7CZ
0FL67DZ	0FLD7ZZ	0FN74ZZ	0FP4XDZ	0FPD30Z	0FRC87Z	0FU50KZ	0FUC4KZ	0FV78ZZ	0FW000Z	0FWB7DZ
0FL67ZZ	0FLD8DZ	0FN77ZZ	0FPB00Z	0FPD31Z	0FRC8JZ	0FU537Z	0FUC87Z	0FV80CZ	0FW002Z	0FWB7JZ
0FL68DZ	0FLD8ZZ	0FN78ZZ	0FPB01Z	0FPD32Z	0FRC8KZ	0FU53JZ	0FUC8JZ	0FV80DZ	0FW003Z	0FWB7KZ
0FL68ZZ	0FLF0CZ	0FN80ZZ	0FPB02Z	0FPD33Z	0FRD87Z	0FU53KZ	0FUC8KZ	0FV80ZZ	0FW00YZ	0FWB7YZ
0FL70CZ	0FLF0DZ	0FN83ZZ	0FPB03Z	0FPD37Z	0FRD8JZ	0FU547Z	0FUD07Z	0FV83CZ	0FW030Z	0FWB80Z
0FL70DZ	0FLF0ZZ	0FN84ZZ	0FPB07Z	0FPD3CZ	0FRD8KZ	0FU54JZ	0FUD0JZ	0FV83DZ	0FW032Z	0FWB82Z
0FL70ZZ	0FLF3CZ	0FN87ZZ	0FPB0CZ	0FPD3DZ	0FRF87Z	0FU54KZ	0FUD0KZ	0FV83ZZ	0FW033Z	0FWB83Z
0FL73CZ	0FLF3DZ	0FN88ZZ	0FPB0DZ	0FPD3JZ	0FRF8JZ	0FU587Z	0FUD37Z	0FV84CZ	0FW03YZ	0FWB87Z
0FL73DZ	0FLF3ZZ	0FN90ZZ	0FPB0JZ	0FPD3KZ	0FRF8KZ	0FU58JZ	0FUD3JZ	0FV84DZ	0FW040Z	0FWB8CZ
0FL73ZZ	0FLF4CZ	0FN93ZZ	0FPB0KZ	0FPD3YZ	0FS70ZZ	0FU58KZ	0FUD3KZ	0FV84ZZ	0FW042Z	0FWB8DZ
0FL74CZ	0FLF4DZ	0FN94ZZ	0FPB0YZ	0FPD40Z	0FS74ZZ	0FU607Z	0FUD47Z	0FV87DZ	0FW043Z	0FWB8JZ
0FL74DZ	0FLF4ZZ	0FN97ZZ	0FPB30Z	0FPD41Z	0FS84ZZ	0FU60JZ	0FUD4JZ	0FV87ZZ	0FW04YZ	0FWB8KZ
0FL74ZZ	0FLF7DZ	0FN98ZZ	0FPB31Z	0FPD42Z	0FS90ZZ	0FU60KZ	0FUD4KZ	0FV88DZ	0FW0X0Z	0FWB8YZ
0FL77DZ	0FLF7ZZ	0FNC0ZZ	0FPB32Z	0FPD43Z	0FS94ZZ	0FU637Z	0FUD87Z	0FV88ZZ	0FW0X2Z	0FWBX0Z
0FL77ZZ	0FLF8DZ	0FNC4ZZ	0FPB33Z	0FPD47Z	0FSC0ZZ	0FU63JZ	0FUD8JZ	0FV90CZ	0FW0X3Z	0FWBX2Z
0FL78DZ	0FLF8ZZ	0FNC7ZZ	0FPB37Z	0FPD4CZ	0FSC4ZZ	0FU63KZ	0FUD8KZ	0FV90DZ	0FW400Z	0FWBX3Z
0FL78ZZ	0FM00ZZ	0FNC8ZZ	0FPB3CZ	0FPD4YZ	0FSD0ZZ	0FU647Z	0FUF07Z	0FV90ZZ	0FW402Z	0FWBX7Z
0FL80CZ	0FM04ZZ	0FND0ZZ	0FPB3DZ	0FPD70Z	0FSD4ZZ	0FU64JZ	0FUF0JZ	0FV93CZ	0FW403Z	0FWBXCZ
0FL80DZ	0FM10ZZ	0FND3ZZ	0FPB3JZ	0FPD72Z	0FSF0ZZ	0FU64KZ	0FUF0KZ	0FV93DZ	0FW40DZ	0FWBXDZ
0FL80ZZ	0FM14ZZ	0FND4ZZ	0FPB3KZ	0FPD73Z	0FSF4ZZ	0FU687Z	0FUF37Z	0FV93ZZ	0FW40YZ	0FWBXJZ
0FL83CZ	0FM20ZZ	0FND7ZZ	0FPB3YZ	0FPD7DZ	0FSG0ZZ	0FU68JZ	0FUF3JZ	0FV94CZ	0FW430Z	0FWBXKZ
0FL83DZ	0FM24ZZ	0FND8ZZ	0FPB40Z	0FPD7YZ	0FSG4ZZ	0FU68KZ	0FUF3KZ	0FV94DZ	0FW432Z	0FWD00Z
0FL83ZZ	0FM40ZZ	0FNF0ZZ	0FPB41Z	0FPD80Z	0FT00ZZ	0FU707Z	0FUF47Z	0FV94ZZ	0FW433Z	0FWD02Z
0FL84CZ	0FM44ZZ	0FNF3ZZ	0FPB42Z	0FPD82Z	0FT04ZZ	0FU70JZ	0FUF4JZ	0FV97DZ	0FW43DZ	0FWD03Z
0FL84DZ	0FM50ZZ	0FNF4ZZ	0FPB43Z	0FPD83Z	0FT10ZZ	0FU70KZ	0FUF4KZ	0FV97ZZ	0FW43YZ	0FWD07Z
0FL84ZZ	0FM54ZZ	0FNF7ZZ	0FPB47Z	0FPD8DZ	0FT14ZZ	0FU737Z	0FUF87Z	0FV98DZ	0FW440Z	0FWD0CZ
0FL87DZ	0FM60ZZ	0FNF8ZZ	0FPB4CZ	0FPD8YZ	0FT20ZZ	0FU73JZ	0FUF8JZ	0FV98ZZ	0FW442Z	0FWD0DZ
0FL87ZZ	0FM64ZZ	0FNG0ZZ	0FPB4DZ	0FPDX0Z	0FT24ZZ	0FU73KZ	0FUF8KZ	0FVC0CZ	0FW443Z	0FWD0JZ
0FL88DZ	0FM70ZZ	0FNG3ZZ	0FPB4JZ	0FPDX1Z	0FT40ZZ	0FU747Z	0FV50CZ	0FVC0DZ	0FW44DZ	0FWD0KZ
0FL88ZZ	0FM74ZZ	0FNG4ZZ	0FPB4KZ	0FPDX2Z	0FT44ZZ	0FU74JZ	0FV50DZ	0FVC0ZZ	0FW44YZ	0FWD0YZ
0FL90CZ	0FM80ZZ	0FNG8ZZ	0FPB4YZ	0FPDX3Z	0FT50ZZ	0FU74KZ	0FV50ZZ	0FVC3CZ	0FW4X0Z	0FWD30Z
0FL90DZ	0FM84ZZ	0FP000Z	0FPB70Z	0FPDXDZ	0FT54ZZ	0FU787Z	0FV53CZ	0FVC3DZ	0FW4X2Z	0FWD32Z
0FL90ZZ	0FM90ZZ	0FP002Z	0FPB71Z	0FPG0YZ	0FT57ZZ	0FU78JZ	0FV53DZ	0FVC3ZZ	0FW4X3Z	0FWD33Z
0FL93CZ	0FM94ZZ		0FPB72Z	0FPG3YZ	0FT58ZZ	0FU78KZ	0FV53ZZ	0FVC4CZ	0FW4XDZ	0FWD37Z
0FL93DZ	0FMC0ZZ		0FPB73Z	0FPG4YZ	0FT60ZZ	0FU807Z	0FV54CZ	0FVC4DZ	0FWB00Z	0FWD3CZ

0FWD3DZ	0G21X0Z	0G5N4ZZ	0G9H30Z	0GCD3ZZ	0GMH4ZZ	0GNM4ZZ	0GQ70ZZ	0GSP4ZZ	0GWKX0Z	0H52XZD
0FWD3JZ	0G21XYZ	0G5P0ZZ	0G9H3ZX	0GCD4ZZ	0GML0ZZ	0GNN0ZZ	0GQ73ZZ	0GSQ0ZZ	0GWR00Z	0H52XZZ
0FWD3KZ	0G25X0Z	0G5P3ZZ	0G9H3ZZ	0GCF0ZZ	0GML4ZZ	0GNN3ZZ	0GQ74ZZ	0GSQ4ZZ	0GWR30Z	0H53XZD
0FWD3YZ	0G25XYZ	0G5P4ZZ	0G9H40Z	0GCF3ZZ	0GMM0ZZ	0GNN4ZZ	0GQ80ZZ	0GSR0ZZ	0GWR40Z	0H53XZZ
0FWD40Z	0G2KX0Z	0G5Q0ZZ	0G9H4ZX	0GCF4ZZ	0GMM4ZZ	0GNP0ZZ	0GQ83ZZ	0GSR4ZZ	0GWRX0Z	0H54XZD
0FWD42Z	0G2KXYZ	0G5Q3ZZ	0G9H4ZZ	0GCG0ZZ	0GMN0ZZ	0GNP3ZZ	0GQ84ZZ	0GT00ZZ	0GWS00Z	0H54XZZ
0FWD43Z	0G2RX0Z	0G5Q4ZZ	0G9K30Z	0GCG3ZZ	0GMN4ZZ	0GNP4ZZ	0GQ90ZZ	0GT04ZZ	0GWS02Z	0H55XZD
0FWD47Z	0G2RXYZ	0G5R0ZZ	0G9K3ZX	0GCG4ZZ	0GMP0ZZ	0GNQ0ZZ	0GQ93ZZ	0GT10ZZ	0GWS03Z	0H55XZZ
0FWD4CZ	0G2SX0Z	0G5R3ZZ	0G9K3ZZ	0GCH0ZZ	0GMP4ZZ	0GNQ3ZZ	0GQ94ZZ	0GT14ZZ	0GWS0YZ	0H56XZD
0FWD4DZ	0G2SXYZ	0G5R4ZZ	0G9K40Z	0GCH3ZZ	0GMQ0ZZ	0GNQ4ZZ	0GQB0ZZ	0GT20ZZ	0GWS30Z	0H56XZZ
0FWD4JZ	0G500ZZ	0G800ZZ	0G9K4ZX	0GCH4ZZ	0GMQ4ZZ	0GNR0ZZ	0GQB3ZZ	0GT24ZZ	0GWS32Z	0H57XZD
0FWD4KZ	0G503ZZ	0G803ZZ	0G9K4ZZ	0GCK0ZZ	0GMR0ZZ	0GNR3ZZ	0GQB4ZZ	0GT30ZZ	0GWS33Z	0H57XZZ
0FWD4YZ	0G504ZZ	0G804ZZ	0G9L30Z	0GCK3ZZ	0GMR4ZZ	0GNR4ZZ	0GQC0ZZ	0GT34ZZ	0GWS3YZ	0H58XZD
0FWD70Z	0G510ZZ	0G810ZZ	0G9L3ZZ	0GCK4ZZ	0GN00ZZ	0GP000Z	0GQC3ZZ	0GT40ZZ	0GWS40Z	0H58XZZ
0FWD72Z	0G513ZZ	0G8J0ZZ	0G9L40Z	0GCL0ZZ	0GN03ZZ	0GP030Z	0GQC4ZZ	0GT44ZZ	0GWS42Z	0H59XZD
0FWD73Z	0G514ZZ	0G8J3ZZ	0G9L4ZZ	0GCL3ZZ	0GN04ZZ	0GP040Z	0GQD0ZZ	0GT60ZZ	0GWS43Z	0H59XZZ
0FWD77Z	0G520ZZ	0G8J4ZZ	0G9M30Z	0GCL4ZZ	0GN10ZZ	0GP0X0Z	0GQD3ZZ	0GT64ZZ	0GWS4YZ	0H5AXZD
0FWD7CZ	0G523ZZ	0G9000Z	0G9M3ZZ	0GCM0ZZ	0GN13ZZ	0GP100Z	0GQD4ZZ	0GT70ZZ	0GWSX0Z	0H5AXZZ
0FWD7DZ	0G524ZZ	0G900ZX	0G9M40Z	0GCM3ZZ	0GN14ZZ	0GP130Z	0GQF0ZZ	0GT74ZZ	0GWSX3Z	0H5BXZD
0FWD7JZ	0G530ZZ	0G900ZZ	0G9M4ZZ	0GCM4ZZ	0GN20ZZ	0GP140Z	0GQF3ZZ	0GT80ZZ	0H0T07Z	0H5BXZZ
0FWD7KZ	0G533ZZ	0G9030Z	0G9N30Z	0GCN0ZZ	0GN23ZZ	0GP1X0Z	0GQF4ZZ	0GT84ZZ	0H0T0JZ	0H5CXZD
0FWD7YZ	0G534ZZ	0G903ZX	0G9N3ZZ	0GCN3ZZ	0GN24ZZ	0GP500Z	0GQG0ZZ	0GT90ZZ	0H0T0KZ	0H5CXZZ
0FWD80Z	0G540ZZ	0G903ZZ	0G9N40Z	0GCN4ZZ	0GN30ZZ	0GP530Z	0GQG3ZZ	0GT94ZZ	0H0T0ZZ	0H5DXZD
0FWD82Z	0G543ZZ	0G9040Z	0G9N4ZZ	0GCP0ZZ	0GN33ZZ	0GP540Z	0GQG4ZZ	0GTB0ZZ	0H0T37Z	0H5DXZZ
0FWD83Z	0G544ZZ	0G904ZX	0G9P30Z	0GCP3ZZ	0GN34ZZ	0GP5X0Z	0GQH0ZZ	0GTB4ZZ	0H0T3JZ	0H5EXZD
0FWD87Z	0G560ZZ	0G904ZZ	0G9P3ZZ	0GCP4ZZ	0GN40ZZ	0GPK00Z	0GQH3ZZ	0GTC0ZZ	0H0T3KZ	0H5EXZZ
0FWD8CZ	0G563ZZ	0G9100Z	0G9P40Z	0GCQ0ZZ	0GN43ZZ	0GPK30Z	0GQH4ZZ	0GTC4ZZ	0H0T3ZZ	0H5FXZD
0FWD8DZ	0G564ZZ	0G910ZX	0G9P4ZZ	0GCQ3ZZ	0GN44ZZ	0GPK40Z	0GQJ0ZZ	0GTD0ZZ	0H0T7Z	0H5FXZZ
0FWD8JZ	0G570ZZ	0G910ZZ	0G9Q30Z	0GCQ4ZZ	0GN60ZZ	0GPKX0Z	0GQJ3ZZ	0GTD4ZZ	0H0TXJZ	0H5GXZD
0FWD8KZ	0G573ZZ	0G9130Z	0G9Q3ZZ	0GCR0ZZ	0GN63ZZ	0GPR00Z	0GQJ4ZZ	0GTF0ZZ	0H0TXKZ	0H5GXZZ
0FWD8YZ	0G574ZZ	0G913ZX	0G9Q40Z	0GCR3ZZ	0GN64ZZ	0GPR30Z	0GQK0ZZ	0GTF4ZZ	0H0TXZZ	0H5HXZD
0FWDX0Z	0G580ZZ	0G913ZZ	0G9Q4ZZ	0GCR4ZZ	0GN70ZZ	0GPR40Z	0GQK3ZZ	0GTG0ZZ	0H0U07Z	0H5HXZZ
0FWDX2Z	0G583ZZ	0G9140Z	0G9R30Z	0GHS02Z	0GN73ZZ	0GPRX0Z	0GQK4ZZ	0GTG4ZZ	0H0U0JZ	0H5JXZD
0FWDX3Z	0G584ZZ	0G9230Z	0G9R3ZZ	0GHS03Z	0GN74ZZ	0GPS00Z	0GQL0ZZ	0GTH0ZZ	0H0U0KZ	0H5JXZZ
0FWDX7Z	0G590ZZ	0G923ZX	0G9R40Z	0GHS0YZ	0GN80ZZ	0GPS02Z	0GQL3ZZ	0GTH4ZZ	0H0U0ZZ	0H5KXZD
0FWDXCZ	0G593ZZ	0G923ZZ	0G9R4ZZ	0GHS32Z	0GN83ZZ	0GPS03Z	0GQL4ZZ	0GTJ0ZZ	0H0U37Z	0H5KXZZ
0FWDXDZ	0G594ZZ	0G924ZX	0GB23ZX	0GHS33Z	0GN84ZZ	0GPS0YZ	0GQM0ZZ	0GTJ4ZZ	0H0U3JZ	0H5LXZD
0FWDXJZ	0G5B0ZZ	0G9330Z	0GB24ZX	0GHS3YZ	0GN90ZZ	0GPS30Z	0GQM3ZZ	0GTK0ZZ	0H0U3KZ	0H5LXZZ
0FWDXKZ	0G5B3ZZ	0G933ZX	0GB33ZX	0GHS42Z	0GN93ZZ	0GPS32Z	0GQM4ZZ	0GTK4ZZ	0H0U3ZZ	0H5MXZD
0FWG00Z	0G5B4ZZ	0G933ZZ	0GB34ZX	0GHS43Z	0GN94ZZ	0GPS33Z	0GQN0ZZ	0GTL0ZZ	0H0UX7Z	0H5MXZZ
0FWG02Z	0G5C0ZZ	0G934ZX	0GB43ZX	0GHS4YZ	0GNB0ZZ	0GPS3YZ	0GQN3ZZ	0GTL4ZZ	0H0UXJZ	0H5NXZD
0FWG03Z	0G5C3ZZ	0G9430Z	0GB44ZX	0GJ00ZZ	0GNB3ZZ	0GPS40Z	0GQN4ZZ	0GTM0ZZ	0H0UXKZ	0H5NXZZ
0FWG0DZ	0G5C4ZZ	0G943ZX	0GBG3ZX	0GJ03ZZ	0GNB4ZZ	0GPS42Z	0GQP0ZZ	0GTM4ZZ	0H0UXZZ	0H5QXZZ
0FWG0YZ	0G5D0ZZ	0G943ZZ	0GBG4ZX	0GJ04ZZ	0GNC0ZZ	0GPS43Z	0GQP3ZZ	0GTN0ZZ	0H0V07Z	0H5RXZZ
0FWG30Z	0G5D3ZZ	0G944ZX	0GBH3ZX	0GJ10ZZ	0GNC3ZZ	0GPS4YZ	0GQP4ZZ	0GTN4ZZ	0H0V0JZ	0H5T0ZZ
0FWG32Z	0G5D4ZZ	0G963ZZ	0GBH4ZX	0GJ13ZZ	0GNC4ZZ	0GPSX0Z	0GQQ0ZZ	0GTP0ZZ	0H0V0KZ	0H5T3ZZ
0FWG33Z	0G5F0ZZ	0G9730Z	0GBJ0ZX	0GJ14ZZ	0GND0ZZ	0GPSX2Z	0GQQ3ZZ	0GTP4ZZ	0H0V0ZZ	0H5T7ZZ
0FWG3DZ	0G5F3ZZ	0G973ZZ	0GBJ0ZZ	0GJ50ZZ	0GND3ZZ	0GPSX3Z	0GQQ4ZZ	0GTQ0ZZ	0H0V37Z	0H5T8ZZ
0FWG3YZ	0G5F4ZZ	0G9830Z	0GBJ3ZX	0GJ53ZZ	0GND4ZZ	0GQ00ZZ	0GQR0ZZ	0GTQ4ZZ	0H0V3JZ	0H5TXZZ
0FWG40Z	0G5G0ZZ	0G983ZZ	0GBJ3ZZ	0GJ54ZZ	0GNF0ZZ	0GQ03ZZ	0GQR3ZZ	0GTR0ZZ	0H0V3KZ	0H5U0ZZ
0FWG42Z	0G5G3ZZ	0G9930Z	0GBJ4ZX	0GJK0ZZ	0GNF3ZZ	0GQ04ZZ	0GQR4ZZ	0GTR4ZZ	0H0V3ZZ	0H82XZZ
0FWG43Z	0G5G4ZZ	0G993ZZ	0GBJ4ZZ	0GJK3ZZ	0GNF4ZZ	0GQ10ZZ	0GS20ZZ	0GW000Z	0H0VX7Z	0H83XZZ
0FWG4DZ	0G5H0ZZ	0G9B30Z	0GC74ZZ	0GJK4ZZ	0GNG0ZZ	0GQ13ZZ	0GS24ZZ	0GW030Z	0H0VXJZ	0H90X0Z
0FWG4YZ	0G5H3ZZ	0G9B3ZZ	0GC80ZZ	0GJR0ZZ	0GNG3ZZ	0GQ14ZZ	0GS30ZZ	0GW040Z	0H0VXKZ	0H90XZX
0FWGX0Z	0G5H4ZZ	0G9C30Z	0GC83ZZ	0GJR3ZZ	0GNG4ZZ	0GQ20ZZ	0GS34ZZ	0GW0X0Z	0H0VXZZ	0H90XZZ
0FWGX2Z	0G5K0ZZ	0G9C3ZZ	0GC84ZZ	0GJR4ZZ	0GNH0ZZ	0GQ23ZZ	0GSG0ZZ	0GW100Z	0H2PX0Z	0H91X0Z
0FWGX3Z	0G5K3ZZ	0G9D30Z	0GC90ZZ	0GJS0ZZ	0GNH3ZZ	0GQ24ZZ	0GSG4ZZ	0GW130Z	0H2PXYZ	0H91XZX
0FWGXDZ	0G5K4ZZ	0G9D3ZZ	0GC93ZZ	0GJS3ZZ	0GNH4ZZ	0GQ30ZZ	0GSH0ZZ	0GW140Z	0H2TX0Z	0H91XZZ
0FY00Z0	0G5L0ZZ	0G9F30Z	0GC94ZZ	0GJS4ZZ	0GNK0ZZ	0GQ33ZZ	0GSH4ZZ	0GW1X0Z	0H2TXYZ	0H92X0Z
0FY00Z1	0G5L3ZZ	0G9F3ZZ	0GCB0ZZ	0GM20ZZ	0GNK3ZZ	0GQ34ZZ	0GSL0ZZ	0GW500Z	0H2UX0Z	0H92XZX
0FY00Z2	0G5L4ZZ	0G9G30Z	0GCB3ZZ	0GM24ZZ	0GNK4ZZ	0GQ40ZZ	0GSL4ZZ	0GW530Z	0H2UXYZ	0H92XZZ
0FYG0Z0	0G5M0ZZ	0G9G3ZX	0GCB4ZZ	0GM30ZZ	0GNL0ZZ	0GQ43ZZ	0GSM0ZZ	0GW540Z	0H50XZD	0H93X0Z
0FYG0Z1	0G5M3ZZ	0G9G3ZZ	0GCC0ZZ	0GM34ZZ	0GNL4ZZ	0GQ44ZZ	0GSM4ZZ	0GW5X0Z	0H50XZZ	0H93XZX
0FYG0Z2	0G5M4ZZ	0G9G40Z	0GCC3ZZ	0GMG0ZZ	0GNL4ZZ	0GQ60ZZ	0GSN0ZZ	0GWK00Z	0H51XZD	0H93XZZ
0G20X0Z	0G5N0ZZ	0G9G4ZZ	0GCC4ZZ	0GMG4ZZ	0GNM0ZZ	0GQ63ZZ	0GSN4ZZ	0GWK30Z	0H51XZZ	0H94X0Z
0G20XYZ	0G5N3ZZ	0G9G4ZZ	0GCD0ZZ	0GMH0ZZ	0GNM3ZZ	0GQ64ZZ	0GSP0ZZ	0GWK40Z		0H94XZX

APPENDIX H: NON-OR NOT AFFECTING MS-DRG ASSIGNMENT

0H94XZZ-0HWT0KZ

0H94XZZ	0H9T7ZZ	0HB2XZZ	0HBVXZZ	0HCV0ZZ	0HHU8YZ	0HMUXZZ	0HPRXKZ	0HPUX1Z	0HR1X73	0HRHXJ4
0H95X0Z	0H9T80Z	0HB3XZX	0HBW0ZX	0HCV3ZZ	0HHUX1Z	0HMVXZZ	0HPSX7Z	0HPUX7Z	0HR1X74	0HRHXJZ
0H95XZX	0H9T8ZX	0HB3XZZ	0HBW0ZZ	0HCV7ZZ	0HHV01Z	0HMWXZZ	0HPSXJZ	0HPUXJZ	0HR1XJ3	0HRHXK3
0H95XZZ	0H9T8ZZ	0HB4XZX	0HBW3ZX	0HCV8ZZ	0HHV0NZ	0HMXXZZ	0HPSXKZ	0HPUXKZ	0HR1XJ4	0HRHXK4
0H96X0Z	0H9TX0Z	0HB5XZX	0HBW3ZZ	0HCVXZZ	0HHV31Z	0HN0XZZ	0HPT00Z	0HQ0XZZ	0HR8XJZ	0HRJX73
0H96XZX	0H9TXZX	0HB6XZX	0HBW7ZX	0HCW0ZZ	0HHV3NZ	0HN1XZZ	0HPT01Z	0HQ1XZZ	0HR8XK3	0HRJX74
0H96XZZ	0H9TXZZ	0HB7XZX	0HBW7ZZ	0HCW3ZZ	0HHV71Z	0HN2XZZ	0HPT07Z	0HQ2XZZ	0HR8XK4	0HRJXJ3
0H97X0Z	0H9U00Z	0HB8XZX	0HBW8ZX	0HCW7ZZ	0HHV7NZ	0HN3XZZ	0HPT0JZ	0HQ3XZZ	0HR9X73	0HRJXJ4
0H97XZX	0H9U0ZZ	0HB9XZX	0HBW8ZZ	0HCW8ZZ	0HHV81Z	0HN4XZZ	0HPT0KZ	0HQ4XZZ	0HR9X74	0HRJXJZ
0H97XZZ	0H9U30Z	0HBAXZX	0HBWXZX	0HCWXZZ	0HHV8NZ	0HN5XZZ	0HPT0NZ	0HQ5XZZ	0HR9XJ3	0HRJXK3
0H98X0Z	0H9U3ZX	0HBBXZX	0HBWXZZ	0HCX0ZZ	0HHVX1Z	0HN6XZZ	0HPT0YZ	0HQ6XZZ	0HR9XJ4	0HRJXK4
0H98XZX	0H9U3ZZ	0HBCXZX	0HBX0ZX	0HCX3ZZ	0HHW01Z	0HN7XZZ	0HPT30Z	0HQ7XZZ	0HR9XJZ	0HRKX73
0H98XZZ	0H9U70Z	0HBCXZZ	0HBX0ZZ	0HCX7ZZ	0HHW0NZ	0HN8XZZ	0HPT31Z	0HQ8XZZ	0HR9XK3	0HRKX74
0H99XZZ	0H9U7ZX	0HBDXZX	0HBX3ZX	0HCX8ZZ	0HHW31Z	0HN9XZZ	0HPT37Z	0HQ9XZZ	0HR9XK4	0HRKXJ3
0H9AX0Z	0H9U7ZZ	0HBDXZZ	0HBX3ZZ	0HCXXZZ	0HHW3NZ	0HNAXZZ	0HPT3JZ	0HQAXZZ	0HRAX73	0HRKXJ4
0H9AXZX	0H9U80Z	0HBEXZX	0HBX7ZX	0HD0XZZ	0HHW71Z	0HNBXZZ	0HPT3KZ	0HQBXZZ	0HRAX74	0HRKXJZ
0H9AXZZ	0H9U8ZX	0HBEXZZ	0HBX7ZZ	0HD1XZZ	0HHW7NZ	0HNCXZZ	0HPT3NZ	0HQCXZZ	0HRAXJ3	0HRKXK3
0H9BX0Z	0H9U8ZZ	0HBFXZX	0HBX8ZX	0HD2XZZ	0HHW81Z	0HNDXZZ	0HPT3YZ	0HQDXZZ	0HRAXJ4	0HRKXK4
0H9BXZX	0H9UX0Z	0HBFXZZ	0HBX8ZZ	0HD3XZZ	0HHW8NZ	0HNEXZZ	0HPT70Z	0HQEXZZ	0HRAXJZ	0HRLX73
0H9BXZZ	0H9UXZX	0HBGXZX	0HBXXZX	0HD4XZZ	0HHWX1Z	0HNFXZZ	0HPT71Z	0HQFXZZ	0HRAXK3	0HRLX74
0H9CX0Z	0H9UXZZ	0HBGXZZ	0HBXXZZ	0HD5XZZ	0HHX01Z	0HNGXZZ	0HPT77Z	0HQGXZZ	0HRAXK4	0HRLXJ3
0H9CXZX	0H9V00Z	0HBHXZX	0HBY0ZX	0HD6XZZ	0HHX0NZ	0HNHXZZ	0HPT7JZ	0HQHXZZ	0HRBX73	0HRLXJ4
0H9CXZZ	0H9V0ZZ	0HBHXZZ	0HBY0ZZ	0HD7XZZ	0HHX31Z	0HNJXZZ	0HPT7KZ	0HQJXZZ	0HRBX74	0HRLXJZ
0H9DX0Z	0H9V30Z	0HBJXZX	0HBY3ZX	0HD8XZZ	0HHX3NZ	0HNKXZZ	0HPT7NZ	0HQKXZZ	0HRBXJ3	0HRLXK3
0H9DXZX	0H9V3ZX	0HBJXZZ	0HBY3ZZ	0HD9XZZ	0HHX71Z	0HNLXZZ	0HPT7YZ	0HQLXZZ	0HRBXJ4	0HRLXK4
0H9DXZZ	0H9V3ZZ	0HBKXZX	0HBY7ZX	0HDAXZZ	0HHX7NZ	0HNMXZZ	0HPT80Z	0HQMXZZ	0HRBXJZ	0HRMX73
0H9EX0Z	0H9V70Z	0HBKXZZ	0HBY7ZZ	0HDBXZZ	0HHX81Z	0HNNXZZ	0HPT81Z	0HQNXZZ	0HRBXK3	0HRMX74
0H9EXZX	0H9V7ZX	0HBLXZX	0HBY8ZX	0HDCXZZ	0HHX8NZ	0HNQXZZ	0HPT87Z	0HQQXZZ	0HRBXK4	0HRMXJ3
0H9EXZZ	0H9V7ZZ	0HBLXZZ	0HBY8ZZ	0HDDXZZ	0HHXX1Z	0HNRXZZ	0HPT8JZ	0HQRXZZ	0HRCX73	0HRMXJ4
0H9FX0Z	0H9V80Z	0HBMXZX	0HBYXZX	0HDEXZZ	0HJPXZZ	0HNT0ZZ	0HPT8KZ	0HQT0ZZ	0HRCX74	0HRMXJZ
0H9FXZX	0H9V8ZX	0HBMXZZ	0HBYXZZ	0HDFXZZ	0HJQXZZ	0HNT3ZZ	0HPT8NZ	0HQT3ZZ	0HRCXJ3	0HRMXK3
0H9FXZZ	0H9V8ZZ	0HBNXZX	0HC0XZZ	0HDGXZZ	0HJRXZZ	0HNT7ZZ	0HPT8YZ	0HQT7ZZ	0HRCXJ4	0HRMXK4
0H9GX0Z	0H9VX0Z	0HBNXZZ	0HC1XZZ	0HDHXZZ	0HJT0ZZ	0HNT8ZZ	0HPTX0Z	0HQT8ZZ	0HRCXJZ	0HRNX73
0H9GXZX	0H9VXZX	0HBQXZX	0HC2XZZ	0HDJXZZ	0HJT3ZZ	0HNTXZZ	0HPTX1Z	0HQTXZZ	0HRCXK3	0HRNX74
0H9GXZZ	0H9VXZZ	0HBQXZZ	0HC3XZZ	0HDKXZZ	0HJT7ZZ	0HNU0ZZ	0HPTX7Z	0HQU0ZZ	0HRCXK4	0HRNXJ3
0H9HX0Z	0H9W00Z	0HBRXZX	0HC4XZZ	0HDLXZZ	0HJT8ZZ	0HNU3ZZ	0HPTXJZ	0HQU3ZZ	0HRDX73	0HRSX7Z
0H9HXZX	0H9W0ZZ	0HBRXZZ	0HC5XZZ	0HDMXZZ	0HJTXZZ	0HNU7ZZ	0HPTXKZ	0HQU7ZZ	0HRDX74	0HSSXZZ
0H9HXZZ	0H9W30Z	0HBT0ZX	0HC6XZZ	0HDNXZZ	0HJU0ZZ	0HNU8ZZ	0HPU00Z	0HQU8ZZ	0HRDXJ3	0HTQXZZ
0H9JX0Z	0H9W3ZX	0HBT0ZZ	0HC7XZZ	0HDQXZZ	0HJU3ZZ	0HNUXZZ	0HPU01Z	0HQUXZZ	0HRDXJ4	0HTRXZZ
0H9JXZX	0H9W3ZZ	0HBT3ZX	0HC8XZZ	0HDRXZZ	0HJU7ZZ	0HNV0ZZ	0HPU07Z	0HQV0ZZ	0HRDXJZ	0HUX7KZ
0H9JXZZ	0H9W70Z	0HBT3ZZ	0HC9XZZ	0HDSXZZ	0HJU8ZZ	0HNV3ZZ	0HPU0JZ	0HQV3ZZ	0HRDXK3	0HUX87Z
0H9KX0Z	0H9W7ZX	0HBT7ZX	0HCAXZZ	0HHPXYZ	0HJUXZZ	0HNV7ZZ	0HPU0KZ	0HQV7ZZ	0HRDXK4	0HUX8JZ
0H9KXZX	0H9W7ZZ	0HBT7ZZ	0HCBXZZ	0HHT01Z	0HM0XZZ	0HNV8ZZ	0HPU0NZ	0HQV8ZZ	0HREX73	0HUX8KZ
0H9KXZZ	0H9W80Z	0HBT8ZX	0HCCXZZ	0HHT0NZ	0HM1XZZ	0HNVXZZ	0HPU0YZ	0HQVXZZ	0HREX74	0HUXX7Z
0H9LX0Z	0H9W8ZX	0HBT8ZZ	0HCDXZZ	0HHT0YZ	0HM2XZZ	0HNW0ZZ	0HPU30Z	0HQW0ZZ	0HREXJ3	0HUXXJZ
0H9LXZX	0H9W8ZZ	0HBTXZX	0HCEXZZ	0HHT31Z	0HM3XZZ	0HNW3ZZ	0HPU31Z	0HQW3ZZ	0HREXJ4	0HUXXKZ
0H9LXZZ	0H9WX0Z	0HBTXZZ	0HCFXZZ	0HHT3NZ	0HM4XZZ	0HNW7ZZ	0HPU37Z	0HQW7ZZ	0HREXJZ	0HWPX0Z
0H9MX0Z	0H9WXZX	0HBU0ZX	0HCGXZZ	0HHT3YZ	0HM5XZZ	0HNW8ZZ	0HPU3JZ	0HQW8ZZ	0HREXK3	0HWPX7Z
0H9MXZX	0H9WXZZ	0HBU0ZZ	0HCHXZZ	0HHT71Z	0HM6XZZ	0HNWXZZ	0HPU3KZ	0HQWXZZ	0HREXK4	0HWPXJZ
0H9MXZZ	0H9X00Z	0HBU3ZX	0HCJXZZ	0HHT7NZ	0HM7XZZ	0HNX0ZZ	0HPU3NZ	0HQX0ZZ	0HRFX73	0HWPXKZ
0H9NX0Z	0H9X0ZZ	0HBU3ZZ	0HCKXZZ	0HHT7YZ	0HM8XZZ	0HNX3ZZ	0HPU3YZ	0HQX3ZZ	0HRFX74	0HWPXYZ
0H9NXZX	0H9X30Z	0HBU7ZX	0HCLXZZ	0HHT81Z	0HM9XZZ	0HNX7ZZ	0HPU70Z	0HQX7ZZ	0HRFXJ3	0HWQX0Z
0H9NXZZ	0H9X3ZX	0HBU7ZZ	0HCMXZZ	0HHT8NZ	0HMAXZZ	0HNX8ZZ	0HPU71Z	0HQX8ZZ	0HRFXJ4	0HWQX7Z
0H9QX0Z	0H9X3ZZ	0HBU8ZX	0HCNXZZ	0HHT8YZ	0HMBXZZ	0HNXXZZ	0HPU77Z	0HQXXZZ	0HRFXJZ	0HWQXJZ
0H9QXZX	0H9X70Z	0HBU8ZZ	0HCQXZZ	0HHTX1Z	0HMCXZZ	0HPPX0Z	0HPU7JZ	0HQY0ZZ	0HRFXK3	0HWQXKZ
0H9QXZZ	0H9X7ZX	0HBUXZX	0HCRXZZ	0HHU01Z	0HMDXZZ	0HPPX7Z	0HPU7KZ	0HQY3ZZ	0HRFXK4	0HWRX0Z
0H9RX0Z	0H9X7ZZ	0HBUXZZ	0HCT0ZZ	0HHU0NZ	0HMEXZZ	0HPPXJZ	0HPU7NZ	0HQY7ZZ	0HRGX73	0HWRX7Z
0H9RXZX	0H9X80Z	0HBV0ZX	0HCT3ZZ	0HHU0YZ	0HMFXZZ	0HPPXKZ	0HPU7YZ	0HQY8ZZ	0HRGX74	0HWRXJZ
0H9RXZZ	0H9X8ZX	0HBV0ZZ	0HCT7ZZ	0HHU31Z	0HMGXZZ	0HPPXYZ	0HPU80Z	0HQYXZZ	0HRGXJ3	0HWRXKZ
0H9T00Z	0H9X8ZZ	0HBV3ZX	0HCT8ZZ	0HHU3NZ	0HMHXZZ	0HPQX0Z	0HPU81Z	0HR0X73	0HRGXJ4	0HWSX7Z
0H9T0ZZ	0H9XX0Z	0HBV3ZZ	0HCTXZZ	0HHU3YZ	0HMJXZZ	0HPQX7Z	0HPU87Z	0HR0X74	0HRGXJZ	0HWSXJZ
0H9T30Z	0H9XXZX	0HBV7ZX	0HCU0ZZ	0HHU71Z	0HMKXZZ	0HPQXJZ	0HPU8JZ	0HR0XJ3	0HRGXK3	0HWSXKZ
0H9T3ZX	0H9XXZZ	0HBV7ZZ	0HCU3ZZ	0HHU7NZ	0HMLXZZ	0HPQXKZ	0HPU8KZ	0HR0XJ4	0HRGXK4	0HWT00Z
0H9T3ZZ	0HB0XZX	0HBV8ZX	0HCU7ZZ	0HHU7YZ	0HMMXZZ	0HPRX0Z	0HPU8NZ	0HR0XJZ	0HRHX73	0HWT07Z
0H9T70Z	0HB1XZX	0HBV8ZZ	0HCU8ZZ	0HHU81Z	0HMNXZZ	0HPRX7Z	0HPU8YZ	0HR0XK3	0HRHX74	0HWT0JZ
0H9T7ZX	0HB2XZX	0HBVXZX	0HCUXZZ	0HHU8NZ	0HMTXZZ	0HPRXJZ	0HPUX0Z	0HR0XK4	0HRHXJ3	0HWT0KZ

0HWT0NZ	0HXEXZZ	0J5C3ZZ	0J8Q3ZZ	0J9C0ZX	0J9Q0ZX	0JC60ZZ	0JH10NZ	0JH808Z	0JHG3NZ	0JNKXZZ
0HWT0YZ	0HXFXZZ	0J5D0ZZ	0J8R0ZZ	0J9C0ZZ	0J9Q0ZZ	0JC63ZZ	0JH13NZ	0JH809Z	0JHG3VZ	0JNLXZZ
0HWT30Z	0HXGXZZ	0J5D3ZZ	0J8R3ZZ	0J9C30Z	0J9Q30Z	0JC70ZZ	0JH40NZ	0JH80AZ	0JHG3WZ	0JNMXZZ
0HWT37Z	0HXHXZZ	0J5F0ZZ	0J8S0ZZ	0J9C3ZX	0J9Q3ZX	0JC73ZZ	0JH43NZ	0JH80BZ	0JHG3XZ	0JNNXZZ
0HWT3JZ	0HXJXZZ	0J5F3ZZ	0J8S3ZZ	0J9C3ZZ	0J9Q3ZZ	0JC80ZZ	0JH50NZ	0JH80CZ	0JHH0HZ	0JNPXZZ
0HWT3KZ	0HXKXZZ	0J5G0ZZ	0J8T0ZZ	0J9D00Z	0J9R00Z	0JC83ZZ	0JH53NZ	0JH80DZ	0JHH0NZ	0JNQXZZ
0HWT3NZ	0HXLXZZ	0J5G3ZZ	0J8T3ZZ	0J9D0ZX	0J9R0ZX	0JC90ZZ	0JH600Z	0JH80EZ	0JHH0VZ	0JNRXZZ
0HWT3YZ	0HXMXZZ	0J5H0ZZ	0J8V0ZZ	0J9D0ZZ	0J9R0ZZ	0JC93ZZ	0JH602Z	0JH80HZ	0JHH0WZ	0JPS00Z
0HWT70Z	0HXNXZZ	0J5H3ZZ	0J8V3ZZ	0J9D30Z	0J9R30Z	0JCB0ZZ	0JH604Z	0JH80MZ	0JHH0XZ	0JPS01Z
0HWT77Z	0J010ZZ	0J5J0ZZ	0J8W0ZZ	0J9D3ZX	0J9R3ZX	0JCB3ZZ	0JH605Z	0JH80NZ	0JHH3HZ	0JPS03Z
0HWT7JZ	0J013ZZ	0J5J3ZZ	0J8W3ZZ	0J9D3ZZ	0J9R3ZZ	0JCC0ZZ	0JH606Z	0JH80PZ	0JHH3NZ	0JPS07Z
0HWT7KZ	0J040ZZ	0J5K0ZZ	0J9000Z	0J9F00Z	0JB00ZX	0JCC3ZZ	0JH607Z	0JH80VZ	0JHH3VZ	0JPS0JZ
0HWT7NZ	0J043ZZ	0J5K3ZZ	0J900ZX	0J9F0ZX	0JB00ZZ	0JCD0ZZ	0JH608Z	0JH80WZ	0JHH3WZ	0JPS0KZ
0HWT7YZ	0J050ZZ	0J5L0ZZ	0J900ZZ	0J9F0ZZ	0JB03ZX	0JCD3ZZ	0JH609Z	0JH80XZ	0JHH3XZ	0JPS0NZ
0HWT80Z	0J053ZZ	0J5L3ZZ	0J9030Z	0J9F30Z	0JB03ZZ	0JCF0ZZ	0JH60AZ	0JH830Z	0JHJ0NZ	0JPS0YZ
0HWT87Z	0J060ZZ	0J5M0ZZ	0J903ZX	0J9F3ZX	0JB10ZX	0JCF3ZZ	0JH60BZ	0JH832Z	0JHJ3NZ	0JPS30Z
0HWT8JZ	0J063ZZ	0J5M3ZZ	0J903ZZ	0J9F3ZZ	0JB10ZZ	0JCG0ZZ	0JH60CZ	0JH834Z	0JHK0NZ	0JPS31Z
0HWT8KZ	0J070ZZ	0J5N0ZZ	0J9100Z	0J9G00Z	0JB13ZX	0JCG3ZZ	0JH60DZ	0JH835Z	0JHK3NZ	0JPS33Z
0HWT8NZ	0J073ZZ	0J5N3ZZ	0J910ZX	0J9G0ZX	0JB40ZX	0JCH0ZZ	0JH60EZ	0JH836Z	0JHL0HZ	0JPS37Z
0HWT8YZ	0J080ZZ	0J5P0ZZ	0J910ZZ	0J9G0ZZ	0JB43ZX	0JCH3ZZ	0JH60HZ	0JH837Z	0JHL3HZ	0JPS3JZ
0HWTX0Z	0J083ZZ	0J5P3ZZ	0J9130Z	0J9G30Z	0JB50ZX	0JCJ0ZZ	0JH60MZ	0JH838Z	0JHM0HZ	0JPS3KZ
0HWTX7Z	0J090ZZ	0J5Q0ZZ	0J913ZX	0J9G3ZX	0JB53ZX	0JCJ3ZZ	0JH60NZ	0JH839Z	0JHM3HZ	0JPS3NZ
0HWTXJZ	0J093ZZ	0J5Q3ZZ	0J913ZZ	0J9G3ZZ	0JB60ZX	0JCK0ZZ	0JH60PZ	0JH83AZ	0JHN0HZ	0JPS3YZ
0HWTXKZ	0J0D0ZZ	0J5R0ZZ	0J9400Z	0J9H00Z	0JB63ZX	0JCK3ZZ	0JH60VZ	0JH83BZ	0JHS03Z	0JPSX0Z
0HWU00Z	0J0D3ZZ	0J5R3ZZ	0J940ZX	0J9H0ZX	0JB70ZX	0JCL0ZZ	0JH60WZ	0JH83CZ	0JHS0YZ	0JPSX1Z
0HWU07Z	0J0F0ZZ	0J800ZZ	0J940ZZ	0J9H0ZZ	0JB73ZX	0JCL3ZZ	0JH60XZ	0JH83DZ	0JHS33Z	0JPSX3Z
0HWU0JZ	0J0F3ZZ	0J803ZZ	0J9430Z	0J9H30Z	0JB80ZX	0JCM0ZZ	0JH630Z	0JH83EZ	0JHS3YZ	0JPT00Z
0HWU0KZ	0J0G0ZZ	0J810ZZ	0J943ZX	0J9H3ZX	0JB83ZX	0JCM3ZZ	0JH632Z	0JH83HZ	0JHT03Z	0JPT01Z
0HWU0NZ	0J0G3ZZ	0J813ZZ	0J943ZZ	0J9H3ZZ	0JB90ZX	0JCN0ZZ	0JH634Z	0JH83MZ	0JHT0YZ	0JPT02Z
0HWU0YZ	0J0H0ZZ	0J840ZZ	0J9500Z	0J9J00Z	0JB93ZX	0JCN3ZZ	0JH635Z	0JH83NZ	0JHT33Z	0JPT03Z
0HWU30Z	0J0H3ZZ	0J843ZZ	0J950ZX	0J9J0ZX	0JBB0ZX	0JCP0ZZ	0JH636Z	0JH83PZ	0JHT3YZ	0JPT07Z
0HWU37Z	0J0L0ZZ	0J850ZZ	0J950ZZ	0J9J0ZZ	0JBB3ZX	0JCP3ZZ	0JH637Z	0JH83VZ	0JHV03Z	0JPT0HZ
0HWU3JZ	0J0L3ZZ	0J853ZZ	0J9530Z	0J9J30Z	0JBC0ZX	0JCQ0ZZ	0JH638Z	0JH83WZ	0JHV0YZ	0JPT0JZ
0HWU3KZ	0J0M0ZZ	0J860ZZ	0J953ZX	0J9J3ZX	0JBC3ZX	0JCQ3ZZ	0JH639Z	0JH83XZ	0JHV33Z	0JPT0KZ
0HWU3NZ	0J0M3ZZ	0J863ZZ	0J953ZZ	0J9J3ZZ	0JBD0ZX	0JCR0ZZ	0JH63AZ	0JH90NZ	0JHV3YZ	0JPT0MZ
0HWU3YZ	0J0N0ZZ	0J870ZZ	0J9600Z	0J9K00Z	0JBD3ZX	0JCR3ZZ	0JH63BZ	0JH93NZ	0JHW03Z	0JPT0NZ
0HWU70Z	0J0N3ZZ	0J873ZZ	0J960ZX	0J9K0ZX	0JBF0ZX	0JDB0ZZ	0JH63CZ	0JHB0NZ	0JHW0YZ	0JPT0VZ
0HWU77Z	0J0P0ZZ	0J880ZZ	0J960ZZ	0J9K0ZZ	0JBF3ZX	0JDB3ZZ	0JH63DZ	0JHB3NZ	0JHW33Z	0JPT0WZ
0HWU7JZ	0J0P3ZZ	0J883ZZ	0J9630Z	0J9K30Z	0JBG0ZX	0JDC0ZZ	0JH63EZ	0JHC0NZ	0JHW3YZ	0JPT0XZ
0HWU7KZ	0J2SX0Z	0J890ZZ	0J963ZX	0J9K3ZX	0JBG3ZX	0JDC3ZZ	0JH63HZ	0JHC3NZ	0JJS0ZZ	0JPT0YZ
0HWU7NZ	0J2SXYZ	0J893ZZ	0J963ZZ	0J9K3ZZ	0JBH0ZX	0JDD0ZZ	0JH63MZ	0JHD0HZ	0JJS3ZZ	0JPT30Z
0HWU7YZ	0J2TX0Z	0J8B0ZZ	0J9700Z	0J9L00Z	0JBH3ZX	0JDD3ZZ	0JH63NZ	0JHD0NZ	0JJSXZZ	0JPT31Z
0HWU80Z	0J2TXYZ	0J8B3ZZ	0J970ZX	0J9L0ZX	0JBJ0ZX	0JDF0ZZ	0JH63PZ	0JHD0VZ	0JJT0ZZ	0JPT32Z
0HWU87Z	0J2VX0Z	0J8C0ZZ	0J970ZZ	0J9L0ZZ	0JBJ3ZX	0JDF3ZZ	0JH63VZ	0JHD0WZ	0JJT3ZZ	0JPT33Z
0HWU8JZ	0J2VXYZ	0J8C3ZZ	0J9730Z	0J9L30Z	0JBK0ZX	0JDG0ZZ	0JH63WZ	0JHD0XZ	0JJTXZZ	0JPT37Z
0HWU8KZ	0J2WX0Z	0J8D0ZZ	0J973ZX	0J9L3ZX	0JBK3ZX	0JDG3ZZ	0JH63XZ	0JHD3HZ	0JJV0ZZ	0JPT3HZ
0HWU8NZ	0J2WXYZ	0J8D3ZZ	0J973ZZ	0J9L3ZZ	0JBL0ZX	0JDH0ZZ	0JH70BZ	0JHD3NZ	0JJV3ZZ	0JPT3JZ
0HWU8YZ	0J500ZZ	0J8F0ZZ	0J9800Z	0J9M00Z	0JBL3ZX	0JDH3ZZ	0JH70CZ	0JHD3VZ	0JJVXZZ	0JPT3KZ
0HWUX0Z	0J503ZZ	0J8F3ZZ	0J980ZX	0J9M0ZX	0JBM0ZX	0JDJ0ZZ	0JH70DZ	0JHD3WZ	0JJW0ZZ	0JPT3MZ
0HWUX7Z	0J510ZZ	0J8G0ZZ	0J980ZZ	0J9M0ZZ	0JBM3ZX	0JDJ3ZZ	0JH70EZ	0JHD3XZ	0JJW3ZZ	0JPT3NZ
0HWUXJZ	0J513ZZ	0J8G3ZZ	0J9830Z	0J9M30Z	0JBN0ZX	0JDK0ZZ	0JH70MZ	0JHF0HZ	0JJWXZZ	0JPT3VZ
0HWUXKZ	0J540ZZ	0J8H0ZZ	0J983ZX	0J9M3ZX	0JBN3ZX	0JDK3ZZ	0JH70NZ	0JHF0NZ	0JN0XZZ	0JPT3WZ
0HX0XZZ	0J543ZZ	0J8H3ZZ	0J983ZZ	0J9M3ZZ	0JBP0ZX	0JDL0ZZ	0JH70VZ	0JHF0VZ	0JN1XZZ	0JPT3XZ
0HX1XZZ	0J550ZZ	0J8J0ZZ	0J9900Z	0J9N00Z	0JBP3ZX	0JDL3ZZ	0JH73BZ	0JHF0WZ	0JN4XZZ	0JPT3YZ
0HX2XZZ	0J553ZZ	0J8J3ZZ	0J990ZX	0J9N0ZX	0JBQ0ZX	0JDM0ZZ	0JH73CZ	0JHF0XZ	0JN5XZZ	0JPTX0Z
0HX3XZZ	0J560ZZ	0J8K0ZZ	0J990ZZ	0J9N0ZZ	0JBQ3ZX	0JDM3ZZ	0JH73DZ	0JHF3HZ	0JN6XZZ	0JPTX1Z
0HX4XZZ	0J563ZZ	0J8K3ZZ	0J9930Z	0J9N30Z	0JBR0ZX	0JDN0ZZ	0JH73EZ	0JHF3NZ	0JN7XZZ	0JPTX2Z
0HX5XZZ	0J570ZZ	0J8L0ZZ	0J993ZX	0J9N3ZX	0JBR3ZX	0JDN3ZZ	0JH73MZ	0JHF3VZ	0JN8XZZ	0JPTX3Z
0HX6XZZ	0J573ZZ	0J8L3ZZ	0J993ZZ	0J9N3ZZ	0JC00ZZ	0JDP0ZZ	0JH73NZ	0JHF3WZ	0JN9XZZ	0JPTXHZ
0HX7XZZ	0J580ZZ	0J8M0ZZ	0J9B00Z	0J9P00Z	0JC03ZZ	0JDP3ZZ	0JH73VZ	0JHF3XZ	0JNBXZZ	0JPTXVZ
0HX8XZZ	0J583ZZ	0J8M3ZZ	0J9B0ZX	0J9P0ZX	0JC10ZZ	0JDQ0ZZ	0JH800Z	0JHG0HZ	0JNCXZZ	0JPTXXZ
0HX9XZZ	0J590ZZ	0J8N0ZZ	0J9B0ZZ	0J9P0ZZ	0JC13ZZ	0JDQ3ZZ	0JH802Z	0JHG0NZ	0JNDXZZ	0JPV00Z
0HXAXZZ	0J593ZZ	0J8N3ZZ	0J9B30Z	0J9P30Z	0JC40ZZ	0JDR0ZZ	0JH804Z	0JHG0VZ	0JNFXZZ	0JPV01Z
0HXBXZZ	0J5B0ZZ	0J8P0ZZ	0J9B3ZX	0J9P3ZX	0JC43ZZ	0JDR3ZZ	0JH805Z	0JHG0WZ	0JNGXZZ	0JPV03Z
0HXCXZZ	0J5B3ZZ	0J8P3ZZ	0J9B3ZZ	0J9P3ZZ	0JC50ZZ	0JH00NZ	0JH806Z	0JHG0XZ	0JNHXZZ	0JPV07Z
0HXDXZZ	0J5C0ZZ	0J8Q0ZZ	0J9C00Z	0J9Q00Z	0JC53ZZ	0JH03NZ	0JH807Z	0JHG3HZ	0JNJXZZ	0JPV0HZ

0JPV0JZ	0JQG0ZZ	0JR93JZ	0JRN3JZ	0JU93JZ	0JX40ZZ	0JXH0ZZ	0K840ZZ	0K8V0ZZ	0K9640Z	0K9G00Z
0JPV0KZ	0JQG3ZZ	0JR93KZ	0JRN3KZ	0JU93KZ	0JX43ZB	0JXH3ZB	0K843ZZ	0K8V3ZZ	0K964ZX	0K9G0ZX
0JPV0NZ	0JQH0ZZ	0JRB07Z	0JRP07Z	0JUB07Z	0JX43ZC	0JXH3ZC	0K844ZZ	0K8V4ZZ	0K964ZZ	0K9G0ZZ
0JPV0VZ	0JQH3ZZ	0JRB0JZ	0JRP0JZ	0JUB0JZ	0JX43ZZ	0JXH3ZZ	0K850ZZ	0K8W0ZZ	0K9700Z	0K9G30Z
0JPV0WZ	0JQJ0ZZ	0JRB0KZ	0JRP0KZ	0JUB0KZ	0JX50ZB	0JXJ0ZB	0K853ZZ	0K8W3ZZ	0K970ZX	0K9G3ZX
0JPV0XZ	0JQJ3ZZ	0JRB37Z	0JRP37Z	0JUB37Z	0JX50ZC	0JXJ0ZC	0K854ZZ	0K8W4ZZ	0K970ZZ	0K9G3ZZ
0JPV0YZ	0JQK0ZZ	0JRB3JZ	0JRP3JZ	0JUB3JZ	0JX50ZZ	0JXJ0ZZ	0K860ZZ	0K9000Z	0K9730Z	0K9G40Z
0JPV30Z	0JQK3ZZ	0JRB3KZ	0JRP3KZ	0JUB3KZ	0JX53ZB	0JXJ3ZB	0K863ZZ	0K900ZX	0K973ZX	0K9G4ZX
0JPV31Z	0JQL0ZZ	0JRC07Z	0JRQ07Z	0JUC07Z	0JX53ZC	0JXJ3ZC	0K864ZZ	0K900ZZ	0K973ZZ	0K9G4ZZ
0JPV33Z	0JQL3ZZ	0JRC0JZ	0JRQ0JZ	0JUC0JZ	0JX53ZZ	0JXJ3ZZ	0K870ZZ	0K9030Z	0K9740Z	0K9H00Z
0JPV37Z	0JQM0ZZ	0JRC0KZ	0JRQ0KZ	0JUC0KZ	0JX60ZB	0JXK0ZB	0K873ZZ	0K903ZX	0K974ZX	0K9H0ZX
0JPV3HZ	0JQM3ZZ	0JRC37Z	0JRQ37Z	0JWS0YZ	0JX60ZC	0JXK0ZC	0K874ZZ	0K903ZZ	0K974ZZ	0K9H0ZZ
0JPV3JZ	0JQN0ZZ	0JRC3JZ	0JRQ3JZ	0JWS3YZ	0JX60ZZ	0JXK0ZZ	0K880ZZ	0K9040Z	0K9800Z	0K9H30Z
0JPV3KZ	0JQN3ZZ	0JRC3KZ	0JRQ3KZ	0JWSX0Z	0JX63ZB	0JXK3ZB	0K883ZZ	0K904ZX	0K980ZX	0K9H3ZX
0JPV3NZ	0JQP0ZZ	0JRD07Z	0JRR07Z	0JWSX3Z	0JX63ZC	0JXK3ZC	0K884ZZ	0K904ZZ	0K980ZZ	0K9H3ZZ
0JPV3VZ	0JQP3ZZ	0JRD0JZ	0JRR0JZ	0JWSX7Z	0JX63ZZ	0JXK3ZZ	0K890ZZ	0K9100Z	0K9830Z	0K9H40Z
0JPV3WZ	0JQQ0ZZ	0JRD0KZ	0JRR0KZ	0JWSXJZ	0JX70ZB	0JXL0ZB	0K893ZZ	0K910ZX	0K983ZX	0K9H4ZX
0JPV3XZ	0JQQ3ZZ	0JRD37Z	0JRR37Z	0JWSXKZ	0JX70ZC	0JXL0ZC	0K894ZZ	0K910ZZ	0K983ZZ	0K9H4ZZ
0JPV3YZ	0JQR0ZZ	0JRD3JZ	0JRR3JZ	0JWSXNZ	0JX70ZZ	0JXL0ZZ	0K8B0ZZ	0K9130Z	0K9840Z	0K9J00Z
0JPVX0Z	0JQR3ZZ	0JRD3KZ	0JRR3KZ	0JWT0YZ	0JX73ZB	0JXL3ZB	0K8B3ZZ	0K913ZX	0K984ZX	0K9J0ZX
0JPVX1Z	0JR007Z	0JRF07Z	0JU007Z	0JWT3YZ	0JX73ZC	0JXL3ZC	0K8B4ZZ	0K913ZZ	0K984ZZ	0K9J0ZZ
0JPVX3Z	0JR00JZ	0JRF0JZ	0JU00JZ	0JWTX0Z	0JX73ZZ	0JXL3ZZ	0K8C0ZZ	0K9140Z	0K9900Z	0K9J30Z
0JPVXHZ	0JR00KZ	0JRF0KZ	0JU00KZ	0JWTX2Z	0JX80ZB	0JXM0ZB	0K8C3ZZ	0K914ZX	0K990ZX	0K9J3ZX
0JPVXVZ	0JR037Z	0JRF37Z	0JU037Z	0JWTX3Z	0JX80ZC	0JXM0ZC	0K8C4ZZ	0K914ZZ	0K990ZZ	0K9J3ZZ
0JPVXXZ	0JR03JZ	0JRF3JZ	0JU03JZ	0JWTX7Z	0JX80ZZ	0JXM0ZZ	0K8D0ZZ	0K9200Z	0K9930Z	0K9J40Z
0JPW00Z	0JR03KZ	0JRF3KZ	0JU03KZ	0JWTXHZ	0JX83ZB	0JXM3ZB	0K8D3ZZ	0K920ZX	0K993ZX	0K9J4ZX
0JPW01Z	0JR107Z	0JRG07Z	0JU107Z	0JWTXJZ	0JX83ZC	0JXM3ZC	0K8D4ZZ	0K920ZZ	0K993ZZ	0K9J4ZZ
0JPW03Z	0JR10JZ	0JRG0JZ	0JU10JZ	0JWTXKZ	0JX83ZZ	0JXM3ZZ	0K8F0ZZ	0K9230Z	0K9940Z	0K9K00Z
0JPW07Z	0JR10KZ	0JRG0KZ	0JU10KZ	0JWTXNZ	0JX90ZB	0JXN0ZB	0K8F3ZZ	0K923ZX	0K994ZX	0K9K0ZX
0JPW0HZ	0JR137Z	0JRG37Z	0JU137Z	0JWTXPZ	0JX90ZC	0JXN0ZC	0K8F4ZZ	0K923ZZ	0K994ZZ	0K9K0ZZ
0JPW0JZ	0JR13JZ	0JRG3JZ	0JU13JZ	0JWTXVZ	0JX90ZZ	0JXN0ZZ	0K8G0ZZ	0K9240Z	0K9B00Z	0K9K30Z
0JPW0KZ	0JR13KZ	0JRG3KZ	0JU13KZ	0JWTXWZ	0JX93ZB	0JXN3ZB	0K8G3ZZ	0K924ZX	0K9B0ZX	0K9K3ZX
0JPW0NZ	0JR407Z	0JRH07Z	0JU407Z	0JWTXXZ	0JX93ZC	0JXN3ZC	0K8G4ZZ	0K924ZZ	0K9B0ZZ	0K9K3ZZ
0JPW0VZ	0JR40JZ	0JRH0JZ	0JU40JZ	0JWV0YZ	0JX93ZZ	0K2XX0Z	0K8H0ZZ	0K9300Z	0K9B30Z	0K9K40Z
0JPW0WZ	0JR40KZ	0JRH0KZ	0JU40KZ	0JWV3YZ	0JXB0ZB	0K2XXYZ	0K8H3ZZ	0K930ZX	0K9B3ZX	0K9K4ZX
0JPW0XZ	0JR437Z	0JRH37Z	0JU437Z	0JWVX0Z	0JXB0ZC	0K2YX0Z	0K8H4ZZ	0K930ZZ	0K9B3ZZ	0K9K4ZZ
0JPW0YZ	0JR43JZ	0JRH3JZ	0JU43JZ	0JWVX3Z	0JXB0ZZ	0K2YXYZ	0K8J0ZZ	0K9330Z	0K9B40Z	0K9L00Z
0JPW30Z	0JR43KZ	0JRH3KZ	0JU43KZ	0JWVX7Z	0JXB3ZB	0K5Q3ZZ	0K8J3ZZ	0K933ZX	0K9B4ZX	0K9L0ZX
0JPW31Z	0JR507Z	0JRJ07Z	0JU507Z	0JWVXHZ	0JXB3ZC	0K5Q4ZZ	0K8J4ZZ	0K933ZZ	0K9B4ZZ	0K9L0ZZ
0JPW33Z	0JR50JZ	0JRJ0JZ	0JU50JZ	0JWVXJZ	0JXB3ZZ	0K5R0ZZ	0K8K0ZZ	0K9340Z	0K9C00Z	0K9L30Z
0JPW37Z	0JR50KZ	0JRJ0KZ	0JU50KZ	0JWVXKZ	0JXC0ZB	0K5R3ZZ	0K8K3ZZ	0K934ZX	0K9C0ZX	0K9L3ZX
0JPW3HZ	0JR537Z	0JRJ37Z	0JU537Z	0JWVXNZ	0JXC0ZC	0K5R4ZZ	0K8K4ZZ	0K934ZZ	0K9C0ZZ	0K9L3ZZ
0JPW3JZ	0JR53JZ	0JRJ3JZ	0JU53JZ	0JWVXVZ	0JXC0ZZ	0K5S0ZZ	0K8L0ZZ	0K9400Z	0K9C30Z	0K9L40Z
0JPW3KZ	0JR53KZ	0JRJ3KZ	0JU53KZ	0JWVXWZ	0JXC3ZB	0K5S3ZZ	0K8L3ZZ	0K940ZX	0K9C3ZX	0K9L4ZX
0JPW3NZ	0JR607Z	0JRK07Z	0JU607Z	0JWVXXZ	0JXC3ZC	0K5S4ZZ	0K8L4ZZ	0K940ZZ	0K9C3ZZ	0K9L4ZZ
0JPW3VZ	0JR60JZ	0JRK0JZ	0JU60JZ	0JWW0YZ	0JXC3ZZ	0K5T0ZZ	0K8M0ZZ	0K9430Z	0K9C40Z	0K9M00Z
0JPW3WZ	0JR60KZ	0JRK0KZ	0JU60KZ	0JWW3YZ	0JXD0ZB	0K5T3ZZ	0K8M3ZZ	0K943ZX	0K9C4ZX	0K9M0ZX
0JPW3XZ	0JR637Z	0JRK37Z	0JU637Z	0JWWX0Z	0JXD0ZC	0K5T4ZZ	0K8M4ZZ	0K943ZZ	0K9C4ZZ	0K9M0ZZ
0JPW3YZ	0JR63JZ	0JRK3JZ	0JU63JZ	0JWWX3Z	0JXD0ZZ	0K5V0ZZ	0K8N0ZZ	0K9440Z	0K9D00Z	0K9M30Z
0JPWX0Z	0JR63KZ	0JRK3KZ	0JU63KZ	0JWWX7Z	0JXD3ZB	0K5V3ZZ	0K8N3ZZ	0K944ZX	0K9D0ZX	0K9M3ZX
0JPWX1Z	0JR707Z	0JRL07Z	0JU707Z	0JWWXHZ	0JXD3ZC	0K5V4ZZ	0K8N4ZZ	0K944ZZ	0K9D0ZZ	0K9M3ZZ
0JPWX3Z	0JR70JZ	0JRL0JZ	0JU70JZ	0JWWXJZ	0JXD3ZZ	0K5W0ZZ	0K8P0ZZ	0K9500Z	0K9D30Z	0K9M40Z
0JPWXHZ	0JR70KZ	0JRL0KZ	0JU70KZ	0JWWXKZ	0JXF0ZB	0K5W3ZZ	0K8P3ZZ	0K950ZX	0K9D3ZX	0K9M4ZX
0JPWXVZ	0JR737Z	0JRL37Z	0JU737Z	0JWWXNZ	0JXF0ZC	0K5W4ZZ	0K8P4ZZ	0K950ZZ	0K9D3ZZ	0K9M4ZZ
0JPWXXZ	0JR73JZ	0JRL3JZ	0JU73JZ	0JWWXVZ	0JXF0ZZ	0K800ZZ	0K8Q0ZZ	0K9530Z	0K9D40Z	0K9N00Z
0JQ83ZZ	0JR73KZ	0JRL3KZ	0JU73KZ	0JWWXWZ	0JXF3ZB	0K803ZZ	0K8Q3ZZ	0K953ZX	0K9D4ZX	0K9N0ZX
0JQ90ZZ	0JR807Z	0JRM07Z	0JU807Z	0JWWXXZ	0JXF3ZC	0K804ZZ	0K8Q4ZZ	0K953ZZ	0K9D4ZZ	0K9N0ZZ
0JQ93ZZ	0JR80JZ	0JRM0JZ	0JU80JZ	0JX03ZZ	0JXF3ZZ	0K810ZZ	0K8R0ZZ	0K9540Z	0K9F00Z	0K9N30Z
0JQB0ZZ	0JR80KZ	0JRM0KZ	0JU80KZ	0JX10ZB	0JXG0ZB	0K813ZZ	0K8R3ZZ	0K954ZX	0K9F0ZX	0K9N3ZX
0JQB3ZZ	0JR837Z	0JRM37Z	0JU837Z	0JX10ZC	0JXG0ZC	0K814ZZ	0K8R4ZZ	0K954ZZ	0K9F0ZZ	0K9N3ZZ
0JQC0ZZ	0JR83JZ	0JRM3JZ	0JU83JZ	0JX10ZZ	0JXG0ZZ	0K820ZZ	0K8S0ZZ	0K9600Z	0K9F30Z	0K9N40Z
0JQC3ZZ	0JR83KZ	0JRM3KZ	0JU83KZ	0JX13ZB	0JXG3ZB	0K823ZZ	0K8S3ZZ	0K960ZX	0K9F3ZX	0K9N4ZX
0JQD0ZZ	0JR907Z	0JRN07Z	0JU907Z	0JX13ZC	0JXG3ZC	0K824ZZ	0K8S4ZZ	0K960ZZ	0K9F3ZZ	0K9N4ZZ
0JQD3ZZ	0JR90JZ	0JRN0JZ	0JU90JZ	0JX13ZZ	0JXG3ZZ	0K830ZZ	0K8T0ZZ	0K9630Z	0K9F40Z	0K9P00Z
0JQF0ZZ	0JR90KZ	0JRN0KZ	0JU90KZ	0JX40ZB	0JXH0ZB	0K833ZZ	0K8T3ZZ	0K963ZX	0K9F4ZX	0K9P0ZX
0JQF3ZZ	0JR937Z	0JRN37Z	0JU937Z	0JX40ZC	0JXH0ZC	0K834ZZ	0K8T4ZZ	0K963ZZ	0K9F4ZZ	0K9P0ZZ

0K9P30Z	0KBQ3ZZ	0KCC0ZZ	0KDH0ZZ	0KMJ4ZZ	0KQG3ZZ	0KR40JZ	0KRH0JZ	0KRV0JZ	0KSW4ZZ	0KU147Z
0K9P3ZX	0KBQ4ZX	0KCC3ZZ	0KDJ0ZZ	0KMK0ZZ	0KQG4ZZ	0KR40KZ	0KRH0KZ	0KRV0KZ	0KT00ZZ	0KU14JZ
0K9P3ZZ	0KBQ4ZZ	0KCC4ZZ	0KDK0ZZ	0KMK4ZZ	0KQH0ZZ	0KR447Z	0KRH47Z	0KRV47Z	0KT04ZZ	0KU14KZ
0K9P40Z	0KBR0ZX	0KCD0ZZ	0KDL0ZZ	0KML0ZZ	0KQH3ZZ	0KR44JZ	0KRH4JZ	0KRV4JZ	0KT10ZZ	0KU207Z
0K9P4ZX	0KBR0ZZ	0KCD3ZZ	0KDM0ZZ	0KML4ZZ	0KQH4ZZ	0KR44KZ	0KRH4KZ	0KRV4KZ	0KT14ZZ	0KU20JZ
0K9P4ZZ	0KBR3ZX	0KCD4ZZ	0KDN0ZZ	0KMM0ZZ	0KQJ0ZZ	0KR507Z	0KRJ07Z	0KRW07Z	0KT20ZZ	0KU20KZ
0K9Q30Z	0KBR3ZZ	0KCF0ZZ	0KDP0ZZ	0KMM4ZZ	0KQJ3ZZ	0KR50JZ	0KRJ0JZ	0KRW0JZ	0KT24ZZ	0KU247Z
0K9Q3ZZ	0KBR4ZX	0KCF3ZZ	0KDQ0ZZ	0KMN0ZZ	0KQJ4ZZ	0KR50KZ	0KRJ0KZ	0KRW0KZ	0KT30ZZ	0KU24JZ
0K9R30Z	0KBR4ZZ	0KCF4ZZ	0KDR0ZZ	0KMN4ZZ	0KQK0ZZ	0KR547Z	0KRJ47Z	0KRW47Z	0KT34ZZ	0KU24KZ
0K9R3ZZ	0KBS0ZX	0KCG0ZZ	0KDS0ZZ	0KMP0ZZ	0KQK3ZZ	0KR54JZ	0KRJ4JZ	0KRW4JZ	0KT40ZZ	0KUM0JZ
0K9S30Z	0KBS0ZZ	0KCG3ZZ	0KDT0ZZ	0KMP4ZZ	0KQK4ZZ	0KR54KZ	0KRJ4KZ	0KRW4KZ	0KT44ZZ	0KUM0KZ
0K9S3ZZ	0KBS3ZX	0KCG4ZZ	0KDV0ZZ	0KMQ0ZZ	0KQL0ZZ	0KR607Z	0KRK07Z	0KS00ZZ	0KT50ZZ	0KUM47Z
0K9T30Z	0KBS3ZZ	0KCH0ZZ	0KDW0ZZ	0KMQ4ZZ	0KQL3ZZ	0KR60JZ	0KRK0JZ	0KS04ZZ	0KT54ZZ	0KUM4JZ
0K9T3ZZ	0KBS4ZX	0KCH3ZZ	0KHX0MZ	0KMR0ZZ	0KQL4ZZ	0KR60KZ	0KRK0KZ	0KS10ZZ	0KT60ZZ	0KUM4KZ
0K9V30Z	0KBS4ZZ	0KCH4ZZ	0KHX0YZ	0KMR4ZZ	0KQM0ZZ	0KR647Z	0KRK47Z	0KS14ZZ	0KT64ZZ	0KUN07Z
0K9V3ZZ	0KBT0ZX	0KCJ0ZZ	0KHX3MZ	0KMS0ZZ	0KQM3ZZ	0KR64JZ	0KRK4JZ	0KS20ZZ	0KT70ZZ	0KUN0JZ
0K9W30Z	0KBT0ZZ	0KCJ3ZZ	0KHX3YZ	0KMS4ZZ	0KQM4ZZ	0KR64KZ	0KRK4KZ	0KS24ZZ	0KT74ZZ	0KUN0KZ
0K9W3ZZ	0KBT3ZX	0KCJ4ZZ	0KHX4MZ	0KMT0ZZ	0KQN0ZZ	0KR707Z	0KRL07Z	0KS30ZZ	0KT80ZZ	0KUN47Z
0KBG3ZZ	0KBT3ZZ	0KCK0ZZ	0KHX4YZ	0KMT4ZZ	0KQN4ZZ	0KR70JZ	0KRL0JZ	0KS34ZZ	0KT84ZZ	0KUN4JZ
0KBG4ZX	0KBT4ZX	0KCK3ZZ	0KHY0MZ	0KMV0ZZ	0KQP0ZZ	0KR70KZ	0KRL0KZ	0KS40ZZ	0KT90ZZ	0KUN4KZ
0KBG4ZZ	0KBT4ZZ	0KCK4ZZ	0KHY0YZ	0KMV4ZZ	0KQP3ZZ	0KR747Z	0KRL47Z	0KS44ZZ	0KT94ZZ	0KUP07Z
0KBH0ZX	0KBV0ZX	0KCL0ZZ	0KHY3MZ	0KMW0ZZ	0KQP4ZZ	0KR74JZ	0KRL4JZ	0KS50ZZ	0KTB0ZZ	0KUP0JZ
0KBH0ZZ	0KBV0ZZ	0KCL3ZZ	0KHY3YZ	0KMW4ZZ	0KQQ0ZZ	0KR74KZ	0KRL4KZ	0KS54ZZ	0KTB4ZZ	0KUP0KZ
0KBH3ZX	0KBV3ZX	0KCL4ZZ	0KHY4MZ	0KN0XZZ	0KQQ3ZZ	0KR807Z	0KRM07Z	0KS60ZZ	0KTC0ZZ	0KUP47Z
0KBH3ZZ	0KBV3ZZ	0KCM0ZZ	0KHY4YZ	0KN1XZZ	0KQQ4ZZ	0KR80JZ	0KRM0JZ	0KS64ZZ	0KTC4ZZ	0KUP4JZ
0KBH4ZX	0KBV4ZX	0KCM3ZZ	0KJX0ZZ	0KN2XZZ	0KQR0ZZ	0KR80KZ	0KRM0KZ	0KS70ZZ	0KTD0ZZ	0KUP4KZ
0KBH4ZZ	0KBV4ZZ	0KCM4ZZ	0KJX3ZZ	0KN3XZZ	0KQR3ZZ	0KR847Z	0KRM47Z	0KS74ZZ	0KTD4ZZ	0KUQ07Z
0KBJ0ZX	0KBW0ZX	0KCN0ZZ	0KJX4ZZ	0KN4XZZ	0KQR4ZZ	0KR84JZ	0KRM4JZ	0KS80ZZ	0KTF0ZZ	0KUQ0JZ
0KBJ0ZZ	0KBW0ZZ	0KCN3ZZ	0KJXXZZ	0KN5XZZ	0KQS0ZZ	0KR84KZ	0KRM4KZ	0KS84ZZ	0KTF4ZZ	0KUQ0KZ
0KBJ3ZX	0KBW3ZX	0KCN4ZZ	0KJY0ZZ	0KN6XZZ	0KQS3ZZ	0KR907Z	0KRN07Z	0KS90ZZ	0KTG0ZZ	0KUQ47Z
0KBJ3ZZ	0KBW3ZZ	0KCP0ZZ	0KJY3ZZ	0KN7XZZ	0KQS4ZZ	0KR90JZ	0KRN0JZ	0KS94ZZ	0KTG4ZZ	0KUQ4JZ
0KBJ4ZX	0KBW4ZX	0KCP3ZZ	0KJY4ZZ	0KN8XZZ	0KQT0ZZ	0KR90KZ	0KRN0KZ	0KSB0ZZ	0KTH0ZZ	0KUQ4KZ
0KBJ4ZZ	0KBW4ZZ	0KCP4ZZ	0KJYXZZ	0KN9XZZ	0KQT3ZZ	0KR947Z	0KRN47Z	0KSB4ZZ	0KTH4ZZ	0KUR07Z
0KBK0ZX	0KC00ZZ	0KCQ0ZZ	0KM00ZZ	0KNBXZZ	0KQT4ZZ	0KR94JZ	0KRN4JZ	0KSC0ZZ	0KTJ0ZZ	0KUR0JZ
0KBK0ZZ	0KC03ZZ	0KCQ3ZZ	0KM04ZZ	0KNCXZZ	0KQV0ZZ	0KR94KZ	0KRN4KZ	0KSC4ZZ	0KTJ4ZZ	0KUR0KZ
0KBK3ZX	0KC04ZZ	0KCQ4ZZ	0KM10ZZ	0KNDXZZ	0KQV3ZZ	0KRB07Z	0KRP07Z	0KSD0ZZ	0KTK0ZZ	0KUR47Z
0KBK3ZZ	0KC10ZZ	0KCR0ZZ	0KM14ZZ	0KNFXZZ	0KQV4ZZ	0KRB0JZ	0KRP0JZ	0KSD4ZZ	0KTK4ZZ	0KUR4JZ
0KBK4ZX	0KC13ZZ	0KCR3ZZ	0KM20ZZ	0KNGXZZ	0KQW0ZZ	0KRB0KZ	0KRP0KZ	0KSF0ZZ	0KTL0ZZ	0KUR4KZ
0KBK4ZZ	0KC14ZZ	0KCR4ZZ	0KM24ZZ	0KNHXZZ	0KQW3ZZ	0KRB47Z	0KRP47Z	0KSF4ZZ	0KTL4ZZ	0KUS07Z
0KBL0ZX	0KC20ZZ	0KCS0ZZ	0KM30ZZ	0KNJXZZ	0KQW4ZZ	0KRB4JZ	0KRP4JZ	0KSG0ZZ	0KTM0ZZ	0KUS0JZ
0KBL0ZZ	0KC23ZZ	0KCS3ZZ	0KM34ZZ	0KNKXZZ	0KR007Z	0KRB4KZ	0KRP4KZ	0KSG4ZZ	0KTM4ZZ	0KUS0KZ
0KBL3ZX	0KC24ZZ	0KCS4ZZ	0KM40ZZ	0KNLXZZ	0KR00JZ	0KRC07Z	0KRQ07Z	0KSH0ZZ	0KTN0ZZ	0KUS47Z
0KBL3ZZ	0KC30ZZ	0KCT0ZZ	0KM44ZZ	0KNMXZZ	0KR00KZ	0KRC0JZ	0KRQ0JZ	0KSH4ZZ	0KTN4ZZ	0KUS4JZ
0KBL4ZX	0KC33ZZ	0KCT3ZZ	0KM50ZZ	0KNNXZZ	0KR047Z	0KRC0KZ	0KRQ0KZ	0KSJ0ZZ	0KTP0ZZ	0KUS4KZ
0KBL4ZZ	0KC34ZZ	0KCT4ZZ	0KM54ZZ	0KNPXZZ	0KR04JZ	0KRC47Z	0KRQ47Z	0KSJ4ZZ	0KTP4ZZ	0KUT07Z
0KBM0ZX	0KC40ZZ	0KCV0ZZ	0KM60ZZ	0KNQXZZ	0KR04KZ	0KRC4JZ	0KRQ4JZ	0KSK0ZZ	0KTQ0ZZ	0KUT0JZ
0KBM0ZZ	0KC43ZZ	0KCV3ZZ	0KM64ZZ	0KNRXZZ	0KR107Z	0KRC4KZ	0KRQ4KZ	0KSK4ZZ	0KTQ4ZZ	0KUT0KZ
0KBM3ZX	0KC44ZZ	0KCV4ZZ	0KM70ZZ	0KNSXZZ	0KR10JZ	0KRD07Z	0KRR07Z	0KSL0ZZ	0KTR0ZZ	0KUT47Z
0KBM3ZZ	0KC50ZZ	0KCW0ZZ	0KM74ZZ	0KNTXZZ	0KR10KZ	0KRD0JZ	0KRR0JZ	0KSL4ZZ	0KTR4ZZ	0KUT4JZ
0KBM4ZX	0KC53ZZ	0KCW3ZZ	0KM80ZZ	0KNVXZZ	0KR147Z	0KRD0KZ	0KRR0KZ	0KSM0ZZ	0KTS0ZZ	0KUT4KZ
0KBM4ZZ	0KC54ZZ	0KCW4ZZ	0KM84ZZ	0KNWXZZ	0KR14JZ	0KRD47Z	0KRR47Z	0KSM4ZZ	0KTS4ZZ	0KUV07Z
0KBN0ZX	0KC60ZZ	0KD00ZZ	0KM90ZZ	0KPX0YZ	0KR14KZ	0KRD4JZ	0KRR4JZ	0KSN0ZZ	0KTT0ZZ	0KUV0JZ
0KBN0ZZ	0KC63ZZ	0KD10ZZ	0KM94ZZ	0KPX3YZ	0KR207Z	0KRD4KZ	0KRR4KZ	0KSN4ZZ	0KTT4ZZ	0KUV0KZ
0KBN3ZX	0KC64ZZ	0KD20ZZ	0KMB0ZZ	0KPX4YZ	0KR20JZ	0KRF07Z	0KRS07Z	0KSP0ZZ	0KTV0ZZ	0KUV47Z
0KBN3ZZ	0KC70ZZ	0KD30ZZ	0KMB4ZZ	0KPXX0Z	0KR20KZ	0KRF0JZ	0KRS0JZ	0KSP4ZZ	0KTV4ZZ	0KUV4JZ
0KBN4ZX	0KC73ZZ	0KD40ZZ	0KMC0ZZ	0KPXXMZ	0KR247Z	0KRF0KZ	0KRS0KZ	0KSQ0ZZ	0KTW0ZZ	0KUV4KZ
0KBN4ZZ	0KC74ZZ	0KD50ZZ	0KMC4ZZ	0KPY0YZ	0KR24JZ	0KRF47Z	0KRS47Z	0KSQ4ZZ	0KTW4ZZ	0KUW07Z
0KBP0ZX	0KC80ZZ	0KD60ZZ	0KMD0ZZ	0KPY3YZ	0KR24KZ	0KRF4JZ	0KRS4JZ	0KSR0ZZ	0KU007Z	0KUW0JZ
0KBP0ZZ	0KC83ZZ	0KD70ZZ	0KMD4ZZ	0KPY4YZ	0KR307Z	0KRF4KZ	0KRS4KZ	0KSR4ZZ	0KU00JZ	0KUW0KZ
0KBP3ZX	0KC84ZZ	0KD80ZZ	0KMF0ZZ	0KPYX0Z	0KR30JZ	0KRG07Z	0KRT07Z	0KSS0ZZ	0KU00KZ	0KUW47Z
0KBP3ZZ	0KC90ZZ	0KD90ZZ	0KMF4ZZ	0KPYXMZ	0KR30KZ	0KRG0JZ	0KRT0JZ	0KSS4ZZ	0KU047Z	0KUW4JZ
0KBP4ZX	0KC93ZZ	0KDB0ZZ	0KMG0ZZ	0KQD4ZZ	0KR347Z	0KRG0KZ	0KRT0KZ	0KST0ZZ	0KU04JZ	0KUW4KZ
0KBP4ZZ	0KC94ZZ	0KDC0ZZ	0KMG4ZZ	0KQF0ZZ	0KR34JZ	0KRG47Z	0KRT47Z	0KST4ZZ	0KU04KZ	0KWX00Z
0KBQ0ZX	0KCB0ZZ	0KDD0ZZ	0KMH0ZZ	0KQF3ZZ	0KR34KZ	0KRG4JZ	0KRT4JZ	0KSV0ZZ	0KU107Z	0KWX07Z
0KBQ0ZZ	0KCB3ZZ	0KDF0ZZ	0KMH4ZZ	0KQF4ZZ	0KR407Z	0KRG4KZ	0KRT4KZ	0KSV4ZZ	0KU10JZ	0KWX0JZ
0KBQ3ZX	0KCB4ZZ	0KDG0ZZ	0KMJ0ZZ	0KQG0ZZ	0KRH07Z	0KRH07Z	0KRV07Z	0KSW0ZZ	0KU10KZ	0KWX0KZ

0KWX0MZ	0KX30Z0	0KXC0Z2	0KXK0ZZ	0KXT0Z2	0L8M0ZZ	0L9430Z	0L9C40Z	0L9M00Z	0L9V30Z	0LB83ZZ	
0KWX0YZ	0KX30Z1	0KXC0ZZ	0KXK4Z0	0KXT0ZZ	0L8M3ZZ	0L943ZX	0L9C4ZX	0L9M0ZX	0L9V3ZX	0LB84ZX	
0KWX30Z	0KX30Z2	0KXC4Z0	0KXK4Z1	0KXT4Z0	0L8M4ZZ	0L943ZZ	0L9C4ZZ	0L9M0ZZ	0L9V3ZZ	0LB84ZZ	
0KWX37Z	0KX30ZZ	0KXC4Z1	0KXK4Z2	0KXT4Z1	0L8N0ZZ	0L9440Z	0L9D00Z	0L9M30Z	0L9V40Z	0LB90ZX	
0KWX3JZ	0KX34Z0	0KXC4Z2	0KXK4Z6	0KXT4Z2	0L8N3ZZ	0L944ZX	0L9D0ZX	0L9M3ZX	0L9V4ZX	0LB90ZZ	
0KWX3KZ	0KX34Z1	0KXC4ZZ	0KXK4ZZ	0KXT4ZZ	0L8N4ZZ	0L944ZZ	0L9D0ZZ	0L9M3ZZ	0L9V4ZZ	0LB93ZX	
0KWX3MZ	0KX34Z2	0KXD0Z0	0KXL0Z0	0KXV0Z0	0L8P0ZZ	0L9500Z	0L9D30Z	0L9M40Z	0L9W00Z	0LB93ZZ	
0KWX3YZ	0KX34ZZ	0KXD0Z1	0KXL0Z1	0KXV0Z1	0L8P3ZZ	0L950ZX	0L9D3ZX	0L9M4ZX	0L9W0ZX	0LB94ZX	
0KWX40Z	0KX40Z0	0KXD0Z2	0KXL0Z2	0KXV0Z2	0L8P4ZZ	0L950ZZ	0L9D3ZZ	0L9M4ZZ	0L9W0ZZ	0LB94ZZ	
0KWX47Z	0KX40Z1	0KXD0ZZ	0KXL0Z6	0KXV0ZZ	0L8Q0ZZ	0L9530Z	0L9D40Z	0L9N00Z	0L9W30Z	0LBB0ZX	
0KWX4JZ	0KX40Z2	0KXD4Z0	0KXL0ZZ	0KXV4Z0	0L8Q3ZZ	0L953ZX	0L9D4ZX	0L9N0ZX	0L9W3ZX	0LBB0ZZ	
0KWX4KZ	0KX40ZZ	0KXD4Z1	0KXL4Z0	0KXV4Z1	0L8Q4ZZ	0L953ZZ	0L9D4ZZ	0L9N0ZZ	0L9W3ZZ	0LBB3ZX	
0KWX4MZ	0KX44Z0	0KXD4Z2	0KXL4Z1	0KXV4Z2	0L8R0ZZ	0L9540Z	0L9F00Z	0L9N30Z	0L9W40Z	0LBB3ZZ	
0KWX4YZ	0KX44Z1	0KXD4ZZ	0KXL4Z2	0KXV4ZZ	0L8R3ZZ	0L954ZX	0L9F0ZX	0L9N3ZX	0L9W4ZX	0LBB4ZX	
0KWXX0Z	0KX44Z2	0KXF0Z0	0KXL4Z6	0KXW0Z0	0L8R4ZZ	0L954ZZ	0L9F0ZZ	0L9N3ZZ	0L9W4ZZ	0LBB4ZZ	
0KWXX7Z	0KX44ZZ	0KXF0Z1	0KXL4ZZ	0KXW0Z1	0L8S0ZZ	0L9600Z	0L9F30Z	0L9N40Z	0LB00ZX	0LBC0ZX	
0KWXXJZ	0KX50Z0	0KXF0Z5	0KXM0Z0	0KXW0Z2	0L8S3ZZ	0L960ZX	0L9F3ZX	0L9N4ZX	0LB00ZZ	0LBC0ZZ	
0KWXXKZ	0KX50Z1	0KXF0Z7	0KXM0Z1	0L2XX0Z	0L8S4ZZ	0L960ZZ	0L9F3ZZ	0L9N4ZZ	0LB03ZX	0LBC3ZX	
0KWXXMZ	0KX50Z2	0KXF0Z8	0KXM0ZZ	0L2XXYZ	0L8T0ZZ	0L9630Z	0L9F40Z	0L9P00Z	0LB03ZZ	0LBC3ZZ	
0KWY00Z	0KX50ZZ	0KXF0Z9	0KXM4Z0	0L2YX0Z	0L8T3ZZ	0L963ZX	0L9F4ZX	0L9P0ZX	0LB04ZX	0LBC4ZX	
0KWY07Z	0KX54Z0	0KXF0ZZ	0KXM4Z1	0L2YXYZ	0L8T4ZZ	0L963ZZ	0L9F4ZZ	0L9P0ZZ	0LB04ZZ	0LBC4ZZ	
0KWY0JZ	0KX54Z1	0KXF4Z0	0KXM4Z2	0L840ZZ	0L8V0ZZ	0L9640Z	0L9G00Z	0L9P30Z	0LB10ZX	0LBD0ZX	
0KWY0KZ	0KX54Z2	0KXF4Z1	0KXM4ZZ	0L843ZZ	0L8V3ZZ	0L964ZX	0L9G0ZX	0L9P3ZX	0LB10ZZ	0LCR0ZZ	
0KWY0MZ	0KX54ZZ	0KXF4Z2	0KXN0Z0	0L844ZZ	0L8V4ZZ	0L964ZZ	0L9G0ZZ	0L9P3ZZ	0LB13ZX	0LCR3ZZ	
0KWY0YZ	0KX60Z0	0KXF4Z5	0KXN0Z1	0L850ZZ	0L8W0ZZ	0L9700Z	0L9G30Z	0L9P40Z	0LB13ZZ	0LCR4ZZ	
0KWY30Z	0KX60Z1	0KXF4Z7	0KXN0Z2	0L853ZZ	0L8W3ZZ	0L970ZX	0L9G3ZX	0L9P4ZX	0LB14ZX	0LCS0ZZ	
0KWY37Z	0KX60Z2	0KXF4Z8	0KXN0ZZ	0L854ZZ	0L8W4ZZ	0L970ZZ	0L9G3ZZ	0L9P4ZZ	0LB14ZZ	0LCS3ZZ	
0KWY3JZ	0KX60ZZ	0KXF4Z9	0KXN4Z0	0L860ZZ	0L9000Z	0L9730Z	0L9G40Z	0L9Q00Z	0LB20ZX	0LCS4ZZ	
0KWY3KZ	0KX64Z0	0KXF4ZZ	0KXN4Z1	0L863ZZ	0L900ZX	0L973ZX	0L9G4ZX	0L9Q0ZX	0LB20ZZ	0LCT0ZZ	
0KWY3MZ	0KX64Z1	0KXG0Z0	0KXN4Z2	0L864ZZ	0L900ZZ	0L973ZZ	0L9G4ZZ	0L9Q0ZZ	0LB23ZX	0LCT3ZZ	
0KWY3YZ	0KX64Z2	0KXG0Z1	0KXN4ZZ	0L870ZZ	0L9030Z	0L9740Z	0L9H00Z	0L9Q30Z	0LB23ZZ	0LCT4ZZ	
0KWY40Z	0KX64ZZ	0KXG0Z2	0KXP0Z0	0L873ZZ	0L903ZX	0L974ZX	0L9H0ZX	0L9Q3ZX	0LB24ZX	0LCV0ZZ	
0KWY47Z	0KX70Z0	0KXG0Z5	0KXP0Z1	0L874ZZ	0L903ZZ	0L974ZZ	0L9H0ZZ	0L9Q3ZZ	0LB24ZZ	0LCV3ZZ	
0KWY4JZ	0KX70Z1	0KXG0Z7	0KXP0Z2	0L880ZZ	0L9040Z	0L9800Z	0L9H30Z	0L9Q40Z	0LB30ZX	0LCV4ZZ	
0KWY4KZ	0KX70Z2	0KXG0Z8	0KXP0ZZ	0L883ZZ	0L904ZX	0L980ZX	0L9H3ZX	0L9Q4ZX	0LB30ZZ	0LCW0ZZ	
0KWY4MZ	0KX70ZZ	0KXG0Z9	0KXP4Z0	0L884ZZ	0L904ZZ	0L980ZZ	0L9H3ZZ	0L9Q4ZZ	0LB33ZX	0LCW3ZZ	
0KWY4YZ	0KX74Z0	0KXG0ZZ	0KXP4Z1	0L890ZZ	0L9100Z	0L9830Z	0L9H40Z	0L9R00Z	0LB33ZZ	0LCW4ZZ	
0KWYX0Z	0KX74Z1	0KXG4Z0	0KXP4Z2	0L893ZZ	0L910ZX	0L983ZX	0L9H4ZX	0L9R0ZX	0LB34ZX	0LD00ZZ	
0KWYX7Z	0KX74Z2	0KXG4Z1	0KXP4ZZ	0L894ZZ	0L910ZZ	0L983ZZ	0L9H4ZZ	0L9R0ZZ	0LB34ZZ	0LD10ZZ	
0KWYXJZ	0KX74ZZ	0KXG4Z2	0KXQ0Z0	0L8B0ZZ	0L9130Z	0L9840Z	0L9J00Z	0L9R30Z	0LB40ZX	0LD20ZZ	
0KWYXKZ	0KX80Z0	0KXG4Z5	0KXQ0Z1	0L8B3ZZ	0L913ZX	0L984ZX	0L9J0ZX	0L9R3ZX	0LB40ZZ	0LD30ZZ	
0KWYXMZ	0KX80Z1	0KXG4Z7	0KXQ0Z2	0L8B4ZZ	0L913ZZ	0L984ZZ	0L9J0ZZ	0L9R3ZZ	0LB43ZX	0LD40ZZ	
0KX00Z0	0KX80Z2	0KXG4Z8	0KXQ0ZZ	0L8C0ZZ	0L9140Z	0L9900Z	0L9J30Z	0L9R40Z	0LB43ZZ	0LD50ZZ	
0KX00Z1	0KX80ZZ	0KXG4Z9	0KXQ4Z0	0L8C3ZZ	0L914ZX	0L990ZX	0L9J3ZX	0L9R4ZX	0LB44ZX	0LD60ZZ	
0KX00Z2	0KX84Z0	0KXG4ZZ	0KXQ4Z1	0L8C4ZZ	0L914ZZ	0L990ZZ	0L9J3ZZ	0L9R4ZZ	0LB44ZZ	0LD70ZZ	
0KX00ZZ	0KX84Z1	0KXH0Z0	0KXQ4Z2	0L8D0ZZ	0L9200Z	0L9930Z	0L9J40Z	0L9S00Z	0LB50ZX	0LD80ZZ	
0KX04Z0	0KX84Z2	0KXH0Z1	0KXQ4ZZ	0L8D3ZZ	0L920ZX	0L993ZX	0L9J4ZX	0L9S0ZX	0LB50ZZ	0LD90ZZ	
0KX04Z1	0KX84ZZ	0KXH0Z2	0KXR0Z0	0L8D4ZZ	0L920ZZ	0L993ZZ	0L9J4ZZ	0L9S0ZZ	0LB53ZX	0LDB0ZZ	
0KX04Z2	0KX90Z0	0KXH0ZZ	0KXR0Z1	0L8F0ZZ	0L9230Z	0L9940Z	0L9K00Z	0L9S30Z	0LB53ZZ	0LDC0ZZ	
0KX04ZZ	0KX90Z1	0KXH4Z0	0KXR0Z2	0L8F3ZZ	0L923ZX	0L994ZX	0L9K0ZX	0L9S3ZX	0LB54ZX	0LDD0ZZ	
0KX10Z0	0KX90Z2	0KXH4Z1	0KXR0ZZ	0L8F4ZZ	0L923ZZ	0L994ZZ	0L9K0ZZ	0L9S3ZZ	0LB54ZZ	0LDF0ZZ	
0KX10Z1	0KX90ZZ	0KXH4Z2	0KXR4Z0	0L8G0ZZ	0L9240Z	0L9B00Z	0L9K30Z	0L9S40Z	0LB60ZX	0LDG0ZZ	
0KX10Z2	0KX94Z0	0KXH4ZZ	0KXR4Z1	0L8G3ZZ	0L924ZX	0L9B0ZX	0L9K3ZX	0L9S4ZX	0LB60ZZ	0LDH0ZZ	
0KX10ZZ	0KX94Z1	0KXJ0Z0	0KXR4Z2	0L8G4ZZ	0L924ZZ	0L9B0ZZ	0L9K3ZZ	0L9S4ZZ	0LB63ZX	0LDJ0ZZ	
0KX14Z0	0KX94Z2	0KXJ0Z1	0KXR4ZZ	0L8H0ZZ	0L9300Z	0L9B30Z	0L9K40Z	0L9T00Z	0LB63ZZ	0LDK0ZZ	
0KX14Z1	0KX94ZZ	0KXJ0Z2	0KXS0Z0	0L8H3ZZ	0L930ZX	0L9B3ZX	0L9K4ZX	0L9T0ZX	0LB64ZX	0LDL0ZZ	
0KX14Z2	0KXB0Z0	0KXJ0ZZ	0KXS0Z1	0L8H4ZZ	0L930ZZ	0L9B3ZZ	0L9K4ZZ	0L9T0ZZ	0LB64ZZ	0LDM0ZZ	
0KX20Z0	0KXB0Z1	0KXJ4Z0	0KXS0Z2	0L8J0ZZ	0L9330Z	0L9B40Z	0L9L00Z	0L9T30Z	0LB70ZX	0LDN0ZZ	
0KX20Z1	0KXB0ZZ	0KXJ4Z1	0KXS0ZZ	0L8J3ZZ	0L933ZX	0L9B4ZX	0L9L0ZX	0L9T3ZX	0LB70ZZ	0LDP0ZZ	
0KX20Z2	0KXB4Z0	0KXJ4Z2	0KXS4Z0	0L8K0ZZ	0L933ZZ	0L9B4ZZ	0L9L0ZZ	0L9T3ZZ	0LB73ZX	0LDQ0ZZ	
0KX20ZZ	0KXB4Z1	0KXJ4ZZ	0KXS4Z1	0L8K3ZZ	0L9340Z	0L9C00Z	0L9L30Z	0L9T40Z	0LB73ZZ	0LDR0ZZ	
0KX24Z0	0KXB4Z2	0KXK0Z0	0KXS4Z2	0L8K4ZZ	0L934ZX	0L9C0ZX	0L9L3ZX	0L9T4ZX	0LB74ZX	0LDS0ZZ	
0KX24Z1	0KXB4ZZ	0KXK0Z1	0KXS4ZZ	0L8L0ZZ	0L934ZZ	0L9C0ZZ	0L9L3ZZ	0L9T4ZZ	0LB74ZZ	0LDT0ZZ	
0KX24Z2	0KXC0Z0	0KXK0Z2	0KXT0Z0	0L8L3ZZ	0L9400Z	0L9C30Z	0L9L40Z	0L9V00Z	0LB80ZX	0LDV0ZZ	
0KX24ZZ	0KXC0Z1	0KXK0Z6	0KXT0Z1	0L8L4ZZ	0L940ZX	0L9C3ZX	0L9L4ZX	0L9V0ZX	0LB80ZZ	0LDW0ZZ	
						0L940ZZ	0L9C3ZZ	0L9L4ZZ	0L9V0ZZ	0LB83ZX	0LHX0YZ

0LHX3YZ	0LMV4ZZ	0LNHXZZ	0LPY07Z	0LQK0ZZ	0LSL4ZZ	0LTR4ZZ	0LU947Z	0LUN47Z	0LWY0JZ	0M804ZZ
0LHX4YZ	0LMW0ZZ	0LNJ0ZZ	0LPY0JZ	0LQK3ZZ	0LSM0ZZ	0LTS0ZZ	0LU94JZ	0LUN4JZ	0LWY0KZ	0M810ZZ
0LHY0YZ	0LMW4ZZ	0LNJ3ZZ	0LPY0KZ	0LQK4ZZ	0LSM4ZZ	0LTS4ZZ	0LU94KZ	0LUN4KZ	0LWY0YZ	0M813ZZ
0LHY3YZ	0LN00ZZ	0LNJ4ZZ	0LPY0YZ	0LQL0ZZ	0LSN0ZZ	0LTT0ZZ	0LUB07Z	0LUP07Z	0LWY30Z	0M814ZZ
0LHY4YZ	0LN03ZZ	0LNJXZZ	0LPY30Z	0LQL3ZZ	0LSN4ZZ	0LTT4ZZ	0LUB0JZ	0LUP0JZ	0LWY37Z	0M820ZZ
0LJX0ZZ	0LN04ZZ	0LNK0ZZ	0LPY37Z	0LQL4ZZ	0LSP0ZZ	0LTV0ZZ	0LUB0KZ	0LUP0KZ	0LWY3JZ	0M823ZZ
0LJX3ZZ	0LN0XZZ	0LNK3ZZ	0LPY3JZ	0LQM0ZZ	0LSP4ZZ	0LTV4ZZ	0LUB47Z	0LUP47Z	0LWY3KZ	0M824ZZ
0LJX4ZZ	0LN10ZZ	0LNK4ZZ	0LPY3KZ	0LQM3ZZ	0LSQ0ZZ	0LTW0ZZ	0LUB4JZ	0LUP4JZ	0LWY3YZ	0M830ZZ
0LJXXZZ	0LN13ZZ	0LNKXZZ	0LPY3YZ	0LQM4ZZ	0LSQ4ZZ	0LTW4ZZ	0LUB4KZ	0LUP4KZ	0LWY40Z	0M833ZZ
0LJY0ZZ	0LN14ZZ	0LNL0ZZ	0LPY40Z	0LQN0ZZ	0LSR0ZZ	0LU007Z	0LUC07Z	0LUQ07Z	0LWY47Z	0M834ZZ
0LJY3ZZ	0LN1XZZ	0LNL3ZZ	0LPY47Z	0LQN3ZZ	0LSR4ZZ	0LU00JZ	0LUC0JZ	0LUQ0JZ	0LWY4JZ	0M840ZZ
0LJY4ZZ	0LN20ZZ	0LNL4ZZ	0LPY4JZ	0LQN4ZZ	0LSS0ZZ	0LU00KZ	0LUC0KZ	0LUQ0KZ	0LWY4KZ	0M843ZZ
0LJYXZZ	0LN23ZZ	0LNLXZZ	0LPY4KZ	0LQP0ZZ	0LSS4ZZ	0LU047Z	0LUC47Z	0LUQ47Z	0LWY4YZ	0M844ZZ
0LM00ZZ	0LN24ZZ	0LNM0ZZ	0LPY4YZ	0LQP3ZZ	0LST0ZZ	0LU04JZ	0LUC4JZ	0LUQ4JZ	0LWYX0Z	0M850ZZ
0LM04ZZ	0LN2XZZ	0LNM3ZZ	0LPYX0Z	0LQP4ZZ	0LST4ZZ	0LU04KZ	0LUC4KZ	0LUQ4KZ	0LWYX7Z	0M853ZZ
0LM10ZZ	0LN30ZZ	0LNM4ZZ	0LQ00ZZ	0LQQ0ZZ	0LSV0ZZ	0LU107Z	0LUD07Z	0LUR07Z	0LWYXJZ	0M854ZZ
0LM14ZZ	0LN33ZZ	0LNMXZZ	0LQ03ZZ	0LQQ3ZZ	0LSV4ZZ	0LU10JZ	0LUD0JZ	0LUR0JZ	0LWYXKZ	0M860ZZ
0LM20ZZ	0LN34ZZ	0LNN0ZZ	0LQ04ZZ	0LQQ4ZZ	0LSW0ZZ	0LU10KZ	0LUD0KZ	0LUR0KZ	0LX00ZZ	0M863ZZ
0LM24ZZ	0LN3XZZ	0LNN3ZZ	0LQ10ZZ	0LQR0ZZ	0LSW4ZZ	0LU147Z	0LUD47Z	0LUR47Z	0LX04ZZ	0M864ZZ
0LM30ZZ	0LN40ZZ	0LNN4ZZ	0LQ13ZZ	0LQR3ZZ	0LT00ZZ	0LU14JZ	0LUD4JZ	0LUR4JZ	0LX10ZZ	0M870ZZ
0LM34ZZ	0LN43ZZ	0LNNXZZ	0LQ14ZZ	0LQR4ZZ	0LT04ZZ	0LU14KZ	0LUD4KZ	0LUR4KZ	0LX14ZZ	0M873ZZ
0LM40ZZ	0LN44ZZ	0LNP0ZZ	0LQ20ZZ	0LQS0ZZ	0LT10ZZ	0LU207Z	0LUF07Z	0LUS07Z	0LX20ZZ	0M874ZZ
0LM44ZZ	0LN4XZZ	0LNP3ZZ	0LQ23ZZ	0LQS3ZZ	0LT14ZZ	0LU20JZ	0LUF0JZ	0LUS0JZ	0M2XX0Z	0M880ZZ
0LM50ZZ	0LN50ZZ	0LNP4ZZ	0LQ24ZZ	0LQS4ZZ	0LT20ZZ	0LU20KZ	0LUF0KZ	0LUS0KZ	0M2XXYZ	0M883ZZ
0LM54ZZ	0LN53ZZ	0LNPXZZ	0LQ30ZZ	0LQT0ZZ	0LT24ZZ	0LU247Z	0LUF47Z	0LUS47Z	0M2YX0Z	0M884ZZ
0LM60ZZ	0LN54ZZ	0LNQ0ZZ	0LQ33ZZ	0LQT3ZZ	0LT30ZZ	0LU24JZ	0LUF4JZ	0LUS4JZ	0M2YXYZ	0M890ZZ
0LM64ZZ	0LN5XZZ	0LNQ3ZZ	0LQ34ZZ	0LQT4ZZ	0LT34ZZ	0LU24KZ	0LUF4KZ	0LUS4KZ	0M5H3ZZ	0M893ZZ
0LM70ZZ	0LN60ZZ	0LNQ4ZZ	0LQ40ZZ	0LQV0ZZ	0LT40ZZ	0LU307Z	0LUG07Z	0LUT07Z	0M5H4ZZ	0M894ZZ
0LM74ZZ	0LN63ZZ	0LNQXZZ	0LQ43ZZ	0LQV3ZZ	0LT44ZZ	0LU30JZ	0LUG0JZ	0LUT0JZ	0M5J0ZZ	0M8B0ZZ
0LM80ZZ	0LN64ZZ	0LNR0ZZ	0LQ44ZZ	0LQV4ZZ	0LT50ZZ	0LU30KZ	0LUG0KZ	0LUT0KZ	0M5J3ZZ	0M8B3ZZ
0LM84ZZ	0LN6XZZ	0LNR3ZZ	0LQ50ZZ	0LQW0ZZ	0LT54ZZ	0LU347Z	0LUG47Z	0LUT47Z	0M5J4ZZ	0M8B4ZZ
0LM90ZZ	0LN70ZZ	0LNR4ZZ	0LQ53ZZ	0LQW3ZZ	0LT60ZZ	0LU34JZ	0LUG4JZ	0LUT4JZ	0M5K0ZZ	0M8C0ZZ
0LM94ZZ	0LN73ZZ	0LNRXZZ	0LQ54ZZ	0LQW4ZZ	0LT64ZZ	0LU34KZ	0LUG4KZ	0LUT4KZ	0M5K3ZZ	0M8C3ZZ
0LMB0ZZ	0LN74ZZ	0LNS0ZZ	0LQ60ZZ	0LR007Z	0LT70ZZ	0LU407Z	0LUH07Z	0LUV07Z	0M5K4ZZ	0M8C4ZZ
0LMB4ZZ	0LN7XZZ	0LNS3ZZ	0LQ63ZZ	0LR00JZ	0LT74ZZ	0LU40JZ	0LUH0JZ	0LUV0JZ	0M5L0ZZ	0M8D0ZZ
0LMC0ZZ	0LN80ZZ	0LNS4ZZ	0LQ64ZZ	0LR00KZ	0LT80ZZ	0LU40KZ	0LUH0KZ	0LUV0KZ	0M5L3ZZ	0M8D3ZZ
0LMC4ZZ	0LN83ZZ	0LNSXZZ	0LQ70ZZ	0LR047Z	0LT84ZZ	0LU447Z	0LUH47Z	0LUV47Z	0M5L4ZZ	0M8D4ZZ
0LMD0ZZ	0LN84ZZ	0LNT0ZZ	0LQ73ZZ	0LT90ZZ	0LU44JZ	0LUH4JZ	0LUV4JZ	0M5M0ZZ	0M8F0ZZ
0LMD4ZZ	0LN8XZZ	0LNT3ZZ	0LQ74ZZ	0LS40ZZ	0LT94ZZ	0LU44KZ	0LUH4KZ	0LUV4KZ	0M5M3ZZ	0M8F3ZZ
0LMF0ZZ	0LN90ZZ	0LNT4ZZ	0LQ80ZZ	0LS44ZZ	0LTB0ZZ	0LU507Z	0LUJ07Z	0LUW07Z	0M5M4ZZ	0M8F4ZZ
0LMF4ZZ	0LN93ZZ	0LNTXZZ	0LQ83ZZ	0LS50ZZ	0LTB4ZZ	0LU50JZ	0LUJ0JZ	0LUW0JZ	0M5N0ZZ	0M8G0ZZ
0LMG0ZZ	0LN94ZZ	0LNV0ZZ	0LQ84ZZ	0LS54ZZ	0LTC0ZZ	0LU50KZ	0LUJ0KZ	0LUW0KZ	0M5N3ZZ	0M8G3ZZ
0LMG4ZZ	0LN9XZZ	0LNV3ZZ	0LQ90ZZ	0LS60ZZ	0LTC4ZZ	0LU547Z	0LUJ47Z	0LUW47Z	0M5N4ZZ	0M8G4ZZ
0LMH0ZZ	0LNB0ZZ	0LNV4ZZ	0LQ93ZZ	0LS64ZZ	0LTD0ZZ	0LU54JZ	0LUJ4JZ	0LUW4JZ	0M5P0ZZ	0M8H0ZZ
0LMH4ZZ	0LNB3ZZ	0LNVXZZ	0LQ94ZZ	0LS70ZZ	0LTD4ZZ	0LU54KZ	0LUJ4KZ	0LUW4KZ	0M5P3ZZ	0M8H3ZZ
0LMJ0ZZ	0LNB4ZZ	0LNW0ZZ	0LQB0ZZ	0LS74ZZ	0LTF0ZZ	0LU607Z	0LUK07Z	0LWX00Z	0M5P4ZZ	0M8H4ZZ
0LMJ4ZZ	0LNBXZZ	0LNW3ZZ	0LQB3ZZ	0LS80ZZ	0LTF4ZZ	0LU60JZ	0LUK0JZ	0LWX07Z	0M5Q0ZZ	0M8J0ZZ
0LMK0ZZ	0LNC0ZZ	0LNW4ZZ	0LQB4ZZ	0LS84ZZ	0LTG0ZZ	0LU60KZ	0LUK0KZ	0LWX0JZ	0M5Q3ZZ	0M8J3ZZ
0LMK4ZZ	0LNC3ZZ	0LNWXZZ	0LQC0ZZ	0LS90ZZ	0LTG4ZZ	0LU647Z	0LUK47Z	0LWX0KZ	0M5Q4ZZ	0M8J4ZZ
0LML0ZZ	0LNC4ZZ	0LPX00Z	0LQC3ZZ	0LS94ZZ	0LTH0ZZ	0LU64JZ	0LUK4JZ	0LWX0YZ	0M5R0ZZ	0M8K0ZZ
0LML4ZZ	0LNCXZZ	0LPX07Z	0LQC4ZZ	0LSB0ZZ	0LTH4ZZ	0LU64KZ	0LUK4KZ	0LWX30Z	0M5R3ZZ	0M8K3ZZ
0LMM0ZZ	0LND0ZZ	0LPX0JZ	0LQD0ZZ	0LSB4ZZ	0LTJ0ZZ	0LU707Z	0LUL07Z	0LWX37Z	0M5R4ZZ	0M8K4ZZ
0LMM4ZZ	0LND3ZZ	0LPX0KZ	0LQD3ZZ	0LSC0ZZ	0LTJ4ZZ	0LU70JZ	0LUL0JZ	0LWX3JZ	0M5S0ZZ	0M8L0ZZ
0LMN0ZZ	0LND4ZZ	0LPX0YZ	0LQD4ZZ	0LSC4ZZ	0LTK0ZZ	0LU70KZ	0LUL0KZ	0LWX3KZ	0M5S3ZZ	0M8L3ZZ
0LMN4ZZ	0LNDXZZ	0LPX30Z	0LQF0ZZ	0LSD0ZZ	0LTK4ZZ	0LU747Z	0LUL47Z	0LWX3YZ	0M5S4ZZ	0M8L4ZZ
0LMP0ZZ	0LNF0ZZ	0LPX37Z	0LQF3ZZ	0LSD4ZZ	0LTL0ZZ	0LU74JZ	0LUL4JZ	0LWX40Z	0M5T0ZZ	0M8M0ZZ
0LMP4ZZ	0LNF3ZZ	0LPX3JZ	0LQF4ZZ	0LSF0ZZ	0LTL4ZZ	0LU74KZ	0LUL4KZ	0LWX47Z	0M5T3ZZ	0M8M3ZZ
0LMQ0ZZ	0LNF4ZZ	0LPX3KZ	0LQG0ZZ	0LSF4ZZ	0LTM0ZZ	0LU807Z	0LUM07Z	0LWX4JZ	0M5T4ZZ	0M8M4ZZ
0LMQ4ZZ	0LNFXZZ	0LPX3YZ	0LQG3ZZ	0LSG0ZZ	0LTM4ZZ	0LU80JZ	0LUM0JZ	0LWX4KZ	0M5V0ZZ	0M8N0ZZ
0LMR0ZZ	0LNG0ZZ	0LPX40Z	0LQG4ZZ	0LSG4ZZ	0LTN0ZZ	0LU80KZ	0LUM0KZ	0LWX4YZ	0M5V3ZZ	0M8N3ZZ
0LMR4ZZ	0LNG3ZZ	0LPX47Z	0LQH0ZZ	0LSH0ZZ	0LTN4ZZ	0LU847Z	0LUM47Z	0LWXX0Z	0M5V4ZZ	0M8N4ZZ
0LMS0ZZ	0LNG4ZZ	0LPX4JZ	0LQH3ZZ	0LSH4ZZ	0LTP0ZZ	0LU84JZ	0LUM4JZ	0LWXX7Z	0M5W0ZZ	0M8P0ZZ
0LMS4ZZ	0LNGXZZ	0LPX4KZ	0LQH4ZZ	0LSJ0ZZ	0LTP4ZZ	0LU84KZ	0LUM4KZ	0LWXXJZ	0M5W3ZZ	0M8P3ZZ
0LMT0ZZ	0LNH0ZZ	0LPX4YZ	0LQJ0ZZ	0LSJ4ZZ	0LTQ0ZZ	0LU907Z	0LUN07Z	0LWXXKZ	0M5W4ZZ	0M8P4ZZ
0LMT4ZZ	0LNH3ZZ	0LPXX0Z	0LQJ3ZZ	0LSK0ZZ	0LTQ4ZZ	0LU90JZ	0LUN0JZ	0LWY00Z	0M800ZZ	0M8Q0ZZ
0LMV0ZZ	0LNH4ZZ	0LPY00Z	0LQJ4ZZ	0LSK4ZZ	0LTR0ZZ	0LU90KZ	0LUN0KZ	0LWY07Z	0M803ZZ	0M8Q3ZZ

APPENDIX H: NON-OR NOT AFFECTING MS-DRG ASSIGNMENT

0M8Q4ZZ-0MQQ0ZZ

0M8Q4ZZ	0M953ZZ	0M9D4ZZ	0M9N0ZZ	0M9W3ZZ	0MBB3ZX	0MBP3ZX	0MM14ZZ	0MN33ZZ	0MNMXZZ	0MQ03ZZ
0M8R0ZZ	0M9540Z	0M9F00Z	0M9N30Z	0M9W40Z	0MBB3ZZ	0MBP3ZZ	0MM20ZZ	0MN34ZZ	0MNN0ZZ	0MQ04ZZ
0M8R3ZZ	0M954ZX	0M9F0ZX	0M9N3ZX	0M9W4ZX	0MBB4ZX	0MBP4ZX	0MM24ZZ	0MN3XZZ	0MNN3ZZ	0MQ10ZZ
0M8R4ZZ	0M954ZZ	0M9F0ZZ	0M9N3ZZ	0M9W4ZZ	0MBB4ZZ	0MBP4ZZ	0MM30ZZ	0MN40ZZ	0MNN4ZZ	0MQ13ZZ
0M8S0ZZ	0M9600Z	0M9F30Z	0M9N40Z	0MB00ZX	0MBC0ZX	0MBQ0ZX	0MM34ZZ	0MN43ZZ	0MNNXZZ	0MQ14ZZ
0M8S3ZZ	0M960ZX	0M9F3ZX	0M9N4ZX	0MB00ZZ	0MBC0ZZ	0MBQ0ZZ	0MM40ZZ	0MN44ZZ	0MNP0ZZ	0MQ20ZZ
0M8S4ZZ	0M960ZZ	0M9F3ZZ	0M9N4ZZ	0MB03ZX	0MBC3ZX	0MBQ3ZX	0MM44ZZ	0MN4XZZ	0MNP3ZZ	0MQ23ZZ
0M8T0ZZ	0M9630Z	0M9F40Z	0M9P00Z	0MB03ZZ	0MBC3ZZ	0MBQ3ZZ	0MM50ZZ	0MN50ZZ	0MNP4ZZ	0MQ24ZZ
0M8T3ZZ	0M963ZX	0M9F4ZX	0M9P0ZX	0MB04ZX	0MBC4ZX	0MBQ4ZX	0MM54ZZ	0MN53ZZ	0MNPXZZ	0MQ30ZZ
0M8T4ZZ	0M963ZZ	0M9F4ZZ	0M9P0ZZ	0MB04ZZ	0MBC4ZZ	0MBQ4ZZ	0MM60ZZ	0MN54ZZ	0MNQ0ZZ	0MQ33ZZ
0M8V0ZZ	0M9640Z	0M9G00Z	0M9P30Z	0MB10ZX	0MBD0ZX	0MBR0ZX	0MM64ZZ	0MN5XZZ	0MNQ3ZZ	0MQ34ZZ
0M8V3ZZ	0M964ZX	0M9G0ZX	0M9P3ZX	0MB10ZZ	0MBD0ZZ	0MBR0ZZ	0MM70ZZ	0MN60ZZ	0MNQ4ZZ	0MQ40ZZ
0M8V4ZZ	0M964ZZ	0M9G0ZZ	0M9P3ZZ	0MB13ZX	0MBD3ZX	0MBR3ZX	0MM74ZZ	0MN63ZZ	0MNQXZZ	0MQ43ZZ
0M8W0ZZ	0M9700Z	0M9G30Z	0M9P40Z	0MB13ZZ	0MBD3ZZ	0MBR3ZZ	0MM80ZZ	0MN64ZZ	0MNR0ZZ	0MQ44ZZ
0M8W3ZZ	0M970ZX	0M9G3ZX	0M9P4ZX	0MB14ZX	0MBD4ZX	0MBR4ZX	0MM84ZZ	0MN6XZZ	0MNR3ZZ	0MQ50ZZ
0M8W4ZZ	0M970ZZ	0M9G3ZZ	0M9P4ZZ	0MB14ZZ	0MBD4ZZ	0MBR4ZZ	0MM90ZZ	0MN70ZZ	0MNR4ZZ	0MQ53ZZ
0M9000Z	0M9730Z	0M9G40Z	0M9Q00Z	0MB20ZX	0MBF0ZX	0MBS0ZX	0MM94ZZ	0MN73ZZ	0MNRXZZ	0MQ54ZZ
0M900ZX	0M973ZX	0M9G4ZX	0M9Q0ZX	0MB20ZZ	0MBF0ZZ	0MBS0ZZ	0MMB0ZZ	0MN74ZZ	0MNS0ZZ	0MQ60ZZ
0M900ZZ	0M973ZZ	0M9G4ZZ	0M9Q0ZZ	0MB23ZX	0MBF3ZX	0MBS3ZX	0MMB4ZZ	0MN7XZZ	0MNS3ZZ	0MQ63ZZ
0M9030Z	0M9740Z	0M9H00Z	0M9Q30Z	0MB23ZZ	0MBF3ZZ	0MBS3ZZ	0MMC0ZZ	0MN80ZZ	0MNS4ZZ	0MQ64ZZ
0M903ZX	0M974ZX	0M9H0ZX	0M9Q3ZX	0MB24ZX	0MBF4ZX	0MBS4ZX	0MMC4ZZ	0MN83ZZ	0MNSXZZ	0MQ70ZZ
0M903ZZ	0M974ZZ	0M9H0ZZ	0M9Q3ZZ	0MB24ZZ	0MBF4ZZ	0MBS4ZZ	0MMD0ZZ	0MN84ZZ	0MNT0ZZ	0MQ73ZZ
0M9040Z	0M9800Z	0M9H30Z	0M9Q40Z	0MB30ZX	0MBG0ZX	0MBT0ZX	0MMD4ZZ	0MN8XZZ	0MNT3ZZ	0MQ74ZZ
0M904ZX	0M980ZX	0M9H3ZX	0M9Q4ZX	0MB30ZZ	0MBG0ZZ	0MBT0ZZ	0MMF0ZZ	0MN90ZZ	0MNT4ZZ	0MQ80ZZ
0M904ZZ	0M980ZZ	0M9H3ZZ	0M9Q4ZZ	0MB33ZX	0MBG3ZX	0MBT3ZX	0MMF4ZZ	0MN93ZZ	0MNTXZZ	0MQ83ZZ
0M9100Z	0M9830Z	0M9H40Z	0M9R00Z	0MB33ZZ	0MBG3ZZ	0MBT3ZZ	0MMG0ZZ	0MN94ZZ	0MNV0ZZ	0MQ84ZZ
0M910ZX	0M983ZX	0M9H4ZX	0M9R0ZX	0MB34ZX	0MBG4ZX	0MBT4ZX	0MMG4ZZ	0MN9XZZ	0MNV3ZZ	0MQ90ZZ
0M910ZZ	0M983ZZ	0M9H4ZZ	0M9R0ZZ	0MB34ZZ	0MBG4ZZ	0MBT4ZZ	0MMH0ZZ	0MNB0ZZ	0MNV4ZZ	0MQ93ZZ
0M9130Z	0M9840Z	0M9J00Z	0M9R30Z	0MB40ZX	0MBH0ZX	0MBV0ZX	0MMH4ZZ	0MNB3ZZ	0MNVXZZ	0MQ94ZZ
0M913ZX	0M984ZX	0M9J0ZX	0M9R3ZX	0MB40ZZ	0MBH0ZZ	0MBV0ZZ	0MMJ0ZZ	0MNB4ZZ	0MNW0ZZ	0MQB0ZZ
0M913ZZ	0M984ZZ	0M9J0ZZ	0M9R3ZZ	0MB43ZX	0MBH3ZX	0MBV3ZX	0MMJ4ZZ	0MNBXZZ	0MNW3ZZ	0MQB3ZZ
0M9140Z	0M9900Z	0M9J30Z	0M9R40Z	0MB43ZZ	0MBH3ZZ	0MBV3ZZ	0MMK0ZZ	0MNC0ZZ	0MNW4ZZ	0MQB4ZZ
0M914ZX	0M990ZX	0M9J3ZX	0M9R4ZX	0MB44ZX	0MBH4ZX	0MBV4ZX	0MMK4ZZ	0MNC3ZZ	0MNWXZZ	0MQC0ZZ
0M914ZZ	0M990ZZ	0M9J3ZZ	0M9R4ZZ	0MB44ZZ	0MBH4ZZ	0MBV4ZZ	0MML0ZZ	0MNC4ZZ	0MPX00Z	0MQC3ZZ
0M9200Z	0M9930Z	0M9J40Z	0M9S00Z	0MB50ZX	0MBJ0ZX	0MBW0ZX	0MML4ZZ	0MNCXZZ	0MPX07Z	0MQC4ZZ
0M920ZX	0M993ZX	0M9J4ZX	0M9S0ZX	0MB50ZZ	0MBJ0ZZ	0MBW0ZZ	0MMM0ZZ	0MND0ZZ	0MPX0JZ	0MQD0ZZ
0M920ZZ	0M993ZZ	0M9J4ZZ	0M9S0ZZ	0MB53ZX	0MBJ3ZX	0MBW3ZX	0MMM4ZZ	0MND3ZZ	0MPX0KZ	0MQD3ZZ
0M9230Z	0M9940Z	0M9K00Z	0M9S30Z	0MB53ZZ	0MBJ3ZZ	0MBW3ZZ	0MMN0ZZ	0MND4ZZ	0MPX0YZ	0MQD4ZZ
0M923ZX	0M994ZX	0M9K0ZX	0M9S3ZX	0MB54ZX	0MBJ4ZX	0MBW4ZX	0MMN4ZZ	0MNDXZZ	0MPX30Z	0MQF0ZZ
0M923ZZ	0M994ZZ	0M9K0ZZ	0M9S3ZZ	0MB54ZZ	0MBJ4ZZ	0MBW4ZZ	0MMP0ZZ	0MNF0ZZ	0MPX37Z	0MQF3ZZ
0M9240Z	0M9B00Z	0M9K30Z	0M9S40Z	0MB60ZX	0MBK0ZX	0MC00ZZ	0MMP4ZZ	0MNF3ZZ	0MPX3JZ	0MQF4ZZ
0M924ZX	0M9B0ZX	0M9K3ZX	0M9S4ZX	0MB60ZZ	0MBK0ZZ	0MC03ZZ	0MMQ0ZZ	0MNF4ZZ	0MPX3KZ	0MQG0ZZ
0M924ZZ	0M9B0ZZ	0M9K3ZZ	0M9S4ZZ	0MB63ZX	0MBK3ZX	0MDT4ZZ	0MMQ4ZZ	0MNFXZZ	0MPX3YZ	0MQG3ZZ
0M9300Z	0M9B30Z	0M9K40Z	0M9T00Z	0MB63ZZ	0MBK3ZZ	0MDV0ZZ	0MMR0ZZ	0MNG0ZZ	0MPX40Z	0MQG4ZZ
0M930ZX	0M9B3ZX	0M9K4ZX	0M9T0ZX	0MB64ZX	0MBK4ZX	0MDV3ZZ	0MMR4ZZ	0MNG3ZZ	0MPX47Z	0MQH0ZZ
0M930ZZ	0M9B3ZZ	0M9K4ZZ	0M9T0ZZ	0MB64ZZ	0MBK4ZZ	0MDV4ZZ	0MMS0ZZ	0MNG4ZZ	0MPX4JZ	0MQH3ZZ
0M9330Z	0M9B40Z	0M9L00Z	0M9T30Z	0MB70ZX	0MBL0ZX	0MDW0ZZ	0MMS4ZZ	0MNGXZZ	0MPX4KZ	0MQJ0ZZ
0M933ZX	0M9B4ZX	0M9L0ZX	0M9T3ZX	0MB70ZZ	0MBL0ZZ	0MDW3ZZ	0MMT0ZZ	0MNH0ZZ	0MPX4YZ	0MQJ3ZZ
0M933ZZ	0M9B4ZZ	0M9L0ZZ	0M9T3ZZ	0MB73ZX	0MBL3ZX	0MDW4ZZ	0MMT4ZZ	0MNH3ZZ	0MPXX0Z	0MQJ4ZZ
0M9340Z	0M9C00Z	0M9L30Z	0M9T40Z	0MB73ZZ	0MBL3ZZ	0MHX0YZ	0MMV0ZZ	0MNH4ZZ	0MPY00Z	0MQK0ZZ
0M934ZX	0M9C0ZX	0M9L3ZX	0M9T4ZX	0MB74ZX	0MBL4ZX	0MHX3YZ	0MMV4ZZ	0MNHXZZ	0MPY07Z	0MQK3ZZ
0M934ZZ	0M9C0ZZ	0M9L3ZZ	0M9T4ZZ	0MB74ZZ	0MBL4ZZ	0MHX4YZ	0MMW0ZZ	0MNJ0ZZ	0MPY0JZ	0MQK4ZZ
0M9400Z	0M9C30Z	0M9L40Z	0M9V00Z	0MB80ZX	0MBM0ZX	0MHY0YZ	0MMW4ZZ	0MNJ3ZZ	0MPY0KZ	0MQL0ZZ
0M940ZX	0M9C3ZX	0M9L4ZX	0M9V0ZX	0MB80ZZ	0MBM0ZZ	0MHY3YZ	0MN00ZZ	0MNJ4ZZ	0MPY0YZ	0MQL3ZZ
0M940ZZ	0M9C3ZZ	0M9L4ZZ	0M9V0ZZ	0MB83ZX	0MBM3ZX	0MHY4YZ	0MN03ZZ	0MNJXZZ	0MPY30Z	0MQL4ZZ
0M9430Z	0M9C40Z	0M9M00Z	0M9V30Z	0MB83ZZ	0MBM3ZZ	0MJX0ZZ	0MN04ZZ	0MNK0ZZ	0MPY37Z	0MQM0ZZ
0M943ZX	0M9C4ZX	0M9M0ZX	0M9V3ZX	0MB84ZX	0MBM4ZX	0MJX3ZZ	0MN0XZZ	0MNK3ZZ	0MPY3JZ	0MQM3ZZ
0M943ZZ	0M9C4ZZ	0M9M0ZZ	0M9V3ZZ	0MB84ZZ	0MBM4ZZ	0MJX4ZZ	0MN10ZZ	0MNK4ZZ	0MPY3KZ	0MQM4ZZ
0M9440Z	0M9D00Z	0M9M30Z	0M9V40Z	0MB90ZX	0MBN0ZX	0MJXXZZ	0MN13ZZ	0MNKXZZ	0MPY3YZ	0MQN0ZZ
0M944ZX	0M9D0ZX	0M9M3ZX	0M9V4ZX	0MB90ZZ	0MBN0ZZ	0MJY0ZZ	0MN14ZZ	0MNL0ZZ	0MPY40Z	0MQN3ZZ
0M944ZZ	0M9D0ZZ	0M9M3ZZ	0M9V4ZZ	0MB93ZX	0MBN3ZX	0MJY3ZZ	0MN1XZZ	0MNL3ZZ	0MPY47Z	0MQN4ZZ
0M9500Z	0M9D30Z	0M9M40Z	0M9W00Z	0MB93ZZ	0MBN3ZZ	0MJY4ZZ	0MN20ZZ	0MNL4ZZ	0MPY4JZ	0MQP0ZZ
0M950ZX	0M9D3ZX	0M9M4ZX	0M9W0ZX	0MB94ZX	0MBN4ZX	0MJYXZZ	0MN23ZZ	0MNLXZZ	0MPY4KZ	0MQP3ZZ
0M950ZZ	0M9D3ZZ	0M9M4ZZ	0M9W0ZZ	0MB94ZZ	0MBN4ZZ	0MM00ZZ	0MN24ZZ	0MNM0ZZ	0MPY4YZ	0MQP4ZZ
0M9530Z	0M9D40Z	0M9N00Z	0M9W30Z	0MBB0ZX	0MBP0ZX	0MM04ZZ	0MN2XZZ	0MNM3ZZ	0MPYX0Z	0MQQ0ZZ
0M953ZX	0M9D4ZX	0M9N0ZX	0M9W3ZX	0MBB0ZZ	0MBP0ZZ	0MM10ZZ	0MN30ZZ	0MNM4ZZ	0MQ00ZZ	0MQQ0ZZ

0MQQ3ZZ	0MR80JZ	0MRM0JZ	0MS64ZZ	0MTC4ZZ	0MU547Z	0MUJ47Z	0MUW47Z	0N850ZZ	0N904ZZ	0N9C0ZZ
0MQQ4ZZ	0MR80KZ	0MRM0KZ	0MS70ZZ	0MTD0ZZ	0MU54JZ	0MUJ4JZ	0MUW4JZ	0N853ZZ	0N9100Z	0N9C30Z
0MQR0ZZ	0MR847Z	0MRM47Z	0MS74ZZ	0MTD4ZZ	0MU54KZ	0MUJ4KZ	0MUW4KZ	0N854ZZ	0N910ZX	0N9C3ZX
0MQR3ZZ	0MR84JZ	0MRM4JZ	0MS80ZZ	0MTF0ZZ	0MU607Z	0MUK07Z	0MWX00Z	0N860ZZ	0N910ZZ	0N9C3ZZ
0MQR4ZZ	0MR84KZ	0MRM4KZ	0MS84ZZ	0MTF4ZZ	0MU60JZ	0MUK0JZ	0MWX07Z	0N863ZZ	0N9130Z	0N9C40Z
0MQS0ZZ	0MR907Z	0MRN07Z	0MS90ZZ	0MTG0ZZ	0MU60KZ	0MUK0KZ	0MWX0JZ	0N864ZZ	0N913ZX	0N9C4ZX
0MQS3ZZ	0MR90JZ	0MRN0JZ	0MS94ZZ	0MTG4ZZ	0MU647Z	0MUK47Z	0MWX0KZ	0N870ZZ	0N913ZZ	0N9C4ZZ
0MQS4ZZ	0MR90KZ	0MRN0KZ	0MSB0ZZ	0MTH0ZZ	0MU64JZ	0MUK4JZ	0MWX0YZ	0N873ZZ	0N9140Z	0N9F00Z
0MQT0ZZ	0MR947Z	0MRN47Z	0MSB4ZZ	0MTH4ZZ	0MU64KZ	0MUK4KZ	0MWX30Z	0N874ZZ	0N914ZX	0N9F0ZX
0MQT3ZZ	0MR94JZ	0MRN4JZ	0MSC0ZZ	0MTJ0ZZ	0MU707Z	0MUL07Z	0MWX37Z	0N8B0ZZ	0N914ZZ	0N9F0ZZ
0MQT4ZZ	0MR94KZ	0MRN4KZ	0MSC4ZZ	0MTJ4ZZ	0MU70JZ	0MUL0JZ	0MWX3YZ	0N8B3ZZ	0N9300Z	0N9F30Z
0MQV0ZZ	0MRB07Z	0MRP07Z	0MSD0ZZ	0MTK0ZZ	0MU70KZ	0MUL0KZ	0MWX4YZ	0N8B4ZZ	0N930ZX	0N9F3ZX
0MQV3ZZ	0MRB0JZ	0MRP0JZ	0MSD4ZZ	0MTK4ZZ	0MU747Z	0MUL47Z	0MWXX0Z	0N8C0ZZ	0N930ZZ	0N9F3ZZ
0MQV4ZZ	0MRB0KZ	0MRP0KZ	0MSF0ZZ	0MTL0ZZ	0MU74JZ	0MUL4JZ	0MWXX7Z	0N8C3ZZ	0N9330Z	0N9F40Z
0MQW0ZZ	0MRB47Z	0MRP47Z	0MSF4ZZ	0MTL4ZZ	0MU74KZ	0MUL4KZ	0MWXXJZ	0N8C4ZZ	0N933ZX	0N9F4ZX
0MQW3ZZ	0MRB4JZ	0MRP4JZ	0MSG0ZZ	0MTM0ZZ	0MU807Z	0MUM07Z	0MWXXKZ	0N8D0ZZ	0N933ZZ	0N9F4ZZ
0MQW4ZZ	0MRB4KZ	0MRP4KZ	0MSG4ZZ	0MTM4ZZ	0MU80JZ	0MUM0JZ	0MWY0YZ	0N8F0ZZ	0N9340Z	0N9G00Z
0MR007Z	0MRC07Z	0MRQ07Z	0MSH0ZZ	0MTN0ZZ	0MU80KZ	0MUM0KZ	0MWY3YZ	0N8F3ZZ	0N934ZX	0N9G0ZX
0MR00JZ	0MRC0JZ	0MRQ0JZ	0MSH4ZZ	0MTN4ZZ	0MU847Z	0MUM47Z	0MWY4YZ	0N8F4ZZ	0N934ZZ	0N9G0ZZ
0MR00KZ	0MRC0KZ	0MRQ0KZ	0MSJ0ZZ	0MTP0ZZ	0MU84JZ	0MUM4JZ	0MWYX0Z	0N8G0ZZ	0N9400Z	0N9G30Z
0MR047Z	0MRC47Z	0MRQ47Z	0MSJ4ZZ	0MTP4ZZ	0MU84KZ	0MUM4KZ	0MWYX7Z	0N8G3ZZ	0N940ZX	0N9G3ZX
0MR04JZ	0MRC4JZ	0MRQ4JZ	0MSK0ZZ	0MTQ0ZZ	0MU907Z	0MUN07Z	0MWYXJZ	0N8G4ZZ	0N940ZZ	0N9G3ZZ
0MR04KZ	0MRC4KZ	0MRQ4KZ	0MSK4ZZ	0MTQ4ZZ	0MU90JZ	0MUN0JZ	0MWYXKZ	0N8H0ZZ	0N9430Z	0N9G40Z
0MR107Z	0MRD07Z	0MRR07Z	0MSL0ZZ	0MTR0ZZ	0MU90KZ	0MUN0KZ	0N20X0Z	0N8H3ZZ	0N943ZX	0N9G4ZX
0MR10JZ	0MRD0JZ	0MRR0JZ	0MSL4ZZ	0MTR4ZZ	0MU947Z	0MUN47Z	0N20XYZ	0N8H4ZZ	0N943ZZ	0N9G4ZZ
0MR10KZ	0MRD0KZ	0MRR0KZ	0MSM0ZZ	0MTS0ZZ	0MU94JZ	0MUN4JZ	0N2BX0Z	0N8J0ZZ	0N9440Z	0N9H00Z
0MR147Z	0MRD47Z	0MRR47Z	0MSM4ZZ	0MTS4ZZ	0MU94KZ	0MUN4KZ	0N2BXYZ	0N8J3ZZ	0N944ZX	0N9H0ZX
0MR14JZ	0MRD4JZ	0MRR4JZ	0MSN0ZZ	0MTT0ZZ	0MUB07Z	0MUP07Z	0N2WX0Z	0N8J4ZZ	0N944ZZ	0N9H0ZZ
0MR14KZ	0MRD4KZ	0MRR4KZ	0MSN4ZZ	0MTT4ZZ	0MUB0JZ	0MUP0JZ	0N2WXYZ	0N8K0ZZ	0N9500Z	0N9H30Z
0MR207Z	0MRF07Z	0MRS07Z	0MSP0ZZ	0MTV0ZZ	0MUB0KZ	0MUP0KZ	0N5L4ZZ	0N8K3ZZ	0N950ZX	0N9H3ZX
0MR20JZ	0MRF0JZ	0MRS0JZ	0MSP4ZZ	0MTV4ZZ	0MUB47Z	0MUP47Z	0N5M0ZZ	0N8K4ZZ	0N950ZZ	0N9H3ZZ
0MR20KZ	0MRF0KZ	0MRS0KZ	0MSQ0ZZ	0MTW0ZZ	0MUB4JZ	0MUP4JZ	0N5M3ZZ	0N8L0ZZ	0N9530Z	0N9H40Z
0MR247Z	0MRF47Z	0MRS47Z	0MSQ4ZZ	0MTW4ZZ	0MUB4KZ	0MUP4KZ	0N5M4ZZ	0N8L3ZZ	0N953ZX	0N9H4ZX
0MR24JZ	0MRF4JZ	0MRS4JZ	0MSR0ZZ	0MU007Z	0MUC07Z	0MUQ07Z	0N5N0ZZ	0N8L4ZZ	0N953ZZ	0N9H4ZZ
0MR24KZ	0MRF4KZ	0MRS4KZ	0MSR4ZZ	0MU00JZ	0MUC0JZ	0MUQ0JZ	0N5N3ZZ	0N8M0ZZ	0N9540Z	0N9J00Z
0MR307Z	0MRG07Z	0MRT07Z	0MSS0ZZ	0MU00KZ	0MUC0KZ	0MUQ0KZ	0N5N4ZZ	0N8M3ZZ	0N954ZX	0N9J0ZX
0MR30JZ	0MRG0JZ	0MRT0JZ	0MSS4ZZ	0MU047Z	0MUC47Z	0MUQ47Z	0N5P0ZZ	0N8M4ZZ	0N954ZZ	0N9J0ZZ
0MR30KZ	0MRG0KZ	0MRT0KZ	0MST0ZZ	0MU04JZ	0MUC4JZ	0MUQ4JZ	0N5P3ZZ	0N8N0ZZ	0N9600Z	0N9J30Z
0MR347Z	0MRG47Z	0MRT47Z	0MST4ZZ	0MU04KZ	0MUC4KZ	0MUQ4KZ	0N5P4ZZ	0N8N3ZZ	0N960ZX	0N9J3ZX
0MR34JZ	0MRG4JZ	0MRT4JZ	0MSV0ZZ	0MU107Z	0MUD07Z	0MUR07Z	0N5Q0ZZ	0N8N4ZZ	0N960ZZ	0N9J3ZZ
0MR34KZ	0MRG4KZ	0MRT4KZ	0MSV4ZZ	0MU10JZ	0MUD0JZ	0MUR0JZ	0N5Q3ZZ	0N8P0ZZ	0N9630Z	0N9J40Z
0MR407Z	0MRH07Z	0MRV07Z	0MSW0ZZ	0MU10KZ	0MUD0KZ	0MUR0KZ	0N5Q4ZZ	0N8P3ZZ	0N963ZX	0N9J4ZX
0MR40JZ	0MRH0JZ	0MRV0JZ	0MSW4ZZ	0MU147Z	0MUD47Z	0MUR47Z	0N5R0ZZ	0N8P4ZZ	0N963ZZ	0N9J4ZZ
0MR40KZ	0MRH0KZ	0MRV0KZ	0MT00ZZ	0MU14JZ	0MUD4JZ	0MUR4JZ	0N5R3ZZ	0N8Q0ZZ	0N9640Z	0N9K00Z
0MR447Z	0MRH47Z	0MRV47Z	0MT04ZZ	0MU14KZ	0MUD4KZ	0MUR4KZ	0N5R4ZZ	0N8Q3ZZ	0N964ZX	0N9K0ZX
0MR44JZ	0MRH4JZ	0MRV4JZ	0MT10ZZ	0MU207Z	0MUF07Z	0MUS07Z	0N5T0ZZ	0N8Q4ZZ	0N964ZZ	0N9K0ZZ
0MR44KZ	0MRH4KZ	0MRV4KZ	0MT14ZZ	0MU20JZ	0MUF0JZ	0MUS0JZ	0N5T3ZZ	0N8R0ZZ	0N9700Z	0N9K30Z
0MR507Z	0MRJ07Z	0MRW07Z	0MT20ZZ	0MU20KZ	0MUF0KZ	0MUS0KZ	0N5T4ZZ	0N8R3ZZ	0N970ZX	0N9K3ZX
0MR50JZ	0MRJ0JZ	0MRW0JZ	0MT24ZZ	0MU247Z	0MUF47Z	0MUS47Z	0N5V0ZZ	0N8R4ZZ	0N970ZZ	0N9K3ZZ
0MR50KZ	0MRJ0KZ	0MRW0KZ	0MT30ZZ	0MU24JZ	0MUF4JZ	0MUS4JZ	0N5V3ZZ	0N8T0ZZ	0N9730Z	0N9K40Z
0MR547Z	0MRJ47Z	0MRW47Z	0MT34ZZ	0MU24KZ	0MUF4KZ	0MUS4KZ	0N5V4ZZ	0N8T3ZZ	0N973ZX	0N9K4ZX
0MR54JZ	0MRJ4JZ	0MRW4JZ	0MT40ZZ	0MU307Z	0MUG07Z	0MUT07Z	0N5X0ZZ	0N8T4ZZ	0N973ZZ	0N9K4ZZ
0MR54KZ	0MRJ4KZ	0MRW4KZ	0MT44ZZ	0MU30JZ	0MUG0JZ	0MUT0JZ	0N5X3ZZ	0N8V0ZZ	0N9740Z	0N9L00Z
0MR607Z	0MRK07Z	0MS00ZZ	0MT50ZZ	0MU30KZ	0MUG0KZ	0MUT0KZ	0N5X4ZZ	0N8V3ZZ	0N974ZX	0N9L0ZX
0MR60JZ	0MRK0JZ	0MS04ZZ	0MT54ZZ	0MU347Z	0MUG47Z	0MUT47Z	0N800ZZ	0N8V4ZZ	0N974ZZ	0N9L0ZZ
0MR60KZ	0MRK0KZ	0MS10ZZ	0MT60ZZ	0MU34JZ	0MUG4JZ	0MUT4JZ	0N803ZZ	0N8X0ZZ	0N9B00Z	0N9L30Z
0MR647Z	0MRK47Z	0MS14ZZ	0MT64ZZ	0MU34KZ	0MUG4KZ	0MUT4KZ	0N804ZZ	0N8X3ZZ	0N9B0ZX	0N9L3ZX
0MR64JZ	0MRK4JZ	0MS20ZZ	0MT70ZZ	0MU407Z	0MUH07Z	0MUV07Z	0N810ZZ	0N8X4ZZ	0N9B0ZZ	0N9L3ZZ
0MR64KZ	0MRK4KZ	0MS24ZZ	0MT74ZZ	0MU40JZ	0MUH0JZ	0MUV0JZ	0N813ZZ	0N9000Z	0N9B30Z	0N9L40Z
0MR707Z	0MRL07Z	0MS30ZZ	0MT80ZZ	0MU40KZ	0MUH0KZ	0MUV0KZ	0N814ZZ	0N900ZX	0N9B3ZX	0N9L4ZX
0MR70JZ	0MRL0JZ	0MS34ZZ	0MT84ZZ	0MU447Z	0MUH47Z	0MUV47Z	0N830ZZ	0N900ZZ	0N9B3ZZ	0N9L4ZZ
0MR70KZ	0MRL0KZ	0MS40ZZ	0MT90ZZ	0MU44JZ	0MUH4JZ	0MUV4JZ	0N833ZZ	0N9030Z	0N9B40Z	0N9M00Z
0MR747Z	0MRL47Z	0MS44ZZ	0MT94ZZ	0MU44KZ	0MUH4KZ	0MUV4KZ	0N834ZZ	0N903ZX	0N9B4ZX	0N9M0ZX
0MR74JZ	0MRL4JZ	0MS50ZZ	0MTB0ZZ	0MU507Z	0MUJ07Z	0MUW07Z	0N840ZZ	0N903ZZ	0N9B4ZZ	0N9M0ZZ
0MR74KZ	0MRL4KZ	0MS54ZZ	0MTB4ZZ	0MU50JZ	0MUJ0JZ	0MUW0JZ	0N843ZZ	0N9040Z	0N9C00Z	0N9M30Z
0MR807Z	0MRM07Z	0MS60ZZ	0MTC0ZZ	0MU50KZ	0MUJ0KZ	0MUW0KZ	0N844ZZ	0N904ZX	0N9C0ZX	0N9M3ZX

0N9M3ZZ	0N9X4ZZ	0NCG0ZZ	0NH034Z	0NHQ04Z	0NNG0ZZ	0NP0X5Z	0NQ63ZZ	0NRF0KZ	0NRN3KZ	0NS04ZZ
0N9M40Z	0NB00ZX	0NCG3ZZ	0NH035Z	0NHQ34Z	0NNG3ZZ	0NP0XMZ	0NR307Z	0NRF37Z	0NRN47Z	0NS0XZZ
0N9M4ZX	0NB00ZZ	0NCG4ZZ	0NH03MZ	0NHQ44Z	0NNG4ZZ	0NP0XSZ	0NR30JZ	0NRF3JZ	0NRN4JZ	0NS104Z
0N9M4ZZ	0NB03ZX	0NCH0ZZ	0NH044Z	0NHR04Z	0NNH0ZZ	0NPB00Z	0NR30KZ	0NRF3KZ	0NRN4KZ	0NS10ZZ
0N9N00Z	0NB03ZZ	0NCH3ZZ	0NH045Z	0NHR05Z	0NNH3ZZ	0NPB04Z	0NR337Z	0NRF47Z	0NRP07Z	0NS134Z
0N9N0ZX	0NB04ZX	0NCH4ZZ	0NH04MZ	0NHR34Z	0NNH4ZZ	0NPB07Z	0NR33JZ	0NRF4JZ	0NRP0JZ	0NS13ZZ
0N9N0ZZ	0NB04ZZ	0NCJ0ZZ	0NH104Z	0NHR35Z	0NNJ0ZZ	0NPB0JZ	0NR33KZ	0NRF4KZ	0NRP0KZ	0NS144Z
0N9N30Z	0NB10ZX	0NCJ3ZZ	0NH134Z	0NHR44Z	0NNJ3ZZ	0NPB0KZ	0NR347Z	0NRG07Z	0NRP37Z	0NS14ZZ
0N9N3ZX	0NB10ZZ	0NCJ4ZZ	0NH144Z	0NHR45Z	0NNJ4ZZ	0NPB0MZ	0NR34JZ	0NRG0JZ	0NRP3JZ	0NS1XZZ
0N9N3ZZ	0NB13ZX	0NCK0ZZ	0NH304Z	0NHT04Z	0NNK0ZZ	0NPB30Z	0NR34KZ	0NRG0KZ	0NRP3KZ	0NS304Z
0N9N40Z	0NB13ZZ	0NCK3ZZ	0NH334Z	0NHT05Z	0NNK3ZZ	0NPB34Z	0NR407Z	0NRG37Z	0NRP47Z	0NS30ZZ
0N9N4ZX	0NB14ZX	0NCK4ZZ	0NH344Z	0NHT34Z	0NNK4ZZ	0NPB37Z	0NR40JZ	0NRG3JZ	0NRP4JZ	0NS334Z
0N9N4ZZ	0NB14ZZ	0NCL0ZZ	0NH404Z	0NHT35Z	0NNL0ZZ	0NPB3JZ	0NR40KZ	0NRG3KZ	0NRP4KZ	0NS33ZZ
0N9P00Z	0NB30ZX	0NCL3ZZ	0NH434Z	0NHT44Z	0NNL3ZZ	0NPB3KZ	0NR437Z	0NRG47Z	0NRQ07Z	0NS344Z
0N9P0ZX	0NB30ZZ	0NCL4ZZ	0NH444Z	0NHT45Z	0NNL4ZZ	0NPB3MZ	0NR43JZ	0NRG4JZ	0NRQ0JZ	0NSB34Z
0N9P0ZZ	0NB33ZX	0NCM0ZZ	0NH504Z	0NHV04Z	0NNM0ZZ	0NPB40Z	0NR43KZ	0NRG4KZ	0NRQ0KZ	0NSB3ZZ
0N9P30Z	0NB33ZZ	0NCM3ZZ	0NH50SZ	0NHV05Z	0NNM3ZZ	0NPB44Z	0NR447Z	0NRH07Z	0NRQ37Z	0NSB44Z
0N9P3ZX	0NB34ZX	0NCM4ZZ	0NH534Z	0NHV34Z	0NNM4ZZ	0NPB47Z	0NR44JZ	0NRH0JZ	0NRQ3JZ	0NSB4ZZ
0N9P3ZZ	0NB34ZZ	0NCN0ZZ	0NH53SZ	0NHV35Z	0NNN0ZZ	0NPB4JZ	0NR44KZ	0NRH0KZ	0NRQ3KZ	0NSBXZZ
0N9P40Z	0NB40ZX	0NCN3ZZ	0NH544Z	0NHV44Z	0NNN3ZZ	0NPB4KZ	0NR507Z	0NRH37Z	0NRQ47Z	0NSC34Z
0N9P4ZX	0NB40ZZ	0NCN4ZZ	0NH54SZ	0NHV45Z	0NNN4ZZ	0NPB4MZ	0NR50JZ	0NRH3JZ	0NRQ4JZ	0NSC3ZZ
0N9P4ZZ	0NB43ZX	0NCP0ZZ	0NH604Z	0NHW0MZ	0NNP0ZZ	0NPBX0Z	0NR50KZ	0NRH3KZ	0NRQ4KZ	0NSC44Z
0N9Q00Z	0NB43ZZ	0NCP3ZZ	0NH60SZ	0NHW3MZ	0NNP3ZZ	0NPBX4Z	0NR537Z	0NRH47Z	0NRR07Z	0NSC4ZZ
0N9Q0ZX	0NB44ZX	0NCP4ZZ	0NH634Z	0NHW4MZ	0NNP4ZZ	0NPBXMZ	0NR53JZ	0NRH4JZ	0NRR0JZ	0NSCXZZ
0N9Q0ZZ	0NB44ZZ	0NCQ0ZZ	0NH63SZ	0NHX04Z	0NNQ0ZZ	0NPW00Z	0NR53KZ	0NRH4KZ	0NRR0KZ	0NSF34Z
0N9Q30Z	0NB50ZX	0NCQ3ZZ	0NH644Z	0NHX34Z	0NNQ3ZZ	0NPW04Z	0NR547Z	0NRJ07Z	0NRR37Z	0NSF3ZZ
0N9Q3ZX	0NB50ZZ	0NCQ4ZZ	0NH64SZ	0NHX44Z	0NNQ4ZZ	0NPW07Z	0NR54JZ	0NRJ0JZ	0NRR3JZ	0NSF44Z
0N9Q3ZZ	0NB53ZX	0NCR0ZZ	0NH704Z	0NJ00ZZ	0NNR0ZZ	0NPW0JZ	0NR54KZ	0NRJ0KZ	0NRR3KZ	0NSF4ZZ
0N9Q40Z	0NB53ZZ	0NCR3ZZ	0NH734Z	0NJ03ZZ	0NNR3ZZ	0NPW0KZ	0NR607Z	0NRJ37Z	0NRR47Z	0NSFXZZ
0N9Q4ZX	0NB54ZX	0NCR4ZZ	0NH744Z	0NJ04ZZ	0NNR4ZZ	0NPW0MZ	0NR60JZ	0NRJ3JZ	0NRR4JZ	0NSG34Z
0N9Q4ZZ	0NB54ZZ	0NCT0ZZ	0NHB04Z	0NJ0XZZ	0NNT0ZZ	0NPW30Z	0NR60KZ	0NRJ3KZ	0NRR4KZ	0NSG3ZZ
0N9R00Z	0NB60ZX	0NCT3ZZ	0NHB0MZ	0NJB0ZZ	0NNT3ZZ	0NPW34Z	0NR637Z	0NRJ47Z	0NRT07Z	0NSG44Z
0N9R0ZX	0NB60ZZ	0NCT4ZZ	0NHB34Z	0NJB3ZZ	0NNT4ZZ	0NPW37Z	0NR63JZ	0NRJ4JZ	0NRT0JZ	0NSG4ZZ
0N9R0ZZ	0NB63ZX	0NCV0ZZ	0NHB3MZ	0NJB4ZZ	0NNV0ZZ	0NPW3JZ	0NR63KZ	0NRJ4KZ	0NRT0KZ	0NSGXZZ
0N9R30Z	0NB63ZZ	0NCV3ZZ	0NHB44Z	0NJBXZZ	0NNV3ZZ	0NPW3KZ	0NR647Z	0NRK07Z	0NRT37Z	0NSH34Z
0N9R3ZX	0NB64ZX	0NCV4ZZ	0NHB4MZ	0NJW0ZZ	0NNV4ZZ	0NPW3MZ	0NR64JZ	0NRK0JZ	0NRT3JZ	0NSH3ZZ
0N9R3ZZ	0NB64ZZ	0NCX0ZZ	0NHC04Z	0NJW3ZZ	0NNX0ZZ	0NPW40Z	0NR64KZ	0NRK0KZ	0NRT3KZ	0NSH44Z
0N9R40Z	0NB70ZX	0NCX3ZZ	0NHC34Z	0NJW4ZZ	0NNX3ZZ	0NPW44Z	0NR707Z	0NRK37Z	0NRT47Z	0NSH4ZZ
0N9R4ZX	0NB70ZZ	0NCX4ZZ	0NHC44Z	0NJWXZZ	0NNX4ZZ	0NPW47Z	0NR70JZ	0NRK3JZ	0NRT4JZ	0NSHXZZ
0N9R4ZZ	0NB73ZX	0NHF04Z	0NN10ZZ	0NPW4JZ	0NR70KZ	0NRK3KZ	0NRT4KZ	0NSJ34Z
0N9T00Z	0NB73ZZ	0ND00ZZ	0NHF34Z	0NN13ZZ	0NP000Z	0NPW4KZ	0NR737Z	0NRK47Z	0NRV07Z	0NSJ3ZZ
0N9T0ZX	0NB74ZX	0ND10ZZ	0NHF44Z	0NN14ZZ	0NP004Z	0NPW4MZ	0NR73JZ	0NRK4JZ	0NRV0JZ	0NSJ44Z
0N9T0ZZ	0NB74ZZ	0ND30ZZ	0NHG04Z	0NN30ZZ	0NP005Z	0NPWX0Z	0NR73KZ	0NRK4KZ	0NRV0KZ	0NSJ4ZZ
0N9T30Z	0NBB0ZX	0ND40ZZ	0NHG34Z	0NN33ZZ	0NP007Z	0NPWX4Z	0NR747Z	0NRL07Z	0NRV37Z	0NSJXZZ
0N9T3ZX	0NBB3ZX	0ND50ZZ	0NHG44Z	0NN34ZZ	0NP00JZ	0NPWXMZ	0NR74JZ	0NRL0JZ	0NRV3JZ	0NSK34Z
0N9T3ZZ	0NBB4ZX	0ND60ZZ	0NHH04Z	0NN40ZZ	0NP00KZ		0NR74KZ	0NRL0KZ	0NRV3KZ	0NSK3ZZ
0N9T40Z	0NBR0ZX	0ND70ZZ	0NHH34Z	0NN43ZZ	0NP00MZ	0NQ00ZZ	0NRB07Z	0NRL37Z	0NRV47Z	0NSK44Z
0N9T4ZX	0NBR3ZX	0NDB0ZZ	0NHH44Z	0NN44ZZ	0NP00NZ	0NQ03ZZ	0NRB0JZ	0NRL3JZ	0NRV4JZ	0NSK4ZZ
0N9T4ZZ	0NBR4ZX	0NDC0ZZ	0NHJ04Z	0NN50ZZ	0NP00SZ	0NQ04ZZ	0NRB0KZ	0NRL3KZ	0NRV4KZ	0NSKXZZ
0N9V00Z	0NBT0ZX	0NDF0ZZ	0NHJ34Z	0NN53ZZ	0NP030Z	0NQ0XZZ	0NRB37Z	0NRL47Z	0NRX07Z	0NSL34Z
0N9V0ZX	0NBT3ZX	0NDG0ZZ	0NHJ44Z	0NN54ZZ	0NP034Z	0NQ10ZZ	0NRB3JZ	0NRL4JZ	0NRX0JZ	0NSL3ZZ
0N9V0ZZ	0NBT4ZX	0NDH0ZZ	0NHK04Z	0NN60ZZ	0NP035Z	0NQ13ZZ	0NRB3KZ	0NRL4KZ	0NRX0KZ	0NSL44Z
0N9V30Z	0NBV0ZX	0NDJ0ZZ	0NHK34Z	0NN63ZZ	0NP037Z	0NQ14ZZ	0NRB47Z	0NRM07Z	0NRX37Z	0NSL4ZZ
0N9V3ZX	0NBV3ZX	0NDK0ZZ	0NHK44Z	0NN64ZZ	0NP03JZ	0NQ1XZZ	0NRB4JZ	0NRM0JZ	0NRX3JZ	0NSLXZZ
0N9V3ZZ	0NBV4ZX	0NDL0ZZ	0NHL04Z	0NN70ZZ	0NP03KZ	0NQ30ZZ	0NRB4KZ	0NRM0KZ	0NRX3KZ	0NSM34Z
0N9V40Z	0NC73ZZ	0NDM0ZZ	0NHL34Z	0NN73ZZ	0NP03MZ	0NQ33ZZ	0NRC07Z	0NRM37Z	0NRX47Z	0NSM3ZZ
0N9V4ZX	0NC74ZZ	0NDN0ZZ	0NHL44Z	0NN74ZZ	0NP03SZ	0NQ34ZZ	0NRC0JZ	0NRM3JZ	0NRX4JZ	0NSM44Z
0N9V4ZZ	0NCB0ZZ	0NDP0ZZ	0NHM04Z	0NNB0ZZ	0NP040Z	0NQ3XZZ	0NRC0KZ	0NRM3KZ	0NRX4KZ	0NSM4ZZ
0N9X00Z	0NCB3ZZ	0NDQ0ZZ	0NHM34Z	0NNB3ZZ	0NP044Z	0NQ40ZZ	0NRC37Z	0NRM47Z	0NS004Z	0NSMXZZ
0N9X0ZX	0NCB4ZZ	0NDR0ZZ	0NHM44Z	0NNB4ZZ	0NP045Z	0NQ43ZZ	0NRC3JZ	0NRM4JZ	0NS005Z	0NSN34Z
0N9X0ZZ	0NCC0ZZ	0NDT0ZZ	0NHN04Z	0NNC0ZZ	0NP047Z	0NQ44ZZ	0NRC3KZ	0NRM4KZ	0NS00ZZ	0NSN3ZZ
0N9X30Z	0NCC3ZZ	0NDV0ZZ	0NHN34Z	0NNC3ZZ	0NP04JZ	0NQ4XZZ	0NRC47Z	0NRN07Z	0NS034Z	0NSN44Z
0N9X3ZX	0NCC4ZZ	0NDX0ZZ	0NHN44Z	0NNC4ZZ	0NP04KZ	0NQ50ZZ	0NRC4JZ	0NRN0JZ	0NS035Z	0NSN4ZZ
0N9X3ZZ	0NCF0ZZ	0NH004Z	0NHP04Z	0NNF0ZZ	0NP04MZ	0NQ53ZZ	0NRC4KZ	0NRN0KZ	0NS03ZZ	0NSNXZZ
0N9X40Z	0NCF3ZZ	0NH005Z	0NHP34Z	0NNF3ZZ	0NP04SZ	0NQ54ZZ	0NRF07Z	0NRN37Z	0NS044Z	0NSP34Z
0N9X4ZX	0NCF4ZZ	0NH00MZ	0NHP44Z	0NNF4ZZ	0NP0X0Z	0NQ5XZZ	0NRF0JZ	0NRN3JZ	0NS045Z	0NSP3ZZ
		0NH00NZ			0NP0X4Z	0NQ60ZZ				

0NSP44Z	0NU13KZ	0NUC4KZ	0NUN0KZ	0NWB3MZ	0P8J3ZZ	0P934ZX	0P9C0ZZ	0P9L3ZX	0P9T4ZX	0PBQ4ZX
0NSP4ZZ	0NU147Z	0NUF07Z	0NUN37Z	0NWB40Z	0P8J4ZZ	0P934ZZ	0P9C0ZZ	0P9L3ZZ	0P9T4ZZ	0PBQ4ZZ
0NSPXZZ	0NU14JZ	0NUF0JZ	0NUN3JZ	0NWB44Z	0P8K0ZZ	0P9400Z	0P9C30Z	0P9L40Z	0P9V00Z	0PBR0ZX
0NSQ34Z	0NU14KZ	0NUF0KZ	0NUN3KZ	0NWB47Z	0P8K3ZZ	0P940ZX	0P9C3ZX	0P9L4ZX	0P9V0ZX	0PBR0ZZ
0NSQ3ZZ	0NU307Z	0NUF37Z	0NUN47Z	0NWB4JZ	0P8K4ZZ	0P940ZZ	0P9C3ZZ	0P9L4ZZ	0P9V0ZZ	0PBR3ZX
0NSQ44Z	0NU30JZ	0NUF3JZ	0NUN4JZ	0NWB4KZ	0P8L0ZZ	0P9430Z	0P9C40Z	0P9M00Z	0P9V30Z	0PBR3ZZ
0NSQ4ZZ	0NU30KZ	0NUF3KZ	0NUN4KZ	0NWB4MZ	0P8L3ZZ	0P943ZX	0P9C4ZX	0P9M0ZX	0P9V3ZX	0PBR4ZX
0NSQXZZ	0NU337Z	0NUF47Z	0NUP07Z	0NWBX0Z	0P8L4ZZ	0P943ZZ	0P9C4ZZ	0P9M0ZZ	0P9V3ZZ	0PBR4ZZ
0NSR34Z	0NU33JZ	0NUF4JZ	0NUP0JZ	0NWBX4Z	0P8M0ZZ	0P9440Z	0P9D00Z	0P9M30Z	0P9V40Z	0PBS0ZX
0NSR35Z	0NU33KZ	0NUF4KZ	0NUP0KZ	0NWBX7Z	0P8M3ZZ	0P944ZX	0P9D0ZX	0P9M3ZX	0P9V4ZX	0PBS0ZZ
0NSR3ZZ	0NU347Z	0NUG07Z	0NUP37Z	0NWBXJZ	0P8M4ZZ	0P944ZZ	0P9D0ZZ	0P9M3ZZ	0P9V4ZZ	0PBS3ZX
0NSR44Z	0NU34JZ	0NUG0JZ	0NUP3JZ	0NWBXKZ	0P8N0ZZ	0P9500Z	0P9D30Z	0P9M40Z	0PB00ZX	0PBS3ZZ
0NSR45Z	0NU34KZ	0NUG0KZ	0NUP3KZ	0NWBXMZ	0P8N3ZZ	0P950ZX	0P9D3ZX	0P9M4ZX	0PB00ZZ	0PBS4ZX
0NSR4ZZ	0NU407Z	0NUG37Z	0NUP47Z	0NWWX0Z	0P8N4ZZ	0P950ZZ	0P9D3ZZ	0P9M4ZZ	0PB03ZX	0PBS4ZZ
0NSRXZZ	0NU40JZ	0NUG3JZ	0NUP4JZ	0NWWX4Z	0P8P0ZZ	0P9530Z	0P9D40Z	0P9N00Z	0PB03ZZ	0PBT0ZX
0NST34Z	0NU40KZ	0NUG3KZ	0NUP4KZ	0NWWX7Z	0P8P3ZZ	0P953ZX	0P9D4ZX	0P9N0ZX	0PBG0ZZ	0PBT0ZZ
0NST35Z	0NU437Z	0NUG47Z	0NUQ07Z	0NWWXJZ	0P8P4ZZ	0P953ZZ	0P9D4ZZ	0P9N0ZZ	0PBG3ZX	0PBT3ZX
0NST3ZZ	0NU43JZ	0NUG4JZ	0NUQ0JZ	0NWWXKZ	0P8Q0ZZ	0P9540Z	0P9F00Z	0P9N30Z	0PBG3ZZ	0PBT3ZZ
0NST44Z	0NU43KZ	0NUG4KZ	0NUQ0KZ	0NWWXMZ	0P8Q3ZZ	0P954ZX	0P9F0ZX	0P9N3ZX	0PBG4ZX	0PBT4ZX
0NST45Z	0NU447Z	0NUH07Z	0NUQ37Z	0P2YX0Z	0P8Q4ZZ	0P954ZZ	0P9F0ZZ	0P9N3ZZ	0PBG4ZZ	0PBT4ZZ
0NST4ZZ	0NU44JZ	0NUH0JZ	0NUQ3JZ	0P2YXYZ	0P8R0ZZ	0P9600Z	0P9F30Z	0P9N40Z	0PBH0ZX	0PBV0ZX
0NSTXZZ	0NU44KZ	0NUH0KZ	0NUQ3KZ	0P813ZZ	0P8R3ZZ	0P960ZX	0P9F3ZX	0P9N4ZX	0PBH0ZZ	0PBV0ZZ
0NSV34Z	0NU507Z	0NUH37Z	0NUQ47Z	0P814ZZ	0P8R4ZZ	0P960ZZ	0P9F3ZZ	0P9N4ZZ	0PBH3ZX	0PBV3ZX
0NSV35Z	0NU50JZ	0NUH3JZ	0NUQ4JZ	0P820ZZ	0P8S0ZZ	0P9630Z	0P9F40Z	0P9P00Z	0PBH3ZZ	0PBV3ZZ
0NSV3ZZ	0NU50KZ	0NUH3KZ	0NUQ4KZ	0P823ZZ	0P8S3ZZ	0P963ZX	0P9F4ZX	0P9P0ZX	0PBH4ZX	0PBV4ZX
0NSV44Z	0NU537Z	0NUH47Z	0NUR07Z	0P824ZZ	0P8S4ZZ	0P963ZZ	0P9F4ZZ	0P9P0ZZ	0PBH4ZZ	0PBV4ZZ
0NSV45Z	0NU53JZ	0NUH4JZ	0NUR0JZ	0P830ZZ	0P8T0ZZ	0P9640Z	0P9G00Z	0P9P30Z	0PBJ0ZX	0PC00ZZ
0NSV4ZZ	0NU53KZ	0NUH4KZ	0NUR0KZ	0P833ZZ	0P8T3ZZ	0P964ZX	0P9G0ZX	0P9P3ZX	0PBJ0ZZ	0PC03ZZ
0NSVXZZ	0NU547Z	0NUJ07Z	0NUR37Z	0P834ZZ	0P8T4ZZ	0P964ZZ	0P9G0ZZ	0P9P3ZZ	0PBJ3ZX	0PC04ZZ
0NSX34Z	0NU54JZ	0NUJ0JZ	0NUR3JZ	0P840ZZ	0P8V0ZZ	0P9700Z	0P9G30Z	0P9P40Z	0PBJ3ZZ	0PC10ZZ
0NSX3ZZ	0NU54KZ	0NUJ0KZ	0NUR3KZ	0P843ZZ	0P8V3ZZ	0P970ZX	0P9G3ZX	0P9P4ZX	0PBJ4ZX	0PC13ZZ
0NSX44Z	0NU607Z	0NUJ37Z	0NUR47Z	0P844ZZ	0P8V4ZZ	0P970ZZ	0P9G3ZZ	0P9P4ZZ	0PBJ4ZZ	0PC14ZZ
0NSX4ZZ	0NU60JZ	0NUJ3JZ	0NUR4JZ	0P850ZZ	0P9000Z	0P9730Z	0P9G40Z	0P9Q00Z	0PBK0ZX	0PC20ZZ
0NSXXZZ	0NU60KZ	0NUJ3KZ	0NUR4KZ	0P853ZZ	0P900ZX	0P973ZX	0P9G4ZX	0P9Q0ZX	0PBK0ZZ	0PC23ZZ
0NT60ZZ	0NU637Z	0NUJ47Z	0NUT07Z	0P854ZZ	0P900ZZ	0P973ZZ	0P9G4ZZ	0P9Q0ZZ	0PBK3ZX	0PC24ZZ
0NT70ZZ	0NU63JZ	0NUJ4JZ	0NUT0JZ	0P860ZZ	0P9030Z	0P9740Z	0P9H00Z	0P9Q30Z	0PBK3ZZ	0PC30ZZ
0NTB0ZZ	0NU63KZ	0NUJ4KZ	0NUT0KZ	0P863ZZ	0P903ZX	0P974ZX	0P9H0ZX	0P9Q3ZX	0PBK4ZX	0PC33ZZ
0NTC0ZZ	0NU647Z	0NUK07Z	0NUT37Z	0P864ZZ	0P903ZZ	0P974ZZ	0P9H0ZZ	0P9Q3ZZ	0PBK4ZZ	0PC34ZZ
0NTF0ZZ	0NU64JZ	0NUK0JZ	0NUT3JZ	0P870ZZ	0P9040Z	0P9800Z	0P9H30Z	0P9Q40Z	0PBL0ZX	0PC40ZZ
0NTG0ZZ	0NU64KZ	0NUK0KZ	0NUT3KZ	0P873ZZ	0P904ZX	0P980ZX	0P9H3ZX	0P9Q4ZX	0PBL0ZZ	0PC43ZZ
0NTH0ZZ	0NU707Z	0NUK37Z	0NUT47Z	0P874ZZ	0P904ZZ	0P980ZZ	0P9H3ZZ	0P9Q4ZZ	0PBL3ZX	0PC44ZZ
0NTJ0ZZ	0NU70JZ	0NUK3JZ	0NUT4JZ	0P880ZZ	0P9100Z	0P9830Z	0P9H40Z	0P9R00Z	0PBL3ZZ	0PC50ZZ
0NTK0ZZ	0NU70KZ	0NUK3KZ	0NUT4KZ	0P883ZZ	0P910ZX	0P983ZX	0P9H4ZX	0P9R0ZX	0PBL4ZX	0PC53ZZ
0NTL0ZZ	0NU737Z	0NUK47Z	0NUV07Z	0P884ZZ	0P910ZZ	0P983ZZ	0P9H4ZZ	0P9R0ZZ	0PBL4ZZ	0PC54ZZ
0NTM0ZZ	0NU73JZ	0NUK4JZ	0NUV0JZ	0P890ZZ	0P9130Z	0P9840Z	0P9J00Z	0P9R30Z	0PBM0ZX	0PC60ZZ
0NTN0ZZ	0NU73KZ	0NUK4KZ	0NUV0KZ	0P893ZZ	0P913ZX	0P984ZX	0P9J0ZX	0P9R3ZX	0PBM0ZZ	0PC63ZZ
0NTP0ZZ	0NU747Z	0NUL07Z	0NUV37Z	0P894ZZ	0P913ZZ	0P984ZZ	0P9J0ZZ	0P9R3ZZ	0PBM3ZX	0PC64ZZ
0NTQ0ZZ	0NU74JZ	0NUL0JZ	0NW0X0Z	0P8B0ZZ	0P9140Z	0P9900Z	0P9J30Z	0P9R40Z	0PBM3ZZ	0PC70ZZ
0NTR0ZZ	0NU74KZ	0NUL0KZ	0NW0X4Z	0P8B3ZZ	0P914ZX	0P990ZX	0P9J3ZX	0P9R4ZX	0PBM4ZX	0PC73ZZ
0NTT0ZZ	0NUB07Z	0NUL37Z	0NW0X5Z	0P8B4ZZ	0P914ZZ	0P990ZZ	0P9J3ZZ	0P9R4ZZ	0PBM4ZZ	0PC74ZZ
0NTV0ZZ	0NUB0JZ	0NUL3JZ	0NW0X7Z	0P8C0ZZ	0P9200Z	0P9930Z	0P9J40Z	0P9S00Z	0PBN0ZX	0PC80ZZ
0NTX0ZZ	0NUB0KZ	0NUL3KZ	0NW0XJZ	0P8C3ZZ	0P920ZX	0P993ZX	0P9J4ZX	0P9S0ZX	0PBN0ZZ	0PC83ZZ
0NU007Z	0NUB37Z	0NUL47Z	0NW0XKZ	0P8C4ZZ	0P920ZZ	0P993ZZ	0P9J4ZZ	0P9S0ZZ	0PBN3ZX	0PC84ZZ
0NU00JZ	0NUB3JZ	0NUL4JZ	0NW0XMZ	0P8D0ZZ	0P9230Z	0P9940Z	0P9K00Z	0P9S30Z	0PBN3ZZ	0PC90ZZ
0NU00KZ	0NUB3KZ	0NUL4KZ	0NW0XSZ	0P8D3ZZ	0P923ZX	0P994ZX	0P9K0ZX	0P9S3ZZ	0PBN4ZX	0PC93ZZ
0NU037Z	0NUB47Z	0NUM07Z	0NWB00Z	0P8D4ZZ	0P923ZZ	0P994ZZ	0P9K0ZZ	0P9S3ZZ	0PBN4ZZ	0PC94ZZ
0NU03JZ	0NUB4JZ	0NUM0JZ	0NWB04Z	0P8F0ZZ	0P9240Z	0P9B00Z	0P9K30Z	0P9S40Z	0PBP0ZX	0PCB0ZZ
0NU03KZ	0NUB4KZ	0NUM0KZ	0NWB07Z	0P8F3ZZ	0P924ZX	0P9B0ZX	0P9K3ZX	0P9S4ZX	0PBP0ZZ	0PCB3ZZ
0NU047Z	0NUC07Z	0NUM37Z	0NWB0JZ	0P8F4ZZ	0P924ZZ	0P9B0ZZ	0P9K3ZZ	0P9S4ZZ	0PBP3ZX	0PCB4ZZ
0NU04JZ	0NUC0JZ	0NUM3JZ	0NWB0KZ	0P8G0ZZ	0P9300Z	0P9B30Z	0P9K40Z	0P9T00Z	0PBP3ZZ	0PCC0ZZ
0NU04KZ	0NUC0KZ	0NUM3KZ	0NWB0MZ	0P8G3ZZ	0P930ZX	0P9B3ZX	0P9K4ZX	0P9T0ZX	0PBP4ZX	0PCC3ZZ
0NU107Z	0NUC37Z	0NUM47Z	0NWB30Z	0P8G4ZZ	0P930ZZ	0P9B3ZZ	0P9K4ZZ	0P9T0ZZ	0PBP4ZZ	0PCC4ZZ
0NU10JZ	0NUC3JZ	0NUM4JZ	0NWB34Z	0P8H0ZZ	0P9330Z	0P9B40Z	0P9L00Z	0P9T30Z	0PBQ0ZX	0PCD0ZZ
0NU10KZ	0NUC3KZ	0NUM4KZ	0NWB37Z	0P8H3ZZ	0P933ZX	0P9B4ZX	0P9L0ZX	0P9T3ZX	0PBQ0ZZ	0PCD3ZZ
0NU137Z	0NUC47Z	0NUN07Z	0NWB3JZ	0P8H4ZZ	0P933ZZ	0P9B4ZZ	0P9L0ZZ	0P9T3ZZ	0PBQ3ZX	0PCD4ZZ
0NU13JZ	0NUC4JZ	0NUN0JZ	0NWB3KZ	0P8J0ZZ	0P9340Z	0P9C00Z	0P9L30Z	0P9T40Z	0PBQ3ZZ	0PCF0ZZ

0PCF3ZZ	0PDT0ZZ	0PHF48Z	0PN14ZZ	0PNR4ZZ	0PP434Z	0PP937Z	0PPF45Z	0PPV04Z	0PQB3ZZ	0PQVXZZ
0PCF4ZZ	0PDV0ZZ	0PHG08Z	0PN20ZZ	0PNS0ZZ	0PP437Z	0PP93KZ	0PPF47Z	0PPV05Z	0PQB4ZZ	0PR007Z
0PCG0ZZ	0PH000Z	0PHG38Z	0PN23ZZ	0PNS3ZZ	0PP43JZ	0PP93KZ	0PPF4JZ	0PPV07Z	0PQBXZZ	0PR00JZ
0PCG3ZZ	0PH004Z	0PHG48Z	0PN24ZZ	0PNS4ZZ	0PP43KZ	0PP944Z	0PPF4KZ	0PPV0JZ	0PQC0ZZ	0PR00KZ
0PCG4ZZ	0PH030Z	0PHH08Z	0PN30ZZ	0PNT0ZZ	0PP444Z	0PP947Z	0PPFX4Z	0PPV0KZ	0PQC3ZZ	0PR037Z
0PCH0ZZ	0PH034Z	0PHH38Z	0PN33ZZ	0PNT3ZZ	0PP447Z	0PP94JZ	0PPFX5Z	0PPV34Z	0PQC4ZZ	0PR03JZ
0PCH3ZZ	0PH040Z	0PHH48Z	0PN34ZZ	0PNT4ZZ	0PP44JZ	0PP94KZ	0PPG04Z	0PPV35Z	0PQCXZZ	0PR03KZ
0PCH4ZZ	0PH044Z	0PHJ08Z	0PN40ZZ	0PNV0ZZ	0PP44KZ	0PP9X4Z	0PPG05Z	0PPV37Z	0PQD0ZZ	0PR047Z
0PCJ0ZZ	0PH104Z	0PHJ38Z	0PN43ZZ	0PNV3ZZ	0PP4X4Z	0PPB04Z	0PPG07Z	0PPV3JZ	0PQD3ZZ	0PR04JZ
0PCJ3ZZ	0PH134Z	0PHJ48Z	0PN44ZZ	0PNV4ZZ	0PP504Z	0PPB07Z	0PPG0JZ	0PPV3KZ	0PQD4ZZ	0PR04KZ
0PCJ4ZZ	0PH144Z	0PHK08Z	0PN50ZZ	0PP004Z	0PP507Z	0PPB0JZ	0PPG0KZ	0PPV44Z	0PQDXZZ	0PR107Z
0PCK0ZZ	0PH204Z	0PHK38Z	0PN53ZZ	0PP007Z	0PP50JZ	0PPB0KZ	0PPG34Z	0PPV45Z	0PQF0ZZ	0PR10JZ
0PCK3ZZ	0PH234Z	0PHK48Z	0PN54ZZ	0PP00JZ	0PP50KZ	0PPB34Z	0PPG35Z	0PPV47Z	0PQF3ZZ	0PR10KZ
0PCK4ZZ	0PH244Z	0PHL08Z	0PN60ZZ	0PP00KZ	0PP534Z	0PPB37Z	0PPG37Z	0PPV4JZ	0PQF4ZZ	0PR137Z
0PCL0ZZ	0PH304Z	0PHL38Z	0PN63ZZ	0PP034Z	0PP537Z	0PPB3JZ	0PPG3JZ	0PPV4KZ	0PQFXZZ	0PR13JZ
0PCL3ZZ	0PH334Z	0PHL48Z	0PN64ZZ	0PP037Z	0PP53JZ	0PPB3KZ	0PPG3KZ	0PPVX4Z	0PQG0ZZ	0PR13KZ
0PCL4ZZ	0PH344Z	0PHN44Z	0PN70ZZ	0PP03JZ	0PP53KZ	0PPB44Z	0PPG44Z	0PPVX5Z	0PQG3ZZ	0PR147Z
0PCM0ZZ	0PH404Z	0PHN45Z	0PN73ZZ	0PP03KZ	0PP544Z	0PPB47Z	0PPG45Z	0PPY00Z	0PQG4ZZ	0PR14JZ
0PCM3ZZ	0PH434Z	0PHP04Z	0PN74ZZ	0PP044Z	0PP547Z	0PPB4JZ	0PPG47Z	0PPY0MZ	0PQGXZZ	0PR14KZ
0PCM4ZZ	0PH444Z	0PHP05Z	0PN80ZZ	0PP047Z	0PP54JZ	0PPB4KZ	0PPG4JZ	0PPY30Z	0PQH0ZZ	0PR207Z
0PCN0ZZ	0PH504Z	0PHP34Z	0PN83ZZ	0PP04JZ	0PP54KZ	0PPBX4Z	0PPG4KZ	0PPY3MZ	0PQH3ZZ	0PR20JZ
0PCN3ZZ	0PH534Z	0PHP35Z	0PN84ZZ	0PP04KZ	0PP5X4Z	0PPC04Z	0PPGX4Z	0PPY40Z	0PQH4ZZ	0PR20KZ
0PCN4ZZ	0PH544Z	0PHP44Z	0PN90ZZ	0PP0X4Z	0PP604Z	0PPC05Z	0PPGX5Z	0PPY4MZ	0PQHXZZ	0PR237Z
0PCP0ZZ	0PH604Z	0PHP45Z	0PN93ZZ	0PP104Z	0PP607Z	0PPC07Z	0PPH04Z	0PPYX0Z	0PQJ0ZZ	0PR23JZ
0PCP3ZZ	0PH634Z	0PHQ04Z	0PN94ZZ	0PP107Z	0PP60JZ	0PPC0JZ	0PPH05Z	0PPYXMZ	0PQJ3ZZ	0PR23KZ
0PCP4ZZ	0PH644Z	0PHQ05Z	0PNB0ZZ	0PP10JZ	0PP60KZ	0PPC0KZ	0PPH07Z	0PQ00ZZ	0PQJ4ZZ	0PR247Z
0PCQ0ZZ	0PH704Z	0PHQ34Z	0PNB3ZZ	0PP10KZ	0PP634Z	0PPC34Z	0PPH0JZ	0PQ03ZZ	0PQJXZZ	0PR24JZ
0PCQ3ZZ	0PH734Z	0PHQ35Z	0PNB4ZZ	0PP134Z	0PP637Z	0PPC35Z	0PPH0KZ	0PQ04ZZ	0PQK0ZZ	0PR24KZ
0PCQ4ZZ	0PH744Z	0PHQ44Z	0PNC0ZZ	0PP137Z	0PP63JZ	0PPC37Z	0PPH34Z	0PQ0XZZ	0PQK3ZZ	0PR307Z
0PCR0ZZ	0PH804Z	0PHQ45Z	0PNC3ZZ	0PP13JZ	0PP63KZ	0PPC3JZ	0PPH35Z	0PQ10ZZ	0PQK4ZZ	0PR30JZ
0PCR3ZZ	0PH834Z	0PHR04Z	0PNC4ZZ	0PP13KZ	0PP644Z	0PPC3KZ	0PPHX4Z	0PQ13ZZ	0PQKXZZ	0PR30KZ
0PCR4ZZ	0PH844Z	0PHR05Z	0PND0ZZ	0PP144Z	0PP647Z	0PPC44Z	0PPHX5Z	0PQ14ZZ	0PQL0ZZ	0PR337Z
0PCS0ZZ	0PH904Z	0PHR34Z	0PND3ZZ	0PP147Z	0PP64JZ	0PPC45Z	0PPJX4Z	0PQ1XZZ	0PQL3ZZ	0PR33JZ
0PCS3ZZ	0PH934Z	0PHR35Z	0PND4ZZ	0PP14JZ	0PP64KZ	0PPC47Z	0PPJX5Z	0PQ20ZZ	0PQL4ZZ	0PR33KZ
0PCS4ZZ	0PH944Z	0PHR44Z	0PNF0ZZ	0PP14KZ	0PP6X4Z	0PPC4JZ	0PPKX4Z	0PQ23ZZ	0PQLXZZ	0PR347Z
0PCT0ZZ	0PHB04Z	0PHR45Z	0PNF3ZZ	0PP1X4Z	0PP704Z	0PPC4KZ	0PPKX5Z	0PQ24ZZ	0PQM0ZZ	0PR34JZ
0PCT3ZZ	0PHB34Z	0PHS04Z	0PNF4ZZ	0PP204Z	0PP707Z	0PPCX4Z	0PPLX4Z	0PQ2XZZ	0PQM3ZZ	0PR34KZ
0PCT4ZZ	0PHB44Z	0PHS05Z	0PNG0ZZ	0PP207Z	0PP70JZ	0PPCX5Z	0PPLX5Z	0PQ30ZZ	0PQM4ZZ	0PR407Z
0PCV0ZZ	0PHC04Z	0PHS34Z	0PNG3ZZ	0PP20JZ	0PP70KZ	0PPD04Z	0PPMX4Z	0PQ33ZZ	0PQMXZZ	0PR40JZ
0PCV3ZZ	0PHC05Z	0PHS35Z	0PNG4ZZ	0PP20KZ	0PP734Z	0PPD05Z	0PPMX5Z	0PQ34ZZ	0PQN0ZZ	0PR40KZ
0PCV4ZZ	0PHC06Z	0PHS44Z	0PNH0ZZ	0PP234Z	0PP737Z	0PPD07Z	0PPNX4Z	0PQ3XZZ	0PQN3ZZ	0PR437Z
0PD00ZZ	0PHC08Z	0PHS45Z	0PNH3ZZ	0PP237Z	0PP73JZ	0PPD0JZ	0PPNX5Z	0PQ40ZZ	0PQN4ZZ	0PR43JZ
0PD10ZZ	0PHC0BZ	0PHT04Z	0PNH4ZZ	0PP23JZ	0PP73KZ	0PPD0KZ	0PPPX4Z	0PQ43ZZ	0PQNXZZ	0PR43KZ
0PD20ZZ	0PHC0CZ	0PHT05Z	0PNJ0ZZ	0PP23KZ	0PP744Z	0PPD34Z	0PPPX5Z	0PQ44ZZ	0PQP0ZZ	0PR447Z
0PD30ZZ	0PHC0DZ	0PHT34Z	0PNJ3ZZ	0PP244Z	0PP747Z	0PPD35Z	0PPQX4Z	0PQ4XZZ	0PQP3ZZ	0PR44JZ
0PD40ZZ	0PHC34Z	0PHT35Z	0PNJ4ZZ	0PP247Z	0PP74JZ	0PPD37Z	0PPQX5Z	0PQ50ZZ	0PQP4ZZ	0PR44KZ
0PD50ZZ	0PHC35Z	0PHT44Z	0PNK0ZZ	0PP24JZ	0PP74KZ	0PPD3JZ	0PPRX4Z	0PQ53ZZ	0PQPXZZ	0PR507Z
0PD60ZZ	0PHC36Z	0PHT45Z	0PNK3ZZ	0PP24KZ	0PP7X4Z	0PPD3KZ	0PPRX5Z	0PQ54ZZ	0PQQ0ZZ	0PR50JZ
0PD70ZZ	0PHC38Z	0PHV04Z	0PNK4ZZ	0PP2X4Z	0PP804Z	0PPD44Z	0PPSX4Z	0PQ5XZZ	0PQQ3ZZ	0PR50KZ
0PD80ZZ	0PHC3BZ	0PHV05Z	0PNL0ZZ	0PP304Z	0PP807Z	0PPD45Z	0PPSX5Z	0PQ60ZZ	0PQQ4ZZ	0PR537Z
0PD90ZZ	0PHC3CZ	0PHV34Z	0PNL3ZZ	0PP307Z	0PP80JZ	0PPD47Z	0PPT05Z	0PQ63ZZ	0PQQXZZ	0PR53JZ
0PDB0ZZ	0PHC3DZ	0PHV35Z	0PNL4ZZ	0PP30JZ	0PP80KZ	0PPD4JZ	0PPT07Z	0PQ64ZZ	0PQR0ZZ	0PR53KZ
0PDC0ZZ	0PHC44Z	0PHV44Z	0PNM0ZZ	0PP30KZ	0PP834Z	0PPD4KZ	0PPT0JZ	0PQ6XZZ	0PQR3ZZ	0PR547Z
0PDD0ZZ	0PHC45Z	0PHV45Z	0PNM3ZZ	0PP334Z	0PP837Z	0PPDX4Z	0PPT0KZ	0PQ70ZZ	0PQR4ZZ	0PR54JZ
0PDF0ZZ	0PHC46Z	0PHY0MZ	0PNM4ZZ	0PP337Z	0PP83JZ	0PPDX5Z	0PPT34Z	0PQ73ZZ	0PQRXZZ	0PR54KZ
0PDG0ZZ	0PHC48Z	0PHY3MZ	0PNN0ZZ	0PP33JZ	0PP83KZ	0PPF04Z	0PPT35Z	0PQ74ZZ	0PQS0ZZ	0PR607Z
0PDH0ZZ	0PHC4BZ	0PHY4MZ	0PNN3ZZ	0PP33KZ	0PP844Z	0PPF05Z	0PPT37Z	0PQ7XZZ	0PQS3ZZ	0PR60JZ
0PDJ0ZZ	0PHC4CZ	0PJY0ZZ	0PNN4ZZ	0PP344Z	0PP847Z	0PPF07Z	0PPT3JZ	0PQ80ZZ	0PQS4ZZ	0PR60KZ
0PDK0ZZ	0PHC4DZ	0PJY3ZZ	0PNP0ZZ	0PP347Z	0PP84JZ	0PPF0JZ	0PPT3KZ	0PQ83ZZ	0PQSXZZ	0PR637Z
0PDL0ZZ	0PHD04Z	0PJY4ZZ	0PNP3ZZ	0PP34JZ	0PP84KZ	0PPF0KZ	0PPT44Z	0PQ84ZZ	0PQT0ZZ	0PR63JZ
0PDM0ZZ	0PHD05Z	0PJYXZZ	0PNP4ZZ	0PP34KZ	0PP8X4Z	0PPF34Z	0PPT45Z	0PQ8XZZ	0PQT3ZZ	0PR63KZ
0PDN0ZZ	0PHD08Z	0PN00ZZ	0PNQ0ZZ	0PP3X4Z	0PP904Z	0PPF35Z	0PPT47Z	0PQ90ZZ	0PQT4ZZ	0PR647Z
0PDP0ZZ	0PHD38Z	0PN03ZZ	0PNQ3ZZ	0PP404Z	0PP907Z	0PPF37Z	0PPT4JZ	0PQ93ZZ	0PQTXZZ	0PR64JZ
0PDQ0ZZ	0PHD48Z	0PN04ZZ	0PNQ4ZZ	0PP407Z	0PP90JZ	0PPF3JZ	0PPT4KZ	0PQ94ZZ	0PQV0ZZ	0PR64KZ
0PDR0ZZ	0PHF08Z	0PN10ZZ	0PNR0ZZ	0PP40JZ	0PP90KZ	0PPF3KZ	0PPTX4Z	0PQ9XZZ	0PQV3ZZ	0PR707Z
0PDS0ZZ	0PHF38Z	0PN13ZZ	0PNR3ZZ	0PP40KZ	0PP934Z	0PPF44Z	0PPTX5Z	0PQB0ZZ	0PQV4ZZ	0PR70JZ

0PR70KZ	0PRG3KZ	0PRP4KZ	0PSG0DZ	0PSK0DZ	0PSP45Z	0PTH0ZZ	0PU607Z	0PW23KZ	0PW647Z	0PWB4KZ
0PR737Z	0PRG47Z	0PS03ZZ	0PSG0ZZ	0PSK0ZZ	0PSP4ZZ	0PTJ0ZZ	0PU60JZ	0PW244Z	0PW64JZ	0PWBX4Z
0PR73JZ	0PRG4JZ	0PS04ZZ	0PSG34Z	0PSK34Z	0PSPXZZ	0PTK0ZZ	0PU60KZ	0PW247Z	0PW64KZ	0PWBX7Z
0PR73KZ	0PRG4KZ	0PS0XZZ	0PSG35Z	0PSK35Z	0PSQ04Z	0PTL0ZZ	0PU637Z	0PW24JZ	0PW6X4Z	0PWBXJZ
0PR747Z	0PRH07Z	0PS13ZZ	0PSG36Z	0PSK36Z	0PSQ05Z	0PTM0ZZ	0PU63JZ	0PW24KZ	0PW6X7Z	0PWBXKZ
0PR74JZ	0PRH0JZ	0PS14ZZ	0PSG3BZ	0PSK3BZ	0PSQ0ZZ	0PTN0ZZ	0PU63KZ	0PW2X4Z	0PW6XJZ	0PWC04Z
0PR74KZ	0PRH0KZ	0PS1XZZ	0PSG3CZ	0PSK3CZ	0PSQ34Z	0PTP0ZZ	0PU647Z	0PW2X7Z	0PW6XKZ	0PWC05Z
0PR807Z	0PRH37Z	0PS23ZZ	0PSG3DZ	0PSK3DZ	0PSQ35Z	0PTQ0ZZ	0PU64JZ	0PW2XJZ	0PW704Z	0PWC07Z
0PR80JZ	0PRH3JZ	0PS24ZZ	0PSG3ZZ	0PSK3ZZ	0PSQ3ZZ	0PTR0ZZ	0PU64KZ	0PW2XKZ	0PW707Z	0PWC0JZ
0PR80KZ	0PRH3KZ	0PS2XZZ	0PSG44Z	0PSK44Z	0PSQ44Z	0PTS0ZZ	0PU707Z	0PW304Z	0PW70JZ	0PWC0KZ
0PR837Z	0PRH47Z	0PS53ZZ	0PSG45Z	0PSK45Z	0PSQ45Z	0PTT0ZZ	0PU70JZ	0PW307Z	0PW70KZ	0PWC34Z
0PR83JZ	0PRH4JZ	0PS54ZZ	0PSG46Z	0PSK46Z	0PSQ4ZZ	0PTV0ZZ	0PU70KZ	0PW30JZ	0PW734Z	0PWC35Z
0PR83KZ	0PRH4KZ	0PS5XZZ	0PSG4BZ	0PSK4BZ	0PSQXZZ	0PU007Z	0PU737Z	0PW30KZ	0PW737Z	0PWC37Z
0PR847Z	0PRJ07Z	0PS63ZZ	0PSG4CZ	0PSK4CZ	0PSR04Z	0PU00JZ	0PU73JZ	0PW334Z	0PW73JZ	0PWC3JZ
0PR84JZ	0PRJ0JZ	0PS64ZZ	0PSG4DZ	0PSK4DZ	0PSR05Z	0PU00KZ	0PU73KZ	0PW337Z	0PW73KZ	0PWC3KZ
0PR84KZ	0PRJ0KZ	0PS6XZZ	0PSG4ZZ	0PSK4ZZ	0PSR0ZZ	0PU037Z	0PU747Z	0PW33JZ	0PW744Z	0PWC44Z
0PR907Z	0PRJ37Z	0PS73ZZ	0PSGXZZ	0PSKXZZ	0PSR34Z	0PU03JZ	0PU74JZ	0PW33KZ	0PW747Z	0PWC45Z
0PR90JZ	0PRJ3JZ	0PS74ZZ	0PSH04Z	0PSL04Z	0PSR35Z	0PU03KZ	0PU74KZ	0PW344Z	0PW74JZ	0PWC47Z
0PR90KZ	0PRJ3KZ	0PS7XZZ	0PSH05Z	0PSL05Z	0PSR3ZZ	0PU047Z	0PU807Z	0PW347Z	0PW74KZ	0PWC4JZ
0PR937Z	0PRJ47Z	0PS83ZZ	0PSH06Z	0PSL06Z	0PSR44Z	0PU04JZ	0PU80JZ	0PW34JZ	0PW7X4Z	0PWC4KZ
0PR93JZ	0PRJ4JZ	0PS84ZZ	0PSH0BZ	0PSL0BZ	0PSR45Z	0PU04KZ	0PU80KZ	0PW34KZ	0PW7X7Z	0PWCX4Z
0PR93KZ	0PRJ4KZ	0PS8XZZ	0PSH0CZ	0PSL0CZ	0PSR4ZZ	0PU107Z	0PU837Z	0PW3X4Z	0PW7XJZ	0PWCX5Z
0PR947Z	0PRK07Z	0PS93ZZ	0PSH0DZ	0PSL0DZ	0PSRXZZ	0PU10JZ	0PU83JZ	0PW3X7Z	0PW7XKZ	0PWCX7Z
0PR94JZ	0PRK0JZ	0PS94ZZ	0PSH0ZZ	0PSL0ZZ	0PSS04Z	0PU10KZ	0PU83KZ	0PW3XJZ	0PW804Z	0PWCXJZ
0PR94KZ	0PRK0KZ	0PS9XZZ	0PSH34Z	0PSL34Z	0PSS05Z	0PU137Z	0PU847Z	0PW3XKZ	0PW807Z	0PWCXKZ
0PRB07Z	0PRK37Z	0PSB3ZZ	0PSH35Z	0PSL35Z	0PSS0ZZ	0PU13JZ	0PU84JZ	0PW404Z	0PW80JZ	0PWD04Z
0PRB0JZ	0PRK3JZ	0PSB4ZZ	0PSH36Z	0PSL36Z	0PSS34Z	0PU13KZ	0PU84KZ	0PW407Z	0PW80KZ	0PWD05Z
0PRB0KZ	0PRK3KZ	0PSBXZZ	0PSH3BZ	0PSL3BZ	0PSS35Z	0PU147Z	0PU907Z	0PW40JZ	0PW834Z	0PWD07Z
0PRB37Z	0PRK47Z	0PSC3ZZ	0PSH3CZ	0PSL3CZ	0PSS3ZZ	0PU14JZ	0PU90JZ	0PW40KZ	0PW837Z	0PWD0JZ
0PRB3JZ	0PRK4JZ	0PSC4ZZ	0PSH3DZ	0PSL3DZ	0PSS44Z	0PU14KZ	0PU90KZ	0PW434Z	0PW83JZ	0PWD0KZ
0PRB3KZ	0PRK4KZ	0PSCXZZ	0PSH3ZZ	0PSL3ZZ	0PSS45Z	0PU207Z	0PU937Z	0PW437Z	0PW83KZ	0PWD34Z
0PRB47Z	0PRL07Z	0PSD3ZZ	0PSH44Z	0PSL44Z	0PSS4ZZ	0PU20JZ	0PU93JZ	0PW43JZ	0PW844Z	0PWD35Z
0PRB4JZ	0PRL0JZ	0PSD45Z	0PSH45Z	0PSL45Z	0PSSXZZ	0PU20KZ	0PU93KZ	0PW43KZ	0PW847Z	0PWD37Z
0PRB4KZ	0PRL0KZ	0PSD46Z	0PSH46Z	0PSL46Z	0PST04Z	0PU237Z	0PU947Z	0PW444Z	0PW84JZ	0PWD3JZ
0PRC07Z	0PRL37Z	0PSD4BZ	0PSH4BZ	0PSL4BZ	0PST05Z	0PU23JZ	0PU94JZ	0PW447Z	0PW84KZ	0PWD3KZ
0PRC0JZ	0PRL3JZ	0PSD4CZ	0PSH4CZ	0PSL4CZ	0PST0ZZ	0PU23KZ	0PU94KZ	0PW44JZ	0PW8X4Z	0PWD44Z
0PRC0KZ	0PRL3KZ	0PSD4DZ	0PSH4DZ	0PSL4DZ	0PST34Z	0PU247Z	0PUB07Z	0PW44KZ	0PW8X7Z	0PWD45Z
0PRC37Z	0PRL47Z	0PSD4ZZ	0PSH4ZZ	0PSL4ZZ	0PST35Z	0PU24JZ	0PUB0JZ	0PW4X4Z	0PW8XJZ	0PWD47Z
0PRC3JZ	0PRL4JZ	0PSDXZZ	0PSHXZZ	0PSLXZZ	0PST3ZZ	0PU24KZ	0PUB0KZ	0PW4X7Z	0PW8XKZ	0PWD4JZ
0PRC3KZ	0PRL4KZ	0PSF04Z	0PSJ04Z	0PSM04Z	0PST44Z	0PU307Z	0PUB37Z	0PW4XJZ	0PW904Z	0PWD4KZ
0PRC47Z	0PRM07Z	0PSF05Z	0PSJ05Z	0PSM05Z	0PST45Z	0PU30JZ	0PUB3JZ	0PW4XKZ	0PW907Z	0PWDX4Z
0PRC4JZ	0PRM0JZ	0PSF06Z	0PSJ06Z	0PSM0ZZ	0PST4ZZ	0PU30KZ	0PUB3KZ	0PW504Z	0PW90JZ	0PWDX5Z
0PRC4KZ	0PRM0KZ	0PSF0BZ	0PSJ0BZ	0PSM34Z	0PSTXZZ	0PU337Z	0PUB47Z	0PW507Z	0PW90KZ	0PWDX7Z
0PRD07Z	0PRM37Z	0PSF0CZ	0PSJ0CZ	0PSM35Z	0PSV04Z	0PU33JZ	0PUB4JZ	0PW50JZ	0PW934Z	0PWDXJZ
0PRD0JZ	0PRM3JZ	0PSF0DZ	0PSJ0DZ	0PSM3ZZ	0PSV05Z	0PU33KZ	0PUB4KZ	0PW50KZ	0PW937Z	0PWDXKZ
0PRD0KZ	0PRM3KZ	0PSF0ZZ	0PSJ0ZZ	0PSM44Z	0PSV0ZZ	0PU347Z	0PUC07Z	0PW534Z	0PW93JZ	0PWF04Z
0PRD37Z	0PRM47Z	0PSF34Z	0PSJ34Z	0PSM45Z	0PSV34Z	0PU34JZ	0PW0X4Z	0PW537Z	0PW93KZ	0PWF05Z
0PRD3JZ	0PRM4JZ	0PSF35Z	0PSJ35Z	0PSM4ZZ	0PSV35Z	0PU34KZ	0PW0X7Z	0PW53JZ	0PW944Z	0PWF07Z
0PRD3KZ	0PRM4KZ	0PSF36Z	0PSJ36Z	0PSMXZZ	0PSV3ZZ	0PU407Z	0PW0XJZ	0PW53KZ	0PW947Z	0PWF0JZ
0PRD47Z	0PRN07Z	0PSF3BZ	0PSJ3BZ	0PSN04Z	0PSV44Z	0PU40JZ	0PW0XKZ	0PW544Z	0PW94JZ	0PWF0KZ
0PRD4JZ	0PRN0JZ	0PSF3CZ	0PSJ3CZ	0PSN05Z	0PSV45Z	0PU40KZ	0PW13KZ	0PW547Z	0PW94KZ	0PWF34Z
0PRD4KZ	0PRN0KZ	0PSF3DZ	0PSJ3DZ	0PSN0ZZ	0PSV4ZZ	0PU437Z	0PW144Z	0PW54JZ	0PW9X4Z	0PWF35Z
0PRF07Z	0PRN37Z	0PSF3ZZ	0PSJ3ZZ	0PSN34Z	0PSVXZZ	0PU43JZ	0PW147Z	0PW54KZ	0PW9X7Z	0PWF37Z
0PRF0JZ	0PRN3JZ	0PSF44Z	0PSJ44Z	0PSN35Z	0PT00ZZ	0PU43KZ	0PW14JZ	0PW5X4Z	0PW9XJZ	0PWF3JZ
0PRF0KZ	0PRN3KZ	0PSF45Z	0PSJ45Z	0PSN3ZZ	0PT10ZZ	0PU447Z	0PW14KZ	0PW5X7Z	0PW9XKZ	0PWF3KZ
0PRF37Z	0PRN47Z	0PSF46Z	0PSJ46Z	0PSN44Z	0PT20ZZ	0PU44JZ	0PW1X4Z	0PW5XJZ	0PWB04Z	0PWF44Z
0PRF3JZ	0PRN4JZ	0PSF4BZ	0PSJ4BZ	0PSN45Z	0PT50ZZ	0PU44KZ	0PW1X7Z	0PW5XKZ	0PWB07Z	0PWF45Z
0PRF3KZ	0PRN4KZ	0PSF4CZ	0PSJ4CZ	0PSN4ZZ	0PT60ZZ	0PU507Z	0PW1XJZ	0PW604Z	0PWB0JZ	0PWF47Z
0PRF47Z	0PRP07Z	0PSF4DZ	0PSJ4DZ	0PSNXZZ	0PT70ZZ	0PU50JZ	0PW1XKZ	0PW607Z	0PWB0KZ	0PWF4JZ
0PRF4JZ	0PRP0JZ	0PSF4ZZ	0PSJ4ZZ	0PSP04Z	0PT80ZZ	0PU50KZ	0PW204Z	0PW60JZ	0PWB34Z	0PWF4KZ
0PRF4KZ	0PRP0KZ	0PSFXZZ	0PSJXZZ	0PSP05Z	0PT90ZZ	0PU537Z	0PW207Z	0PW60KZ	0PWB37Z	0PWFX4Z
0PRG07Z	0PRP37Z	0PSG04Z	0PSK04Z	0PSP0ZZ	0PTB0ZZ	0PU53JZ	0PW20JZ	0PW634Z	0PWB3JZ	0PWFX5Z
0PRG0JZ	0PRP3JZ	0PSG05Z	0PSK05Z	0PSP34Z	0PTC0ZZ	0PU53KZ	0PW20KZ	0PW637Z	0PWB3KZ	0PWFX7Z
0PRG0KZ	0PRP3KZ	0PSG06Z	0PSK06Z	0PSP35Z	0PTD0ZZ	0PU547Z	0PW234Z	0PW63JZ	0PWB44Z	0PWFXJZ
0PRG37Z	0PRP47Z	0PSG0BZ	0PSK0BZ	0PSP3ZZ	0PTF0ZZ	0PU54JZ	0PW237Z	0PW63KZ	0PWB47Z	0PWFXKZ
0PRG3JZ	0PRP4JZ	0PSG0CZ	0PSK0CZ	0PSP44Z	0PTG0ZZ	0PU54KZ	0PW23JZ	0PW644Z	0PWB4JZ	0PWG04Z

0PWG05Z	0PWK37Z	0PWN4JZ	0PWRXKZ	0PWY4MZ	0Q5N3ZZ	0Q8K3ZZ	0Q9N0ZZ	0QB34ZZ	0QBG4ZZ	0QC14ZZ
0PWG07Z	0PWK3JZ	0PWN4KZ	0PWS04Z	0PWYX0Z	0Q5N4ZZ	0Q8K4ZZ	0Q9N30Z	0QB40ZX	0QBH0ZX	0QC20ZZ
0PWG0JZ	0PWK3KZ	0PWNX4Z	0PWS05Z	0PWYXMZ	0Q5P0ZZ	0Q8L0ZZ	0Q9N3ZX	0QB40ZZ	0QBH0ZZ	0QC23ZZ
0PWG0KZ	0PWK44Z	0PWNX5Z	0PWS07Z	0Q2YX0Z	0Q5P3ZZ	0Q8L3ZZ	0Q9N3ZZ	0QB43ZX	0QBH3ZX	0QC24ZZ
0PWG34Z	0PWK45Z	0PWNX7Z	0PWS0JZ	0Q2YXYZ	0Q5P4ZZ	0Q8L4ZZ	0Q9N40Z	0QB43ZZ	0QBH3ZZ	0QD00ZZ
0PWG35Z	0PWK47Z	0PWNXJZ	0PWS0KZ	0Q500ZZ	0Q5Q0ZZ	0Q8M0ZZ	0Q9N4ZX	0QB44ZX	0QBH4ZX	0QD10ZZ
0PWG37Z	0PWK4JZ	0PWNXKZ	0PWS34Z	0Q503ZZ	0Q5Q3ZZ	0Q8M3ZZ	0Q9N4ZZ	0QB44ZZ	0QBH4ZZ	0QD20ZZ
0PWG3JZ	0PWK4KZ	0PWP04Z	0PWS35Z	0Q504ZZ	0Q5Q4ZZ	0Q8M4ZZ	0Q9P00Z	0QB50ZX	0QBJ0ZX	0QD30ZZ
0PWG3KZ	0PWKX4Z	0PWP05Z	0PWS37Z	0Q510ZZ	0Q5R0ZZ	0Q8N0ZZ	0Q9P0ZX	0QB50ZZ	0QBJ0ZZ	0QD40ZZ
0PWG44Z	0PWKX5Z	0PWP07Z	0PWS3JZ	0Q513ZZ	0Q5R3ZZ	0Q9030Z	0Q9P0ZZ	0QB53ZX	0QBJ3ZX	0QD50ZZ
0PWG45Z	0PWKX7Z	0PWP0JZ	0PWS3KZ	0Q514ZZ	0Q5R4ZZ	0Q903ZZ	0Q9P30Z	0QB53ZZ	0QBJ3ZZ	0QD60ZZ
0PWG47Z	0PWKXJZ	0PWP0KZ	0PWS44Z	0Q520ZZ	0Q5S0ZZ	0Q9130Z	0Q9P3ZX	0QB54ZX	0QBJ4ZX	0QD70ZZ
0PWG4JZ	0PWKXKZ	0PWP34Z	0PWS45Z	0Q523ZZ	0Q5S3ZZ	0Q913ZZ	0Q9P3ZZ	0QB54ZZ	0QBJ4ZZ	0QD80ZZ
0PWG4KZ	0PWL04Z	0PWP35Z	0PWS47Z	0Q524ZZ	0Q5S4ZZ	0Q9230Z	0Q9P40Z	0QB60ZX	0QBK0ZX	0QD90ZZ
0PWGX4Z	0PWL05Z	0PWP37Z	0PWS4JZ	0Q530ZZ	0Q800ZZ	0Q923ZZ	0Q9P4ZX	0QB60ZZ	0QBK0ZZ	0QDB0ZZ
0PWGX5Z	0PWL07Z	0PWP3JZ	0PWS4KZ	0Q533ZZ	0Q803ZZ	0Q9330Z	0Q9P4ZZ	0QB63ZX	0QBK3ZX	0QDC0ZZ
0PWGX7Z	0PWL0JZ	0PWP3KZ	0PWSX4Z	0Q534ZZ	0Q804ZZ	0Q933ZZ	0Q9Q00Z	0QB63ZZ	0QBK3ZZ	0QDD0ZZ
0PWGXJZ	0PWL0KZ	0PWP44Z	0PWSX5Z	0Q540ZZ	0Q810ZZ	0Q9430Z	0Q9Q0ZX	0QB64ZX	0QBK4ZX	0QDF0ZZ
0PWGXKZ	0PWL34Z	0PWP45Z	0PWSX7Z	0Q543ZZ	0Q813ZZ	0Q943ZZ	0Q9Q0ZZ	0QB64ZZ	0QBK4ZZ	0QDG0ZZ
0PWH04Z	0PWL35Z	0PWP47Z	0PWSXJZ	0Q544ZZ	0Q814ZZ	0Q9530Z	0Q9Q30Z	0QB70ZX	0QBL0ZX	0QDH0ZZ
0PWH05Z	0PWL37Z	0PWP4JZ	0PWSXKZ	0Q550ZZ	0Q820ZZ	0Q953ZZ	0Q9Q3ZX	0QB70ZZ	0QBL0ZZ	0QDJ0ZZ
0PWH07Z	0PWL3JZ	0PWP4KZ	0PWT04Z	0Q553ZZ	0Q823ZZ	0Q9630Z	0Q9Q3ZZ	0QB73ZX	0QBL3ZX	0QDK0ZZ
0PWH0JZ	0PWL3KZ	0PWPX4Z	0PWT05Z	0Q554ZZ	0Q824ZZ	0Q963ZZ	0Q9Q40Z	0QB73ZZ	0QBL3ZZ	0QDL0ZZ
0PWH0KZ	0PWL44Z	0PWPX5Z	0PWT07Z	0Q560ZZ	0Q830ZZ	0Q9730Z	0Q9Q4ZX	0QB74ZX	0QBL4ZX	0QDM0ZZ
0PWH34Z	0PWL45Z	0PWPX7Z	0PWT0JZ	0Q563ZZ	0Q833ZZ	0Q973ZZ	0Q9Q4ZZ	0QB74ZZ	0QBL4ZZ	0QDN0ZZ
0PWH35Z	0PWL47Z	0PWPXJZ	0PWT0KZ	0Q564ZZ	0Q834ZZ	0Q9830Z	0Q9R00Z	0QB80ZX	0QBM0ZX	0QDP0ZZ
0PWH37Z	0PWL4JZ	0PWPXKZ	0PWT34Z	0Q570ZZ	0Q840ZZ	0Q983ZZ	0Q9R0ZX	0QB80ZZ	0QBM0ZZ	0QDQ0ZZ
0PWH3JZ	0PWL4KZ	0PWQ04Z	0PWT35Z	0Q573ZZ	0Q843ZZ	0Q9930Z	0Q9R0ZZ	0QB83ZX	0QBM3ZX	0QDR0ZZ
0PWH3KZ	0PWLX4Z	0PWQ05Z	0PWT37Z	0Q574ZZ	0Q844ZZ	0Q993ZZ	0Q9R30Z	0QB83ZZ	0QBM3ZZ	0QDS0ZZ
0PWH44Z	0PWLX5Z	0PWQ07Z	0PWT3JZ	0Q580ZZ	0Q850ZZ	0Q9B30Z	0Q9R3ZX	0QB84ZX	0QBM4ZX	0QH608Z
0PWH45Z	0PWLX7Z	0PWQ0JZ	0PWT3KZ	0Q583ZZ	0Q853ZZ	0Q9B3ZZ	0Q9R3ZZ	0QB84ZZ	0QBM4ZZ	0QH638Z
0PWH47Z	0PWLXJZ	0PWQ0KZ	0PWT44Z	0Q584ZZ	0Q854ZZ	0Q9C30Z	0Q9R40Z	0QB90ZX	0QBN0ZX	0QH648Z
0PWH4JZ	0PWLXKZ	0PWQ34Z	0PWT45Z	0Q590ZZ	0Q860ZZ	0Q9C3ZZ	0Q9R4ZX	0QB90ZZ	0QBN0ZZ	0QH708Z
0PWH4KZ	0PWM04Z	0PWQ35Z	0PWT47Z	0Q593ZZ	0Q863ZZ	0Q9D30Z	0Q9R4ZZ	0QB93ZX	0QBN3ZX	0QH738Z
0PWHX4Z	0PWM05Z	0PWQ37Z	0PWT4JZ	0Q594ZZ	0Q864ZZ	0Q9D3ZZ	0Q9S00Z	0QB93ZZ	0QBN3ZZ	0QH746Z
0PWHX5Z	0PWM07Z	0PWQ3JZ	0PWT4KZ	0Q5B0ZZ	0Q870ZZ	0Q9F30Z	0Q9S0ZX	0QB94ZX	0QBN4ZX	0QH748Z
0PWHX7Z	0PWM0JZ	0PWQ3KZ	0PWTX4Z	0Q5B3ZZ	0Q873ZZ	0Q9F3ZZ	0Q9S0ZZ	0QB94ZZ	0QBN4ZZ	0QH74BZ
0PWHXJZ	0PWM0KZ	0PWQ44Z	0PWTX5Z	0Q5B4ZZ	0Q874ZZ	0Q9G30Z	0Q9S30Z	0QBB0ZX	0QBP0ZX	0QH74CZ
0PWHXKZ	0PWM34Z	0PWQ45Z	0PWTX7Z	0Q5C0ZZ	0Q880ZZ	0Q9G3ZZ	0Q9S3ZX	0QBB0ZZ	0QBP0ZZ	0QH74DZ
0PWJ04Z	0PWM35Z	0PWQ47Z	0PWTXJZ	0Q5C3ZZ	0Q883ZZ	0Q9H30Z	0Q9S3ZZ	0QBB3ZX	0QBP3ZX	0QH804Z
0PWJ05Z	0PWM37Z	0PWQ4JZ	0PWTXKZ	0Q5C4ZZ	0Q884ZZ	0Q9H3ZZ	0Q9S40Z	0QBB3ZZ	0QBP3ZZ	0QH805Z
0PWJ07Z	0PWM3JZ	0PWQ4KZ	0PWV04Z	0Q5D0ZZ	0Q890ZZ	0Q9J30Z	0Q9S4ZX	0QBB4ZX	0QBP4ZX	0QH806Z
0PWJ0JZ	0PWM3KZ	0PWQX4Z	0PWV05Z	0Q5D3ZZ	0Q893ZZ	0Q9J3ZZ	0Q9S4ZZ	0QBB4ZZ	0QBP4ZZ	0QH808Z
0PWJ0KZ	0PWM44Z	0PWQX5Z	0PWV07Z	0Q5D4ZZ	0Q894ZZ	0Q9K30Z	0QB00ZX	0QBC0ZX	0QBQ0ZX	0QH80BZ
0PWJ34Z	0PWM45Z	0PWQX7Z	0PWV0JZ	0Q5F0ZZ	0Q8B0ZZ	0Q9K3ZZ	0QB00ZZ	0QBC0ZZ	0QBQ0ZZ	0QH80CZ
0PWJ35Z	0PWM47Z	0PWQXJZ	0PWV0KZ	0Q5F3ZZ	0Q8B3ZZ	0Q9K4ZZ	0QB03ZX	0QBC3ZX	0QBQ3ZX	0QH80DZ
0PWJ37Z	0PWM4JZ	0PWQXKZ	0PWV34Z	0Q5F4ZZ	0Q8B4ZZ	0Q9L00Z	0QB03ZZ	0QBC3ZZ	0QBQ3ZZ	0QH834Z
0PWJ3JZ	0PWM4KZ	0PWR04Z	0PWV35Z	0Q5G0ZZ	0Q8C0ZZ	0Q9L0ZX	0QB04ZX	0QBC4ZX	0QBQ4ZZ	0QH835Z
0PWJ3KZ	0PWMX4Z	0PWR05Z	0PWV37Z	0Q5G3ZZ	0Q8C3ZZ	0Q9L0ZZ	0QB04ZZ	0QBC4ZZ	0QBR0ZX	0QH836Z
0PWJ44Z	0PWMX5Z	0PWR07Z	0PWV3JZ	0Q5G4ZZ	0Q8C4ZZ	0Q9L30Z	0QB10ZX	0QBD0ZX	0QBR0ZZ	0QH838Z
0PWJ45Z	0PWMX7Z	0PWR0JZ	0PWV3KZ	0Q5H0ZZ	0Q8D0ZZ	0Q9L3ZX	0QB10ZZ	0QBD0ZZ	0QBR3ZX	0QH83BZ
0PWJ47Z	0PWMXJZ	0PWR0KZ	0PWV44Z	0Q5H3ZZ	0Q8D3ZZ	0Q9L3ZZ	0QB13ZX	0QBD3ZX	0QBR3ZZ	0QH83CZ
0PWJ4JZ	0PWMXKZ	0PWR34Z	0PWV45Z	0Q5H4ZZ	0Q8D4ZZ	0Q9L40Z	0QB13ZZ	0QBD3ZZ	0QBR4ZX	0QH83DZ
0PWJ4KZ	0PWN04Z	0PWR35Z	0PWV47Z	0Q5J0ZZ	0Q8F0ZZ	0Q9L4ZX	0QB14ZX	0QBD4ZX	0QBR4ZZ	0QH844Z
0PWJX4Z	0PWN05Z	0PWR37Z	0PWV4JZ	0Q5J3ZZ	0Q8F3ZZ	0Q9L4ZZ	0QB14ZZ	0QBD4ZZ	0QBS0ZX	0QH845Z
0PWJX5Z	0PWN07Z	0PWR3JZ	0PWV4KZ	0Q5J4ZZ	0Q8F4ZZ	0Q9M00Z	0QB20ZX	0QBF0ZX	0QBS0ZZ	0QH846Z
0PWJX7Z	0PWN0JZ	0PWR3KZ	0PWVX4Z	0Q5K0ZZ	0Q8G0ZZ	0Q9M0ZX	0QB20ZZ	0QBF0ZZ	0QBS3ZX	0QH848Z
0PWJXJZ	0PWN0KZ	0PWR44Z	0PWVX5Z	0Q5K3ZZ	0Q8G3ZZ	0Q9M0ZZ	0QB23ZX	0QBF3ZX	0QBS3ZZ	0QH84BZ
0PWJXKZ	0PWN34Z	0PWR45Z	0PWVX7Z	0Q5K4ZZ	0Q8G4ZZ	0Q9M30Z	0QB23ZZ	0QBF3ZZ	0QBS4ZX	0QH84CZ
0PWK04Z	0PWN35Z	0PWR47Z	0PWVXJZ	0Q5L0ZZ	0Q8H0ZZ	0Q9M3ZX	0QB24ZX	0QBF4ZX	0QBS4ZZ	0QH84DZ
0PWK05Z	0PWN37Z	0PWR4JZ	0PWVXKZ	0Q5L3ZZ	0Q8H3ZZ	0Q9M3ZZ	0QB24ZZ	0QBF4ZZ	0QC00ZZ	0QH904Z
0PWK07Z	0PWN3JZ	0PWR4KZ	0PWY00Z	0Q5L4ZZ	0Q8H4ZZ	0Q9M40Z	0QB30ZX	0QBG0ZX	0QC03ZZ	0QH905Z
0PWK0JZ	0PWN3KZ	0PWRX4Z	0PWY0MZ	0Q5M0ZZ	0Q8J0ZZ	0Q9M4ZX	0QB30ZZ	0QBG0ZZ	0QC04ZZ	0QH906Z
0PWK0KZ	0PWN44Z	0PWRX5Z	0PWY30Z	0Q5M3ZZ	0Q8J3ZZ	0Q9M4ZZ	0QB33ZX	0QBG3ZX	0QC10ZZ	0QH908Z
0PWK34Z	0PWN45Z	0PWRX7Z	0PWY3MZ	0Q5M4ZZ	0Q8J4ZZ	0Q9N00Z	0QB33ZZ	0QBG3ZZ	0QC13ZZ	0QH90BZ
0PWK35Z	0PWN47Z	0PWRXJZ	0PWY40Z	0Q5N0ZZ	0Q8K0ZZ	0Q9N0ZX	0QB34ZX	0QBG4ZX	0QC13ZZ	0QH90CZ

0QH90DZ	0QHF35Z	0QHK04Z	0QJY0ZZ	0QNN4ZZ	0QPF34Z	0QPK0JZ	0QPP05Z	0QPY3MZ	0QQH3ZZ	0QRM4JZ
0QH934Z	0QHF44Z	0QHK05Z	0QJY3ZZ	0QNP0ZZ	0QPF35Z	0QPK0KZ	0QPP07Z	0QPY40Z	0QQH4ZZ	0QRM4KZ
0QH935Z	0QHF45Z	0QHK06Z	0QJY4ZZ	0QNP3ZZ	0QPF37Z	0QPK34Z	0QPP0JZ	0QPY4MZ	0QQHXZZ	0QRN07Z
0QH936Z	0QHG04Z	0QHK08Z	0QJYXZZ	0QNP4ZZ	0QPF3JZ	0QPK35Z	0QPP0KZ	0QPYX0Z	0QQJ0ZZ	0QRN0JZ
0QH938Z	0QHG05Z	0QHK0BZ	0QN00ZZ	0QNQ0ZZ	0QPF3KZ	0QPK37Z	0QPP34Z	0QPYXMZ	0QQJ3ZZ	0QRN0KZ
0QH93BZ	0QHG06Z	0QHK0CZ	0QN03ZZ	0QNQ3ZZ	0QPF44Z	0QPK3JZ	0QPP35Z	0QQ00ZZ	0QQJ4ZZ	0QRN37Z
0QH93CZ	0QHG08Z	0QHK0DZ	0QN04ZZ	0QNQ4ZZ	0QPF45Z	0QPK3KZ	0QPP37Z	0QQ03ZZ	0QQJXZZ	0QRN3JZ
0QH93DZ	0QHG0BZ	0QHK34Z	0QN10ZZ	0QNR0ZZ	0QPF47Z	0QPK44Z	0QPP3JZ	0QQ04ZZ	0QQK0ZZ	0QRN3KZ
0QH944Z	0QHG0CZ	0QHK35Z	0QN13ZZ	0QNR3ZZ	0QPF4JZ	0QPK45Z	0QPP3KZ	0QQ0XZZ	0QQK3ZZ	0QRN47Z
0QH945Z	0QHG0DZ	0QHK36Z	0QN14ZZ	0QNR4ZZ	0QPF4KZ	0QPK47Z	0QPP44Z	0QQ10ZZ	0QQK4ZZ	0QRN4JZ
0QH946Z	0QHG34Z	0QHK38Z	0QN20ZZ	0QNS0ZZ	0QPFX4Z	0QPK4JZ	0QPP45Z	0QQ13ZZ	0QQKXZZ	0QRN4KZ
0QH948Z	0QHG35Z	0QHK3BZ	0QN23ZZ	0QNS3ZZ	0QPFX5Z	0QPK4KZ	0QPP47Z	0QQ14ZZ	0QQL0ZZ	0QRP07Z
0QH94BZ	0QHG36Z	0QHK3CZ	0QN24ZZ	0QNS4ZZ	0QPG04Z	0QPKX4Z	0QPP4JZ	0QQ1XZZ	0QQL3ZZ	0QRP0JZ
0QH94CZ	0QHG38Z	0QHK3DZ	0QN30ZZ	0QP004Z	0QPG05Z	0QPKX5Z	0QPP4KZ	0QQ20ZZ	0QQL4ZZ	0QRP0KZ
0QH94DZ	0QHG3BZ	0QHK44Z	0QN33ZZ	0QP007Z	0QPG07Z	0QPL04Z	0QPPX4Z	0QQ23ZZ	0QQLXZZ	0QRP37Z
0QHB04Z	0QHG3CZ	0QHK45Z	0QN34ZZ	0QP00JZ	0QPG0JZ	0QPL05Z	0QPPX5Z	0QQ24ZZ	0QQM0ZZ	0QRP3JZ
0QHB05Z	0QHG3DZ	0QHK46Z	0QN40ZZ	0QP00KZ	0QPG0KZ	0QPL07Z	0QPQ04Z	0QQ2XZZ	0QQM3ZZ	0QRP3KZ
0QHB06Z	0QHG44Z	0QHK48Z	0QN43ZZ	0QP034Z	0QPG34Z	0QPL0JZ	0QPQ05Z	0QQ30ZZ	0QQM4ZZ	0QRP47Z
0QHB08Z	0QHG45Z	0QHK4BZ	0QN44ZZ	0QP037Z	0QPG35Z	0QPL0KZ	0QPQ07Z	0QQ33ZZ	0QQMXZZ	0QRP4JZ
0QHB0BZ	0QHG46Z	0QHK4CZ	0QN50ZZ	0QP03JZ	0QPG37Z	0QPL34Z	0QPQ0JZ	0QQ34ZZ	0QQN0ZZ	0QRP4KZ
0QHB0CZ	0QHG48Z	0QHK4DZ	0QN53ZZ	0QP0X4Z	0QPG3JZ	0QPL35Z	0QPQ0KZ	0QQ3XZZ	0QQN3ZZ	0QRQ07Z
0QHB0DZ	0QHG4BZ	0QHL04Z	0QN54ZZ	0QP1X4Z	0QPG3KZ	0QPL37Z	0QPQ34Z	0QQ40ZZ	0QQNXZZ	0QRQ0JZ
0QHB34Z	0QHG4CZ	0QHL05Z	0QN60ZZ	0QP2X4Z	0QPG44Z	0QPL3JZ	0QPQ35Z	0QQ43ZZ	0QQP0ZZ	0QRQ0KZ
0QHB35Z	0QHG4DZ	0QHL34Z	0QN63ZZ	0QP2X5Z	0QPG45Z	0QPL3KZ	0QPQ37Z	0QQ44ZZ	0QQP3ZZ	0QRQ37Z
0QHB36Z	0QHH04Z	0QHL35Z	0QN64ZZ	0QP3X4Z	0QPG47Z	0QPL44Z	0QPQ3JZ	0QQ4XZZ	0QQP4ZZ	0QRQ3JZ
0QHB38Z	0QHH05Z	0QHL44Z	0QN70ZZ	0QP3X5Z	0QPG4JZ	0QPL45Z	0QPQ3KZ	0QQ50ZZ	0QQPXZZ	0QRQ3KZ
0QHB3BZ	0QHH06Z	0QHL45Z	0QN73ZZ	0QP4X4Z	0QPG4KZ	0QPL47Z	0QPQ44Z	0QQ53ZZ	0QQQ0ZZ	0QRQ47Z
0QHB3CZ	0QHH08Z	0QHM04Z	0QN74ZZ	0QP5X4Z	0QPGX4Z	0QPL4JZ	0QPQ45Z	0QQ54ZZ	0QQQ3ZZ	0QRQ4JZ
0QHB3DZ	0QHH0BZ	0QHM05Z	0QN80ZZ	0QP6X4Z	0QPGX5Z	0QPL4KZ	0QPQ47Z	0QQ5XZZ	0QQQ4ZZ	0QRQ4KZ
0QHB44Z	0QHH0CZ	0QHM34Z	0QN83ZZ	0QP6X5Z	0QPH04Z	0QPLX4Z	0QPQ4JZ	0QQ60ZZ	0QQQXZZ	0QRR07Z
0QHB45Z	0QHH0DZ	0QHM35Z	0QN84ZZ	0QP7X4Z	0QPH05Z	0QPLX5Z	0QPQ4KZ	0QQ63ZZ	0QQR0ZZ	0QRR0JZ
0QHB46Z	0QHH34Z	0QHM44Z	0QN90ZZ	0QP7X5Z	0QPH07Z	0QPM04Z	0QPQX4Z	0QQ64ZZ	0QQR3ZZ	0QRR0KZ
0QHB48Z	0QHH35Z	0QHM45Z	0QN93ZZ	0QP8X4Z	0QPH0JZ	0QPM05Z	0QPQX5Z	0QQ6XZZ	0QQR4ZZ	0QRR37Z
0QHB4BZ	0QHH36Z	0QHN04Z	0QN94ZZ	0QP8X5Z	0QPH0KZ	0QPM07Z	0QPR04Z	0QQ70ZZ	0QQRXZZ	0QRR3JZ
0QHB4CZ	0QHH38Z	0QHN05Z	0QNB0ZZ	0QP9X4Z	0QPH34Z	0QPM0JZ	0QPR05Z	0QQ73ZZ	0QQS0ZZ	0QRR3KZ
0QHB4DZ	0QHH3BZ	0QHN34Z	0QNB3ZZ	0QP9X5Z	0QPH35Z	0QPM0KZ	0QPR07Z	0QQ74ZZ	0QQS3ZZ	0QRR47Z
0QHC04Z	0QHH3CZ	0QHN35Z	0QNB4ZZ	0QPBX4Z	0QPH37Z	0QPM34Z	0QPR0JZ	0QQ7XZZ	0QQS4ZZ	0QRR4JZ
0QHC05Z	0QHH3DZ	0QHN44Z	0QNC0ZZ	0QPBX5Z	0QPH3JZ	0QPM35Z	0QPR0KZ	0QQ80ZZ	0QQSXZZ	0QRR4KZ
0QHC06Z	0QHH44Z	0QHN45Z	0QNC3ZZ	0QPC45Z	0QPH3KZ	0QPM37Z	0QPR34Z	0QQ83ZZ	0QR007Z	0QRS07Z
0QHC08Z	0QHH45Z	0QHP04Z	0QNC4ZZ	0QPC47Z	0QPH44Z	0QPM3JZ	0QPR35Z	0QQ84ZZ	0QR00JZ	0QRS0JZ
0QHC0BZ	0QHH46Z	0QHP05Z	0QND0ZZ	0QPC4JZ	0QPH45Z	0QPM3KZ	0QPR37Z	0QQ8XZZ	0QR00KZ	0QRS0KZ
0QHC0CZ	0QHH48Z	0QHP34Z	0QND3ZZ	0QPC4KZ	0QPH47Z	0QPM44Z	0QPR3JZ	0QQ90ZZ	0QR037Z	0QRS37Z
0QHC0DZ	0QHH4BZ	0QHP35Z	0QND4ZZ	0QPCX4Z	0QPH4KZ	0QPM45Z	0QPR3KZ	0QQ93ZZ	0QR03JZ	0QRS3JZ
0QHC34Z	0QHH4CZ	0QHP44Z	0QNF0ZZ	0QPCX5Z	0QPH4KZ	0QPM47Z	0QPR44Z	0QQ94ZZ	0QRK37Z	0QRS3KZ
0QHC35Z	0QHH4DZ	0QHP45Z	0QNF3ZZ	0QPD04Z	0QPHX4Z	0QPM4JZ	0QPR45Z	0QQ9XZZ	0QRK3JZ	0QRS47Z
0QHC36Z	0QHJ04Z	0QHQ04Z	0QNF4ZZ	0QPD05Z	0QPHX5Z	0QPM4KZ	0QPR47Z	0QQB0ZZ	0QRK3KZ	0QRS4JZ
0QHC38Z	0QHJ05Z	0QHQ05Z	0QNG0ZZ	0QPD07Z	0QPJ04Z	0QPMX4Z	0QPR4JZ	0QQB3ZZ	0QRK47Z	0QRS4KZ
0QHC3BZ	0QHJ06Z	0QHQ34Z	0QNG3ZZ	0QPD0JZ	0QPJ05Z	0QPMX5Z	0QPR4KZ	0QQB4ZZ	0QRK4JZ	0QS004Z
0QHC3CZ	0QHJ08Z	0QHQ35Z	0QNG4ZZ	0QPD0KZ	0QPJ07Z	0QPN04Z	0QPRX4Z	0QQBXZZ	0QRK4KZ	0QS00ZZ
0QHC3DZ	0QHJ0BZ	0QHQ44Z	0QNH0ZZ	0QPD34Z	0QPJ0JZ	0QPN05Z	0QPRX5Z	0QQC0ZZ	0QRL07Z	0QS034Z
0QHC44Z	0QHJ0CZ	0QHQ45Z	0QNH3ZZ	0QPD35Z	0QPJ0KZ	0QPN07Z	0QPS04Z	0QQC3ZZ	0QRL0JZ	0QS03ZZ
0QHC45Z	0QHJ0DZ	0QHR04Z	0QNH4ZZ	0QPD37Z	0QPJ34Z	0QPN0JZ	0QPS07Z	0QQC4ZZ	0QRL0KZ	0QS044Z
0QHC46Z	0QHJ34Z	0QHR05Z	0QNJ0ZZ	0QPD3JZ	0QPJ35Z	0QPN0KZ	0QPS0JZ	0QQCXZZ	0QRL37Z	0QS04ZZ
0QHC48Z	0QHJ35Z	0QHR34Z	0QNJ3ZZ	0QPD3KZ	0QPJ37Z	0QPN34Z	0QPS0KZ	0QQD0ZZ	0QRL3JZ	0QS0XZZ
0QHC4BZ	0QHJ36Z	0QHR35Z	0QNJ4ZZ	0QPD44Z	0QPJ3JZ	0QPN35Z	0QPS34Z	0QQD3ZZ	0QRL3KZ	0QS104Z
0QHC4CZ	0QHJ38Z	0QHR44Z	0QNK0ZZ	0QPD45Z	0QPJ3KZ	0QPN37Z	0QPS37Z	0QQD4ZZ	0QRL47Z	0QS10ZZ
0QHC4DZ	0QHJ3BZ	0QHR45Z	0QNK3ZZ	0QPD47Z	0QPJ44Z	0QPN3JZ	0QPS3JZ	0QQDXZZ	0QRL4JZ	0QS134Z
0QHD04Z	0QHJ3CZ	0QHS04Z	0QNK4ZZ	0QPD4JZ	0QPJ45Z	0QPN3KZ	0QPS3KZ	0QQF0ZZ	0QRL4KZ	0QS13ZZ
0QHD05Z	0QHJ3DZ	0QHS05Z	0QNL0ZZ	0QPD4KZ	0QPJ47Z	0QPN44Z	0QPS44Z	0QQF3ZZ	0QRM07Z	0QS144Z
0QHD34Z	0QHJ44Z	0QHS34Z	0QNL3ZZ	0QPDX4Z	0QPJ4JZ	0QPN45Z	0QPS47Z	0QQF4ZZ	0QRM0JZ	0QS14ZZ
0QHD35Z	0QHJ45Z	0QHS35Z	0QNL4ZZ	0QPDX5Z	0QPJ4KZ	0QPN47Z	0QPS4JZ	0QQFXZZ	0QRM0KZ	0QS1XZZ
0QHD44Z	0QHJ46Z	0QHS44Z	0QNM0ZZ	0QPF04Z	0QPJX4Z	0QPN4JZ	0QPS4KZ	0QQG0ZZ	0QRM37Z	0QS204Z
0QHD45Z	0QHJ48Z	0QHS45Z	0QNM3ZZ	0QPF05Z	0QPJX5Z	0QPN4KZ	0QPSX4Z	0QQG3ZZ	0QRM3JZ	0QS205Z
0QHF04Z	0QHJ4BZ	0QHY0MZ	0QNM4ZZ	0QPF07Z	0QPK04Z	0QPNX4Z	0QPY00Z	0QQG4ZZ	0QRM3KZ	0QS20ZZ
0QHF05Z	0QHJ4CZ	0QHY3MZ	0QNN0ZZ	0QPF0JZ	0QPK05Z	0QPNX5Z	0QPY0MZ	0QQGXZZ	0QRM47Z	0QS234Z
0QHF34Z	0QHJ4DZ	0QHY4MZ	0QNN3ZZ	0QPF0KZ	0QPK07Z	0QPP04Z	0QPY30Z	0QQH0ZZ	0QRM47Z	0QS235Z

0QS23ZZ	0QS745Z	0QSB45Z	0QSG4BZ	0QU10JZ	0QU83JZ	0QUH4JZ	0QUR0JZ	0QW2X7Z	0QW645Z	0QW9X7Z
0QS244Z	0QS746Z	0QSB46Z	0QSG4CZ	0QU10KZ	0QU83KZ	0QUH4KZ	0QUR0KZ	0QW2XJZ	0QW647Z	0QW9XJZ
0QS245Z	0QS74BZ	0QSB4BZ	0QSG4DZ	0QU137Z	0QU847Z	0QUJ07Z	0QUR37Z	0QW2XKZ	0QW64JZ	0QW9XKZ
0QS24ZZ	0QS74CZ	0QSB4CZ	0QSG4ZZ	0QU13JZ	0QU84JZ	0QUJ0JZ	0QUR3JZ	0QW304Z	0QW64KZ	0QWB04Z
0QS2XZZ	0QS74DZ	0QSB4DZ	0QSGXZZ	0QU13KZ	0QU84KZ	0QUJ0KZ	0QUR3KZ	0QW305Z	0QW6X4Z	0QWB05Z
0QS304Z	0QS74ZZ	0QSB4ZZ	0QSH04Z	0QU147Z	0QU907Z	0QUJ37Z	0QUR47Z	0QW307Z	0QW6X5Z	0QWB07Z
0QS305Z	0QS7XZZ	0QSBXZZ	0QSH05Z	0QU14JZ	0QU90JZ	0QUJ3JZ	0QUR4JZ	0QW30JZ	0QW6X7Z	0QWB0JZ
0QS30ZZ	0QS804Z	0QSC04Z	0QSH06Z	0QU14KZ	0QU90KZ	0QUJ3KZ	0QUR4KZ	0QW30KZ	0QW6XJZ	0QWB0KZ
0QS334Z	0QS805Z	0QSC05Z	0QSH0BZ	0QU207Z	0QU937Z	0QUJ47Z	0QUS07Z	0QW334Z	0QW6XKZ	0QWB34Z
0QS335Z	0QS806Z	0QSC06Z	0QSH0CZ	0QU20JZ	0QU93JZ	0QUJ4JZ	0QUS0JZ	0QW335Z	0QW704Z	0QWB35Z
0QS33ZZ	0QS80BZ	0QSC0BZ	0QSH0DZ	0QU20KZ	0QU93KZ	0QUJ4KZ	0QUS0KZ	0QW337Z	0QW705Z	0QWB37Z
0QS344Z	0QS80CZ	0QSC0CZ	0QSH0ZZ	0QU237Z	0QU947Z	0QUK07Z	0QUS37Z	0QW33JZ	0QW707Z	0QWB3JZ
0QS345Z	0QS80DZ	0QSC0DZ	0QSH34Z	0QU23JZ	0QU94JZ	0QUK0JZ	0QUS3JZ	0QW33KZ	0QW70JZ	0QWB3KZ
0QS34ZZ	0QS80ZZ	0QSC0ZZ	0QSH35Z	0QU23KZ	0QU94KZ	0QUK0KZ	0QUS3KZ	0QW344Z	0QW70KZ	0QWB44Z
0QS3XZZ	0QS834Z	0QSC34Z	0QSH3ZZ	0QU247Z	0QUB07Z	0QUK37Z	0QUS47Z	0QW345Z	0QW734Z	0QWB45Z
0QS404Z	0QS835Z	0QSC35Z	0QSH4ZZ	0QU24JZ	0QUB0JZ	0QUK3JZ	0QUS4JZ	0QW347Z	0QW735Z	0QWB47Z
0QS40ZZ	0QS836Z	0QSC36Z	0QSHXZZ	0QU24KZ	0QUB0KZ	0QUK3KZ	0QUS4KZ	0QW34JZ	0QW737Z	0QWB4JZ
0QS434Z	0QS83BZ	0QSC3BZ	0QSJ3ZZ	0QU307Z	0QUB37Z	0QUK47Z	0QW004Z	0QW34KZ	0QW73JZ	0QWB4KZ
0QS43ZZ	0QS83CZ	0QSC3CZ	0QSJ4ZZ	0QU30JZ	0QUB3JZ	0QUK4JZ	0QW007Z	0QW3X4Z	0QW73KZ	0QWBX4Z
0QS444Z	0QS83DZ	0QSC3DZ	0QSJXZZ	0QU30KZ	0QUB3KZ	0QUK4KZ	0QW00JZ	0QW3X5Z	0QW744Z	0QWBX5Z
0QS44ZZ	0QS83ZZ	0QSC3ZZ	0QSK3ZZ	0QU337Z	0QUB47Z	0QUL07Z	0QW00KZ	0QW3X7Z	0QW745Z	0QWBX7Z
0QS4XZZ	0QS844Z	0QSC44Z	0QSK4ZZ	0QU33JZ	0QUB4JZ	0QUL0JZ	0QW034Z	0QW3XJZ	0QW747Z	0QWBXJZ
0QS504Z	0QS845Z	0QSC45Z	0QSKXZZ	0QU33KZ	0QUB4KZ	0QUL0KZ	0QW037Z	0QW3XKZ	0QW74JZ	0QWBXKZ
0QS50ZZ	0QS846Z	0QSC46Z	0QSL3ZZ	0QU347Z	0QUC07Z	0QUL37Z	0QW03JZ	0QW404Z	0QW74KZ	0QWC04Z
0QS534Z	0QS84BZ	0QSC4BZ	0QSL4ZZ	0QU34JZ	0QUC0JZ	0QUL3JZ	0QW03KZ	0QW407Z	0QW7X4Z	0QWC05Z
0QS53ZZ	0QS84CZ	0QSC4CZ	0QSLXZZ	0QU34KZ	0QUC0KZ	0QUL3KZ	0QW044Z	0QW40JZ	0QW7X5Z	0QWC07Z
0QS544Z	0QS84DZ	0QSC4DZ	0QSM3ZZ	0QU407Z	0QUC37Z	0QUL47Z	0QW047Z	0QW40KZ	0QW7X7Z	0QWC0JZ
0QS54ZZ	0QS84ZZ	0QSC4ZZ	0QSM4ZZ	0QU40JZ	0QUC3JZ	0QUL4JZ	0QW04JZ	0QW434Z	0QW7XJZ	0QWC0KZ
0QS5XZZ	0QS8XZZ	0QSCXZZ	0QSMXZZ	0QU40KZ	0QUC3KZ	0QUL4KZ	0QW04KZ	0QW437Z	0QW7XKZ	0QWC34Z
0QS604Z	0QS904Z	0QSD04Z	0QSN042	0QU437Z	0QUC47Z	0QUM07Z	0QW0X4Z	0QW43JZ	0QW804Z	0QWC35Z
0QS605Z	0QS905Z	0QSD05Z	0QSN052	0QU43JZ	0QUC4JZ	0QUM0JZ	0QW0X7Z	0QW43KZ	0QW805Z	0QWC37Z
0QS606Z	0QS906Z	0QSD0ZZ	0QSN0Z2	0QU43KZ	0QUC4KZ	0QUM0KZ	0QW0XJZ	0QW444Z	0QW807Z	0QWC3JZ
0QS60BZ	0QS90BZ	0QSD34Z	0QSN342	0QU447Z	0QUD07Z	0QUM37Z	0QW0XKZ	0QW447Z	0QW80JZ	0QWC3KZ
0QS60CZ	0QS90CZ	0QSD35Z	0QSN352	0QU44JZ	0QUD0JZ	0QUM3JZ	0QW104Z	0QW44JZ	0QW80KZ	0QWC44Z
0QS60DZ	0QS90DZ	0QSD3ZZ	0QSN3Z2	0QU44KZ	0QUD0KZ	0QUM3KZ	0QW107Z	0QW44KZ	0QW834Z	0QWC45Z
0QS60ZZ	0QS90ZZ	0QSD44Z	0QSN3ZZ	0QU507Z	0QUD37Z	0QUM47Z	0QW10JZ	0QW4X4Z	0QW835Z	0QWC47Z
0QS634Z	0QS934Z	0QSD45Z	0QSN442	0QU50JZ	0QUD3JZ	0QUM4JZ	0QW10KZ	0QW4X7Z	0QW837Z	0QWC4JZ
0QS635Z	0QS935Z	0QSD4ZZ	0QSN452	0QU50KZ	0QUD3KZ	0QUM4KZ	0QW134Z	0QW4XJZ	0QW83JZ	0QWC4KZ
0QS636Z	0QS936Z	0QSDXZZ	0QSN4Z2	0QU537Z	0QUD47Z	0QUN07Z	0QW137Z	0QW4XKZ	0QW83KZ	0QWCX4Z
0QS63BZ	0QS93BZ	0QSF04Z	0QSN4ZZ	0QU53JZ	0QUD4JZ	0QUN0JZ	0QW13JZ	0QW504Z	0QW844Z	0QWCX5Z
0QS63CZ	0QS93CZ	0QSF05Z	0QSNXZ2	0QU53KZ	0QUD4KZ	0QUN0KZ	0QW13KZ	0QW507Z	0QW845Z	0QWCX7Z
0QS63DZ	0QS93DZ	0QSF0ZZ	0QSNXZZ	0QU547Z	0QUF07Z	0QUN37Z	0QW144Z	0QW50JZ	0QW847Z	0QWCXJZ
0QS63ZZ	0QS93ZZ	0QSF34Z	0QSP042	0QU54JZ	0QUF0JZ	0QUN3JZ	0QW147Z	0QW50KZ	0QW84JZ	0QWCXKZ
0QS644Z	0QS944Z	0QSF35Z	0QSP052	0QU54KZ	0QUF0KZ	0QUN3KZ	0QW14JZ	0QW534Z	0QW84KZ	0QWD04Z
0QS645Z	0QS945Z	0QSF3ZZ	0QSP0Z2	0QU607Z	0QUF37Z	0QUN47Z	0QW14KZ	0QW537Z	0QW8X4Z	0QWD05Z
0QS646Z	0QS946Z	0QSF44Z	0QSP342	0QU60JZ	0QUF3JZ	0QUN4JZ	0QW1X4Z	0QW53JZ	0QW8X5Z	0QWD07Z
0QS64BZ	0QS94BZ	0QSF45Z	0QSP352	0QU60KZ	0QUF3KZ	0QUN4KZ	0QW1X7Z	0QW53KZ	0QW8X7Z	0QWD0JZ
0QS64CZ	0QS94CZ	0QSF4ZZ	0QSP3Z2	0QU637Z	0QUF47Z	0QUP07Z	0QW1XJZ	0QW544Z	0QW8XJZ	0QWD0KZ
0QS64DZ	0QS94DZ	0QSFXZZ	0QSP3ZZ	0QU63JZ	0QUF4JZ	0QUP0JZ	0QW1XKZ	0QW547Z	0QW8XKZ	0QWD34Z
0QS64ZZ	0QS94ZZ	0QSG04Z	0QSP442	0QU63KZ	0QUF4KZ	0QUP0KZ	0QW204Z	0QW54JZ	0QW904Z	0QWD35Z
0QS6XZZ	0QS9XZZ	0QSG05Z	0QSP452	0QU647Z	0QUG07Z	0QUP37Z	0QW205Z	0QW54KZ	0QW905Z	0QWD37Z
0QS704Z	0QSB04Z	0QSG06Z	0QSP4Z2	0QU64JZ	0QUG0JZ	0QUP3JZ	0QW207Z	0QW5X4Z	0QW907Z	0QWD3JZ
0QS705Z	0QSB05Z	0QSG0BZ	0QSP4ZZ	0QU64KZ	0QUG0KZ	0QUP3KZ	0QW20JZ	0QW5X7Z	0QW90JZ	0QWD3KZ
0QS706Z	0QSB06Z	0QSG0CZ	0QSPXZ2	0QU707Z	0QUG37Z	0QUP47Z	0QW20KZ	0QW5XJZ	0QW90KZ	0QWD44Z
0QS70BZ	0QSB0BZ	0QSG0DZ	0QSPXZZ	0QU70JZ	0QUG3JZ	0QUP4JZ	0QW234Z	0QW5XKZ	0QW934Z	0QWD45Z
0QS70CZ	0QSB0CZ	0QSG0ZZ	0QSQ3ZZ	0QU70KZ	0QUG3KZ	0QUP4KZ	0QW235Z	0QW604Z	0QW935Z	0QWD47Z
0QS70DZ	0QSB0DZ	0QSG34Z	0QSQ4ZZ	0QU737Z	0QUG47Z	0QUQ07Z	0QW237Z	0QW605Z	0QW937Z	0QWD4JZ
0QS70ZZ	0QSB0ZZ	0QSG35Z	0QSQXZZ	0QU73JZ	0QUG4JZ	0QUQ0JZ	0QW23JZ	0QW607Z	0QW93JZ	0QWD4KZ
0QS734Z	0QSB34Z	0QSG36Z	0QSR3ZZ	0QU73KZ	0QUG4KZ	0QUQ0KZ	0QW23KZ	0QW60JZ	0QW93KZ	0QWDX4Z
0QS735Z	0QSB35Z	0QSG3BZ	0QSR4ZZ	0QU747Z	0QUH07Z	0QUQ37Z	0QW244Z	0QW60KZ	0QW944Z	0QWDX5Z
0QS736Z	0QSB36Z	0QSG3CZ	0QSRXZZ	0QU74JZ	0QUH0JZ	0QUQ3JZ	0QW245Z	0QW634Z	0QW945Z	0QWDX7Z
0QS73BZ	0QSB3BZ	0QSG3DZ	0QU03KZ	0QU74KZ	0QUH0KZ	0QUQ3KZ	0QW247Z	0QW635Z	0QW947Z	0QWDXJZ
0QS73CZ	0QSB3CZ	0QSG3ZZ	0QU047Z	0QU807Z	0QUH37Z	0QUQ47Z	0QW24JZ	0QW637Z	0QW94JZ	0QWDXKZ
0QS73DZ	0QSB3DZ	0QSG44Z	0QU04JZ	0QU80JZ	0QUH3JZ	0QUQ4JZ	0QW24KZ	0QW63JZ	0QW94KZ	0QWF04Z
0QS73ZZ	0QSB3ZZ	0QSG45Z	0QU04KZ	0QU80KZ	0QUH3KZ	0QUQ4KZ	0QW2X4Z	0QW63KZ	0QW9X4Z	0QWF05Z
0QS744Z	0QSB44Z	0QSG46Z	0QU107Z	0QU837Z	0QUH47Z	0QUR07Z	0QW2X5Z	0QW644Z	0QW9X5Z	0QWF07Z

0QWF0JZ	0R553ZZ	0R953ZX	0R9E4ZX	0R9N0ZX	0R9V3ZX	0RBA0ZZ	0RBM0ZZ	0RC03ZZ	0RCR3ZZ	0RG24Z0
0QWFX4Z	0R554ZZ	0R953ZZ	0R9E4ZZ	0R9N0ZZ	0R9V3ZZ	0RBA3ZX	0RBM3ZX	0RC04ZZ	0RCR4ZZ	0RG24Z1
0QWFX5Z	0R593ZZ	0R9540Z	0R9F00Z	0R9N30Z	0R9V40Z	0RBA3ZZ	0RBM3ZZ	0RC10ZZ	0RCS0ZZ	0RG24ZJ
0QWFX7Z	0R594ZZ	0R954ZX	0R9F0ZX	0R9N3ZX	0R9V4ZX	0RBA4ZX	0RBM4ZX	0RC13ZZ	0RCS4ZZ	0RG4070
0QWFXJZ	0R5B3ZZ	0R954ZZ	0R9F0ZZ	0R9N3ZZ	0R9V4ZZ	0RBA4ZZ	0RBM4ZZ	0RC14ZZ	0RCT0ZZ	0RG4071
0QWFXKZ	0R5B4ZZ	0R9600Z	0R9F30Z	0R9N40Z	0R9W00Z	0RBB0ZX	0RBN0ZX	0RC30ZZ	0RCT3ZZ	0RG407J
0QWGX4Z	0R5R3ZZ	0R960ZX	0R9F3ZX	0R9N4ZX	0R9W0ZX	0RBB0ZZ	0RBN0ZZ	0RC33ZZ	0RCT4ZZ	0RG40A0
0QWGX5Z	0R5R4ZZ	0R960ZZ	0R9F3ZZ	0R9N4ZZ	0R9W0ZZ	0RBB3ZX	0RBN3ZX	0RC34ZZ	0RCU0ZZ	0RG40AJ
0QWGX7Z	0R5S0ZZ	0R9630Z	0R9F40Z	0R9P00Z	0R9W30Z	0RBB3ZZ	0RBN3ZZ	0RC40ZZ	0RCU3ZZ	0RG40J0
0QWGXJZ	0R5S3ZZ	0R963ZX	0R9F4ZX	0R9P0ZX	0R9W3ZX	0RBB4ZX	0RBN4ZX	0RC43ZZ	0RCU4ZZ	0RG40J1
0QWGXKZ	0R5S4ZZ	0R963ZZ	0R9F4ZZ	0R9P0ZZ	0R9W3ZZ	0RBB4ZZ	0RBN4ZZ	0RC44ZZ	0RCV0ZZ	0RG40JJ
0QWHX4Z	0R5T0ZZ	0R9640Z	0R9G00Z	0R9P30Z	0R9W40Z	0RBC0ZX	0RBP0ZX	0RC50ZZ	0RCV3ZZ	0RG40K0
0QWHX5Z	0R5T3ZZ	0R964ZX	0R9G0ZX	0R9P3ZX	0R9W4ZX	0RBC0ZZ	0RBP0ZZ	0RC53ZZ	0RCV4ZZ	0RG40K1
0QWHX7Z	0R5T4ZZ	0R964ZZ	0R9G0ZZ	0R9P3ZZ	0R9W4ZZ	0RBC3ZX	0RBP3ZX	0RC54ZZ	0RCW0ZZ	0RG40KJ
0QWHXJZ	0R5U0ZZ	0R9900Z	0R9G30Z	0R9P40Z	0R9X00Z	0RBC3ZZ	0RBP3ZZ	0RC60ZZ	0RCW3ZZ	0RG40Z0
0QWHXKZ	0R5U3ZZ	0R990ZX	0R9G3ZX	0R9P4ZX	0R9X0ZX	0RBC4ZX	0RBP4ZX	0RC63ZZ	0RCW4ZZ	0RG40Z1
0QWJX4Z	0R5U4ZZ	0R990ZZ	0R9G3ZZ	0R9P4ZZ	0R9X0ZZ	0RBC4ZZ	0RBP4ZZ	0RC64ZZ	0RCX0ZZ	0RG40ZJ
0QWJX5Z	0R5V0ZZ	0R9930Z	0R9G40Z	0R9Q00Z	0R9X30Z	0RBD0ZX	0RBQ0ZX	0RC90ZZ	0RCX3ZZ	0RG4370
0QWJX7Z	0R5V3ZZ	0R993ZX	0R9G4ZX	0R9Q0ZX	0R9X3ZX	0RBD0ZZ	0RBQ0ZZ	0RC93ZZ	0RCX4ZZ	0RG4371
0QWJXJZ	0R5V4ZZ	0R993ZZ	0R9G4ZZ	0R9Q0ZZ	0R9X3ZZ	0RBD3ZX	0RBQ3ZX	0RC94ZZ	0RG0070	0RG437J
0QWJXKZ	0R5W0ZZ	0R9940Z	0R9H00Z	0R9Q30Z	0R9X40Z	0RBD3ZZ	0RBQ3ZZ	0RCA0ZZ	0RG0071	0RG43A0
0QWKX4Z	0R5W3ZZ	0R994ZX	0R9H0ZX	0R9Q3ZX	0R9X4ZX	0RBD4ZX	0RBQ4ZX	0RCA3ZZ	0RG007J	0RG43AJ
0QWKX5Z	0R5W4ZZ	0R994ZZ	0R9H0ZZ	0R9Q3ZZ	0R9X4ZZ	0RBD4ZZ	0RBQ4ZZ	0RCA4ZZ	0RG00A0	0RG43J0
0QWKX7Z	0R5X0ZZ	0R9A00Z	0R9H30Z	0R9Q40Z	0RB00ZX	0RBE0ZX	0RBR0ZX	0RCB0ZZ	0RG00AJ	0RG43J1
0QWKXJZ	0R5X3ZZ	0R9A0ZX	0R9H3ZX	0R9Q4ZX	0RB00ZZ	0RBE0ZZ	0RBR0ZZ	0RCB3ZZ	0RG00J0	0RG43K0
0QWKXKZ	0R5X4ZZ	0R9A0ZZ	0R9H3ZZ	0R9Q4ZZ	0RB03ZX	0RBE3ZX	0RBR3ZX	0RCB4ZZ	0RG00J1	0RG43K1
0QWLX4Z	0R9000Z	0R9A30Z	0R9H40Z	0R9R00Z	0RB03ZZ	0RBE3ZZ	0RBR3ZZ	0RCC0ZZ	0RG00JJ	0RG43KJ
0QWLX5Z	0R900ZX	0R9A3ZX	0R9H4ZX	0R9R0ZX	0RB04ZX	0RBE4ZX	0RBR4ZX	0RCC3ZZ	0RG00K0	0RG43Z0
0QWLX7Z	0R900ZZ	0R9A3ZZ	0R9H4ZZ	0R9R0ZZ	0RB04ZZ	0RBE4ZZ	0RBR4ZZ	0RCC4ZZ	0RG00K1	0RG43Z1
0QWLXJZ	0R9030Z	0R9A40Z	0R9J00Z	0R9R30Z	0RB10ZX	0RBF0ZX	0RBS0ZX	0RCD0ZZ	0RG00KJ	0RG43ZJ
0QWLXKZ	0R903ZX	0R9A4ZX	0R9J0ZX	0R9R3ZX	0RB10ZZ	0RBF0ZZ	0RBS0ZZ	0RCD3ZZ	0RG00Z0	0RG4470
0QWMX4Z	0R903ZZ	0R9A4ZZ	0R9J0ZZ	0R9R3ZZ	0RB13ZX	0RBF3ZX	0RBS3ZX	0RCD4ZZ	0RG00Z1	0RG4471
0QWMX5Z	0R9040Z	0R9B00Z	0R9J30Z	0R9R40Z	0RB13ZZ	0RBF3ZZ	0RBS3ZZ	0RCE0ZZ	0RG00ZJ	0RG447J
0QWMX7Z	0R904ZX	0R9B0ZX	0R9J3ZX	0R9R4ZX	0RB14ZX	0RBF4ZX	0RBS4ZX	0RCE3ZZ	0RG0370	0RG44A0
0QWMXJZ	0R904ZZ	0R9B0ZZ	0R9J3ZZ	0R9R4ZZ	0RB14ZZ	0RBF4ZZ	0RBS4ZZ	0RCE4ZZ	0RG0371	0RG44AJ
0QWMXKZ	0R9100Z	0R9B30Z	0R9J40Z	0R9S00Z	0RB30ZX	0RBG0ZX	0RBT0ZX	0RCF0ZZ	0RG037J	0RG44J0
0QWNX4Z	0R910ZX	0R9B3ZX	0R9J4ZX	0R9S0ZX	0RB30ZZ	0RBG0ZZ	0RBT0ZZ	0RCF3ZZ	0RG03A0	0RG44J1
0QWNX5Z	0R910ZZ	0R9B3ZZ	0R9J4ZZ	0R9S0ZZ	0RB33ZX	0RBG3ZX	0RBT3ZX	0RCF4ZZ	0RG03AJ	0RG44JJ
0QWNX7Z	0R9130Z	0R9B40Z	0R9K00Z	0R9S30Z	0RB33ZZ	0RBG3ZZ	0RBT3ZZ	0RCG0ZZ	0RG03J0	0RG44K0
0QWNXJZ	0R913ZX	0R9B4ZX	0R9K0ZX	0R9S3ZX	0RB34ZX	0RBG4ZX	0RBT4ZX	0RCG3ZZ	0RG03J1	0RG44K1
0QWNXKZ	0R913ZZ	0R9B4ZZ	0R9K0ZZ	0R9S3ZZ	0RB34ZZ	0RBG4ZZ	0RBT4ZZ	0RCG4ZZ	0RG03JJ	0RG44KJ
0QWPX4Z	0R9140Z	0R9C00Z	0R9K30Z	0R9S40Z	0RB40ZX	0RBH0ZX	0RBU0ZX	0RCH0ZZ	0RG03K0	0RG44Z0
0QWPX5Z	0R914ZX	0R9C0ZX	0R9K3ZX	0R9S4ZX	0RB40ZZ	0RBH0ZZ	0RBU0ZZ	0RCH3ZZ	0RG03K1	0RG44Z1
0QWPX7Z	0R914ZZ	0R9C0ZZ	0R9K3ZZ	0R9S4ZZ	0RB43ZX	0RBH3ZX	0RBU3ZX	0RCH4ZZ	0RG03KJ	0RG44ZJ
0QWPXJZ	0R9300Z	0R9C30Z	0R9K40Z	0R9T00Z	0RB43ZZ	0RBH3ZZ	0RBU3ZZ	0RCJ0ZZ	0RG03Z0	0RG6070
0QWPXKZ	0R930ZX	0R9C3ZX	0R9K4ZX	0R9T0ZX	0RB44ZX	0RBH4ZX	0RBU4ZX	0RCJ3ZZ	0RG03Z1	0RG6071
0QWQX4Z	0R930ZZ	0R9C3ZZ	0R9K4ZZ	0R9T0ZZ	0RB44ZZ	0RBH4ZZ	0RBU4ZZ	0RCJ4ZZ	0RG03ZJ	0RG607J
0QWQX5Z	0R9330Z	0R9C40Z	0R9L00Z	0R9T30Z	0RB50ZX	0RBJ0ZX	0RBV0ZX	0RCK0ZZ	0RG0470	0RG60A0
0QWQX7Z	0R933ZX	0R9C4ZX	0R9L0ZX	0R9T3ZX	0RB50ZZ	0RBJ0ZZ	0RBV0ZZ	0RCK3ZZ	0RG0471	0RG60AJ
0QWQXJZ	0R933ZZ	0R9C4ZZ	0R9L0ZZ	0R9T3ZZ	0RB53ZX	0RBJ3ZX	0RBV3ZX	0RCK4ZZ	0RG23K1	0RG60J0
0QWQXKZ	0R9340Z	0R9D00Z	0R9L30Z	0R9T40Z	0RB53ZZ	0RBJ3ZZ	0RBV3ZZ	0RCL0ZZ	0RG23KJ	0RG60J1
0QWRX4Z	0R934ZX	0R9D0ZX	0R9L3ZX	0R9T4ZX	0RB54ZX	0RBJ4ZX	0RBV4ZX	0RCL3ZZ	0RG23Z0	0RG60JJ
0QWRX5Z	0R934ZZ	0R9D0ZZ	0R9L3ZZ	0R9T4ZZ	0RB54ZZ	0RBJ4ZZ	0RBV4ZZ	0RCL4ZZ	0RG23Z1	0RG60K0
0QWRX7Z	0R9400Z	0R9D30Z	0R9L40Z	0R9U00Z	0RB60ZX	0RBK0ZX	0RBW0ZX	0RCM0ZZ	0RG23ZJ	0RG60K1
0QWRXJZ	0R940ZX	0R9D3ZX	0R9L4ZX	0R9U0ZX	0RB60ZZ	0RBK0ZZ	0RBW0ZZ	0RCM3ZZ	0RG2470	0RG60KJ
0QWRXKZ	0R940ZZ	0R9D3ZZ	0R9L4ZZ	0R9U0ZZ	0RB63ZX	0RBK3ZX	0RBW3ZX	0RCM4ZZ	0RG2471	0RG60Z0
0QWSX4Z	0R9430Z	0R9D40Z	0R9M00Z	0R9U30Z	0RB63ZZ	0RBK3ZZ	0RBW3ZZ	0RCN0ZZ	0RG247J	0RG60Z1
0QWSX7Z	0R943ZX	0R9D4ZX	0R9M0ZX	0R9U3ZX	0RB64ZX	0RBK4ZX	0RBW4ZX	0RCN3ZZ	0RG24A0	0RG60ZJ
0QWSXJZ	0R943ZZ	0R9D4ZZ	0R9M0ZZ	0R9U3ZZ	0RB64ZZ	0RBK4ZZ	0RBW4ZZ	0RCN4ZZ	0RG24AJ	0RG6370
0QWSXKZ	0R9440Z	0R9E00Z	0R9M30Z	0R9U40Z	0RB90ZX	0RBL0ZX	0RBX0ZX	0RCP0ZZ	0RG24J0	0RG6371
0QWYX0Z	0R944ZX	0R9E0ZX	0R9M3ZX	0R9U4ZX	0RB90ZZ	0RBL0ZZ	0RBX0ZZ	0RCP3ZZ	0RG24J1	0RG637J
0QWYXMZ	0R944ZZ	0R9E0ZZ	0R9M3ZZ	0R9U4ZZ	0RB93ZX	0RBL3ZX	0RBX3ZX	0RCP4ZZ	0RG24JJ	0RG63A0
0R2YX0Z	0R9500Z	0R9E30Z	0R9M40Z	0R9V00Z	0RB93ZZ	0RBL3ZZ	0RBX3ZZ	0RCQ0ZZ	0RG24K0	0RG63AJ
0R2YXYZ	0R950ZX	0R9E3ZX	0R9M4ZX	0R9V0ZX	0RB94ZX	0RBL4ZX	0RBX4ZX	0RCQ3ZZ	0RG24K1	0RG63J0
0R533ZZ	0R950ZZ	0R9E3ZZ	0R9M4ZZ	0R9V0ZZ	0RB94ZZ	0RBL4ZZ	0RBX4ZZ	0RCQ4ZZ	0RG24KJ	0RG63J1
0R534ZZ	0R9530Z	0R9E40Z	0R9N00Z	0R9V30Z	0RBA0ZX	0RBM0ZX	0RC00ZZ	0RCR0ZZ		

0RG63JJ	0RGA3KJ	0RGF0KZ	0RGK3ZZ	0RGP34Z	0RGT04Z	0RHC38Z	0RHK48Z	0RHR34Z	0RHW48Z	0RJG3ZZ
0RG63K0	0RGA3Z0	0RGF0ZZ	0RGK44Z	0RGP35Z	0RGT05Z	0RHC43Z	0RHL03Z	0RHR35Z	0RHX03Z	0RJG4ZZ
0RG63K1	0RGA3Z1	0RGF34Z	0RGK47Z	0RGP37Z	0RGT07Z	0RHC44Z	0RHL04Z	0RHR38Z	0RHX04Z	0RJGXZZ
0RG63KJ	0RGA3ZJ	0RGF37Z	0RGK4JZ	0RGP3JZ	0RGT0JZ	0RHC48Z	0RHL05Z	0RHR43Z	0RHX05Z	0RJH0ZZ
0RG63Z0	0RGA470	0RGF3JZ	0RGK4KZ	0RGP3KZ	0RGT0KZ	0RHD03Z	0RHL08Z	0RHR44Z	0RHX08Z	0RJH3ZZ
0RG63Z1	0RGA471	0RGF3KZ	0RGK4ZZ	0RGP3ZZ	0RH003Z	0RHD04Z	0RHL33Z	0RHR45Z	0RHX33Z	0RJH4ZZ
0RG63ZJ	0RGA47J	0RGF3ZZ	0RGL04Z	0RGP44Z	0RH008Z	0RHD08Z	0RHL34Z	0RHR48Z	0RHX34Z	0RJHXZZ
0RG6470	0RGA4A0	0RGF44Z	0RGL05Z	0RGP45Z	0RH033Z	0RHD33Z	0RHL35Z	0RHS03Z	0RHX35Z	0RJJ0ZZ
0RG6471	0RGA4AJ	0RGF47Z	0RGL07Z	0RGP47Z	0RH038Z	0RHD34Z	0RHL38Z	0RHS04Z	0RHX38Z	0RJJ3ZZ
0RG647J	0RGA4J0	0RGF4JZ	0RGL0JZ	0RGP4JZ	0RH043Z	0RHD38Z	0RHL43Z	0RHS05Z	0RHX43Z	0RJJ4ZZ
0RG64A0	0RGA4J1	0RGF4KZ	0RGL0KZ	0RGP4KZ	0RH048Z	0RHD43Z	0RHL44Z	0RHS08Z	0RHX44Z	0RJJK0ZZ
0RG64AJ	0RGA4JJ	0RGF4ZZ	0RGL0ZZ	0RGP4ZZ	0RH103Z	0RHD44Z	0RHL45Z	0RHS33Z	0RHX45Z	0RJK0ZZ
0RG64J0	0RGA4K0	0RGG04Z	0RGL34Z	0RGQ04Z	0RH108Z	0RHD48Z	0RHL48Z	0RHS34Z	0RHX48Z	0RJK3ZZ
0RG64J1	0RGA4K1	0RGG07Z	0RGL35Z	0RGQ05Z	0RH133Z	0RHE03Z	0RHM03Z	0RHS35Z	0RJ00ZZ	0RJK4ZZ
0RG64JJ	0RGA4KJ	0RGG0JZ	0RGL37Z	0RGQ07Z	0RH138Z	0RHE04Z	0RHM04Z	0RHS38Z	0RJ03ZZ	0RJKXZZ
0RG64K0	0RGA4Z0	0RGG0KZ	0RGL3JZ	0RGQ0JZ	0RH143Z	0RHE08Z	0RHM05Z	0RHS43Z	0RJ04ZZ	0RJL0ZZ
0RG64K1	0RGA4Z1	0RGG0ZZ	0RGL3KZ	0RGQ0KZ	0RH148Z	0RHE33Z	0RHM08Z	0RHS44Z	0RJ0XZZ	0RJL3ZZ
0RG64KJ	0RGA4ZJ	0RGG34Z	0RGL3ZZ	0RGQ0ZZ	0RH303Z	0RHE34Z	0RHM33Z	0RHS45Z	0RJ10ZZ	0RJL4ZZ
0RG64Z0	0RGC04Z	0RGG37Z	0RGL44Z	0RGQ34Z	0RH333Z	0RHE38Z	0RHM34Z	0RHS48Z	0RJ13ZZ	0RJLXZZ
0RG64Z1	0RGC07Z	0RGG3JZ	0RGL45Z	0RGQ35Z	0RH343Z	0RHE43Z	0RHM35Z	0RHT03Z	0RJ14ZZ	0RJM0ZZ
0RG64ZJ	0RGC0JZ	0RGG3KZ	0RGL47Z	0RGQ37Z	0RH403Z	0RHE44Z	0RHM38Z	0RHT04Z	0RJ1XZZ	0RJM3ZZ
0RG7070	0RGC0KZ	0RGG3ZZ	0RGL4JZ	0RGQ3JZ	0RH408Z	0RHE48Z	0RHM43Z	0RHT05Z	0RJ30ZZ	0RJM4ZZ
0RG7071	0RGC0ZZ	0RGG44Z	0RGL4KZ	0RGQ3KZ	0RH433Z	0RHF03Z	0RHM44Z	0RHT08Z	0RJ33ZZ	0RJMXZZ
0RG707J	0RGC34Z	0RGG47Z	0RGL4ZZ	0RGQ3ZZ	0RH438Z	0RHF04Z	0RHM45Z	0RHT33Z	0RJ34ZZ	0RJN0ZZ
0RG70A0	0RGC37Z	0RGG4JZ	0RGM04Z	0RGQ44Z	0RH443Z	0RHF08Z	0RHM48Z	0RHT34Z	0RJ3XZZ	0RJN3ZZ
0RG70AJ	0RGC3JZ	0RGG4KZ	0RGM05Z	0RGQ45Z	0RH448Z	0RHF33Z	0RHN03Z	0RHT35Z	0RJ40ZZ	0RJN4ZZ
0RG70J0	0RGC3KZ	0RGG4ZZ	0RGM07Z	0RGQ47Z	0RH503Z	0RHF34Z	0RHN04Z	0RHT38Z	0RJ43ZZ	0RJNXZZ
0RG70J1	0RGC3ZZ	0RGH04Z	0RGM0JZ	0RGQ4JZ	0RH533Z	0RHF38Z	0RHN05Z	0RHT43Z	0RJ44ZZ	0RJP0ZZ
0RG70JJ	0RGC44Z	0RGH07Z	0RGM0KZ	0RGQ4KZ	0RH543Z	0RHF43Z	0RHN08Z	0RHT44Z	0RJ4XZZ	0RJP3ZZ
0RG70K0	0RGC47Z	0RGH0JZ	0RGM0ZZ	0RGQ4ZZ	0RH603Z	0RHF44Z	0RHN33Z	0RHT45Z	0RJ50ZZ	0RJP4ZZ
0RG70K1	0RGC4JZ	0RGH0KZ	0RGM34Z	0RGR04Z	0RH608Z	0RHF48Z	0RHN34Z	0RHT48Z	0RJ53ZZ	0RJPXZZ
0RG70KJ	0RGC4KZ	0RGH0ZZ	0RGM35Z	0RGR05Z	0RH633Z	0RHG03Z	0RHN35Z	0RHU04Z	0RJ54ZZ	0RJQ0ZZ
0RG70Z0	0RGC4ZZ	0RGH34Z	0RGM37Z	0RGR07Z	0RH638Z	0RHG04Z	0RHN38Z	0RHU05Z	0RJ5XZZ	0RJQ3ZZ
0RG70Z1	0RGD04Z	0RGH37Z	0RGM3JZ	0RGR0JZ	0RH643Z	0RHG08Z	0RHN43Z	0RHU08Z	0RJ60ZZ	0RJQ4ZZ
0RG70ZJ	0RGD07Z	0RGH3JZ	0RGM3KZ	0RGR0KZ	0RH648Z	0RHG33Z	0RHN44Z	0RHU33Z	0RJ63ZZ	0RJQXZZ
0RG7370	0RGD0JZ	0RGH3KZ	0RGM3ZZ	0RGR0ZZ	0RH64CZ	0RHG34Z	0RHN45Z	0RHU34Z	0RJ64ZZ	0RJR0ZZ
0RG7371	0RGD0KZ	0RGH3ZZ	0RGM44Z	0RGR34Z	0RH64DZ	0RHG38Z	0RHN48Z	0RHU35Z	0RJ6XZZ	0RJR3ZZ
0RG737J	0RGD0ZZ	0RGH44Z	0RGM45Z	0RGR35Z	0RH903Z	0RHG43Z	0RHP03Z	0RHU38Z	0RJ90ZZ	0RJR4ZZ
0RG73A0	0RGD34Z	0RGH47Z	0RGM47Z	0RGR37Z	0RH933Z	0RHG44Z	0RHP04Z	0RHU43Z	0RJ93ZZ	0RJRXZZ
0RG73AJ	0RGD37Z	0RGH4JZ	0RGM4JZ	0RGR3JZ	0RH943Z	0RHG48Z	0RHP05Z	0RHU44Z	0RJ94ZZ	0RJS0ZZ
0RG73J0	0RGD3JZ	0RGH4KZ	0RGM4KZ	0RGR3KZ	0RHA03Z	0RHH03Z	0RHP08Z	0RHU45Z	0RJ9XZZ	0RJS3ZZ
0RG73J1	0RGD3KZ	0RGH4ZZ	0RGM4ZZ	0RGR3ZZ	0RHA04Z	0RHH04Z	0RHP33Z	0RHU48Z	0RJA0ZZ	0RJS4ZZ
0RG73JJ	0RGD3ZZ	0RGJ04Z	0RGN04Z	0RGR44Z	0RHA08Z	0RHH08Z	0RHP34Z	0RHV03Z	0RJA3ZZ	0RJSXZZ
0RG73K0	0RGD44Z	0RGJ07Z	0RGN05Z	0RGR45Z	0RHA0BZ	0RHH33Z	0RHP35Z	0RHV04Z	0RJA4ZZ	0RJT0ZZ
0RG73K1	0RGD47Z	0RGJ0JZ	0RGN07Z	0RGR47Z	0RHA0CZ	0RHH34Z	0RHP38Z	0RHV05Z	0RJAXZZ	0RJT3ZZ
0RG73KJ	0RGD4JZ	0RGJ0KZ	0RGN0JZ	0RGR4JZ	0RHA0DZ	0RHH38Z	0RHP43Z	0RHV08Z	0RJB0ZZ	0RJT4ZZ
0RG73Z0	0RGD4KZ	0RGJ0ZZ	0RGN0KZ	0RGR4KZ	0RHA33Z	0RHH43Z	0RHP44Z	0RHV33Z	0RJB3ZZ	0RJTXZZ
0RG73Z1	0RGD4ZZ	0RGJ34Z	0RGN0ZZ	0RGR4ZZ	0RHA34Z	0RHH44Z	0RHP45Z	0RHV34Z	0RJB4ZZ	0RJU0ZZ
0RG73ZJ	0RGE04Z	0RGJ37Z	0RGN34Z	0RGS04Z	0RHA38Z	0RHH48Z	0RHP48Z	0RHV35Z	0RJBXZZ	0RJU3ZZ
0RG7470	0RGE07Z	0RGJ3JZ	0RGN35Z	0RGS05Z	0RHA3BZ	0RHJ03Z	0RHQ03Z	0RHV38Z	0RJC0ZZ	0RJU4ZZ
0RG7471	0RGE0JZ	0RGJ3KZ	0RGN37Z	0RGS07Z	0RHA3CZ	0RHJ04Z	0RHQ04Z	0RHV43Z	0RJC3ZZ	0RJUXZZ
0RG747J	0RGE0KZ	0RGJ3ZZ	0RGN3JZ	0RGS0JZ	0RHA3DZ	0RHJ08Z	0RHQ05Z	0RHV44Z	0RJC4ZZ	0RJV0ZZ
0RG74A0	0RGE0ZZ	0RGJ44Z	0RGN3KZ	0RGS0KZ	0RHA43Z	0RHJ33Z	0RHQ08Z	0RHV45Z	0RJCXZZ	0RJV3ZZ
0RGA0Z0	0RGE34Z	0RGJ47Z	0RGN3ZZ	0RGS0ZZ	0RHA44Z	0RHJ34Z	0RHQ33Z	0RHV48Z	0RJD0ZZ	0RJV4ZZ
0RGA0Z1	0RGE37Z	0RGJ4JZ	0RGN44Z	0RGS34Z	0RHA48Z	0RHJ38Z	0RHQ34Z	0RHW03Z	0RJD3ZZ	0RJVXZZ
0RGA0ZJ	0RGE3JZ	0RGJ4KZ	0RGN45Z	0RGS35Z	0RHA4BZ	0RHJ43Z	0RHQ35Z	0RHW04Z	0RJD4ZZ	0RJW0ZZ
0RGA370	0RGE3KZ	0RGJ4ZZ	0RGN47Z	0RGS37Z	0RHA4CZ	0RHJ44Z	0RHQ38Z	0RHW05Z	0RJDXZZ	0RJW3ZZ
0RGA371	0RGE3ZZ	0RGK04Z	0RGN4JZ	0RGS3JZ	0RHA4DZ	0RHJ48Z	0RHQ43Z	0RHW08Z	0RJE0ZZ	0RJW4ZZ
0RGA37J	0RGE44Z	0RGK07Z	0RGN4KZ	0RGS3KZ	0RHB03Z	0RHK03Z	0RHQ44Z	0RHW33Z	0RJE3ZZ	0RJWXZZ
0RGA3A0	0RGE47Z	0RGK0JZ	0RGN4ZZ	0RGS3ZZ	0RHB33Z	0RHK04Z	0RHQ45Z	0RHW34Z	0RJE4ZZ	0RJX0ZZ
0RGA3AJ	0RGE4JZ	0RGK0KZ	0RGP04Z	0RGS44Z	0RHB43Z	0RHK08Z	0RHQ48Z	0RHW35Z	0RJEXZZ	0RJX3ZZ
0RGA3J0	0RGE4KZ	0RGK0ZZ	0RGP05Z	0RGS45Z	0RHC03Z	0RHK33Z	0RHR03Z	0RHW38Z	0RJF0ZZ	0RJX4ZZ
0RGA3J1	0RGE4ZZ	0RGK34Z	0RGP07Z	0RGS47Z	0RHC04Z	0RHK34Z	0RHR04Z	0RHW43Z	0RJF3ZZ	0RJXXZZ
0RGA3JJ	0RGF04Z	0RGK37Z	0RGP0JZ	0RGS4JZ	0RHC08Z	0RHK38Z	0RHR05Z	0RHW44Z	0RJF4ZZ	0RN00ZZ
0RGA3K0	0RGF07Z	0RGK3JZ	0RGP0KZ	0RGS4KZ	0RHC33Z	0RHK43Z	0RHR08Z	0RHW45Z	0RJFXZZ	0RN03ZZ
0RGA3K1	0RGF0JZ	0RGK3KZ	0RGP0ZZ	0RGS4ZZ	0RHC34Z	0RHK44Z	0RHR33Z	0RHW48Z	0RJG0ZZ	0RN04ZZ

0RN0XZZ	0RNL3ZZ	0RP047Z	0RP43JZ	0RP93KZ	0RPF30Z	0RPN3KZ	0RPQX3Z	0RPT0KZ	0RPV43Z	0RPXX5Z
0RN10ZZ	0RNL4ZZ	0RP048Z	0RP43KZ	0RP940Z	0RPF33Z	0RPN40Z	0RPQX4Z	0RPT30Z	0RPV44Z	0RQ00ZZ
0RN13ZZ	0RNLXZZ	0RP04AZ	0RP440Z	0RP943Z	0RPF38Z	0RPN43Z	0RPQX5Z	0RPT33Z	0RPV45Z	0RQ03ZZ
0RN14ZZ	0RNM0ZZ	0RP04JZ	0RP443Z	0RP947Z	0RPF48Z	0RPN44Z	0RPR00Z	0RPT34Z	0RPV47Z	0RQ04ZZ
0RN1XZZ	0RNM3ZZ	0RP04KZ	0RP444Z	0RP94JZ	0RPFX0Z	0RPN45Z	0RPR03Z	0RPT35Z	0RPV48Z	0RQ0XZZ
0RN30ZZ	0RNM4ZZ	0RP0X0Z	0RP447Z	0RP94KZ	0RPFX3Z	0RPN47Z	0RPR04Z	0RPT37Z	0RPV4JZ	0RQ10ZZ
0RN33ZZ	0RNMXZZ	0RP0X3Z	0RP448Z	0RP9X0Z	0RPFX4Z	0RPN48Z	0RPR05Z	0RPT38Z	0RPV4KZ	0RQ13ZZ
0RN34ZZ	0RNN0ZZ	0RP0X4Z	0RP44AZ	0RP9X3Z	0RPG08Z	0RPN4JZ	0RPR07Z	0RPT3JZ	0RPVX0Z	0RQ14ZZ
0RN3XZZ	0RNN3ZZ	0RP100Z	0RP44JZ	0RPA00Z	0RPG30Z	0RPN4KZ	0RPR08Z	0RPT3KZ	0RPVX3Z	0RQ1XZZ
0RN40ZZ	0RNN4ZZ	0RP103Z	0RP44KZ	0RPA03Z	0RPG33Z	0RPNX0Z	0RPR0JZ	0RPT40Z	0RPVX4Z	0RQ30ZZ
0RN43ZZ	0RNNXZZ	0RP104Z	0RP4X0Z	0RPA04Z	0RPG38Z	0RPNX3Z	0RPR0KZ	0RPT43Z	0RPVX5Z	0RQ33ZZ
0RN44ZZ	0RNP0ZZ	0RP107Z	0RP4X3Z	0RPA07Z	0RPG48Z	0RPNX4Z	0RPR30Z	0RPT44Z	0RPW00Z	0RQ34ZZ
0RN4XZZ	0RNP3ZZ	0RP108Z	0RP4X4Z	0RPA08Z	0RPGX0Z	0RPNX5Z	0RPR33Z	0RPT45Z	0RPW03Z	0RQ3XZZ
0RN50ZZ	0RNP4ZZ	0RP10AZ	0RP500Z	0RPA0AZ	0RPGX3Z	0RPP00Z	0RPR34Z	0RPT47Z	0RPW04Z	0RQ40ZZ
0RN53ZZ	0RNPXZZ	0RP10JZ	0RP503Z	0RPA0JZ	0RPGX4Z	0RPP03Z	0RPR35Z	0RPT48Z	0RPW05Z	0RQ43ZZ
0RN54ZZ	0RNQ0ZZ	0RP10KZ	0RP507Z	0RPA0KZ	0RPH08Z	0RPP04Z	0RPR37Z	0RPT4JZ	0RPW07Z	0RQ44ZZ
0RN5XZZ	0RNQ3ZZ	0RP130Z	0RP50JZ	0RPA30Z	0RPH30Z	0RPP05Z	0RPR38Z	0RPT4KZ	0RPW08Z	0RQ4XZZ
0RN60ZZ	0RNQ4ZZ	0RP133Z	0RP50KZ	0RPA33Z	0RPH33Z	0RPP07Z	0RPR3JZ	0RPTX0Z	0RPW0JZ	0RQ50ZZ
0RN63ZZ	0RNQXZZ	0RP134Z	0RP530Z	0RPA34Z	0RPH38Z	0RPP08Z	0RPR3KZ	0RPTX3Z	0RPW0KZ	0RQ53ZZ
0RN64ZZ	0RNR0ZZ	0RP137Z	0RP533Z	0RPA37Z	0RPH48Z	0RPP0JZ	0RPR40Z	0RPTX4Z	0RPW30Z	0RQ54ZZ
0RN6XZZ	0RNR3ZZ	0RP138Z	0RP537Z	0RPA38Z	0RPHX0Z	0RPP0KZ	0RPR43Z	0RPTX5Z	0RPW33Z	0RQ5XZZ
0RN90ZZ	0RNR4ZZ	0RP13AZ	0RP53JZ	0RPA3AZ	0RPHX3Z	0RPP30Z	0RPR44Z	0RPU00Z	0RPW34Z	0RQ60ZZ
0RN93ZZ	0RNRXZZ	0RP13JZ	0RP53KZ	0RPA3JZ	0RPHX4Z	0RPP33Z	0RPR45Z	0RPU03Z	0RPW35Z	0RQ63ZZ
0RN94ZZ	0RNS0ZZ	0RP13KZ	0RP540Z	0RPA3KZ	0RPJ08Z	0RPP34Z	0RPR47Z	0RPU04Z	0RPW37Z	0RQ64ZZ
0RN9XZZ	0RNS3ZZ	0RP140Z	0RP543Z	0RPA40Z	0RPJ30Z	0RPP35Z	0RPR48Z	0RPU05Z	0RPW38Z	0RQ6XZZ
0RNA0ZZ	0RNS4ZZ	0RP143Z	0RP547Z	0RPA43Z	0RPJ33Z	0RPP37Z	0RPR4JZ	0RPU07Z	0RPW3JZ	0RQ90ZZ
0RNA3ZZ	0RNSXZZ	0RP144Z	0RP54JZ	0RPA44Z	0RPJ38Z	0RPP38Z	0RPR4KZ	0RPU08Z	0RPW3KZ	0RQ93ZZ
0RNA4ZZ	0RNT0ZZ	0RP147Z	0RP54KZ	0RPA47Z	0RPJ48Z	0RPP3JZ	0RPRX0Z	0RPU0JZ	0RPW40Z	0RQ94ZZ
0RNAXZZ	0RNT3ZZ	0RP148Z	0RP5X0Z	0RPA48Z	0RPJX0Z	0RPP3KZ	0RPRX3Z	0RPU0KZ	0RPW43Z	0RQ9XZZ
0RNB0ZZ	0RNT4ZZ	0RP14AZ	0RP5X3Z	0RPA4AZ	0RPJX3Z	0RPP40Z	0RPRX4Z	0RPU30Z	0RPW44Z	0RQA0ZZ
0RNB3ZZ	0RNTXZZ	0RP14JZ	0RP600Z	0RPA4JZ	0RPJX4Z	0RPP43Z	0RPRX5Z	0RPU33Z	0RPW45Z	0RQA3ZZ
0RNB4ZZ	0RNU0ZZ	0RP14KZ	0RP603Z	0RPA4KZ	0RPK08Z	0RPP44Z	0RPS00Z	0RPU34Z	0RPW47Z	0RQA4ZZ
0RNBXZZ	0RNU3ZZ	0RP1X0Z	0RP604Z	0RPAX0Z	0RPK30Z	0RPP45Z	0RPS03Z	0RPU35Z	0RPW48Z	0RQAXZZ
0RNC0ZZ	0RNU4ZZ	0RP1X3Z	0RP607Z	0RPAX3Z	0RPK33Z	0RPP47Z	0RPS04Z	0RPU37Z	0RPW4JZ	0RQB0ZZ
0RNC3ZZ	0RNUXZZ	0RP1X4Z	0RP608Z	0RPAX4Z	0RPK38Z	0RPP48Z	0RPS05Z	0RPU38Z	0RPW4KZ	0RQB3ZZ
0RNC4ZZ	0RNV0ZZ	0RP300Z	0RP60AZ	0RPB00Z	0RPK48Z	0RPP4JZ	0RPS07Z	0RPU3JZ	0RPWX0Z	0RQB4ZZ
0RNCXZZ	0RNV3ZZ	0RP303Z	0RP60JZ	0RPB03Z	0RPKX0Z	0RPP4KZ	0RPS08Z	0RPU3KZ	0RPWX3Z	0RQBXZZ
0RND0ZZ	0RNV4ZZ	0RP307Z	0RP60KZ	0RPB07Z	0RPKX3Z	0RPPX0Z	0RPS0JZ	0RPU40Z	0RPWX4Z	0RQC0ZZ
0RND3ZZ	0RNVXZZ	0RP30JZ	0RP630Z	0RPB0JZ	0RPKX4Z	0RPPX3Z	0RPS0KZ	0RPU43Z	0RPWX5Z	0RQC3ZZ
0RND4ZZ	0RNW0ZZ	0RP30KZ	0RP633Z	0RPB30Z	0RPL08Z	0RPPX4Z	0RPS30Z	0RPU44Z	0RPX00Z	0RQC4ZZ
0RNDXZZ	0RNW3ZZ	0RP330Z	0RP634Z	0RPB33Z	0RPL30Z	0RPPX5Z	0RPS33Z	0RPU45Z	0RPX03Z	0RQCXZZ
0RNE0ZZ	0RNW4ZZ	0RP333Z	0RP637Z	0RPBX0Z	0RPL33Z	0RPQ00Z	0RPS34Z	0RPU47Z	0RPX04Z	0RQD0ZZ
0RNE3ZZ	0RNWXZZ	0RP337Z	0RP638Z	0RPBX3Z	0RPL38Z	0RPQ03Z	0RPS35Z	0RPU48Z	0RPX05Z	0RQD3ZZ
0RNE4ZZ	0RNX0ZZ	0RP33JZ	0RP63AZ	0RPC08Z	0RPL48Z	0RPQ04Z	0RPS37Z	0RPU4JZ	0RPX07Z	0RQD4ZZ
0RNEXZZ	0RNX3ZZ	0RP33KZ	0RP63JZ	0RPC30Z	0RPLX0Z	0RPQ05Z	0RPS38Z	0RPU4KZ	0RPX08Z	0RQDXZZ
0RNF0ZZ	0RNX4ZZ	0RP340Z	0RP63KZ	0RPC33Z	0RPLX3Z	0RPQ07Z	0RPS3JZ	0RPUX0Z	0RPX0JZ	0RQE0ZZ
0RNF3ZZ	0RNXXZZ	0RP343Z	0RP640Z	0RPC38Z	0RPLX4Z	0RPQ08Z	0RPS3KZ	0RPUX3Z	0RPX0KZ	0RQE3ZZ
0RNF4ZZ	0RP000Z	0RP347Z	0RP643Z	0RPC48Z	0RPLX5Z	0RPQ0JZ	0RPS40Z	0RPUX4Z	0RPX30Z	0RQE4ZZ
0RNFXZZ	0RP003Z	0RP34JZ	0RP644Z	0RPCX0Z	0RPM08Z	0RPQ0KZ	0RPS43Z	0RPUX5Z	0RPX33Z	0RQEXZZ
0RNG0ZZ	0RP004Z	0RP34KZ	0RP647Z	0RPCX3Z	0RPM30Z	0RPQ30Z	0RPS44Z	0RPV00Z	0RPX34Z	0RQF0ZZ
0RNG3ZZ	0RP007Z	0RP3X0Z	0RP648Z	0RPD08Z	0RPM33Z	0RPQ33Z	0RPS45Z	0RPV03Z	0RPX35Z	0RQF3ZZ
0RNG4ZZ	0RP008Z	0RP3X3Z	0RP64AZ	0RPD30Z	0RPM38Z	0RPQ34Z	0RPS47Z	0RPV04Z	0RPX37Z	0RQF4ZZ
0RNGXZZ	0RP00AZ	0RP400Z	0RP64JZ	0RPD33Z	0RPM48Z	0RPQ35Z	0RPS48Z	0RPV05Z	0RPX38Z	0RQFXZZ
0RNH0ZZ	0RP00JZ	0RP403Z	0RP64KZ	0RPD38Z	0RPMX0Z	0RPQ37Z	0RPS4JZ	0RPV07Z	0RPX3JZ	0RQG0ZZ
0RNH3ZZ	0RP00KZ	0RP404Z	0RP6X0Z	0RPD48Z	0RPMX3Z	0RPQ38Z	0RPS4KZ	0RPV08Z	0RPX3KZ	0RQG3ZZ
0RNH4ZZ	0RP030Z	0RP407Z	0RP6X3Z	0RPDX0Z	0RPMX4Z	0RPQ3JZ	0RPSX0Z	0RPV0JZ	0RPX40Z	0RQG4ZZ
0RNHXZZ	0RP033Z	0RP408Z	0RP6X4Z	0RPDX3Z	0RPMX5Z	0RPQ3KZ	0RPSX3Z	0RPV0KZ	0RPX43Z	0RQGXZZ
0RNJ0ZZ	0RP034Z	0RP40AZ	0RP900Z	0RPE08Z	0RPN08Z	0RPQ40Z	0RPSX4Z	0RPV30Z	0RPX44Z	0RQH0ZZ
0RNJ3ZZ	0RP037Z	0RP40JZ	0RP903Z	0RPE30Z	0RPN0KZ	0RPQ43Z	0RPSX5Z	0RPV33Z	0RPX45Z	0RQH3ZZ
0RNJ4ZZ	0RP038Z	0RP40KZ	0RP907Z	0RPE33Z	0RPN30Z	0RPQ44Z	0RPT00Z	0RPV34Z	0RPX47Z	0RQH4ZZ
0RNJXZZ	0RP03AZ	0RP430Z	0RP90JZ	0RPE38Z	0RPN33Z	0RPQ45Z	0RPT03Z	0RPV35Z	0RPX48Z	0RQHXZZ
0RNK0ZZ	0RP03JZ	0RP433Z	0RP90KZ	0RPE48Z	0RPN34Z	0RPQ47Z	0RPT04Z	0RPV37Z	0RPX4JZ	0RQJ0ZZ
0RNK3ZZ	0RP03KZ	0RP434Z	0RP930Z	0RPEX0Z	0RPN35Z	0RPQ48Z	0RPT05Z	0RPV38Z	0RPX4KZ	0RQJ3ZZ
0RNK4ZZ	0RP040Z	0RP437Z	0RP933Z	0RPEX3Z	0RPN37Z	0RPQ4JZ	0RPT07Z	0RPV3JZ	0RPXX0Z	0RQJ4ZZ
0RNKXZZ	0RP043Z	0RP438Z	0RP937Z	0RPEX4Z	0RPN38Z	0RPQ4KZ	0RPT08Z	0RPV3KZ	0RPXX3Z	0RQJXZZ
0RNL0ZZ	0RP044Z	0RP43AZ	0RP93JZ	0RPF08Z	0RPN3JZ	0RPQX0Z	0RPT0JZ	0RPV40Z	0RPXX4Z	0RQK0ZZ

0RQK3ZZ	0RR607Z	0RSE4ZZ	0RSPX4Z	0RSX34Z	0RU507Z	0RUE37Z	0RUM47Z	0RW3XJZ	0RWB33Z	0RWDX7Z
0RQK4ZZ	0RR60JZ	0RSEX4Z	0RSPX5Z	0RSX35Z	0RU50JZ	0RUE3JZ	0RUM4JZ	0RW3XKZ	0RWB37Z	0RWDX8Z
0RQKXZZ	0RR60KZ	0RSEXZZ	0RSPXZZ	0RSX3ZZ	0RU50KZ	0RUE3KZ	0RUM4KZ	0RW4X0Z	0RWB3JZ	0RWDXJZ
0RQL0ZZ	0RR907Z	0RSF34Z	0RSQ34Z	0RSX44Z	0RU537Z	0RUE47Z	0RUN07Z	0RW4X3Z	0RWB3KZ	0RWDXKZ
0RQL3ZZ	0RR90JZ	0RSF3ZZ	0RSQ35Z	0RSX45Z	0RU53JZ	0RUE4JZ	0RUN0JZ	0RW4X7Z	0RWB40Z	0RWE00Z
0RQL4ZZ	0RR90KZ	0RSF44Z	0RSQ3ZZ	0RSX4ZZ	0RU53KZ	0RUE4KZ	0RUN0KZ	0RW4X8Z	0RWB43Z	0RWE03Z
0RQLXZZ	0RRA07Z	0RSF4ZZ	0RSQ44Z	0RSXX4Z	0RU547Z	0RUF07Z	0RUN37Z	0RW4XAZ	0RWB47Z	0RWE04Z
0RQM0ZZ	0RRA0JZ	0RSFX4Z	0RSQ45Z	0RSXX5Z	0RU54JZ	0RUF0JZ	0RUN3JZ	0RW4XJZ	0RWB4JZ	0RWE07Z
0RQM3ZZ	0RRA0KZ	0RSFXZZ	0RSQ4ZZ	0RSXXZZ	0RU54KZ	0RUF0KZ	0RUN3KZ	0RW4XKZ	0RWB4KZ	0RWE08Z
0RQM4ZZ	0RRB07Z	0RSG34Z	0RSQX4Z	0RTB0ZZ	0RU607Z	0RUF37Z	0RUN47Z	0RW5X0Z	0RWBX0Z	0RWE0JZ
0RQMXZZ	0RRB0JZ	0RSG3ZZ	0RSQX5Z	0RTC0ZZ	0RU60JZ	0RUF3JZ	0RUN4JZ	0RW5X3Z	0RWBX3Z	0RWE0KZ
0RQN0ZZ	0RRB0KZ	0RSG44Z	0RSQXZZ	0RTD0ZZ	0RU60KZ	0RUF3KZ	0RUN4KZ	0RW5X7Z	0RWBX7Z	0RWE30Z
0RQN3ZZ	0RRC07Z	0RSG4ZZ	0RSR34Z	0RTE0ZZ	0RU637Z	0RUF47Z	0RUP07Z	0RW5XJZ	0RWBXJZ	0RWE33Z
0RQN4ZZ	0RRC0JZ	0RSGX4Z	0RSR35Z	0RTF0ZZ	0RU63JZ	0RUF4JZ	0RUP0JZ	0RW5XKZ	0RWBXKZ	0RWE34Z
0RQNXZZ	0RRC0KZ	0RSGXZZ	0RSR3ZZ	0RTG0ZZ	0RU63KZ	0RUF4KZ	0RUP0KZ	0RW6X0Z	0RWC00Z	0RWE37Z
0RQP0ZZ	0RRD07Z	0RSH34Z	0RSR44Z	0RTH0ZZ	0RU647Z	0RUG07Z	0RUP37Z	0RW6X3Z	0RWC03Z	0RWE38Z
0RQP3ZZ	0RRD0JZ	0RSH3ZZ	0RSR45Z	0RTJ0ZZ	0RU64JZ	0RUG0JZ	0RUP3JZ	0RW6X4Z	0RWC04Z	0RWE3JZ
0RQP4ZZ	0RRD0KZ	0RSH44Z	0RSR4ZZ	0RTK0ZZ	0RU64KZ	0RUG0KZ	0RUP3KZ	0RW6X7Z	0RWC07Z	0RWE3KZ
0RQPXZZ	0RRE07Z	0RSH4ZZ	0RSRX4Z	0RTL0ZZ	0RU907Z	0RUG37Z	0RUP47Z	0RW6X8Z	0RWC08Z	0RWE40Z
0RQQ0ZZ	0RRE0JZ	0RSHX4Z	0RSRX5Z	0RTM0ZZ	0RU90JZ	0RUG3JZ	0RUP4JZ	0RW6XAZ	0RWC0JZ	0RWE43Z
0RQQ3ZZ	0RRE0KZ	0RSHXZZ	0RSRXZZ	0RTN0ZZ	0RU90KZ	0RUG3KZ	0RUP4KZ	0RW6XJZ	0RWC0KZ	0RWE44Z
0RQQ4ZZ	0RS034Z	0RSJ34Z	0RSS34Z	0RTP0ZZ	0RU937Z	0RUG47Z	0RUQ07Z	0RW6XKZ	0RWC30Z	0RWE47Z
0RQQXZZ	0RS03ZZ	0RSJ3ZZ	0RSS35Z	0RTQ0ZZ	0RU93JZ	0RUG4JZ	0RUQ0JZ	0RW9X0Z	0RWC33Z	0RWE48Z
0RQR0ZZ	0RS044Z	0RSJ44Z	0RSS3ZZ	0RTR0ZZ	0RU93KZ	0RUG4KZ	0RUQ0KZ	0RW9X3Z	0RWC34Z	0RWE4JZ
0RQR3ZZ	0RS04ZZ	0RSJ4ZZ	0RSS44Z	0RTS0ZZ	0RU947Z	0RUH07Z	0RUQ37Z	0RW9X7Z	0RWC37Z	0RWE4KZ
0RQR4ZZ	0RS0X4Z	0RSJX4Z	0RSS45Z	0RTT0ZZ	0RU94JZ	0RUH0JZ	0RUQ3JZ	0RW9XJZ	0RWC38Z	0RWEX0Z
0RQRXZZ	0RS0XZZ	0RSJXZZ	0RSS4ZZ	0RTU0ZZ	0RU94KZ	0RUH0KZ	0RUQ3KZ	0RW9XKZ	0RWC3JZ	0RWEX3Z
0RQS0ZZ	0RS134Z	0RSK34Z	0RSSX4Z	0RTV0ZZ	0RUA07Z	0RUH37Z	0RUQ47Z	0RWA00Z	0RWC3KZ	0RWEX4Z
0RQS3ZZ	0RS13ZZ	0RSK3ZZ	0RSSX5Z	0RTW0ZZ	0RUA0JZ	0RUH3JZ	0RUQ4JZ	0RWA03Z	0RWC40Z	0RWEX7Z
0RQS4ZZ	0RS144Z	0RSK44Z	0RSSXZZ	0RTX0ZZ	0RUA0KZ	0RUH3KZ	0RUQ4KZ	0RWA04Z	0RWC43Z	0RWEX8Z
0RQSXZZ	0RS14ZZ	0RSK4ZZ	0RST34Z	0RU007Z	0RUA37Z	0RUH47Z	0RUR07Z	0RWA07Z	0RWC44Z	0RWEXJZ
0RQT0ZZ	0RS1X4Z	0RSKX4Z	0RST35Z	0RU00JZ	0RUA3JZ	0RUH4JZ	0RUR0JZ	0RWA08Z	0RWC47Z	0RWEXKZ
0RQT3ZZ	0RS1XZZ	0RSKXZZ	0RST3ZZ	0RU00KZ	0RUA3KZ	0RUH4KZ	0RUR0KZ	0RWA0AZ	0RWC48Z	0RWF00Z
0RQT4ZZ	0RS434Z	0RSL34Z	0RST44Z	0RU037Z	0RUA47Z	0RUJ07Z	0RUR37Z	0RWA0JZ	0RWC4JZ	0RWF03Z
0RQTXZZ	0RS43ZZ	0RSL35Z	0RST45Z	0RU03JZ	0RUA4JZ	0RUJ0JZ	0RUR3JZ	0RWA0KZ	0RWC4KZ	0RWF04Z
0RQU0ZZ	0RS444Z	0RSL3ZZ	0RST4ZZ	0RU03KZ	0RUA4KZ	0RUJ0KZ	0RUR3KZ	0RWA30Z	0RWCX0Z	0RWF07Z
0RQU3ZZ	0RS44ZZ	0RSL44Z	0RSTX4Z	0RU047Z	0RUB07Z	0RUJ37Z	0RUR47Z	0RWA33Z	0RWCX3Z	0RWF08Z
0RQU4ZZ	0RS4X4Z	0RSL45Z	0RSTX5Z	0RU04JZ	0RUB0JZ	0RUJ3JZ	0RUR4JZ	0RWA34Z	0RWCX4Z	0RWF0JZ
0RQUXZZ	0RS4XZZ	0RSL4ZZ	0RSTXZZ	0RU04KZ	0RUB0KZ	0RUJ3KZ	0RUR4KZ	0RWA37Z	0RWCX7Z	0RWF0KZ
0RQV0ZZ	0RS634Z	0RSLX4Z	0RSU34Z	0RU107Z	0RUB37Z	0RUJ47Z	0RUS07Z	0RWA38Z	0RWCX8Z	0RWF30Z
0RQV3ZZ	0RS63ZZ	0RSLX5Z	0RSU35Z	0RU10JZ	0RUB3JZ	0RUJ4JZ	0RUS0JZ	0RWA3AZ	0RWCXJZ	0RWF33Z
0RQV4ZZ	0RS644Z	0RSLXZZ	0RSU3ZZ	0RU10KZ	0RUB3KZ	0RUJ4KZ	0RUS0KZ	0RWA3JZ	0RWCXKZ	0RWF34Z
0RQVXZZ	0RS64ZZ	0RSM34Z	0RSU44Z	0RU137Z	0RUB47Z	0RUK07Z	0RUS37Z	0RWA3KZ	0RWD00Z	0RWF37Z
0RQW0ZZ	0RS6X4Z	0RSM35Z	0RSU45Z	0RU13JZ	0RUB4JZ	0RUK0JZ	0RUS3JZ	0RWA40Z	0RWD03Z	0RWF38Z
0RQW3ZZ	0RS6XZZ	0RSM3ZZ	0RSU4ZZ	0RU13KZ	0RUB4KZ	0RUK0KZ	0RUS3KZ	0RWA43Z	0RWD04Z	0RWF3JZ
0RQW4ZZ	0RSA34Z	0RSM44Z	0RSUX4Z	0RU147Z	0RUC07Z	0RUK37Z	0RUS4JZ	0RWA44Z	0RWD07Z	0RWF3KZ
0RQWXZZ	0RSA3ZZ	0RSM45Z	0RSUX5Z	0RU14JZ	0RUC0JZ	0RUK3JZ	0RUS4JZ	0RWA47Z	0RWD08Z	0RWF40Z
0RQX0ZZ	0RSA44Z	0RSM4ZZ	0RSUXZZ	0RU14KZ	0RUC0KZ	0RUK3KZ	0RW0X0Z	0RWA48Z	0RWD0JZ	0RWF43Z
0RQX3ZZ	0RSA4ZZ	0RSMX4Z	0RSV34Z	0RU307Z	0RUC37Z	0RUK47Z	0RW0X3Z	0RWA4AZ	0RWD0KZ	0RWF44Z
0RQX4ZZ	0RSAX4Z	0RSMX5Z	0RSV35Z	0RU30JZ	0RUC3JZ	0RUK4JZ	0RW0X4Z	0RWA4JZ	0RWD30Z	0RWF47Z
0RQXXZZ	0RSAXZZ	0RSMXZZ	0RSV3ZZ	0RU30KZ	0RUC3KZ	0RUK4KZ	0RW0X7Z	0RWA4KZ	0RWD33Z	0RWF48Z
0RR007Z	0RSC34Z	0RSN34Z	0RSV44Z	0RU337Z	0RUC47Z	0RUL07Z	0RW0X8Z	0RWAX0Z	0RWD34Z	0RWF4JZ
0RR00JZ	0RSC3ZZ	0RSN35Z	0RSV45Z	0RU33JZ	0RUC4JZ	0RUL0JZ	0RW0XAZ	0RWAX3Z	0RWD37Z	0RWF4KZ
0RR00KZ	0RSC44Z	0RSN3ZZ	0RSV4ZZ	0RU33KZ	0RUC4KZ	0RUL0KZ	0RW0XJZ	0RWAX4Z	0RWD38Z	0RWFX0Z
0RR107Z	0RSC4ZZ	0RSN44Z	0RSVX4Z	0RU347Z	0RUD07Z	0RUL37Z	0RW0XKZ	0RWAX7Z	0RWD3JZ	0RWFX3Z
0RR10JZ	0RSCX4Z	0RSN45Z	0RSVX5Z	0RU34JZ	0RUD0JZ	0RUL3JZ	0RW1X0Z	0RWAX8Z	0RWD3KZ	0RWFX4Z
0RR10KZ	0RSCXZZ	0RSN4ZZ	0RSVXZZ	0RU34KZ	0RUD0KZ	0RUL3KZ	0RW1X3Z	0RWAXAZ	0RWD40Z	0RWFX7Z
0RR307Z	0RSD34Z	0RSNX4Z	0RSW34Z	0RU407Z	0RUD37Z	0RUL47Z	0RW1X4Z	0RWAXJZ	0RWD43Z	0RWFX8Z
0RR30JZ	0RSD3ZZ	0RSNX5Z	0RSW35Z	0RU40JZ	0RUD3JZ	0RUL4JZ	0RW1X7Z	0RWAXKZ	0RWD44Z	0RWFXJZ
0RR30KZ	0RSD44Z	0RSNXZZ	0RSW3ZZ	0RU40KZ	0RUD3KZ	0RUL4KZ	0RW1X8Z	0RWB00Z	0RWD47Z	0RWFXKZ
0RR407Z	0RSD4ZZ	0RSP34Z	0RSW44Z	0RU437Z	0RUD47Z	0RUM07Z	0RW1XAZ	0RWB03Z	0RWD48Z	0RWG00Z
0RR40JZ	0RSDX4Z	0RSP35Z	0RSW45Z	0RU43JZ	0RUD4JZ	0RUM0JZ	0RW1XJZ	0RWB07Z	0RWD4JZ	0RWG03Z
0RR40KZ	0RSDXZZ	0RSP3ZZ	0RSW4ZZ	0RU43KZ	0RUD4KZ	0RUM0KZ	0RW1XKZ	0RWB0JZ	0RWD4KZ	0RWG04Z
0RR507Z	0RSE34Z	0RSP44Z	0RSWX4Z	0RU447Z	0RUE07Z	0RUM37Z	0RW3X0Z	0RWB0KZ	0RWDX0Z	0RWG07Z
0RR50JZ	0RSE3ZZ	0RSP45Z	0RSWX5Z	0RU44JZ	0RUE0JZ	0RUM3JZ	0RW3X3Z	0RWB30Z	0RWDX3Z	0RWG08Z
0RR50KZ	0RSE44Z	0RSP4ZZ	0RSWXZZ	0RU44KZ	0RUE0KZ	0RUM3KZ	0RW3X7Z	0RWB30Z	0RWDX4Z	0RWG0JZ

0RWG0KZ	0RWJ44Z	0RWLX4Z	0RWNX7Z	0RWQXJZ	0RWT00Z	0RWWX8Z	0S964ZX	0S9G0ZX	0S9P3ZX	0SB94ZX
0RWG30Z	0RWJ47Z	0RWLX5Z	0RWNX8Z	0RWQXKZ	0RWT03Z	0RWWXJZ	0S964ZZ	0S9G0ZZ	0S9P3ZZ	0SB94ZZ
0RWG33Z	0RWJ48Z	0RWLX7Z	0RWNXJZ	0RWR00Z	0RWT04Z	0RWWXKZ	0S9700Z	0S9G30Z	0S9P40Z	0SBB0ZX
0RWG34Z	0RWJ4JZ	0RWLX8Z	0RWNXKZ	0RWR03Z	0RWT05Z	0RWXX0Z	0S970ZX	0S9G3ZX	0S9P4ZX	0SBB0ZZ
0RWG37Z	0RWJ4KZ	0RWLXJZ	0RWP00Z	0RWR04Z	0RWT07Z	0RWXX3Z	0S970ZZ	0S9G3ZZ	0S9P4ZZ	0SBB3ZX
0RWG38Z	0RWJX0Z	0RWLXKZ	0RWP03Z	0RWR05Z	0RWT08Z	0RWXX4Z	0S9730Z	0S9G40Z	0S9Q00Z	0SBB3ZZ
0RWG3JZ	0RWJX3Z	0RWM00Z	0RWP04Z	0RWR07Z	0RWT0JZ	0RWXX5Z	0S973ZX	0S9G4ZX	0S9Q0ZX	0SBB4ZX
0RWG3KZ	0RWJX4Z	0RWM03Z	0RWP05Z	0RWR08Z	0RWT0KZ	0RWXX7Z	0S973ZZ	0S9G4ZZ	0S9Q0ZZ	0SBB4ZZ
0RWG40Z	0RWJX7Z	0RWM04Z	0RWP07Z	0RWR0JZ	0RWT30Z	0RWXX8Z	0S9740Z	0S9H00Z	0S9Q30Z	0SBC0ZX
0RWG43Z	0RWJX8Z	0RWM05Z	0RWP08Z	0RWR0KZ	0RWT33Z	0RWXXJZ	0S974ZX	0S9H0ZX	0S9Q3ZX	0SBC0ZZ
0RWG44Z	0RWJXJZ	0RWM07Z	0RWP0JZ	0RWR30Z	0RWT34Z	0RWXXKZ	0S974ZZ	0S9H0ZZ	0S9Q3ZZ	0SBC3ZX
0RWG47Z	0RWJXKZ	0RWM08Z	0RWP0KZ	0RWR33Z	0RWT35Z	0S2YX0Z	0S9800Z	0S9H30Z	0S9Q40Z	0SBC3ZZ
0RWG48Z	0RWK00Z	0RWM0JZ	0RWP30Z	0RWR34Z	0RWT37Z	0S2YXYZ	0S980ZX	0S9H3ZX	0S9Q4ZX	0SBC4ZX
0RWG4JZ	0RWK03Z	0RWM0KZ	0RWP33Z	0RWR35Z	0RWT38Z	0S5Q4ZZ	0S980ZZ	0S9H3ZZ	0S9Q4ZZ	0SBC4ZZ
0RWG4KZ	0RWK04Z	0RWM30Z	0RWP34Z	0RWR37Z	0RWT3JZ	0S9000Z	0S9830Z	0S9H40Z	0SB00ZX	0SBD0ZX
0RWGX0Z	0RWK07Z	0RWM33Z	0RWP35Z	0RWR38Z	0RWT3KZ	0S900ZX	0S983ZX	0S9H4ZX	0SB00ZZ	0SBD0ZZ
0RWGX3Z	0RWK08Z	0RWM34Z	0RWP37Z	0RWR3JZ	0RWT40Z	0S900ZZ	0S983ZZ	0S9H4ZZ	0SB03ZX	0SBD3ZX
0RWGX4Z	0RWK0JZ	0RWM35Z	0RWP38Z	0RWR3KZ	0RWT43Z	0S9030Z	0S9840Z	0S9J00Z	0SB03ZZ	0SBD3ZZ
0RWGX7Z	0RWK0KZ	0RWM37Z	0RWP3JZ	0RWR40Z	0RWT44Z	0S903ZX	0S984ZX	0S9J0ZX	0SB04ZX	0SBD4ZX
0RWGX8Z	0RWK30Z	0RWM38Z	0RWP3KZ	0RWR43Z	0RWT45Z	0S903ZZ	0S984ZZ	0S9J0ZZ	0SB04ZZ	0SBD4ZZ
0RWGXJZ	0RWK33Z	0RWM3JZ	0RWP40Z	0RWR44Z	0RWT47Z	0S9040Z	0S9900Z	0S9J30Z	0SB20ZX	0SBF0ZX
0RWGXKZ	0RWK34Z	0RWM3KZ	0RWP43Z	0RWR45Z	0RWT48Z	0S904ZX	0S990ZX	0S9J3ZX	0SB20ZZ	0SBF0ZZ
0RWH00Z	0RWK37Z	0RWM40Z	0RWP44Z	0RWR47Z	0RWT4JZ	0S904ZZ	0S990ZZ	0S9J3ZZ	0SB23ZX	0SBF3ZX
0RWH03Z	0RWK38Z	0RWM43Z	0RWP45Z	0RWR48Z	0RWT4KZ	0S9200Z	0S9930Z	0S9J40Z	0SB23ZZ	0SBF3ZZ
0RWH04Z	0RWK3JZ	0RWM44Z	0RWP47Z	0RWR4JZ	0RWTX0Z	0S920ZX	0S993ZX	0S9J4ZX	0SB24ZX	0SBF4ZX
0RWH07Z	0RWK3KZ	0RWM45Z	0RWP48Z	0RWR4KZ	0RWTX3Z	0S920ZZ	0S993ZZ	0S9J4ZZ	0SB24ZZ	0SBF4ZZ
0RWH08Z	0RWK40Z	0RWM47Z	0RWP4JZ	0RWRX0Z	0RWTX4Z	0S9230Z	0S9940Z	0S9K00Z	0SB30ZX	0SBG0ZX
0RWH0JZ	0RWK43Z	0RWM48Z	0RWP4KZ	0RWRX3Z	0RWTX5Z	0S923ZX	0S994ZX	0S9K0ZX	0SB30ZZ	0SBG0ZZ
0RWH0KZ	0RWK44Z	0RWM4JZ	0RWPX0Z	0RWRX4Z	0RWTX7Z	0S923ZZ	0S994ZZ	0S9K0ZZ	0SB33ZX	0SBG3ZX
0RWH30Z	0RWK47Z	0RWM4KZ	0RWPX3Z	0RWRX5Z	0RWTX8Z	0S9240Z	0S9B00Z	0S9K30Z	0SB33ZZ	0SBG3ZZ
0RWH33Z	0RWK48Z	0RWMX0Z	0RWPX4Z	0RWRX7Z	0RWTXJZ	0S924ZX	0S9B0ZX	0S9K3ZX	0SB34ZX	0SBG4ZX
0RWH34Z	0RWK4JZ	0RWMX3Z	0RWPX5Z	0RWRX8Z	0RWTXKZ	0S924ZZ	0S9B0ZZ	0S9K3ZZ	0SB34ZZ	0SBG4ZZ
0RWH37Z	0RWK4KZ	0RWMX4Z	0RWPX7Z	0RWRXJZ	0RWU00Z	0S9300Z	0S9B30Z	0S9K40Z	0SB40ZX	0SBH0ZX
0RWH38Z	0RWKX0Z	0RWMX5Z	0RWPX8Z	0RWRXKZ	0RWU03Z	0S930ZX	0S9B3ZX	0S9K4ZX	0SB40ZZ	0SBH0ZZ
0RWH3JZ	0RWKX3Z	0RWMX7Z	0RWPXJZ	0RWS00Z	0RWU04Z	0S930ZZ	0S9B3ZZ	0S9K4ZZ	0SB43ZX	0SBH3ZX
0RWH3KZ	0RWKX4Z	0RWMX8Z	0RWPXKZ	0RWS03Z	0RWU05Z	0S9330Z	0S9B40Z	0S9L00Z	0SB43ZZ	0SBH3ZZ
0RWH40Z	0RWKX7Z	0RWMXJZ	0RWQ00Z	0RWS04Z	0RWU07Z	0S933ZX	0S9B4ZX	0S9L0ZX	0SB44ZX	0SBH4ZX
0RWH43Z	0RWKX8Z	0RWMXKZ	0RWQ03Z	0RWS05Z	0RWU08Z	0S933ZZ	0S9B4ZZ	0S9L0ZZ	0SB44ZZ	0SBH4ZZ
0RWH44Z	0RWKXJZ	0RWN00Z	0RWQ04Z	0RWS07Z	0RWU0JZ	0S9340Z	0S9C00Z	0S9L30Z	0SB50ZX	0SBJ0ZX
0RWH47Z	0RWKXKZ	0RWN03Z	0RWQ05Z	0RWS08Z	0RWU0KZ	0S934ZX	0S9C0ZX	0S9L3ZX	0SB50ZZ	0SBJ0ZZ
0RWH48Z	0RWL00Z	0RWN04Z	0RWQ07Z	0RWS0JZ	0RWU30Z	0S934ZZ	0S9C0ZZ	0S9L3ZZ	0SB53ZX	0SBJ3ZX
0RWH4JZ	0RWL03Z	0RWN05Z	0RWQ08Z	0RWS0KZ	0RWU33Z	0S9400Z	0S9C30Z	0S9L40Z	0SB53ZZ	0SBJ3ZZ
0RWH4KZ	0RWL04Z	0RWN07Z	0RWQ0JZ	0RWS30Z	0RWU34Z	0S940ZX	0S9C3ZX	0S9L4ZX	0SB54ZX	0SBJ4ZX
0RWHX0Z	0RWL05Z	0RWN08Z	0RWQ0KZ	0RWS33Z	0RWU35Z	0S940ZZ	0S9C3ZZ	0S9L4ZZ	0SB54ZZ	0SBJ4ZZ
0RWHX3Z	0RWL07Z	0RWN0JZ	0RWQ30Z	0RWS34Z	0RWU37Z	0S9430Z	0S9C40Z	0S9M00Z	0SB60ZX	0SBK0ZX
0RWHX4Z	0RWL08Z	0RWN0KZ	0RWQ33Z	0RWS35Z	0RWUX0Z	0S943ZX	0S9C4ZX	0S9M0ZX	0SB60ZZ	0SBK0ZZ
0RWHX7Z	0RWL0JZ	0RWN30Z	0RWQ34Z	0RWS37Z	0RWUX3Z	0S943ZZ	0S9C4ZZ	0S9M0ZZ	0SB63ZX	0SBK3ZX
0RWHX8Z	0RWL0KZ	0RWN33Z	0RWQ35Z	0RWS38Z	0RWUX4Z	0S9440Z	0S9D00Z	0S9M30Z	0SB63ZZ	0SBK3ZZ
0RWHXJZ	0RWL30Z	0RWN34Z	0RWQ37Z	0RWS3JZ	0RWUX5Z	0S944ZX	0S9D0ZX	0S9M3ZX	0SB64ZX	0SBK4ZX
0RWHXKZ	0RWL33Z	0RWN35Z	0RWQ38Z	0RWS3KZ	0RWUX7Z	0S944ZZ	0S9D0ZZ	0S9M3ZZ	0SB64ZZ	0SBK4ZZ
0RWJ00Z	0RWL34Z	0RWN37Z	0RWQ3JZ	0RWS40Z	0RWUX8Z	0S9500Z	0S9D30Z	0S9M40Z	0SB70ZX	0SBL0ZX
0RWJ03Z	0RWL35Z	0RWN38Z	0RWQ3KZ	0RWS43Z	0RWUXJZ	0S950ZX	0S9D3ZX	0S9M4ZX	0SB70ZZ	0SBL0ZZ
0RWJ04Z	0RWL37Z	0RWN3JZ	0RWQ40Z	0RWS44Z	0RWUXKZ	0S950ZZ	0S9D3ZZ	0S9M4ZZ	0SB73ZX	0SBL3ZX
0RWJ07Z	0RWL38Z	0RWN3KZ	0RWQ43Z	0RWS45Z	0RWVX0Z	0S9530Z	0S9D40Z	0S9N00Z	0SB73ZZ	0SBL3ZZ
0RWJ08Z	0RWL3JZ	0RWN40Z	0RWQ44Z	0RWS47Z	0RWVX3Z	0S953ZX	0S9D4ZX	0S9N0ZX	0SB74ZX	0SBL4ZX
0RWJ0JZ	0RWL3KZ	0RWN43Z	0RWQ45Z	0RWS48Z	0RWVX4Z	0S953ZZ	0S9D4ZZ	0S9N0ZZ	0SB74ZZ	0SBL4ZZ
0RWJ0KZ	0RWL40Z	0RWN44Z	0RWQ47Z	0RWS4JZ	0RWVX5Z	0S9540Z	0S9F00Z	0S9N30Z	0SB80ZX	0SBM0ZX
0RWJ30Z	0RWL43Z	0RWN45Z	0RWQ48Z	0RWS4KZ	0RWVX7Z	0S954ZX	0S9F0ZX	0S9N3ZX	0SB80ZZ	0SBM0ZZ
0RWJ33Z	0RWL44Z	0RWN47Z	0RWQ4JZ	0RWSX0Z	0RWVX8Z	0S954ZZ	0S9F0ZZ	0S9N3ZZ	0SB83ZX	0SBM3ZX
0RWJ34Z	0RWL45Z	0RWN48Z	0RWQ4KZ	0RWSX3Z	0RWVXJZ	0S9600Z	0S9F30Z	0S9N40Z	0SB83ZZ	0SBM3ZZ
0RWJ37Z	0RWL47Z	0RWN4JZ	0RWQX0Z	0RWSX4Z	0RWVXKZ	0S960ZX	0S9F3ZX	0S9N4ZX	0SB84ZX	0SBM4ZX
0RWJ38Z	0RWL48Z	0RWN4KZ	0RWQX3Z	0RWSX5Z	0RWWX0Z	0S960ZZ	0S9F3ZZ	0S9N4ZZ	0SB84ZZ	0SBM4ZZ
0RWJ3JZ	0RWL4JZ	0RWNX0Z	0RWQX4Z	0RWSX7Z	0RWWX3Z	0S9630Z	0S9F40Z	0S9P00Z	0SB90ZX	0SBN0ZX
0RWJ3KZ	0RWL4KZ	0RWNX3Z	0RWQX5Z	0RWSX8Z	0RWWX4Z	0S963ZX	0S9F4ZX	0S9P0ZX	0SB90ZZ	0SBN0ZZ
0RWJ40Z	0RWLX0Z	0RWNX4Z	0RWQX7Z	0RWSXJZ	0RWWX5Z	0S963ZZ	0S9F4ZZ	0S9P0ZZ	0SB93ZX	0SBN3ZX
0RWJ43Z	0RWLX3Z	0RWNX5Z	0RWQX8Z	0RWSXKZ	0RWWX7Z	0S9640Z	0S9G00Z	0S9P30Z	0SB93ZZ	0SBN3ZZ

0SBN4ZX	0SCL3ZZ	0SG10KJ	0SG844Z	0SGD35Z	0SH038Z	0SHB38Z	0SHJ04Z	0SHP38Z	0SJF3ZZ	0SN7XZZ
0SBN4ZZ	0SCL4ZZ	0SG34AJ	0SG847Z	0SGD37Z	0SH043Z	0SHB43Z	0SHJ05Z	0SHP43Z	0SJF4ZZ	0SN80ZZ
0SBP0ZX	0SCM0ZZ	0SG34J0	0SG84JZ	0SGD3JZ	0SH048Z	0SHB44Z	0SHJ08Z	0SHP44Z	0SJFXZZ	0SN83ZZ
0SBP0ZZ	0SCM3ZZ	0SG34J1	0SG84KZ	0SGD3KZ	0SH203Z	0SHB45Z	0SHJ33Z	0SHP45Z	0SJG0ZZ	0SN84ZZ
0SBP3ZX	0SCM4ZZ	0SG34JJ	0SG84ZZ	0SGD3ZZ	0SH208Z	0SHB48Z	0SHJ34Z	0SHP48Z	0SJG3ZZ	0SN8XZZ
0SBP3ZZ	0SCN0ZZ	0SG34K0	0SG904Z	0SGD44Z	0SH233Z	0SHC03Z	0SHJ35Z	0SHQ03Z	0SJG4ZZ	0SN90ZZ
0SBP4ZX	0SCN3ZZ	0SG34K1	0SG905Z	0SGD45Z	0SH238Z	0SHC04Z	0SHJ38Z	0SHQ04Z	0SJGXZZ	0SN93ZZ
0SBP4ZZ	0SCN4ZZ	0SG34KJ	0SG907Z	0SGD47Z	0SH243Z	0SHC05Z	0SHJ43Z	0SHQ05Z	0SJH0ZZ	0SN94ZZ
0SBQ0ZX	0SCP0ZZ	0SG34Z0	0SG90JZ	0SGD4JZ	0SH248Z	0SHC08Z	0SHJ44Z	0SHQ08Z	0SJH3ZZ	0SN9XZZ
0SBQ0ZZ	0SCP3ZZ	0SG34Z1	0SG90KZ	0SGD4KZ	0SH303Z	0SHC33Z	0SHJ45Z	0SHQ33Z	0SJH4ZZ	0SNB0ZZ
0SBQ3ZX	0SCP4ZZ	0SG34ZJ	0SG90ZZ	0SGD4ZZ	0SH308Z	0SHC34Z	0SHJ48Z	0SHQ34Z	0SJHXZZ	0SNB3ZZ
0SBQ3ZZ	0SCQ0ZZ	0SG504Z	0SG934Z	0SGF04Z	0SH333Z	0SHC35Z	0SHK03Z	0SHQ35Z	0SJJ0ZZ	0SNB4ZZ
0SBQ4ZX	0SCQ3ZZ	0SG507Z	0SG935Z	0SGF05Z	0SH338Z	0SHC38Z	0SHK04Z	0SHQ38Z	0SJJ3ZZ	0SNBXZZ
0SBQ4ZZ	0SCQ4ZZ	0SG50JZ	0SG937Z	0SGF07Z	0SH343Z	0SHC43Z	0SHK05Z	0SHQ43Z	0SJJ4ZZ	0SNC0ZZ
0SC00ZZ	0SG0070	0SG50KZ	0SG93JZ	0SGF0JZ	0SH348Z	0SHC44Z	0SHK08Z	0SHQ44Z	0SJJXZZ	0SNC3ZZ
0SC03ZZ	0SG0071	0SG50ZZ	0SG93KZ	0SGF0KZ	0SH403Z	0SHC45Z	0SHK33Z	0SHQ45Z	0SJK0ZZ	0SNC4ZZ
0SC04ZZ	0SG007J	0SG534Z	0SG93ZZ	0SGF0ZZ	0SH408Z	0SHC48Z	0SHK34Z	0SHQ48Z	0SJK3ZZ	0SNCXZZ
0SC20ZZ	0SG00A0	0SG537Z	0SG944Z	0SGF34Z	0SH433Z	0SHD03Z	0SHK35Z	0SJ00ZZ	0SJK4ZZ	0SND0ZZ
0SC23ZZ	0SG00AJ	0SG53JZ	0SG945Z	0SGF35Z	0SH438Z	0SHD04Z	0SHK38Z	0SJ03ZZ	0SJKXZZ	0SND3ZZ
0SC24ZZ	0SG00J0	0SG53KZ	0SG947Z	0SGF37Z	0SH443Z	0SHD05Z	0SHK43Z	0SJ04ZZ	0SJL0ZZ	0SND4ZZ
0SC30ZZ	0SG00J1	0SG53ZZ	0SG94JZ	0SGF3JZ	0SH448Z	0SHD08Z	0SHK44Z	0SJ0XZZ	0SJL3ZZ	0SNDXZZ
0SC33ZZ	0SG00JJ	0SG544Z	0SG94KZ	0SGF3KZ	0SH503Z	0SHD33Z	0SHK45Z	0SJ20ZZ	0SJL4ZZ	0SNF0ZZ
0SC34ZZ	0SG00K0	0SG547Z	0SG94ZZ	0SGF3ZZ	0SH508Z	0SHD34Z	0SHK48Z	0SJ23ZZ	0SJLXZZ	0SNF3ZZ
0SC40ZZ	0SG00K1	0SG54JZ	0SGB04Z	0SGF44Z	0SH533Z	0SHD35Z	0SHL03Z	0SJ24ZZ	0SJM0ZZ	0SNF4ZZ
0SC43ZZ	0SG00KJ	0SGB05Z	0SGB05Z	0SGF45Z	0SH538Z	0SHD38Z	0SHL04Z	0SJ2XZZ	0SJM3ZZ	0SNFXZZ
0SC44ZZ	0SG00Z0	0SG54ZZ	0SGB07Z	0SGF47Z	0SH543Z	0SHD43Z	0SHL05Z	0SJ30ZZ	0SJM4ZZ	0SNG0ZZ
0SC50ZZ	0SG00Z1	0SG604Z	0SGB0JZ	0SGF4JZ	0SH548Z	0SHD44Z	0SHL08Z	0SJ33ZZ	0SJMXZZ	0SNG3ZZ
0SC53ZZ	0SG00ZJ	0SG607Z	0SGB0KZ	0SGF4KZ	0SH603Z	0SHD45Z	0SHL33Z	0SJ34ZZ	0SJN0ZZ	0SNG4ZZ
0SC54ZZ	0SG0370	0SG60JZ	0SGB0ZZ	0SGF4ZZ	0SH608Z	0SHD48Z	0SHL34Z	0SJ3XZZ	0SJN3ZZ	0SNGXZZ
0SC60ZZ	0SG0371	0SG60KZ	0SGB34Z	0SGG04Z	0SH633Z	0SHF03Z	0SHL35Z	0SJ40ZZ	0SJN4ZZ	0SNH0ZZ
0SC63ZZ	0SG037J	0SG60ZZ	0SGB35Z	0SGG05Z	0SH638Z	0SHF04Z	0SHL38Z	0SJ43ZZ	0SJNXZZ	0SNH3ZZ
0SC64ZZ	0SG03A0	0SG634Z	0SGB37Z	0SGG07Z	0SH643Z	0SHF05Z	0SHL43Z	0SJ44ZZ	0SJP0ZZ	0SNH4ZZ
0SC70ZZ	0SG03AJ	0SG637Z	0SGB3JZ	0SGG0JZ	0SH648Z	0SHF08Z	0SHL44Z	0SJ4XZZ	0SJP3ZZ	0SNHXZZ
0SC73ZZ	0SG03J0	0SG63JZ	0SGB3KZ	0SGG0KZ	0SH703Z	0SHF33Z	0SHL45Z	0SJ50ZZ	0SJP4ZZ	0SNJ0ZZ
0SC74ZZ	0SG03J1	0SG63KZ	0SGB3ZZ	0SGG0ZZ	0SH708Z	0SHF34Z	0SHL48Z	0SJ53ZZ	0SJPXZZ	0SNJ3ZZ
0SC80ZZ	0SG03JJ	0SG63ZZ	0SGB44Z	0SGG34Z	0SH733Z	0SHF35Z	0SHM03Z	0SJ54ZZ	0SJQ0ZZ	0SNJ4ZZ
0SC83ZZ	0SG03K0	0SG644Z	0SGB45Z	0SGG35Z	0SH738Z	0SHF38Z	0SHM04Z	0SJ5XZZ	0SJQ3ZZ	0SNJXZZ
0SC84ZZ	0SG03K1	0SG647Z	0SGB47Z	0SGG37Z	0SH743Z	0SHF43Z	0SHM05Z	0SJ60ZZ	0SJQ4ZZ	0SNK0ZZ
0SC90ZZ	0SG03KJ	0SG64JZ	0SGB4JZ	0SGG3JZ	0SH748Z	0SHF44Z	0SHM08Z	0SJ63ZZ	0SJQXZZ	0SNK3ZZ
0SC93ZZ	0SG03Z0	0SG64KZ	0SGB4KZ	0SGG3KZ	0SH803Z	0SHF45Z	0SHM33Z	0SJ64ZZ	0SN00ZZ	0SNK4ZZ
0SC94ZZ	0SG03Z1	0SG64ZZ	0SGB4ZZ	0SGG3ZZ	0SH808Z	0SHF48Z	0SHM34Z	0SJ6XZZ	0SN03ZZ	0SNKXZZ
0SCB0ZZ	0SG03ZJ	0SG704Z	0SGC04Z	0SGG44Z	0SH833Z	0SHG03Z	0SHM35Z	0SJ70ZZ	0SN04ZZ	0SNL0ZZ
0SCB3ZZ	0SG0470	0SG707Z	0SGC05Z	0SGG45Z	0SH834Z	0SHG04Z	0SHM38Z	0SJ73ZZ	0SN0XZZ	0SNL3ZZ
0SCB4ZZ	0SG0471	0SG70JZ	0SGC07Z	0SGG47Z	0SH838Z	0SHG05Z	0SHM43Z	0SJ74ZZ	0SN20ZZ	0SNL4ZZ
0SCC0ZZ	0SG047J	0SG70KZ	0SGC0JZ	0SGG4JZ	0SH843Z	0SHG08Z	0SHM44Z	0SJ7XZZ	0SN23ZZ	0SNLXZZ
0SCC3ZZ	0SG04A0	0SG70ZZ	0SGC0KZ	0SGG4KZ	0SH844Z	0SHG33Z	0SHM45Z	0SJ80ZZ	0SN24ZZ	0SNM0ZZ
0SCC4ZZ	0SG04AJ	0SG734Z	0SGC0ZZ	0SGG4ZZ	0SH848Z	0SHG34Z	0SHM48Z	0SJ83ZZ	0SN2XZZ	0SNM3ZZ
0SCD0ZZ	0SG04J0	0SG737Z	0SGC34Z	0SGH04Z	0SH903Z	0SHG35Z	0SHN03Z	0SJ84ZZ	0SN30ZZ	0SNM4ZZ
0SCD3ZZ	0SG04J1	0SG73JZ	0SGC35Z	0SGH05Z	0SH904Z	0SHG38Z	0SHN04Z	0SJ8XZZ	0SN33ZZ	0SNMXZZ
0SCD4ZZ	0SG04JJ	0SG73KZ	0SGC37Z	0SGH07Z	0SH905Z	0SHG43Z	0SHN05Z	0SJ90ZZ	0SN34ZZ	0SNN0ZZ
0SCF0ZZ	0SG04K0	0SG73ZZ	0SGC3JZ	0SGH0JZ	0SH908Z	0SHG44Z	0SHN08Z	0SJ93ZZ	0SN3XZZ	0SNN3ZZ
0SCF3ZZ	0SG04K1	0SG744Z	0SGC3KZ	0SGH0KZ	0SH933Z	0SHG45Z	0SHN33Z	0SJ94ZZ	0SN40ZZ	0SNN4ZZ
0SCF4ZZ	0SG04KJ	0SG747Z	0SGC3ZZ	0SGH0ZZ	0SH934Z	0SHG48Z	0SHN34Z	0SJ9XZZ	0SN43ZZ	0SNNXZZ
0SCG0ZZ	0SG04Z0	0SG74JZ	0SGC44Z	0SGH34Z	0SH935Z	0SHH03Z	0SHN35Z	0SJB0ZZ	0SN44ZZ	0SNP0ZZ
0SCG3ZZ	0SG04Z1	0SG74KZ	0SGC45Z	0SGH35Z	0SH938Z	0SHH04Z	0SHN38Z	0SJB3ZZ	0SN4XZZ	0SNP3ZZ
0SCG4ZZ	0SG04ZJ	0SG74ZZ	0SGC47Z	0SGH37Z	0SH943Z	0SHH05Z	0SHN43Z	0SJB4ZZ	0SN50ZZ	0SNP4ZZ
0SCH0ZZ	0SG1070	0SG804Z	0SGC4JZ	0SGH3JZ	0SH944Z	0SHH08Z	0SHN44Z	0SJBXZZ	0SN53ZZ	0SNPXZZ
0SCH3ZZ	0SG1071	0SG807Z	0SGC4KZ	0SGH3KZ	0SH945Z	0SHH33Z	0SHN45Z	0SJC0ZZ	0SN54ZZ	0SNQ0ZZ
0SCH4ZZ	0SG107J	0SG80JZ	0SGC4ZZ	0SGH3ZZ	0SH948Z	0SHH34Z	0SHN48Z	0SJC3ZZ	0SN5XZZ	0SNQ3ZZ
0SCJ0ZZ	0SG10A0	0SG80KZ	0SGD04Z	0SGH44Z	0SHB03Z	0SHH35Z	0SHP03Z	0SJC4ZZ	0SN60ZZ	0SNQ4ZZ
0SCJ3ZZ	0SG10AJ	0SG80ZZ	0SGD05Z	0SGH45Z	0SHB04Z	0SHH38Z	0SHP04Z	0SJCXZZ	0SN63ZZ	0SNQXZZ
0SCJ4ZZ	0SG10J0	0SG834Z	0SGD07Z	0SGH47Z	0SHB05Z	0SHH43Z	0SHP05Z	0SJD0ZZ	0SN64ZZ	0SP000Z
0SCK0ZZ	0SG10J1	0SG837Z	0SGD0JZ	0SGH4JZ	0SHB08Z	0SHH44Z	0SHP08Z	0SJD3ZZ	0SN6XZZ	0SP003Z
0SCK3ZZ	0SG10JJ	0SG83JZ	0SGD0KZ	0SH003Z	0SHB33Z	0SHH45Z	0SHP33Z	0SJD4ZZ	0SN70ZZ	0SP004Z
0SCK4ZZ	0SG10K0	0SG83KZ	0SGD0ZZ	0SH008Z	0SHB34Z	0SHH48Z	0SHP34Z	0SJDXZZ	0SN73ZZ	0SP007Z
0SCL0ZZ	0SG10K1	0SG83ZZ	0SGD34Z	0SH033Z	0SHB35Z	0SHJ03Z	0SHP35Z	0SJF0ZZ	0SN74ZZ	0SP008Z

0SP00AZ	0SP400Z	0SP703Z	0SP943Z	0SPC45Z	0SPKX3Z	0SPQ44Z	0SQB4ZZ	0SR60JZ	0SRC0J9	0SRR019
0SP00JZ	0SP403Z	0SP704Z	0SP944Z	0SPC47Z	0SPKX4Z	0SPQ45Z	0SQBXZZ	0SR60KZ	0SRC0JA	0SRR01A
0SP00KZ	0SP407Z	0SP707Z	0SP945Z	0SPC48Z	0SPKX5Z	0SPQ47Z	0SQC0ZZ	0SR707Z	0SRC0JZ	0SRR01Z
0SP030Z	0SP40JZ	0SP708Z	0SP947Z	0SPC4JC	0SPL08Z	0SPQ48Z	0SQC3ZZ	0SR70JZ	0SRC0KZ	0SRR039
0SP033Z	0SP40KZ	0SP70JZ	0SP948Z	0SPC4JZ	0SPL30Z	0SPQ4JZ	0SQC4ZZ	0SR70KZ	0SRC0L9	0SRR03A
0SP034Z	0SP430Z	0SP70KZ	0SP94JZ	0SPC4KZ	0SPL33Z	0SPQ4KZ	0SQCXZZ	0SR807Z	0SRC0LA	0SRR03Z
0SP037Z	0SP433Z	0SP730Z	0SP94KZ	0SPCX0Z	0SPL38Z	0SPQX0Z	0SQD0ZZ	0SR80JZ	0SRC0LZ	0SRR07Z
0SP038Z	0SP437Z	0SP733Z	0SP9X0Z	0SPCX3Z	0SPL48Z	0SPQX3Z	0SQD3ZZ	0SR80KZ	0SRD069	0SRR0J9
0SP03AZ	0SP43JZ	0SP734Z	0SP9X3Z	0SPCX4Z	0SPLX0Z	0SPQX4Z	0SQD4ZZ	0SR9019	0SRD06A	0SRR0JA
0SP03JZ	0SP43KZ	0SP737Z	0SP9X4Z	0SPCX5Z	0SPLX3Z	0SPQX5Z	0SQDXZZ	0SR901A	0SRD06Z	0SRR0JZ
0SP03KZ	0SP440Z	0SP738Z	0SP9X5Z	0SPD00Z	0SPLX4Z	0SPR0JZ	0SQF0ZZ	0SR901Z	0SRD07Z	0SS034Z
0SP040Z	0SP443Z	0SP73JZ	0SPA0JZ	0SPD03Z	0SPLX5Z	0SPR3JZ	0SQF3ZZ	0SR9029	0SRD0J9	0SS03ZZ
0SP043Z	0SP447Z	0SP73KZ	0SPA3JZ	0SPD04Z	0SPM08Z	0SPR4JZ	0SQF4ZZ	0SR902A	0SRD0JA	0SS044Z
0SP044Z	0SP44JZ	0SP740Z	0SPA4JZ	0SPD05Z	0SPM30Z	0SPS0JZ	0SQFXZZ	0SR902Z	0SRD0JZ	0SS04ZZ
0SP047Z	0SP44KZ	0SP743Z	0SPB00Z	0SPD07Z	0SPM33Z	0SPS3JZ	0SQG0ZZ	0SR9039	0SRD0KZ	0SS0X4Z
0SP048Z	0SP4X0Z	0SP744Z	0SPB03Z	0SPD08Z	0SPM38Z	0SPS4JZ	0SQG3ZZ	0SR903A	0SRD0L9	0SS0XZZ
0SP04AZ	0SP4X3Z	0SP747Z	0SPB04Z	0SPD09Z	0SPM48Z	0SPT0JZ	0SQG4ZZ	0SR903Z	0SRD0LA	0SS334Z
0SP04JZ	0SP500Z	0SP748Z	0SPB05Z	0SPD0JC	0SPMX0Z	0SPT3JZ	0SQGXZZ	0SR9049	0SRD0LZ	0SS33ZZ
0SP04KZ	0SP503Z	0SP74JZ	0SPB07Z	0SPD30Z	0SPMX3Z	0SPT4JZ	0SQH0ZZ	0SR904A	0SRE009	0SS344Z
0SP0X0Z	0SP504Z	0SP74KZ	0SPB08Z	0SPD33Z	0SPMX4Z	0SPU0JZ	0SQH3ZZ	0SR904Z	0SRE00A	0SS34ZZ
0SP0X3Z	0SP507Z	0SP7X0Z	0SPB09Z	0SPDX0Z	0SPMX5Z	0SPU3JZ	0SQH4ZZ	0SR9069	0SRE00Z	0SS3X4Z
0SP0X4Z	0SP508Z	0SP7X3Z	0SPB0BZ	0SPDX3Z	0SPN08Z	0SPU4JZ	0SQHXZZ	0SR906A	0SRE019	0SS3XZZ
0SP200Z	0SP50JZ	0SP7X4Z	0SPB0JZ	0SPDX4Z	0SPN30Z	0SPV0JZ	0SQJ0ZZ	0SR906Z	0SRE01A	0SS534Z
0SP203Z	0SP50KZ	0SP800Z	0SPB0KZ	0SPDX5Z	0SPN33Z	0SPV3JZ	0SQJ3ZZ	0SR907Z	0SRE01Z	0SS53ZZ
0SP207Z	0SP530Z	0SP803Z	0SPB30Z	0SPF08Z	0SPN38Z	0SPV4JZ	0SQJ4ZZ	0SR90J9	0SRE039	0SS544Z
0SP20JZ	0SP533Z	0SP804Z	0SPB33Z	0SPF30Z	0SPN48Z	0SPW0JZ	0SQJXZZ	0SR90JA	0SRE03A	0SS54ZZ
0SP20KZ	0SP534Z	0SP807Z	0SPB34Z	0SPF33Z	0SPNX0Z	0SPW3JZ	0SQK0ZZ	0SR90JZ	0SRE03Z	0SS5X4Z
0SP230Z	0SP537Z	0SP808Z	0SPB35Z	0SPF38Z	0SPNX3Z	0SPW4JZ	0SQK3ZZ	0SR90KZ	0SRE07Z	0SS5XZZ
0SP233Z	0SP538Z	0SP80JZ	0SPB37Z	0SPF48Z	0SPNX4Z	0SQ00ZZ	0SQK4ZZ	0SRA009	0SRE0J9	0SS634Z
0SP237Z	0SP53JZ	0SP80KZ	0SPB38Z	0SPFX0Z	0SPNX5Z	0SQ03ZZ	0SQKXZZ	0SRA00A	0SRE0JA	0SS63ZZ
0SP23JZ	0SP53KZ	0SP830Z	0SPB3JZ	0SPFX3Z	0SPP08Z	0SQ04ZZ	0SQL0ZZ	0SRA00Z	0SRE0JZ	0SS644Z
0SP23KZ	0SP540Z	0SP833Z	0SPB3KZ	0SPFX4Z	0SPP30Z	0SQ0XZZ	0SQL3ZZ	0SRA019	0SRE0KZ	0SS64ZZ
0SP240Z	0SP543Z	0SP834Z	0SPB40Z	0SPFX5Z	0SPP33Z	0SQ20ZZ	0SQL4ZZ	0SRA01A	0SRF07Z	0SS6X4Z
0SP243Z	0SP544Z	0SP837Z	0SPB43Z	0SPG08Z	0SPP38Z	0SQ23ZZ	0SQLXZZ	0SRA01Z	0SRF0J9	0SS6XZZ
0SP247Z	0SP547Z	0SP838Z	0SPB44Z	0SPG30Z	0SPP3JZ	0SQ24ZZ	0SQM0ZZ	0SRA039	0SRF0JA	0SS734Z
0SP24JZ	0SP548Z	0SP83JZ	0SPB45Z	0SPG33Z	0SPP3KZ	0SQ2XZZ	0SQM3ZZ	0SRA03A	0SRF0JZ	0SS73ZZ
0SP24KZ	0SP54JZ	0SP83KZ	0SPB47Z	0SPG38Z	0SPP40Z	0SQ30ZZ	0SQM4ZZ	0SRA03Z	0SRF0KZ	0SS744Z
0SP2X0Z	0SP54KZ	0SP840Z	0SPB48Z	0SPG48Z	0SPP43Z	0SQ33ZZ	0SQMXZZ	0SRA07Z	0SRG07Z	0SS74ZZ
0SP2X3Z	0SP5X0Z	0SP843Z	0SPB4JZ	0SPGX0Z	0SPP44Z	0SQ34ZZ	0SQN0ZZ	0SRA0J9	0SRG0J9	0SS7X4Z
0SP300Z	0SP5X3Z	0SP844Z	0SPB4KZ	0SPGX3Z	0SPP45Z	0SQ3XZZ	0SQN3ZZ	0SRA0JA	0SRG0JZ	0SS7XZZ
0SP303Z	0SP5X4Z	0SP847Z	0SPBX0Z	0SPGX4Z	0SPP47Z	0SQ40ZZ	0SQN4ZZ	0SRA0JZ	0SRG0KZ	0SS834Z
0SP304Z	0SP600Z	0SP848Z	0SPBX3Z	0SPGX5Z	0SPP48Z	0SQ43ZZ	0SQNXZZ	0SRA0KZ	0SRH07Z	0SS83ZZ
0SP307Z	0SP603Z	0SP84JZ	0SPBX4Z	0SPH08Z	0SPP4JZ	0SQ44ZZ	0SQP0ZZ	0SRB019	0SRH0JZ	0SS844Z
0SP308Z	0SP604Z	0SP84KZ	0SPBX5Z	0SPH30Z	0SPP4KZ	0SQ4XZZ	0SQP3ZZ	0SRB01A	0SRH0KZ	0SS84ZZ
0SP30AZ	0SP607Z	0SP8X0Z	0SPC00Z	0SPH33Z	0SPPX0Z	0SQ50ZZ	0SQP4ZZ	0SRB01Z	0SRJ07Z	0SS8X4Z
0SP30JZ	0SP608Z	0SP8X3Z	0SPC03Z	0SPH38Z	0SPPX3Z	0SQ53ZZ	0SQPXZZ	0SRB029	0SRJ0JZ	0SS8XZZ
0SP30KZ	0SP60JZ	0SP8X4Z	0SPC04Z	0SPH48Z	0SPPX4Z	0SQ54ZZ	0SQQ0ZZ	0SRB02A	0SRJ0KZ	0SS934Z
0SP330Z	0SP60KZ	0SP900Z	0SPC05Z	0SPHX0Z	0SPPX5Z	0SQ5XZZ	0SQQ3ZZ	0SRB02Z	0SRK07Z	0SS935Z
0SP333Z	0SP630Z	0SP903Z	0SPC07Z	0SPHX3Z	0SPQ00Z	0SQ60ZZ	0SQQ4ZZ	0SRB039	0SRK0JZ	0SS93ZZ
0SP334Z	0SP633Z	0SP904Z	0SPC08Z	0SPHX4Z	0SPQ03Z	0SQ63ZZ	0SQQXZZ	0SRB03A	0SRK0KZ	0SS944Z
0SP337Z	0SP634Z	0SP905Z	0SPC09Z	0SPHX5Z	0SPQ04Z	0SQ64ZZ	0SR007Z	0SRB03Z	0SRL07Z	0SS945Z
0SP338Z	0SP637Z	0SP907Z	0SPC0JC	0SPJ08Z	0SPQ05Z	0SQ6XZZ	0SR00JZ	0SRB049	0SRL0JZ	0SS94ZZ
0SP33AZ	0SP638Z	0SP908Z	0SPC0JZ	0SPJ30Z	0SPQ07Z	0SQ70ZZ	0SR00KZ	0SRB04A	0SRL0KZ	0SS9X4Z
0SP33JZ	0SP63JZ	0SP909Z	0SPC0KZ	0SPJ33Z	0SPQ08Z	0SQ73ZZ	0SR207Z	0SRB04Z	0SRM07Z	0SS9X5Z
0SP33KZ	0SP63KZ	0SP90BZ	0SPC30Z	0SPJ38Z	0SPQ0JZ	0SQ74ZZ	0SR20JZ	0SRB069	0SRM0JZ	0SS9XZZ
0SP340Z	0SP640Z	0SP90JZ	0SPC33Z	0SPJ48Z	0SPQ0KZ	0SQ7XZZ	0SR20KZ	0SRB06A	0SRM0KZ	0SSB34Z
0SP343Z	0SP643Z	0SP90KZ	0SPC34Z	0SPJX0Z	0SPQ30Z	0SQ80ZZ	0SR307Z	0SRB06Z	0SRN07Z	0SSB35Z
0SP344Z	0SP644Z	0SP930Z	0SPC35Z	0SPJX3Z	0SPQ33Z	0SQ83ZZ	0SR30JZ	0SRB07Z	0SRN0JZ	0SSB3Z
0SP347Z	0SP647Z	0SP933Z	0SPC37Z	0SPJX4Z	0SPQ34Z	0SQ84ZZ	0SR30KZ	0SRB0J9	0SRN0KZ	0SSB44Z
0SP348Z	0SP648Z	0SP934Z	0SPC38Z	0SPJX5Z	0SPQ35Z	0SQ8XZZ	0SR407Z	0SRB0JA	0SRP07Z	0SSB45Z
0SP34AZ	0SP64JZ	0SP935Z	0SPC3JC	0SPK08Z	0SPQ37Z	0SQ90ZZ	0SR40JZ	0SRB0JZ	0SRP0JZ	0SSB4Z
0SP34JZ	0SP64KZ	0SP937Z	0SPC3JZ	0SPK30Z	0SPQ38Z	0SQ93ZZ	0SR40KZ	0SRB0KZ	0SRP0KZ	0SSBX4Z
0SP34KZ	0SP6X0Z	0SP938Z	0SPC3KZ	0SPK33Z	0SPQ3JZ	0SQ94ZZ	0SR507Z	0SRC069	0SRQ07Z	0SSBX5Z
0SP3X0Z	0SP6X3Z	0SP93JZ	0SPC40Z	0SPK38Z	0SPQ3KZ	0SQ9XZZ	0SR50JZ	0SRC06A	0SRQ0JZ	0SSBXZZ
0SP3X3Z	0SP6X4Z	0SP93KZ	0SPC43Z	0SPK48Z	0SPQ40Z	0SQB0ZZ	0SR50KZ	0SRC06Z	0SRQ0KZ	0SSC34Z
0SP3X4Z	0SP700Z	0SP940Z	0SPC44Z	0SPKX0Z	0SPQ43Z	0SQB3ZZ	0SR607Z	0SRC07Z	0SRQ0KZ	0SSC35Z

0SSC3ZZ	0SSL4ZZ	0SU50JZ	0SUC3KZ	0SUL3JZ	0SW043Z	0SW3XKZ	0SW647Z	0SW8XKZ	0SWBX3Z	0SWD45Z
0SSC44Z	0SSLX4Z	0SU50KZ	0SUC47Z	0SUL3KZ	0SW044Z	0SW400Z	0SW648Z	0SW900Z	0SWBX4Z	0SWDX0Z
0SSC45Z	0SSLX5Z	0SU537Z	0SUC4JZ	0SUL47Z	0SW047Z	0SW403Z	0SW64JZ	0SW903Z	0SWBX7Z	0SWDX3Z
0SSC4ZZ	0SSLXZZ	0SU53JZ	0SUC4KZ	0SUL4JZ	0SW048Z	0SW407Z	0SW64KZ	0SW904Z	0SWBX8Z	0SWDX4Z
0SSCX4Z	0SSM34Z	0SU53KZ	0SUD07Z	0SUL4KZ	0SW04AZ	0SW40JZ	0SW6X0Z	0SW905Z	0SWBXJZ	0SWDX5Z
0SSCX5Z	0SSM35Z	0SU547Z	0SUD09C	0SUM07Z	0SW04JZ	0SW40KZ	0SW6X3Z	0SW907Z	0SWBXKZ	0SWDX7Z
0SSCXZZ	0SSM3ZZ	0SU54JZ	0SUD09Z	0SUM0JZ	0SW04KZ	0SW430Z	0SW6X4Z	0SW908Z	0SWC00Z	0SWDX8Z
0SSD34Z	0SSM44Z	0SU54KZ	0SUD0JZ	0SUM0KZ	0SW0X0Z	0SW433Z	0SW6X7Z	0SW909Z	0SWC03Z	0SWDXJC
0SSD35Z	0SSM45Z	0SU607Z	0SUD0KZ	0SUM37Z	0SW0X3Z	0SW437Z	0SW6X8Z	0SW90BZ	0SWC04Z	0SWDXJZ
0SSD3ZZ	0SSM4ZZ	0SU60JZ	0SUD37Z	0SUM3JZ	0SW0X4Z	0SW43JZ	0SW6XJZ	0SW90JZ	0SWC05Z	0SWDXKZ
0SSD44Z	0SSMX4Z	0SU60KZ	0SUD3JZ	0SUM3KZ	0SW0X7Z	0SW43KZ	0SW6XKZ	0SW90KZ	0SWC07Z	0SWEXJZ
0SSD45Z	0SSMX5Z	0SU637Z	0SUD3KZ	0SUM47Z	0SW0X8Z	0SW440Z	0SW700Z	0SW930Z	0SWC08Z	0SWFX0Z
0SSD4ZZ	0SSMXZZ	0SU63JZ	0SUD47Z	0SUM4JZ	0SW0XAZ	0SW443Z	0SW703Z	0SW933Z	0SWC09Z	0SWFX3Z
0SSDX4Z	0SSN34Z	0SU63KZ	0SUD4JZ	0SUM4KZ	0SW0XJZ	0SW447Z	0SW704Z	0SW934Z	0SWC0JC	0SWFX4Z
0SSDX5Z	0SSN35Z	0SU647Z	0SUD4KZ	0SUN07Z	0SW0XKZ	0SW44JZ	0SW707Z	0SW935Z	0SWC0JZ	0SWFX5Z
0SSDXZZ	0SSN3ZZ	0SU64JZ	0SUE09Z	0SUN0JZ	0SW200Z	0SW44KZ	0SW708Z	0SW937Z	0SWC0KZ	0SWFX7Z
0SSF34Z	0SSN44Z	0SU64KZ	0SUE0BZ	0SUN0KZ	0SW203Z	0SW4X0Z	0SW70JZ	0SW938Z	0SWC30Z	0SWFX8Z
0SSF35Z	0SSN45Z	0SU707Z	0SUF07Z	0SUN37Z	0SW207Z	0SW4X3Z	0SW70KZ	0SW93JZ	0SWC33Z	0SWFXJZ
0SSF3ZZ	0SSN4ZZ	0SU70JZ	0SUF0JZ	0SUN3JZ	0SW20JZ	0SW4X7Z	0SW730Z	0SW93KZ	0SWC34Z	0SWFXKZ
0SSF44Z	0SSNX4Z	0SU70KZ	0SUF0KZ	0SUN3KZ	0SW20KZ	0SW4XJZ	0SW733Z	0SW940Z	0SWC35Z	0SWGX0Z
0SSF45Z	0SSNX5Z	0SU737Z	0SUF37Z	0SUN47Z	0SW230Z	0SW4XKZ	0SW734Z	0SW943Z	0SWC37Z	0SWGX3Z
0SSF4ZZ	0SSNXZZ	0SU73JZ	0SUF3JZ	0SUN4JZ	0SW233Z	0SW500Z	0SW737Z	0SW944Z	0SWC38Z	0SWGX4Z
0SSFX4Z	0SSP34Z	0SU73KZ	0SUF3KZ	0SUN4KZ	0SW237Z	0SW503Z	0SW738Z	0SW947Z	0SWC3JC	0SWGX5Z
0SSFX5Z	0SSP35Z	0SU747Z	0SUF47Z	0SUP07Z	0SW23JZ	0SW504Z	0SW73JZ	0SW948Z	0SWC3JZ	0SWGX7Z
0SSFXZZ	0SSP3ZZ	0SU74JZ	0SUF4JZ	0SUP0JZ	0SW23KZ	0SW507Z	0SW73KZ	0SW94JZ	0SWC3KZ	0SWGX8Z
0SSG34Z	0SSP44Z	0SU74KZ	0SUF4KZ	0SUP0KZ	0SW240Z	0SW508Z	0SW740Z	0SW94KZ	0SWC40Z	0SWGXJZ
0SSG35Z	0SSP45Z	0SU807Z	0SUG07Z	0SUP37Z	0SW243Z	0SW50JZ	0SW743Z	0SW9X0Z	0SWC43Z	0SWGXKZ
0SSG3ZZ	0SSP4ZZ	0SU80JZ	0SUG0JZ	0SUP3JZ	0SW247Z	0SW50KZ	0SW744Z	0SW9X3Z	0SWC44Z	0SWHX0Z
0SSG44Z	0SSPX4Z	0SU80KZ	0SUG0KZ	0SUP3KZ	0SW24JZ	0SW530Z	0SW747Z	0SW9X4Z	0SWC45Z	0SWHX3Z
0SSG45Z	0SSPX5Z	0SU837Z	0SUG37Z	0SUP47Z	0SW24KZ	0SW533Z	0SW748Z	0SW9X5Z	0SWC47Z	0SWHX4Z
0SSG4ZZ	0SSPXZZ	0SU83JZ	0SUG3JZ	0SUP4JZ	0SW2X0Z	0SW534Z	0SW74JZ	0SW9X7Z	0SWC48Z	0SWHX5Z
0SSGX4Z	0SSQ34Z	0SU83KZ	0SUG3KZ	0SUP4KZ	0SW2X3Z	0SW537Z	0SW74KZ	0SW9X8Z	0SWC4JC	0SWHX7Z
0SSGX5Z	0SSQ35Z	0SU847Z	0SUG47Z	0SUQ07Z	0SW2X7Z	0SW538Z	0SW7X0Z	0SW9XJZ	0SWC4JZ	0SWHX8Z
0SSGXZZ	0SSQ3ZZ	0SU84JZ	0SUG4JZ	0SUQ0JZ	0SW2XJZ	0SW53JZ	0SW7X3Z	0SW9XKZ	0SWC4KZ	0SWHXJZ
0SSH34Z	0SSQ44Z	0SU84KZ	0SUG4KZ	0SUQ0KZ	0SW2XKZ	0SW53KZ	0SW7X4Z	0SWA0JZ	0SWCX0Z	0SWHXKZ
0SSH35Z	0SSQ45Z	0SU907Z	0SUH07Z	0SUQ37Z	0SW300Z	0SW540Z	0SW7X7Z	0SWA3JZ	0SWCX3Z	0SWJX0Z
0SSH3ZZ	0SSQ4ZZ	0SU909Z	0SUH0JZ	0SUQ3JZ	0SW303Z	0SW543Z	0SW7X8Z	0SWA4JZ	0SWCX4Z	0SWJX3Z
0SSH44Z	0SSQX4Z	0SU90BZ	0SUH0KZ	0SUQ3KZ	0SW304Z	0SW544Z	0SW7XJZ	0SWAXJZ	0SWCX5Z	0SWJX4Z
0SSH45Z	0SSQX5Z	0SU90JZ	0SUH37Z	0SUQ47Z	0SW307Z	0SW547Z	0SW7XKZ	0SWB00Z	0SWCX7Z	0SWJX5Z
0SSH4ZZ	0SSQXZZ	0SU90KZ	0SUH3JZ	0SUQ4JZ	0SW308Z	0SW548Z	0SW800Z	0SWB03Z	0SWCX8Z	0SWJX7Z
0SSHX4Z	0SU20KZ	0SU937Z	0SUH3KZ	0SUQ4KZ	0SW30AZ	0SW54JZ	0SW803Z	0SWB04Z	0SWCXJC	0SWJX8Z
0SSHX5Z	0SU237Z	0SU93JZ	0SUH47Z	0SUR09Z	0SW30JZ	0SW54KZ	0SW804Z	0SWB05Z	0SWCXJZ	0SWJXJZ
0SSHXZZ	0SU23JZ	0SU93KZ	0SUH4JZ	0SUR0BZ	0SW30KZ	0SW5X0Z	0SW807Z	0SWB07Z	0SWCXKZ	0SWJXKZ
0SSJ34Z	0SU23KZ	0SU947Z	0SUH4KZ	0SUS09Z	0SW330Z	0SW5X3Z	0SW808Z	0SWB08Z	0SWD00Z	0SWKX0Z
0SSJ35Z	0SU247Z	0SU94JZ	0SUJ07Z	0SUS0BZ	0SW333Z	0SW5X4Z	0SW80JZ	0SWB09Z	0SWD03Z	0SWKX3Z
0SSJ3ZZ	0SU24JZ	0SU94KZ	0SUJ0JZ	0SUT09Z	0SW334Z	0SW5X7Z	0SW80KZ	0SWB0BZ	0SWD04Z	0SWKX5Z
0SSJ44Z	0SU24KZ	0SUA09Z	0SUJ0KZ	0SUU09Z	0SW337Z	0SW5X8Z	0SW830Z	0SWB0JZ	0SWD05Z	0SWKX7Z
0SSJ45Z	0SU307Z	0SUA0BZ	0SUJ37Z	0SUV09Z	0SW338Z	0SW5XJZ	0SW833Z	0SWB0KZ	0SWD07Z	0SWKX8Z
0SSJ4ZZ	0SU30JZ	0SUB07Z	0SUJ3JZ	0SUW09Z	0SW33AZ	0SW5XKZ	0SW834Z	0SWB30Z	0SWD08Z	0SWKXJZ
0SSJX4Z	0SU30KZ	0SUB09Z	0SUJ3KZ	0SW000Z	0SW33JZ	0SW600Z	0SW837Z	0SWB33Z	0SWD09Z	0SWKXKZ
0SSJX5Z	0SU337Z	0SUB0BZ	0SUJ47Z	0SW003Z	0SW33KZ	0SW603Z	0SW838Z	0SWB34Z	0SWD0JC	0SWLX0Z
0SSJXZZ	0SU33JZ	0SUB0JZ	0SUJ4JZ	0SW004Z	0SW340Z	0SW604Z	0SW83JZ	0SWB35Z	0SWD0JZ	0SWLX3Z
0SSK34Z	0SU33KZ	0SUB0KZ	0SUJ4KZ	0SW007Z	0SW343Z	0SW607Z	0SW83KZ	0SWB37Z	0SWD0KZ	0SWLX4Z
0SSK35Z	0SU347Z	0SUB37Z	0SUK07Z	0SW008Z	0SW344Z	0SW608Z	0SW840Z	0SWB38Z	0SWD30Z	0SWLX5Z
0SSK3ZZ	0SU34JZ	0SUB3JZ	0SUK0JZ	0SW00AZ	0SW347Z	0SW60JZ	0SW843Z	0SWB3JZ	0SWD33Z	0SWLX7Z
0SSK44Z	0SU34KZ	0SUB3KZ	0SUK0KZ	0SW00JZ	0SW348Z	0SW60KZ	0SW844Z	0SWB3KZ	0SWD34Z	0SWLX8Z
0SSK45Z	0SU407Z	0SUB47Z	0SUK37Z	0SW00KZ	0SW34AZ	0SW630Z	0SW847Z	0SWB40Z	0SWD35Z	0SWLXJZ
0SSK4ZZ	0SU40JZ	0SUB4JZ	0SUK3JZ	0SW030Z	0SW34JZ	0SW633Z	0SW848Z	0SWB43Z	0SWD37Z	0SWLXKZ
0SSKX4Z	0SU40KZ	0SUB4KZ	0SUK3KZ	0SW033Z	0SW34KZ	0SW634Z	0SW84JZ	0SWB44Z	0SWD38Z	0SWMX0Z
0SSKX5Z	0SU437Z	0SUC07Z	0SUK47Z	0SW034Z	0SW3X0Z	0SW637Z	0SW84KZ	0SWB45Z	0SWD3JC	0SWMX3Z
0SSKXZZ	0SU43JZ	0SUC09C	0SUK4JZ	0SW037Z	0SW3X3Z	0SW638Z	0SW8X0Z	0SWB47Z	0SWD3JZ	0SWMX4Z
0SSL34Z	0SU43KZ	0SUC09Z	0SUK4KZ	0SW038Z	0SW3X4Z	0SW63JZ	0SW8X3Z	0SWB48Z	0SWD3KZ	0SWMX5Z
0SSL35Z	0SU447Z	0SUC0JZ	0SUL07Z	0SW03AZ	0SW3X7Z	0SW63KZ	0SW8X4Z	0SWB4JZ	0SWD40Z	0SWMX7Z
0SSL3ZZ	0SU44JZ	0SUC0KZ	0SUL0JZ	0SW03JZ	0SW3X8Z	0SW640Z	0SW8X7Z	0SWB4KZ	0SWD43Z	0SWMX8Z
0SSL44Z	0SU44KZ	0SUC37Z	0SUL0KZ	0SW03KZ	0SW3XAZ	0SW643Z	0SW8X8Z	0SWBX0Z	0SWD44Z	0SWMXJZ
0SSL45Z	0SU507Z	0SUC3JZ	0SUL37Z	0SW040Z	0SW3XJZ	0SW644Z	0SW8XJZ	0SWBX0Z		

0SWMXKZ	0SWQ34Z	0T130K3	0T14079	0T144Z3	0T174KA	0T184KB	0T564ZZ	0T783DZ	0T9730Z	0TB73ZZ
0SWN33Z	0SWQ35Z	0T130K4	0T1407A	0T144Z4	0T174KB	0T184KC	0T567ZZ	0T783ZZ	0T973ZX	0TB74ZX
0SWN34Z	0SWQ37Z	0T130K6	0T1407B	0T144Z6	0T174KC	0T184KD	0T568ZZ	0T784DZ	0T973ZZ	0TB74ZZ
0SWN35Z	0SWQ38Z	0T130K7	0T1407C	0T144Z7	0T174KD	0T184Z6	0T570ZZ	0T784ZZ	0T9740Z	0TB77ZX
0SWN37Z	0SWQ3JZ	0T130K8	0T1407D	0T144Z8	0T174Z6	0T184Z7	0T573ZZ	0T787DZ	0T974ZX	0TB77ZZ
0SWN38Z	0SWQ3KZ	0T130K9	0T140J3	0T144Z9	0T174Z7	0T184Z8	0T574ZZ	0T787ZZ	0T9770Z	0TB78ZX
0SWN3JZ	0SWQ40Z	0T130KA	0T140J4	0T144ZA	0T174Z8	0T184Z9	0T577ZZ	0T788DZ	0T977ZX	0TB78ZZ
0SWN3KZ	0SWQ43Z	0T130KB	0T140J6	0T144ZB	0T174Z9	0T184ZA	0T578ZZ	0T788ZZ	0T9780Z	0TBB0ZX
0SWN40Z	0SWQ44Z	0T130KC	0T140J7	0T144ZC	0T174ZA	0T184ZB	0T5B0ZZ	0T7B0DZ	0T978ZX	0TBB0ZZ
0SWN43Z	0SWQ45Z	0T130KD	0T140J8	0T144ZD	0T174ZB	0T184ZC	0T5B3ZZ	0T7B0ZZ	0T9800Z	0TBB3ZX
0SWN44Z	0SWQ47Z	0T130Z3	0T140J9	0T16076	0T174ZC	0T184ZD	0T5B4ZZ	0T7B3DZ	0T9830Z	0TBB3ZZ
0SWN45Z	0SWQ48Z	0T130Z4	0T140JA	0T16077	0T174ZD	0T1B079	0T5B7ZZ	0T7B3ZZ	0T983ZX	0TBB4ZX
0SWN47Z	0SWQ4JZ	0T130Z6	0T140JB	0T16078	0T18076	0T1B07C	0T5B8ZZ	0T7C0DZ	0T983ZZ	0TBB4ZZ
0SWN48Z	0SWQ4KZ	0T130Z7	0T140JC	0T16079	0T18077	0T1B07D	0T5C0ZZ	0T7C0ZZ	0T9840Z	0TBB7ZX
0SWN4JZ	0SWQX0Z	0T130Z8	0T140JD	0T1607A	0T18078	0T1B0J9	0T5C3ZZ	0T7C3DZ	0T984ZX	0TBB7ZZ
0SWN4KZ	0SWQX3Z	0T130Z9	0T140K3	0T1607B	0T18079	0T1B0JC	0T5C4ZZ	0T7C3ZZ	0T9870Z	0TBB8ZX
0SWNX0Z	0SWQX4Z	0T130ZA	0T140K4	0T1607C	0T1807A	0T1B0JD	0T5C7ZZ	0T7C4DZ	0T987ZX	0TBB8ZZ
0SWNX3Z	0SWQX5Z	0T130ZB	0T140K6	0T1607D	0T1807B	0T1B0K9	0T5C8ZZ	0T7C4ZZ	0T9880Z	0TBC0ZX
0SWNX4Z	0SWQX7Z	0T130ZC	0T140K7	0T160J6	0T1807C	0T1B0KC	0T5D0ZZ	0T7C7DZ	0T988ZX	0TBC0ZZ
0SWNX5Z	0SWQX8Z	0T130ZD	0T140K8	0T160J7	0T1807D	0T1B0KD	0T5D3ZZ	0T7C7ZZ	0T9B30Z	0TBC3ZX
0SWNX7Z	0SWQXJZ	0T133JD	0T140K9	0T160J8	0T180J6	0T1B0Z9	0T5D4ZZ	0T7C8DZ	0T9B3ZZ	0TBC3ZZ
0SWNX8Z	0SWQXKZ	0T13473	0T140KA	0T160J9	0T180J7	0T1B0ZC	0T5D7ZZ	0T7C8ZZ	0T9B40Z	0TBC4ZX
0SWNXJZ	0SWR0JZ	0T13474	0T140KB	0T160JA	0T180J8	0T1B0ZD	0T5D8ZZ	0T7D0DZ	0T9B4ZZ	0TBC4ZZ
0SWNXKZ	0SWR3JZ	0T13476	0T140KC	0T160JB	0T180J9	0T1B3JD	0T5DXZZ	0T7D3DZ	0T9B70Z	0TBC7ZX
0SWP00Z	0SWR4JZ	0T13477	0T140KD	0T160JC	0T180JA	0T1B479	0T730DZ	0T7D4DZ	0T9B7ZZ	0TBC7ZZ
0SWP03Z	0SWRXJZ	0T13478	0T140Z3	0T160JD	0T180JB	0T1B47C	0T730ZZ	0T7D7DZ	0T9B80Z	0TBC8ZX
0SWP04Z	0SWS0JZ	0T13479	0T140Z4	0T160K6	0T180JC	0T1B47D	0T733DZ	0T7D7ZZ	0T9B8ZZ	0TBC8ZZ
0SWP05Z	0SWS3JZ	0T1347A	0T140Z6	0T160K7	0T180JD	0T1B4J9	0T733ZZ	0T7D8DZ	0T9C30Z	0TBD0ZX
0SWP07Z	0SWS4JZ	0T1347B	0T140Z7	0T160K8	0T180K6	0T1B4JC	0T734DZ	0T7D8ZZ	0T9C3ZZ	0TBD0ZZ
0SWP08Z	0SWSXJZ	0T1347C	0T140Z8	0T160K9	0T180K7	0T1B4JD	0T734ZZ	0T9030Z	0T9C40Z	0TBD3ZX
0SWP0JZ	0SWT0JZ	0T1347D	0T140Z9	0T160KA	0T180K8	0T1B4K9	0T737DZ	0T903ZX	0T9C4ZZ	0TBD3ZZ
0SWP0KZ	0SWT3JZ	0T134J3	0T140ZA	0T160KB	0T180K9	0T1B4KC	0T737ZZ	0T903ZZ	0T9C70Z	0TBD4ZX
0SWP30Z	0SWT4JZ	0T134J4	0T140ZB	0T160KC	0T180KA	0T1B4KD	0T738DZ	0T904ZX	0T9C7ZZ	0TBD4ZZ
0SWP33Z	0SWTXJZ	0T134J6	0T140ZC	0T160KD	0T180KB	0T1B4Z9	0T738ZZ	0T904ZZ	0T9C80Z	0TBD7ZX
0SWP34Z	0SWU0JZ	0T134J7	0T140ZD	0T160Z6	0T180KC	0T1B4ZC	0T740DZ	0T907ZX	0T9C8ZZ	0TBD7ZZ
0SWP35Z	0SWU3JZ	0T134J8	0T143JD	0T160Z7	0T180KD	0T1B4ZD	0T740ZZ	0T908ZX	0T9D0ZX	0TBD8ZX
0SWP37Z	0SWU4JZ	0T134J9	0T14473	0T160Z8	0T180Z6	0T25X0Z	0T743DZ	0T9130Z	0T9D30Z	0TBD8ZZ
0SWP38Z	0SWUXJZ	0T134JA	0T14474	0T160Z9	0T180Z7	0T25XYZ	0T743ZZ	0T913ZX	0T9D3ZX	0TBDXZX
0SWP3JZ	0SWV0JZ	0T134JB	0T14476	0T160ZA	0T180Z8	0T29X0Z	0T744DZ	0T913ZZ	0T9D3ZZ	0TBDXZZ
0SWP3KZ	0SWV3JZ	0T134JC	0T14477	0T160ZB	0T180Z9	0T29XYZ	0T744ZZ	0T914ZX	0T9D4ZZ	0TC00ZZ
0SWP40Z	0SWV4JZ	0T134JD	0T14478	0T160ZC	0T180ZA	0T2BX0Z	0T747DZ	0T914ZZ	0T9D7ZZ	0TC03ZZ
0SWP43Z	0SWVXJZ	0T134K3	0T14479	0T160ZD	0T180ZB	0T2BXYZ	0T747ZZ	0T917ZX	0T9D8ZX	0TC04ZZ
0SWP44Z	0SWW0JZ	0T134K4	0T1447A	0T163JD	0T180ZC	0T2DX0Z	0T748DZ	0T918ZX	0T9DXZX	0TC07ZZ
0SWP45Z	0SWW3JZ	0T134K6	0T1447B	0T16476	0T180ZD	0T2DXYZ	0T748ZZ	0T933ZX	0TB03ZX	0TC08ZZ
0SWP47Z	0SWW4JZ	0T134K7	0T1447C	0T16477	0T183JD	0T500ZZ	0T760DZ	0T933ZZ	0TB04ZX	0TC10ZZ
0SWP48Z	0SWWXJZ	0T134K8	0T1447D	0T16478	0T18476	0T503ZZ	0T760ZZ	0T934ZX	0TB07ZX	0TC13ZZ
0SWP4JZ	0T13073	0T134K9	0T144J3	0T16479	0T18477	0T504ZZ	0T763DZ	0T934ZZ	0TB08ZX	0TC14ZZ
0SWP4KZ	0T13074	0T134KA	0T144J4	0T1647A	0T18478	0T507ZZ	0T763ZZ	0T937ZX	0TB13ZX	0TC17ZZ
0SWPX0Z	0T13076	0T134KB	0T144J6	0T1647B	0T18479	0T508ZZ	0T764DZ	0T938ZX	0TB14ZX	0TC18ZZ
0SWPX3Z	0T13077	0T134KC	0T144J7	0T1647C	0T1847A	0T510ZZ	0T764ZZ	0T943ZX	0TB17ZX	0TC30ZZ
0SWPX4Z	0T13078	0T134KD	0T144J8	0T1647D	0T1847B	0T513ZZ	0T767DZ	0T943ZZ	0TB18ZX	0TC33ZZ
0SWPX5Z	0T13079	0T134Z3	0T144J9	0T164J6	0T1847C	0T514ZZ	0T767ZZ	0T944ZX	0TB33ZX	0TC34ZZ
0SWPX7Z	0T1307A	0T134Z4	0T144JA	0T164J7	0T1847D	0T517ZZ	0T768DZ	0T944ZZ	0TB34ZX	0TC37ZZ
0SWPX8Z	0T1307B	0T134Z6	0T144JB	0T164J8	0T184J6	0T518ZZ	0T768ZZ	0T947ZX	0TB37ZX	0TC38ZZ
0SWPXJZ	0T1307C	0T134Z7	0T144JC	0T164J9	0T184J7	0T530ZZ	0T770DZ	0T948ZX	0TB38ZX	0TC40ZZ
0SWPXKZ	0T1307D	0T134Z8	0T144JD	0T164JA	0T184J8	0T533ZZ	0T770ZZ	0T9600Z	0TB43ZX	0TC43ZZ
0SWQ00Z	0T130J3	0T134Z9	0T144K3	0T164JB	0T184J9	0T534ZZ	0T773DZ	0T9630Z	0TB44ZX	0TC44ZZ
0SWQ03Z	0T130J4	0T134ZA	0T144K4	0T164JC	0T184JA	0T537ZZ	0T773ZZ	0T963ZX	0TB47ZX	0TC47ZZ
0SWQ04Z	0T130J6	0T134ZB	0T144K6	0T164JD	0T184JB	0T538ZZ	0T774DZ	0T963ZZ	0TB48ZX	0TC48ZZ
0SWQ05Z	0T130J7	0T134ZC	0T144K7	0T164K6	0T184JC	0T540ZZ	0T774ZZ	0T9640Z	0TB63ZX	0TC60ZZ
0SWQ07Z	0T130J8	0T134ZD	0T144K8	0T164K7	0T184JD	0T543ZZ	0T777DZ	0T964ZX	0TB64ZX	0TC63ZZ
0SWQ08Z	0T130J9	0T14073	0T144K9	0T164K8	0T184K6	0T544ZZ	0T777ZZ	0T9670Z	0TB67ZX	0TC64ZZ
0SWQ0JZ	0T130JA	0T14074	0T144KA	0T164K9	0T184K7	0T547ZZ	0T778DZ	0T967ZX	0TB68ZX	0TC67ZZ
0SWQ0KZ	0T130JB	0T14076	0T144KB	0T164KA	0T184K8	0T548ZZ	0T778ZZ	0T9680Z	0TB70ZX	0TC68ZZ
0SWQ30Z	0T130JC	0T14077	0T144KC	0T174K8	0T184K9	0T560ZZ	0T780DZ	0T968ZX	0TB70ZZ	0TC70ZZ
0SWQ33Z	0T130JD	0T14078	0T144KD	0T174K9	0T184KA	0T563ZZ	0T780ZZ	0T9700Z	0TB73ZX	0TC73ZZ

0TC74ZZ	0TFDXZZ	0THD02Z	0TL44CZ	0TLD4DZ	0TP5XDZ	0TQ40ZZ	0TR68KZ	0TS80ZZ	0TU607Z	0TW5XJZ
0TC77ZZ	0TH502Z	0THD03Z	0TL44DZ	0TLD4ZZ	0TP90YZ	0TQ43ZZ	0TR707Z	0TS84ZZ	0TU60JZ	0TW5XKZ
0TC78ZZ	0TH503Z	0THD0LZ	0TL44ZZ	0TLD7DZ	0TP93YZ	0TQ44ZZ	0TR70JZ	0TSB0ZZ	0TU60KZ	0TW90YZ
0TCB0ZZ	0TH50YZ	0THD0YZ	0TL47DZ	0TLD7ZZ	0TP94YZ	0TQ47ZZ	0TR70KZ	0TSB4ZZ	0TU647Z	0TW93YZ
0TCB3ZZ	0TH532Z	0THD32Z	0TL47ZZ	0TLD8DZ	0TP970Z	0TQ48ZZ	0TR747Z	0TSC0ZZ	0TU64JZ	0TW94YZ
0TCB4ZZ	0TH533Z	0THD33Z	0TL48DZ	0TLD8ZZ	0TP972Z	0TQ60ZZ	0TR74JZ	0TSC4ZZ	0TU64KZ	0TW97YZ
0TCB7ZZ	0TH53YZ	0THD3LZ	0TL48ZZ	0TLDXCZ	0TP973Z	0TQ63ZZ	0TR74KZ	0TSD0ZZ	0TU677Z	0TW980Z
0TCB8ZZ	0TH542Z	0THD3YZ	0TL60CZ	0TLDXDZ	0TP97DZ	0TQ64ZZ	0TR777Z	0TSD4ZZ	0TU67JZ	0TW982Z
0TCC0ZZ	0TH543Z	0THD42Z	0TL60DZ	0TLDXZZ	0TP97YZ	0TQ67ZZ	0TR77JZ	0TT00ZZ	0TU67KZ	0TW983Z
0TCC3ZZ	0TH54YZ	0THD43Z	0TL60ZZ	0TM00ZZ	0TP980Z	0TQ68ZZ	0TR77KZ	0TT04ZZ	0TU687Z	0TW987Z
0TCC4ZZ	0TH572Z	0THD4LZ	0TL63CZ	0TM04ZZ	0TP982Z	0TQ70ZZ	0TR787Z	0TT10ZZ	0TU68JZ	0TW98CZ
0TCC7ZZ	0TH573Z	0THD4YZ	0TL63DZ	0TM10ZZ	0TP983Z	0TQ73ZZ	0TR78JZ	0TT14ZZ	0TU68KZ	0TW98DZ
0TCC8ZZ	0TH57YZ	0THD72Z	0TL63ZZ	0TM14ZZ	0TP98DZ	0TQ74ZZ	0TR78KZ	0TT20ZZ	0TU707Z	0TW98JZ
0TCD0ZZ	0TH582Z	0THD73Z	0TL64CZ	0TM20ZZ	0TP98YZ	0TQ77ZZ	0TRB07Z	0TT24ZZ	0TU70JZ	0TW98KZ
0TCD3ZZ	0TH583Z	0THD7LZ	0TL64DZ	0TM24ZZ	0TP9X0Z	0TQ78ZZ	0TRB0JZ	0TT30ZZ	0TU70KZ	0TW98MZ
0TCD4ZZ	0TH58YZ	0THD7YZ	0TL64ZZ	0TM30ZZ	0TP9X2Z	0TQB0ZZ	0TRB0KZ	0TT34ZZ	0TU747Z	0TW98YZ
0TCD7ZZ	0TH902Z	0THD82Z	0TL67DZ	0TM34ZZ	0TP9X3Z	0TQB3ZZ	0TRB47Z	0TT37ZZ	0TU74JZ	0TW9X0Z
0TCD8ZZ	0TH903Z	0THD83Z	0TL67ZZ	0TM40ZZ	0TP9XDZ	0TQB4ZZ	0TRB4JZ	0TT38ZZ	0TU74KZ	0TW9X2Z
0TCDXZZ	0TH90MZ	0THD8LZ	0TL68DZ	0TM44ZZ	0TPB0YZ	0TQB7ZZ	0TRB4KZ	0TT40ZZ	0TU777Z	0TW9X3Z
0TD00ZZ	0TH90YZ	0THD8YZ	0TL68ZZ	0TM60ZZ	0TPB3YZ	0TQB8ZZ	0TRB77Z	0TT44ZZ	0TU77JZ	0TW9X7Z
0TD03ZZ	0TH932Z	0THDX2Z	0TL70CZ	0TM64ZZ	0TPB4YZ	0TQC0ZZ	0TRB7JZ	0TT47ZZ	0TU77KZ	0TW9XCZ
0TD04ZZ	0TH933Z	0THDX3Z	0TL70DZ	0TM70ZZ	0TPB70Z	0TQC3ZZ	0TRB7KZ	0TT48ZZ	0TU787Z	0TW9XDZ
0TD10ZZ	0TH93MZ	0THDXLZ	0TL70ZZ	0TM74ZZ	0TPB72Z	0TQC4ZZ	0TRB87Z	0TT60ZZ	0TU78JZ	0TW9XJZ
0TD13ZZ	0TH93YZ	0TJ50ZZ	0TL73CZ	0TM80ZZ	0TPB73Z	0TQC7ZZ	0TRB8JZ	0TT64ZZ	0TU78KZ	0TW9XKZ
0TD14ZZ	0TH942Z	0TJ53ZZ	0TL73DZ	0TM84ZZ	0TPB7DZ	0TQC8ZZ	0TRB8KZ	0TT67ZZ	0TUB07Z	0TW9XMZ
0TF30ZZ	0TH943Z	0TJ54ZZ	0TL73ZZ	0TMB0ZZ	0TPB7YZ	0TQD0ZZ	0TRC07Z	0TT68ZZ	0TUB0JZ	0TWB00Z
0TF33ZZ	0TH94MZ	0TJ57ZZ	0TL74CZ	0TMB4ZZ	0TPB80Z	0TQD3ZZ	0TRC0JZ	0TT70ZZ	0TUB0KZ	0TWB02Z
0TF34ZZ	0TH94YZ	0TJ58ZZ	0TL74DZ	0TMC0ZZ	0TPB82Z	0TQD4ZZ	0TRC0KZ	0TT74ZZ	0TUB47Z	0TWB03Z
0TF37ZZ	0TH972Z	0TJ5XZZ	0TL74ZZ	0TMC4ZZ	0TPB83Z	0TQD7ZZ	0TRC47Z	0TT77ZZ	0TUB4JZ	0TWB07Z
0TF38ZZ	0TH973Z	0TJ90ZZ	0TL77DZ	0TMD0ZZ	0TPB8DZ	0TQD8ZZ	0TRC4JZ	0TT78ZZ	0TUB4KZ	0TWB0CZ
0TF3XZZ	0TH97MZ	0TJ93ZZ	0TL77ZZ	0TMD4ZZ	0TPB8YZ	0TQDXZZ	0TRC4KZ	0TTB0ZZ	0TUB77Z	0TWB0DZ
0TF40ZZ	0TH97YZ	0TJ94ZZ	0TL78DZ	0TN00ZZ	0TPBX0Z	0TR307Z	0TRC77Z	0TTB4ZZ	0TUB7JZ	0TWB0JZ
0TF43ZZ	0TH982Z	0TJ97ZZ	0TL78ZZ	0TN03ZZ	0TPBX2Z	0TR30JZ	0TRC7JZ	0TTB7ZZ	0TUB7KZ	0TWB0KZ
0TF44ZZ	0TH983Z	0TJ98ZZ	0TLB0CZ	0TN04ZZ	0TPBX3Z	0TR30KZ	0TRC7KZ	0TTB8ZZ	0TUB87Z	0TWB0LZ
0TF47ZZ	0TH98MZ	0TJ9XZZ	0TLB0DZ	0TN07ZZ	0TPBXDZ	0TR347Z	0TRC87Z	0TTC0ZZ	0TUB8JZ	0TWB0MZ
0TF48ZZ	0TH98YZ	0TJB0ZZ	0TLB0ZZ	0TN08ZZ	0TPBXLZ	0TR34JZ	0TRC8JZ	0TTC4ZZ	0TUB8KZ	0TWB0YZ
0TF4XZZ	0THB02Z	0TJB3ZZ	0TLB3CZ	0TN10ZZ	0TPD0YZ	0TR34KZ	0TRC8KZ	0TTC7ZZ	0TUC07Z	0TWB30Z
0TF60ZZ	0THB03Z	0TJB4ZZ	0TLB3DZ	0TN13ZZ	0TPD3YZ	0TR377Z	0TRD07Z	0TTC8ZZ	0TUC0JZ	0TWB32Z
0TF63ZZ	0THB0LZ	0TJB7ZZ	0TLB3ZZ	0TN14ZZ	0TPD4YZ	0TR37JZ	0TRD0JZ	0TTD0ZZ	0TUC0KZ	0TWB33Z
0TF64ZZ	0THB0MZ	0TJB8ZZ	0TLB4CZ	0TN17ZZ	0TPD70Z	0TR37KZ	0TRD0KZ	0TTD4ZZ	0TUC47Z	0TWB37Z
0TF67ZZ	0THB0YZ	0TJBXZZ	0TLB4DZ	0TN18ZZ	0TPD72Z	0TR387Z	0TRD47Z	0TTD7ZZ	0TUC4JZ	0TWB3CZ
0TF68ZZ	0THB32Z	0TJD0ZZ	0TLB4ZZ	0TN30ZZ	0TPD73Z	0TR38JZ	0TRD4JZ	0TTD8ZZ	0TUC4KZ	0TWB3DZ
0TF6XZZ	0THB33Z	0TJD3ZZ	0TLB7DZ	0TN33ZZ	0TPD7DZ	0TR38KZ	0TRD4KZ	0TU307Z	0TUC77Z	0TWB3JZ
0TF70ZZ	0THB3LZ	0TJD7ZZ	0TLB7ZZ	0TN34ZZ	0TPD7YZ	0TR407Z	0TRD77Z	0TU30JZ	0TUC7JZ	0TWB3KZ
0TF73ZZ	0THB3MZ	0TJD8ZZ	0TLB8DZ	0TN37ZZ	0TPD80Z	0TR40JZ	0TRD7JZ	0TU30KZ	0TUC7KZ	0TWB3LZ
0TF74ZZ	0THB3YZ	0TJDXZZ	0TLB8ZZ	0TN38ZZ	0TPD82Z	0TR40KZ	0TRD7KZ	0TU347Z	0TUC87Z	0TWB3MZ
0TF77ZZ	0THB42Z	0TL30CZ	0TLC0CZ	0TN40ZZ	0TPD83Z	0TR447Z	0TRD87Z	0TU34JZ	0TUC8JZ	0TWB3YZ
0TF78ZZ	0THB43Z	0TL30DZ	0TLC0DZ	0TN43ZZ	0TPD8DZ	0TR44JZ	0TRD8JZ	0TU34KZ	0TUC8KZ	0TWB40Z
0TF7XZZ	0THB4LZ	0TL30ZZ	0TLC0ZZ	0TN44ZZ	0TPD8YZ	0TR44KZ	0TRD8KZ	0TU377Z	0TUD07Z	0TWB42Z
0TFB0ZZ	0THB4MZ	0TL33CZ	0TLC3CZ	0TN47ZZ	0TPDX0Z	0TR477Z	0TRDX7Z	0TU37JZ	0TUD0JZ	0TWB43Z
0TFB3ZZ	0THB4YZ	0TL33DZ	0TLC3DZ	0TP50YZ	0TPDX2Z	0TR47JZ	0TRDXJZ	0TU37KZ	0TUD0KZ	0TWB47Z
0TFB4ZZ	0THB72Z	0TL33ZZ	0TLC3ZZ	0TP53YZ	0TPDX3Z	0TR47KZ	0TRDXKZ	0TU387Z	0TUD47Z	0TWB4CZ
0TFB7ZZ	0THB73Z	0TL34CZ	0TLC4CZ	0TP54YZ	0TPDXDZ	0TR487Z	0TS00ZZ	0TU38JZ	0TUD4JZ	0TWB4DZ
0TFB8ZZ	0THB7LZ	0TL34DZ	0TLC4DZ	0TP570Z	0TQ04ZZ	0TR48JZ	0TS04ZZ	0TU38KZ	0TUD4KZ	0TWB4JZ
0TFBXZZ	0THB7MZ	0TL34ZZ	0TLC4ZZ	0TP572Z	0TQ07ZZ	0TR48KZ	0TS10ZZ	0TU407Z	0TUD77Z	0TWB4KZ
0TFC0ZZ	0THB7YZ	0TL37DZ	0TLC7DZ	0TP573Z	0TQ08ZZ	0TR607Z	0TS14ZZ	0TU40JZ	0TW50YZ	0TWB4LZ
0TFC3ZZ	0THB82Z	0TL37ZZ	0TLC7ZZ	0TP57DZ	0TQ10ZZ	0TR60JZ	0TS20ZZ	0TU40KZ	0TW53YZ	0TWB4MZ
0TFC4ZZ	0THB83Z	0TL38DZ	0TLC8DZ	0TP57YZ	0TQ13ZZ	0TR60KZ	0TS24ZZ	0TU447Z	0TW54YZ	0TWB4YZ
0TFC7ZZ	0THB8LZ	0TL38ZZ	0TLC8ZZ	0TP580Z	0TQ14ZZ	0TR647Z	0TS30ZZ	0TU44JZ	0TW57YZ	0TWB70Z
0TFC8ZZ	0THB8MZ	0TL40CZ	0TLD0CZ	0TP582Z	0TQ17ZZ	0TR64JZ	0TS34ZZ	0TU44KZ	0TW58YZ	0TWB72Z
0TFCXZZ	0THB8YZ	0TL40DZ	0TLD0DZ	0TP583Z	0TQ18ZZ	0TR64KZ	0TS40ZZ	0TU477Z	0TW5X0Z	0TWB73Z
0TFD0ZZ	0THC0LZ	0TL40ZZ	0TLD0ZZ	0TP58DZ	0TQ30ZZ	0TR677Z	0TS44ZZ	0TU47JZ	0TW5X2Z	0TWB77Z
0TFD3ZZ	0THC3LZ	0TL43CZ	0TLD3CZ	0TP58YZ	0TQ33ZZ	0TR67JZ	0TS60ZZ	0TU47KZ	0TW5X3Z	0TWB7CZ
0TFD4ZZ	0THC4LZ	0TL43DZ	0TLD3DZ	0TP5X0Z	0TQ34ZZ	0TR67KZ	0TS64ZZ	0TU487Z	0TW5X7Z	0TWB7DZ
0TFD7ZZ	0THC7LZ	0TL43ZZ	0TLD3ZZ	0TP5X2Z	0TQ37ZZ	0TR687Z	0TS70ZZ	0TU48JZ	0TW5XCZ	0TWB7JZ
0TFD8ZZ	0THC8LZ	0TL43ZZ	0TLD4CZ	0TP5X3Z	0TQ38ZZ	0TR68JZ	0TS74ZZ	0TU48KZ	0TW5XDZ	0TWB7KZ

0TWB7LZ	0TWD83Z	0U164K6	0U5F7ZZ	0U7C7DZ	0U91XZZ	0U977ZX	0UC04ZZ	0UCMXZZ	0UHD73Z	0UL63DZ
0TWB7MZ	0TWD87Z	0U164K9	0U5F8ZZ	0U7C7ZZ	0U9200Z	0U977ZZ	0UC08ZZ	0UDB7ZX	0UHD7YZ	0UL63ZZ
0TWB7YZ	0TWD8CZ	0U164Z5	0U5G0ZZ	0U7C8DZ	0U920ZX	0U9780Z	0UC10ZZ	0UDB7ZZ	0UHD83Z	0UL64CZ
0TWB80Z	0TWD8DZ	0U164Z6	0U5G3ZZ	0U7C8ZZ	0U920ZZ	0U978ZX	0UC13ZZ	0UDB8ZX	0UHD8YZ	0UL64DZ
0TWB82Z	0TWD8JZ	0U164Z9	0U5G4ZZ	0U7G0DZ	0U9230Z	0U978ZZ	0UC14ZZ	0UDB8ZZ	0UHF7GZ	0UL64ZZ
0TWB83Z	0TWD8KZ	0U23X0Z	0U5G7ZZ	0U7G0DZ	0U923ZX	0U9900Z	0UC18ZZ	0UDN0ZZ	0UHF8GZ	0UL67DZ
0TWB7BZ	0TWD8LZ	0U23XYZ	0U5G8ZZ	0U7G0ZZ	0U923ZZ	0U990ZX	0UC20ZZ	0UDN3ZZ	0UHG01Z	0UL67ZZ
0TWB8CZ	0TWD8YZ	0U28X0Z	0U5GXZZ	0U7G3DZ	0U9240Z	0U990ZZ	0UC23ZZ	0UDN4ZZ	0UHG31Z	0UL68DZ
0TWB8DZ	0TWDX0Z	0U28XYZ	0U5J0ZZ	0U7G3ZZ	0U924ZX	0U9930Z	0UC24ZZ	0UF50ZZ	0UHG41Z	0UL68ZZ
0TWB8JZ	0TWDX2Z	0U2DX0Z	0U5JXZZ	0U7G4DZ	0U924ZZ	0U993ZX	0UC28ZZ	0UF53ZZ	0UHG71Z	0UL70CZ
0TWB8KZ	0TWDX3Z	0U2DXHZ	0U5K0ZZ	0U7G4ZZ	0U9280Z	0U993ZZ	0UC40ZZ	0UF54ZZ	0UHG7GZ	0UL70DZ
0TWB8LZ	0TWDX7Z	0U2DXYZ	0U5K3ZZ	0U7G7DZ	0U928ZX	0U9940Z	0UC43ZZ	0UF57ZZ	0UHG81Z	0UL70ZZ
0TWB8MZ	0TWDXCZ	0U2HX0Z	0U5K4ZZ	0U7G7ZZ	0U928ZZ	0U994ZX	0UC44ZZ	0UF58ZZ	0UHG8GZ	0UL73CZ
0TWB8YZ	0TWDXDZ	0U2HXGZ	0U5K7ZZ	0U7G8DZ	0U92XZZ	0U994ZZ	0UC48ZZ	0UF5XZZ	0UHGX1Z	0UL73DZ
0TWBX0Z	0TWDXJZ	0U2HXYZ	0U5K8ZZ	0U7G8ZZ	0U9400Z	0U9970Z	0UC50ZZ	0UF60ZZ	0UHH03Z	0UL73ZZ
0TWBX2Z	0TWDXKZ	0U2MX0Z	0U5KXZZ	0U7K0DZ	0U940ZX	0U997ZX	0UC53ZZ	0UF63ZZ	0UHH0YZ	0UL74CZ
0TWBX3Z	0TWDXLZ	0U2MXYZ	0U5L0ZZ	0U7K0ZZ	0U940ZZ	0U997ZZ	0UC54ZZ	0UF64ZZ	0UHH33Z	0UL74DZ
0TWBX7Z	0TY00Z0	0U500ZZ	0U5LXZZ	0U7K3DZ	0U9430Z	0U9980Z	0UC57ZZ	0UF67ZZ	0UHH3YZ	0UL74ZZ
0TWBXCZ	0TY00Z1	0U503ZZ	0U5M0ZZ	0U7K3ZZ	0U943ZX	0U998ZX	0UC58ZZ	0UF68ZZ	0UHH43Z	0UL77DZ
0TWBXDZ	0TY00Z2	0U504ZZ	0U5MXZZ	0U7K4DZ	0U943ZZ	0U998ZZ	0UC60ZZ	0UF6XZZ	0UHH4YZ	0UL77ZZ
0TWBXJZ	0TY10Z0	0U508ZZ	0U750DZ	0U7K4ZZ	0U9440Z	0U9C00Z	0UC63ZZ	0UF70ZZ	0UHH73Z	0UL78DZ
0TWBXKZ	0TY10Z1	0U510ZZ	0U750ZZ	0U7K7DZ	0U944ZX	0U9C0ZX	0UC64ZZ	0UF73ZZ	0UHH7YZ	0UL78ZZ
0TWBXLZ	0TY10Z2	0U513ZZ	0U753DZ	0U7K7ZZ	0U944ZZ	0U9C30Z	0UC67ZZ	0UF74ZZ	0UHH83Z	0ULF7DZ
0TWBXMZ	0U15075	0U514ZZ	0U753ZZ	0U7K8DZ	0U9480Z	0U9C3ZZ	0UC68ZZ	0UF77ZZ	0UHH8YZ	0ULF7ZZ
0TWD00Z	0U15076	0U518ZZ	0U754DZ	0U7K8ZZ	0U948ZX	0U9F30Z	0UC70ZZ	0UF78ZZ	0UJ30ZZ	0ULF8DZ
0TWD02Z	0U15079	0U520ZZ	0U754ZZ	0U7KXDZ	0U948ZZ	0U9F3ZZ	0UC73ZZ	0UF7XZZ	0UJ33ZZ	0ULF8ZZ
0TWD03Z	0U150J5	0U523ZZ	0U757DZ	0U7KXZZ	0U9500Z	0U9F40Z	0UC74ZZ	0UF90ZZ	0UJ34ZZ	0ULG7DZ
0TWD07Z	0U150J6	0U524ZZ	0U757ZZ	0U800ZZ	0U950ZX	0U9F4ZZ	0UC77ZZ	0UF93ZZ	0UJ38ZZ	0ULG7ZZ
0TWD0CZ	0U150J9	0U528ZZ	0U758DZ	0U803ZZ	0U950ZZ	0U9G30Z	0UC78ZZ	0UF94ZZ	0UJ3XZZ	0ULG8DZ
0TWD0DZ	0U150K5	0U540ZZ	0U758ZZ	0U804ZZ	0U9530Z	0U9G3ZZ	0UC90ZZ	0UF97ZZ	0UJ80ZZ	0ULG8ZZ
0TWD0JZ	0U150K6	0U543ZZ	0U760DZ	0U810ZZ	0U953ZX	0U9K00Z	0UC93ZZ	0UF98ZZ	0UJ83ZZ	0UM00ZZ
0TWD0KZ	0U150K9	0U544ZZ	0U760ZZ	0U813ZZ	0U953ZZ	0U9K0ZZ	0UC94ZZ	0UF9XZZ	0UJ84ZZ	0UM04ZZ
0TWD0LZ	0U150Z5	0U548ZZ	0U763DZ	0U814ZZ	0U9540Z	0U9K30Z	0UC97ZZ	0UH303Z	0UJ87ZZ	0UM10ZZ
0TWD0YZ	0U150Z6	0U550ZZ	0U763ZZ	0U820ZZ	0U954ZX	0U9K3ZZ	0UC98ZZ	0UH30YZ	0UJ88ZZ	0UM14ZZ
0TWD30Z	0U150Z9	0U553ZZ	0U764DZ	0U823ZZ	0U954ZZ	0U9K40Z	0UCB0ZZ	0UH333Z	0UJ8XZZ	0UM20ZZ
0TWD32Z	0U15475	0U554ZZ	0U764ZZ	0U824ZZ	0U9570Z	0U9K4ZZ	0UCB3ZZ	0UH33YZ	0UJD0ZZ	0UM24ZZ
0TWD33Z	0U15476	0U557ZZ	0U767DZ	0U840ZZ	0U957ZX	0U9K70Z	0UCB4ZZ	0UH343Z	0UJD3ZZ	0UM40ZZ
0TWD37Z	0U15479	0U558ZZ	0U767ZZ	0U843ZZ	0U957ZZ	0U9K7ZZ	0UCB7ZZ	0UH34YZ	0UJD4ZZ	0UM44ZZ
0TWD3CZ	0U154J5	0U560ZZ	0U768DZ	0U844ZZ	0U9580Z	0U9K80Z	0UCB8ZZ	0UH37YZ	0UJD7ZZ	0UM50ZZ
0TWD3DZ	0U154J6	0U563ZZ	0U768ZZ	0U8K7ZZ	0U958ZX	0U9K8ZZ	0UCC0ZZ	0UH38YZ	0UJD8ZZ	0UM54ZZ
0TWD3JZ	0U154J9	0U564ZZ	0U770DZ	0U8K8ZZ	0U958ZZ	0U9KX0Z	0UCC3ZZ	0UH803Z	0UJDXZZ	0UM60ZZ
0TWD3KZ	0U154K5	0U567ZZ	0U770ZZ	0U8KXZZ	0U9600Z	0U9KXZZ	0UCC4ZZ	0UH80YZ	0UJH0ZZ	0UM64ZZ
0TWD3LZ	0U154K6	0U568ZZ	0U773DZ	0U9000Z	0U960ZX	0U9L00Z	0UCC7ZZ	0UH833Z	0UJH3ZZ	0UM70ZZ
0TWD3YZ	0U154K9	0U570ZZ	0U773ZZ	0U900ZX	0U960ZZ	0U9L0ZZ	0UCC8ZZ	0UH83YZ	0UJH4ZZ	0UM74ZZ
0TWD40Z	0U154Z5	0U573ZZ	0U774DZ	0U900ZZ	0U9630Z	0U9LX0Z	0UCF0ZZ	0UH843Z	0UJH7ZZ	0UM90ZZ
0TWD42Z	0U154Z6	0U574ZZ	0U774ZZ	0U9030Z	0U963ZX	0U9LXZZ	0UCF3ZZ	0UH84YZ	0UJH8ZZ	0UM94ZZ
0TWD43Z	0U154Z9	0U577ZZ	0U777DZ	0U903ZX	0U963ZZ	0UBK3ZX	0UCF4ZZ	0UH873Z	0UJHXZZ	0UMC0ZZ
0TWD47Z	0U16075	0U578ZZ	0U777ZZ	0U903ZZ	0U9640Z	0UBK3ZZ	0UCF7ZZ	0UH87YZ	0UJM0ZZ	0UMC4ZZ
0TWD4CZ	0U16076	0U590ZZ	0U778DZ	0U904ZX	0U964ZX	0UBK4ZX	0UCF8ZZ	0UH883Z	0UJMXZZ	0UMF0ZZ
0TWD4DZ	0U16079	0U593ZZ	0U778ZZ	0U904ZZ	0U964ZZ	0UBK4ZZ	0UCG0ZZ	0UH88YZ	0UL50CZ	0UMF4ZZ
0TWD4JZ	0U160J5	0U594ZZ	0U790DZ	0U9080Z	0U9670Z	0UBK7ZX	0UCG3ZZ	0UH90HZ	0UL50DZ	0UMG0ZZ
0TWD4KZ	0U160J6	0U597ZZ	0U790ZZ	0U908ZX	0U967ZX	0UBK7ZZ	0UCG4ZZ	0UH97HZ	0UL50ZZ	0UMG4ZZ
0TWD4LZ	0U160J9	0U598ZZ	0U793DZ	0U908ZZ	0U967ZZ	0UBK8ZX	0UCG7ZZ	0UH98HZ	0UL53CZ	0UMJXZZ
0TWD4YZ	0U160K5	0U5B0ZZ	0U793ZZ	0U90XZZ	0U9680Z	0UBK8ZZ	0UCG8ZZ	0UHC01Z	0UL53DZ	0UMK0ZZ
0TWD70Z	0U160K6	0U5B3ZZ	0U794DZ	0U9100Z	0U968ZX	0UBKXZX	0UCGXZZ	0UHC31Z	0UL53ZZ	0UMK4ZZ
0TWD72Z	0U160K9	0U5B4ZZ	0U794ZZ	0U910ZX	0U968ZZ	0UBKXZZ	0UCJ0ZZ	0UHC41Z	0UL54CZ	0UMKXZZ
0TWD73Z	0U160Z5	0U5B7ZZ	0U797DZ	0U910ZZ	0U9700Z	0UBL0ZX	0UCJXZZ	0UHC71Z	0UL54DZ	0UMMXZZ
0TWD77Z	0U160Z6	0U5B8ZZ	0U797ZZ	0U9130Z	0U970ZX	0UBL0ZZ	0UCK0ZZ	0UHC7HZ	0UL54ZZ	0UN00ZZ
0TWD7CZ	0U160Z9	0U5C0ZZ	0U798DZ	0U913ZX	0U970ZZ	0UBLXZX	0UCK3ZZ	0UHC81Z	0UL57DZ	0UN03ZZ
0TWD7DZ	0U16475	0U5C3ZZ	0U798ZZ	0U913ZZ	0U9730Z	0UBLXZZ	0UCK4ZZ	0UHC8HZ	0UL57ZZ	0UN04ZZ
0TWD7JZ	0U16476	0U5C4ZZ	0U7C0DZ	0U9140Z	0U973ZX	0UBM0ZX	0UCK7ZZ	0UHD03Z	0UL58DZ	0UN08ZZ
0TWD7KZ	0U16479	0U5C7ZZ	0U7C0ZZ	0U914ZX	0U973ZZ	0UBM0ZZ	0UCK8ZZ	0UHD0YZ	0UL58ZZ	0UN10ZZ
0TWD7LZ	0U164J5	0U5C8ZZ	0U7C3DZ	0U914ZZ	0U9740Z	0UBMXZX	0UCKXZZ	0UHD33Z	0UL60CZ	0UN13ZZ
0TWD7YZ	0U164J6	0U5F0ZZ	0U7C3ZZ	0U9180Z	0U974ZX	0UBMXZZ	0UCL0ZZ	0UHD3YZ	0UL60DZ	0UN14ZZ
0TWD80Z	0U164J9	0U5F3ZZ	0U7C4DZ	0U918ZX	0U974ZZ	0UC00ZZ	0UCLXZZ	0UHD43Z	0UL60ZZ	0UN18ZZ
0TWD82Z	0U164K5	0U5F4ZZ	0U7C4ZZ	0U918ZZ	0U9770Z	0UC03ZZ	0UCM0ZZ	0UHD4YZ	0UL63CZ	0UN20ZZ

0UN23ZZ	0UP3X0Z	0UPD41Z	0UT04ZZ	0UU407Z	0UUGX7Z	0UW837Z	0UWD4YZ	0UWMXJZ	0V953ZX	0V9H3ZX
0UN24ZZ	0UP3X3Z	0UPD43Z	0UT07ZZ	0UU40JZ	0UUGXJZ	0UW83CZ	0UWD70Z	0UWMXKZ	0V953ZZ	0V9H3ZZ
0UN28ZZ	0UP800Z	0UPD47Z	0UT08ZZ	0UU40KZ	0UUGXKZ	0UW83DZ	0UWD71Z	0V24X0Z	0V9540Z	0V9H40Z
0UN40ZZ	0UP803Z	0UPD4CZ	0UT0FZZ	0UU447Z	0UUJ07Z	0UW83JZ	0UWD73Z	0V24XYZ	0V954ZX	0V9H4ZX
0UN43ZZ	0UP807Z	0UPD4YZ	0UT10ZZ	0UU44JZ	0UUJ0JZ	0UW83KZ	0UWD77Z	0V28X0Z	0V954ZZ	0V9H4ZZ
0UN44ZZ	0UP80CZ	0UPD70Z	0UT14ZZ	0UU44KZ	0UUJX7Z	0UW83YZ	0UWD7CZ	0V28XYZ	0V95X0Z	0V9J0ZX
0UN48ZZ	0UP80DZ	0UPD73Z	0UT17ZZ	0UU507Z	0UUJXJZ	0UW840Z	0UWD7DZ	0V2DX0Z	0V95XXZ	0V9J30Z
0UN50ZZ	0UP80JZ	0UPD7CZ	0UT18ZZ	0UU50JZ	0UUJXKZ	0UW843Z	0UWD7HZ	0V2DXYZ	0V95XZZ	0V9J3ZX
0UN53ZZ	0UP80KZ	0UPD7DZ	0UT1FZZ	0UU50KZ	0UUK07Z	0UW847Z	0UWD7JZ	0V2MX0Z	0V9600Z	0V9J3ZZ
0UN54ZZ	0UP80YZ	0UPD7HZ	0UT20ZZ	0UU547Z	0UUK0JZ	0UW84CZ	0UWD7KZ	0V2MXYZ	0V960ZX	0V9J4ZX
0UN57ZZ	0UP830Z	0UPD7YZ	0UT24ZZ	0UU54JZ	0UUK0KZ	0UW84DZ	0UWD7YZ	0V2RX0Z	0V960ZZ	0V9K0ZX
0UN58ZZ	0UP833Z	0UPD80Z	0UT27ZZ	0UU54KZ	0UUK47Z	0UW84JZ	0UWD80Z	0V2RXYZ	0V9630Z	0V9K30Z
0UN60ZZ	0UP837Z	0UPD83Z	0UT28ZZ	0UU577Z	0UUK4JZ	0UW84KZ	0UWD81Z	0V2SX0Z	0V963ZX	0V9K3ZX
0UN63ZZ	0UP83CZ	0UPD8CZ	0UT2FZZ	0UU57JZ	0UUK4KZ	0UW84YZ	0UWD83Z	0V2SXYZ	0V963ZZ	0V9K3ZZ
0UN64ZZ	0UP83DZ	0UPD8DZ	0UT40ZZ	0UU57KZ	0UUK77Z	0UW870Z	0UWD87Z	0V550ZZ	0V9640Z	0V9K4ZX
0UN67ZZ	0UP83JZ	0UPD8HZ	0UT44ZZ	0UU587Z	0UUK7JZ	0UW873Z	0UWD8CZ	0V553ZZ	0V964ZX	0V9L0ZX
0UN68ZZ	0UP83KZ	0UPD8YZ	0UT47ZZ	0UU58JZ	0UUK7KZ	0UW877Z	0UWD8DZ	0V554ZZ	0V964ZZ	0V9L30Z
0UN70ZZ	0UP83YZ	0UPDX0Z	0UT48ZZ	0UU58KZ	0UUK87Z	0UW87CZ	0UWD8HZ	0V55XZZ	0V9700Z	0V9L3ZX
0UN73ZZ	0UP840Z	0UPDX3Z	0UT50ZZ	0UU607Z	0UUK8JZ	0UW87DZ	0UWD8JZ	0V5F8ZZ	0V970ZX	0V9L3ZZ
0UN74ZZ	0UP843Z	0UPDXDZ	0UT54ZZ	0UU60JZ	0UUK8KZ	0UW87JZ	0UWD8KZ	0V5G8ZZ	0V970ZZ	0V9L4ZX
0UN77ZZ	0UP847Z	0UPDXHZ	0UT57ZZ	0UU60KZ	0UUKX7Z	0UW87KZ	0UWD8YZ	0V5H8ZZ	0V9730Z	0V9N00Z
0UN78ZZ	0UP84CZ	0UPH0YZ	0UT58ZZ	0UU647Z	0UUKXJZ	0UW87YZ	0UWDX0Z	0V5J8ZZ	0V973ZX	0V9N0ZX
0UN90ZZ	0UP84DZ	0UPH3YZ	0UT5FZZ	0UU64JZ	0UUKXKZ	0UW880Z	0UWDX3Z	0V5K8ZZ	0V973ZZ	0V9N0ZZ
0UN93ZZ	0UP84JZ	0UPH4YZ	0UT60ZZ	0UU64KZ	0UUM07Z	0UW883Z	0UWDX7Z	0V5L8ZZ	0V9740Z	0V9N30Z
0UN94ZZ	0UP84KZ	0UPH70Z	0UT64ZZ	0UU677Z	0UUM0JZ	0UW887Z	0UWDXCZ	0V5N0ZZ	0V974ZX	0V9N3ZX
0UN97ZZ	0UP84YZ	0UPH73Z	0UT67ZZ	0UU67JZ	0UUM0KZ	0UW88CZ	0UWDXDZ	0V5N3ZZ	0V974ZZ	0V9N3ZZ
0UN98ZZ	0UP870Z	0UPH7DZ	0UT68ZZ	0UU67KZ	0UUMX7Z	0UW88DZ	0UWDXHZ	0V5N4ZZ	0V9930Z	0V9N40Z
0UNC0ZZ	0UP873Z	0UPH7YZ	0UT6FZZ	0UU687Z	0UUMXJZ	0UW88JZ	0UWDXJZ	0V5N8ZZ	0V993ZX	0V9N4ZX
0UNC3ZZ	0UP877Z	0UPH80Z	0UT70ZZ	0UU68JZ	0UUMXKZ	0UW88KZ	0UWDXKZ	0V5P0ZZ	0V993ZZ	0V9N4ZZ
0UNC4ZZ	0UP87CZ	0UPH83Z	0UT74ZZ	0UU68KZ	0UVC0CZ	0UW88YZ	0UWH00Z	0V5P3ZZ	0V9940Z	0V9P00Z
0UNC7ZZ	0UP87DZ	0UPH8DZ	0UT77ZZ	0UU707Z	0UVC0DZ	0UW8X0Z	0UWH01Z	0V5P4ZZ	0V994ZX	0V9P0ZX
0UNC8ZZ	0UP87JZ	0UPH8YZ	0UT78ZZ	0UU70JZ	0UVC0ZZ	0UW8X3Z	0UWH03Z	0V5P8ZZ	0V994ZZ	0V9P0ZZ
0UNF0ZZ	0UP87KZ	0UPHX0Z	0UT7FZZ	0UU70KZ	0UVC3CZ	0UW8X7Z	0UWH07Z	0V5Q0ZZ	0V9B30Z	0V9P30Z
0UNF3ZZ	0UP87YZ	0UPHX1Z	0UT90ZL	0UU747Z	0UVC3DZ	0UW8XCZ	0UWH0DZ	0V5Q3ZZ	0V9B3ZX	0V9P3ZX
0UNF4ZZ	0UP880Z	0UPHX3Z	0UT90ZZ	0UU74JZ	0UVC3ZZ	0UW8XDZ	0UWH0JZ	0V5Q4ZZ	0V9B3ZZ	0V9P3ZZ
0UNF7ZZ	0UP883Z	0UPHXDZ	0UT94ZL	0UU74KZ	0UVC4CZ	0UW8XJZ	0UWH0KZ	0V5Q8ZZ	0V9B40Z	0V9P40Z
0UNF8ZZ	0UP887Z	0UPMX0Z	0UT94ZZ	0UU777Z	0UVC4DZ	0UW8XKZ	0UWH0YZ	0V9030Z	0V9B4ZX	0V9P4ZX
0UNG0ZZ	0UP88CZ	0UQ08ZZ	0UT97ZL	0UU77JZ	0UVC4ZZ	0UWD00Z	0UWH30Z	0V903ZX	0V9B4ZZ	0V9P4ZZ
0UNG3ZZ	0UP88DZ	0UQ18ZZ	0UT97ZZ	0UU77KZ	0UVC7DZ	0UWD01Z	0UWH31Z	0V903ZZ	0V9C30Z	0V9Q00Z
0UNG4ZZ	0UP88JZ	0UQ28ZZ	0UT98ZL	0UU787Z	0UVC7ZZ	0UWD03Z	0UWH33Z	0V9040Z	0V9C3ZX	0V9Q0ZX
0UNG7ZZ	0UP88KZ	0UQ48ZZ	0UT98ZZ	0UU78JZ	0UVC8DZ	0UWD07Z	0UWH37Z	0V904ZX	0V9C3ZZ	0V9Q0ZZ
0UNG8ZZ	0UP88YZ	0US08ZZ	0UT9FZL	0UU78KZ	0UVC8ZZ	0UWD0CZ	0UWH3DZ	0V904ZZ	0V9C40Z	0V9Q30Z
0UNGXZZ	0UP8X0Z	0US18ZZ	0UT9FZZ	0UUF07Z	0UW300Z	0UWD0DZ	0UWH3JZ	0V907ZX	0V9C4ZX	0V9Q3ZX
0UNJ0ZZ	0UP8X3Z	0US28ZZ	0UTC0ZZ	0UUF0JZ	0UW303Z	0UWD0HZ	0UWH3KZ	0V908ZX	0V9C4ZZ	0V9Q3ZZ
0UNJXZZ	0UP8XDZ	0US48ZZ	0UTC4ZZ	0UUF0KZ	0UW30YZ	0UWD0JZ	0UWH3YZ	0V9130Z	0V9F00Z	0V9Q40Z
0UNK0ZZ	0UPD00Z	0US58ZZ	0UTC7ZZ	0UUF47Z	0UW330Z	0UWD0KZ	0UWH40Z	0V913ZX	0V9F0ZX	0V9Q4ZX
0UNK3ZZ	0UPD01Z	0US68ZZ	0UTC8ZZ	0UUF4JZ	0UW333Z	0UWD0YZ	0UWH41Z	0V913ZZ	0V9F0ZZ	0V9Q4ZZ
0UNK4ZZ	0UPD03Z	0US74ZZ	0UTF0ZZ	0UUF4KZ	0UW33YZ	0UWD30Z	0UWH43Z	0V9140Z	0V9F30Z	0V9S30Z
0UNK7ZZ	0UPD07Z	0US78ZZ	0UTF4ZZ	0UUF77Z	0UW340Z	0UWD31Z	0UWH47Z	0V914ZX	0V9F3ZX	0V9S3ZZ
0UNK8ZZ	0UPD0CZ	0US90ZZ	0UTF7ZZ	0UUF7JZ	0UW343Z	0UWD33Z	0UWH4DZ	0V914ZZ	0V9F3ZZ	0V9T30Z
0UNKXZZ	0UPD0DZ	0US94ZZ	0UTF8ZZ	0UUF7KZ	0UW34YZ	0UWD37Z	0UWH4JZ	0V9230Z	0V9F40Z	0V9T3ZZ
0UNL0ZZ	0UPD0HZ	0US97ZZ	0UTG0ZZ	0UUF87Z	0UW37YZ	0UWD3CZ	0UWH4KZ	0V923ZX	0V9F4ZX	0VB03ZX
0UNLXZZ	0UPD0JZ	0US98ZZ	0UTG4ZZ	0UUF8JZ	0UW38YZ	0UWD3DZ	0UWH4YZ	0V923ZZ	0V9F4ZZ	0VB04ZX
0UNM0ZZ	0UPD0KZ	0US9XZZ	0UTG7ZZ	0UUF8KZ	0UW3X0Z	0UWD3HZ	0UWH70Z	0V9240Z	0V9G00Z	0VB07ZX
0UNMXZZ	0UPD0YZ	0USC0ZZ	0UTG8ZZ	0UUG07Z	0UW3X3Z	0UWD3JZ	0UWH71Z	0V924ZX	0V9G0ZX	0VB08ZX
0UP300Z	0UPD30Z	0USC4ZZ	0UTJ0ZZ	0UUG0JZ	0UW3X0Z	0UWD3KZ	0UWH73Z	0V924ZZ	0V9G0ZZ	0VB13ZX
0UP303Z	0UPD31Z	0USC8ZZ	0UTJXZZ	0UUG0KZ	0UW800Z	0UWD3YZ	0UWH7YZ	0V9330Z	0V9G30Z	0VB14ZX
0UP30YZ	0UPD33Z	0USF0ZZ	0UTK0ZZ	0UUG47Z	0UW803Z	0UWD40Z	0UWH8YZ	0V933ZX	0V9G3ZX	0VB23ZX
0UP330Z	0UPD37Z	0USF4ZZ	0UTK4ZZ	0UUG4JZ	0UW807Z	0UWD41Z	0UWHX0Z	0V933ZZ	0V9G3ZZ	0VB24ZX
0UP333Z	0UPD3CZ	0USF8ZZ	0UTK7ZZ	0UUG4KZ	0UW80CZ	0UWD43Z	0UWHX3Z	0V9340Z	0V9G40Z	0VB33ZX
0UP33YZ	0UPD3DZ	0USG0ZZ	0UTK8ZZ	0UUG77Z	0UW80DZ	0UWD47Z	0UWHX7Z	0V934ZX	0V9G4ZX	0VB34ZX
0UP340Z	0UPD3HZ	0USG4ZZ	0UTKXZZ	0UUG7JZ	0UW80JZ	0UWD4CZ	0UWHXDZ	0V934ZZ	0V9G4ZZ	0VB50ZX
0UP343Z	0UPD3JZ	0USG7ZZ	0UTL0ZZ	0UUG7KZ	0UW80KZ	0UWD4DZ	0UWHXJZ	0V9500Z	0V9H00Z	0VB50ZZ
0UP34YZ	0UPD3KZ	0USG8ZZ	0UTLXZZ	0UUG87Z	0UW80YZ	0UWD4HZ	0UWHXKZ	0V950ZX	0V9H0ZX	0VB53ZX
0UP37YZ	0UPD3YZ	0USGXZZ	0UTM0ZZ	0UUG8JZ	0UW830Z	0UWD4JZ	0UWMX0Z	0V950ZZ	0V9H0ZZ	0VB53ZZ
0UP38YZ	0UPD40Z	0UT00ZZ	0UTMXZZ	0UUG8KZ	0UW833Z	0UWD4KZ	0UWMX7Z	0V9530Z	0V9H30Z	0VB54ZX

0VB54ZZ	0VBQ4ZZ	0VCL0ZZ	0VHR0YZ	0VLH0CZ	0VN00ZZ	0VNQ3ZZ	0VP84YZ	0VPM4KZ	0VPS0YZ	0VQG4ZZ
0VB5XZX	0VBQ8ZX	0VCL3ZZ	0VHR33Z	0VLH0DZ	0VN03ZZ	0VNQ4ZZ	0VP870Z	0VPM4YZ	0VPS30Z	0VQG8ZZ
0VB5XZZ	0VBQ8ZZ	0VCL4ZZ	0VHR3YZ	0VLH0ZZ	0VN04ZZ	0VNQ8ZZ	0VP873Z	0VPM70Z	0VPS33Z	0VQH0ZZ
0VB60ZX	0VBS0ZZ	0VCN0ZZ	0VHR43Z	0VLH3CZ	0VN07ZZ	0VNS0ZZ	0VP877Z	0VPM73Z	0VPS37Z	0VQH3ZZ
0VB63ZX	0VBS3ZX	0VCN3ZZ	0VHR4YZ	0VLH3DZ	0VN08ZZ	0VNS4ZZ	0VP87JZ	0VPM77Z	0VPS3JZ	0VQH4ZZ
0VB64ZX	0VBS3ZZ	0VCN4ZZ	0VHR73Z	0VLH3ZZ	0VN10ZZ	0VNSXZZ	0VP87KZ	0VPM7CZ	0VPS3KZ	0VQH8ZZ
0VB70ZX	0VBS4ZX	0VCP0ZZ	0VHR7YZ	0VLH4CZ	0VN13ZZ	0VNT0ZZ	0VP87YZ	0VPM7JZ	0VPS3YZ	0VQJ0ZZ
0VB73ZX	0VBS4ZZ	0VCP3ZZ	0VHR83Z	0VLH4DZ	0VN14ZZ	0VNT3ZZ	0VP880Z	0VPM7KZ	0VPS40Z	0VQJ3ZZ
0VB74ZX	0VBSXZX	0VCP4ZZ	0VHR8YZ	0VLH4ZZ	0VN20ZZ	0VNT4ZZ	0VP883Z	0VPM7YZ	0VPS43Z	0VQJ4ZZ
0VB93ZX	0VBSXZZ	0VCQ0ZZ	0VHS03Z	0VLH8CZ	0VN23ZZ	0VNTXZZ	0VP887Z	0VPM80Z	0VPS47Z	0VQJ8ZZ
0VB94ZX	0VBT0ZX	0VCQ3ZZ	0VHS0YZ	0VLH8DZ	0VN24ZZ	0VP400Z	0VP88JZ	0VPM83Z	0VPS4JZ	0VQK0ZZ
0VBB3ZX	0VBT0ZZ	0VCQ4ZZ	0VHS33Z	0VLH8ZZ	0VN30ZZ	0VP401Z	0VP88KZ	0VPM87Z	0VPS4KZ	0VQK3ZZ
0VBB4ZX	0VBT3ZX	0VCS0ZZ	0VHS3YZ	0VLN0CZ	0VN33ZZ	0VP403Z	0VP88YZ	0VPM8CZ	0VPS4YZ	0VQK4ZZ
0VBC3ZX	0VBT3ZZ	0VCS3ZZ	0VHS43Z	0VLN0DZ	0VN34ZZ	0VP407Z	0VP8X0Z	0VPM8JZ	0VPS70Z	0VQK8ZZ
0VBC4ZX	0VBT4ZX	0VCS4ZZ	0VHS4YZ	0VLN0ZZ	0VN50ZZ	0VP40JZ	0VP8X3Z	0VPM8KZ	0VPS73Z	0VQL0ZZ
0VBF0ZX	0VBT4ZZ	0VCSXZZ	0VHS7YZ	0VLN3CZ	0VN53ZZ	0VP40KZ	0VPD00Z	0VPM8YZ	0VPS77Z	0VQL3ZZ
0VBF3ZX	0VBTXZX	0VCT0ZZ	0VHS8YZ	0VLN3DZ	0VN54ZZ	0VP40YZ	0VPD03Z	0VPMX0Z	0VPS7JZ	0VQL4ZZ
0VBF4ZX	0VBTXZZ	0VCT3ZZ	0VHSX3Z	0VLN3ZZ	0VN5XZZ	0VP430Z	0VPD07Z	0VPMX3Z	0VPS7KZ	0VQL8ZZ
0VBF8ZX	0VC00ZZ	0VCT4ZZ	0VJ40ZZ	0VLN4CZ	0VN60ZZ	0VP431Z	0VPD0JZ	0VPR00Z	0VPS7YZ	0VQN0ZZ
0VBF8ZZ	0VC03ZZ	0VCTXZZ	0VJ43ZZ	0VLN4DZ	0VN63ZZ	0VP433Z	0VPD0KZ	0VPR03Z	0VPS80Z	0VQN3ZZ
0VBG0ZX	0VC04ZZ	0VH001Z	0VJ44ZZ	0VLN4ZZ	0VN64ZZ	0VP437Z	0VPD0YZ	0VPR07Z	0VPS83Z	0VQN4ZZ
0VBG3ZX	0VC07ZZ	0VH031Z	0VJ4XZZ	0VLN8CZ	0VN70ZZ	0VP43JZ	0VPD30Z	0VPR0CZ	0VPS87Z	0VQN8ZZ
0VBG4ZX	0VC08ZZ	0VH041Z	0VJ80ZZ	0VLN8DZ	0VN73ZZ	0VP43KZ	0VPD33Z	0VPR0DZ	0VPS8JZ	0VQP0ZZ
0VBG8ZX	0VC10ZZ	0VH071Z	0VJ83ZZ	0VLN8ZZ	0VN74ZZ	0VP43YZ	0VPD37Z	0VPR0JZ	0VPS8KZ	0VQP3ZZ
0VBG8ZZ	0VC13ZZ	0VH081Z	0VJ84ZZ	0VLP0CZ	0VN90ZZ	0VP440Z	0VPD3JZ	0VPR0KZ	0VPS8YZ	0VQP4ZZ
0VBH0ZX	0VC14ZZ	0VH403Z	0VJ8XZZ	0VLP0DZ	0VN93ZZ	0VP441Z	0VPD3KZ	0VPR0YZ	0VPSX0Z	0VQP8ZZ
0VBH3ZX	0VC20ZZ	0VH40YZ	0VJD0ZZ	0VLP0ZZ	0VN94ZZ	0VP443Z	0VPD3YZ	0VPR30Z	0VPSX3Z	0VQQ0ZZ
0VBH4ZX	0VC23ZZ	0VH433Z	0VJD3ZZ	0VLP3CZ	0VNB0ZZ	0VP447Z	0VPD40Z	0VPR33Z	0VQ00ZZ	0VQQ3ZZ
0VBH8ZX	0VC24ZZ	0VH43YZ	0VJD4ZZ	0VLP3DZ	0VNB3ZZ	0VP44JZ	0VPD43Z	0VPR37Z	0VQ03ZZ	0VQQ4ZZ
0VBH8ZZ	0VC30ZZ	0VH443Z	0VJDXZZ	0VLP3ZZ	0VNB4ZZ	0VP44KZ	0VPD47Z	0VPR3CZ	0VQ04ZZ	0VQQ8ZZ
0VBJ0ZX	0VC33ZZ	0VH44YZ	0VJM0ZZ	0VLP4CZ	0VNC0ZZ	0VP44YZ	0VPD4JZ	0VPR3DZ	0VQ07ZZ	0VQS0ZZ
0VBJ3ZX	0VC34ZZ	0VH473Z	0VJM3ZZ	0VLP4DZ	0VNC3ZZ	0VP470Z	0VPD4KZ	0VPR3JZ	0VQ08ZZ	0VQS3ZZ
0VBJ4ZX	0VC50ZZ	0VH47YZ	0VJM4ZZ	0VLP4ZZ	0VNC4ZZ	0VP471Z	0VPD4YZ	0VPR3KZ	0VQ10ZZ	0VQS4ZZ
0VBJ8ZX	0VC53ZZ	0VH483Z	0VJMXZZ	0VLP8CZ	0VNF0ZZ	0VP473Z	0VPD70Z	0VPR3YZ	0VQ13ZZ	0VQSXZZ
0VBJ8ZZ	0VC54ZZ	0VH48YZ	0VJR0ZZ	0VLP8DZ	0VNF3ZZ	0VP477Z	0VPD73Z	0VPR40Z	0VQ14ZZ	0VQT0ZZ
0VBK0ZX	0VC5XZZ	0VH803Z	0VJR3ZZ	0VLP8ZZ	0VNF4ZZ	0VP47JZ	0VPD77Z	0VPR43Z	0VQ20ZZ	0VQT3ZZ
0VBK3ZX	0VC60ZZ	0VH80YZ	0VJR4ZZ	0VLQ0CZ	0VNF8ZZ	0VP47KZ	0VPD7JZ	0VPR47Z	0VQ23ZZ	0VQT4ZZ
0VBK4ZX	0VC63ZZ	0VH833Z	0VJRXZZ	0VLQ0DZ	0VNG0ZZ	0VP47YZ	0VPD7KZ	0VPR4CZ	0VQ24ZZ	0VQTXZZ
0VBK8ZX	0VC64ZZ	0VH83YZ	0VJS0ZZ	0VLQ0ZZ	0VNG3ZZ	0VP480Z	0VPD7YZ	0VPR4DZ	0VQ30ZZ	0VR90JZ
0VBK8ZZ	0VC70ZZ	0VH843Z	0VJS3ZZ	0VLQ3CZ	0VNG4ZZ	0VP481Z	0VPD80Z	0VPR4JZ	0VQ33ZZ	0VRB0JZ
0VBL0ZX	0VC73ZZ	0VH84YZ	0VJS4ZZ	0VLQ3DZ	0VNG8ZZ	0VP483Z	0VPD83Z	0VPR4KZ	0VQ34ZZ	0VRC0JZ
0VBL3ZX	0VC74ZZ	0VH873Z	0VJSXZZ	0VLQ3ZZ	0VNH0ZZ	0VP487Z	0VPD87Z	0VPR4YZ	0VQ50ZZ	0VS90ZZ
0VBL4ZX	0VC90ZZ	0VH87YZ	0VLF0CZ	0VLQ4CZ	0VNH3ZZ	0VP48JZ	0VPD8JZ	0VPR70Z	0VQ53ZZ	0VS93ZZ
0VBL8ZX	0VC93ZZ	0VH883Z	0VLF0DZ	0VLQ4DZ	0VNH4ZZ	0VP48KZ	0VPD8KZ	0VPR73Z	0VQ54ZZ	0VS94ZZ
0VBL8ZZ	0VC94ZZ	0VH88YZ	0VLF0ZZ	0VLQ4ZZ	0VNH8ZZ	0VP48YZ	0VPD8YZ	0VPR77Z	0VQ5XZZ	0VS98ZZ
0VBN0ZX	0VCB0ZZ	0VHD03Z	0VLF3CZ	0VLQ8CZ	0VNJ0ZZ	0VP4X0Z	0VPDX0Z	0VPR7CZ	0VQ60ZZ	0VSB0ZZ
0VBN0ZZ	0VCB3ZZ	0VHD0YZ	0VLF3DZ	0VLQ8DZ	0VNJ3ZZ	0VP4X1Z	0VPDX3Z	0VPR7DZ	0VQ63ZZ	0VSB3ZZ
0VBN3ZX	0VCB4ZZ	0VHD33Z	0VLF3ZZ	0VLQ8ZZ	0VNJ4ZZ	0VP4X3Z	0VPM00Z	0VPR7JZ	0VQ64ZZ	0VSB4ZZ
0VBN3ZZ	0VCC0ZZ	0VHD3YZ	0VLF4CZ	0VM5XZZ	0VNJ8ZZ	0VP800Z	0VPM03Z	0VPR7KZ	0VQ70ZZ	0VSB8ZZ
0VBN4ZX	0VCC3ZZ	0VHD43Z	0VLF4DZ	0VM60ZZ	0VNK0ZZ	0VP803Z	0VPM07Z	0VPR7YZ	0VQ73ZZ	0VSC0ZZ
0VBN4ZZ	0VCC4ZZ	0VHD4YZ	0VLF4ZZ	0VM64ZZ	0VNK3ZZ	0VP807Z	0VPM0CZ	0VPR80Z	0VQ74ZZ	0VSC3ZZ
0VBN8ZX	0VCF0ZZ	0VHD73Z	0VLF8CZ	0VM70ZZ	0VNK4ZZ	0VP80JZ	0VPM0JZ	0VPR83Z	0VQ90ZZ	0VSC4ZZ
0VBN8ZZ	0VCF3ZZ	0VHD7YZ	0VLF8DZ	0VM74ZZ	0VNK8ZZ	0VP80KZ	0VPM0KZ	0VPR87Z	0VQ93ZZ	0VSC8ZZ
0VBP0ZX	0VCF4ZZ	0VHD83Z	0VLF8ZZ	0VM90ZZ	0VNL0ZZ	0VP80YZ	0VPM0YZ	0VPR8CZ	0VQ94ZZ	0VSF0ZZ
0VBP0ZZ	0VCG0ZZ	0VHD8YZ	0VLG0CZ	0VM94ZZ	0VNL3ZZ	0VP830Z	0VPM30Z	0VPR8DZ	0VQB0ZZ	0VSF3ZZ
0VBP3ZX	0VCG3ZZ	0VHM03Z	0VLG0DZ	0VMB0ZZ	0VNL4ZZ	0VP833Z	0VPM33Z	0VPR8JZ	0VQB3ZZ	0VSF4ZZ
0VBP3ZZ	0VCG4ZZ	0VHM0YZ	0VLG0ZZ	0VMB4ZZ	0VNL8ZZ	0VP837Z	0VPM37Z	0VPR8KZ	0VQB4ZZ	0VSF8ZZ
0VBP4ZX	0VCH0ZZ	0VHM33Z	0VLG3CZ	0VMC0ZZ	0VNN0ZZ	0VP83JZ	0VPM3CZ	0VPR8YZ	0VQC0ZZ	0VSG0ZZ
0VBP4ZZ	0VCH3ZZ	0VHM3YZ	0VLG3DZ	0VMC4ZZ	0VNN3ZZ	0VP83KZ	0VPM3JZ	0VPRX0Z	0VQC3ZZ	0VSG3ZZ
0VBP8ZX	0VCH4ZZ	0VHM43Z	0VLG3ZZ	0VMF0ZZ	0VNN4ZZ	0VP83YZ	0VPM3KZ	0VPRX3Z	0VQC4ZZ	0VSG4ZZ
0VBP8ZZ	0VCJ0ZZ	0VHM4YZ	0VLG4CZ	0VMF4ZZ	0VNN8ZZ	0VP840Z	0VPM3YZ	0VPRXDZ	0VQF0ZZ	0VSG8ZZ
0VBQ0ZX	0VCJ3ZZ	0VHM73Z	0VLG4DZ	0VMG0ZZ	0VNP0ZZ	0VP843Z	0VPM40Z	0VPS00Z	0VQF3ZZ	0VSH0ZZ
0VBQ0ZZ	0VCJ4ZZ	0VHM7YZ	0VLG4ZZ	0VMG4ZZ	0VNP3ZZ	0VP847Z	0VPM43Z	0VPS03Z	0VQF4ZZ	0VSH3ZZ
0VBQ3ZX	0VCK0ZZ	0VHM83Z	0VLG8CZ	0VMH0ZZ	0VNP4ZZ	0VP84JZ	0VPM47Z	0VPS07Z	0VQF8ZZ	0VSH4ZZ
0VBQ3ZZ	0VCK3ZZ	0VHM8YZ	0VLG8DZ	0VMH4ZZ	0VNP8ZZ	0VP84KZ	0VPM4CZ	0VPS0JZ	0VQG0ZZ	0VSH8ZZ
0VBQ4ZX	0VCK4ZZ	0VHR03Z	0VLG8ZZ	0VMSXZZ	0VNQ0ZZ	0VP84ZZ	0VPM4JZ	0VPS0KZ	0VQG3ZZ	0VT00ZZ

0VT04ZZ	0VU30KZ	0VW4X7Z	0VWR0YZ	0W003JZ	0W084ZZ	0W190J9	0W29XYZ	0W3G3ZZ	0W9C30Z	0W9M30Z
0VT07ZZ	0VU347Z	0VW4XJZ	0VWR30Z	0W003KZ	0W0F07Z	0W190JB	0W2BX0Z	0W3P8ZZ	0W9C3ZX	0W9M3ZX
0VT08ZZ	0VU34JZ	0VW4XKZ	0VWR33Z	0W003ZZ	0W0F0JZ	0W190JG	0W2BXYZ	0W8NXZZ	0W9C3ZZ	0W9M3ZZ
0VT10ZZ	0VU34KZ	0VW800Z	0VWR37Z	0W0047Z	0W0F0KZ	0W190JJ	0W2CX0Z	0W9000Z	0W9C4ZX	0W9M40Z
0VT14ZZ	0VU387Z	0VW803Z	0VWR3CZ	0W004JZ	0W0F0ZZ	0W190JY	0W2CXYZ	0W900ZX	0W9D30Z	0W9M4ZX
0VT20ZZ	0VU38JZ	0VW807Z	0VWR3DZ	0W004KZ	0W0F37Z	0W193J4	0W2DX0Z	0W900ZZ	0W9D3ZX	0W9M4ZZ
0VT24ZZ	0VU38KZ	0VW80JZ	0VWR3JZ	0W004ZZ	0W0F3JZ	0W194J4	0W2DXYZ	0W9030Z	0W9D3ZZ	0W9N00Z
0VT30ZZ	0VU507Z	0VW80KZ	0VWR3KZ	0W0207Z	0W0F3KZ	0W194J9	0W2FX0Z	0W903ZX	0W9D40Z	0W9N0ZX
0VT34ZZ	0VU50JZ	0VW80YZ	0VWR3YZ	0W020JZ	0W0F3ZZ	0W194JB	0W2FXYZ	0W903ZZ	0W9D4ZX	0W9N0ZX
0VT50ZZ	0VU50KZ	0VW830Z	0VWR40Z	0W020KZ	0W0F47Z	0W194JG	0W2GX0Z	0W9040Z	0W9D4ZZ	0W9N30Z
0VT54ZZ	0VU547Z	0VW833Z	0VWR43Z	0W020ZZ	0W0F4JZ	0W194JJ	0W2GXYZ	0W904ZX	0W9F0ZX	0W9N3ZX
0VT5XZZ	0VU54JZ	0VW837Z	0VWR47Z	0W0237Z	0W0F4KZ	0W194JY	0W2HX0Z	0W904ZZ	0W9F0ZZ	0W9N3ZZ
0VT60ZZ	0VU54KZ	0VW83JZ	0VWR4CZ	0W023JZ	0W0F4ZZ	0W1B0J4	0W2HXYZ	0W9130Z	0W9F30Z	0W9N40Z
0VT64ZZ	0VU5X7Z	0VW83KZ	0VWR4DZ	0W023KZ	0W0K07Z	0W1B0J9	0W2JX0Z	0W913ZX	0W9F3ZX	0W9N4ZX
0VT70ZZ	0VU5XJZ	0VW83YZ	0VWR4JZ	0W023ZZ	0W0K0JZ	0W1B0JB	0W2JXYZ	0W913ZZ	0W9F3ZZ	0W9N4ZZ
0VT74ZZ	0VU5XKZ	0VW840Z	0VWR4KZ	0W0247Z	0W0K0KZ	0W1B0JG	0W2KX0Z	0W9140Z	0W9F40Z	0WB00ZX
0VT90ZZ	0VU607Z	0VW843Z	0VWR4YZ	0W024JZ	0W0K0ZZ	0W1B0JJ	0W2KXYZ	0W914ZX	0W9F4ZX	0WB00ZZ
0VT94ZZ	0VU60JZ	0VW847Z	0VWR70Z	0W024KZ	0W0K37Z	0W1B0JY	0W2LX0Z	0W914ZZ	0W9F4ZZ	0WB03ZX
0VTB0ZZ	0VU60KZ	0VW84JZ	0VWR73Z	0W024ZZ	0W0K3JZ	0W1B3J4	0W2LXYZ	0W920ZX	0W9G00Z	0WB03ZZ
0VTB4ZZ	0VU647Z	0VW84KZ	0VWR77Z	0W0407Z	0W0K3KZ	0W1B4J4	0W2MX0Z	0W9230Z	0W9G0ZX	0WB04ZX
0VTC0ZZ	0VU64JZ	0VW84YZ	0VWR7CZ	0W040JZ	0W0K3ZZ	0W1B4J9	0W2MXYZ	0W923ZX	0W9G0ZZ	0WB04ZZ
0VTC4ZZ	0VU64KZ	0VW870Z	0VWR7DZ	0W040KZ	0W0K47Z	0W1B4JB	0W2NX0Z	0W923ZZ	0W9G30Z	0WB0XZX
0VTF0ZZ	0VU687Z	0VW873Z	0VWR7JZ	0W040ZZ	0W0K4JZ	0W1B4JG	0W2NXYZ	0W924ZX	0W9G3ZX	0WB0XZZ
0VTF4ZZ	0VU68JZ	0VW877Z	0VWR7KZ	0W0437Z	0W0K4KZ	0W1B4JJ	0W300ZZ	0W930ZX	0W9G3ZZ	0WB20ZX
0VTG0ZZ	0VU68KZ	0VW87JZ	0VWR7YZ	0W043JZ	0W0K4ZZ	0W1B4JY	0W303ZZ	0W9330Z	0W9G40Z	0WB20ZZ
0VTG4ZZ	0VU707Z	0VW87KZ	0VWR80Z	0W043KZ	0W0L07Z	0W1G0J4	0W304ZZ	0W933ZX	0W9G4ZX	0WB23ZX
0VTH0ZZ	0VU787Z	0VW87YZ	0VWR83Z	0W043ZZ	0W0L0JZ	0W1G0J9	0W310ZZ	0W933ZZ	0W9G4ZZ	0WB23ZZ
0VTH4ZZ	0VU78JZ	0VW880Z	0VWR87Z	0W0447Z	0W0L0KZ	0W1G0JB	0W313ZZ	0W934ZX	0W9H00Z	0WB24ZX
0VTJ0ZZ	0VU78KZ	0VW883Z	0VWR8CZ	0W044JZ	0W0L0ZZ	0W1G0JG	0W314ZZ	0W940ZX	0W9H0ZX	0WB24ZZ
0VTJ4ZZ	0VUF87Z	0VW887Z	0VWR8DZ	0W044KZ	0W0L37Z	0W1G0JJ	0W320ZZ	0W9430Z	0W9H0ZZ	0WB2XZX
0VTK0ZZ	0VUF8JZ	0VW88JZ	0VWR8JZ	0W044ZZ	0W0L3JZ	0W1G0JY	0W323ZZ	0W943ZX	0W9H30Z	0WB2XZZ
0VTK4ZZ	0VUF8KZ	0VW88KZ	0VWR8KZ	0W0507Z	0W0L3KZ	0W1G3J4	0W324ZZ	0W943ZZ	0W9H3ZX	0WB30ZX
0VTL0ZZ	0VUG87Z	0VW88YZ	0VWR8YZ	0W050JZ	0W0L3ZZ	0W1G4J4	0W330ZZ	0W944ZX	0W9H3ZZ	0WB30ZZ
0VTL4ZZ	0VUG8JZ	0VW8X0Z	0VWRX0Z	0W050KZ	0W0L47Z	0W1G4J9	0W333ZZ	0W950ZX	0W9H40Z	0WB33ZX
0VTN0ZZ	0VUG8KZ	0VW8X3Z	0VWRX3Z	0W050ZZ	0W0L4JZ	0W1G4JB	0W334ZZ	0W9530Z	0W9H4ZX	0WB33ZZ
0VTN4ZZ	0VUH87Z	0VW8X7Z	0VWRX7Z	0W0537Z	0W0L4KZ	0W1G4JG	0W337ZZ	0W953ZX	0W9H4ZZ	0WB34ZX
0VTP0ZZ	0VUH8JZ	0VW8XJZ	0VWRXCZ	0W053JZ	0W0L4ZZ	0W1G4JJ	0W338ZZ	0W953ZZ	0W9J00Z	0WB34ZZ
0VTP4ZZ	0VUH8KZ	0VW8XKZ	0VWRXDZ	0W053KZ	0W0M07Z	0W1G4JY	0W33XZZ	0W954ZX	0W9J0ZX	0WB3XZX
0VTQ0ZZ	0VUJ87Z	0VWD0YZ	0VWRXJZ	0W053ZZ	0W0M0JZ	0W1J0J4	0W340ZZ	0W960ZX	0W9J0ZZ	0WB3XZZ
0VTQ4ZZ	0VUJ8JZ	0VWD3YZ	0VWRXKZ	0W0547Z	0W0M0KZ	0W1J0J9	0W343ZZ	0W9630Z	0W9J30Z	0WB40ZX
0VTS0ZZ	0VUJ8KZ	0VWD4YZ	0VWS0YZ	0W054JZ	0W0M0ZZ	0W1J0JB	0W344ZZ	0W963ZX	0W9J3ZX	0WB40ZZ
0VTS4ZZ	0VUK87Z	0VWD7YZ	0VWS3YZ	0W054KZ	0W0M37Z	0W1J0JG	0W350ZZ	0W963ZZ	0W9J3ZZ	0WB43ZX
0VTSXZZ	0VUK8JZ	0VWD8YZ	0VWS4KZ	0W054ZZ	0W0M3JZ	0W1J0JJ	0W353ZZ	0W964ZX	0W9J40Z	0WB43ZZ
0VTT0ZZ	0VUK8KZ	0VWDX0Z	0VWS4YZ	0W0607Z	0W0M3KZ	0W1J0JY	0W354ZZ	0W9800Z	0W9J4ZX	0WB44ZX
0VTT4ZZ	0VUL87Z	0VWDX3Z	0VWS70Z	0W060JZ	0W0M3ZZ	0W1J3J4	0W360ZZ	0W980ZX	0W9J4ZZ	0WB44ZZ
0VTTXZZ	0VUL8JZ	0VWDX7Z	0VWS73Z	0W060ZZ	0W0M47Z	0W1J4J4	0W363ZZ	0W980ZZ	0W9K00Z	0WB4XZX
0VU107Z	0VUL8KZ	0VWDXJZ	0VWS77Z	0W0637Z	0W0M4JZ	0W1J4J9	0W364ZZ	0W9830Z	0W9K0ZX	0WB4XZZ
0VU10JZ	0VUN87Z	0VWDXKZ	0VWS7JZ	0W063JZ	0W0M4KZ	0W1J4JB	0W380ZZ	0W983ZX	0W9K0ZZ	0WB50ZX
0VU10KZ	0VUN8JZ	0VWM0YZ	0VWS7KZ	0W063KZ	0W0M4ZZ	0W1J4JG	0W383ZZ	0W983ZZ	0W9K30Z	0WB50ZZ
0VU147Z	0VUN8KZ	0VWM3YZ	0VWS7YZ	0W063ZZ	0W0N07Z	0W1J4JJ	0W384ZZ	0W9840Z	0W9K3ZX	0WB53ZX
0VU14JZ	0VUP87Z	0VWM4YZ	0VWS80Z	0W0647Z	0W0N0JZ	0W1J4JY	0W390ZZ	0W984ZX	0W9K3ZZ	0WB53ZZ
0VU14KZ	0VUP8JZ	0VWM7YZ	0VWS83Z	0W064JZ	0W0N0KZ	0W20X0Z	0W393ZZ	0W984ZZ	0W9K40Z	0WB54ZX
0VU187Z	0VUP8KZ	0VWM8YZ	0VWS87Z	0W064KZ	0W0N0ZZ	0W20XYZ	0W394ZZ	0W9900Z	0W9K4ZX	0WB54ZZ
0VU18JZ	0VUQ87Z	0VWMX0Z	0VWS8JZ	0W064ZZ	0W0N37Z	0W21X0Z	0W3B0ZZ	0W990ZX	0W9K4ZZ	0WB5XZX
0VU18KZ	0VUQ8JZ	0VWMX3Z	0VWS8KZ	0W0807Z	0W0N3JZ	0W21XYZ	0W3B3ZZ	0W990ZZ	0W9L00Z	0WB5XZZ
0VU207Z	0VUQ8KZ	0VWMX7Z	0VWS8YZ	0W080JZ	0W0N3KZ	0W22X0Z	0W3B4ZZ	0W9930Z	0W9L0ZX	0WB60ZX
0VU20JZ	0VUSX7Z	0VWMXCZ	0VWSX0Z	0W080KZ	0W0N3ZZ	0W22XYZ	0W3C0ZZ	0W993ZX	0W9L0ZZ	0WB60ZZ
0VU20KZ	0VUSXJZ	0VWMXJZ	0VWSX3Z	0W080ZZ	0W0N47Z	0W24X0Z	0W3C3ZZ	0W993ZZ	0W9L30Z	0WB63ZX
0VU247Z	0VUSXKZ	0VWMXKZ	0VWSX7Z	0W0837Z	0W0N4JZ	0W24XYZ	0W3C4ZZ	0W994ZX	0W9L3ZX	0WB63ZZ
0VU24JZ	0VW40YZ	0VWR00Z	0VWSXJZ	0W083JZ	0W0N4KZ	0W25X0Z	0W3D0ZZ	0W9B00Z	0W9L3ZZ	0WB64ZX
0VU24KZ	0VW43YZ	0VWR03Z	0VWSXKZ	0W083KZ	0W0N4ZZ	0W25XYZ	0W3D3ZZ	0W9B0ZX	0W9L40Z	0WB64ZZ
0VU287Z	0VW44YZ	0VWR07Z	0W0007Z	0W083ZZ	0W110J9	0W26X0Z	0W3D4ZZ	0W9B0ZZ	0W9L4ZZ	0WB6XZ2
0VU28JZ	0VW47YZ	0VWR0CZ	0W000JZ	0W0847Z	0W110JB	0W26XYZ	0W3F0ZZ	0W9B30Z	0W9L4ZZ	0WB6XZX
0VU28KZ	0VW48YZ	0VWR0DZ	0W000KZ	0W084JZ	0W110JG	0W28X0Z	0W3F3ZZ	0W9B3ZX	0W9M00Z	0WB6XZZ
0VU307Z	0VW4X0Z	0VWR0JZ	0W000ZZ	0W084KZ	0W110JJ	0W28XYZ	0W3F4ZZ	0W9B3ZZ	0W9M0ZZ	0WB80ZX
0VU30JZ	0VW4X3Z	0VWR0KZ	0W0037Z	0W084KZ	0W190J4	0W29X0Z	0W3G0ZZ	0W9B4ZX	0W9M0ZZ	0WB80ZZ

0WB83ZX	0WC3XZZ	0WFCXZZ	0WHP83Z	0WJL4ZZ	0WP10JZ	0WP4X3Z	0WP80KZ	0WPC30Z	0WPG03Z	0WPK47Z
0WB83ZZ	0WC90ZZ	0WFD0ZZ	0WHP8YZ	0WJLXZZ	0WP10YZ	0WP4X7Z	0WP80YZ	0WPC31Z	0WPG0JZ	0WPK4JZ
0WB84ZX	0WC93ZZ	0WFD3ZZ	0WHQ03Z	0WJM0ZZ	0WP130Z	0WP4XJZ	0WP830Z	0WPC33Z	0WPG0YZ	0WPK4KZ
0WB84ZZ	0WC94ZZ	0WFD4ZZ	0WHQ0YZ	0WJM3ZZ	0WP131Z	0WP4XKZ	0WP831Z	0WPC37Z	0WPG30Z	0WPK4YZ
0WB8XZX	0WC9XZZ	0WFDXZZ	0WHQ73Z	0WJM4ZZ	0WP133Z	0WP4XYZ	0WP833Z	0WPC3JZ	0WPG31Z	0WPKX0Z
0WB8XZZ	0WCB0ZZ	0WFG0ZZ	0WHQ7YZ	0WJMXZZ	0WP13JZ	0WP500Z	0WP837Z	0WPC3KZ	0WPG3JZ	0WPKX1Z
0WBC0ZX	0WCB3ZZ	0WFG3ZZ	0WHQ83Z	0WJN0ZZ	0WP13YZ	0WP501Z	0WP83JZ	0WPC3YZ	0WPG3YZ	0WPKX3Z
0WBC0ZZ	0WCB4ZZ	0WFG4ZZ	0WHQ8YZ	0WJN3ZZ	0WP140Z	0WP503Z	0WP83KZ	0WPC40Z	0WPG40Z	0WPKX7Z
0WBC3ZX	0WCBXZZ	0WFGXZZ	0WHR03Z	0WJN4ZZ	0WP141Z	0WP507Z	0WP83YZ	0WPC41Z	0WPG41Z	0WPKXJZ
0WBC3ZZ	0WCC0ZZ	0WFJ0ZZ	0WHR0YZ	0WJNXZZ	0WP143Z	0WP50JZ	0WP840Z	0WPC43Z	0WPG43Z	0WPKXKZ
0WBC4ZX	0WCC3ZZ	0WFJ3ZZ	0WHR33Z	0WJP0ZZ	0WP14JZ	0WP50KZ	0WP841Z	0WPC47Z	0WPG4JZ	0WPKXYZ
0WBC4ZZ	0WCC4ZZ	0WFJ4ZZ	0WHR3YZ	0WJP3ZZ	0WP14YZ	0WP50YZ	0WP843Z	0WPC4JZ	0WPG4YZ	0WPL00Z
0WBF0ZX	0WCCXZZ	0WFJXZZ	0WHR43Z	0WJP4ZZ	0WP1X0Z	0WP530Z	0WP847Z	0WPC4KZ	0WPGX0Z	0WPL01Z
0WBF0ZZ	0WCD0ZZ	0WFP0ZZ	0WHR4YZ	0WJP7ZZ	0WP1X1Z	0WP531Z	0WP84JZ	0WPC4YZ	0WPGX1Z	0WPL03Z
0WBF3ZX	0WCD3ZZ	0WFP3ZZ	0WHR73Z	0WJP8ZZ	0WP1X3Z	0WP533Z	0WP84KZ	0WPCX0Z	0WPGX3Z	0WPL07Z
0WBF3ZZ	0WCD4ZZ	0WFP4ZZ	0WHR7YZ	0WJQ0ZZ	0WP200Z	0WP537Z	0WP84YZ	0WPCX1Z	0WPH00Z	0WPL0JZ
0WBF4ZX	0WCDXZZ	0WFP7ZZ	0WHR83Z	0WJQ3ZZ	0WP201Z	0WP53JZ	0WP8X0Z	0WPCX3Z	0WPH01Z	0WPL0KZ
0WBF4ZZ	0WCG0ZZ	0WFP8ZZ	0WHR8YZ	0WJQ4ZZ	0WP203Z	0WP53KZ	0WP8X1Z	0WPCX7Z	0WPH03Z	0WPL0YZ
0WBFXZ2	0WCG3ZZ	0WFPXZZ	0WJ03ZZ	0WJQ7ZZ	0WP207Z	0WP53YZ	0WP8X3Z	0WPCXJZ	0WPH0YZ	0WPL30Z
0WBFXZX	0WCG4ZZ	0WFQ0ZZ	0WJ04ZZ	0WJQ8ZZ	0WP20JZ	0WP540Z	0WP8X7Z	0WPCXKZ	0WPH30Z	0WPL31Z
0WBFXZZ	0WCGXZZ	0WFQ3ZZ	0WJ0XZZ	0WJR0ZZ	0WP20KZ	0WP541Z	0WP8XJZ	0WPCXYZ	0WPH31Z	0WPL33Z
0WBH0ZX	0WCH0ZZ	0WFQ4ZZ	0WJ23ZZ	0WJR3ZZ	0WP20YZ	0WP543Z	0WP8XKZ	0WPD00Z	0WPH33Z	0WPL37Z
0WBH0ZZ	0WCH3ZZ	0WFQ7ZZ	0WJ24ZZ	0WJR4ZZ	0WP230Z	0WP547Z	0WP8XYZ	0WPD01Z	0WPH3YZ	0WPL3JZ
0WBH3ZX	0WCH4ZZ	0WFQ8ZZ	0WJ2XZZ	0WJR7ZZ	0WP231Z	0WP54JZ	0WP900Z	0WPD03Z	0WPH40Z	0WPL3KZ
0WBH3ZZ	0WCHXZZ	0WFQXZZ	0WJ30ZZ	0WJR8ZZ	0WP233Z	0WP54KZ	0WP901Z	0WPD0YZ	0WPH41Z	0WPL3YZ
0WBH4ZX	0WCJ0ZZ	0WFR0ZZ	0WJ33ZZ	0WM20ZZ	0WP237Z	0WP54YZ	0WP903Z	0WPD30Z	0WPH4YZ	0WPL40Z
0WBH4ZZ	0WCJ3ZZ	0WFR3ZZ	0WJ34ZZ	0WM40ZZ	0WP23JZ	0WP5X0Z	0WP90JZ	0WPD31Z	0WPHX0Z	0WPL41Z
0WBK0ZX	0WCJ4ZZ	0WFR4ZZ	0WJ3XZZ	0WM50ZZ	0WP23KZ	0WP5X1Z	0WP90YZ	0WPD33Z	0WPHX1Z	0WPL43Z
0WBK0ZZ	0WCJXZZ	0WFR7ZZ	0WJ43ZZ	0WM60ZZ	0WP23YZ	0WP5X3Z	0WP930Z	0WPD3YZ	0WPHX3Z	0WPL47Z
0WBK3ZX	0WCP0ZZ	0WFR8ZZ	0WJ44ZZ	0WM80ZZ	0WP240Z	0WP5X7Z	0WP931Z	0WPD40Z	0WPJ00Z	0WPL4JZ
0WBK3ZZ	0WCP3ZZ	0WFRXZZ	0WJ4XZZ	0WMF0ZZ	0WP241Z	0WP5XJZ	0WP933Z	0WPD41Z	0WPJ01Z	0WPL4KZ
0WBK4ZX	0WCP4ZZ	0WH001Z	0WJ53ZZ	0WMK0ZZ	0WP243Z	0WP5XKZ	0WP93JZ	0WPD43Z	0WPJ03Z	0WPL4YZ
0WBK4ZZ	0WCP7ZZ	0WH003Z	0WJ54ZZ	0WML0ZZ	0WP247Z	0WP5XYZ	0WP93YZ	0WPD4YZ	0WPJ0JZ	0WPLX0Z
0WBKXZX	0WCP8ZZ	0WH00YZ	0WJ5XZZ	0WMM0ZZ	0WP24JZ	0WP600Z	0WP940Z	0WPDX0Z	0WPJ0YZ	0WPLX1Z
0WBKXZZ	0WCPXZZ	0WH031Z	0WJ63ZZ	0WMN0ZZ	0WP24KZ	0WP601Z	0WP941Z	0WPDX1Z	0WPJ30Z	0WPLX3Z
0WBL0ZX	0WCQ0ZZ	0WH033Z	0WJ6XZZ	0WP000Z	0WP24YZ	0WP603Z	0WP943Z	0WPDX3Z	0WPJ31Z	0WPLX7Z
0WBL0ZZ	0WCQ3ZZ	0WH03YZ	0WJ83ZZ	0WP001Z	0WP2X0Z	0WP607Z	0WP94JZ	0WPF00Z	0WPJ33Z	0WPLXJZ
0WBL3ZX	0WCQ4ZZ	0WH041Z	0WJ8XZZ	0WP003Z	0WP2X1Z	0WP60JZ	0WP94YZ	0WPF01Z	0WPJ3JZ	0WPLXKZ
0WBL3ZZ	0WCQ7ZZ	0WH103Z	0WJ93ZZ	0WP007Z	0WP2X3Z	0WP60KZ	0WP9X0Z	0WPF03Z	0WPJ3YZ	0WPLXYZ
0WBL4ZX	0WCQ8ZZ	0WH133Z	0WJB3ZZ	0WP00JZ	0WP2X7Z	0WP60YZ	0WP9X1Z	0WPF07Z	0WPJ40Z	0WPM00Z
0WBL4ZZ	0WCQXZZ	0WH143Z	0WJB4ZZ	0WP00KZ	0WP2XJZ	0WP630Z	0WP9X3Z	0WPF0JZ	0WPJ41Z	0WPM01Z
0WBLXZX	0WCR0ZZ	0WH803Z	0WJC0ZZ	0WP00YZ	0WP2XKZ	0WP631Z	0WPB00Z	0WPF0KZ	0WPJ43Z	0WPM03Z
0WBLXZZ	0WCR3ZZ	0WH80YZ	0WJC3ZZ	0WP030Z	0WP2XYZ	0WP633Z	0WPB01Z	0WPF0YZ	0WPJ4JZ	0WPM07Z
0WBM0ZX	0WCR4ZZ	0WH833Z	0WJC4ZZ	0WP031Z	0WP400Z	0WP637Z	0WPB03Z	0WPF30Z	0WPJ4YZ	0WPM0JZ
0WBM0ZZ	0WCR7ZZ	0WH83YZ	0WJD0ZZ	0WP033Z	0WP401Z	0WP63JZ	0WPB0JZ	0WPF31Z	0WPJX0Z	0WPM0KZ
0WBM3ZX	0WCR8ZZ	0WH843Z	0WJD3ZZ	0WP037Z	0WP403Z	0WP63KZ	0WPB0YZ	0WPF33Z	0WPJX1Z	0WPM0YZ
0WBM3ZZ	0WCRXZZ	0WH84YZ	0WJD4ZZ	0WP03JZ	0WP407Z	0WP63YZ	0WPB30Z	0WPF37Z	0WPJX3Z	0WPM30Z
0WBM4ZX	0WF10ZZ	0WH903Z	0WJF0ZZ	0WP03KZ	0WP40JZ	0WP640Z	0WPB31Z	0WPF3JZ	0WPK00Z	0WPM31Z
0WBM4ZZ	0WF13ZZ	0WH90YZ	0WJF3ZZ	0WP03YZ	0WP40KZ	0WP641Z	0WPB33Z	0WPF3KZ	0WPK01Z	0WPM33Z
0WBMXZX	0WF14ZZ	0WH933Z	0WJF4ZZ	0WP040Z	0WP40YZ	0WP643Z	0WPB3JZ	0WPF3YZ	0WPK03Z	0WPM37Z
0WBMXZZ	0WF1XZZ	0WH93YZ	0WJFXZZ	0WP041Z	0WP430Z	0WP647Z	0WPB3YZ	0WPF40Z	0WPK07Z	0WPM3JZ
0WBN0ZX	0WF30ZZ	0WH943Z	0WJG0ZZ	0WP043Z	0WP431Z	0WP64JZ	0WPB40Z	0WPF41Z	0WPK0JZ	0WPM3KZ
0WBN0ZZ	0WF33ZZ	0WH94YZ	0WJG3ZZ	0WP047Z	0WP433Z	0WP64KZ	0WPB41Z	0WPF43Z	0WPK0KZ	0WPM3YZ
0WBN3ZX	0WF34ZZ	0WHB03Z	0WJG4ZZ	0WP04JZ	0WP437Z	0WP64YZ	0WPB43Z	0WPF47Z	0WPK0YZ	0WPM40Z
0WBN3ZZ	0WF3XZZ	0WHB0YZ	0WJH0ZZ	0WP04KZ	0WP43JZ	0WP6X0Z	0WPB4JZ	0WPF4JZ	0WPK30Z	0WPM41Z
0WBN4ZX	0WF90ZZ	0WHB33Z	0WJH3ZZ	0WP04YZ	0WP43KZ	0WP6X1Z	0WPB4YZ	0WPF4KZ	0WPK31Z	0WPM43Z
0WBN4ZZ	0WF93ZZ	0WHB3YZ	0WJH4ZZ	0WP0X0Z	0WP43YZ	0WP6X3Z	0WPBX0Z	0WPF4YZ	0WPK33Z	0WPM47Z
0WBNXZX	0WF94ZZ	0WHB43Z	0WJJ0ZZ	0WP0X1Z	0WP440Z	0WP6X7Z	0WPBX1Z	0WPFX0Z	0WPK37Z	0WPM4JZ
0WBNXZZ	0WF9XZZ	0WHB4YZ	0WJJ3ZZ	0WP0X3Z	0WP441Z	0WP6XJZ	0WPBX3Z	0WPFX1Z	0WPK3JZ	0WPM4KZ
0WC10ZZ	0WFB0ZZ	0WHP0YZ	0WJJ4ZZ	0WP0X7Z	0WP443Z	0WP6XKZ	0WPC00Z	0WPFX3Z	0WPK3KZ	0WPM4YZ
0WC13ZZ	0WFB3ZZ	0WHP33Z	0WJK0ZZ	0WP0XJZ	0WP447Z	0WP6XYZ	0WPC01Z	0WPFX7Z	0WPK3YZ	0WPMX0Z
0WC14ZZ	0WFB4ZZ	0WHP3YZ	0WJK3ZZ	0WP0XKZ	0WP44JZ	0WP800Z	0WPC03Z	0WPFXJZ	0WPK40Z	0WPMX1Z
0WC1XZZ	0WFBXZZ	0WHP43Z	0WJK4ZZ	0WP0XYZ	0WP44KZ	0WP801Z	0WPC07Z	0WPFXKZ	0WPK41Z	0WPMX3Z
0WC30ZZ	0WFC0ZZ	0WHP4YZ	0WJKXZZ	0WP100Z	0WP44YZ	0WP803Z	0WPC0JZ	0WPFXYZ	0WPK43Z	0WPMX7Z
0WC33ZZ	0WFC3ZZ	0WHP73Z	0WJL0ZZ	0WP101Z	0WP4X0Z	0WP807Z	0WPC0KZ	0WPG00Z	0WPG01Z	0WPMXJZ
0WC34ZZ	0WFC4ZZ	0WHP7YZ	0WJL3ZZ	0WP103Z	0WP4X1Z	0WP80JZ	0WPC0YZ	0WPG01Z		0WPMXKZ

0WPMXYZ	0WPR03Z	0WQN0ZZ	0WW80KZ	0WWCX7Z	0WWH31Z	0WWL30Z	0WWN47Z	0WY20Z1	0X073JZ	0X0D4ZZ
0WPN00Z	0WPR0YZ	0WQN3ZZ	0WW80YZ	0WWCXJZ	0WWH33Z	0WWL31Z	0WWN4JZ	0X0207Z	0X073KZ	0X0F07Z
0WPN01Z	0WPR31Z	0WQN4ZZ	0WW830Z	0WWCXKZ	0WWH3YZ	0WWL33Z	0WWN4KZ	0X020JZ	0X073ZZ	0X0F0JZ
0WPN03Z	0WPR33Z	0WQNXZZ	0WW831Z	0WWCXYZ	0WWH40Z	0WWL37Z	0WWN4YZ	0X020KZ	0X0747Z	0X0F0KZ
0WPN07Z	0WPR3YZ	0WU007Z	0WW833Z	0WWD3YZ	0WWH41Z	0WWL3JZ	0WWNX0Z	0X020ZZ	0X074JZ	0X0F0ZZ
0WPN0JZ	0WPR41Z	0WU00JZ	0WW837Z	0WWD40Z	0WWH43Z	0WWL3KZ	0WWNX1Z	0X0237Z	0X074KZ	0X0F37Z
0WPN0KZ	0WPR43Z	0WU00KZ	0WW83JZ	0WWD41Z	0WWH4YZ	0WWL3YZ	0WWNX3Z	0X023JZ	0X074ZZ	0X0F3JZ
0WPN0YZ	0WPR4YZ	0WU047Z	0WW83KZ	0WWD43Z	0WWHX0Z	0WWL40Z	0WWNX7Z	0X023KZ	0X0807Z	0X0F3KZ
0WPN30Z	0WPR71Z	0WU04JZ	0WW83YZ	0WWD4YZ	0WWHX1Z	0WWL41Z	0WWNXJZ	0X023ZZ	0X080JZ	0X0F3ZZ
0WPN31Z	0WPR73Z	0WU04KZ	0WW840Z	0WWDX0Z	0WWHX3Z	0WWL43Z	0WWNXKZ	0X0247Z	0X080KZ	0X0F47Z
0WPN33Z	0WPR7YZ	0WU207Z	0WW841Z	0WWDX1Z	0WWHXYZ	0WWL47Z	0WWNXYZ	0X024JZ	0X080ZZ	0X0F4JZ
0WPN37Z	0WPR81Z	0WU20JZ	0WW843Z	0WWDX3Z	0WWJ00Z	0WWL4JZ	0WWP01Z	0X024KZ	0X0837Z	0X0F4KZ
0WPN3JZ	0WPR83Z	0WU20KZ	0WW847Z	0WWDXYZ	0WWJ01Z	0WWL4KZ	0WWP03Z	0X024ZZ	0X083JZ	0X0F4ZZ
0WPN3KZ	0WPR8YZ	0WU247Z	0WW84JZ	0WWF00Z	0WWJ03Z	0WWL4YZ	0WWP0YZ	0X0307Z	0X083KZ	0X0G07Z
0WPN3YZ	0WPRX1Z	0WU24JZ	0WW84KZ	0WWF01Z	0WWJ0JZ	0WWLX0Z	0WWP31Z	0X030JZ	0X0847Z	0X0G0JZ
0WPN40Z	0WPRX3Z	0WU24KZ	0WW84YZ	0WWF03Z	0WWJ0YZ	0WWLX1Z	0WWP33Z	0X030KZ	0X084JZ	0X0G0KZ
0WPN41Z	0WPRXYZ	0WU407Z	0WW8X0Z	0WWF07Z	0WWJ30Z	0WWLX3Z	0WWP3YZ	0X030ZZ	0X084KZ	0X0G0ZZ
0WPN43Z	0WQ00ZZ	0WU40JZ	0WW8X1Z	0WWF0JZ	0WWJ31Z	0WWLX7Z	0WWP41Z	0X0337Z	0X084ZZ	0X0G37Z
0WPN47Z	0WQ03ZZ	0WU40KZ	0WW8X3Z	0WWF0KZ	0WWJ33Z	0WWLXJZ	0WWP43Z	0X033JZ	0X0907Z	0X0G3JZ
0WPN4JZ	0WQ04ZZ	0WU447Z	0WW8X7Z	0WWF0YZ	0WWJ3JZ	0WWLXKZ	0WWP4YZ	0X033KZ	0X090JZ	0X0G3KZ
0WPN4KZ	0WQ0XZZ	0WU44JZ	0WW8XJZ	0WWF30Z	0WWJ3YZ	0WWLXYZ	0WWP71Z	0X033ZZ	0X090KZ	0X0G3ZZ
0WPN4YZ	0WQ20ZZ	0WW0X0Z	0WW8XKZ	0WWF31Z	0WWJ40Z	0WWM00Z	0WWP73Z	0X0347Z	0X090ZZ	0X0G47Z
0WPNX0Z	0WQ23ZZ	0WW0X1Z	0WW8XYZ	0WWF33Z	0WWJ41Z	0WWM01Z	0WWP7YZ	0X034JZ	0X0937Z	0X0G4JZ
0WPNX1Z	0WQ24ZZ	0WW0X3Z	0WW900Z	0WWF37Z	0WWJ43Z	0WWM03Z	0WWP81Z	0X034KZ	0X093JZ	0X0G4KZ
0WPNX3Z	0WQ2XZZ	0WW0X7Z	0WW901Z	0WWF3JZ	0WWJ4JZ	0WWM07Z	0WWP83Z	0X034ZZ	0X093KZ	0X0G4ZZ
0WPNX7Z	0WQ30ZZ	0WW0XJZ	0WW903Z	0WWF3KZ	0WWJ4YZ	0WWM0JZ	0WWP8YZ	0X0407Z	0X093ZZ	0X0H07Z
0WPNXJZ	0WQ33ZZ	0WW0XKZ	0WW90JZ	0WWF3YZ	0WWJX0Z	0WWM0KZ	0WWPX1Z	0X040JZ	0X0947Z	0X0H0JZ
0WPNXKZ	0WQ34ZZ	0WW0XYZ	0WW90YZ	0WWF40Z	0WWJX1Z	0WWM0YZ	0WWPX3Z	0X040KZ	0X094JZ	0X0H0KZ
0WPNXYZ	0WQ3XZZ	0WW1X0Z	0WW930Z	0WWF41Z	0WWJX3Z	0WWM30Z	0WWPXYZ	0X040ZZ	0X094KZ	0X0H0ZZ
0WPP01Z	0WQ40ZZ	0WW1X1Z	0WW931Z	0WWF43Z	0WWJXJZ	0WWM31Z	0WWQ01Z	0X0437Z	0X094ZZ	0X0H37Z
0WPP03Z	0WQ43ZZ	0WW1X3Z	0WW933Z	0WWF47Z	0WWJXYZ	0WWM33Z	0WWQ03Z	0X043JZ	0X0B07Z	0X0H3JZ
0WPP0YZ	0WQ44ZZ	0WW1XJZ	0WW93JZ	0WWF4JZ	0WWK00Z	0WWM37Z	0WWQ0YZ	0X043KZ	0X0B0JZ	0X0H3KZ
0WPP31Z	0WQ4XZZ	0WW1XYZ	0WW93YZ	0WWF4KZ	0WWK01Z	0WWM3JZ	0WWQ31Z	0X043ZZ	0X0B0KZ	0X0H3ZZ
0WPP33Z	0WQ50ZZ	0WW2X0Z	0WW940Z	0WWF4YZ	0WWK03Z	0WWM3KZ	0WWQ33Z	0X0447Z	0X0B0ZZ	0X0H47Z
0WPP3YZ	0WQ53ZZ	0WW2X1Z	0WW941Z	0WWFX0Z	0WWK07Z	0WWM3YZ	0WWQ3YZ	0X044JZ	0X0B37Z	0X0H4JZ
0WPP41Z	0WQ54ZZ	0WW2X3Z	0WW943Z	0WWFX1Z	0WWK0JZ	0WWM40Z	0WWQ41Z	0X044KZ	0X0B3JZ	0X0H4KZ
0WPP43Z	0WQ5XZZ	0WW2X7Z	0WW94JZ	0WWFX3Z	0WWK0KZ	0WWM41Z	0WWQ43Z	0X044ZZ	0X0B3KZ	0X0H4ZZ
0WPP4YZ	0WQ60ZZ	0WW2XJZ	0WW94YZ	0WWFX7Z	0WWK0YZ	0WWM43Z	0WWQ4YZ	0X0507Z	0X0B3ZZ	0X26X0Z
0WPP71Z	0WQ63ZZ	0WW2XKZ	0WW9X0Z	0WWFXJZ	0WWK30Z	0WWM47Z	0WWQ71Z	0X050JZ	0X0B3ZZ	0X26XYZ
0WPP73Z	0WQ64ZZ	0WW2XYZ	0WW9X1Z	0WWFXKZ	0WWK31Z	0WWM4JZ	0WWQ73Z	0X050KZ	0X0B47Z	0X27X0Z
0WPP7YZ	0WQ6XZ2	0WW4X0Z	0WW9X3Z	0WWFXYZ	0WWK33Z	0WWM4KZ	0WWQ7YZ	0X050ZZ	0X0B4JZ	0X27XYZ
0WPP81Z	0WQ6XZZ	0WW4X1Z	0WW9XJZ	0WWG00Z	0WWK37Z	0WWM4YZ	0WWQ81Z	0X0537Z	0X0B4KZ	0X320ZZ
0WPP83Z	0WQ80ZZ	0WW4X3Z	0WW9XYZ	0WWG01Z	0WWK3JZ	0WWMX0Z	0WWQ83Z	0X053JZ	0X0B4ZZ	0X323ZZ
0WPP8YZ	0WQ83ZZ	0WW4X7Z	0WWB00Z	0WWG03Z	0WWK3KZ	0WWMX1Z	0WWQ8YZ	0X053KZ	0X0C07Z	0X324ZZ
0WPPX1Z	0WQ84ZZ	0WW4XJZ	0WWB01Z	0WWG0JZ	0WWK3YZ	0WWMX3Z	0WWQX1Z	0X053ZZ	0X0C0JZ	0X330ZZ
0WPPX3Z	0WQ8XZZ	0WW4XKZ	0WWB03Z	0WWG0YZ	0WWK40Z	0WWMX7Z	0WWQX3Z	0X0547Z	0X0C0KZ	0X333ZZ
0WPPXYZ	0WQC0ZZ	0WW4XYZ	0WWB0JZ	0WWG30Z	0WWK41Z	0WWMXJZ	0WWQXYZ	0X054JZ	0X0C0ZZ	0X334ZZ
0WPQ01Z	0WQC3ZZ	0WW5X0Z	0WWB0YZ	0WWG31Z	0WWK43Z	0WWMXKZ	0WWR01Z	0X054KZ	0X0C37Z	0X340ZZ
0WPQ03Z	0WQC4ZZ	0WW5X1Z	0WWB30Z	0WWG33Z	0WWK47Z	0WWMXYZ	0WWR03Z	0X054ZZ	0X0C3JZ	0X343ZZ
0WPQ0YZ	0WQF0ZZ	0WW5X3Z	0WWB31Z	0WWG3JZ	0WWK4JZ	0WWN00Z	0WWR0YZ	0X0607Z	0X0C3KZ	0X344ZZ
0WPQ31Z	0WQF3ZZ	0WW5X7Z	0WWB33Z	0WWG3YZ	0WWK4KZ	0WWN01Z	0WWR31Z	0X060JZ	0X0C3ZZ	0X350ZZ
0WPQ33Z	0WQF4ZZ	0WW5XJZ	0WWB3JZ	0WWG40Z	0WWK4YZ	0WWN03Z	0WWR33Z	0X060KZ	0X0C47Z	0X353ZZ
0WPQ3YZ	0WQFXZ2	0WW5XKZ	0WWB3YZ	0WWG41Z	0WWKX0Z	0WWN07Z	0WWR3YZ	0X060ZZ	0X0C4JZ	0X354ZZ
0WPQ41Z	0WQFXZZ	0WW5XYZ	0WWB40Z	0WWG43Z	0WWKX1Z	0WWN0JZ	0WWR41Z	0X0637Z	0X0C4KZ	0X360ZZ
0WPQ43Z	0WQK0ZZ	0WW6X0Z	0WWB41Z	0WWG4JZ	0WWKX3Z	0WWN0KZ	0WWR43Z	0X063JZ	0X0C4ZZ	0X363ZZ
0WPQ4YZ	0WQK3ZZ	0WW6X1Z	0WWB43Z	0WWG4YZ	0WWKX7Z	0WWN0YZ	0WWR4YZ	0X063KZ	0X0D07Z	0X364ZZ
0WPQ71Z	0WQK4ZZ	0WW6X3Z	0WWB4JZ	0WWGX0Z	0WWKXJZ	0WWN30Z	0WWR71Z	0X063ZZ	0X0D0JZ	0X370ZZ
0WPQ73Z	0WQKXZZ	0WW6X7Z	0WWB4YZ	0WWGX1Z	0WWKXKZ	0WWN31Z	0WWR73Z	0X0647Z	0X0D0KZ	0X373ZZ
0WPQ7YZ	0WQL0ZZ	0WW6XJZ	0WWBX0Z	0WWGX3Z	0WWKXYZ	0WWN33Z	0WWR7YZ	0X064JZ	0X0D0ZZ	0X374ZZ
0WPQ81Z	0WQL3ZZ	0WW6XKZ	0WWBX1Z	0WWGXJZ	0WWL00Z	0WWN37Z	0WWR81Z	0X064KZ	0X0D37Z	0X380ZZ
0WPQ83Z	0WQL4ZZ	0WW6XYZ	0WWBX3Z	0WWGXYZ	0WWL01Z	0WWN3JZ	0WWR83Z	0X064ZZ	0X0D3JZ	0X383ZZ
0WPQ8YZ	0WQLXZZ	0WW800Z	0WWBXJZ	0WWH00Z	0WWL03Z	0WWN3KZ	0WWR8YZ	0X0707Z	0X0D3KZ	0X384ZZ
0WPQX1Z	0WQM0ZZ	0WW801Z	0WWBXYZ	0WWH01Z	0WWL07Z	0WWN3YZ	0WWRX1Z	0X070JZ	0X0D3ZZ	0X390ZZ
0WPQX3Z	0WQM3ZZ	0WW803Z	0WWCX0Z	0WWH03Z	0WWL0JZ	0WWN40Z	0WWRX3Z	0X070KZ	0X0D47Z	0X393ZZ
0WPQXYZ	0WQM4ZZ	0WW807Z	0WWCX1Z	0WWH0YZ	0WWL0KZ	0WWN41Z	0WWRXYZ	0X070ZZ	0X0D4JZ	0X394ZZ
0WPR01Z	0WQMXZZ	0WW80JZ	0WWCX3Z	0WWH30Z	0WWL0YZ	0WWN43Z	0WY20Z0	0X0737Z	0X0D4KZ	0X3B0ZZ

0X3B3ZZ	0X954ZZ	0X9F0ZZ	0XB54ZZ	0XBJ4ZZ	0XH83YZ	0XHH4YZ	0XJFXZZ	0XP6X0Z	0XQ9XZZ	0XUR4KZ
0X6N0Z2	0X9600Z	0X9F30Z	0XB60ZX	0XBK0ZX	0XH841Z	0XHJ01Z	0XJG0ZZ	0XP6X1Z	0XQB0ZZ	0XUS07Z
0X6N0Z3	0X960ZX	0X9F3ZX	0XB60ZZ	0XBK0ZZ	0XH843Z	0XHJ03Z	0XJG3ZZ	0XP6X3Z	0XQB4ZZ	0XUS0JZ
0X6P0Z0	0X960ZZ	0X9F3ZZ	0XB63ZX	0XBK3ZX	0XH84YZ	0XHJ0YZ	0XJG4ZZ	0XP6X7Z	0XQBXZZ	0XUS0KZ
0X6P0Z1	0X9630Z	0X9F40Z	0XB63ZZ	0XBK3ZZ	0XH901Z	0XHJ31Z	0XJGXZZ	0XP6XJZ	0XQC0ZZ	0XUS47Z
0X6P0Z2	0X963ZX	0X9F4ZX	0XB64ZX	0XBK4ZX	0XH903Z	0XHJ33Z	0XJH0ZZ	0XP6XKZ	0XQC3ZZ	0XUS4JZ
0X6P0Z3	0X963ZZ	0X9F4ZZ	0XB64ZZ	0XBK4ZZ	0XH90YZ	0XHJ3YZ	0XJH3ZZ	0XP6XYZ	0XQC4ZZ	0XUS4KZ
0X6Q0Z0	0X9640Z	0X9G00Z	0XB70ZX	0XH201Z	0XH931Z	0XHJ41Z	0XJH4ZZ	0XP700Z	0XQCXZZ	0XUT07Z
0X6Q0Z1	0X964ZX	0X9G0ZX	0XB70ZZ	0XH203Z	0XH933Z	0XHJ43Z	0XJHXZZ	0XP701Z	0XQD0ZZ	0XUT0JZ
0X6Q0Z2	0X964ZZ	0X9G0ZZ	0XB73ZX	0XH20YZ	0XH93YZ	0XHJ4YZ	0XJJ0ZZ	0XP703Z	0XQD3ZZ	0XUT0KZ
0X6Q0Z3	0X9700Z	0X9G30Z	0XB73ZZ	0XH231Z	0XH941Z	0XHK01Z	0XJJ3ZZ	0XP707Z	0XQD4ZZ	0XUT47Z
0X6R0Z0	0X970ZX	0X9G3ZX	0XB74ZX	0XH233Z	0XH943Z	0XHK03Z	0XJJ4ZZ	0XP70JZ	0XQDXZZ	0XUT4JZ
0X6R0Z1	0X970ZZ	0X9G3ZZ	0XB74ZZ	0XH23YZ	0XH94YZ	0XHK0YZ	0XJJXZZ	0XP70KZ	0XQF0ZZ	0XUT4KZ
0X6R0Z2	0X9730Z	0X9G40Z	0XB80ZX	0XH241Z	0XHB01Z	0XHK31Z	0XJK0ZZ	0XP70YZ	0XQF3ZZ	0XUV07Z
0X6R0Z3	0X973ZX	0X9G4ZX	0XB80ZZ	0XH243Z	0XHB03Z	0XHK33Z	0XJK3ZZ	0XP730Z	0XQF4ZZ	0XUV0JZ
0X6S0Z0	0X973ZZ	0X9G4ZZ	0XB83ZX	0XH24YZ	0XHB0YZ	0XHK3YZ	0XJK4ZZ	0XP731Z	0XQFXZZ	0XUV0KZ
0X6S0Z1	0X9740Z	0X9H00Z	0XB83ZZ	0XH301Z	0XHB31Z	0XHK41Z	0XJKXZZ	0XP733Z	0XQG0ZZ	0XUV47Z
0X6S0Z2	0X974ZX	0X9H0ZX	0XB84ZX	0XH303Z	0XHB33Z	0XHK43Z	0XM00ZZ	0XP737Z	0XQG3ZZ	0XUV4JZ
0X6S0Z3	0X974ZZ	0X9H0ZZ	0XB84ZZ	0XH30YZ	0XHB3YZ	0XHK4YZ	0XM10ZZ	0XP73JZ	0XQG4ZZ	0XUV4KZ
0X6T0Z0	0X9800Z	0X9H30Z	0XB90ZX	0XH331Z	0XHB41Z	0XJ20ZZ	0XM20ZZ	0XP73KZ	0XQGXZZ	0XUW07Z
0X6T0Z1	0X980ZX	0X9H3ZX	0XB90ZZ	0XH333Z	0XHB43Z	0XJ23ZZ	0XM30ZZ	0XP73YZ	0XQH0ZZ	0XUW0JZ
0X6T0Z2	0X980ZZ	0X9H3ZZ	0XB93ZX	0XH33YZ	0XHB4YZ	0XJ24ZZ	0XM40ZZ	0XP740Z	0XQH3ZZ	0XUW0KZ
0X6T0Z3	0X9830Z	0X9H40Z	0XB93ZZ	0XH341Z	0XHC01Z	0XJ2XZZ	0XM50ZZ	0XP741Z	0XQH4ZZ	0XUW47Z
0X6V0Z0	0X983ZX	0X9H4ZX	0XB94ZX	0XH343Z	0XHC03Z	0XJ30ZZ	0XM60ZZ	0XP743Z	0XQHXZZ	0XUW4JZ
0X6V0Z1	0X983ZZ	0X9H4ZZ	0XB94ZZ	0XH34YZ	0XHC0YZ	0XJ33ZZ	0XM70ZZ	0XP747Z	0XQJ0ZZ	0XUW4KZ
0X6V0Z2	0X9840Z	0X9J00Z	0XBB0ZX	0XH401Z	0XHC31Z	0XJ34ZZ	0XM80ZZ	0XP74JZ	0XQJ3ZZ	0XW600Z
0X6V0Z3	0X984ZX	0X9J0ZX	0XBB0ZZ	0XH403Z	0XHC33Z	0XJ3XZZ	0XM90ZZ	0XP74KZ	0XUK0KZ	0XW603Z
0X6W0Z0	0X984ZZ	0X9J0ZZ	0XBB3ZX	0XH40YZ	0XHC3YZ	0XJ40ZZ	0XMB0ZZ	0XP74YZ	0XUK47Z	0XW607Z
0X6W0Z1	0X9900Z	0X9J30Z	0XBB3ZZ	0XH431Z	0XHC41Z	0XJ43ZZ	0XMC0ZZ	0XP7X0Z	0XUK4JZ	0XW60JZ
0X6W0Z2	0X990ZX	0X9J3ZX	0XBB4ZX	0XH433Z	0XHC43Z	0XJ44ZZ	0XMD0ZZ	0XP7X1Z	0XUK4KZ	0XW60KZ
0X6W0Z3	0X990ZZ	0X9J3ZZ	0XBB4ZZ	0XH43YZ	0XHC4YZ	0XJ4XZZ	0XMF0ZZ	0XP7X3Z	0XUL07Z	0XW60YZ
0X9200Z	0X9930Z	0X9J40Z	0XBC0ZX	0XH441Z	0XHD01Z	0XJ50ZZ	0XMG0ZZ	0XP7X7Z	0XUL0JZ	0XW630Z
0X920ZX	0X993ZX	0X9J4ZX	0XBC0ZZ	0XH443Z	0XHD03Z	0XJ53ZZ	0XMH0ZZ	0XP7XJZ	0XUL0KZ	0XW633Z
0X920ZZ	0X993ZZ	0X9J4ZZ	0XBC3ZX	0XH44YZ	0XHD0YZ	0XJ54ZZ	0XMJ0ZZ	0XP7XKZ	0XUL47Z	0XW637Z
0X9230Z	0X9940Z	0X9K00Z	0XBC3ZZ	0XH501Z	0XHD31Z	0XJ5XZZ	0XMK0ZZ	0XP7XYZ	0XUL4JZ	0XW63JZ
0X923ZX	0X994ZX	0X9K0ZX	0XBC4ZX	0XH503Z	0XHD33Z	0XJ60ZZ	0XML0ZZ	0XQ20ZZ	0XUL4KZ	0XW63KZ
0X923ZZ	0X994ZZ	0X9K0ZZ	0XBC4ZZ	0XH50YZ	0XHD3YZ	0XJ63ZZ	0XMM0ZZ	0XQ23ZZ	0XUM07Z	0XW63YZ
0X9240Z	0X9B00Z	0X9K30Z	0XBD0ZX	0XH531Z	0XHD41Z	0XJ64ZZ	0XMN0ZZ	0XQ24ZZ	0XUM0JZ	0XW640Z
0X924ZX	0X9B0ZX	0X9K3ZX	0XBD0ZZ	0XH533Z	0XHD43Z	0XJ6XZZ	0XMP0ZZ	0XQ2XZZ	0XUM0KZ	0XW643Z
0X924ZZ	0X9B0ZZ	0X9K3ZZ	0XBD3ZX	0XH53YZ	0XHD4YZ	0XJ70ZZ	0XMQ0ZZ	0XQ30ZZ	0XUM47Z	0XW647Z
0X9300Z	0X9B30Z	0X9K40Z	0XBD3ZZ	0XH541Z	0XHF01Z	0XJ73ZZ	0XMR0ZZ	0XQ33ZZ	0XUM4JZ	0XW64JZ
0X930ZX	0X9B3ZX	0X9K4ZX	0XBD4ZX	0XH543Z	0XHF03Z	0XJ74ZZ	0XMS0ZZ	0XQ34ZZ	0XUM4KZ	0XW64KZ
0X930ZZ	0X9B3ZZ	0X9K4ZZ	0XBD4ZZ	0XH54YZ	0XHF0YZ	0XJ7XZZ	0XMT0ZZ	0XQ3XZZ	0XUM4KZ	0XW64YZ
0X9330Z	0X9B40Z	0XB20ZX	0XBF0ZX	0XH601Z	0XHF31Z	0XJ80ZZ	0XMV0ZZ	0XQ40ZZ	0XUN07Z	0XW6X0Z
0X933ZX	0X9B4ZX	0XB20ZZ	0XBF0ZZ	0XH603Z	0XHF33Z	0XJ83ZZ	0XMW0ZZ	0XQ43ZZ	0XUN0JZ	0XW6X3Z
0X933ZZ	0X9B4ZZ	0XB23ZX	0XBF3ZX	0XH60YZ	0XHF3YZ	0XJ84ZZ	0XP600Z	0XQ44ZZ	0XUN0KZ	0XW6X7Z
0X9340Z	0X9C00Z	0XB23ZZ	0XBF3ZZ	0XH631Z	0XHF41Z	0XJ8XZZ	0XP601Z	0XQ4XZZ	0XUN47Z	0XW6XJZ
0X934ZX	0X9C0ZX	0XB24ZX	0XBF4ZX	0XH633Z	0XHF43Z	0XJ90ZZ	0XP603Z	0XQ50ZZ	0XUN4JZ	0XW6XKZ
0X934ZZ	0X9C0ZZ	0XB24ZZ	0XBF4ZZ	0XH63YZ	0XHF4YZ	0XJ93ZZ	0XP607Z	0XQ53ZZ	0XUN4KZ	0XW6XYZ
0X9400Z	0X9C30Z	0XB30ZX	0XBG0ZX	0XH641Z	0XHG01Z	0XJ94ZZ	0XP60JZ	0XQ54ZZ	0XUP07Z	0XW700Z
0X940ZX	0X9C3ZX	0XB30ZZ	0XBG0ZZ	0XH643Z	0XHG03Z	0XJ9XZZ	0XP60KZ	0XQ5XZZ	0XUP0JZ	0XW703Z
0X940ZZ	0X9C3ZZ	0XB33ZX	0XBG3ZX	0XH64YZ	0XHG0YZ	0XJB0ZZ	0XP60YZ	0XQ60ZZ	0XUP0KZ	0XW707Z
0X9430Z	0X9C40Z	0XB33ZZ	0XBG3ZZ	0XH701Z	0XHG31Z	0XJB3ZZ	0XP630Z	0XQ63ZZ	0XUP47Z	0XW70JZ
0X943ZX	0X9C4ZX	0XB34ZX	0XBG4ZX	0XH703Z	0XHG33Z	0XJB4ZZ	0XP631Z	0XQ64ZZ	0XUP4JZ	0XW70KZ
0X943ZZ	0X9C4ZZ	0XB34ZZ	0XBG4ZZ	0XH70YZ	0XHG3YZ	0XJBXZZ	0XP633Z	0XQ6XZZ	0XUP4KZ	0XW70YZ
0X9440Z	0X9D00Z	0XB40ZX	0XBH0ZX	0XH731Z	0XHG41Z	0XJC0ZZ	0XP637Z	0XQ70ZZ	0XUQ07Z	0XW730Z
0X944ZX	0X9D0ZX	0XB40ZZ	0XBH0ZZ	0XH733Z	0XHG43Z	0XJC3ZZ	0XP63JZ	0XQ73ZZ	0XUQ0JZ	0XW733Z
0X944ZZ	0X9D0ZZ	0XB43ZX	0XBH3ZX	0XH73YZ	0XHG4YZ	0XJC4ZZ	0XP63KZ	0XQ74ZZ	0XUQ0KZ	0XW737Z
0X9500Z	0X9D30Z	0XB43ZZ	0XBH3ZZ	0XH741Z	0XHH01Z	0XJCXZZ	0XP63YZ	0XQ7XZZ	0XUQ47Z	0XW73JZ
0X950ZX	0X9D3ZX	0XB44ZX	0XBH4ZX	0XH743Z	0XHH03Z	0XJD0ZZ	0XP640Z	0XQ80ZZ	0XUQ4JZ	0XW73KZ
0X950ZZ	0X9D3ZZ	0XB44ZZ	0XBH4ZZ	0XH74YZ	0XHH0YZ	0XJD3ZZ	0XP641Z	0XQ83ZZ	0XUQ4KZ	0XW73YZ
0X9530Z	0X9D40Z	0XB50ZX	0XBJ0ZX	0XH801Z	0XHH31Z	0XJD4ZZ	0XP643Z	0XQ84ZZ	0XUR07Z	0XW740Z
0X953ZX	0X9D4ZX	0XB50ZZ	0XBJ0ZZ	0XH803Z	0XHH33Z	0XJDXZZ	0XP647Z	0XQ8XZZ	0XUR0JZ	0XW743Z
0X953ZZ	0X9D4ZZ	0XB53ZX	0XBJ3ZX	0XH80YZ	0XHH3YZ	0XJF0ZZ	0XP64JZ	0XQ90ZZ	0XUR0KZ	0XW747Z
0X9540Z	0X9F00Z	0XB53ZZ	0XBJ3ZZ	0XH831Z	0XHH41Z	0XJF3ZZ	0XP64KZ	0XQ93ZZ	0XUR47Z	0XW74JZ
0X954ZX	0X9F0ZX	0XB54ZX	0XBJ4ZX	0XH833Z	0XHH43Z	0XJF4ZZ	0XP64YZ	0XQ94ZZ	0XUR4JZ	0XW74KZ

0XW74YZ	0Y0C3JZ	0Y0J4ZZ	0Y6P0Z1	0Y9600Z	0Y9F30Z	0Y9N40Z	0YBF3ZZ	0YJJ4ZZ	0YPB37Z	0YQF0ZZ
0XW7X0Z	0Y0C3KZ	0Y0K07Z	0Y6P0Z2	0Y960ZX	0Y9F3ZX	0Y9N4ZX	0YBF4ZX	0YJJXZZ	0YPB3JZ	0YQF3ZZ
0XW7X3Z	0Y0C3ZZ	0Y0K0JZ	0Y6P0Z3	0Y960ZZ	0Y9F3ZZ	0Y9N4ZZ	0YBF4ZZ	0YJK3ZZ	0YPB3KZ	0YQF4ZZ
0XW7X7Z	0Y0C47Z	0Y0K0KZ	0Y6Q0Z0	0Y9630Z	0Y9F40Z	0YB00ZX	0YBG0ZX	0YJK4ZZ	0YPB3YZ	0YQFXZZ
0XW7XJZ	0Y0C4JZ	0Y0K37Z	0Y6Q0Z1	0Y963ZX	0Y9F4ZX	0YB00ZZ	0YBG0ZZ	0YJKXZZ	0YPB40Z	0YQG0ZZ
0XW7XKZ	0Y0C4KZ	0Y0K3JZ	0Y6Q0Z3	0Y963ZZ	0Y9F4ZZ	0YB03ZX	0YBG3ZX	0YJL3ZZ	0YPB41Z	0YQG3ZZ
0XW7XYZ	0Y0C4ZZ	0Y0K3KZ	0Y6R0Z0	0Y9640Z	0Y9G00Z	0YB03ZZ	0YBG3ZZ	0YJL4ZZ	0YPB43Z	0YQG4ZZ
0XXN0ZL	0Y0D07Z	0Y0K3ZZ	0Y6R0Z1	0Y964ZX	0Y9G0ZX	0YB04ZX	0YBG4ZX	0YJLXZZ	0YPB47Z	0YQGXZZ
0XXP0ZM	0Y0D0JZ	0Y0K47Z	0Y6R0Z2	0Y964ZZ	0Y9G0ZZ	0YB04ZZ	0YBG4ZZ	0YJM3ZZ	0YPB4JZ	0YQH0ZZ
0XYJ0Z0	0Y0D0KZ	0Y0K4JZ	0Y6R0Z3	0Y9700Z	0Y9G30Z	0YB10ZX	0YBH0ZX	0YJM4ZZ	0YPB4KZ	0YQH3ZZ
0XYJ0Z1	0Y0D0ZZ	0Y0K4KZ	0Y6S0Z0	0Y970ZX	0Y9G3ZX	0YB10ZZ	0YBH0ZZ	0YJMXZZ	0YPB4YZ	0YQH4ZZ
0XYK0Z0	0Y0D37Z	0Y0K4ZZ	0Y6S0Z1	0Y970ZZ	0Y9G3ZZ	0YB13ZX	0YBH3ZX	0YJN3ZZ	0YPBX0Z	0YQHXZZ
0XYK0Z1	0Y0D3JZ	0Y0L07Z	0Y6S0Z2	0Y9730Z	0Y9G40Z	0YB13ZZ	0YBH3ZZ	0YJN4ZZ	0YPBX1Z	0YQJ0ZZ
0Y0007Z	0Y0D3KZ	0Y0L0JZ	0Y6S0Z3	0Y973ZX	0Y9G4ZX	0YB14ZX	0YBH4ZX	0YJNXZZ	0YPBX3Z	0YQJ3ZZ
0Y000JZ	0Y0D3ZZ	0Y0L0KZ	0Y6T0Z0	0Y973ZZ	0Y9G4ZZ	0YB14ZZ	0YBH4ZZ	0YMK0ZZ	0YPBX7Z	0YQJ4ZZ
0Y000KZ	0Y0D47Z	0Y0L0ZZ	0Y6T0Z1	0Y9740Z	0Y9H00Z	0YB50ZX	0YBJ0ZX	0YML0ZZ	0YPBXJZ	0YQJXZZ
0Y000ZZ	0Y0D4JZ	0Y0L37Z	0Y6T0Z2	0Y974ZX	0Y9H0ZX	0YB50ZZ	0YBJ0ZZ	0YMM0ZZ	0YPBXKZ	0YQK0ZZ
0Y0037Z	0Y0D4KZ	0Y0L3JZ	0Y6T0Z3	0Y974ZZ	0Y9H0ZZ	0YB53ZX	0YBJ3ZX	0YMN0ZZ	0YPBXYZ	0YQK3ZZ
0Y003JZ	0Y0D4ZZ	0Y0L3KZ	0Y6U0Z0	0Y9800Z	0Y9H30Z	0YB53ZZ	0YBJ3ZZ	0YMP0ZZ	0YQ00ZZ	0YQK4ZZ
0Y003KZ	0Y0F07Z	0Y0L3ZZ	0Y6U0Z1	0Y980ZX	0Y9H3ZX	0YB54ZX	0YBJ4ZX	0YMQ0ZZ	0YQ03ZZ	0YQKXZZ
0Y003ZZ	0Y0F0JZ	0Y0L47Z	0Y6U0Z2	0Y980ZZ	0Y9H3ZZ	0YB54ZZ	0YBK0ZX	0YMR0ZZ	0YQ04ZZ	0YQL0ZZ
0Y0047Z	0Y0F0KZ	0Y0L4JZ	0Y6U0Z3	0Y9830Z	0Y9H40Z	0YB60ZX	0YBK3ZX	0YMS0ZZ	0YQ0XZZ	0YQL3ZZ
0Y004JZ	0Y0F0ZZ	0Y0L4KZ	0Y6V0Z0	0Y983ZX	0Y9H4ZX	0YB60ZZ	0YBK4ZX	0YMT0ZZ	0YQ10ZZ	0YQL4ZZ
0Y004KZ	0Y0F37Z	0Y0L4ZZ	0Y6V0Z1	0Y983ZZ	0Y9H4ZZ	0YB63ZX	0YBL0ZX	0YMU0ZZ	0YQ13ZZ	0YQLXZZ
0Y004ZZ	0Y0F3JZ	0Y29X0Z	0Y6V0Z2	0Y9840Z	0Y9J00Z	0YB63ZZ	0YBL3ZX	0YMV0ZZ	0YQ14ZZ	0YQM0ZZ
0Y0107Z	0Y0F3KZ	0Y29XYZ	0Y6V0Z3	0Y984ZX	0Y9J0ZX	0YB64ZX	0YBL4ZX	0YMW0ZZ	0YQ1XZZ	0YQM3ZZ
0Y010JZ	0Y0F3ZZ	0Y2BX0Z	0Y6W0Z0	0Y984ZZ	0Y9J0ZZ	0YB64ZZ	0YBM0ZX	0YMX0ZZ	0YQ50ZZ	0YQM4ZZ
0Y010KZ	0Y0F47Z	0Y2BXYZ	0Y6W0Z1	0Y9900Z	0Y9J30Z	0YB70ZX	0YBM3ZX	0YMY0ZZ	0YQ53ZZ	0YQMXZZ
0Y010ZZ	0Y0F4JZ	0Y300ZZ	0Y6W0Z2	0Y990ZX	0Y9J3ZX	0YB70ZZ	0YBM4ZX	0YP900Z	0YQ54ZZ	0YQN0ZZ
0Y0137Z	0Y0F4KZ	0Y303ZZ	0Y6W0Z3	0Y990ZZ	0Y9J3ZZ	0YB73ZX	0YBN0ZX	0YP901Z	0YQ5XZZ	0YQN3ZZ
0Y013JZ	0Y0F4ZZ	0Y304ZZ	0Y6X0Z0	0Y9930Z	0Y9J40Z	0YB73ZZ	0YBN3ZX	0YP903Z	0YQ60ZZ	0YQN4ZZ
0Y013KZ	0Y0G07Z	0Y310ZZ	0Y6X0Z1	0Y993ZX	0Y9J4ZX	0YB74ZX	0YBN4ZX	0YP907Z	0YQ63ZZ	0YQNXZZ
0Y013ZZ	0Y0G0JZ	0Y313ZZ	0Y6X0Z2	0Y993ZZ	0Y9J4ZZ	0YB74ZZ	0YJ03ZZ	0YP90JZ	0YQ64ZZ	0YQP0ZZ
0Y0147Z	0Y0G0KZ	0Y314ZZ	0Y6X0Z3	0Y9940Z	0Y9K00Z	0YB80ZX	0YJ04ZZ	0YP90KZ	0YQ6XZZ	0YQP3ZZ
0Y014JZ	0Y0G0ZZ	0Y350ZZ	0Y6Y0Z0	0Y994ZX	0Y9K0ZX	0YB80ZZ	0YJ0XZZ	0YP90YZ	0YQ70ZZ	0YQP4ZZ
0Y014KZ	0Y0G37Z	0Y353ZZ	0Y6Y0Z1	0Y994ZZ	0Y9K0ZZ	0YB83ZX	0YJ13ZZ	0YP930Z	0YQ73ZZ	0YQPXZZ
0Y014ZZ	0Y0G3JZ	0Y354ZZ	0Y6Y0Z2	0Y9B00Z	0Y9K30Z	0YB83ZZ	0YJ14ZZ	0YP931Z	0YQ74ZZ	0YQQ0ZZ
0Y0907Z	0Y0G3KZ	0Y360ZZ	0Y6Y0Z3	0Y9B0ZX	0Y9K3ZX	0YB84ZX	0YJ1XZZ	0YP933Z	0YQ7XZZ	0YQQ3ZZ
0Y090JZ	0Y0G3ZZ	0Y363ZZ	0Y9000Z	0Y9B0ZZ	0Y9K3ZZ	0YB84ZZ	0YJ5XZZ	0YP937Z	0YQ80ZZ	0YQQ4ZZ
0Y090KZ	0Y0G47Z	0Y364ZZ	0Y900ZX	0Y9B30Z	0Y9K40Z	0YB90ZX	0YJ6XZZ	0YP93JZ	0YQ83ZZ	0YQQXZZ
0Y090ZZ	0Y0G4JZ	0Y370ZZ	0Y900ZZ	0Y9B3ZX	0Y9K4ZX	0YB90ZZ	0YJ7XZZ	0YP93KZ	0YQ84ZZ	0YQR0ZZ
0Y0937Z	0Y0G4KZ	0Y373ZZ	0Y9030Z	0Y9B3ZZ	0Y9K4ZZ	0YB93ZX	0YJ8XZZ	0YP93YZ	0YQ8XZZ	0YQR3ZZ
0Y093JZ	0Y0G4ZZ	0Y374ZZ	0Y903ZX	0Y9B40Z	0Y9L00Z	0YB93ZZ	0YJ93ZZ	0YP940Z	0YQ90ZZ	0YQR4ZZ
0Y093KZ	0Y0H07Z	0Y380ZZ	0Y903ZZ	0Y9B4ZX	0Y9L0ZX	0YB94ZX	0YJ94ZZ	0YP941Z	0YQ93ZZ	0YQRXZZ
0Y093ZZ	0Y0H0JZ	0Y383ZZ	0Y9040Z	0Y9B4ZZ	0Y9L0ZZ	0YB94ZZ	0YJ9XZZ	0YP943Z	0YQ94ZZ	0YQS0ZZ
0Y0947Z	0Y0H0KZ	0Y384ZZ	0Y904ZX	0Y9C00Z	0Y9L30Z	0YBB0ZX	0YJAXZZ	0YP947Z	0YQ9XZZ	0YQS3ZZ
0Y094JZ	0Y0H0ZZ	0Y390ZZ	0Y904ZZ	0Y9C0ZX	0Y9L3ZX	0YBB0ZZ	0YJB3ZZ	0YP94JZ	0YQA0ZZ	0YQS4ZZ
0Y094KZ	0Y0H37Z	0Y393ZZ	0Y9100Z	0Y9C0ZZ	0Y9L3ZZ	0YBB3ZZ	0YJB4ZZ	0YP94KZ	0YQA3ZZ	0YQSXZZ
0Y094ZZ	0Y0H3JZ	0Y394ZZ	0Y910ZX	0Y9C30Z	0Y9L40Z	0YBB3ZZ	0YJBXZZ	0YP94YZ	0YQA4ZZ	0YQT0ZZ
0Y0B07Z	0Y0H3KZ	0Y3B0ZZ	0Y910ZZ	0Y9C3ZX	0Y9L4ZX	0YBB4ZX	0YJC3ZZ	0YP9X0Z	0YQAXZZ	0YQT3ZZ
0Y0B0JZ	0Y0H3ZZ	0Y3B3ZZ	0Y9130Z	0Y9C3ZZ	0Y9L4ZZ	0YBB4ZZ	0YJC4ZZ	0YP9X1Z	0YQB0ZZ	0YQT4ZZ
0Y0B0KZ	0Y0H47Z	0Y3B3ZZ	0Y913ZX	0Y9C40Z	0Y9M00Z	0YBC0ZX	0YJCXZZ	0YP9X3Z	0YQB3ZZ	0YQTXZZ
0Y0B0ZZ	0Y0H4JZ	0Y3B4ZZ	0Y913ZZ	0Y9C4ZX	0Y9M0ZX	0YBC0ZZ	0YJD3ZZ	0YP9X7Z	0YQB4ZZ	0YQU0ZZ
0Y0B37Z	0Y0H4KZ	0Y3C0ZZ	0Y9140Z	0Y9C4ZZ	0Y9M0ZZ	0YBC3ZX	0YJD4ZZ	0YP9XJZ	0YQBXZZ	0YQU3ZZ
0Y0B3JZ	0Y0H4ZZ	0Y3C3ZZ	0Y914ZX	0Y9D00Z	0Y9M30Z	0YBC3ZZ	0YJDXZZ	0YP9XKZ	0YQC0ZZ	0YQU4ZZ
0Y0B3KZ	0Y0J07Z	0Y3C4ZZ	0Y914ZZ	0Y9D0ZX	0Y9M3ZX	0YBC4ZX	0YJEXZZ	0YP9XYZ	0YQC3ZZ	0YQUXZZ
0Y0B3ZZ	0Y0J0JZ	0Y6N0Z5	0Y9500Z	0Y9D0ZZ	0Y9M3ZZ	0YBC4ZZ	0YJF3ZZ	0YPB00Z	0YQC4ZZ	0YQV0ZZ
0Y0B47Z	0Y0J0KZ	0Y6N0Z6	0Y950ZX	0Y9D30Z	0Y9M40Z	0YBD0ZX	0YJF4ZZ	0YPB01Z	0YQCXZZ	0YQV3ZZ
0Y0B4JZ	0Y0J0ZZ	0Y6N0Z7	0Y950ZZ	0Y9D3ZX	0Y9M4ZX	0YBD0ZZ	0YJFXZZ	0YPB03Z	0YQD0ZZ	0YQV4ZZ
0Y0B4KZ	0Y0J37Z	0Y6N0Z8	0Y9530Z	0Y9D3ZZ	0Y9M4ZZ	0YBD3ZX	0YJG3ZZ	0YPB07Z	0YQD3ZZ	0YQVXZZ
0Y0B4ZZ	0Y0J3JZ	0Y6N0Z9	0Y953ZX	0Y9D40Z	0Y9N00Z	0YBD3ZZ	0YJG4ZZ	0YPB0JZ	0YQD4ZZ	0YQW0ZZ
0Y0C07Z	0Y0J3KZ	0Y6N0ZB	0Y953ZZ	0Y9D4ZX	0Y9N0ZX	0YBD4ZX	0YJGXZZ	0YPB0KZ	0YQDXZZ	0YQW3ZZ
0Y0C0JZ	0Y0J3ZZ	0Y6N0ZC	0Y9540Z	0Y9D4ZZ	0Y9N0ZZ	0YBD4ZZ	0YJH3ZZ	0YPB0YZ	0YQE0ZZ	0YQW4ZZ
0Y0C0KZ	0Y0J47Z	0Y6N0ZD	0Y954ZX	0Y9F00Z	0Y9N30Z	0YBF0ZX	0YJH4ZZ	0YPB30Z	0YQE3ZZ	0YQWXZZ
0Y0C0ZZ	0Y0J4JZ	0Y6N0ZF	0Y954ZZ	0Y9F0ZX	0Y9N3ZX	0YBF0ZZ	0YJHXZZ	0YPB31Z	0YQE4ZZ	0YQX0ZZ
0Y0C37Z	0Y0J4KZ	0Y6P0Z0	0Y954ZZ	0Y9F0ZZ	0Y9N3ZZ	0YBF3ZX	0YJJ3ZZ	0YPB33Z	0YQEXZZ	0YQX3ZZ

0YQX4ZZ	0YUD07Z	0YUQ07Z	0YW940Z	10908ZD	10Q00YV	10Q04ZE	2W00X3Z	2W07X5Z	2W0EXYZ	2W0NX2Z
0YQXXZZ	0YUD0JZ	0YUQ0JZ	0YW943Z	10908ZU	10Q00YY	10Q04ZF	2W00X4Z	2W07X6Z	2W0FX0Z	2W0NX3Z
0YQY0ZZ	0YUD0KZ	0YUQ0KZ	0YW947Z	10A00ZZ	10Q00ZE	10Q04ZG	2W00X5Z	2W07X7Z	2W0FX1Z	2W0NX4Z
0YQY3ZZ	0YUD47Z	0YUQ47Z	0YW94JZ	10A03ZZ	10Q00ZF	10Q04ZH	2W00X6Z	2W07XYZ	2W0FX3Z	2W0NX5Z
0YQY4ZZ	0YUD4JZ	0YUQ4JZ	0YW94KZ	10A04ZZ	10Q00ZG	10Q04ZJ	2W00X7Z	2W08X0Z	2W0FX4Z	2W0NX7Z
0YQYXZZ	0YUD4KZ	0YUQ4KZ	0YW94YZ	10A07Z6	10Q00ZH	10Q04ZK	2W00XYZ	2W08X1Z	2W0FX5Z	2W0NXYZ
0YU007Z	0YUE07Z	0YUR07Z	0YW9X0Z	10A07ZW	10Q00ZJ	10Q04ZL	2W01X0Z	2W08X2Z	2W0FX6Z	2W0PX0Z
0YU00JZ	0YUE0JZ	0YUR0JZ	0YW9X3Z	10A07ZX	10Q00ZK	10Q04ZM	2W01X1Z	2W08X3Z	2W0FX7Z	2W0PX1Z
0YU00KZ	0YUE0KZ	0YUR0KZ	0YW9X7Z	10A07ZZ	10Q00ZL	10Q04ZN	2W01X2Z	2W08X4Z	2W0FXYZ	2W0PX2Z
0YU047Z	0YUE47Z	0YUR47Z	0YW9XJZ	10A08ZZ	10Q00ZM	10Q04ZP	2W01X3Z	2W08X5Z	2W0GX0Z	2W0PX3Z
0YU04JZ	0YUE4JZ	0YUR4JZ	0YW9XKZ	10D00Z0	10Q00ZN	10Q04ZQ	2W01X4Z	2W08X6Z	2W0GX1Z	2W0PX4Z
0YU04KZ	0YUE4KZ	0YUR4KZ	0YW9XYZ	10D00Z1	10Q00ZP	10Q04ZR	2W01X5Z	2W08X7Z	2W0GX2Z	2W0PX5Z
0YU107Z	0YUF07Z	0YUS07Z	0YWB00Z	10D00Z2	10Q00ZQ	10Q04ZS	2W01X6Z	2W08XYZ	2W0GX3Z	2W0PX6Z
0YU10JZ	0YUF0JZ	0YUS0JZ	0YWB03Z	10D07Z3	10Q00ZR	10Q04ZT	2W01X7Z	2W09X0Z	2W0GX4Z	2W0PX7Z
0YU10KZ	0YUF0KZ	0YUS0KZ	0YWB07Z	10D07Z4	10Q00ZS	10Q04ZV	2W01X9Z	2W09X1Z	2W0GX5Z	2W0PXYZ
0YU147Z	0YUF47Z	0YUS47Z	0YWB0JZ	10D07Z5	10Q00ZT	10Q04ZY	2W01XYZ	2W09X2Z	2W0GX6Z	2W0QX0Z
0YU14JZ	0YUF4JZ	0YUS4JZ	0YWB0KZ	10D07Z6	10Q00ZV	10Q07YE	2W02X0Z	2W09X3Z	2W0GX7Z	2W0QX1Z
0YU14KZ	0YUF4KZ	0YUS4KZ	0YWB0YZ	10D07Z7	10Q00ZY	10Q07YF	2W02X1Z	2W09X4Z	2W0GXYZ	2W0QX2Z
0YU507Z	0YUG07Z	0YUT07Z	0YWB30Z	10D07Z8	10Q03YE	10Q07YG	2W02X2Z	2W09X5Z	2W0HX0Z	2W0QX3Z
0YU50JZ	0YUG0JZ	0YUT0JZ	0YWB33Z	10D17Z9	10Q03YF	10Q07YH	2W02X3Z	2W09X6Z	2W0HX1Z	2W0QX4Z
0YU50KZ	0YUG0KZ	0YUT0KZ	0YWB37Z	10D17ZZ	10Q03YG	10Q07YJ	2W02X4Z	2W09X7Z	2W0HX2Z	2W0QX5Z
0YU547Z	0YUG47Z	0YUT47Z	0YWB3JZ	10D18Z9	10Q03YH	10Q07YK	2W02X5Z	2W09XYZ	2W0HX3Z	2W0QX6Z
0YU54JZ	0YUG4JZ	0YUT4JZ	0YWB3KZ	10D18ZZ	10Q03YJ	10Q07YL	2W02X6Z	2W0AX0Z	2W0HX4Z	2W0QX7Z
0YU54KZ	0YUG4KZ	0YUT4KZ	0YWB3YZ	10D27ZZ	10Q03YK	10Q07YM	2W02X7Z	2W0AX1Z	2W0HX5Z	2W0QXYZ
0YU607Z	0YUH07Z	0YUU07Z	0YWB40Z	10D28ZZ	10Q03YL	10Q07YN	2W02XYZ	2W0AX2Z	2W0HX6Z	2W0RX0Z
0YU60JZ	0YUH0JZ	0YUU0JZ	0YWB43Z	10E0XZZ	10Q03YM	10Q07YP	2W03X0Z	2W0AX3Z	2W0HX7Z	2W0RX1Z
0YU60KZ	0YUH0KZ	0YUU0KZ	0YWB47Z	10H003Z	10Q03YN	10Q07YQ	2W03X1Z	2W0AX4Z	2W0HXYZ	2W0RX2Z
0YU647Z	0YUH47Z	0YUU47Z	0YWB4JZ	10H00YZ	10Q03YP	10Q07YR	2W03X2Z	2W0AX5Z	2W0JX0Z	2W0RX3Z
0YU64JZ	0YUH4JZ	0YUU4JZ	0YWB4KZ	10H073Z	10Q03YQ	10Q07YS	2W03X3Z	2W0AX6Z	2W0JX1Z	2W0RX4Z
0YU64KZ	0YUH4KZ	0YUU4KZ	0YWB4YZ	10H07YZ	10Q03YR	10Q07YT	2W03X4Z	2W0AX7Z	2W0JX2Z	2W0RX5Z
0YU707Z	0YUJ07Z	0YUV07Z	0YWBX0Z	10J00ZZ	10Q03YS	10Q07YV	2W03X5Z	2W0AXYZ	2W0JX3Z	2W0RX6Z
0YU70JZ	0YUJ0JZ	0YUV0JZ	0YWBX3Z	10J03ZZ	10Q03YT	10Q07YY	2W03X6Z	2W0BX0Z	2W0JX4Z	2W0RX7Z
0YU70KZ	0YUJ0KZ	0YUV0KZ	0YWBX7Z	10J04ZZ	10Q03YV	10Q07ZE	2W03X7Z	2W0BX1Z	2W0JX5Z	2W0RXYZ
0YU747Z	0YUJ47Z	0YUV47Z	0YWBXJZ	10J07ZZ	10Q03YY	10Q07ZF	2W03XYZ	2W0BX2Z	2W0JX6Z	2W0SX0Z
0YU74JZ	0YUJ4JZ	0YUV4JZ	0YWBXKZ	10J08ZZ	10Q03ZE	10Q07ZG	2W04X0Z	2W0BX3Z	2W0JX7Z	2W0SX1Z
0YU74KZ	0YUJ4KZ	0YUV4KZ	0YWBXYZ	10J0XZZ	10Q03ZF	10Q07ZH	2W04X1Z	2W0BX4Z	2W0JXYZ	2W0SX2Z
0YU807Z	0YUK07Z	0YUW07Z	102073Z	10J10ZZ	10Q03ZG	10Q07ZJ	2W04X2Z	2W0BX5Z	2W0KX0Z	2W0SX3Z
0YU80JZ	0YUK0JZ	0YUW0JZ	10207YZ	10J13ZZ	10Q03ZH	10Q07ZK	2W04X3Z	2W0BX6Z	2W0KX1Z	2W0SX4Z
0YU80KZ	0YUK0KZ	0YUW0KZ	10900Z9	10J14ZZ	10Q03ZJ	10Q07ZL	2W04X4Z	2W0BX7Z	2W0KX2Z	2W0SX5Z
0YU847Z	0YUK47Z	0YUW47Z	10900ZA	10J17ZZ	10Q03ZK	10Q07ZM	2W04X5Z	2W0BXYZ	2W0KX3Z	2W0SX6Z
0YU84JZ	0YUK4JZ	0YUW4JZ	10900ZB	10J18ZZ	10Q03ZL	10Q07ZN	2W04X6Z	2W0CX0Z	2W0KX4Z	2W0SX7Z
0YU84KZ	0YUK4KZ	0YUW4KZ	10900ZC	10J1XZZ	10Q03ZM	10Q07ZP	2W04X7Z	2W0CX1Z	2W0KX5Z	2W0SXYZ
0YU907Z	0YUL07Z	0YUX07Z	10900ZD	10J20ZZ	10Q03ZN	10Q07ZQ	2W04XYZ	2W0CX2Z	2W0KX6Z	2W0TX0Z
0YU90JZ	0YUL0JZ	0YUX0JZ	10900ZU	10J23ZZ	10Q03ZP	10Q07ZR	2W05X0Z	2W0CX3Z	2W0KX7Z	2W0TX1Z
0YU90KZ	0YUL0KZ	0YUX0KZ	10903Z9	10J24ZZ	10Q03ZQ	10Q07ZS	2W05X1Z	2W0CX4Z	2W0KXYZ	2W0TX2Z
0YU947Z	0YUL47Z	0YUX47Z	10903ZA	10J27ZZ	10Q03ZR	10Q07ZT	2W05X3Z	2W0CX5Z	2W0LX0Z	2W0TX3Z
0YU94JZ	0YUL4JZ	0YUX4JZ	10903ZB	10J28ZZ	10Q03ZS	10Q07ZV	2W05X4Z	2W0CX6Z	2W0LX1Z	2W0TX4Z
0YU94KZ	0YUL4KZ	0YUX4KZ	10903ZC	10J2XZZ	10Q03ZT	10Q07ZY	2W05X5Z	2W0CX7Z	2W0LX2Z	2W0TX5Z
0YUA07Z	0YUM07Z	0YUY07Z	10903ZD	10P003Z	10Q03ZV	10Q08YE	2W05X6Z	2W0CXYZ	2W0LX3Z	2W0TX6Z
0YUA0JZ	0YUM0JZ	0YUY0JZ	10903ZU	10P00YZ	10Q03ZY	10Q08YF	2W05X7Z	2W0DX0Z	2W0LX4Z	2W0TX7Z
0YUA0KZ	0YUM0KZ	0YUY0KZ	10904Z9	10P073Z	10Q04YE	10Q08YG	2W05XYZ	2W0DX1Z	2W0LX5Z	2W0TXYZ
0YUA47Z	0YUM47Z	0YUY47Z	10904ZA	10P07YZ	10Q04YF	10Q08YH	2W06X0Z	2W0DX2Z	2W0LX6Z	2W0UX0Z
0YUA4JZ	0YUM4JZ	0YUY4JZ	10904ZB	10Q00YE	10Q04YG	10Q08YJ	2W06X1Z	2W0DX3Z	2W0LX7Z	2W0UX1Z
0YUA4KZ	0YUM4KZ	0YUY4KZ	10904ZC	10Q00YF	10Q04YH	10Q08YK	2W06X2Z	2W0DX4Z	2W0LXYZ	2W0UX2Z
0YUB07Z	0YUN07Z	0YW900Z	10904ZD	10Q00YG	10Q04YJ	10Q08YL	2W06X3Z	2W0DX5Z	2W0MX0Z	2W0UX3Z
0YUB0JZ	0YUN0JZ	0YW903Z	10904ZU	10Q00YH	10Q04YK	10Q08YM	2W06X4Z	2W0DX6Z	2W0MX1Z	2W0UX4Z
0YUB0KZ	0YUN0KZ	0YW907Z	10907Z9	10Q00YJ	10Q04YL	10Q08YN	2W06X5Z	2W0DX7Z	2W0MX2Z	2W0UX5Z
0YUB47Z	0YUN47Z	0YW90JZ	10907ZA	10Q00YK	10Q04YM	10Q08YP	2W06X6Z	2W0DXYZ	2W0MX3Z	2W0UX6Z
0YUB4JZ	0YUN4JZ	0YW90KZ	10907ZB	10Q00YL	10Q04YN	10Q08YQ	2W06X7Z	2W0EX0Z	2W0MX4Z	2W0UX7Z
0YUB4KZ	0YUN4KZ	0YW90YZ	10907ZC	10Q00YM	10Q04YP	10Q08YR	2W06XYZ	2W0EX1Z	2W0MX5Z	2W0UXYZ
0YUC07Z	0YUP07Z	0YW930Z	10907ZD	10Q00YN	10Q04YQ	10Q08YS	2W07X0Z	2W0EX2Z	2W0MX6Z	2W0VX0Z
0YUC0JZ	0YUP0JZ	0YW933Z	10907ZU	10Q00YP	10Q04YR	10Q08YT	2W07X1Z	2W0EX3Z	2W0MX7Z	2W0VX1Z
0YUC0KZ	0YUP0KZ	0YW937Z	10908Z9	10Q00YQ	10Q04YS	10S0XZZ	2W07X2Z	2W0EX4Z	2W0MXYZ	2W0VX2Z
0YUC47Z	0YUP47Z	0YW93JZ	10908ZA	10Q00YR	10Q04YT	2W00X0Z	2W07X3Z	2W0EX5Z	2W0NX0Z	2W0VX3Z
0YUC4JZ	0YUP4JZ	0YW93KZ	10908ZB	10Q00YS	10Q04YV	2W00X1Z	2W07X4Z	2W0EX6Z	2W0NX0Z	2W0VX4Z
0YUC4KZ	0YUP4KZ	0YW93YZ	10908ZC	10Q00YT	10Q04YY	2W00X2Z	2W07X4Z	2W0EX7Z	2W0NX1Z	

2W0VX5Z	2W22X4Z	2W39X2Z	2W3RXYZ	2W52X0Z	2W59X3Z	2W5GX6Z	2W5QX0Z	2W66X0Z	30230AZ	30233V0
2W0VX6Z	2W23X4Z	2W39X3Z	2W3SX1Z	2W52X1Z	2W59X4Z	2W5GX7Z	2W5QX1Z	2W66XZZ	30230G0	30233V1
2W0VX7Z	2W24X4Z	2W39XYZ	2W3SX2Z	2W52X2Z	2W59X5Z	2W5GXYZ	2W5QX2Z	2W67X0Z	30230G2	30233W0
2W0VXYZ	2W25X4Z	2W3AX1Z	2W3SX3Z	2W52X3Z	2W59X6Z	2W5HX0Z	2W5QX3Z	2W67XZZ	30230G3	30233W1
2W10X6Z	2W26X4Z	2W3AX2Z	2W3SXYZ	2W52X4Z	2W59X7Z	2W5HX1Z	2W5QX4Z	2W68X0Z	30230G4	30233X0
2W10X7Z	2W27X4Z	2W3AX3Z	2W3TX1Z	2W52X5Z	2W59XYZ	2W5HX2Z	2W5QX5Z	2W68XZZ	30230H0	30233X2
2W11X6Z	2W28X4Z	2W3AXYZ	2W3TX2Z	2W52X6Z	2W5AX0Z	2W5HX3Z	2W5QX6Z	2W69X0Z	30230H1	30233X3
2W11X7Z	2W29X4Z	2W3BX1Z	2W3TX3Z	2W52X7Z	2W5AX1Z	2W5HX4Z	2W5QX7Z	2W69XZZ	30230J0	30233X4
2W12X6Z	2W2AX4Z	2W3BX2Z	2W3TXYZ	2W52XYZ	2W5AX2Z	2W5HX5Z	2W5QXYZ	2W6AX0Z	30230J1	30233Y0
2W12X7Z	2W2BX4Z	2W3BX3Z	2W3UX1Z	2W53X0Z	2W5AX3Z	2W5HX6Z	2W5RX0Z	2W6AXZZ	30230K0	30233Y2
2W13X6Z	2W2CX4Z	2W3BXYZ	2W3UX2Z	2W53X1Z	2W5AX4Z	2W5HX7Z	2W5RX1Z	2W6BX0Z	30230K1	30233Y3
2W13X7Z	2W2DX4Z	2W3CX1Z	2W3UX3Z	2W53X2Z	2W5AX5Z	2W5HXYZ	2W5RX2Z	2W6BXZZ	30230L0	30233Y4
2W14X6Z	2W2EX4Z	2W3CX2Z	2W3UXYZ	2W53X3Z	2W5AX6Z	2W5JX0Z	2W5RX3Z	2W6CX0Z	30230L1	30240AZ
2W14X7Z	2W2FX4Z	2W3CX3Z	2W3VX1Z	2W53X4Z	2W5AX7Z	2W5JX1Z	2W5RX4Z	2W6CXZZ	30230M0	30240G0
2W15X6Z	2W2GX4Z	2W3CXYZ	2W3VX2Z	2W53X5Z	2W5AXYZ	2W5JX2Z	2W5RX5Z	2W6DX0Z	30230M1	30240G2
2W15X7Z	2W2HX4Z	2W3DX1Z	2W3VX3Z	2W53X6Z	2W5BX0Z	2W5JX3Z	2W5RX6Z	2W6DXZZ	30230N0	30240G3
2W16X6Z	2W2JX4Z	2W3DX2Z	2W3VXYZ	2W53X7Z	2W5BX1Z	2W5JX4Z	2W5RX7Z	2W6EX0Z	30230N1	30240G4
2W16X7Z	2W2KX4Z	2W3DX3Z	2W40X5Z	2W53XYZ	2W5BX2Z	2W5JX5Z	2W5RXYZ	2W6EXZZ	30230P0	30240H0
2W17X6Z	2W2LX4Z	2W3DXYZ	2W41X5Z	2W54X0Z	2W5BX3Z	2W5JX6Z	2W5SX0Z	2W6FX0Z	30230P1	30240H1
2W17X7Z	2W2MX4Z	2W3EX1Z	2W42X5Z	2W54X1Z	2W5BX4Z	2W5JX7Z	2W5SX1Z	2W6FXZZ	30230Q0	30240J0
2W18X6Z	2W2NX4Z	2W3EX2Z	2W43X5Z	2W54X2Z	2W5BX5Z	2W5JXYZ	2W5SX2Z	2W6GX0Z	30230Q1	30240J1
2W18X7Z	2W2PX4Z	2W3EX3Z	2W44X5Z	2W54X3Z	2W5BX6Z	2W5KX0Z	2W5SX3Z	2W6GXZZ	30230R0	30240K0
2W19X6Z	2W2QX4Z	2W3EXYZ	2W45X5Z	2W54X4Z	2W5BX7Z	2W5KX1Z	2W5SX4Z	2W6HX0Z	30230R1	30240K1
2W19X7Z	2W2RX4Z	2W3FX1Z	2W46X5Z	2W54X5Z	2W5BXYZ	2W5KX2Z	2W5SX5Z	2W6HXZZ	30230S0	30240L0
2W1AX6Z	2W2SX4Z	2W3FX2Z	2W47X5Z	2W54X6Z	2W5CX0Z	2W5KX3Z	2W5SX6Z	2W6JX0Z	30230S1	30240L1
2W1AX7Z	2W2TX4Z	2W3FX3Z	2W48X5Z	2W54X7Z	2W5CX1Z	2W5KX4Z	2W5SX7Z	2W6JXZZ	30230T0	30240M0
2W1BX6Z	2W2UX4Z	2W3FXYZ	2W49X5Z	2W54XYZ	2W5CX2Z	2W5KX5Z	2W5SXYZ	2W6KX0Z	30230T1	30240M1
2W1BX7Z	2W2VX4Z	2W3GX1Z	2W4AX5Z	2W55X0Z	2W5CX3Z	2W5KX6Z	2W5TX0Z	2W6KXZZ	30230V0	30240N0
2W1CX6Z	2W30X1Z	2W3GX2Z	2W4BX5Z	2W55X1Z	2W5CX4Z	2W5KX7Z	2W5TX1Z	2W6LX0Z	30230V1	30240N1
2W1CX7Z	2W30X2Z	2W3GX3Z	2W4CX5Z	2W55X2Z	2W5CX5Z	2W5KXYZ	2W5TX2Z	2W6LXZZ	30230W0	30240P0
2W1DX6Z	2W30X3Z	2W3GXYZ	2W4DX5Z	2W55X3Z	2W5CX6Z	2W5LX0Z	2W5TX3Z	2W6MX0Z	30230W1	30240P1
2W1DX7Z	2W30XYZ	2W3HX1Z	2W4EX5Z	2W55X4Z	2W5CX7Z	2W5LX1Z	2W5TX4Z	2W6MXZZ	30230X0	30240Q0
2W1EX6Z	2W31X1Z	2W3HX2Z	2W4FX5Z	2W55X5Z	2W5CXYZ	2W5LX2Z	2W5TX5Z	2W6NX0Z	30230X2	30240Q1
2W1EX7Z	2W31X2Z	2W3HX3Z	2W4GX5Z	2W55X6Z	2W5DX0Z	2W5LX3Z	2W5TX6Z	2W6NXZZ	30230X3	30240R0
2W1FX6Z	2W31X3Z	2W3HXYZ	2W4HX5Z	2W55X7Z	2W5DX1Z	2W5LX4Z	2W5TX7Z	2W6PX0Z	30230X4	30240R1
2W1FX7Z	2W31X9Z	2W3JX1Z	2W4JX5Z	2W55XYZ	2W5DX2Z	2W5LX5Z	2W5TXYZ	2W6PXZZ	30230Y0	30240S0
2W1GX6Z	2W31XYZ	2W3JX2Z	2W4KX5Z	2W56X0Z	2W5DX3Z	2W5LX6Z	2W5UX0Z	2W6QX0Z	30230Y2	30240S1
2W1GX7Z	2W32X1Z	2W3JX3Z	2W4LX5Z	2W56X1Z	2W5DX4Z	2W5LX7Z	2W5UX1Z	2W6QXZZ	30230Y3	30240T0
2W1HX6Z	2W32X2Z	2W3JXYZ	2W4MX5Z	2W56X2Z	2W5DX5Z	2W5LXYZ	2W5UX2Z	2W6RX0Z	30230Y4	30240T1
2W1HX7Z	2W32X3Z	2W3KX1Z	2W4NX5Z	2W56X3Z	2W5DX6Z	2W5MX0Z	2W5UX3Z	2W6RXZZ	30233AZ	30240V0
2W1JX6Z	2W32XYZ	2W3KX2Z	2W4PX5Z	2W56X4Z	2W5DX7Z	2W5MX1Z	2W5UX4Z	2W6SX0Z	30233G0	30240V1
2W1JX7Z	2W33X1Z	2W3KX3Z	2W4QX5Z	2W56X5Z	2W5DXYZ	2W5MX2Z	2W5UX5Z	2W6SXZZ	30233G2	30240W0
2W1KX6Z	2W33X2Z	2W3KXYZ	2W4RX5Z	2W56X6Z	2W5EX0Z	2W5MX3Z	2W5UX6Z	2W6TX0Z	30233G3	30240W1
2W1KX7Z	2W33X3Z	2W3LX1Z	2W4SX5Z	2W56X7Z	2W5EX1Z	2W5MX4Z	2W5UX7Z	2W6TXZZ	30233G4	30240X0
2W1LX6Z	2W33XYZ	2W3LX2Z	2W4TX5Z	2W56XYZ	2W5EX2Z	2W5MX5Z	2W5UXYZ	2W6UX0Z	30233H0	30240X2
2W1LX7Z	2W34X1Z	2W3LX3Z	2W4UX5Z	2W57X0Z	2W5EX3Z	2W5MX6Z	2W5VX0Z	2W6UXZZ	30233H1	30240X3
2W1MX6Z	2W34X2Z	2W3LXYZ	2W4VX5Z	2W57X1Z	2W5EX4Z	2W5MX7Z	2W5VX1Z	2W6VX0Z	30233J0	30240X4
2W1MX7Z	2W34X3Z	2W3MX1Z	2W50X0Z	2W57X2Z	2W5EX5Z	2W5MXYZ	2W5VX2Z	2W6VXZZ	30233J1	30240Y0
2W1NX6Z	2W34XYZ	2W3MX2Z	2W50X1Z	2W57X3Z	2W5EX6Z	2W5NX0Z	2W5VX3Z	2Y00X5Z	30233K0	30240Y2
2W1NX7Z	2W35X1Z	2W3MX3Z	2W50X2Z	2W57X4Z	2W5EX7Z	2W5NX1Z	2W5VX4Z	2Y01X5Z	30233K1	30240Y3
2W1PX6Z	2W35X2Z	2W3MXYZ	2W50X3Z	2W57X5Z	2W5EXYZ	2W5NX2Z	2W5VX5Z	2Y02X5Z	30233L0	30240Y4
2W1PX7Z	2W35X3Z	2W3NX1Z	2W50X4Z	2W57X6Z	2W5FX0Z	2W5NX3Z	2W5VX6Z	2Y03X5Z	30233L1	30243AZ
2W1QX6Z	2W35XYZ	2W3NX2Z	2W50X5Z	2W57X7Z	2W5FX1Z	2W5NX4Z	2W5VX7Z	2Y04X5Z	30233M0	30243G0
2W1QX7Z	2W36X1Z	2W3NX3Z	2W50X6Z	2W57XYZ	2W5FX2Z	2W5NX5Z	2W5VXYZ	2Y05X5Z	30233M1	30243G2
2W1RX6Z	2W36X2Z	2W3NXYZ	2W50X7Z	2W58X0Z	2W5FX3Z	2W5NX6Z	2W60X0Z	2Y40X5Z	30233N0	30243G3
2W1RX7Z	2W36X3Z	2W3PX1Z	2W50XYZ	2W58X1Z	2W5FX4Z	2W5NX7Z	2W60XZZ	2Y41X5Z	30233N1	30243G4
2W1SX6Z	2W36XYZ	2W3PX2Z	2W51X0Z	2W58X2Z	2W5FX5Z	2W5NXYZ	2W61X0Z	2Y42X5Z	30233P0	30243H0
2W1SX7Z	2W37X1Z	2W3PX3Z	2W51X1Z	2W58X3Z	2W5FX6Z	2W5PX0Z	2W61XZZ	2Y43X5Z	30233P1	30243H1
2W1TX6Z	2W37X2Z	2W3PXYZ	2W51X2Z	2W58X4Z	2W5FX7Z	2W5PX1Z	2W62X0Z	2Y44X5Z	30233Q0	30243J0
2W1TX7Z	2W37X3Z	2W3QX1Z	2W51X3Z	2W58X5Z	2W5FXYZ	2W5PX2Z	2W62XZZ	2Y45X5Z	30233Q1	30243J1
2W1UX6Z	2W37XYZ	2W3QX2Z	2W51X4Z	2W58X6Z	2W5GX0Z	2W5PX3Z	2W63X0Z	2Y50X5Z	30233R0	30243K0
2W1UX7Z	2W38X1Z	2W3QX3Z	2W51X5Z	2W58X7Z	2W5GX1Z	2W5PX4Z	2W63XZZ	2Y51X5Z	30233R1	30243K1
2W1VX6Z	2W38X2Z	2W3QXYZ	2W51X6Z	2W58XYZ	2W5GX2Z	2W5PX5Z	2W64X0Z	2Y52X5Z	30233S0	30243L0
2W1VX7Z	2W38X3Z	2W3RX1Z	2W51X7Z	2W59X0Z	2W5GX3Z	2W5PX6Z	2W64XZZ	2Y53X5Z	30233S1	30243L1
2W20X4Z	2W38XYZ	2W3RX2Z	2W51X9Z	2W59X1Z	2W5GX4Z	2W5PX7Z	2W65X0Z	2Y54X5Z	30233T0	30243M0
2W21X4Z	2W39X1Z	2W3RX3Z	2W51XYZ	2W59X2Z	2W5GX5Z	2W5PXYZ	2W65XZZ	2Y55X5Z	30233T1	30243M1

30243N0	30253M0	30263N0	3E0132A	3E033GC	3E043WL	3E060GC	3E093BZ	3E0BXKZ	3E0D73Z	3E0E8BZ
30243N1	30253M1	30263N1	3E0133Z	3E033GN	3E043XZ	3E060GN	3E093GC	3E0BXNZ	3E0D74Z	3E0E8GC
30243P0	30253N0	30263P0	3E01340	3E033GQ	3E05003	3E060HZ	3E093HZ	3E0BXTZ	3E0D76Z	3E0E8HZ
30243P1	30253N1	30263P1	3E0134Z	3E033HZ	3E05005	3E060KZ	3E093KZ	3E0C304	3E0D77Z	3E0E8KZ
30243Q0	30253P0	30263Q0	3E0136Z	3E033KZ	3E0500M	3E060NZ	3E093NZ	3E0C305	3E0D7BZ	3E0E8NZ
30243Q1	30253P1	30263Q1	3E0137Z	3E033NZ	3E0500P	3E060PZ	3E093TZ	3E0C30M	3E0D7GC	3E0E8SF
30243R0	30253Q0	30263R0	3E013BZ	3E033PZ	3E05016	3E060RZ	3E09705	3E0C328	3E0D7HZ	3E0E8TZ
30243R1	30253Q1	30263R1	3E013GC	3E033RZ	3E05028	3E060TZ	3E0970M	3E0C329	3E0D7KZ	3E0F304
30243S0	30253R0	30263S0	3E013HZ	3E033TZ	3E05029	3E060VG	3E09728	3E0C33Z	3E0D7NZ	3E0F305
30243S1	30253R1	30263S1	3E013KZ	3E033VG	3E0503Z	3E060VH	3E09729	3E0C3BZ	3E0D7RZ	3E0F30M
30243T0	30253S0	30263T0	3E013NZ	3E033VH	3E0504Z	3E060VJ	3E0973Z	3E0C3GC	3E0D7TZ	3E0F328
30243T1	30253S1	30263T1	3E013TZ	3E033VJ	3E0506Z	3E060WK	3E0974Z	3E0C3HZ	3E0DX04	3E0F329
30243V0	30253T0	30263V0	3E013VG	3E033WK	3E0507Z	3E060WL	3E097BZ	3E0C3KZ	3E0DX05	3E0F33Z
30243V1	30253T1	30263V1	3E013VJ	3E033WL	3E050FZ	3E060XZ	3E097GC	3E0C3MZ	3E0DX0M	3E0F36Z
30243W0	30253V0	30263W0	3E02305	3E033XZ	3E050GC	3E06303	3E097HZ	3E0C3NZ	3E0DX28	3E0F37Z
30243W1	30253V1	30263W1	3E0230M	3E04003	3E050GN	3E06305	3E097KZ	3E0C3SF	3E0DX29	3E0F3BZ
30243X0	30253W0	30263X0	3E02328	3E04005	3E050HZ	3E0630M	3E097NZ	3E0C3TZ	3E0DX3Z	3E0F3GC
30243X2	30253W1	30263X1	3E02329	3E0400M	3E050KZ	3E0630P	3E097TZ	3E0C704	3E0DX4Z	3E0F3HZ
30243X3	30253X0	30263Y0	3E0233Z	3E0400P	3E050NZ	3E06316	3E09X05	3E0C705	3E0DX6Z	3E0F3KZ
30243X4	30253X1	30263Y1	3E0234Z	3E04016	3E050PZ	3E06328	3E09X0M	3E0C70M	3E0DX7Z	3E0F3NZ
30243Y0	30253Y0	30273H1	3E0236Z	3E04028	3E050RZ	3E06329	3E09X28	3E0C728	3E0DXBZ	3E0F3SD
30243Y2	30253Y1	30273J1	3E0237Z	3E04029	3E050TZ	3E0633Z	3E09X29	3E0C729	3E0DXGC	3E0F3SF
30243Y3	30260G0	30273K1	3E023BZ	3E0403Z	3E050VG	3E0634Z	3E09X3Z	3E0C73Z	3E0DXHZ	3E0F3TZ
30243Y4	30260G1	30273L1	3E023GC	3E0404Z	3E050VH	3E0636Z	3E09X4Z	3E0C7BZ	3E0DXKZ	3E0F4GC
30250G0	30260H0	30273M1	3E023HZ	3E0406Z	3E050VJ	3E0637Z	3E09XBZ	3E0C7GC	3E0DXNZ	3E0F704
30250G1	30260H1	30273N1	3E023KZ	3E0407Z	3E050WK	3E063FZ	3E09XGC	3E0C7HZ	3E0DXRZ	3E0F705
30250H0	30260J0	30273P1	3E023NZ	3E040FZ	3E050WL	3E063GC	3E09XHZ	3E0C7KZ	3E0DXTZ	3E0F70M
30250H1	30260J1	30273Q1	3E023TZ	3E040GC	3E050XZ	3E063GN	3E09XKZ	3E0C7MZ	3E0E304	3E0F728
30250J0	30260K0	30273R1	3E03003	3E040GN	3E05303	3E063HZ	3E09XNZ	3E0C7NZ	3E0E305	3E0F729
30250J1	30260K1	30273S1	3E03005	3E040HZ	3E05305	3E063KZ	3E09XTZ	3E0C7SF	3E0E30M	3E0F73Z
30250K0	30260L0	30273T1	3E0300M	3E040KZ	3E0530M	3E063NZ	3E0A305	3E0C7TZ	3E0E328	3E0F76Z
30250K1	30260L1	30273V1	3E0300P	3E040NZ	3E0530P	3E063PZ	3E0A30M	3E0CX04	3E0E329	3E0F77Z
30250L0	30260M0	30273W1	3E03016	3E040PZ	3E05316	3E063RZ	3E0A3GC	3E0CX05	3E0E33Z	3E0F7BZ
30250L1	30260M1	30277H1	3E03028	3E040RZ	3E05328	3E063TZ	3E0B304	3E0CX0M	3E0E36Z	3E0F7GC
30250M0	30260N0	30277J1	3E03029	3E040TZ	3E05329	3E063VG	3E0B305	3E0CX28	3E0E37Z	3E0F7HZ
30250M1	30260N1	30277K1	3E0303Z	3E040VG	3E0533Z	3E063VH	3E0B30M	3E0CX29	3E0E3BZ	3E0F7KZ
30250N0	30260P0	30277L1	3E0304Z	3E040VH	3E0534Z	3E063VJ	3E0B328	3E0CX3Z	3E0E3GC	3E0F7NZ
30250N1	30260P1	30277M1	3E0306Z	3E040VJ	3E0536Z	3E063WK	3E0B329	3E0CXBZ	3E0E3HZ	3E0F7SD
30250P0	30260Q0	30277N1	3E0307Z	3E040WK	3E0537Z	3E063WL	3E0B33Z	3E0CXGC	3E0E3KZ	3E0F7SF
30250P1	30260Q1	30277P1	3E030FZ	3E040WL	3E053FZ	3E063XZ	3E0B3BZ	3E0CXHZ	3E0E3NZ	3E0F7TZ
30250Q0	30260R0	30277Q1	3E030GC	3E040XZ	3E053GC	3E07016	3E0B3GC	3E0CXKZ	3E0E3SF	3E0F804
30250Q1	30260R1	30277R1	3E030GN	3E04303	3E053GN	3E07017	3E0B3HZ	3E0CXMZ	3E0E3TZ	3E0F805
30250R0	30260S0	30277S1	3E030HZ	3E04305	3E053HZ	3E070GC	3E0B3KZ	3E0CXNZ	3E0E4GC	3E0F80M
30250R1	30260S1	30277T1	3E030KZ	3E0430M	3E053KZ	3E070KZ	3E0B3NZ	3E0CXSF	3E0E704	3E0F828
30250S0	30260T0	30277V1	3E030NZ	3E0430P	3E053NZ	3E070PZ	3E0B3TZ	3E0CXTZ	3E0E705	3E0F829
30250S1	30260T1	30277W1	3E030PZ	3E04316	3E053PZ	3E07316	3E0B704	3E0D304	3E0E70M	3E0F83Z
30250T0	30260V0	30280B1	3E030RZ	3E04328	3E053RZ	3E07317	3E0B705	3E0D305	3E0E728	3E0F86Z
30250T1	30260V1	30283B1	3E030TZ	3E04329	3E053TZ	3E073GC	3E0B70M	3E0D30M	3E0E729	3E0F87Z
30250V0	30260W0	3C1ZX8Z	3E030VG	3E0433Z	3E053VG	3E073KZ	3E0B728	3E0D328	3E0E73Z	3E0F8BZ
30250V1	30260W1	3E00X05	3E030VH	3E0434Z	3E053VH	3E073PZ	3E0B729	3E0D329	3E0E76Z	3E0F8GC
30250W0	30260X0	3E00X0M	3E030VJ	3E0436Z	3E053VJ	3E074GC	3E0B73Z	3E0D33Z	3E0E77Z	3E0F8HZ
30250W1	30260X1	3E00X28	3E030WK	3E0437Z	3E053WK	3E08016	3E0B7BZ	3E0D34Z	3E0E7BZ	3E0F8KZ
30250X0	30260Y0	3E00X29	3E030WL	3E043FZ	3E053WL	3E080GC	3E0B7GC	3E0D36Z	3E0E7GC	3E0F8NZ
30250X1	30260Y1	3E00X3Z	3E030XZ	3E043GC	3E053XZ	3E080KZ	3E0B7HZ	3E0D37Z	3E0E7HZ	3E0F8SD
30250Y0	30263G0	3E00X4Z	3E03303	3E043GN	3E06003	3E080PZ	3E0B7KZ	3E0D3BZ	3E0E7KZ	3E0F8SF
30250Y1	30263G1	3E00XBZ	3E03305	3E043GQ	3E06005	3E08316	3E0B7NZ	3E0D3GC	3E0E7NZ	3E0F8TZ
30253G0	30263H0	3E00XGC	3E0330M	3E043HZ	3E0600M	3E083GC	3E0B7TZ	3E0D3HZ	3E0E7SF	3E0G304
30253G1	30263H1	3E00XKZ	3E0330P	3E043KZ	3E0600P	3E083KZ	3E0BX04	3E0D3KZ	3E0E7TZ	3E0G305
30253H0	30263J0	3E00XMZ	3E03316	3E043NZ	3E06016	3E083PZ	3E0BX05	3E0D3NZ	3E0E804	3E0G30M
30253H1	30263J1	3E00XNZ	3E03328	3E043PZ	3E06028	3E084GC	3E0BX0M	3E0D3RZ	3E0E805	3E0G328
30253J0	30263K0	3E00XTZ	3E03329	3E043RZ	3E06029	3E09305	3E0BX28	3E0D3TZ	3E0E80M	3E0G329
30253J1	30263K1	3E0102A	3E0333Z	3E043TZ	3E0603Z	3E0930M	3E0BX29	3E0D704	3E0E828	3E0G32Z
30253K0	30263L0	3E01305	3E0334Z	3E043VG	3E0604Z	3E09328	3E0BX3Z	3E0D705	3E0E829	3E0G36Z
30253K1	30263L1	3E0130M	3E0336Z	3E043VH	3E0606Z	3E09329	3E0BXBZ	3E0D70M	3E0E83Z	3E0G37Z
30253L0	30263M0	3E01328	3E0337Z	3E043VJ	3E0607Z	3E0933Z	3E0BXGC	3E0D728	3E0E86Z	3E0G3BZ
30253L1	30263M1	3E01329	3E033FZ	3E043WK	3E060FZ	3E0934Z	3E0BXHZ	3E0D729	3E0E87Z	3E0G3GC

3E0G3HZ	3E0H7TZ	3E0K329	3E0M304	3E0N8SF	3E0Q0AZ	3E0S3NZ	3E0Y36Z	3E1M38X	4A023HZ	4A040J1
3E0G3KZ	3E0H804	3E0K33Z	3E0M305	3E0N8TZ	3E0Q0BZ	3E0S3SF	3E0Y37Z	3E1M38Z	4A023PZ	4A040J2
3E0G3NZ	3E0H805	3E0K36Z	3E0M30M	3E0P05Z	3E0Q0E0	3E0S3TZ	3E0Y3BZ	3E1M39Z	4A0274Z	4A040J3
3E0G3SF	3E0H80M	3E0K37Z	3E0M328	3E0P304	3E0Q0E1	3E0S7SF	3E0Y3GC	3E1N38X	4A0279Z	4A040R1
3E0G3TZ	3E0H828	3E0K3BZ	3E0M329	3E0P305	3E0Q0GC	3E0T33Z	3E0Y3HZ	3E1N38Z	4A027CZ	4A04350
3E0G4GC	3E0H829	3E0K3GC	3E0M33Z	3E0P30M	3E0Q0HZ	3E0T3BZ	3E0Y3KZ	3E1N78X	4A027FZ	4A04351
3E0G704	3E0H83Z	3E0K3HZ	3E0M35Z	3E0P328	3E0Q0KZ	3E0T3GC	3E0Y3NZ	3E1N78Z	4A027HZ	4A04352
3E0G705	3E0H86Z	3E0K3KZ	3E0M36Z	3E0P329	3E0Q0NZ	3E0T3TZ	3E0Y3SF	3E1N88X	4A027N6	4A04353
3E0G70M	3E0H87Z	3E0K3NZ	3E0M37Z	3E0P33Z	3E0Q0SF	3E0U028	3E0Y3TZ	3E1N88Z	4A027N7	4A043B0
3E0G728	3E0H8BZ	3E0K3SF	3E0M3BZ	3E0P35Z	3E0Q0TZ	3E0U029	3E0Y4GC	3E1P38X	4A027N8	4A043B1
3E0G729	3E0H8GC	3E0K3TZ	3E0M3GC	3E0P36Z	3E0Q304	3E0U0GB	3E0Y704	3E1P38Z	4A027PZ	4A043B2
3E0G73Z	3E0H8HZ	3E0K4GC	3E0M3HZ	3E0P37Z	3E0Q30M	3E0U304	3E0Y705	3E1P78X	4A0284Z	4A043B3
3E0G76Z	3E0H8KZ	3E0K704	3E0M3KZ	3E0P3BZ	3E0Q328	3E0U305	3E0Y70M	3E1P78Z	4A0289Z	4A043J0
3E0G77Z	3E0H8NZ	3E0K705	3E0M3NZ	3E0P3GC	3E0Q329	3E0U30M	3E0Y7SF	3E1P88X	4A028CZ	4A043J1
3E0G7BZ	3E0H8SF	3E0K70M	3E0M3SF	3E0P3HZ	3E0Q33Z	3E0U328	3E1038X	3E1P88Z	4A028FZ	4A043J2
3E0G7GC	3E0H8TZ	3E0K728	3E0M3TZ	3E0P3KZ	3E0Q36Z	3E0U329	3E1038Z	3E1Q38X	4A028HZ	4A043J3
3E0G7HZ	3E0J304	3E0K729	3E0M45Z	3E0P3LZ	3E0Q37Z	3E0U33Z	3E10X8X	3E1Q38Z	4A028N6	4A043R1
3E0G7KZ	3E0J305	3E0K73Z	3E0M4GC	3E0P3NZ	3E0Q3AZ	3E0U36Z	3E10X8Z	3E1R38X	4A028N7	4A04X51
3E0G7NZ	3E0J30M	3E0K76Z	3E0M704	3E0P3Q0	3E0Q3BZ	3E0U37Z	3E1938X	3E1R38Z	4A028N8	4A04XB1
3E0G7SF	3E0J328	3E0K77Z	3E0M705	3E0P3Q1	3E0Q3E0	3E0U3BZ	3E1938Z	3E1S38X	4A028PZ	4A04XJ1
3E0G7TZ	3E0J329	3E0K7BZ	3E0M70M	3E0P3SF	3E0Q3E1	3E0U3GB	3E1978X	3E1S38Z	4A02X4A	4A04XR1
3E0G804	3E0J33Z	3E0K7GC	3E0M7SF	3E0P3TZ	3E0Q3GC	3E0U3GC	3E1978Z	3E1U38X	4A02X4Z	4A05XLZ
3E0G805	3E0J36Z	3E0K7HZ	3E0N304	3E0P3VZ	3E0Q3HZ	3E0U3HZ	3E1988X	3E1U38Z	4A02X9Z	4A0605Z
3E0G80M	3E0J37Z	3E0K7KZ	3E0N305	3E0P45Z	3E0Q3KZ	3E0U3KZ	3E1988Z	3E1Y38X	4A02XCZ	4A060BZ
3E0G828	3E0J3BZ	3E0K7NZ	3E0N30M	3E0P4GC	3E0Q3NZ	3E0U3NZ	3E1B38X	3E1Y38Z	4A02XFZ	4A0635Z
3E0G829	3E0J3GC	3E0K7SF	3E0N328	3E0P704	3E0Q3SF	3E0U3SF	3E1B38Z	4A0002Z	4A02XHZ	4A063BZ
3E0G83Z	3E0J3HZ	3E0K7TZ	3E0N329	3E0P705	3E0Q3TZ	3E0U3TZ	3E1B78X	4A0004Z	4A02XM4	4A0675Z
3E0G86Z	3E0J3KZ	3E0K804	3E0N33Z	3E0P70M	3E0Q704	3E0U4GC	3E1B78Z	4A000BZ	4A02XPX	4A067BZ
3E0G87Z	3E0J3NZ	3E0K805	3E0N36Z	3E0P728	3E0Q70M	3E0V0GB	3E1B88X	4A0034Z	4A02XPZ	4A0685Z
3E0G8BZ	3E0J3SF	3E0K80M	3E0N37Z	3E0P729	3E0Q7SF	3E0V305	3E1B88Z	4A003BD	4A03051	4A068BZ
3E0G8GC	3E0J3TZ	3E0K828	3E0N3BZ	3E0P73Z	3E0R0AZ	3E0V30M	3E1C38X	4A003KD	4A03053	4A07X0Z
3E0G8HZ	3E0J4GC	3E0K829	3E0N3GC	3E0P76Z	3E0R0E0	3E0V328	3E1C38Z	4A003RD	4A0305C	4A07X7Z
3E0G8KZ	3E0J704	3E0K83Z	3E0N3HZ	3E0P77Z	3E0R0E1	3E0V329	3E1CX8X	4A0074Z	4A030B1	4A07XBZ
3E0G8NZ	3E0J705	3E0K86Z	3E0N3KZ	3E0P7BZ	3E0R303	3E0V33Z	3E1CX8Z	4A007BD	4A030B3	4A08X0Z
3E0G8SF	3E0J70M	3E0K87Z	3E0N3NZ	3E0P7GC	3E0R304	3E0V36Z	3E1F38X	4A007KD	4A030BC	4A0971Z
3E0G8TZ	3E0J728	3E0K8BZ	3E0N3SF	3E0P7HZ	3E0R305	3E0V37Z	3E1F38Z	4A007RD	4A030BF	4A0975Z
3E0H304	3E0J729	3E0K8GC	3E0N3TZ	3E0P7KZ	3E0R30M	3E0V3BZ	3E1F78X	4A0084Z	4A030H1	4A097CZ
3E0H305	3E0J73Z	3E0K8HZ	3E0N4GC	3E0P7LZ	3E0R328	3E0V3GB	3E1F78Z	4A008BD	4A030J1	4A097DZ
3E0H30M	3E0J76Z	3E0K8KZ	3E0N704	3E0P7NZ	3E0R329	3E0V3GC	3E1F88X	4A008KD	4A030J3	4A097LZ
3E0H328	3E0J77Z	3E0K8NZ	3E0N705	3E0P7Q0	3E0R33Z	3E0V3HZ	3E1F88Z	4A008RD	4A030JC	4A097MZ
3E0H329	3E0J7BZ	3E0K8SF	3E0N70M	3E0P7Q1	3E0R36Z	3E0V3KZ	3E1G38X	4A00X2Z	4A030R1	4A0981Z
3E0H33Z	3E0J7GC	3E0K8TZ	3E0N728	3E0P7SF	3E0R37Z	3E0V3NZ	3E1G38Z	4A00X4Z	4A03351	4A0985Z
3E0H36Z	3E0J7HZ	3E0L05Z	3E0N729	3E0P7TZ	3E0R3AZ	3E0V3TZ	3E1G78X	4A01029	4A03353	4A098CZ
3E0H37Z	3E0J7KZ	3E0L304	3E0N73Z	3E0P7VZ	3E0R3BZ	3E0W305	3E1G78Z	4A0102B	4A0335C	4A098DZ
3E0H3BZ	3E0J7NZ	3E0L305	3E0N76Z	3E0P804	3E0R3E0	3E0W30M	3E1G88X	4A0104Z	4A033B1	4A098LZ
3E0H3GC	3E0J7SF	3E0L30M	3E0N77Z	3E0P805	3E0R3E1	3E0W328	3E1G88Z	4A01329	4A033B3	4A098MZ
3E0H3HZ	3E0J7TZ	3E0L328	3E0N7BZ	3E0P80M	3E0R3GC	3E0W329	3E1H38X	4A0132B	4A033BC	4A09X1Z
3E0H3KZ	3E0J804	3E0L329	3E0N7GC	3E0P828	3E0R3HZ	3E0W33Z	3E1H38Z	4A0134Z	4A033BF	4A09X5Z
3E0H3NZ	3E0J805	3E0L33Z	3E0N7HZ	3E0P829	3E0R3KZ	3E0W36Z	3E1H78X	4A01729	4A033H1	4A09XCZ
3E0H3SF	3E0J80M	3E0L35Z	3E0N7KZ	3E0P83Z	3E0R3NZ	3E0W37Z	3E1H78Z	4A0172B	4A033J1	4A09XDZ
3E0H3TZ	3E0J828	3E0L36Z	3E0N7NZ	3E0P86Z	3E0R3SF	3E0W3BZ	3E1H88X	4A0174Z	4A033J3	4A09XLZ
3E0H4GC	3E0J829	3E0L37Z	3E0N7SF	3E0P87Z	3E0R3TZ	3E0W3GC	3E1H88Z	4A01829	4A033JC	4A09XMZ
3E0H704	3E0J83Z	3E0L3BZ	3E0N7TZ	3E0P8BZ	3E0R7SF	3E0W3HZ	3E1J38X	4A0182B	4A033R1	4A0B78Z
3E0H705	3E0J86Z	3E0L3GC	3E0N804	3E0P8GC	3E0S303	3E0W3KZ	3E1J38Z	4A0184Z	4A03X51	4A0B7BZ
3E0H70M	3E0J87Z	3E0L3HZ	3E0N805	3E0P8HZ	3E0S304	3E0W3NZ	3E1J78X	4A01X29	4A03XB1	4A0B7GZ
3E0H728	3E0J8BZ	3E0L3KZ	3E0N80M	3E0P8KZ	3E0S305	3E0W3TZ	3E1J78Z	4A01X2B	4A03XH1	4A0B88Z
3E0H729	3E0J8GC	3E0L3NZ	3E0N828	3E0P8NZ	3E0S30M	3E0X33Z	3E1J88X	4A01X4Z	4A03XJ1	4A0B8BZ
3E0H73Z	3E0J8HZ	3E0L3SF	3E0N829	3E0P8SF	3E0S328	3E0X3BZ	3E1J88Z	4A0204Z	4A03XR1	4A0B8GZ
3E0H76Z	3E0J8KZ	3E0L3TZ	3E0N83Z	3E0P8TZ	3E0S329	3E0X3GC	3E1K38X	4A0209Z	4A04050	4A0C35Z
3E0H77Z	3E0J8NZ	3E0L45Z	3E0N86Z	3E0Q004	3E0S33Z	3E0X3TZ	3E1K38Z	4A020CZ	4A04051	4A0C3BZ
3E0H7BZ	3E0J8SF	3E0L4GC	3E0N87Z	3E0Q00M	3E0S36Z	3E0Y304	3E1K78X	4A020FZ	4A04052	4A0C45Z
3E0H7GC	3E0J8TZ	3E0L704	3E0N8BZ	3E0Q028	3E0S37Z	3E0Y305	3E1K78Z	4A020HZ	4A04053	4A0C4BZ
3E0H7HZ	3E0K304	3E0L705	3E0N8GC	3E0Q029	3E0S3BZ	3E0Y30M	3E1K88X	4A020PZ	4A040B0	4A0C75Z
3E0H7KZ	3E0K305	3E0L70M	3E0N8HZ	3E0Q03Z	3E0S3GC	3E0Y328	3E1K88Z	4A0234Z	4A040B1	4A0C7BZ
3E0H7NZ	3E0K30M	3E0L7SF	3E0N8KZ	3E0Q06Z	3E0S3HZ	3E0Y329	3E1L38X	4A0239Z	4A040B2	4A0C85Z
3E0H7SF	3E0K328	3E0M05Z	3E0N8NZ	3E0Q07Z	3E0S3KZ	3E0Y33Z	3E1L38Z	4A023CZ	4A040B3	4A0C8BZ
									4A040J0	

4A0D73Z	4A1134G	4A13XH1	4A1D83Z	5A1221Z	7W01X0Z	7W07X6Z	8E0XXBG	9WB5XFZ	B02810Z	B212YZZ
4A0D75Z	4A1134Z	4A13XJ1	4A1D85Z	5A1223Z	7W01X1Z	7W07X7Z	8E0XXBH	9WB5XGZ	B0281ZZ	B213010
4A0D7BZ	4A11729	4A13XR1	4A1D8BZ	5A15223	7W01X2Z	7W07X8Z	8E0XXBZ	9WB5XHZ	B028Y0Z	B2130ZZ
4A0D7DZ	4A1172B	4A14050	4A1D8DZ	5A19054	7W01X3Z	7W07X9Z	8E0XXCZ	9WB5XJZ	B028YZZ	B213110
4A0D7LZ	4A1174G	4A14051	4A1D8LZ	5A1C00Z	7W01X4Z	7W08X0Z	8E0XXY8	9WB5XKZ	B028ZZZ	B2131ZZ
4A0D83Z	4A1174Z	4A14052	4A1GXSH	5A1C60Z	7W01X5Z	7W08X1Z	8E0Y0CZ	9WB5XLZ	B02900Z	B213Y10
4A0D85Z	4A11829	4A14053	4A1H74Z	5A1D70Z	7W01X6Z	7W08X2Z	8E0Y3CZ	9WB6XBZ	B0290ZZ	B213YZZ
4A0D8BZ	4A1182B	4A140B0	4A1H7CZ	5A1D80Z	7W01X7Z	7W08X3Z	8E0Y4CZ	9WB6XCZ	B02910Z	B2140ZZ
4A0D8DZ	4A1184G	4A140B1	4A1H7FZ	5A1D90Z	7W01X8Z	7W08X4Z	8E0YXBF	9WB6XDZ	B0291ZZ	B2141ZZ
4A0D8LZ	4A1184Z	4A140B2	4A1H7HZ	5A2204Z	7W01X9Z	7W08X5Z	8E0YXBG	9WB6XFZ	B029Y0Z	B214YZZ
4A0F33Z	4A11X29	4A140B3	4A1H84Z	6A0Z0ZZ	7W02X0Z	7W08X6Z	8E0YXBH	9WB6XGZ	B029YZZ	B2150ZZ
4A0FX3Z	4A11X2B	4A140J0	4A1H8CZ	6A0Z1ZZ	7W02X1Z	7W08X7Z	8E0YXBZ	9WB6XHZ	B029ZZZ	B2151ZZ
4A0H74Z	4A11X4G	4A140J1	4A1H8FZ	6A150ZZ	7W02X2Z	7W08X8Z	8E0YXCZ	9WB6XJZ	B02B00Z	B215YZZ
4A0H7CZ	4A11X4Z	4A140J2	4A1H8HZ	6A151ZZ	7W02X3Z	7W08X9Z	8E0YXY8	9WB6XKZ	B02B0ZZ	B2160ZZ
4A0H7FZ	4A1204Z	4A140J3	4A1HX4Z	6A210ZZ	7W02X4Z	7W09X0Z	8E0ZXY1	9WB6XLZ	B02B10Z	B2161ZZ
4A0H7HZ	4A1209Z	4A140R0	4A1HXCZ	6A211ZZ	7W02X5Z	7W09X1Z	8E0ZXY4	9WB7XBZ	B02B1ZZ	B216YZZ
4A0H84Z	4A120CZ	4A140R2	4A1HXFZ	6A220ZZ	7W02X6Z	7W09X2Z	8E0ZXY5	9WB7XCZ	B02BY0Z	B2170ZZ
4A0H8CZ	4A120FZ	4A140R3	4A1HXHZ	6A221ZZ	7W02X7Z	7W09X3Z	8E0ZXY6	9WB7XDZ	B02BYZZ	B2171ZZ
4A0H8FZ	4A120HZ	4A14350	4A1J72Z	6A3Z0ZZ	7W02X8Z	7W09X4Z	9WB0XBZ	9WB7XFZ	B02BZZZ	B217YZZ
4A0H8HZ	4A1234Z	4A14351	4A1J74Z	6A3Z1ZZ	7W02X9Z	7W09X5Z	9WB0XCZ	9WB7XGZ	B030Y0Z	B2180ZZ
4A0HX4Z	4A1239Z	4A14352	4A1J7BZ	6A4Z0ZZ	7W03X0Z	7W09X6Z	9WB0XDZ	9WB7XHZ	B030YZZ	B2181ZZ
4A0HXCZ	4A123CZ	4A14353	4A1J82Z	6A4Z1ZZ	7W03X1Z	7W09X7Z	9WB0XFZ	9WB7XJZ	B030ZZZ	B218YZZ
4A0HXFZ	4A123FZ	4A143B0	4A1J84Z	6A550Z0	7W03X2Z	7W09X8Z	9WB0XGZ	9WB7XKZ	B039Y0Z	B21F0ZZ
4A0HXHZ	4A123HZ	4A143B1	4A1J8BZ	6A550Z1	7W03X3Z	7W09X9Z	9WB0XHZ	9WB7XLZ	B039YZZ	B21F1ZZ
4A0J72Z	4A1274Z	4A143B2	4A1JX2Z	6A550Z2	7W03X4Z	8C01X6J	9WB0XJZ	9WB8XBZ	B039ZZZ	B21FYZZ
4A0J74Z	4A1279Z	4A143B3	4A1JX4Z	6A550Z3	7W03X5Z	8C01X6L	9WB0XKZ	9WB8XCZ	B03BY0Z	B22100Z
4A0J7BZ	4A127CZ	4A143J0	4A1JXBZ	6A550ZT	7W03X6Z	8C02X6K	9WB0XLZ	9WB8XDZ	B03BYZZ	B2210ZZ
4A0J82Z	4A127FZ	4A143J1	4A1Z7KZ	6A550ZV	7W03X7Z	8C02X6L	9WB1XBZ	9WB8XFZ	B03BZZZ	B22110Z
4A0J84Z	4A127HZ	4A143J2	4A1ZXKZ	6A551Z0	7W03X8Z	8E01XY7	9WB1XCZ	9WB8XGZ	B03CY0Z	B2211ZZ
4A0J8BZ	4A1284Z	4A143J3	4A1ZXQZ	6A551Z1	7W03X9Z	8E023DZ	9WB1XDZ	9WB8XHZ	B03CYZZ	B221Y0Z
4A0JX2Z	4A1289Z	4A143R0	4B00XVZ	6A551Z2	7W04X0Z	8E090CZ	9WB1XFZ	9WB8XJZ	B03CZZZ	B221YZZ
4A0JX4Z	4A128CZ	4A143R2	4B01XVZ	6A551Z3	7W04X1Z	8E093CZ	9WB1XGZ	9WB8XKZ	B040ZZZ	B221Z2Z
4A0JXBZ	4A128FZ	4A143R3	4B02XSZ	6A551ZT	7W04X2Z	8E094CZ	9WB1XHZ	9WB8XLZ	B04BZZZ	B221ZZZ
4A0Z76Z	4A128HZ	4A14X51	4B02XTZ	6A551ZV	7W04X3Z	8E097CZ	9WB1XJZ	9WB9XBZ	B204YZZ	B22300Z
4A0Z7KZ	4A12X45	4A14XB1	4B09XSZ	6A600ZZ	7W04X4Z	8E098CZ	9WB1XKZ	9WB9XCZ	B2050ZZ	B2230ZZ
4A0ZX6Z	4A12X4Z	4A14XJ1	4B0FXVZ	6A601ZZ	7W04X5Z	8E09XBF	9WB1XLZ	9WB9XDZ	B2051ZZ	B22310Z
4A0ZXKZ	4A12X9Z	4A1605Z	5A02110	6A650ZZ	7W04X6Z	8E09XBG	9WB2XBZ	9WB9XFZ	B205YZZ	B2231ZZ
4A0ZXQZ	4A12XCZ	4A160BZ	5A02115	6A651ZZ	7W04X7Z	8E09XBH	9WB2XCZ	9WB9XGZ	B2060ZZ	B223Y0Z
4A1002Z	4A12XFZ	4A1635Z	5A02116	6A750Z4	7W04X8Z	8E09XBZ	9WB2XDZ	9WB9XHZ	B2061ZZ	B223YZZ
4A1004G	4A12XHZ	4A163BZ	5A0211D	6A750Z5	7W04X9Z	8E09XCZ	9WB2XFZ	9WB9XJZ	B206YZZ	B223Z2Z
4A1004Z	4A12XM4	4A1675Z	5A02210	6A750Z6	7W05X0Z	8E09XY8	9WB2XGZ	9WB9XKZ	B2070ZZ	B223ZZZ
4A100BZ	4A12XSH	4A167BZ	5A02215	6A750Z7	7W05X1Z	8E0H300	9WB2XHZ	9WB9XLZ	B2071ZZ	B22600Z
4A1034G	4A13051	4A1685Z	5A02216	6A750ZZ	7W05X2Z	8E0H30Z	9WB2XJZ	B00B0ZZ	B207YZZ	B2260ZZ
4A1034Z	4A13053	4A168BZ	5A0221D	6A751Z4	7W05X3Z	8E0HX62	9WB2XKZ	B00B1ZZ	B2080ZZ	B22610Z
4A103BD	4A1305C	4A1971Z	5A05121	6A751Z5	7W05X4Z	8E0HXY9	9WB2XLZ	B00BYZZ	B2081ZZ	B2261ZZ
4A103KD	4A130B1	4A1975Z	5A0512C	6A751Z6	7W05X5Z	8E0KX1Z	9WB3XBZ	B00BZZZ	B208YZZ	B226Y0Z
4A103RD	4A130B3	4A197CZ	5A05221	6A751Z7	7W05X6Z	8E0KXY7	9WB3XCZ	B01B0ZZ	B20F0ZZ	B226YZZ
4A1074G	4A130BC	4A197DZ	5A0522C	6A751Z9	7W05X7Z	8E0UXY7	9WB3XDZ	B01B1ZZ	B20F1ZZ	B226Z2Z
4A1074Z	4A130H1	4A197LZ	5A0920Z	6A800ZZ	7W05X8Z	8E0VX1C	9WB3XFZ	B01BYZZ	B20FYZZ	B226ZZZ
4A107BD	4A130J1	4A19X1Z	5A09357	6A801ZZ	7W05X9Z	8E0VX1D	9WB3XGZ	B01BZZZ	B210010	B231Y0Z
4A107KD	4A130J3	4A19X5Z	5A09358	6A930ZZ	7W06X0Z	8E0VX63	9WB3XHZ	B02000Z	B2100ZZ	B231YZZ
4A107RD	4A130JC	4A19XCZ	5A09359	6A931ZZ	7W06X1Z	8E0W0CZ	9WB3XJZ	B0200ZZ	B210110	B231ZZZ
4A1084G	4A130R1	4A19XDZ	5A0935B	6AB50BZ	7W06X2Z	8E0W3CZ	9WB3XKZ	B02010Z	B2101ZZ	B233Y0Z
4A1084Z	4A13351	4A19XLZ	5A0935Z	6ABB0BZ	7W06X3Z	8E0W4CZ	9WB3XLZ	B0201ZZ	B210Y10	B233YZZ
4A108BD	4A13353	4A1B78Z	5A09457	6ABF0BZ	7W06X4Z	8E0W7CZ	9WB4XBZ	B020Y0Z	B210YZZ	B233ZZZ
4A108KD	4A1335C	4A1B7BZ	5A09458	6ABT0BZ	7W06X5Z	8E0W8CZ	9WB4XCZ	B020YZZ	B211010	B236Y0Z
4A108RD	4A133B1	4A1B7GZ	5A09459	7W00X0Z	7W06X6Z	8E0WXBF	9WB4XDZ	B020ZZZ	B2110ZZ	B236YZZ
4A10X2Z	4A133B3	4A1B88Z	5A0945B	7W00X1Z	7W06X7Z	8E0WXBG	9WB4XFZ	B02700Z	B211110	B236ZZZ
4A10X4G	4A133BC	4A1B8BZ	5A0945Z	7W00X2Z	7W06X8Z	8E0WXBH	9WB4XGZ	B0270ZZ	B2111ZZ	B240YZZ
4A10X4Z	4A133H1	4A1B8GZ	5A09557	7W00X3Z	7W06X9Z	8E0WXBZ	9WB4XHZ	B02710Z	B211Y10	B240ZZ3
4A11029	4A133J1	4A1BXSH	5A09558	7W00X4Z	7W07X0Z	8E0WXCZ	9WB4XJZ	B0271ZZ	B211YZZ	B240ZZ4
4A1102B	4A133J3	4A1D73Z	5A09559	7W00X5Z	7W07X1Z	8E0WXY8	9WB4XKZ	B027Y0Z	B212010	B240ZZZ
4A1104G	4A133JC	4A1D75Z	5A0955B	7W00X6Z	7W07X2Z	8E0X0CZ	9WB4XLZ	B027YZZ	B2120ZZ	B241YZZ
4A1104Z	4A133R1	4A1D7BZ	5A0955Z	7W00X7Z	7W07X3Z	8E0X3CZ	9WB5XBZ	B027ZZZ	B212110	B241ZZ3
4A11329	4A13X51	4A1D7DZ	5A12012	7W00X8Z	7W07X4Z	8E0X4CZ	9WB5XCZ	B02800Z	B2121ZZ	B241ZZ4
4A1132B	4A13XB1	4A1D7LZ	5A1213Z	7W00X9Z	7W07X5Z	8E0XXBF	9WB5XDZ	B0280ZZ	B212Y10	B241ZZZ

B244YZZ	B30BYZZ	B310Y10	B31B010	B31M1ZZ	B328Z2Z	B347ZZ3	B410010	B41B1ZZ	B42FYZZ	B44NZZ3
B244ZZ3	B30BZZZ	B310YZZ	B31B0ZZ	B31MY10	B328ZZZ	B347ZZZ	B4100ZZ	B41BY10	B42FZ2Z	B44NZZZ
B244ZZ4	B30C0ZZ	B310ZZZ	B31B110	B31MYZZ	B32G0ZZ	B348ZZ3	B410110	B41BYZZ	B42FZZZ	B5000ZZ
B244ZZZ	B30C1ZZ	B311010	B31B1ZZ	B31MZZZ	B32G1ZZ	B348ZZZ	B4101ZZ	B41BZZZ	B42G0ZZ	B5001ZZ
B245YZZ	B30CYZZ	B3110ZZ	B31BY10	B31N010	B32GYZZ	B34HZZ3	B410Y10	B41C010	B42G1ZZ	B500YZZ
B245ZZ3	B30CZZZ	B311110	B31BYZZ	B31N0ZZ	B32GZ2Z	B34HZZZ	B410YZZ	B41C0ZZ	B42GYZZ	B5010ZZ
B245ZZ4	B30D0ZZ	B3111ZZ	B31BZZZ	B31N110	B32GZZZ	B34JZZ3	B410ZZZ	B41C1ZZ	B42GZ2Z	B5011ZZ
B245ZZZ	B30D1ZZ	B311Y10	B31C010	B31N1ZZ	B32R0ZZ	B34JZZZ	B412010	B41CY10	B42GZZZ	B501YZZ
B246YZZ	B30DYZZ	B311YZZ	B31C0ZZ	B31NY10	B32R1ZZ	B34KZZ3	B4120ZZ	B41CYZZ	B42H0ZZ	B5020ZZ
B246ZZ3	B30DZZZ	B311ZZZ	B31C110	B31NYZZ	B32RYZZ	B34KZZZ	B412110	B41CZZZ	B42H1ZZ	B5021ZZ
B246ZZ4	B30F0ZZ	B312010	B31C1ZZ	B31NZZZ	B32RZ2Z	B34RZZ3	B4121ZZ	B41D010	B42HYZZ	B502YZZ
B246ZZZ	B30F1ZZ	B3120ZZ	B31CY10	B31P010	B32RZZZ	B34RZZZ	B412Y10	B41D0ZZ	B42HZ2Z	B5030ZZ
B24BYZZ	B30FYZZ	B312110	B31CYZZ	B31P0ZZ	B32S0ZZ	B34SZZ3	B412YZZ	B41D110	B42HZZZ	B5031ZZ
B24BZZ3	B30FZZZ	B3121ZZ	B31CZZZ	B31P110	B32S1ZZ	B34SZZZ	B412ZZZ	B41D1ZZ	B42M0ZZ	B503YZZ
B24BZZ4	B30G0ZZ	B312Y10	B31D010	B31P1ZZ	B32SYZZ	B34TZZ3	B413010	B41DY10	B42M1ZZ	B5040ZZ
B24BZZZ	B30G1ZZ	B312YZZ	B31D0ZZ	B31PY10	B32SZ2Z	B34TZZZ	B4130ZZ	B41DYZZ	B42MYZZ	B5041ZZ
B24CYZZ	B30GYZZ	B312ZZZ	B31D110	B31PYZZ	B32SZZZ	B34VZZ3	B413110	B41DZZZ	B42MZ2Z	B504YZZ
B24CZZ3	B30GZZZ	B313010	B31D1ZZ	B31PZZZ	B32T0ZZ	B34VZZZ	B4131ZZ	B41F010	B42MZZZ	B5050ZZ
B24CZZ4	B30H0ZZ	B3130ZZ	B31DY10	B31Q010	B32T1ZZ	B4000ZZ	B413Y10	B41F0ZZ	B430Y0Z	B5051ZZ
B24CZZZ	B30H1ZZ	B313110	B31DYZZ	B31Q0ZZ	B32TYZZ	B4001ZZ	B413YZZ	B41F110	B430YZZ	B505YZZ
B24DYZZ	B30HYZZ	B3131ZZ	B31DZZZ	B31Q110	B32TZ2Z	B400YZZ	B413ZZZ	B41F1ZZ	B430ZZZ	B5060ZZ
B24DZZ3	B30HZZZ	B313Y10	B31F010	B31Q1ZZ	B32TZZZ	B4020ZZ	B414010	B41FY10	B431Y0Z	B5061ZZ
B24DZZ4	B30J0ZZ	B313YZZ	B31F0ZZ	B31QY10	B330Y0Z	B4021ZZ	B4140ZZ	B41FYZZ	B431YZZ	B506YZZ
B24DZZZ	B30J1ZZ	B313ZZZ	B31F110	B31QYZZ	B330YZZ	B402YZZ	B414110	B41FZZZ	B431ZZZ	B5070ZZ
B3000ZZ	B30JYZZ	B314010	B31F1ZZ	B31QZZZ	B330ZZZ	B4030ZZ	B4141ZZ	B41G010	B434Y0Z	B5071ZZ
B3001ZZ	B30JZZZ	B3140ZZ	B31FY10	B31R010	B335Y0Z	B4031ZZ	B414Y10	B41G0ZZ	B434YZZ	B507YZZ
B300YZZ	B30K0ZZ	B314110	B31FYZZ	B31R0ZZ	B335YZZ	B403YZZ	B414YZZ	B41G110	B434ZZZ	B5080ZZ
B300ZZZ	B30K1ZZ	B3141ZZ	B31FZZZ	B31R110	B335ZZZ	B4040ZZ	B414ZZZ	B41G1ZZ	B438Y0Z	B5081ZZ
B3010ZZ	B30KYZZ	B314Y10	B31G010	B31R1ZZ	B338Y0Z	B4041ZZ	B415010	B41GY10	B438YZZ	B508YZZ
B3011ZZ	B30KZZZ	B314YZZ	B31G0ZZ	B31RY10	B338YZZ	B404YZZ	B4150ZZ	B41GYZZ	B438ZZZ	B5090ZZ
B301YZZ	B30L0ZZ	B314ZZZ	B31G110	B31RYZZ	B338ZZZ	B4050ZZ	B415110	B41GZZZ	B43CY0Z	B5091ZZ
B301ZZZ	B30L1ZZ	B315010	B31G1ZZ	B31RZZZ	B33GY0Z	B4051ZZ	B4151ZZ	B41J010	B43CYZZ	B509YZZ
B3020ZZ	B30LYZZ	B3150ZZ	B31GY10	B31S010	B33GYZZ	B405YZZ	B415Y10	B41J0ZZ	B43CZZZ	B50B0ZZ
B3021ZZ	B30LZZZ	B315110	B31GYZZ	B31S0ZZ	B33GZZZ	B4060ZZ	B415YZZ	B41J110	B43FY0Z	B50B1ZZ
B302YZZ	B30M0ZZ	B3151ZZ	B31GZZZ	B31S110	B33HY0Z	B4061ZZ	B415ZZZ	B41J1ZZ	B43FYZZ	B50BYZZ
B302ZZZ	B30M1ZZ	B315Y10	B31H010	B31S1ZZ	B33HYZZ	B406YZZ	B416010	B41JY10	B43FZZZ	B50C0ZZ
B3030ZZ	B30MYZZ	B315YZZ	B31H0ZZ	B31SY10	B33HZZZ	B4070ZZ	B4160ZZ	B41JYZZ	B43GY0Z	B50C1ZZ
B3031ZZ	B30MZZZ	B315ZZZ	B31H110	B31SYZZ	B33JY0Z	B4071ZZ	B416110	B41JZZZ	B43GYZZ	B50CYZZ
B303YZZ	B30N0ZZ	B316010	B31H1ZZ	B31SZZZ	B33JYZZ	B407YZZ	B4161ZZ	B4200ZZ	B43GZZZ	B50D0ZZ
B303ZZZ	B30N1ZZ	B3160ZZ	B31HY10	B31T010	B33JZZZ	B4080ZZ	B416Y10	B4201ZZ	B43HY0Z	B50D1ZZ
B3040ZZ	B30NYZZ	B316110	B31HYZZ	B31T0ZZ	B33KY0Z	B4081ZZ	B416YZZ	B420YZZ	B43HYZZ	B50DYZZ
B3041ZZ	B30NZZZ	B3161ZZ	B31HZZZ	B31T110	B33KYZZ	B408YZZ	B416ZZZ	B420Z2Z	B43HZZZ	B50F0ZZ
B304YZZ	B30P0ZZ	B316Y10	B31J010	B31T1ZZ	B33KZZZ	B4090ZZ	B417010	B420ZZZ	B440ZZ3	B50F1ZZ
B304ZZZ	B30P1ZZ	B316YZZ	B31J0ZZ	B31TY10	B33MY0Z	B4091ZZ	B4170ZZ	B4210ZZ	B440ZZZ	B50FYZZ
B3050ZZ	B30PYZZ	B316ZZZ	B31J110	B31TYZZ	B33MYZZ	B409YZZ	B417110	B4211ZZ	B444ZZ3	B50G0ZZ
B3051ZZ	B30PZZZ	B317010	B31J1ZZ	B31TZZZ	B33MZZZ	B40B0ZZ	B4171ZZ	B421YZZ	B444ZZZ	B50G1ZZ
B305YZZ	B30Q0ZZ	B3170ZZ	B31JY10	B31U010	B33QY0Z	B40B1ZZ	B417Y10	B421Z2Z	B445ZZ3	B50GYZZ
B305ZZZ	B30Q1ZZ	B317110	B31JYZZ	B31U0ZZ	B33QYZZ	B40BYZZ	B417YZZ	B421ZZZ	B445ZZZ	B50H0ZZ
B3060ZZ	B30QYZZ	B3171ZZ	B31JZZZ	B31U110	B33QZZZ	B40C0ZZ	B417ZZZ	B4240ZZ	B446ZZ3	B50H1ZZ
B3061ZZ	B30QZZZ	B317Y10	B31K010	B31U1ZZ	B33RY0Z	B40C1ZZ	B418010	B4241ZZ	B446ZZZ	B50HYZZ
B306YZZ	B30R0ZZ	B317YZZ	B31K0ZZ	B31UY10	B33RYZZ	B40CYZZ	B4180ZZ	B424YZZ	B447ZZ3	B50J0ZZ
B306ZZZ	B30R1ZZ	B317ZZZ	B31K110	B31UYZZ	B33RZZZ	B40D0ZZ	B418110	B424Z2Z	B447ZZZ	B50J1ZZ
B3070ZZ	B30RYZZ	B318010	B31K1ZZ	B31UZZZ	B340ZZ3	B40D1ZZ	B4181ZZ	B424ZZZ	B448ZZ3	B50JYZZ
B3071ZZ	B30RZZZ	B3180ZZ	B31KY10	B3200ZZ	B340ZZZ	B40DYZZ	B418Y10	B4280ZZ	B448ZZZ	B50K0ZZ
B307YZZ	B30S0ZZ	B318110	B31KYZZ	B3201ZZ	B341ZZ3	B40F0ZZ	B418YZZ	B4281ZZ	B44BZZ3	B50K1ZZ
B307ZZZ	B30S1ZZ	B3181ZZ	B31KZZZ	B320YZZ	B341ZZZ	B40F1ZZ	B418ZZZ	B428YZZ	B44BZZZ	B50KYZZ
B3080ZZ	B30SYZZ	B318Y10	B31L010	B320Z2Z	B342ZZ3	B40FYZZ	B419010	B428Z2Z	B44FZZ3	B50L0ZZ
B3081ZZ	B30SZZZ	B318YZZ	B31L0ZZ	B320ZZZ	B342ZZZ	B40G0ZZ	B4190ZZ	B428ZZZ	B44FZZZ	B50L1ZZ
B308YZZ	B30T0ZZ	B318ZZZ	B31L110	B3250ZZ	B343ZZ3	B40G1ZZ	B419110	B42C0ZZ	B44GZZ3	B50LYZZ
B308ZZZ	B30T1ZZ	B319010	B31L1ZZ	B3251ZZ	B343ZZZ	B40GYZZ	B4191ZZ	B42C1ZZ	B44GZZZ	B50M0ZZ
B3090ZZ	B30TYZZ	B3190ZZ	B31LY10	B325YZZ	B344ZZ3	B40J0ZZ	B419Y10	B42CYZZ	B44HZZ3	B50M1ZZ
B3091ZZ	B30TZZZ	B319110	B31LYZZ	B325Z2Z	B344ZZZ	B40J1ZZ	B419YZZ	B42CZ2Z	B44HZZZ	B50MYZZ
B309YZZ	B310010	B3191ZZ	B31LZZZ	B325ZZZ	B345ZZ3	B40JYZZ	B419ZZZ	B42CZZZ	B44KZZ3	B50N0ZZ
B309ZZZ	B3100ZZ	B319Y10	B31M010	B3280ZZ	B345ZZZ	B40M0ZZ	B41B010	B42F0ZZ	B44KZZZ	B50N1ZZ
B30B0ZZ	B310110	B319YZZ	B31M0ZZ	B3281ZZ	B346ZZ3	B40M1ZZ	B41B0ZZ	B42F1ZZ	B44LZZ3	B50NYZZ
B30B1ZZ	B3101ZZ	B319ZZZ	B31M110	B328YZZ	B346ZZZ	B40MYZZ	B41B110		B44LZZZ	B50P0ZZ

B50P1ZZ	B515ZZA	B51G0ZA	B51Q1ZA	B529Y0Z	B52RZ2Z	B543ZZ3	B7080ZZ	B9060ZZ	B92FY0Z	BB290ZZ
B50PYZZ	B515ZZZ	B51G0ZZ	B51Q1ZZ	B529YZZ	B52RZZZ	B543ZZA	B7081ZZ	B9061ZZ	B92FYZZ	BB2910Z
B50Q0ZZ	B5160ZA	B51G1ZA	B51QYZA	B529Z2Z	B52S00Z	B543ZZZ	B708YZZ	B906YZZ	B92FZZZ	BB291ZZ
B50Q1ZZ	B5160ZZ	B51G1ZZ	B51QYZZ	B529ZZZ	B52S0ZZ	B544ZZ3	B7090ZZ	B9070ZZ	B92J00Z	BB29Y0Z
B50QYZZ	B5161ZA	B51GYZA	B51QZZA	B52F00Z	B52S10Z	B544ZZA	B7091ZZ	B9071ZZ	B92J0ZZ	BB29ZZZ
B50R0ZZ	B5161ZZ	B51GYZZ	B51QZZZ	B52F0ZZ	B52S1ZZ	B544ZZZ	B709YZZ	B907YZZ	B92J10Z	BB2F00Z
B50R1ZZ	B516YZA	B51GZZA	B51R0ZA	B52F10Z	B52SY0Z	B546ZZ3	B70B0ZZ	B9080ZZ	B92J1ZZ	BB2F0ZZ
B50RYZZ	B516YZZ	B51GZZZ	B51R0ZZ	B52F1ZZ	B52SYZZ	B546ZZA	B70B1ZZ	B9081ZZ	B92JY0Z	BB2F10Z
B50S0ZZ	B516ZZA	B51H0ZA	B51R1ZA	B52FY0Z	B52SZ2Z	B546ZZZ	B70BYZZ	B908YZZ	B92JYZZ	BB2F1ZZ
B50S1ZZ	B516ZZZ	B51H0ZZ	B51R1ZZ	B52FYZZ	B52SZZZ	B547ZZ3	B70C0ZZ	B9090ZZ	B92JZZZ	BB2FY0Z
B50SYZZ	B5170ZA	B51H1ZA	B51RYZA	B52FZ2Z	B52T00Z	B547ZZA	B70C1ZZ	B9091ZZ	B930Y0Z	BB2FYZZ
B50T0ZZ	B5170ZZ	B51H1ZZ	B51RYZZ	B52FZZZ	B52T0ZZ	B547ZZZ	B70CYZZ	B909YZZ	B930YZZ	BB2FZZZ
B50T1ZZ	B5171ZA	B51HYZA	B51RZZA	B52G00Z	B52T10Z	B548ZZ3	B8000ZZ	B90B0ZZ	B930ZZZ	BB3GY0Z
B50TYZZ	B5171ZZ	B51HYZZ	B51RZZZ	B52G0ZZ	B52T1ZZ	B548ZZA	B8001ZZ	B90B1ZZ	B932Y0Z	BB3GYZZ
B50V0ZZ	B517YZA	B51HZZA	B51S0ZA	B52G10Z	B52TY0Z	B548ZZZ	B800YZZ	B90BYZZ	B932YZZ	BB3GZZZ
B50V1ZZ	B517YZZ	B51HZZZ	B51S0ZZ	B52G1ZZ	B52TYZZ	B549ZZ3	B8010ZZ	B90C0ZZ	B932ZZZ	BB4BZZZ
B50VYZZ	B517ZZA	B51J0ZA	B51S1ZA	B52GY0Z	B52TZ2Z	B549ZZA	B8011ZZ	B90C1ZZ	B936Y0Z	BB4CZZZ
B50W0ZZ	B517ZZZ	B51J0ZZ	B51S1ZZ	B52GYZZ	B52TZZZ	B549ZZZ	B801YZZ	B90CYZZ	B936YZZ	BD11YZZ
B50W1ZZ	B5180ZA	B51J1ZA	B51SYZA	B52GZ2Z	B531Y0Z	B54BZZ3	B8020ZZ	B90D0ZZ	B936ZZZ	BD11ZZZ
B50WYZZ	B5180ZZ	B51J1ZZ	B51SYZZ	B52GZZZ	B531YZZ	B54BZZA	B8021ZZ	B90D1ZZ	B939Y0Z	BD12YZZ
B5100ZA	B5181ZA	B51JYZA	B51SZZA	B52H00Z	B531ZZZ	B54BZZZ	B802YZZ	B90DYZZ	B939YZZ	BD12ZZZ
B5100ZZ	B5181ZZ	B51JYZZ	B51SZZZ	B52H0ZZ	B532Y0Z	B54CZZ3	B803ZZZ	B90FZZZ	B939ZZZ	BD13YZZ
B5101ZA	B518YZA	B51JZZA	B51T0ZA	B52H10Z	B532YZZ	B54CZZA	B804ZZZ	B90HZZZ	B93DY0Z	BD13ZZZ
B5101ZZ	B518YZZ	B51JZZZ	B51T0ZZ	B52H1ZZ	B532ZZZ	B54CZZZ	B805ZZZ	B91GYZZ	B93DYZZ	BD14YZZ
B510YZA	B518ZZA	B51K0ZA	B51T1ZA	B52HY0Z	B535Y0Z	B54DZZ3	B806ZZZ	B91GZZZ	B93DZZZ	BD14ZZZ
B510YZZ	B518ZZZ	B51K0ZZ	B51T1ZZ	B52HYZZ	B535YZZ	B54DZZA	B807ZZZ	B91JYZZ	B93FY0Z	BD15YZZ
B510ZZA	B5190ZA	B51K1ZA	B51TYZA	B52HZ2Z	B535ZZZ	B54DZZZ	B82500Z	B91JZZZ	B93FYZZ	BD15ZZZ
B510ZZZ	B5190ZZ	B51K1ZZ	B51TYZZ	B52HZZZ	B538Y0Z	B54JZZ3	B8250ZZ	B92000Z	B93FZZZ	BD16YZZ
B5110ZA	B5191ZA	B51KYZA	B51TZZA	B52J00Z	B538YZZ	B54JZZA	B82510Z	B9200ZZ	B93JY0Z	BD16ZZZ
B5110ZZ	B5191ZZ	B51KYZZ	B51TZZZ	B52J0ZZ	B538ZZZ	B54JZZZ	B8251ZZ	B92010Z	B93JYZZ	BD19YZZ
B5111ZA	B519YZA	B51KZZA	B51V0ZA	B52J10Z	B539Y0Z	B54KZZ3	B825Y0Z	B9201ZZ	B93JZZZ	BD19ZZZ
B5111ZZ	B519YZZ	B51KZZZ	B51V0ZZ	B52J1ZZ	B539YZZ	B54KZZA	B825YZZ	B920Y0Z	BB07YZZ	BD1BYZZ
B511YZA	B519ZZA	B51L0ZA	B51V1ZA	B52JY0Z	B539ZZZ	B54KZZZ	B825ZZZ	B920YZZ	BB08YZZ	BD1BZZZ
B511YZZ	B519ZZZ	B51L0ZZ	B51V1ZZ	B52JYZZ	B53BY0Z	B54LZZ3	B82600Z	B920ZZZ	BB09YZZ	BD2400Z
B511ZZA	B51B0ZA	B51L1ZA	B51VYZA	B52JZ2Z	B53BYZZ	B54LZZA	B8260ZZ	B92200Z	BB0DZZZ	BD240ZZ
B511ZZZ	B51B0ZZ	B51L1ZZ	B51VYZZ	B52JZZZ	B53BZZZ	B54LZZZ	B82610Z	B9220ZZ	BB12ZZZ	BD2410Z
B5120ZA	B51B1ZA	B51LYZA	B51VZZA	B52K00Z	B53CY0Z	B54MZZ3	B8261ZZ	B92210Z	BB13ZZZ	BD241ZZ
B5120ZZ	B51B1ZZ	B51LYZZ	B51VZZZ	B52K0ZZ	B53CYZZ	B54MZZA	B826Y0Z	B9221ZZ	BB14ZZZ	BD24Y0Z
B5121ZA	B51BYZA	B51LZZA	B51W0ZA	B52K10Z	B53CZZZ	B54MZZZ	B826YZZ	B922Y0Z	BB16ZZZ	BD24YZZ
B5121ZZ	B51BYZZ	B51LZZZ	B51W0ZZ	B52K1ZZ	B53DY0Z	B54NZZ3	B826ZZZ	B922YZZ	BB17YZZ	BD24ZZZ
B512YZA	B51BZZA	B51M0ZA	B51W1ZA	B52KY0Z	B53DYZZ	B54NZZA	B82700Z	B922ZZZ	BB18YZZ	BD41ZZZ
B512YZZ	B51BZZZ	B51M0ZZ	B51W1ZZ	B52KYZZ	B53DZZZ	B54NZZZ	B8270ZZ	B92600Z	BB19YZZ	BD42ZZZ
B512ZZA	B51C0ZA	B51M1ZA	B51WYZA	B52KZ2Z	B53HY0Z	B54PZZ3	B82710Z	B9260ZZ	BB1CZZZ	BD47ZZZ
B512ZZZ	B51C0ZZ	B51M1ZZ	B51WYZZ	B52KZZZ	B53HYZZ	B54PZZA	B8271ZZ	B92610Z	BB1DZZZ	BD48ZZZ
B5130ZA	B51C1ZA	B51MYZA	B51WZZA	B52L00Z	B53HZZZ	B54PZZZ	B827Y0Z	B9261ZZ	BB2400Z	BD49ZZZ
B5130ZZ	B51C1ZZ	B51MYZZ	B51WZZZ	B52L0ZZ	B53LY0Z	B54TZZ3	B827YZZ	B926Y0Z	BB240ZZ	BD4CZZZ
B5131ZA	B51CYZA	B51MZZA	B52200Z	B52L10Z	B53LYZZ	B54TZZA	B827ZZZ	B926YZZ	BB2410Z	BF000ZZ
B5131ZZ	B51CYZZ	B51MZZZ	B5220ZZ	B52L1ZZ	B53LZZZ	B54TZZZ	B835Y0Z	B926ZZZ	BB241ZZ	BF001ZZ
B513YZA	B51CZZA	B51N0ZA	B52210Z	B52LY0Z	B53MY0Z	B7000ZZ	B835YZZ	B92900Z	BB24Y0Z	BF00YZZ
B513YZZ	B51CZZZ	B51N0ZZ	B5221ZZ	B52LYZZ	B53MYZZ	B7001ZZ	B835ZZZ	B9290ZZ	BB24YZZ	BF030ZZ
B513ZZA	B51D0ZA	B51N1ZA	B522Y0Z	B52LZ2Z	B53MZZZ	B700YZZ	B836Y0Z	B92910Z	BB24ZZZ	BF031ZZ
B513ZZZ	B51D0ZZ	B51N1ZZ	B522YZZ	B52LZZZ	B53NY0Z	B7010ZZ	B836YZZ	B9291ZZ	BB2700Z	BF03YZZ
B5140ZA	B51D1ZA	B51NYZA	B522Z2Z	B52Q00Z	B53NYZZ	B7011ZZ	B836ZZZ	B929Y0Z	BB270ZZ	BF0C0ZZ
B5140ZZ	B51D1ZZ	B51NYZZ	B522ZZZ	B52Q0ZZ	B53NZZZ	B701YZZ	B837Y0Z	B929YZZ	BB2710Z	BF0C1ZZ
B5141ZA	B51DYZA	B51NZZA	B52800Z	B52Q10Z	B53PY0Z	B7040ZZ	B837YZZ	B929ZZZ	BB271ZZ	BF0CYZZ
B5141ZZ	B51DYZZ	B51NZZZ	B5280ZZ	B52Q1ZZ	B53PYZZ	B7041ZZ	B837ZZZ	B92D00Z	BB27Y0Z	BF100ZZ
B514YZA	B51DZZA	B51P0ZA	B52810Z	B52QY0Z	B53PZZZ	B704YZZ	B845ZZZ	B92D0ZZ	BB27YZZ	BF101ZZ
B514YZZ	B51DZZZ	B51P0ZZ	B5281ZZ	B52QYZZ	B53SY0Z	B7050ZZ	B846ZZZ	B92D10Z	BB27ZZZ	BF10YZZ
B514ZZA	B51F0ZA	B51P1ZA	B528Y0Z	B52QZ2Z	B53SYZZ	B7051ZZ	B847ZZZ	B92D1ZZ	BB2800Z	BF110ZZ
B514ZZZ	B51F0ZZ	B51P1ZZ	B528YZZ	B52QZZZ	B53SZZZ	B705YZZ	B902ZZZ	B92DY0Z	BB280ZZ	BF111ZZ
B5150ZA	B51F1ZA	B51PYZA	B528Z2Z	B52R00Z	B53TY0Z	B7060ZZ	B9040ZZ	B92DYZZ	BB2810Z	BF11YZZ
B5150ZZ	B51F1ZZ	B51PYZZ	B528ZZZ	B52R0ZZ	B53TYZZ	B7061ZZ	B9041ZZ	B92DZZZ	BB281ZZ	BF120ZZ
B5151ZA	B51FYZA	B51PZZA	B52900Z	B52R10Z	B53TZZZ	B706YZZ	B904YZZ	B92F00Z	BB28Y0Z	BF121ZZ
B5151ZZ	B51FYZZ	B51PZZZ	B5290ZZ	B52R1ZZ	B53VY0Z	B7070ZZ	B9050ZZ	B92F0ZZ	BB28YZZ	BF12YZZ
B515YZA	B51FZZA	B51Q0ZA	B52910Z	B52RY0Z	B53VYZZ	B7071ZZ	B9051ZZ	B92F10Z	BB28ZZZ	BF130ZZ
B515YZZ	B51FZZZ	B51Q0ZZ	B5291ZZ	B52RYZZ	B53VZZZ	B707YZZ	B905YZZ	B92F1ZZ	BB2900Z	

BF131ZZ	BG2400Z	BH42ZZZ	BN23ZZZ	BP0PZZZ	BP23ZZZ	BP2MZZZ	BP3HYZZ	BQ0PZZZ	BQ240ZZ	BQ2V0ZZ
BF13YZZ	BG240ZZ	BH47ZZZ	BN250ZZ	BP0RZZZ	BP240ZZ	BP2N0ZZ	BP3HZZZ	BQ0QZZZ	BQ241ZZ	BQ2V1ZZ
BF140ZZ	BG2410Z	BH48ZZZ	BN251ZZ	BP0SZZZ	BP241ZZ	BP2N1ZZ	BP3JY0Z	BQ0VZZZ	BQ24YZZ	BQ2VYZZ
BF141ZZ	BG241ZZ	BH49ZZZ	BN25YZZ	BP0XZZZ	BP24YZZ	BP2NYZZ	BP3JYZZ	BQ0WZZZ	BQ24ZZZ	BQ2VZZZ
BF14YZZ	BG24Y0Z	BH4BZZZ	BN25ZZZ	BP0YZZZ	BP24ZZZ	BP2NZZZ	BP3JZZZ	BQ0X0ZZ	BQ270ZZ	BQ2W0ZZ
BF180ZZ	BG24YZZ	BH4CZZZ	BN260ZZ	BP10ZZZ	BP250ZZ	BP2P0ZZ	BP3KY0Z	BQ0X1ZZ	BQ271ZZ	BQ2W1ZZ
BF181ZZ	BG24ZZZ	BL30Y0Z	BN261ZZ	BP11ZZZ	BP251ZZ	BP2P1ZZ	BP3KYZZ	BQ0XYZZ	BQ27YZZ	BQ2WYZZ
BF18YZZ	BG32Y0Z	BL30YZZ	BN26YZZ	BP12ZZZ	BP25YZZ	BP2PYZZ	BP3KZZZ	BQ0Y0ZZ	BQ27ZZZ	BQ2WZZZ
BF2500Z	BG32YZZ	BL30ZZZ	BN26ZZZ	BP13ZZZ	BP25ZZZ	BP2PZZZ	BP3LY0Z	BQ0Y1ZZ	BQ280ZZ	BQ2X0ZZ
BF250ZZ	BG32ZZZ	BL31Y0Z	BN290ZZ	BP14ZZZ	BP260ZZ	BP2Q0ZZ	BP3LYZZ	BQ0YYZZ	BQ281ZZ	BQ2X1ZZ
BF2510Z	BG33Y0Z	BL31YZZ	BN291ZZ	BP15ZZZ	BP261ZZ	BP2Q1ZZ	BP3LZZZ	BQ100ZZ	BQ28YZZ	BQ2XYZZ
BF251ZZ	BG33YZZ	BL31ZZZ	BN29YZZ	BP16ZZZ	BP26YZZ	BP2QYZZ	BP3MY0Z	BQ101ZZ	BQ28ZZZ	BQ2XZZZ
BF25Y0Z	BG33ZZZ	BL32Y0Z	BN29ZZZ	BP17ZZZ	BP26ZZZ	BP2QZZZ	BP3MYZZ	BQ10YZZ	BQ2B0ZZ	BQ2Y0ZZ
BF25YZZ	BG34Y0Z	BL32YZZ	BN2F0ZZ	BP180ZZ	BP270ZZ	BP2R0ZZ	BP3MZZZ	BQ10ZZZ	BQ2B1ZZ	BQ2Y1ZZ
BF25ZZZ	BG34YZZ	BL32ZZZ	BN2F1ZZ	BP181ZZ	BP271ZZ	BP2R1ZZ	BP48ZZ1	BQ110ZZ	BQ2BYZZ	BQ2YYZZ
BF2600Z	BG34ZZZ	BL33Y0Z	BN2FYZZ	BP18YZZ	BP27YZZ	BP2RYZZ	BP48ZZZ	BQ111ZZ	BQ2C0ZZ	BQ2YZZZ
BF260ZZ	BG40ZZZ	BL33YZZ	BN2FZZZ	BP18ZZZ	BP27ZZZ	BP2RZZZ	BP49ZZ1	BQ11YZZ	BQ2C1ZZ	BQ30Y0Z
BF2610Z	BG41ZZZ	BL33ZZZ	BN39YZZ	BP190ZZ	BP280ZZ	BP2S0ZZ	BP49ZZZ	BQ11ZZZ	BQ2CYZZ	BQ30YZZ
BF261ZZ	BG42ZZZ	BL40ZZZ	BN39ZZZ	BP191ZZ	BP281ZZ	BP2S1ZZ	BP4GZZ1	BQ13ZZZ	BQ2D0ZZ	BQ30ZZZ
BF26Y0Z	BG43ZZZ	BL41ZZZ	BP00ZZZ	BP19YZZ	BP28YZZ	BP2SYZZ	BP4GZZZ	BQ14ZZZ	BQ2D1ZZ	BQ31Y0Z
BF26YZZ	BG44ZZZ	BL42ZZZ	BP01ZZZ	BP19ZZZ	BP28ZZZ	BP2SZZZ	BP4HZZ1	BQ170ZZ	BQ2DYZZ	BQ31YZZ
BF26ZZZ	BH00ZZZ	BL43ZZZ	BP02ZZZ	BP1AZZZ	BP290ZZ	BP2T0ZZ	BP4HZZZ	BQ171ZZ	BQ2DZZZ	BQ31ZZZ
BF2700Z	BH01ZZZ	BN00ZZZ	BP03ZZZ	BP1BZZZ	BP291ZZ	BP2T1ZZ	BP4LZZ1	BQ17YZZ	BQ2F0ZZ	BQ33Y0Z
BF270ZZ	BH02ZZZ	BN01ZZZ	BP04ZZZ	BP1C0ZZ	BP29YZZ	BP2TYZZ	BP4LZZZ	BQ17ZZZ	BQ2F1ZZ	BQ33YZZ
BF2710Z	BH030ZZ	BN02ZZZ	BP05ZZZ	BP1C1ZZ	BP29ZZZ	BP2TZZZ	BP4MZZ1	BQ180ZZ	BQ2FYZZ	BQ33ZZZ
BF271ZZ	BH031ZZ	BN03ZZZ	BP06ZZZ	BP1CYZZ	BP2A0ZZ	BP2U0ZZ	BP4MZZZ	BQ181ZZ	BQ2FZZZ	BQ34Y0Z
BF27Y0Z	BH03YZZ	BN04ZZZ	BP07ZZZ	BP1D0ZZ	BP2A1ZZ	BP2U1ZZ	BP4NZZ1	BQ18YZZ	BQ2G0ZZ	BQ34YZZ
BF27YZZ	BH03ZZZ	BN05ZZZ	BP080ZZ	BP1D1ZZ	BP2AYZZ	BP2UYZZ	BP4NZZZ	BQ18ZZZ	BQ2G1ZZ	BQ34ZZZ
BF27ZZZ	BH040ZZ	BN06ZZZ	BP081ZZ	BP1DYZZ	BP2AZZZ	BP2UZZZ	BP4PZZ1	BQ1DZZZ	BQ2GYZZ	BQ37Y0Z
BF2C00Z	BH041ZZ	BN070ZZ	BP08YZZ	BP1EZZZ	BP2B0ZZ	BP2V0ZZ	BP4PZZZ	BQ1FZZZ	BQ2GZZZ	BQ37YZZ
BF2C0ZZ	BH04YZZ	BN071ZZ	BP08ZZZ	BP1FZZZ	BP2B1ZZ	BP2V1ZZ	BQ000ZZ	BQ1G0ZZ	BQ2H0ZZ	BQ37ZZZ
BF2C10Z	BH04ZZZ	BN07YZZ	BP090ZZ	BP1G0ZZ	BP2BYZZ	BP2VYZZ	BQ001ZZ	BQ1G1ZZ	BQ2H1ZZ	BQ38Y0Z
BF2C1ZZ	BH050ZZ	BN07ZZZ	BP091ZZ	BP1G1ZZ	BP2BZZZ	BP2VZZZ	BQ00YZZ	BQ1GYZZ	BQ2HYZZ	BQ38YZZ
BF2CY0Z	BH051ZZ	BN080ZZ	BP09YZZ	BP1GYZZ	BP2CZZZ	BP2W0ZZ	BQ00ZZ1	BQ1GZZZ	BQ2HZZZ	BQ38ZZZ
BF2CYZZ	BH05YZZ	BN081ZZ	BP09ZZZ	BP1H0ZZ	BP2DZZZ	BP2W1ZZ	BQ00ZZZ	BQ1H0ZZ	BQ2J0ZZ	BQ3DY0Z
BF2CZZZ	BH05ZZZ	BN08YZZ	BP0AZZZ	BP1H1ZZ	BP2E0ZZ	BP2WYZZ	BQ010ZZ	BQ1H1ZZ	BQ2J1ZZ	BQ3DYZZ
BF35Y0Z	BH060ZZ	BN08ZZZ	BP0BZZZ	BP1HYZZ	BP2E1ZZ	BP2X0ZZ	BQ011ZZ	BQ1HYZZ	BQ2JYZZ	BQ3DZZZ
BF35YZZ	BH061ZZ	BN090ZZ	BP0C0ZZ	BP1JZZZ	BP2EYZZ	BP2X1ZZ	BQ01YZZ	BQ1HZZZ	BQ2JZZZ	BQ3FY0Z
BF35ZZZ	BH06YZZ	BN091ZZ	BP0C1ZZ	BP1KZZZ	BP2EZZZ	BP2XYZZ	BQ01ZZ1	BQ1JZZZ	BQ2K0ZZ	BQ3FYZZ
BF36Y0Z	BH06ZZZ	BN09YZZ	BP0CYZZ	BP1L0ZZ	BP2F0ZZ	BP2XZZZ	BQ01ZZZ	BQ1KZZZ	BQ2K1ZZ	BQ3FZZZ
BF36YZZ	BH30Y0Z	BN09ZZZ	BP0CZZZ	BP1L1ZZ	BP2F1ZZ	BP2Y0ZZ	BQ03ZZ1	BQ1LZZZ	BQ2KYZZ	BQ3GY0Z
BF36ZZZ	BH30YZZ	BN0BZZZ	BP0D0ZZ	BP1LYZZ	BP2FYZZ	BP2Y1ZZ	BQ03ZZZ	BQ1MZZZ	BQ2KZZZ	BQ3GYZZ
BF37Y0Z	BH30ZZZ	BN0CZZZ	BP0D1ZZ	BP1LZZZ	BP2FZZZ	BP2YYZZ	BQ04ZZ1	BQ1PZZZ	BQ2L0ZZ	BQ3GZZZ
BF37YZZ	BH31Y0Z	BN0DZZZ	BP0DYZZ	BP1M0ZZ	BP2G0ZZ	BP2YZZZ	BQ04ZZZ	BQ1QZZZ	BQ2L1ZZ	BQ3HY0Z
BF37ZZZ	BH31YZZ	BN0GZZZ	BP0DZZZ	BP1M1ZZ	BP2G1ZZ	BP38Y0Z	BQ070ZZ	BQ1VZZZ	BQ2LYZZ	BQ3HYZZ
BF40ZZZ	BH31ZZZ	BN0HZZZ	BP0EZZZ	BP1MYZZ	BP2GYZZ	BP38YZZ	BQ071ZZ	BQ1WZZZ	BQ2LZZZ	BQ3HZZZ
BF42ZZZ	BH32Y0Z	BN0JZZZ	BP0FZZZ	BP1MZZZ	BP2GZZZ	BP38ZZZ	BQ07YZZ	BQ1X0ZZ	BQ2M0ZZ	BQ3JY0Z
BF43ZZZ	BH32YZZ	BN170ZZ	BP0G0ZZ	BP1NZZZ	BP2H0ZZ	BP39Y0Z	BQ07ZZZ	BQ1X1ZZ	BQ2M1ZZ	BQ3JYZZ
BF45ZZZ	BH32ZZZ	BN171ZZ	BP0G1ZZ	BP1PZZZ	BP2H1ZZ	BP39YZZ	BQ080ZZ	BQ1XYZZ	BQ2MYZZ	BQ3JZZZ
BF46ZZZ	BH3DY0Z	BN17YZZ	BP0GYZZ	BP1RZZZ	BP2HYZZ	BP39ZZZ	BQ081ZZ	BQ1XZZZ	BQ2MZZZ	BQ3KY0Z
BF47ZZZ	BH3DYZZ	BN17ZZZ	BP0GZZZ	BP1SZZZ	BP2HZZZ	BP3CY0Z	BQ08YZZ	BQ1Y0ZZ	BQ2P0ZZ	BQ3KYZZ
BF4CZZZ	BH3DZZZ	BN180ZZ	BP0H0ZZ	BP1XZZZ	BP2J0ZZ	BP3CYZZ	BQ08ZZZ	BQ1Y1ZZ	BQ2P1ZZ	BQ3KZZZ
BG2200Z	BH3FY0Z	BN181ZZ	BP0H1ZZ	BP1YZZZ	BP2J1ZZ	BP3CZZZ	BQ0DZZZ	BQ1YYZZ	BQ2PYZZ	BQ3LY0Z
BG220ZZ	BH3FYZZ	BN18YZZ	BP0HYZZ	BP200ZZ	BP2JYZZ	BP3DY0Z	BQ0FZZZ	BQ1YZZZ	BQ2PZZZ	BQ3LYZZ
BG2210Z	BH3FZZZ	BN18ZZZ	BP0HZZZ	BP201ZZ	BP2JZZZ	BP3DYZZ	BQ0G0ZZ	BQ200ZZ	BQ2Q0ZZ	BQ3LZZZ
BG221ZZ	BH3GY0Z	BN190ZZ	BP0JZZZ	BP20YZZ	BP2K0ZZ	BP3DZZZ	BQ0G1ZZ	BQ201ZZ	BQ2Q1ZZ	BQ3MY0Z
BG22Y0Z	BH3GYZZ	BN191ZZ	BP0KZZZ	BP210ZZ	BP2K1ZZ	BP3EY0Z	BQ0GYZZ	BQ20YZZ	BQ2QYZZ	BQ3MYZZ
BG22YZZ	BH3GZZZ	BN19YZZ	BP0L0ZZ	BP211ZZ	BP2KYZZ	BP3EYZZ	BQ0GZZZ	BQ20ZZZ	BQ2QZZZ	BQ3MZZZ
BG22ZZZ	BH3HY0Z	BN19ZZZ	BP0L1ZZ	BP21YZZ	BP2KZZZ	BP3EZZZ	BQ0H0ZZ	BQ210ZZ	BQ2R0ZZ	BQ3PY0Z
BG2300Z	BH3HYZZ	BN200ZZ	BP0LYZZ	BP220ZZ	BP2L0ZZ	BP3FY0Z	BQ0H1ZZ	BQ211ZZ	BQ2R1ZZ	BQ3PYZZ
BG230ZZ	BH3HZZZ	BN201ZZ	BP0LZZZ	BP221ZZ	BP2L1ZZ	BP3FYZZ	BQ0HYZZ	BQ21YZZ	BQ2RYZZ	BQ3PZZZ
BG2310Z	BH3JY0Z	BN20YZZ	BP0M0ZZ	BP22YZZ	BP2LYZZ	BP3FZZZ	BQ0HZZZ	BQ21ZZZ	BQ2RZZZ	BQ3QY0Z
BG231ZZ	BH3JYZZ	BN20ZZZ	BP0M1ZZ	BP22ZZZ	BP2LZZZ	BP3GY0Z	BQ0JZZZ	BQ230ZZ	BQ2S0ZZ	BQ3QYZZ
BG23Y0Z	BH3JZZZ	BN230ZZ	BP0MYZZ	BP230ZZ	BP2M0ZZ	BP3GYZZ	BQ0KZZZ	BQ231ZZ	BQ2S1ZZ	BQ3QZZZ
BG23YZZ	BH40ZZZ	BN231ZZ	BP0MZZZ	BP231ZZ	BP2M1ZZ	BP3GZZZ	BQ0LZZZ	BQ23YZZ	BQ2SYZZ	BQ3VY0Z
BG23ZZZ	BH41ZZZ	BN23YZZ	BP0NZZZ	BP23YZZ	BP2MYZZ	BP3HY0Z	BQ0MZZZ	BQ23ZZZ	BQ2SZZZ	BQ3VYZZ

BQ3VZZZ	BR13ZZZ	BR2D1ZZ	BT07ZZZ	BT200ZZ	BU021ZZ	BU45YZZ	BW0BZZZ	BW2F10Z	C010YZZ	C713YZZ
BQ3WY0Z	BR140ZZ	BR2DYZZ	BT080ZZ	BT2010Z	BU02YZZ	BU45ZZZ	BW0CZZZ	BW2F1ZZ	C015DZZ	C7151ZZ
BQ3WYZZ	BR141ZZ	BR2DZZZ	BT081ZZ	BT201ZZ	BU060ZZ	BU46YZZ	BW0JZZZ	BW2FY0Z	C015YZZ	C715YZZ
BQ3WZZZ	BR14YZZ	BR2F0ZZ	BT08YZZ	BT20Y0Z	BU061ZZ	BU46ZZZ	BW0KZZZ	BW2FYZZ	C01YYZZ	C71D1ZZ
BQ40ZZZ	BR14ZZZ	BR2F1ZZ	BT08ZZZ	BT20YZZ	BU06YZZ	BU4CYZZ	BW0LZZZ	BW2FZZZ	C0201ZZ	C71DYZZ
BQ41ZZZ	BR150ZZ	BR2FYZZ	BT0B0ZZ	BT20ZZZ	BU080ZZ	BU4CZZZ	BW0MZZZ	BW2G00Z	C020FZZ	C71J1ZZ
BQ42ZZZ	BR151ZZ	BR2FZZZ	BT0B1ZZ	BT2100Z	BU081ZZ	BV000ZZ	BW110ZZ	BW2G0ZZ	C020SZZ	C71JYZZ
BQ47ZZZ	BR15YZZ	BR30Y0Z	BT0BYZZ	BT210ZZ	BU08YZZ	BV001ZZ	BW111ZZ	BW2G10Z	C020YZZ	C71K1ZZ
BQ48ZZZ	BR15ZZZ	BR30YZZ	BT0BZZZ	BT2110Z	BU090ZZ	BV00YZZ	BW11YZZ	BW2G1ZZ	C025DZZ	C71KYZZ
BQ49ZZZ	BR160ZZ	BR30ZZZ	BT0C0ZZ	BT211ZZ	BU091ZZ	BV010ZZ	BW11ZZZ	BW2GY0Z	C025YZZ	C71L1ZZ
BR00ZZ1	BR161ZZ	BR31Y0Z	BT0C1ZZ	BT21Y0Z	BU09YZZ	BV011ZZ	BW190ZZ	BW2GYZZ	C02YYZZ	C71LYZZ
BR00ZZZ	BR16YZZ	BR31YZZ	BT0CYZZ	BT21YZZ	BU100ZZ	BV01YZZ	BW191ZZ	BW2GZZZ	C030BZZ	C71M1ZZ
BR010ZZ	BR16ZZZ	BR31ZZZ	BT0CZZZ	BT21ZZZ	BU101ZZ	BV020ZZ	BW19YZZ	BW30Y0Z	C030KZZ	C71MYZZ
BR011ZZ	BR170ZZ	BR32Y0Z	BT100ZZ	BT2200Z	BU10YZZ	BV021ZZ	BW19ZZZ	BW30YZZ	C030MZZ	C71N1ZZ
BR01YZZ	BR171ZZ	BR32YZZ	BT101ZZ	BT220ZZ	BU10ZZZ	BV02YZZ	BW1C0ZZ	BW30ZZZ	C030YZZ	C71NYZZ
BR01ZZZ	BR17YZZ	BR32ZZZ	BT10YZZ	BT2210Z	BU110ZZ	BV030ZZ	BW1C1ZZ	BW33Y0Z	C03YYZZ	C71P1ZZ
BR020ZZ	BR17ZZZ	BR33Y0Z	BT10ZZZ	BT221ZZ	BU111ZZ	BV031ZZ	BW1CYZZ	BW33YZZ	C050VZZ	C71PYZZ
BR021ZZ	BR180ZZ	BR33YZZ	BT110ZZ	BT22Y0Z	BU11YZZ	BV03YZZ	BW1CZZZ	BW38Y0Z	C050YZZ	C71YYZZ
BR02YZZ	BR181ZZ	BR33ZZZ	BT111ZZ	BT22YZZ	BU11ZZZ	BV050ZZ	BW1J0ZZ	BW38YZZ	C05YYZZ	C7221ZZ
BR02ZZZ	BR18YZZ	BR37Y0Z	BT11YZZ	BT22ZZZ	BU120ZZ	BV051ZZ	BW1J1ZZ	BW38ZZZ	C2161ZZ	C722YZZ
BR030ZZ	BR18ZZZ	BR37YZZ	BT11ZZZ	BT2300Z	BU121ZZ	BV05YZZ	BW1JYZZ	BW3FY0Z	C216YZZ	C72YYZZ
BR031ZZ	BR190ZZ	BR37ZZZ	BT120ZZ	BT230ZZ	BU12YZZ	BV060ZZ	BW1JZZZ	BW3FYZZ	C21G1ZZ	C7551ZZ
BR03YZZ	BR191ZZ	BR39Y0Z	BT121ZZ	BT2310Z	BU12ZZZ	BV061ZZ	BW2000Z	BW3FZZZ	C21GDZZ	C755YZZ
BR03ZZZ	BR19YZZ	BR39YZZ	BT12YZZ	BT231ZZ	BU160ZZ	BV06YZZ	BW200ZZ	BW3GY0Z	C21GSZZ	C75D1ZZ
BR040ZZ	BR19ZZZ	BR39ZZZ	BT12ZZZ	BT23Y0Z	BU161ZZ	BV080ZZ	BW2010Z	BW3GYZZ	C21GYZZ	C75DYZZ
BR041ZZ	BR1B0ZZ	BR3CY0Z	BT130ZZ	BT23YZZ	BU16YZZ	BV081ZZ	BW201ZZ	BW3GZZZ	C21GZZZ	C75J1ZZ
BR04YZZ	BR1B1ZZ	BR3CYZZ	BT131ZZ	BT23ZZZ	BU16ZZZ	BV08YZZ	BW20Y0Z	BW3HY0Z	C21YYZZ	C75JYZZ
BR04ZZZ	BR1BYZZ	BR3CZZZ	BT13YZZ	BT2900Z	BU180ZZ	BV100ZZ	BW20YZZ	BW3HYZZ	C2261ZZ	C75K1ZZ
BR050ZZ	BR1BZZZ	BR3FY0Z	BT13ZZZ	BT290ZZ	BU181ZZ	BV101ZZ	BW20ZZZ	BW3HZZZ	C226YZZ	C75KYZZ
BR051ZZ	BR1C0ZZ	BR3FYZZ	BT140ZZ	BT2910Z	BU18YZZ	BV10YZZ	BW2100Z	BW3PY0Z	C22G1ZZ	C75L1ZZ
BR05YZZ	BR1C1ZZ	BR3FZZZ	BT141ZZ	BT291ZZ	BU18ZZZ	BV10ZZZ	BW210ZZ	BW3PYZZ	C22GDZZ	C75LYZZ
BR05ZZZ	BR1CYZZ	BR40ZZZ	BT14YZZ	BT29Y0Z	BU190ZZ	BV180ZZ	BW2110Z	BW3PZZZ	C22GKZZ	C75M1ZZ
BR060ZZ	BR1CZZZ	BR47ZZZ	BT14ZZZ	BT29YZZ	BU191ZZ	BV181ZZ	BW211ZZ	BW40ZZZ	C22GSZZ	C75MYZZ
BR061ZZ	BR1D0ZZ	BR49ZZZ	BT150ZZ	BT29ZZZ	BU19YZZ	BV18YZZ	BW21Y0Z	BW41ZZZ	C22GYZZ	C75N1ZZ
BR06YZZ	BR1D1ZZ	BR4FZZZ	BT151ZZ	BT30Y0Z	BU19ZZZ	BV18ZZZ	BW21YZZ	BW4FZZZ	C22GZZZ	C75NYZZ
BR06ZZZ	BR1DYZZ	BT000ZZ	BT15YZZ	BT30YZZ	BU33Y0Z	BV2300Z	BW21ZZZ	BW4GZZZ	C22YYZZ	C75P1ZZ
BR07ZZ1	BR1DZZZ	BT001ZZ	BT15ZZZ	BT30ZZZ	BU33YZZ	BV230ZZ	BW2300Z	BY30Y0Z	C23GKZZ	C75PYZZ
BR07ZZZ	BR1F0ZZ	BT00YZZ	BT160ZZ	BT31Y0Z	BU33ZZZ	BV2310Z	BW230ZZ	BY30YZZ	C23GMZZ	C75YYZZ
BR08ZZZ	BR1F1ZZ	BT00ZZZ	BT161ZZ	BT31YZZ	BU34Y0Z	BV231ZZ	BW2310Z	BY30ZZZ	C23GQZZ	C7631ZZ
BR09ZZ1	BR1FYZZ	BT010ZZ	BT16YZZ	BT31ZZZ	BU34YZZ	BV23Y0Z	BW231ZZ	BY31Y0Z	C23GRZZ	C7637ZZ
BR09ZZZ	BR1FZZZ	BT011ZZ	BT16ZZZ	BT32Y0Z	BU34ZZZ	BV23YZZ	BW24Y0Z	BY31YZZ	C23GYZZ	C763CZZ
BR0BZZZ	BR1G0ZZ	BT01YZZ	BT170ZZ	BT32YZZ	BU35Y0Z	BV23ZZZ	BW24YZZ	BY31ZZZ	C23YYZZ	C763DZZ
BR0CZZZ	BR1G1ZZ	BT01ZZZ	BT171ZZ	BT32ZZZ	BU35YZZ	BV30Y0Z	BW24ZZZ	BY32Y0Z	C2561ZZ	C763HZZ
BR0D0ZZ	BR1GYZZ	BT020ZZ	BT17YZZ	BT33Y0Z	BU35ZZZ	BV30YZZ	BW2500Z	BY32YZZ	C256YZZ	C763WZZ
BR0D1ZZ	BR1GZZZ	BT021ZZ	BT17ZZZ	BT33YZZ	BU36Y0Z	BV30ZZZ	BW250ZZ	BY32ZZZ	C25YYZZ	C763YZZ
BR0DYZZ	BR1H0ZZ	BT02YZZ	BT1B0ZZ	BT33ZZZ	BU36YZZ	BV33Y0Z	BW2510Z	BY33Y0Z	C51B1ZZ	C76YYZZ
BR0DZZZ	BR1H1ZZ	BT02ZZZ	BT1B1ZZ	BT39Y0Z	BU36ZZZ	BV33YZZ	BW251ZZ	BY33YZZ	C51BYZZ	C8191ZZ
BR0FZZZ	BR1HYZZ	BT030ZZ	BT1BYZZ	BT39YZZ	BU39Y0Z	BV33ZZZ	BW25Y0Z	BY33ZZZ	C51C1ZZ	C819YZZ
BR0GZZ1	BR1HZZZ	BT031ZZ	BT1BZZZ	BT39ZZZ	BU39YZZ	BV34Y0Z	BW25YZZ	BY34Y0Z	C51CYZZ	C81YYZZ
BR0GZZZ	BR200ZZ	BT03YZZ	BT1C0ZZ	BT40ZZZ	BU39ZZZ	BV34YZZ	BW25ZZZ	BY34YZZ	C51D1ZZ	C91B1ZZ
BR0HZZZ	BR201ZZ	BT03ZZZ	BT1C1ZZ	BT41ZZZ	BU3BY0Z	BV34ZZZ	BW2800Z	BY34ZZZ	C51DYZZ	C91BYZZ
BR100ZZ	BR20YZZ	BT040ZZ	BT1CYZZ	BT42ZZZ	BU3BYZZ	BV35Y0Z	BW280ZZ	BY35Y0Z	C51N1ZZ	C91YYZZ
BR101ZZ	BR20ZZZ	BT041ZZ	BT1CZZZ	BT43ZZZ	BU3BZZZ	BV35YZZ	BW2810Z	BY35YZZ	C51NYZZ	CB121ZZ
BR10YZZ	BR270ZZ	BT04YZZ	BT1D0ZZ	BT45ZZZ	BU3CY0Z	BV35ZZZ	BW281ZZ	BY35ZZZ	C51P1ZZ	CB129ZZ
BR10ZZZ	BR271ZZ	BT04ZZZ	BT1D1ZZ	BT46ZZZ	BU3CYZZ	BV36Y0Z	BW28Y0Z	BY36Y0Z	C51PYZZ	CB12TZZ
BR110ZZ	BR27YZZ	BT050ZZ	BT1DYZZ	BT47ZZZ	BU3CZZZ	BV36YZZ	BW28YZZ	BY36YZZ	C51Q1ZZ	CB12VZZ
BR111ZZ	BR27ZZZ	BT051ZZ	BT1DZZZ	BT48ZZZ	BU40YZZ	BV36ZZZ	BW28ZZZ	BY36ZZZ	C51QYZZ	CB12YZZ
BR11YZZ	BR290ZZ	BT05YZZ	BT1F0ZZ	BT49ZZZ	BU40ZZZ	BV37Y0Z	BW2900Z	BY47ZZZ	C51R1ZZ	CB1YYZZ
BR11ZZZ	BR291ZZ	BT05ZZZ	BT1F1ZZ	BT4JZZZ	BU41YZZ	BV37YZZ	BW290ZZ	BY48ZZZ	C51RYZZ	CB221ZZ
BR120ZZ	BR29YZZ	BT060ZZ	BT1FYZZ	BU000ZZ	BU41ZZZ	BV37ZZZ	BW2910Z	BY49ZZZ	C51YYZZ	CB229ZZ
BR121ZZ	BR29ZZZ	BT061ZZ	BT1FZZZ	BU001ZZ	BU42YZZ	BV44ZZZ	BW291ZZ	BY4BZZZ	C7101ZZ	CB22YZZ
BR12YZZ	BR2C0ZZ	BT06YZZ	BT1G0ZZ	BU00YZZ	BU42ZZZ	BV49ZZZ	BW29Y0Z	BY4CZZZ	C710DZZ	CB2YYZZ
BR12ZZZ	BR2C1ZZ	BT06ZZZ	BT1G1ZZ	BU010ZZ	BU43YZZ	BV4BZZZ	BW29YZZ	BY4DZZZ	C710YZZ	CB32KZZ
BR130ZZ	BR2CYZZ	BT070ZZ	BT1GYZZ	BU011ZZ	BU43ZZZ	BW00ZZZ	BW29ZZZ	BY4FZZZ	C7121ZZ	CB32YZZ
BR131ZZ	BR2CZZZ	BT071ZZ	BT1GZZZ	BU01YZZ	BU44YZZ	BW01ZZZ	BW2F00Z	BY4GZZZ	C712YZZ	CB3YYZZ
BR13YZZ	BR2D0ZZ	BT07YZZ	BT2000Z	BU020ZZ	BU44ZZZ	BW03ZZZ	BW2F0ZZ	C0101ZZ	C713DZZ	CD151ZZ

CD15DZZ	CP11YZZ	CT231ZZ	CW1JLZZ	CW2BYZZ	D0000ZZ	D016BCZ	D7030ZZ	D711B7Z	D71797Z	D7Y7FZZ
CD15YZZ	CP141ZZ	CT23YZZ	CW1JSZZ	CW2D1ZZ	D0001ZZ	D016BYZ	D7031ZZ	D711B8Z	D71798Z	D7Y88ZZ
CD171ZZ	CP14YZZ	CT2YYZZ	CW1JYZZ	CW2DDZZ	D0002ZZ	D01797Z	D7032ZZ	D711B9Z	D71799Z	D7Y8FZZ
CD17DZZ	CP151ZZ	CT631ZZ	CW1M1ZZ	CW2DFZZ	D0003Z0	D01798Z	D7033Z0	D711BBZ	D7179BZ	D8000ZZ
CD17YZZ	CP15YZZ	CT63FZZ	CW1MDZZ	CW2DGZZ	D0003ZZ	D01799Z	D7033ZZ	D711BCZ	D7179CZ	D8001ZZ
CD1YYZZ	CP161ZZ	CT63GZZ	CW1MFZZ	CW2DKZZ	D0004ZZ	D0179BZ	D7034ZZ	D711BYZ	D7179YZ	D8002ZZ
CD271ZZ	CP16YZZ	CT63HZZ	CW1MGZZ	CW2DLZZ	D0005ZZ	D0179CZ	D7035ZZ	D71297Z	D717B7Z	D8003Z0
CD27DZZ	CP171ZZ	CT63YZZ	CW1MLZZ	CW2DSZZ	D0006ZZ	D0179YZ	D7036ZZ	D71298Z	D717B8Z	D8003ZZ
CD27YZZ	CP17YZZ	CT6YYZZ	CW1MSZZ	CW2DYZZ	D0010ZZ	D017B7Z	D7040ZZ	D71299Z	D717B9Z	D8004ZZ
CD2YYZZ	CP181ZZ	CV191ZZ	CW1MYZZ	CW2J1ZZ	D0011ZZ	D017B8Z	D7041ZZ	D7129BZ	D717BBZ	D8005ZZ
CF141ZZ	CP18YZZ	CV19YZZ	CW1N1ZZ	CW2JDZZ	D0012ZZ	D017B9Z	D7042ZZ	D7129CZ	D717BCZ	D8006ZZ
CF14YZZ	CP191ZZ	CV1YYZZ	CW1NDZZ	CW2JFZZ	D0013Z0	D017BBZ	D7043Z0	D7129YZ	D717BYZ	D81097Z
CF151ZZ	CP19YZZ	CW101ZZ	CW1NFZZ	CW2JGZZ	D0013ZZ	D017BCZ	D7043ZZ	D712B7Z	D71897Z	D81098Z
CF15YZZ	CP1B1ZZ	CW10DZZ	CW1NGZZ	CW2JKZZ	D0014ZZ	D017BYZ	D7044ZZ	D712B8Z	D71898Z	D81099Z
CF161ZZ	CP1BYZZ	CW10FZZ	CW1NLZZ	CW2JLZZ	D0015ZZ	D020DZZ	D7045ZZ	D712B9Z	D71899Z	D8109BZ
CF16YZZ	CP1C1ZZ	CW10GZZ	CW1NSZZ	CW2JSZZ	D0016ZZ	D020HZZ	D7046ZZ	D712BBZ	D7189BZ	D8109CZ
CF1C1ZZ	CP1CYZZ	CW10LZZ	CW1NYZZ	CW2JYZZ	D0060ZZ	D020JZZ	D7050ZZ	D712BCZ	D7189CZ	D8109YZ
CF1CYZZ	CP1D1ZZ	CW10SZZ	CW1YYZZ	CW2M1ZZ	D0061ZZ	D021DZZ	D7051ZZ	D712BYZ	D7189YZ	D810B7Z
CF1YYZZ	CP1DYZZ	CW10YZZ	CW1ZZZZ	CW2MDZZ	D0062ZZ	D021HZZ	D7052ZZ	D71397Z	D718B7Z	D810B8Z
CF241ZZ	CP1F1ZZ	CW111ZZ	CW201ZZ	CW2MFZZ	D0063Z0	D021JZZ	D7053Z0	D71398Z	D718B8Z	D810B9Z
CF24YZZ	CP1FYZZ	CW11DZZ	CW20DZZ	CW2MGZZ	D0063ZZ	D026DZZ	D7053ZZ	D71399Z	D718B9Z	D810BBZ
CF251ZZ	CP1YYZZ	CW11FZZ	CW20FZZ	CW2MKZZ	D0064ZZ	D026HZZ	D7054ZZ	D7139BZ	D718BBZ	D810BCZ
CF25YZZ	CP1Z1ZZ	CW11GZZ	CW20GZZ	CW2MLZZ	D0065ZZ	D026JZZ	D7055ZZ	D7139CZ	D718BCZ	D810BYZ
CF261ZZ	CP1ZYZZ	CW11LZZ	CW20KZZ	CW2MSZZ	D0066ZZ	D027DZZ	D7056ZZ	D7139YZ	D718BYZ	D820DZZ
CF26YZZ	CP211ZZ	CW11SZZ	CW20LZZ	CW2MYZZ	D0070ZZ	D027HZZ	D7060ZZ	D713B7Z	D720DZZ	D820HZZ
CF2YYZZ	CP21YZZ	CW11YZZ	CW20SZZ	CW2YYZZ	D0071ZZ	D027JZZ	D7061ZZ	D713B8Z	D720HZZ	D820JZZ
CG111ZZ	CP221ZZ	CW131ZZ	CW20YZZ	CW3NYZZ	D0072ZZ	D0Y07ZZ	D7062ZZ	D713B9Z	D720JZZ	D8Y07ZZ
CG11SZZ	CP22YZZ	CW13DZZ	CW211ZZ	CW501ZZ	D0073Z0	D0Y08ZZ	D7063Z0	D713BBZ	D721DZZ	D8Y08ZZ
CG11YZZ	CP231ZZ	CW13FZZ	CW21DZZ	CW50DZZ	D0073ZZ	D0Y0FZZ	D7063ZZ	D713BCZ	D721HZZ	D8Y0FZZ
CG121ZZ	CP23YZZ	CW13GZZ	CW21FZZ	CW50YZZ	D0074ZZ	D0Y0KZZ	D7064ZZ	D713BYZ	D721JZZ	D9000ZZ
CG12FZZ	CP241ZZ	CW13KZZ	CW21GZZ	CW511ZZ	D0075ZZ	D0Y17ZZ	D7065ZZ	D71497Z	D722DZZ	D9001ZZ
CG12GZZ	CP24YZZ	CW13LZZ	CW21KZZ	CW51DZZ	D0076ZZ	D0Y18ZZ	D7066ZZ	D71498Z	D722HZZ	D9002ZZ
CG12YZZ	CP261ZZ	CW13SZZ	CW21LZZ	CW51YZZ	D01097Z	D0Y1FZZ	D7070ZZ	D71499Z	D722JZZ	D9003Z0
CG14GZZ	CP26YZZ	CW13YZZ	CW21SZZ	CW531ZZ	D01098Z	D0Y1KZZ	D7071ZZ	D7149BZ	D723DZZ	D9003ZZ
CG14YZZ	CP271ZZ	CW141ZZ	CW21YZZ	CW53DZZ	D01099Z	D0Y67ZZ	D7072ZZ	D7149CZ	D723HZZ	D9004ZZ
CG1YYZZ	CP27YZZ	CW14DZZ	CW231ZZ	CW53YZZ	D0109BZ	D0Y68ZZ	D7073Z0	D7149YZ	D723JZZ	D9005ZZ
CG211ZZ	CP281ZZ	CW14FZZ	CW23DZZ	CW541ZZ	D0109CZ	D0Y6FZZ	D7073ZZ	D714B7Z	D724DZZ	D9006ZZ
CG21SZZ	CP28YZZ	CW14GZZ	CW23FZZ	CW54DZZ	D0109YZ	D0Y6KZZ	D7074ZZ	D714B8Z	D724HZZ	D9010ZZ
CG21YZZ	CP291ZZ	CW14LZZ	CW23GZZ	CW54YZZ	D010B7Z	D0Y77ZZ	D7075ZZ	D714B9Z	D724JZZ	D9011ZZ
CG2YYZZ	CP29YZZ	CW14SZZ	CW23KZZ	CW561ZZ	D010B8Z	D0Y78ZZ	D7076ZZ	D714BBZ	D725DZZ	D9012ZZ
CG421ZZ	CP2B1ZZ	CW14YZZ	CW23LZZ	CW56DZZ	D010B9Z	D0Y7FZZ	D7080ZZ	D714BCZ	D725HZZ	D9013Z0
CG42FZZ	CP2BYZZ	CW161ZZ	CW23SZZ	CW56YZZ	D010BBZ	D0Y7KZZ	D7081ZZ	D714BYZ	D725JZZ	D9013ZZ
CG42GZZ	CP2C1ZZ	CW16DZZ	CW23YZZ	CW5B1ZZ	D010BCZ	D7000ZZ	D7082ZZ	D71597Z	D726DZZ	D9014ZZ
CG42YZZ	CP2CYZZ	CW16FZZ	CW241ZZ	CW5BDZZ	D010BYZ	D7001ZZ	D7083Z0	D71598Z	D726HZZ	D9015ZZ
CG4YYZZ	CP2D1ZZ	CW16GZZ	CW24DZZ	CW5BYZZ	D01197Z	D7002ZZ	D7083ZZ	D71599Z	D726JZZ	D9016ZZ
CH101ZZ	CP2DYZZ	CW16LZZ	CW24FZZ	CW5D1ZZ	D01198Z	D7003Z0	D7084ZZ	D7159BZ	D727DZZ	D9030ZZ
CH10SZZ	CP2F1ZZ	CW16SZZ	CW24GZZ	CW5DDZZ	D01199Z	D7003ZZ	D7085ZZ	D7159CZ	D727HZZ	D9031ZZ
CH10YZZ	CP2FYZZ	CW16YZZ	CW24KZZ	CW5DYZZ	D0119BZ	D7004ZZ	D7086ZZ	D7159YZ	D727JZZ	D9032ZZ
CH111ZZ	CP2G1ZZ	CW1B1ZZ	CW24LZZ	CW5J1ZZ	D0119CZ	D7005ZZ	D71097Z	D715B7Z	D728DZZ	D9033Z0
CH11SZZ	CP2GYZZ	CW1BDZZ	CW24SZZ	CW5JDZZ	D0119YZ	D7006ZZ	D71098Z	D715B8Z	D728HZZ	D9033ZZ
CH11YZZ	CP2H1ZZ	CW1BFZZ	CW24YZZ	CW5JYZZ	D011B7Z	D7010ZZ	D71099Z	D715B9Z	D728JZZ	D9034ZZ
CH121ZZ	CP2HYZZ	CW1BGZZ	CW261ZZ	CW5M1ZZ	D011B8Z	D7011ZZ	D7109BZ	D715BBZ	D7Y08ZZ	D9035ZZ
CH12SZZ	CP2J1ZZ	CW1BLZZ	CW26DZZ	CW5MDZZ	D011B9Z	D7012ZZ	D7109CZ	D715BCZ	D7Y0FZZ	D9036ZZ
CH12YZZ	CP2JYZZ	CW1BSZZ	CW26FZZ	CW5MYZZ	D011BBZ	D7013Z0	D7109YZ	D715BYZ	D7Y18ZZ	D9040ZZ
CH1YYZZ	CP2YYZZ	CW1BYZZ	CW26GZZ	CW70NZZ	D011BCZ	D7013ZZ	D710B7Z	D71697Z	D7Y1FZZ	D9041ZZ
CH201ZZ	CP55ZZZ	CW1D1ZZ	CW26KZZ	CW70YZZ	D011BYZ	D7014ZZ	D710B8Z	D71698Z	D7Y28ZZ	D9042ZZ
CH20SZZ	CP5NZZZ	CW1DDZZ	CW26LZZ	CW73NZZ	D01697Z	D7015ZZ	D710B9Z	D71699Z	D7Y2FZZ	D9043Z0
CH20YZZ	CP5PZZZ	CW1DFZZ	CW26SZZ	CW73YZZ	D01698Z	D7016ZZ	D710BBZ	D7169BZ	D7Y38ZZ	D9043ZZ
CH211ZZ	CP5YYZZ	CW1DGZZ	CW26YZZ	CW7GGZZ	D01699Z	D7020ZZ	D710BCZ	D7169CZ	D7Y3FZZ	D9044ZZ
CH21SZZ	CT131ZZ	CW1DLZZ	CW2B1ZZ	CW7GYZZ	D0169BZ	D7021ZZ	D710BYZ	D7169YZ	D7Y48ZZ	D9045ZZ
CH21YZZ	CT13FZZ	CW1DSZZ	CW2BDZZ	CW7N8ZZ	D0169CZ	D7022ZZ	D71197Z	D716B7Z	D7Y4FZZ	D9046ZZ
CH221ZZ	CT13GZZ	CW1DYZZ	CW2BFZZ	CW7NGZZ	D0169YZ	D7023Z0	D71198Z	D716B8Z	D7Y58ZZ	D9050ZZ
CH22SZZ	CT13YZZ	CW1J1ZZ	CW2BGZZ	CW7NNZZ	D016B7Z	D7023ZZ	D71199Z	D716B9Z	D7Y5FZZ	D9051ZZ
CH22YZZ	CT1H1ZZ	CW1JDZZ	CW2BKZZ	CW7NPZZ	D016B8Z	D7024ZZ	D7119BZ	D716BBZ	D7Y68ZZ	D9052ZZ
CH2YYZZ	CT1HYZZ	CW1JFZZ	CW2BLZZ	CW7NYZZ	D016B9Z	D7025ZZ	D7119CZ	D716BCZ	D7Y6FZZ	D9053Z0
CP111ZZ	CT1YYZZ	CW1JGZZ	CW2BSZZ	CW7YYZZ	D016BBZ	D7026ZZ	D7119YZ	D716BYZ	D7Y78ZZ	D9053ZZ

D9054ZZ	D910B8Z	D91798Z	D91FB8Z	D9YB8ZZ	DB086ZZ	DB179YZ	DBY8FZZ	DD10B9Z	DD1799Z	DDY8FZZ
D9055ZZ	D910B9Z	D91799Z	D91FB9Z	D9YBCZZ	DB1097Z	DB17B7Z	DBY8KZZ	DD10BBZ	DD179BZ	DDY8KZZ
D9056ZZ	D910BBZ	D9179BZ	D91FBBZ	D9YBFZZ	DB1098Z	DB17B8Z	DD000ZZ	DD10BCZ	DD179CZ	DF000ZZ
D9060ZZ	D910BCZ	D9179CZ	D91FBCZ	D9YCCZZ	DB1099Z	DB17B9Z	DD001ZZ	DD10BYZ	DD179YZ	DF001ZZ
D9061ZZ	D910BYZ	D9179YZ	D91FBYZ	D9YCFZZ	DB109BZ	DB17BBZ	DD002ZZ	DD1197Z	DD17B7Z	DF002ZZ
D9062ZZ	D91197Z	D917B7Z	D920DZZ	D9YD7ZZ	DB109CZ	DB17BCZ	DD003Z0	DD1198Z	DD17B8Z	DF003Z0
D9063Z0	D91198Z	D917B8Z	D920HZZ	D9YD8ZZ	DB109YZ	DB17BYZ	DD003ZZ	DD1199Z	DD17B9Z	DF003ZZ
D9063ZZ	D91199Z	D917B9Z	D920JZZ	D9YDCZZ	DB10B7Z	DB1897Z	DD004ZZ	DD119BZ	DD17BBZ	DF004ZZ
D9064ZZ	D9119BZ	D917BBZ	D921DZZ	D9YDFZZ	DB10B8Z	DB1898Z	DD005ZZ	DD119CZ	DD17BCZ	DF005ZZ
D9065ZZ	D9119CZ	D917BCZ	D921HZZ	D9YF7ZZ	DB10B9Z	DB1899Z	DD006ZZ	DD119YZ	DD17BYZ	DF006ZZ
D9066ZZ	D9119YZ	D917BYZ	D921JZZ	D9YF8ZZ	DB10BBZ	DB189BZ	DD010ZZ	DD11B7Z	DD20DZZ	DF010ZZ
D9070ZZ	D911B7Z	D91897Z	D924DZZ	DB000ZZ	DB10BCZ	DB189CZ	DD011ZZ	DD11B8Z	DD20HZZ	DF011ZZ
D9071ZZ	D911B8Z	D91898Z	D924HZZ	DB001ZZ	DB10BYZ	DB189YZ	DD012ZZ	DD11B9Z	DD20JZZ	DF012ZZ
D9072ZZ	D911B9Z	D91899Z	D924JZZ	DB002ZZ	DB1197Z	DB18B7Z	DD013Z0	DD11BBZ	DD21DZZ	DF013Z0
D9073Z0	D911BBZ	D9189BZ	D925DZZ	DB003Z0	DB1198Z	DB18B8Z	DD013ZZ	DD11BCZ	DD21HZZ	DF013ZZ
D9073ZZ	D911BCZ	D9189CZ	D925HZZ	DB003ZZ	DB1199Z	DB18B9Z	DD014ZZ	DD11BYZ	DD21JZZ	DF014ZZ
D9074ZZ	D911BYZ	D9189YZ	D925JZZ	DB004ZZ	DB119BZ	DB18BBZ	DD015ZZ	DD1297Z	DD22DZZ	DF015ZZ
D9075ZZ	D91397Z	D918B7Z	D926DZZ	DB005ZZ	DB119CZ	DB18BCZ	DD016ZZ	DD1298Z	DD22HZZ	DF016ZZ
D9076ZZ	D91398Z	D918B8Z	D926HZZ	DB006ZZ	DB119YZ	DB18BYZ	DD020ZZ	DD1299Z	DD22JZZ	DF020ZZ
D9080ZZ	D91399Z	D918B9Z	D926JZZ	DB010ZZ	DB11B7Z	DB20DZZ	DD021ZZ	DD129BZ	DD23DZZ	DF021ZZ
D9081ZZ	D9139BZ	D918BBZ	D927DZZ	DB011ZZ	DB11B8Z	DB20HZZ	DD022ZZ	DD129CZ	DD23HZZ	DF022ZZ
D9082ZZ	D9139CZ	D918BCZ	D927HZZ	DB012ZZ	DB11B9Z	DB20JZZ	DD023Z0	DD129YZ	DD23JZZ	DF023Z0
D9083Z0	D9139YZ	D918BYZ	D927JZZ	DB013Z0	DB11BBZ	DB21DZZ	DD023ZZ	DD12B7Z	DD24DZZ	DF023ZZ
D9083ZZ	D913B7Z	D91997Z	D928DZZ	DB013ZZ	DB11BCZ	DB21HZZ	DD024ZZ	DD12B8Z	DD24HZZ	DF024ZZ
D9084ZZ	D913B8Z	D91998Z	D928HZZ	DB014ZZ	DB11BYZ	DB21JZZ	DD025ZZ	DD12B9Z	DD24JZZ	DF025ZZ
D9085ZZ	D913B9Z	D91999Z	D928JZZ	DB015ZZ	DB1297Z	DB22DZZ	DD026ZZ	DD12BBZ	DD25DZZ	DF026ZZ
D9086ZZ	D913BBZ	D9199BZ	D929DZZ	DB016ZZ	DB1298Z	DB22HZZ	DD030ZZ	DD12BCZ	DD25HZZ	DF030ZZ
D9090ZZ	D913BCZ	D9199CZ	D929HZZ	DB020ZZ	DB1299Z	DB22JZZ	DD031ZZ	DD12BYZ	DD25JZZ	DF031ZZ
D9091ZZ	D913BYZ	D9199YZ	D929JZZ	DB021ZZ	DB129BZ	DB25DZZ	DD032ZZ	DD1397Z	DD27DZZ	DF032ZZ
D9092ZZ	D91497Z	D919B7Z	D92BDZZ	DB022ZZ	DB129CZ	DB25HZZ	DD033Z0	DD1398Z	DD27HZZ	DF033Z0
D9093Z0	D91498Z	D919B8Z	D92BHZZ	DB023Z0	DB129YZ	DB25JZZ	DD033ZZ	DD1399Z	DD27JZZ	DF033ZZ
D9093ZZ	D91499Z	D919B9Z	D92BJZZ	DB023ZZ	DB12B7Z	DB26DZZ	DD034ZZ	DD139BZ	DDY07ZZ	DF034ZZ
D9094ZZ	D9149BZ	D919BBZ	D92CDZZ	DB024ZZ	DB12B8Z	DB26HZZ	DD035ZZ	DD139CZ	DDY08ZZ	DF035ZZ
D9095ZZ	D9149CZ	D919BCZ	D92CHZZ	DB025ZZ	DB12B9Z	DB26JZZ	DD036ZZ	DD139YZ	DDY0FZZ	DF036ZZ
D9096ZZ	D9149YZ	D919BYZ	D92CJZZ	DB026ZZ	DB12BBZ	DB27DZZ	DD040ZZ	DD13B7Z	DDY0KZZ	DF1097Z
D90B0ZZ	D914B7Z	D91B97Z	D92DDZZ	DB050ZZ	DB12BCZ	DB27HZZ	DD041ZZ	DD13B8Z	DDY17ZZ	DF1098Z
D90B1ZZ	D914B8Z	D91B98Z	D92DHZZ	DB051ZZ	DB12BYZ	DB27JZZ	DD042ZZ	DD13B9Z	DDY18ZZ	DF1099Z
D90B2ZZ	D914B9Z	D91B99Z	D92DJZZ	DB052ZZ	DB1597Z	DB28DZZ	DD043Z0	DD13BBZ	DDY1CZZ	DF109BZ
D90B3Z0	D914BBZ	D91B9BZ	D9Y07ZZ	DB053Z0	DB1598Z	DB28HZZ	DD043ZZ	DD13BCZ	DDY1FZZ	DF109CZ
D90B3ZZ	D914BCZ	D91B9CZ	D9Y08ZZ	DB053ZZ	DB1599Z	DB28JZZ	DD044ZZ	DD13BYZ	DDY1KZZ	DF109YZ
D90B4ZZ	D914BYZ	D91B9YZ	D9Y0FZZ	DB054ZZ	DB159BZ	DBY07ZZ	DD045ZZ	DD1497Z	DDY27ZZ	DF10B7Z
D90B5ZZ	D91597Z	D91BB7Z	D9Y17ZZ	DB055ZZ	DB159CZ	DBY08ZZ	DD046ZZ	DD1498Z	DDY28ZZ	DF10B8Z
D90B6ZZ	D91598Z	D91BB8Z	D9Y18ZZ	DB056ZZ	DB159YZ	DBY0FZZ	DD050ZZ	DD1499Z	DDY2CZZ	DF10B9Z
D90D0ZZ	D91599Z	D91BB9Z	D9Y1FZZ	DB060ZZ	DB15B7Z	DBY0KZZ	DD051ZZ	DD149BZ	DDY2FZZ	DF10BBZ
D90D1ZZ	D9159BZ	D91BBBZ	D9Y37ZZ	DB061ZZ	DB15B8Z	DBY17ZZ	DD052ZZ	DD149CZ	DDY2KZZ	DF10BCZ
D90D2ZZ	D9159CZ	D91BBCZ	D9Y38ZZ	DB062ZZ	DB15B9Z	DBY18ZZ	DD053Z0	DD149YZ	DDY37ZZ	DF10BYZ
D90D3Z0	D9159YZ	D91BBYZ	D9Y47ZZ	DB063Z0	DB15BBZ	DBY1FZZ	DD053ZZ	DD14B7Z	DDY38ZZ	DF1197Z
D90D3ZZ	D915B7Z	D91D97Z	D9Y48ZZ	DB063ZZ	DB15BCZ	DBY1KZZ	DD054ZZ	DD14B8Z	DDY3CZZ	DF1198Z
D90D4ZZ	D915B8Z	D91D98Z	D9Y4CZZ	DB064ZZ	DB15BYZ	DBY27ZZ	DD055ZZ	DD14B9Z	DDY3FZZ	DF1199Z
D90D5ZZ	D915B9Z	D91D99Z	D9Y4FZZ	DB065ZZ	DB1697Z	DBY28ZZ	DD056ZZ	DD14BBZ	DDY3KZZ	DF119BZ
D90D6ZZ	D915BBZ	D91D9BZ	D9Y57ZZ	DB066ZZ	DB1698Z	DBY2FZZ	DD070ZZ	DD14BCZ	DDY47ZZ	DF119CZ
D90F0ZZ	D915BCZ	D91D9CZ	D9Y58ZZ	DB070ZZ	DB1699Z	DBY2KZZ	DD071ZZ	DD14BYZ	DDY48ZZ	DF119YZ
D90F1ZZ	D915BYZ	D91D9YZ	D9Y5FZZ	DB071ZZ	DB169BZ	DBY57ZZ	DD072ZZ	DD1597Z	DDY4CZZ	DF11B7Z
D90F2ZZ	D91697Z	D91DB7Z	D9Y67ZZ	DB072ZZ	DB169CZ	DBY58ZZ	DD073Z0	DD1598Z	DDY4FZZ	DF11B8Z
D90F3Z0	D91698Z	D91DB8Z	D9Y68ZZ	DB073Z0	DB169YZ	DBY5FZZ	DD073ZZ	DD1599Z	DDY4KZZ	DF11B9Z
D90F3ZZ	D91699Z	D91DB9Z	D9Y6FZZ	DB073ZZ	DB16B7Z	DBY5KZZ	DD074ZZ	DD159BZ	DDY57ZZ	DF11BBZ
D90F4ZZ	D9169BZ	D91DBBZ	D9Y77ZZ	DB074ZZ	DB16B8Z	DBY67ZZ	DD075ZZ	DD159CZ	DDY58ZZ	DF11BCZ
D90F5ZZ	D9169CZ	D91DBCZ	D9Y78ZZ	DB075ZZ	DB16B9Z	DBY68ZZ	DD076ZZ	DD159YZ	DDY5CZZ	DF11BYZ
D90F6ZZ	D9169YZ	D91DBYZ	D9Y7FZZ	DB076ZZ	DB16BBZ	DBY6FZZ	DD1097Z	DD15B7Z	DDY5FZZ	DF1297Z
D91097Z	D916B7Z	D91F97Z	D9Y87ZZ	DB080ZZ	DB16BCZ	DBY6KZZ	DD1098Z	DD15B8Z	DDY5KZZ	DF1298Z
D91098Z	D916B8Z	D91F98Z	D9Y88ZZ	DB081ZZ	DB16BYZ	DBY77ZZ	DD1099Z	DD15B9Z	DDY77ZZ	DF1299Z
D91099Z	D916B9Z	D91F99Z	D9Y8FZZ	DB082ZZ	DB1797Z	DBY78ZZ	DD109BZ	DD15BBZ	DDY78ZZ	DF129BZ
D9109BZ	D916BBZ	D91F9BZ	D9Y97ZZ	DB083Z0	DB1798Z	DBY7FZZ	DD109CZ	DD15BCZ	DDY7CZZ	DF129CZ
D9109CZ	D916BCZ	D91F9CZ	D9Y98ZZ	DB083ZZ	DB1799Z	DBY7KZZ	DD109YZ	DD15BYZ	DDY7FZZ	DF129YZ
D9109YZ	D916BYZ	D91F9YZ	D9Y9FZZ	DB084ZZ	DB179BZ	DBY87ZZ	DD10B7Z	DD1797Z	DDY7KZZ	DF12B7Z
D910B7Z	D91797Z	D91FB7Z	D9YB7ZZ	DB085ZZ	DB179CZ	DBY88ZZ	DD10B8Z	DD1798Z	DDY8CZZ	DF12B8Z

DF12B9Z	DG023ZZ	DG1598Z	DH072ZZ	DM012ZZ	DP043ZZ	DPY37ZZ	DT10B8Z	DU011ZZ	DV003Z0	DW034ZZ
DF12BBZ	DG025ZZ	DG1599Z	DH073Z0	DM013Z0	DP044ZZ	DPY38ZZ	DT10B9Z	DU012ZZ	DV003ZZ	DW035ZZ
DF12BCZ	DG026ZZ	DG159BZ	DH073ZZ	DM013ZZ	DP045ZZ	DPY3FZZ	DT10BBZ	DU013Z0	DV004ZZ	DW036ZZ
DF12BYZ	DG040ZZ	DG159CZ	DH074ZZ	DM014ZZ	DP046ZZ	DPY47ZZ	DT10BCZ	DU013ZZ	DV005ZZ	DW040ZZ
DF1397Z	DG041ZZ	DG159YZ	DH075ZZ	DM015ZZ	DP050ZZ	DPY48ZZ	DT10BYZ	DU014ZZ	DV006ZZ	DW041ZZ
DF1398Z	DG042ZZ	DG15B7Z	DH076ZZ	DM016ZZ	DP051ZZ	DPY4FZZ	DT1197Z	DU015ZZ	DV010ZZ	DW042ZZ
DF1399Z	DG043Z0	DG15B8Z	DH080ZZ	DM1097Z	DP052ZZ	DPY57ZZ	DT1198Z	DU016ZZ	DV011ZZ	DW043Z0
DF139BZ	DG043ZZ	DG15B9Z	DH081ZZ	DM1098Z	DP053Z0	DPY58ZZ	DT1199Z	DU020ZZ	DV012ZZ	DW043ZZ
DF139CZ	DG045ZZ	DG15BBZ	DH082ZZ	DM1099Z	DP053ZZ	DPY5FZZ	DT119BZ	DU021ZZ	DV013Z0	DW044ZZ
DF139YZ	DG046ZZ	DG15BCZ	DH083Z0	DM109BZ	DP054ZZ	DPY67ZZ	DT119CZ	DU022ZZ	DV013ZZ	DW045ZZ
DF13B7Z	DG050ZZ	DG15BYZ	DH083ZZ	DM109CZ	DP055ZZ	DPY68ZZ	DT119YZ	DU023Z0	DV014ZZ	DW046ZZ
DF13B8Z	DG051ZZ	DG20DZZ	DH084ZZ	DM109YZ	DP056ZZ	DPY6FZZ	DT11B7Z	DU023ZZ	DV015ZZ	DW050ZZ
DF13B9Z	DG052ZZ	DGY07ZZ	DH085ZZ	DM10B7Z	DP060ZZ	DPY77ZZ	DT11B8Z	DU024ZZ	DV016ZZ	DW051ZZ
DF13BBZ	DG053Z0	DGY08ZZ	DH086ZZ	DM10B8Z	DP061ZZ	DPY78ZZ	DT11B9Z	DU025ZZ	DV1097Z	DW052ZZ
DF13BCZ	DG053ZZ	DGY0FZZ	DH090ZZ	DM10B9Z	DP062ZZ	DPY7FZZ	DT11BBZ	DU026ZZ	DV1098Z	DW053Z0
DF13BYZ	DG055ZZ	DGY0KZZ	DH091ZZ	DM10BBZ	DP063Z0	DPY87ZZ	DT11BCZ	DU1097Z	DV1099Z	DW053ZZ
DF20DZZ	DG056ZZ	DGY17ZZ	DH092ZZ	DM10BCZ	DP063ZZ	DPY88ZZ	DT11BYZ	DU1098Z	DV109BZ	DW054ZZ
DF20HZZ	DG1097Z	DGY18ZZ	DH093Z0	DM10BYZ	DP064ZZ	DPY8FZZ	DT1297Z	DU1099Z	DV109CZ	DW055ZZ
DF20JZZ	DG1098Z	DGY1FZZ	DH093ZZ	DM1197Z	DP065ZZ	DPY97ZZ	DT1298Z	DU109BZ	DV109YZ	DW056ZZ
DF21DZZ	DG1099Z	DGY1KZZ	DH094ZZ	DM1198Z	DP066ZZ	DPY98ZZ	DT1299Z	DU109CZ	DV10B7Z	DW060ZZ
DF21HZZ	DG109BZ	DGY27ZZ	DH095ZZ	DM1199Z	DP070ZZ	DPY9FZZ	DT129BZ	DU109YZ	DV10B8Z	DW061ZZ
DF21JZZ	DG109CZ	DGY28ZZ	DH096ZZ	DM119BZ	DP071ZZ	DPYB7ZZ	DT129CZ	DU10B7Z	DV10B9Z	DW062ZZ
DF22DZZ	DG109YZ	DGY2FZZ	DH0B0ZZ	DM119CZ	DP072ZZ	DPYB8ZZ	DT129YZ	DU10B8Z	DV10BBZ	DW063Z0
DF22HZZ	DG10B7Z	DGY2KZZ	DH0B1ZZ	DM119YZ	DP073Z0	DPYBFZZ	DT12B7Z	DU10B9Z	DV10BCZ	DW063ZZ
DF22JZZ	DG10B8Z	DGY47ZZ	DH0B2ZZ	DM11B7Z	DP073ZZ	DPYC7ZZ	DT12B8Z	DU10BBZ	DV10BYZ	DW064ZZ
DF23DZZ	DG10B9Z	DGY48ZZ	DH0B3Z0	DM11B8Z	DP074ZZ	DPYC8ZZ	DT12B9Z	DU10BCZ	DV1197Z	DW065ZZ
DF23HZZ	DG10BBZ	DGY4FZZ	DH0B3ZZ	DM11B9Z	DP075ZZ	DPYCFZZ	DT12BBZ	DU10BYZ	DV1198Z	DW066ZZ
DF23JZZ	DG10BCZ	DGY4KZZ	DH0B4ZZ	DM11BBZ	DP076ZZ	DT000ZZ	DT12BCZ	DU1197Z	DV1199Z	DW1197Z
DFY07ZZ	DG10BYZ	DGY57ZZ	DH0B5ZZ	DM11BCZ	DP080ZZ	DT001ZZ	DT12BYZ	DU1198Z	DV119BZ	DW1198Z
DFY08ZZ	DG1197Z	DGY58ZZ	DH0B6ZZ	DM11BYZ	DP081ZZ	DT002ZZ	DT1397Z	DU1199Z	DV119CZ	DW1199Z
DFY0CZZ	DG1198Z	DGY5FZZ	DHY27ZZ	DMY07ZZ	DP082ZZ	DT003Z0	DT1398Z	DU119BZ	DV119YZ	DW119BZ
DFY0FZZ	DG1199Z	DGY5KZZ	DHY28ZZ	DMY08ZZ	DP083Z0	DT003ZZ	DT1399Z	DU119CZ	DV11B7Z	DW119CZ
DFY0KZZ	DG119BZ	DH020ZZ	DHY2FZZ	DMY0FZZ	DP083ZZ	DT004ZZ	DT139BZ	DU119YZ	DV11B8Z	DW119YZ
DFY17ZZ	DG119CZ	DH021ZZ	DHY37ZZ	DMY0KZZ	DP084ZZ	DT005ZZ	DT139CZ	DU11B7Z	DV11B9Z	DW11B7Z
DFY18ZZ	DG119YZ	DH022ZZ	DHY38ZZ	DMY17ZZ	DP085ZZ	DT006ZZ	DT139YZ	DU11B8Z	DV11BBZ	DW11B8Z
DFY1CZZ	DG11B7Z	DH023Z0	DHY3FZZ	DMY18ZZ	DP086ZZ	DT010ZZ	DT13B7Z	DU11B9Z	DV11BCZ	DW11B9Z
DFY1FZZ	DG11B8Z	DH023ZZ	DHY47ZZ	DMY1FZZ	DP090ZZ	DT011ZZ	DT13B8Z	DU11BBZ	DV11BYZ	DW11BBZ
DFY1KZZ	DG11B9Z	DH024ZZ	DHY48ZZ	DMY1KZZ	DP091ZZ	DT012ZZ	DT13B9Z	DU11BCZ	DVY07ZZ	DW11BCZ
DFY27ZZ	DG11BBZ	DH025ZZ	DHY4FZZ	DP000ZZ	DP092ZZ	DT013Z0	DT13BBZ	DU11BYZ	DVY08ZZ	DW11BYZ
DFY28ZZ	DG11BCZ	DH026ZZ	DHY5FZZ	DP001ZZ	DP093Z0	DT013ZZ	DT13BCZ	DU1297Z	DVY0CZZ	DW1297Z
DFY2CZZ	DG11BYZ	DH030ZZ	DHY67ZZ	DP002ZZ	DP093ZZ	DT014ZZ	DT13BYZ	DU1298Z	DVY0FZZ	DW1298Z
DFY2FZZ	DG1297Z	DH031ZZ	DHY68ZZ	DP003Z0	DP094ZZ	DT015ZZ	DTY07ZZ	DU1299Z	DVY0KZZ	DW1299Z
DFY2KZZ	DG1298Z	DH032ZZ	DHY6FZZ	DP003ZZ	DP095ZZ	DT016ZZ	DTY08ZZ	DU129BZ	DVY17ZZ	DW129BZ
DFY37ZZ	DG1299Z	DH033Z0	DHY77ZZ	DP004ZZ	DP096ZZ	DT020ZZ	DTY0CZZ	DU129CZ	DVY18ZZ	DW129CZ
DFY38ZZ	DG129BZ	DH033ZZ	DHY78ZZ	DP005ZZ	DP0B0ZZ	DT021ZZ	DTY0FZZ	DU129YZ	DVY1FZZ	DW129YZ
DFY3CZZ	DG129CZ	DH034ZZ	DHY7FZZ	DP006ZZ	DP0B1ZZ	DT022ZZ	DTY17ZZ	DU12B7Z	DW010ZZ	DW12B7Z
DFY3FZZ	DG129YZ	DH035ZZ	DHY87ZZ	DP020ZZ	DP0B2ZZ	DT023Z0	DTY18ZZ	DU12B8Z	DW011ZZ	DW12B8Z
DFY3KZZ	DG12B7Z	DH036ZZ	DHY88ZZ	DP021ZZ	DP0B3Z0	DT023ZZ	DTY1CZZ	DU12B9Z	DW012ZZ	DW12B9Z
DG000ZZ	DG12B8Z	DH040ZZ	DHY8FZZ	DP022ZZ	DP0B3ZZ	DT024ZZ	DTY1FZZ	DU12BBZ	DW013Z0	DW12BBZ
DG001ZZ	DG12B9Z	DH041ZZ	DHY97ZZ	DP023Z0	DP0B4ZZ	DT025ZZ	DTY27ZZ	DU12BCZ	DW013ZZ	DW12BCZ
DG002ZZ	DG12BBZ	DH042ZZ	DHY98ZZ	DP023ZZ	DP0B5ZZ	DT026ZZ	DTY28ZZ	DU12BYZ	DW014ZZ	DW12BYZ
DG003Z0	DG12BCZ	DH043Z0	DHY9FZZ	DP024ZZ	DP0B6ZZ	DT030ZZ	DTY2CZZ	DUY07ZZ	DW015ZZ	DW1397Z
DG003ZZ	DG12BYZ	DH043ZZ	DHYB7ZZ	DP025ZZ	DP0C0ZZ	DT031ZZ	DTY2FZZ	DUY08ZZ	DW016ZZ	DW1398Z
DG005ZZ	DG1497Z	DH044ZZ	DHYB8ZZ	DP026ZZ	DP0C1ZZ	DT032ZZ	DTY37ZZ	DUY0CZZ	DW020ZZ	DW1399Z
DG006ZZ	DG1498Z	DH045ZZ	DHYBFZZ	DP030ZZ	DP0C2ZZ	DT033Z0	DTY38ZZ	DUY0FZZ	DW021ZZ	DW139BZ
DG010ZZ	DG1499Z	DH046ZZ	DHYCFZZ	DP031ZZ	DP0C3Z0	DT033ZZ	DTY3CZZ	DUY17ZZ	DW022ZZ	DW139CZ
DG011ZZ	DG149BZ	DH060ZZ	DM000ZZ	DP032ZZ	DP0C3ZZ	DT034ZZ	DTY3FZZ	DUY18ZZ	DW023Z0	DW139YZ
DG012ZZ	DG149CZ	DH061ZZ	DM001ZZ	DP033Z0	DP0C4ZZ	DT035ZZ	DU000ZZ	DUY1CZZ	DW023ZZ	DW13B7Z
DG013Z0	DG149YZ	DH062ZZ	DM002ZZ	DP033ZZ	DP0C5ZZ	DT036ZZ	DU001ZZ	DUY1FZZ	DW024ZZ	DW13B8Z
DG013ZZ	DG14B7Z	DH063Z0	DM003Z0	DP034ZZ	DP0C6ZZ	DT1097Z	DU002ZZ	DUY27ZZ	DW025ZZ	DW13B9Z
DG015ZZ	DG14B8Z	DH063ZZ	DM003ZZ	DP035ZZ	DPY07ZZ	DT1098Z	DU003Z0	DUY28ZZ	DW026ZZ	DW13BBZ
DG016ZZ	DG14B9Z	DH064ZZ	DM004ZZ	DP036ZZ	DPY08ZZ	DT1099Z	DU003ZZ	DUY2CZZ	DW030ZZ	DW13BCZ
DG020ZZ	DG14BBZ	DH065ZZ	DM005ZZ	DP040ZZ	DPY0FZZ	DT109BZ	DU004ZZ	DUY2FZZ	DW031ZZ	DW13BYZ
DG021ZZ	DG14BCZ	DH066ZZ	DM006ZZ	DP041ZZ	DPY27ZZ	DT109CZ	DU005ZZ	DV000ZZ	DW032ZZ	DW1697Z
DG022ZZ	DG14BYZ	DH070ZZ	DM010ZZ	DP042ZZ	DPY28ZZ	DT109YZ	DU006ZZ	DV001ZZ	DW033Z0	DW1698Z
DG023Z0	DG1597Z	DH071ZZ	DM011ZZ	DP043Z0	DPY2FZZ	DT10B7Z	DU010ZZ	DV002ZZ	DW033ZZ	DW1699Z

DW169BZ	F0123ZZ	F01J5YZ	F0209YZ	F02Z4EZ	F06Z5ZZ	F0706CZ	F0726GZ	F0766ZZ	F07D3EZ	F07G3ZZ
DW169CZ	F0124ZZ	F01J5ZZ	F0209ZZ	F02Z4FZ	F06Z6KZ	F0706DZ	F0726HZ	F0776BZ	F07D3FZ	F07G6BZ
DW169YZ	F0125YZ	F01J6YZ	F020DYZ	F02Z4UZ	F06Z6MZ	F0706EZ	F0726UZ	F0776CZ	F07D3UZ	F07G6CZ
DW16B7Z	F0125ZZ	F01J6ZZ	F020DZZ	F02Z4ZZ	F06Z6PZ	F0706FZ	F0726YZ	F0776DZ	F07D3YZ	F07G6DZ
DW16B8Z	F0126YZ	F01K0EZ	F021DYZ	F02Z5KZ	F06Z6YZ	F0706GZ	F0726ZZ	F0776EZ	F07D3ZZ	F07G6EZ
DW16B9Z	F0126ZZ	F01K0FZ	F021DZZ	F02Z5MZ	F06Z6ZZ	F0706HZ	F0727ZZ	F0776FZ	F07D6BZ	F07G6FZ
DW16BBZ	F012GZZ	F01K0UZ	F022DYZ	F02Z5NZ	F06Z74Z	F0706UZ	F0730EZ	F0776GZ	F07D6CZ	F07G6GZ
DW16BCZ	F0130EZ	F01K0YZ	F022DZZ	F02Z5PZ	F06Z7KZ	F0706YZ	F0730FZ	F0776HZ	F07D6DZ	F07G6HZ
DW16BYZ	F0130FZ	F01K0ZZ	F023DYZ	F02Z5QZ	F06Z7NZ	F0706ZZ	F0730UZ	F0776UZ	F07D6EZ	F07G6UZ
DWY17ZZ	F0130UZ	F01K1ZZ	F023DZZ	F02Z5SZ	F06Z7QZ	F0707ZZ	F0730YZ	F0776YZ	F07D6FZ	F07G6YZ
DWY18ZZ	F0130YZ	F01K5YZ	F024GCZ	F02Z5YZ	F06Z7SZ	F0710EZ	F0730ZZ	F0776ZZ	F07D6GZ	F07G6ZZ
DWY1FZZ	F0130ZZ	F01K5ZZ	F024GGZ	F02Z5ZZ	F06Z7TZ	F0710FZ	F0731EZ	F0786BZ	F07D6HZ	F07G7ZZ
DWY27ZZ	F0131ZZ	F01K6YZ	F024GYZ	F02Z6ZZ	F06Z7YZ	F0710UZ	F0731FZ	F0786CZ	F07D6UZ	F07H0EZ
DWY28ZZ	F0133ZZ	F01K6ZZ	F024GZZ	F02Z8YZ	F06Z7ZZ	F0710YZ	F0731UZ	F0786DZ	F07D6YZ	F07H0FZ
DWY2FZZ	F0134ZZ	F01L0EZ	F025GCZ	F02Z8ZZ	F06Z8KZ	F0710ZZ	F0731YZ	F0786EZ	F07D6ZZ	F07H0UZ
DWY37ZZ	F0135YZ	F01L0FZ	F025GGZ	F02ZBEZ	F06Z8NZ	F0711EZ	F0731ZZ	F0786FZ	F07D7ZZ	F07H0YZ
DWY38ZZ	F0135ZZ	F01L0UZ	F025GYZ	F02ZBFZ	F06Z8PZ	F0711FZ	F0732EZ	F0786GZ	F07F0EZ	F07H0ZZ
DWY3FZZ	F0136YZ	F01L0YZ	F025GZZ	F02ZBUZ	F06Z8QZ	F0711UZ	F0732FZ	F0786HZ	F07F0FZ	F07H1EZ
DWY47ZZ	F0136ZZ	F01L0ZZ	F026GCZ	F02ZBYZ	F06Z8SZ	F0711YZ	F0732UZ	F0786UZ	F07F0UZ	F07H1FZ
DWY48ZZ	F013GZZ	F01L1ZZ	F026GGZ	F02ZBZZ	F06Z8TZ	F0711ZZ	F0732YZ	F0786YZ	F07F0YZ	F07H1UZ
DWY4FZZ	F01D0EZ	F01L5YZ	F026GYZ	F02ZCEZ	F06Z8YZ	F0712EZ	F0732ZZ	F0786ZZ	F07F0ZZ	F07H1YZ
DWY57ZZ	F01D0FZ	F01L5ZZ	F026GZZ	F02ZCFZ	F06Z8ZZ	F0712FZ	F0733EZ	F0796BZ	F07F1EZ	F07H1ZZ
DWY58ZZ	F01D0UZ	F01L6YZ	F0277EZ	F02ZCUZ	F06Z9KZ	F0712UZ	F0733FZ	F0796CZ	F07F1FZ	F07H2EZ
DWY5FZZ	F01D0YZ	F01L6ZZ	F0277GZ	F02ZCYZ	F06Z9PZ	F0712YZ	F0733UZ	F0796DZ	F07F1UZ	F07H2FZ
DWY5GDZ	F01D0ZZ	F01M0EZ	F0277UZ	F02ZCZZ	F06Z9YZ	F0712ZZ	F0733YZ	F0796EZ	F07F1YZ	F07H2UZ
DWY5GFZ	F01D1ZZ	F01M0FZ	F0277YZ	F02ZFYZ	F06Z9ZZ	F0713EZ	F0733ZZ	F0796FZ	F07F1ZZ	F07H2YZ
DWY5GGZ	F01D5YZ	F01M0UZ	F0277ZZ	F02ZFZZ	F06ZBKZ	F0713FZ	F0736BZ	F0796GZ	F07F2EZ	F07H2ZZ
DWY5GHZ	F01D5ZZ	F01M0YZ	F027GCZ	F02ZHEZ	F06ZBLZ	F0713UZ	F0736CZ	F0796HZ	F07F2FZ	F07H3EZ
DWY5GYZ	F01D6YZ	F01M0ZZ	F027GGZ	F02ZHFZ	F06ZBMZ	F0713YZ	F0736DZ	F0796UZ	F07F2UZ	F07H3FZ
DWY67ZZ	F01D6ZZ	F01M1ZZ	F027GYZ	F02ZHGZ	F06ZBPZ	F0713ZZ	F0736EZ	F0796YZ	F07F2YZ	F07H3UZ
DWY68ZZ	F01F0EZ	F01M5YZ	F027GZZ	F02ZHUZ	F06ZBYZ	F0716BZ	F0736FZ	F0796ZZ	F07F2ZZ	F07H3YZ
DWY6FZZ	F01F0FZ	F01M5ZZ	F028GCZ	F02ZHYZ	F06ZBZZ	F0716CZ	F0736GZ	F07B6BZ	F07F3EZ	F07H3ZZ
F00ZWZZ	F01F0UZ	F01M6YZ	F028GGZ	F02ZHZZ	F06ZCKZ	F0716DZ	F0736HZ	F07B6CZ	F07F3FZ	F07H6BZ
F00ZXZZ	F01F0YZ	F01M6ZZ	F028GYZ	F0636KZ	F06ZCNZ	F0716EZ	F0736UZ	F07B6DZ	F07F3UZ	F07H6CZ
F0100EZ	F01F0ZZ	F01N0EZ	F028GZZ	F0636MZ	F06ZCPZ	F0716FZ	F0736YZ	F07B6EZ	F07F3YZ	F07H6DZ
F0100FZ	F01F1ZZ	F01N0FZ	F029GCZ	F0636PZ	F06ZCSZ	F0716GZ	F0736ZZ	F07B6FZ	F07F3ZZ	F07H6EZ
F0100UZ	F01F5YZ	F01N0UZ	F029GGZ	F0636YZ	F06ZCTZ	F0716HZ	F0737ZZ	F07B6GZ	F07F6BZ	F07H6FZ
F0100YZ	F01F5ZZ	F01N0YZ	F029GYZ	F0636ZZ	F06ZCVZ	F0716UZ	F0746BZ	F07B6HZ	F07F6CZ	F07H6GZ
F0100ZZ	F01F6YZ	F01N0ZZ	F029GZZ	F06Z0KZ	F06ZCYZ	F0716YZ	F0746CZ	F07B6UZ	F07F6DZ	F07H6HZ
F0101ZZ	F01F6ZZ	F01Z2KZ	F02BGCZ	F06Z0MZ	F06ZCZZ	F0716ZZ	F0746DZ	F07B6YZ	F07F6EZ	F07H6UZ
F0103ZZ	F01G0EZ	F01Z2MZ	F02BGGZ	F06Z0PZ	F06ZDMZ	F0717ZZ	F0746EZ	F07B6ZZ	F07F6FZ	F07H6YZ
F0104ZZ	F01G0FZ	F01Z2NZ	F02BGYZ	F06Z0YZ	F06ZDTZ	F0720EZ	F0746FZ	F07C6BZ	F07F6GZ	F07H6ZZ
F0105YZ	F01G0UZ	F01Z2PZ	F02BGZZ	F06Z0ZZ	F06ZDVZ	F0720FZ	F0746GZ	F07C6CZ	F07F6HZ	F07H7ZZ
F0105ZZ	F01G0YZ	F01Z2QZ	F02C7EZ	F06Z1KZ	F06ZDYZ	F0720UZ	F0746HZ	F07C6DZ	F07F6UZ	F07J0EZ
F0106YZ	F01G0ZZ	F01Z2SZ	F02C7GZ	F06Z1ZZ	F06ZDZZ	F0720YZ	F0746UZ	F07C6EZ	F07F6YZ	F07J0FZ
F0106ZZ	F01G1ZZ	F01Z2YZ	F02C7UZ	F06Z2KZ	F0700EZ	F0720ZZ	F0746YZ	F07C6FZ	F07F6ZZ	F07J0UZ
F010GZZ	F01G5YZ	F01Z2ZZ	F02C7YZ	F06Z2ZZ	F0700FZ	F0721EZ	F0746ZZ	F07C6GZ	F07F7ZZ	F07J0YZ
F0110EZ	F01G5ZZ	F01Z77Z	F02C7ZZ	F06Z3KZ	F0700UZ	F0721FZ	F0756BZ	F07C6UZ	F07G0EZ	F07J0ZZ
F0110FZ	F01G6YZ	F01Z9JZ	F02CGCZ	F06Z3MZ	F0700YZ	F0721UZ	F0756CZ	F07C6YZ	F07G0FZ	F07J1EZ
F0110UZ	F01G6ZZ	F01ZBEZ	F02CGGZ	F06Z3PZ	F0700ZZ	F0721YZ	F0756DZ	F07C6ZZ	F07G0UZ	F07J1FZ
F0110YZ	F01H0EZ	F01ZBFZ	F02CGYZ	F06Z3YZ	F0701EZ	F0721ZZ	F0756EZ	F07D0EZ	F07G0YZ	F07J1UZ
F0110ZZ	F01H0FZ	F01ZBUZ	F02CGZZ	F06Z3ZZ	F0701FZ	F0722EZ	F0756FZ	F07D0FZ	F07G0ZZ	F07J1YZ
F0111ZZ	F01H0UZ	F01ZBZZ	F02Z0EZ	F06Z4KZ	F0701UZ	F0722FZ	F0756GZ	F07D0UZ	F07G1EZ	F07J1ZZ
F0113ZZ	F01H0YZ	F01ZCEZ	F02Z0FZ	F06Z4PZ	F0701YZ	F0722UZ	F0756HZ	F07D0YZ	F07G1FZ	F07J2EZ
F0114ZZ	F01H0ZZ	F01ZCFZ	F02Z0UZ	F06Z4QZ	F0701ZZ	F0722YZ	F0756UZ	F07D0ZZ	F07G1UZ	F07J2FZ
F0115YZ	F01H1ZZ	F01ZCUZ	F02Z0ZZ	F06Z4TZ	F0702EZ	F0722ZZ	F0756YZ	F07D1EZ	F07G1YZ	F07J2UZ
F0115ZZ	F01H5YZ	F01ZCZZ	F02Z1EZ	F06Z4YZ	F0702FZ	F0723EZ	F0756ZZ	F07D1FZ	F07G1ZZ	F07J2YZ
F0116YZ	F01H5ZZ	F01ZDEZ	F02Z1FZ	F06Z4ZZ	F0702UZ	F0723FZ	F0766BZ	F07D1UZ	F07G2EZ	F07J2ZZ
F0116ZZ	F01H6YZ	F01ZDFZ	F02Z1UZ	F06Z5KZ	F0702YZ	F0723UZ	F0766CZ	F07D1YZ	F07G2FZ	F07J3EZ
F011GZZ	F01H6ZZ	F01ZDUZ	F02Z1ZZ	F06Z5LZ	F0702ZZ	F0723YZ	F0766DZ	F07D1ZZ	F07G2UZ	F07J3FZ
F0120EZ	F01J0EZ	F01ZDYZ	F02Z2YZ	F06Z5MZ	F0703EZ	F0723ZZ	F0766EZ	F07D2EZ	F07G2YZ	F07J3UZ
F0120FZ	F01J0FZ	F01ZDZZ	F02Z2ZZ	F06Z5NZ	F0703FZ	F0726BZ	F0766FZ	F07D2FZ	F07G2ZZ	F07J3YZ
F0120UZ	F01J0UZ	F01ZFEZ	F02Z3EZ	F06Z5PZ	F0703UZ	F0726CZ	F0766GZ	F07D2UZ	F07G3EZ	F07J3ZZ
F0120YZ	F01J0YZ	F01ZFFZ	F02Z3FZ	F06Z5QZ	F0703YZ	F0726DZ	F0766HZ	F07D2YZ	F07G3FZ	F07J6BZ
F0120ZZ	F01J0ZZ	F01ZFUZ	F02Z3UZ	F06Z5SZ	F0703ZZ	F0726EZ	F0766UZ	F07D2ZZ	F07G3UZ	F07J6CZ
F0121ZZ	F01J1ZZ	F01ZFZZ	F02Z3ZZ	F06Z5YZ	F0706BZ	F0726FZ	F0766YZ	F07D2ZZ	F07G3YZ	F07J6DZ

F07J6EZ	F07K6UZ	F07M0EZ	F07N1ZZ	F13Z71Z	F13ZMZZ	F14Z2LZ	F15Z18Z	GZB1ZZZ	X2C1361	XRGC0F3
F07J6FZ	F07K6YZ	F07M0FZ	F0DZ8ZZ	F13Z7KZ	F13ZN6Z	F14Z2PZ	F15Z1ZZ	GZB2ZZZ	X2C2361	XRGD092
F07J6GZ	F07K6ZZ	F07M0UZ	F0DZ9EZ	F13Z7ZZ	F13ZNZZ	F14Z2ZZ	F15Z28Z	GZB3ZZZ	X2C3361	XRGD0F3
F07J6HZ	F07K7ZZ	F07M0YZ	F0DZ9FZ	F13Z83Z	F13ZP1Z	F14Z31Z	F15Z2ZZ	GZB4ZZZ	X2RF032	XW03321
F07J6UZ	F07L0EZ	F07M0ZZ	F0DZ9UZ	F13Z84Z	F13ZP2Z	F14Z32Z	F15Z38Z	GZC9ZZZ	X2RF332	XW03331
F07J6YZ	F07L0FZ	F07M1EZ	F0DZ9ZZ	F13Z8ZZ	F13ZP4Z	F14Z33Z	F15Z3ZZ	GZFZZZZ	X2RF432	XW03341
F07J6ZZ	F07L0UZ	F07M1FZ	F13Z00Z	F13Z91Z	F13ZP9Z	F14Z34Z	F15Z48Z	GZGZZZZ	XHRPXL2	XW03351
F07J7ZZ	F07L0YZ	F07M1UZ	F13Z01Z	F13Z92Z	F13ZPKZ	F14Z35Z	F15Z4ZZ	GZHZZZZ	XK02303	XW03372
F07K0EZ	F07L0ZZ	F07M1YZ	F13Z02Z	F13Z9ZZ	F13ZPLZ	F14Z3KZ	F15Z58Z	GZJZZZZ	XNS0032	XW03392
F07K0FZ	F07L1EZ	F07M1ZZ	F13Z03Z	F13ZB1Z	F13ZPPZ	F14Z3LZ	F15Z5ZZ	HZ2ZZZZ	XNS3032	XW033A3
F07K0UZ	F07L1FZ	F07M2EZ	F13Z08Z	F13ZB2Z	F13ZPZZ	F14Z3PZ	F15Z68Z	HZ3CZZZ	XNS3332	XW033B3
F07K0YZ	F07L1UZ	F07M2FZ	F13Z09Z	F13ZBZZ	F13ZQKZ	F14Z3ZZ	F15Z6ZZ	HZ4CZZZ	XNS4032	XW033C3
F07K0ZZ	F07L1YZ	F07M2UZ	F13Z0ZZ	F13ZC1Z	F13ZQPZ	F14Z41Z	F15Z75Z	HZ63ZZZ	XNS4332	XW033F3
F07K1EZ	F07L1ZZ	F07M2YZ	F13Z10Z	F13ZC2Z	F13ZQYZ	F14Z42Z	F15Z7ZZ	HZ80ZZZ	XR2G021	XW04321
F07K1FZ	F07L2EZ	F07M2ZZ	F13Z11Z	F13ZCZZ	F13ZQZZ	F14Z43Z	F14Z44Z	HZ81ZZZ	XR2H021	XW04331
F07K1UZ	F07L2FZ	F07M3EZ	F13Z12Z	F13ZD3Z	F14Z01Z	F14Z44Z	F14Z4KZ	HZ82ZZZ	XRG0092	XW04341
F07K1YZ	F07L2UZ	F07M3FZ	F13Z1ZZ	F13ZD4Z	F14Z02Z	F14Z4KZ	F14Z4LZ	HZ83ZZZ	XRG00F3	XW04351
F07K1ZZ	F07L2YZ	F07M3UZ	F13Z20Z	F13ZDZZ	F14Z03Z	F14Z4LZ	F14Z4ZZ	HZ84ZZZ	XRG1092	XW04372
F07K2EZ	F07L2ZZ	F07M3YZ	F13Z21Z	F13ZF3Z	F14Z04Z	F14Z4ZZ	F14Z51Z	HZ85ZZZ	XRG10F3	XW04392
F07K2FZ	F07L3EZ	F07M3ZZ	F13Z22Z	F13ZF4Z	F14Z05Z	F14Z51Z	F14Z52Z	HZ86ZZZ	XRG2092	XW043A3
F07K2UZ	F07L3FZ	F07M6BZ	F13Z2ZZ	F13ZFZZ	F14Z07Z	F14Z52Z	F14Z53Z	HZ87ZZZ	XRG20F3	XW043B3
F07K2YZ	F07L3UZ	F07M6CZ	F13Z31Z	F13ZG3Z	F14Z09Z	F14Z53Z	F14Z54Z	HZ88ZZZ	XRG4092	XW043C3
F07K2ZZ	F07L3YZ	F07M6DZ	F13Z32Z	F13ZG4Z	F14Z0KZ	F14Z54Z	F14Z55Z	HZ89ZZZ	XRG40F3	XW043F3
F07K3EZ	F07L3ZZ	F07M6EZ	F13Z3ZZ	F13ZGZZ	F14Z0LZ	F14Z55Z	F14Z5KZ	HZ90ZZZ	XRG6092	XW0DX82
F07K3FZ	F07L6BZ	F07M6FZ	F13Z41Z	F13ZH3Z	F14Z0PZ	F14Z5KZ	F14Z5LZ	HZ91ZZZ	XRG60F3	XY0VX83
F07K3UZ	F07L6CZ	F07M6GZ	F13Z42Z	F13ZH4Z	F14Z0YZ	F14Z5LZ	F14Z5ZZ	HZ92ZZZ	XRG7092	
F07K3YZ	F07L6DZ	F07M6HZ	F13Z4KZ	F13ZHZZ	F14Z0ZZ	F14Z5ZZ	F14Z65Z	HZ93ZZZ	XRG70F3	
F07K3ZZ	F07L6EZ	F07M6UZ	F13Z4ZZ	F13ZJ3Z	F14Z15Z	F14Z65Z	F14Z6ZZ	HZ94ZZZ	XRG8092	
F07K6BZ	F07L6FZ	F07M6YZ	F13Z51Z	F13ZJ4Z	F14Z1ZZ	F14Z6ZZ	F14Z70Z	HZ95ZZZ	XRG80F3	
F07K6CZ	F07L6GZ	F07M6ZZ	F13Z52Z	F13ZJZZ	F14Z21Z	F14Z70Z	F14Z7ZZ	HZ96ZZZ	XRGA092	
F07K6DZ	F07L6HZ	F07M7ZZ	F13Z5KZ	F13ZK7Z	F14Z22Z	F14Z7ZZ	F14Z85Z	HZ97ZZZ	XRGA0F3	
F07K6EZ	F07L6UZ	F07N1EZ	F13Z5ZZ	F13ZKZZ	F14Z23Z	F14Z85Z	F14Z8ZZ	HZ98ZZZ	XRGB092	
F07K6FZ	F07L6YZ	F07N1FZ	F13Z61Z	F13ZL7Z	F14Z24Z	F14Z8ZZ	F15Z08Z	HZ99ZZZ	XRGB0F3	
F07K6GZ	F07L6ZZ	F07N1UZ	F13Z62Z	F13ZLZZ	F14Z25Z	F15Z08Z	F15Z0ZZ	X2A5312	XRGC092	
F07K6HZ	F07L7ZZ	F07N1YZ	F13Z6ZZ	F13ZM6Z	F14Z2KZ	F15Z0ZZ	GZB0ZZZ	X2C0361	XRGC092	

NOTES

NOTES

NOTES

NOTES

NOTES

NOTES